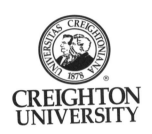

Medical Complications During Pregnancy

MEDICAL COMPLICATIONS DURING PREGNANCY

SIXTH EDITION

Gerard N. Burrow, M.D.
David Paige Smith Professor Emeritus of Medicine
Yale University School of Medicine
New Haven, Connecticut

Thomas P. Duffy, M.D.
Professor of Internal Medicine, Hematology
Yale University School of Medicine
New Haven, Connecticut

Joshua A. Copel, M.D.
Professor of Obstetrics, Gynecology &
    Reproductive Sciences, and of Pediatrics
Yale University School of Medicine
New Haven, Connecticut

ELSEVIER
SAUNDERS

ELSEVIER
SAUNDERS

The Curtis Center
170 S Independence Mall W 300 E
Philadelphia, PA 19106

MEDICAL COMPLICATIONS DURING PREGNANCY, Sixth Edition   ISBN 0-7216-0435-8
Copyright © 2004, 1999, 1995, 1988, 1982, 1975 by Elsevier Inc.

Library of Congress Cataloging-in-Publication Data
Medical complications during pregnancy/[edited by] Gerard N. Burrow, Thomas P.
  Duffy, Joshua A. Copel.–6th ed.
    p. ; cm.
  Includes bibliographical references and index.
  ISBN 0-7216-0435-8
   1. Pregnancy—Complications. I. Burrow, Gerard N. II. Duffy, Thomas P. III.
Copel, Joshua A.
  [DNLM: 1. Pregnancy Complications. 2. Pregnancy, High-Risk. WQ 240 M486 2004]
  RG571.M4 2004
  618.3–dc22   2004046719

Acquisitions Editor: Thomas H. Moore
Developmental Editor: Alison Nastasi
Project Manager: Joan Nikelsky
Design Coordinator: Gene Harris

Printed in the United States of America

Last digit is the print number: 9 8 7 6 5 4 3 2 1

FOR THE 500,000 WOMEN
IN DEVELOPING COUNTRIES
WHO DIE EACH YEAR
IN PREGNANCY OR CHILDBIRTH
BUT SHOULDN'T

CONTRIBUTORS

Jean T. Abbott, MD
Associate Professor, Division of Emergency Medicine, and Attending Physician, Emergency Department, University of Colorado Health Sciences Center; Denver, Colorado
Emergency Management of the Obstetric Patient

Phyllis August, MD, MPH
Professor of Medicine, Obstetrics and Gynecology in Medicine, and Public Health, Weill Medical College of Cornell University; Attending Physician, New York Presbyterian Hospital, New York, New York
Hypertensive Disorders in Pregnancy

Gerard N. Burrow, MD
David Paige Smith Professor Emeritus of Medicine, Department of Medicine, and Dean Emeritus, Yale University School of Medicine, New Haven, Connecticut
Thyroid Disease during Pregnancy
Pituitary and Adrenal Disorders of Pregnancy

Barbara Burtness, MD
Associate Professor and Director, Gastrointestinal Oncology, Department of Internal Medicine, Yale University School of Medicine; Attending Physician, Department of Internal Medicine, Yale–New Haven Hospital, New Haven, Connecticut
Neoplastic Diseases

Teresa Caulin-Glaser, MD
Associate Director of Preventive Cardiology, McConnell Heart Health Center-OhioHealth, Columbus, Ohio
Pregnancy and Cardiovascular Disease

Peter K. Chang, MD
Clinical Instructor, Gastroenterology, Mount Sinai School of Medicine, New York, New York
Gastrointestinal Complications

David A. Clark, MD, PhD
Professor Emeritus, Departments of Medicine, Molecular Medicine and Pathology, and Obstetrics and Gynecology, McMaster University, Hamilton; Professor of Medicine, Institute of Medical Sciences, University of Toronto, Toronto; Staff Physician, Department of Medicine, Hamilton Health Sciences, Hamilton, Ontario, Canada
Immunology of Pregnancy

Joshua A. Copel, MD
Professor of Obstetrics, Gynecology & Reproductive Sciences, and of Pediatrics, Yale University School of Medicine; Attending Physician, Yale–New Haven Hospital, New Haven, Connecticut
Obstetric Management of the High-Risk Patient

Kathryn Czarkowski, MA
Director of Clinical Services, Yale Behavioral Gynecology Program, Department of Psychiatry, Yale University School of Medicine, New Haven, Connecticut
Psychiatric Complications

James O. Donaldson, MD
Professor of Neurology, University of Connecticut School of Medicine, Farmington, Connecticut
Neurologic Complications

Thomas P. Duffy, MD
Professor of Internal Medicine, Hematology, Yale University School of Medicine; Attending Physician, Yale-New Haven Hospital, New Haven, Connecticut
Hematologic Aspects of Pregnancy
Neurologic Complications

C. Neill Epperson, MD
Assistant Professor of Psychiatry and Obstetrics/Gynecology and Director, Yale Behavioral Gynecology Program, Yale University School of Medicine; Attending Physician, Yale–New Haven Hospital and Connecticut Mental Health Center, New Haven, Connecticut
Psychiatric Complications

Harold J. Fallon, MD, MRCP
Dean Emeritus, University of Alabama School of Medicine, Birmingham, Alabama; Home Secretary, Institute of Medicine, Washington, D.C.
The Effects of Pregnancy on the Liver

Peter R. Garner, MD, FRCP(C) (deceased)
Professor of Obstetrics and Gynecology and Professor of Medicine, University of Ottawa, Ottawa, Ontario, Canada
Pituitary and Adrenal Disorders of Pregnancy

Lauren H. Golden, MD
Postdoctoral Fellow–Endocrinology, Section of Endocrinology, Department of Internal Medicine, Yale University School of Medicine, New Haven, Connecticut
Thyroid Disease during Pregnancy

John P. Hayslett, MD
Professor of Medicine (Nephrology) and Obstetrics and Gynecology, Department of Medicine, Yale University School of Medicine; Attending Physician, Yale–New Haven Hospital, New Haven, Connecticut
Renal Disease in Pregnancy

Debra Houry, MD, MPH
Assistant Professor, Department of Emergency Medicine, and Associate Director, Center for Injury Control, Emory University; Attending Physician, Emergency Department, Emory University Hospital and Grady Memorial Hospital, Atlanta, Georgia
Emergency Management of the Obstetric Patient

Karl L. Insogna, MD
Professor of Medicine, Yale University School of Medicine, New Haven, Connecticut
Calcium Homeostasis and Disorders of Calcium Metabolism during Pregnancy and Lactation

Anne B. Kenshole, MB, FRCPC, FACP
Professor Emeritus, Departments of Medicine and Obstetrics, University of Toronto; Staff Physician and Consultant to the South Central Ontario Regional High Risk Pregnancy Service, Sunnybrook and Women's Health Sciences Center, Toronto, Ontario, Canada
Diabetes and Pregnancy

Marie Louise Landry, MD
Professor, Department of Laboratory Medicine, Yale University School of Medicine; Director, Clinical Virology Laboratory, Yale–New Haven Hospital, New Haven, Connecticut
Viral Infections

Carl A. Laskin, MD, FRCPC
Associate Professor of Medicine, Obstetrics and Gynecology, and Immunology, Division of Rheumatology, Department of Medicine, University of Toronto; Consultant, Division of Rheumatology, Department of Medicine, University Health Network, and Department of Medicine and Obstetrics and Gynecology, Mount Sinai Hospital, Toronto, Ontario, Canada
Pregnancy and the Rheumatic Diseases

Richard V. Lee
Professor of Medicine, Pediatrics, and Obstetrics and Adjunct Professor of Anthropology, Social and Preventive Medicine, State University of New York at Buffalo School of Medicine, Buffalo, New York
Substance Abuse

Urania Magriples, MD
Associate Professor and Association Division Director, Maternal-Fetal Medicine, Department of Obstetrics and Gynecology, Yale University School of Medicine; Attending Physician, Yale–New Haven Hospital, New Haven, Connecticut
Obstetric Management of the High-Risk Patient

Jess Mandel, MD
Associate Professor of Medicine, Department of Medicine, Division of Pulmonary, Critical Care, and Occupational Medicine, and Assistant Dean, Office of Student Affairs and Curriculum, University of Iowa, Roy J. and Lucille A. Carver College of Medicine; Co-Director, Pulmonary Hypertension Program, University of Iowa Hospitals and Clinics, Iowa City, Iowa
Pulmonary Diseases

Urszula S. Masiukiewicz, MD
Assistant Professor, Department of Medicine, Yale University School of Medicine, New Haven, Connecticut
Calcium Homeostasis and Disorders of Calcium Metabolism during Pregnancy and Lactation

Ellen D. Mason
Internal Medicine Consultant, Department of Obstetrics and Gynecology, John H. Stroger, Jr., Hospital of Cook County, Chicago, Illinois
Substance Abuse

Mark R. Mercurio, MD
Associate Clinical Professor, Department of Pediatrics, Yale University School of Medicine, New Haven; Attending Neonatologist and Co-chair, Hospital Ethics Committee, Yale–New Haven Hospital, New Haven; Attending Neonatologist and Chair, Hospital Ethics Committee, Lawrence and Memorial Hospital, New London, Connecticut
Ethical Issues in Obstetrics

Peter McPhedran, MD
Professor of Laboratory Medicine and Internal Medicine, Yale University School of Medicine; Director, Clinical Hematology Laboratory, and Attending Physician, Yale–New Haven Hospital, New Haven, Connecticut
Venous Thromboembolism during Pregnancy

Caroline A. Riely, MD
Professor, Medicine and Pediatrics, and Attending Physician, Gastroenterology, University of Tennessee Health Science Center, Memphis, Tennessee
The Effects of Pregnancy on the Liver

Cheryl F. Rosen, MD, FRCPC
Associate Professor, Division of Dermatology, Department of Medicine, University of Toronto; Head, Division of Dermatology, Toronto Western Hospital, Toronto, Ontario, Canada
The Skin in Pregnancy

Maria C. Savoia, MD
Vice Dean for Medical Education and Professor of Medicine, University of California, San Diego, School of Medicine, La Jolla, California
Bacterial, Fungal, and Parasitic Disease

Margretta R. Seashore, MD
Professor of Genetics and Pediatrics, Yale University School of Medicine; Attending Physician, Department of Pediatrics, Yale–New Haven Hospital, New Haven, Connecticut
Clinical Genetics

John F. Setaro, MD
Associate Professor of Medicine and Director, Cardiovascular Disease Prevention Center, Section of Cardiovascular Medicine, Department of Internal Medicine, Yale University School of Medicine; Attending Physician, Department of Medicine, Yale-New Haven Hospital, New Haven, Connecticut
Pregnancy and Cardiovascular Disease

Adam F. Steinlauf, MD
Clinical Instructor, Gastroenterology, Mount Sinai School of Medicine; Clinical Assistant, Mount Sinai Medical Center, New York, New York
Gastrointestinal Complications

Morris Traube, MD, JD
Professor of Medicine and Director of Clinical Affairs, Section of Digestive Diseases, Yale University School of Medicine; Director, Gastrointestinal Procedure Center, Yale–New Haven Hospital, New Haven, Connecticut
Gastrointestinal Complications

Steven E. Weinberger, MD
Professor of Medicine and Faculty Associate Dean for Education, Harvard Medical School; Executive Vice Chair, Department of Medicine, Beth Israel Deaconess Medical Center, Boston, Massachusetts
Pulmonary Diseases

PREFACE

For the sixth edition of *Medical Complications During Pregnancy,* an obstetrician, Joshua A. Copel, has joined the Editors; this addition is long overdue. The basic concept of the book was based on the necessity for the internist and the obstetrician to care for the pregnant woman with medical problems together, often with, in addition, the neonatologist. As Vice Chair for Obstetrics in the Department of Obstetrics, Gynecology & Reproductive Sciences at Yale University School of Medicine, Dr. Copel is particularly well suited for such a role.

Another tenet of the book has been a commitment to keep the book as current as possible by adding new authors and new chapters to adequately cover the field. In the fifth edition, chapters on immunology and on emergency management of the obstetric patient were added to reflect concerns or progress in the field. As a consequence of the availability of new diagnostic and therapeutic modalities, obstetricians are increasingly asked to make difficult ethical decisions. A new chapter in bioethics has been added in the sixth edition, as has a chapter on the psychiatric consequences of pregnancy. New chapters have been written on obstetric care, calcium disorders, diabetes mellitus, rheumatic diseases, and dermatology.

Despite these changes, the basic purpose of the book continues to be to provide answers to clinical questions of physicians caring for pregnant women. Emphasis has been placed on evidence-based medicine, in which the effect of the disease process on pregnancy and the effect of the pregnancy on the disease are examined. There has also been an effort to provide the pathophysiologic foundation on which to base diagnostic and therapeutic measures.

Modern medicine has enabled more women to survive both acute and chronic illnesses that in the past would have resulted in death or such severe disability as to preclude childbearing. As more of these women become pregnant, the need for collaborative care by general obstetricians, specialists in high-risk pregnancy, and internists will only increase. Our purpose in this book is to provide a template for that care and some common ground: a set of information that is useful for physicians from different disciplines who join together to care for pregnant women with complex medical problems.

GERARD N. BURROW, MD
THOMAS P. DUFFY, MD
JOSHUA A. COPEL, MD

CONTENTS

Obstetric Management of the High-Risk Patient

Urania Magriples and Joshua A. Copel

Throughout the developed world in the 20th century, improvements in blood banking, antibiotics, the treatment of hypertension, and the advent of safe alternatives to general anesthesia have led to a reduction in maternal and fetal mortality and morbidity. Coupled with improvements in the understanding of maternal-fetal pathophysiology and with awareness of how changes in maternal physiology affect fetal growth and development, these developments have led to the awareness of high-risk pregnancy as the care of two patients: the mother and fetus. A pregnancy may be considered high risk because of maternal or fetal conditions, but the outcomes are often intimately linked.

Prenatal care in most of the 20th century was designed to identify hypertensive complications of pregnancy and to expedite the care of women with preeclampsia. In the 1980s and 1990s, there was an increased emphasis on early management of women at risk for prematurity, although efforts to delay preterm delivery have, as a whole, been disappointing. Also, since the mid-1970s, a new subspecialty of maternal-fetal medicine has emerged, attracting physicians trained in obstetrics with 2 to 3 years of additional education in the management of women and fetuses during complicated pregnancies.

The normal increase during pregnancy of both blood volume and cardiac output is well tolerated in normal women but may lead to heart failure in a patient with a fixed cardiac lesion or output, such as mitral stenosis or cardiomyopathy. Poor maintenance of cardiac output subsequently affects uterine and fetal perfusion and, therefore, fetal growth. The physiologic nadir of blood pressure in the first and second trimesters with physiologic elevation in the third trimester often makes it difficult to distinguish preeclampsia from exacerbation of chronic hypertension, and this dilemma is even more complicated for women with systemic lupus erythematosus, who may chronically have proteinuria, a hallmark of preeclampsia. Ultimately, if hypertension is not controlled by hospitalization and medication regardless of the diagnosis, it will lead to a need for delivery. The normal physiologic changes

during pregnancy are profound but generally well tolerated by most pregnant women and are completely reversible. Those that are of primary interest are reviewed in Table 1–1. The objective of this chapter is to refine these concepts as well as review the obstetric management and recent technologic advances in the care of these complicated pregnancies.

PRECONCEPTION COUNSELING

The physician taking care of women has the opportunity to have an impact not only on the lives of women but also on the lives of their children. Preconception care is essential in minimizing exposure to drugs and teratogens, maximizing nutritional status, and identifying medical conditions that may either affect pregnancy or be influenced by it.[1–3]

In the United States, more than 150,000 birth defects and more than 500,000 infant deaths, spontaneous abortions, stillbirths, and miscarriages each year result from defective fetal development.[4] It is estimated that 1% to 5% of congenital anomalies may be drug or chemical related. Factors that determine a drug's effect on the fetus include dosage, duration, and time of exposure, as well as drug metabolism, concurrent use of other drugs, genetic susceptibility, and placental transfer. There is a critical period of embryonic development from the 3rd through 12th weeks, when the embryo is undergoing organogenesis. Before this time, exposures tend either to cause abortion or to have no effect at all (known as the "all-or-none phenomenon"). After the 12th week, effects are generally limited to growth and neural development.

Preconception counseling should be the mainstay of women's health care. Therefore, all physicians who care for women of reproductive age need to be aware of the potential influence of disease and medications on pregnancy and make their patients aware of this impact. The effect of teratogens often occurs prior to the recognition of pregnancy. Examples of recognized teratogens and their associated malformations are listed in Table 1–2. Infectious agents

TABLE 1–1 Physiologic Changes of Pregnancy

Organ System	Change	Clinical Correlate
Hematologic		
Blood volume	Increases by 45%	"Dilutional anemia"
Plasma volume	Increases	—
Red cell volume	Increases by 250-450 mL	—
Iron requirements	Increase	Iron deficiency common
White blood cell count	Increases to 12,000 cells/mm³ (higher in stress or labor)	Diagnosis of infection difficult
Fibrinogen, plasminogen, factors VII, VIII, and X	Increase	Increased risk of venous thrombosis
Platelets	Increase turnover	Normal > 100,000
	Increase aggregation	More EDTA-induced clumping; manual platelet count needed to evaluate thrombocytopenia
C-reactive protein	Increases	Not useful as marker of acute infection
Sedimentation rate	Increases	Not useful as marker of acute infection
Cardiovascular		
ECG	Left axis deviation	Nonspecific T wave changes
Chest radiograph	Superior, lateral, and anterior displacement of heart by enlarging uterus	Enlarged cardiac silhouette straightened left heart border
Cardiac output	Increases by 30% to 50%	Systolic ejection murmurs common
	Increased end-diastolic dimensions	
	Myocardial hypertrophy	No long-term effect
Stroke volume	Increases	Increased cardiac work
Heart rate	Increases	Palpitations common; increase in premature atrial contractions; increase in arrhythmias
Blood pressure	Decreases in 1st and 2nd trimesters	Patient may need to decrease antihypertensive medications
	Increases to baseline in 3rd trimester	Increase in antihypertensive medication requirements
		Difficulty in distinguishing chronic hypertension from preeclampsia
Renal		
Kidney length	Increases by 1.5 cm	None
Ureters	Dilate	Right > left
Bladder	Relaxes	Increased dead space, increased risk of urinary tract infections and pyelonephritis
		Need for prophylaxis with recurrent urinary tract infections or pyelonephritis
		Frequent follow-up for women with history of urinary tract infections
Renal plasma flow	Increases by 50%	—
Glomerular filtration	Increases by 50%	Increased clearance of medications; difficulty attaining therapeutic levels, need to adjust dosing interval
Proteinuria	Increases	Underlying proteinuria worsens with pregnancy; symptoms from protein loss more common in pregnancy
Glycosuria	Increases	Poor indicator of diabetes in pregnancy
Alimentary		
Gastric emptying	Delayed	Heartburn, reflux
Sphincter tone	Decreases	Reflux
Motility	Decreases	Constipation, bloating
Gallbladder	Increase in residual volume	Increased risk of sludge and gallstones
	Decrease in emptying	Increase in symptoms with fatty diet
Cholesterol level	Doubles	Do not check in pregnancy
Binding protein levels	Increase	Increase in requirements of protein-bound medications
Transferrin level	Increases	—
Albumin level	Decreases	None
Alkaline phosphatase level	Increases (placental origin)	Unreliable test of liver disease
Transaminase levels	Unchanged	—
Drug metabolism	Increases	Close monitoring of drug levels

(Continued)

TABLE 1–1   Physiologic Changes of Pregnancy—cont'd

Organ System	Change	Clinical Correlate
Pulmonary		
Minute ventilation	Increases	Subjective shortness of breath Mild respiratory alkalosis
Total lung capacity	Decreases by 5%	None
Expiratory reserve volume	Decreases by 20%	Less dead space, more efficient ventilation
Tidal volume	Increases by 40%	—
Vital capacity	Unchanged	—
Inspiratory reserve volume	Unchanged	Unchanged
FEV_1	Unchanged	Decrease not explained by pregnancy
Pao_2	Unchanged	Hypoxemia abnormal
Integumentary		
Skin		
Hyperpigmentation	Increases	Linea nigra Mask of pregnancy Increase in nevi
Sweat glands	Increase production	Increase in sweating and acne

ECG, electrocardiogram; EDTA, ethylenediaminetetraacetic acid; FEV_1, forced expiratory volume in 1 second; Pao_2, partial pressure of arterial oxygen.

TABLE 1–2   Teratogenic Agents

Agent	Clinical Effect
Alcohol*	Fetal alcohol syndrome: cardiac abnormalities (ASD, VSD), characteristic facies, IUGR, maxillary hypoplasia, mental retardation, microcephaly
Methotrexate (antifolate)	Abnormal cranial ossification, cleft palate, hydrocephaly, IUGR and postnatal growth abnormalities, mental retardation, microcephaly, neural tube defects, reduction of derivatives of first branchial arch
Androgens	Masculinization of the female fetus
Angiotensin-converting enzyme inhibitors	Fetal and neonatal death, IUGR, neonatal anuria secondary to renal failure, oligohydramnios, pulmonary hypoplasia, skull hypoplasia (second and third trimester exposure)
Cocaine	Cardiac abnormalities, dislocated hip, facial clefts, musculoskeletal malformations, pyloric stenosis, respiratory malformations, ventriculomegaly
Cyclophosphamide	Cleft palate, eye abnormalities, skeletal and limb abnormalities (first trimester exposure)
Diethylstilbestrol	Cervical and uterine anomalies
Diphenylhydantoin	Cardiac abnormalities, cleft lip/palate, hypoplastic nails and distal phalanges, IUGR, mental retardation, microcephaly
External radiation (>5 rad)	Eye anomalies, IUGR, mental retardation, microcephaly
Hyperthermia	Neural tube defects
Indomethacin	Oligohydramnios, prenatal ductus arteriosus closure (reversible) (second and third trimester exposure)
Iodine deficiency and inorganic iodides	Deafness, fetal goiter, mental retardation
Isotretinoin	Cardiovascular, CNS and ear anomalies, cleft lip/palate
Lead	CNS abnormalities, microcephaly
Lithium carbonate	Ebstein anomaly of the tricuspid valve
Methimazole	Aplasia cutis
Methylmercury	Blindness, deafness, IUGR, microcephaly, neonatal seizures, poor muscle tone
Naphthalene	Hemolysis in G6PD-deficient infants
Nicotine	IUGR, increased incidence of sudden infant death syndrome
Penicillamine	Cutis laxa, joint hyperflexibility
Quinine (high dose)	Ototoxicity
Streptomycin	Ototoxicity
Tegretol	Cardiac abnormalities, developmental delay, fingernail hypoplasia, minor craniofacial defects
Tetracycline	Bone and tooth staining, dental enamel hypoplasia
Thalidomide	Cardiac defects, ear and nasal anomalies, gastrointestinal atresias and stenosis, limb reduction deformities
Trimethadione	Cardiac and CNS anomalies; developmental delay; high, arched palate; irregular teeth; IUGR; low-set ears; V-shaped eyebrows
Valproic acid	Cardiac abnormalities, dysmorphic facies, IUGR, neural tube defects
Warfarin	Anomalies of eyes, hands, and neck; CNS anomalies and hemorrhage; IUGR; nasal hypoplasia; stippling of secondary epiphyses

*Data are based on chronic use (10-12 drinks/day) associated with 30% incidence. Less known about lower amounts.
ASD, atrial septal defect; CNS, central nervous system; G6PD, glucose-6-phosphate dehydrogenase; IUGR, intrauterine growth restriction; VSD, ventricular septal defect.

can also cause maldevelopment in the human (Table 1-3). The lethal or developmental effects may be the result of mitotic inhibition, direct cytotoxicity, or necrosis. Inflammatory responses to infection can lead to metaplasia, scarring, or calcification, which lead to further damage.

Awareness of the need to optimize a medical condition before pregnancy is crucial, because many disease mechanisms are profoundly sensitive to the physiologic and hormonal changes in pregnancy. Routine health care maintenance for women with significant medical illnesses, such as pacemaker replacement and battery changes, stress testing, and appropriate medication changes and testing are best done before pregnancy.

Chronic maternal conditions are associated with an increased risk of teratogenicity. For example, diabetes increases the risk of a fetal abnormality by twofold to threefold.[5] There is still considerable controversy about whether the abnormalities are caused by only hyperglycemia or by the changes in pH and free fatty acids as well as the presence of hypoglycemia and ketosis.[6,7] Despite this debate, multiple studies have demonstrated that diabetic mothers with hemoglobin A_{1c} levels greater than 7.5 have a twofold increased risk of congenital malformations, and the risk is greater with increasing hemoglobin A_{1c} levels.[8,9] There are major cost savings associated with preconception diabetic care; these savings are secondary predominantly to a decrease in congenital anomalies.[10-13]

In mothers with phenylketonuria, levels of phenylalanine higher than 20 mg/dL are associated with a 90% incidence of congenital malformations in their fetuses, whereas levels lower than 16 mg/dL are associated with a 20% incidence.[14] Control of phenylalanine levels throughout the pregnancy is necessary to minimize the ongoing risk of abnormal fetal brain development throughout gestation. This often requires input from a nutritionist as well as close monitoring of blood levels.

In mothers with seizures, there is a twofold to threefold increased incidence of congenital anomalies in fetuses regardless of whether the mothers are taking antiseizure medications.[15] This baseline risk of teratogenicity is further increased by the medications used for treatment of the disorder. However, the risk of uncontrolled seizures for the mother and fetus far outweighs the potential medication risk. Phenylhydantoin is associated with an increased risk of cleft lip/palate and congenital heart disease, as well as a malformation sequence seen in up to 30% of exposed infants, known as the *fetal hydantoin syndrome*.[16,17] The disorder consists of growth restriction, mental retardation, nail hypoplasia, and a variety of craniofacial abnormalities. Trimethadione and carbamazepine have also been reported to produce similar defects, and valproic acid and carbamazepine exposure result in a significantly higher risk of neural tube defects.[18-21] The malformations seen are similar because the breakdown products of many of the medications and their interference with folate metabolism are the primary mechanisms of teratogenicity.[22,23] Elevated levels of oxidative metabolites, which are normally eliminated by the enzyme epoxide hydroxylase, have been associated with an increase in malformations. Unfortunately, predisposition to low enzyme levels may be genetically predetermined; thus, women who have one child with a malformation are more likely to have another affected child.[24] Studies have shown that exposure to higher doses, as well as to multiple medications, increases the fetal risk.[25] Barbiturates seem to have the least risk of teratogenicity and therefore may represent the safest medication to use if control of seizures can be obtained before conception. Folate requirements increase in pregnancy, and women taking antiepileptic medications who plan to become pregnant should begin taking supplemental folate. Careful monitoring of drug levels is necessary because protein binding, metabolism, and excretion of medications all increase in pregnancy.

ANTEPARTUM CARE

Routine obstetric care entails detailed medical, surgical, and family histories and a risk factor assessment based on the intake interview. In patients without risk factors, monthly visits are performed in the first and second trimesters with monitoring of blood pressure, weight,

TABLE 1-3	Fetal Effects of Infectious Agents in Humans
Agent	**Clinical Effect**
Cytomegalovirus	IUGR, mental retardation, microcephaly, chorioretinitis, deafness, hydrocephalus, intracranial hemorrhage and calcification, seizures, cerebral palsy, hepatosplenomegaly, chronic hepatitis, thrombocytopenia, anemia, death
Herpes simplex	IUGR, encephalitis, seizures, conjunctivitis, pulmonary disease, vesicular lesions, hepatosplenomegaly, hepatitis, anemia, thrombocytopenia, death
Parvovirus B19	Anemia secondary to bone marrow suppression, myocarditis, hydrops
Rubella	IUGR, mental retardation, microcephaly, deafness, cataracts, glaucoma, cardiovascular anomalies, hepatosplenomegaly, thrombocytopenia, purpura
Syphilis	Hepatosplenomegaly, hypotonia, rhinorrhea, periostitis, rash
Toxoplasmosis	IUGR, mental retardation, microcephaly, hydrocephalus, cerebral calcifications, seizures, chorioretinitis, hepatosplenomegaly, hydrops
Varicella	Mental retardation, seizures, cataracts, microphthalmia, optic atrophy, chorioretinitis, hepatosplenomegaly, cutaneous scars
Venezuelan equine encephalitis	Hydrocephalus, porencephaly, cataracts, microphthalmia

IUGR, intrauterine growth restriction.

an assessment of signs and symptoms of preterm labor, and evaluation of fetal growth by fundal height measurement. Monitoring is generally more frequent in the third trimester and in high-risk pregnancies, although standards have not been established. The basic laboratory tests recommended for all pregnant women are listed in Table 1–4. Monitoring of drug levels is performed more frequently in pregnancy because of the increase in liver metabolism, volume of distribution, and glomerular filtration rate, as well as changes in binding and binding proteins. Monitoring of thyroid function in the setting of thyroid disease is performed more frequently in pregnancy because of increased binding of thyroid hormone, increases in metabolism, and increases in hormone requirements. The need for thyroid hormone replacement in hypothyroidism almost doubles in pregnancy. Thyroid function also needs to be monitored closely in the postpartum period as hormone requirements return to baseline.

Thorough patient and family histories often reveal risk factors for genetically transmissible diseases. Women with a history of a stillbirth should receive genetic counseling because a stillborn fetus has a 6% to 11% risk of having a chromosomal abnormality. Couples with a history of three or more pregnancy losses or prolonged infertility have up to a 6% risk of a chromosomal abnormality. A previous child with a chromosomal abnormality or congenital malformation likewise puts the parents at increased risk with future pregnancies.[26]

Ethnicity is also important, because certain groups carry a higher risk for genetic diseases. Caucasians have a 1:20 risk of carrying a recessive gene for cystic fibrosis. Mutation analysis is informative in up to 90% of Caucasian

carriers and should be offered to all patients.[27] Individuals of Mediterranean descent have a 1:12 risk of being carriers of the β-thalassemia gene.[28] The mean corpuscular volume is useful as a screening test for thalassemia trait. Ashkenazi Jews, who have a 1:30 risk of carrying the gene for Tay-Sachs disease and a 1:40 risk of carrying the gene for Canavan's disease, should be offered testing for these carrier states, preferably before pregnancy because the testing for Tay-Sachs is more complex during pregnancy as a result of changes in hexosaminidase A activity.[29] The carrier rate for sickle cell disease is 1:12 among African-Americans.[30] When both parents are carriers of any of these autosomal recessive diseases, the chance of having an affected child is 25%, and prenatal testing should be offered.

Although the risk of Down's syndrome (trisomy 21) is highest in women aged 35 or older, the majority of affected infants are born to women younger than 35, inasmuch as they represent a larger percentage of the childbearing population. Prenatal screening on the basis of age alone detects only 30% of these infants; thus screening for maternal serum markers has been used to increase detection.[31] Maternal serum α-fetoprotein (AFP) is the major early fetal serum protein. It enters the amniotic fluid via fetal renal excretion, transudation through skin, and open lesions such as spina bifida and ventral wall defects. An elevated maternal serum level is frequently found with open neural tube and ventral wall defects, twin gestations, intrauterine fetal demise, and pregnancies at risk for growth restriction and fetal demise.[32-34] In contrast, a low maternal serum level of AFP has been associated with an increased risk of trisomy 21 and other autosomal trisomies. Maternal serum AFP testing in women younger than 35 detects an additional 25% of

---

TABLE 1–4   Basic Laboratory Tests

Complete blood cell count (registration and third trimester)
Blood type and antibody screen (indirect Coombs titer)
Hepatitis B surface antigen
Hemoglobin electrophoresis (need not be repeated if previously documented in record)
VDRL or RPR (if positive, test further with FTA-ABS)
Rubella titer
HIV*
Papanicolaou smear
Cervical cultures for gonorrhea and chlamydia (culture or PCR)
Urinalysis (culture if >5 WBCs/hpf or positive leukocyte esterase finding)
One hour 50 gram glucose challenge (28 weeks, or earlier if risk factors)
Three-hour 100-g glucose test (if 1-hour test result is abnormal)
Quadruple screen (maternal serum α-fetoprotein, human chorionic gonadotropin, estriol, and inhibin) (15-20 weeks)*
Genetic testing*
Ultrasonography*
Group B streptococcal swab from vagina and rectum (35-37 weeks)

Routine visit
Weight
Blood pressure
Urine dipstick tests for protein, glucose
Estimation of fetal growth and position by fundal height and palpation
Auscultation of fetal heart
Brief physical examination, including reflex testing and check for edema
Determination of symptoms of preterm labor (contractions, rupture of membranes, bleeding)
Cervical examination if necessary

*Tests generally recommended but necessitating patient counseling to determine appropriateness.
FTA-ABS, fluorescent treponemal antibody absorption (test); HIV, human immunodeficiency virus; hpf, high-power field; PCR, polymerase chain reaction; RPR, rapid plasma reagin (test); VDRL, Venereal Disease Research Laboratory (test); WBC, white blood cell.

pregnancies affected by Down's syndrome, with a 5% false-positive rate (i.e., in 5% of women with normal pregnancies, the risk of trisomy 21 is thought to be higher than the 1:270 risk in a 35-year-old woman). Maternal serum concentrations of human chorionic gonadotropin tend to be higher than normal, and those of unconjugated estriol are lower, in the presence of fetal Down's syndrome. The additional use of these markers along with maternal serum AFP ("triple screen") improves the detection rate of Down's syndrome to 67%, with a 7.2% false-positive rate.[35,36] The addition of the use of inhibin A ("quadruple test") has improved the detection of Down's syndrome to 74% with no change in the false-positive rate. In the first trimester, the combination of pregnancy-associated plasma protein A, free β-human chorionic gonadotropin, maternal serum AFP, and unconjugated estriol can yield a 70% detection rate, and an even higher rate is achieved when the nuchal thickness is measured between 11 and 14 weeks (Fig. 1–1).[37]

Ultrasonography has been used as a screening tool in the detection of neural tube and ventral wall defects in women with elevated maternal serum AFP; when performed by an experienced clinician, it has a very high sensitivity and specificity (Fig. 1–2).[38-40] Routine ultrasonography in all obstetric patients remains a controversial issue in the United States, but if the parents desire information on prenatal diagnosis of congenital anomalies, then second trimester ultrasonography at a facility with extensive experience in the identification of fetal anomalies is certainly advisable.[41-47] The addition of ultrasound detection of nuchal translucency to first trimester serum testing increases the detection of Down's syndrome to 88% and offers couples the best noninvasive screening available to date. Definitive testing for fetal karyotype requires an invasive procedure and can be obtained by chorionic villus sampling (CVS) or amniocentesis. CVS is essentially a placental biopsy and allows for determination of the fetal karyotype as well as extraction of DNA for detection of many genetic diseases.[48,49] It can be performed transcervically or transabdominally with ultrasound guidance of the biopsy catheter or needle, depending on the location of the placenta. Advantages of CVS are that it can be performed in the first trimester (10 to 12 weeks) and results are generally available in less than a week. Thus, pregnancy termination, if desired, is a less complicated and more private procedure. CVS has a procedure-related miscarriage rate of 0.5% to 1%. In some centers, concern was raised about an excess of transverse distal limb abnormalities; however, if there is any association, it is clustered primarily among procedures performed at less than 10 weeks' gestation.[50] Ultrasonographically guided amniocentesis can be performed after 15 weeks' gestation; the procedure-related miscarriage rate is estimated at 0.5%. Amniocytes are extracted from the amniotic fluid and can take 1 to 2 weeks to grow in culture in order to yield fetal DNA and a karyotype. Amniotic fluid can also be assessed for levels of AFP and acetylcholinesterase, both of which are increased when the integrity of the fetal integument is interrupted, as in spina bifida, anencephaly, or ventral wall defects. The availability of both polymerase chain reaction testing and culture of amniotic fluid has made the diagnosis of fetal viral and bacterial infections more accurate.[51-53] Because of the gestational age at which the procedure is performed, as well as the length of time necessary in tissue culture, termination of pregnancy after amniocentesis must be performed by either dilation and evacuation, a more complex procedure than in the first trimester, or induction of labor with prostaglandin. Fluorescent in situ hybridization specifically for chromosomes 21, 13, and 18 and for the sex chromosomes has allowed more rapid diagnosis of the more common trisomies.[54]

Amniocentesis is also used in the third trimester for verification of lung maturity. The predominant constituent of amniotic fluid is fetal urine, which the fetus swallows and "breathes." The phospholipids or surfactants in the lung act as the emulsifying agents that keep the alveoli open. Lung secretions exit the trachea into the amniotic fluid cavity, and therefore the assessment of the ratio of lecithin/sphingomyelin or the presence of phosphatidylglycerol by

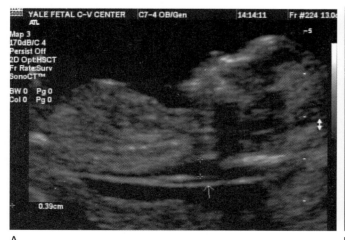
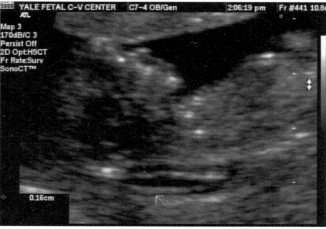

A   B

Figure 1–1. Screening for aneuploidy by nuchal translucency measurement. **A**, Normal nuchal translucency. Sagittal view of fetus with *calipers* on nuchal translucency. *Arrow* depicts normal unfused amniotic membrane. **B**, Abnormal nuchal translucency. Sagittal view of fetus with *calipers* on nuchal translucency. *Arrow* depicts normal unfused amniotic membrane.

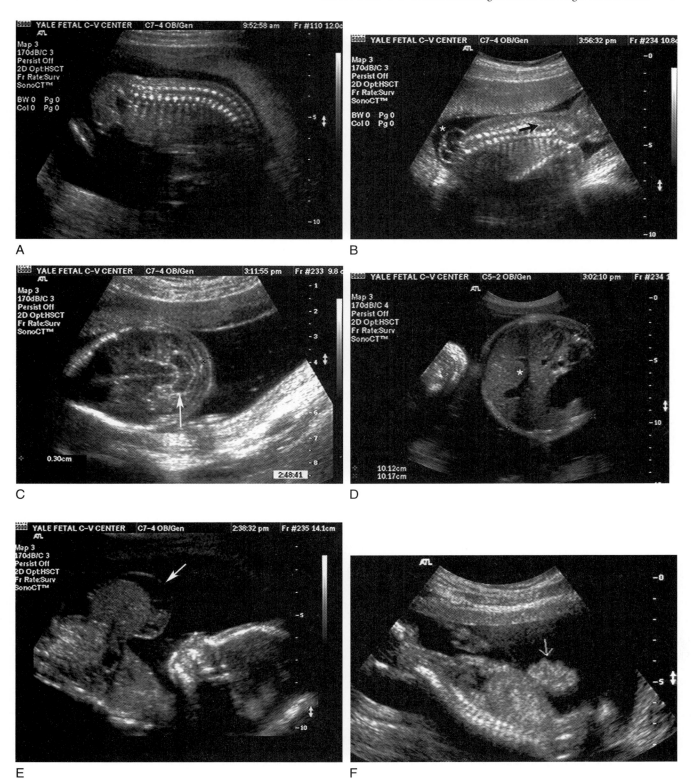

Figure 1–2. Screening for abnormalities with ultrasonography. **A**, Normal sagittal view of the spine with normal skin integrity overlying the bony vertebrae. **B**, Spina bifida. *Arrow* indicates normal portion of thoracic spine. *Asterisk* indicates lumbar meningomyelocele with splaying of vertebrae. **C**, Intracranial findings associated with spina bifida. *Calipers* indicate normal nuchal thickness measurement (less than 6 mm). *Arrow* shows "banana sign," which is the effect of the Arnold-Chiari malformation on the cerebellum with tethering of the cerebellum and obliteration of the cisterna magna. **D**, Normal abdominal circumference. *Calipers* indicate skin margins at the level of the umbilical vein (*asterisk*). **E**, Omphalocele. Sagittal view of the fetus; *arrow* indicates membrane-covered omphalocele with liver inside it. **F**, Gastroschisis. Sagittal view of the fetus; *arrow* indicates free loops of bowel in the amniotic fluid.

amniocentesis enables the determination of lung maturity in cases of elective delivery.[55] The relative ease of access to amniotic fluid and the discovery that fetal urine, like a urinalysis in an adult, can offer a reflection of the fetal status led to the use of amniocentesis in the assessment of fetal anemia in Rh isoimmunization and other blood group incompatibilities.[56] The presence of antibodies that cross the placenta to the fetus in the Rh-sensitized mother leads to hemolytic disease of the fetus and fetal hyperbilirubinemia. The byproducts of hemoglobin degradation are assessed through spectrophotometric analysis of bilirubin pigment in the amniotic fluid, and graphs for the indirect assessment of fetal anemia are thus widely available. Since 1990, this indirect but invasive method of assessment of anemia has been replaced by direct fetal assessment through percutaneous umbilical blood sampling. Fetal blood sampling under ultrasonographic guidance has allowed access to the fetus for assessment of anemia and thrombocytopenia, as well as other biochemical parameters and karyotype, and has become the route for treatment of the anemic fetus through direct transfusion, which has revolutionized the treatment of isoimmunization.[57-59]

Although the use of routine ultrasonography in uncomplicated pregnancies may be controversial, its use in high-risk pregnancies has improved the diagnosis of complications. Accurate determination of gestational age is crucial because interventions for prematurity and postmaturity are dependent on accurate dating. Fetal growth disturbances are increased in diseases that affect uterine blood flow. Commonly used obstetric dating criteria are listed in Table 1–5. First trimester determination of gestational age gives the most accurate prediction of gestational age (±5 days), but measurements in the second trimester still offer projections of dating to within 10 days and also enable assessment of fetal anatomy. Sonographic studies performed in the third trimester cannot be used for accurate determination of gestational age, because there can be a discrepancy of up to 3 weeks. Once an estimated due date is determined by ultrasonography, it should not be altered by later ultrasonograms, because this will make the diagnosis of a growth aberration more difficult. Ultrasonography is key in the determination of aberrant growth patterns and often aids in the timing of delivery. It provides information not only about the fetal size but also about behavior and blood flow. With decreasing uteroplacental perfusion, there are changes in distribution of blood flow, which are thought to be protective to more vital organs. Centralization of blood flow allows delivery of oxygenated blood to the head, heart, and adrenal glands, and it is equivalent to the compensatory process seen in adults in shock. This leads to maintenance of fetal head growth and brain function and has led to the term *brain-sparing* or asymmetric *intrauterine growth restriction,* in which the fetal head growth is maintained but the abdominal circumference lags as a result of the decrease in liver size from reduced glycogen stores. Symmetrical growth restriction is thought to be a process more inherent to the fetus whether the fetal size is genetically predetermined ("constitutionally small"); is affected by early toxicity, viral infection, or chromosomal aberrations; or is a more severe manifestation of early growth restriction. When symmetric growth restriction results from placental factors, it represents a lack or reversal of the normal compensatory changes and is an ominous sign.

Uteroplacental factors are the cause of approximately half of cases of intrauterine growth restriction (defined as growth less than the 10th percentile by gestational age), although morbidity is generally seen once growth is below the fifth percentile.[60] Changes in blood flow through the placenta affect the amount of blood received by the fetus. The decrease in blood flow to the fetus and shunting of blood away from the fetal kidneys to more vital organs leads to decrease in fetal urine production, which is manifested as decreased amniotic fluid or oligohydramnios. Therefore, a quick determination of the amniotic fluid volume aids in the assessment of fetal well-being. With decreasing fetal pH and oxygen levels, fetal movements also decrease, first by conservation of breathing movements and eventually with loss of movement and tone. These parameters, along with monitoring of the fetal heart rate (nonstress test), constitute the biophysical profile (BPP). The fetal behavioral assessment of the BPP developed by Manning and colleagues[61] provides insight into the fetal status. The developed scoring system is presented in Table 1–6. A low score has been demonstrated to be correlated with asphyxia both in low- and high-risk

---

TABLE 1–5　Gestational Dating Criteria

Criterion	Dating Accuracy	Clinical Correlate
Last menstrual period	2 weeks	Not useful if cycles are irregular; only 60% of women can accurately date pregnancy by menstrual dates
First-trimester uterine size	2 weeks	Dependent on operator skill and maternal habitus
Second and third trimester uterine size	8 weeks	Dependent on operator skill, maternal habitus, uterine and fetal size, and fetal position
Fetal heart tone auscultation	2 weeks	Dependent on maternal habitus, may be auscultated at 12 weeks with Doppler stethoscope
Fundal height measurements	3 weeks	Dependent on maternal habitus
First trimester ultrasonography	5 days	Crown-rump length performed at 6 to 12 weeks; accuracy improved with vaginal ultrasonography
Second trimester ultrasonography	10-14 days	Biometry obtained at 15 to 22 weeks
Third trimester ultrasonography	21 days	Biometry obtained after 22 weeks

TABLE 1–6   Biophysical Profile Scoring

Biophysical Component	Finding	Score if Normal
Breathing	Breathing for at least 30 seconds' duration	2
Body movements	Three or more body/limb movements	2
Tone	One or more episode of active extension with return to flexion of limbs or trunk; hand opening and closing	2
Amniotic fluid	At least one pocket of 2 cm	2
Fetal heart rate	Two episodes or more of fetal heart rate acceleration of ≥15 bpm and of at least 15 seconds' duration	2

Score	Interpretation and Management
10/10	Normal infant, low risk for chronic asphyxia
	Repeat test weekly or twice weekly if diabetic or post term
8/10	Normal infant, low risk for chronic asphyxia
	Repeat test weekly or twice weekly
	Deliver if amniotic fluid is decreased at >36 weeks
6/10	Suspected chronic asphyxia
	Repeat test in 4-6 hours
4/10	Suspected chronic asphyxia
	Deliver if amniotic fluid is decreased at >36 weeks
	Consider in utero resuscitation if infant is extremely premature
0-2/10	Strong suspicion of asphyxia
	Attempt in utero resuscitation only with careful intensive fetal monitoring
	If score remains <4, deliver if fetus is sufficiently mature to survive

Adapted from Manning FA, Platt LD, Sipos L: Antepartum fetal evaluation: Development of a fetal biophysical profile. Am J Obstet Gynecol 1980;136:787-795.
bpm, beats per minute.

pregnancies, and management based on use of the system has been shown to significantly lower perinatal morbidity and mortality. In the initial prospective clinical trial of 1184 patients at high risk, the BPP was used to determine the timing of delivery; its use was found to result in a corrected perinatal mortality rate (PMR) of 5 per 1000 (historical controls had a PMR of 40.5 per 1000).[62] This research was expanded to include 12,620 patients, which yielded a PMR of 1.9 in 1000. The false-negative rate, defined as a stillbirth within 1 week of a normal test result, is less than 1 in 1000 births.[63] The BPP has become an invaluable tool in monitoring pregnancies at risk for increased fetal morbidity.

The changes in blood flow previously described can also be assessed through Doppler flow-velocity waveform analysis of the fetus. The systolic-to-diastolic (S/D) characteristics of the Doppler waveform of the umbilical artery are a reflection of impedance to flow in the fetal-placental circulation. With increasing gestational age, the placenta normally becomes an organ of low impedance secondary to extensive branching of highly compliant vessels. Therefore, in normal gestation, diastolic flow increases and the S/D ratio falls. With increased impedance to flow, lower diastolic velocities are seen, which results in elevated S/D ratios (Fig. 1–3). As the resistance increases, diastolic flow eventually stops and then reverses. In gestations complicated with intrauterine growth restriction, approximately 60% to 74% have high umbilical artery S/D ratios.[64] Fetuses with abnormal Doppler waveforms have a higher incidence of perinatal asphyxia and death than do those with normal flow characteristics. Fetuses with no or reversed end-diastolic flow have a high incidence of heart rate decelerations and death within the subsequent 7 to 14 days.[65] The centralization of blood flow with redistribution of cerebral blood flow seen in growth restriction has led to the use of

middle cerebral artery (MCA) waveforms as an adjunct to umbilical cord Doppler analysis. Usually a decrease in umbilical artery diastolic velocity is accompanied by an increase in MCA diastolic velocity, which indicates cerebral vasodilation.[66-68] The loss of the expected increase in cerebral diastolic flow is a prognosticator of poor fetal outcome.

Serial growth ultrasonograms allow clinicians to establish a pattern of growth very similar to the growth curves established in routine pediatric care, in which maintenance of a pattern of growth is important. A downward trend in growth percentile, together with changes in fetal heart rate testing, fetal behavioral profile, and blood flow velocity waveforms are used to aid in the timing of delivery. Many fetuses with growth restriction and abnormal Doppler waveforms tolerate labor poorly, as they have little reserve to compensate for the decrease in uteroplacental blood flow normally associated with uterine contractions. Unfortunately, assessment of maternal risk factors lacks sensitivity and specificity in the detection of growth restriction. Clinical indicators such as fundal height assessment are dependent on maternal habitus, as well as fetal position, amniotic fluid volume, and uterine size and position. This has led to use of third trimester ultrasonography in screening pregnancies at increased risk for growth aberrations secondary to fetal and maternal factors.

MCA Doppler analysis has also revolutionized the management of the Rh-sensitized pregnancy, inasmuch as anemic fetuses have an increase in MCA peak systolic velocity.[69,70] Normal values for MCA peak velocities across the second and third trimesters are available.[71] This allows more specific timing of invasive procedures such as transfusion before the development of fetal hydrops or compromise. It also limits the number of invasive procedures needed, thereby limiting further sensitization.

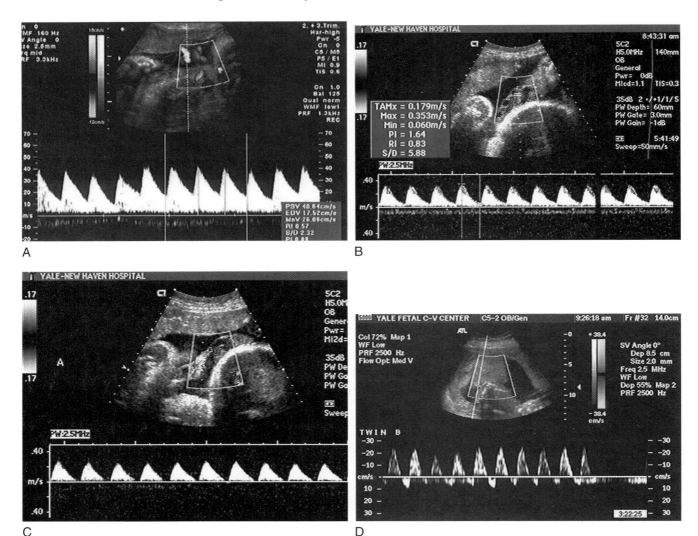

Figure 1–3. Doppler flow velocity waveforms. **A**, Normal systolic/diastolic (S/D) ratio of the umbilical artery. **B**, Elevated S/D ratio with decreasing diastolic flow. **C**, Absence of end-diastolic flow. **D**, Reversed end-diastolic flow.

PRETERM LABOR

Despite a concerted effort to diagnose and treat preterm labor, there has been little change in the rates of prematurity since the early 1980s. This is probably because of the diverse causes of preterm labor. Prematurity prevention efforts have focused on screening and identification of women with risk factors for prematurity, patient education, and tocolysis once labor begins. Unfortunately, most prevention studies lack sensitivity and specificity. Risk scoring systems based on social, behavioral, medical, obstetric, and demographic risk factors have been found to be of variable use, depending on the population screened. Most series report a sensitivity of 50% and a positive predictive value of 20% to 25% for preterm birth.[72,73] In the past, home uterine activity monitoring had been advocated as a method of early detection of contractions, thus theoretically allowing for the benefits of tocolysis before advanced cervical dilation. With this technology, the patient at home applies a contraction monitor, and contractions are recorded and

transmitted to a central receiving station for analysis via modem. A nurse subsequently discusses the transmission with the patient by telephone. Randomized control trials of home uterine activity monitoring have failed to demonstrate any improvement in gestational age at delivery or birth weight in comparison with close telephone contact without monitoring.[74-76]

More recently, fetal fibronectin and cervical ultrasonography have been used to stratify risk of preterm delivery. Fetal fibronectin is a protein produced by the fetal membranes, which is found near the interface of the fetal membranes and decidua. It is likely to be the adhesive that keeps the placental unit intact and is commonly found in vaginal secretions in the first trimester and at term. Its presence before 35 weeks is correlated with increase in relative risk of preterm delivery.[77-80] Quantitative assays have demonstrated an increase in risk with increasing values; unfortunately, the positive predictive value in singleton gestations is only 3%. Although it is a poor predictor of preterm delivery, its negative predictive value is greater than 99%, which makes it a useful tool in distinguishing true preterm labor from clinically insignificant contractions, thus potentially limiting aggressive tocolysis and hospitalization in patients with negative screens. Transvaginal ultrasonography of cervical length has also been used in both symptomatic and asymptomatic patients to predict relative risk of preterm delivery because it provides an objective and reproducible assessment of effacement and dilation. A sonographically determined shortened cervical length alone or in conjunction with a positive fetal fibronectin has been demonstrated to increase the risk of preterm delivery (Fig. 1–4).

Studies have suggested that regardless of the cause, contractions are a response to an inflammatory process within the decidua that leads to an increase in prostaglandins E_2 and F_2 and cytokines.[81,82] This inflammatory process can be initiated by a wide variety of agents, including infection, hemorrhage, and hypoxia. Therefore, it is not surprising that studies have not been able to demonstrate a significant effect of tocolysis as either prophylaxis against or treatment for preterm delivery, because the precipitant of labor may not be comparable between groups compared. Studies of tocolysis with β-sympathomimetic agents (such as terbutaline and ritodrine) have documented prolongation

of pregnancy for up to 48 hours but no change in the rate of preterm delivery.[83,84] Therefore, treatment is often limited for 48 hours to enable the use of antenatal corticosteroids, which have been demonstrated to decrease the risk of neonatal respiratory distress syndrome and intraventricular hemorrhage.[85,86] Intravenous tocolysis has not been beneficial in prospective randomized trials conducted in women with preterm premature rupture of membranes.[87] Antibiotic therapy has been demonstrated to decrease the risk of neonatal infection in preterm premature rupture of membranes, as well as to prolong the period before the onset of labor without increasing the maternal morbidity.[88]

β-Sympathomimetic agents such as ritodrine and terbutaline are used in the oral, subcutaneous, and intravenous forms. Side effects of these agents are more common when they are used intravenously and include tachycardia, arrhythmias, pulmonary edema, increased cardiac output, myocardial ischemia, decreased serum potassium levels, and hyperglycemia. These side effects are often dose limiting and can be exacerbated by the use of excessive intravenous fluids, infection, or the concomitant use of magnesium sulfate.[89]

Magnesium sulfate is commonly used in many centers for both tocolysis and seizure prophylaxis in preeclampsia.

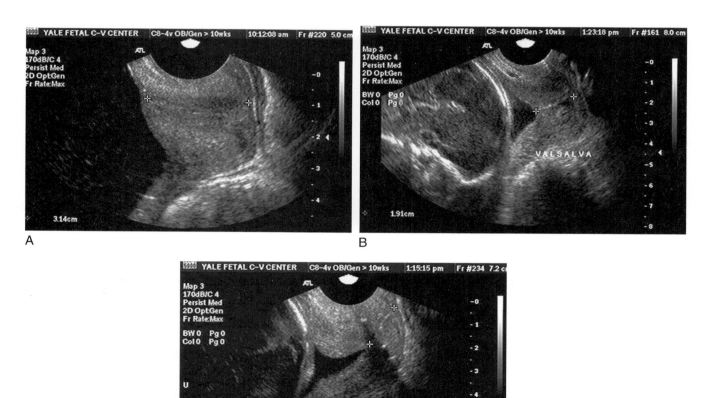

Figure 1–4. Transvaginal ultrasound of the cervix. **A**, Normal cervical length. *Calipers* mark the internal and external os. **B**, Shortening of the cervix with Valsalva maneuver. **C**, Shortening of the cervix with funneling of the internal os. This represents the amniotic membranes prolapsing through the internal os of the cervix.

Several prospective studies have compared its effects with those of β-adrenergic agents and found it to be similar.[90] Its major toxicity is fluid overload and pulmonary edema. Therapeutic tocolysis is usually achieved at levels of 4.5 to 6.5 mg/dL. Magnesium toxicity begins with lethargy and nausea at magnesium levels of 6.5 to 7.0 mg/dL; respiratory depression begins at about 8 mg/dL, and cardiac arrest occurs at 10 mg/dL. Close monitoring of input and output, as well as of reflexes, symptoms, and magnesium levels, is vital, particularly in patients with compromised renal function. Indomethacin has also been used as a tocolytic and has been demonstrated to be more effective than placebo.[91] It has minimal maternal side effects and can be given both orally and rectally. However, fetal side effects preclude its long-term use. These effects include premature closure of the ductus arteriosus, pulmonary hypertension, and oligohydramnios, which occur more commonly with administration longer than 48 hours and in fetuses of gestational ages of more than 32 weeks.[92] A short course of indomethacin failed to demonstrate any sequelae in a long-term follow-up study of treated infants.[93] Therefore, it is an option for short-term use and is useful in the setting of emergency or late cervical cerclage.

The calcium channel blocker nifedipine was compared with ritodrine in a randomized trial and was shown to have a comparable effect.[94] It was also demonstrated to have fewer side effects and has the advantage of being orally administered. Care must be taken in using it concomitantly with magnesium sulfate because of the compounded effect on calcium channels and the potential for affecting cardiac output. The long-term effects of calcium channel blockers as tocolytics have not been evaluated systematically in neonates.

Resuscitation of the preterm infant is optimized by delivery at a tertiary center with a neonatology team present. Although measures of fetal well-being, such as the nonstress test, can be more difficult to obtain in premature infants, the judicious use of fetal heart rate variability with electronic fetal monitoring, the use of prophylactic amnioinfusion (replacement of fluid in the amniotic cavity with preterm rupture of membranes) to decrease the risk of cord compression and the relatively small size of the infant often allow for a successful vaginal delivery if the infant is in the vertex position. Concerns arise in vaginal delivery of the premature or growth-restricted infant from a breech position because of the relative size discrepancy between the head and body and the risk of head entrapment through an incompletely dilated cervix. The benefits of cesarean section to the very premature fetus must be balanced with the risks to the mother and should be weighed with counseling on neonatal survival and long-term morbidity.

Decisions for timing and mode of delivery are generally based on maternal and fetal testing, as well as gestational age. Women with stable medical conditions and fetuses who are tolerating the intrauterine environment without evidence of compromise by antenatal testing are allowed to continue to term and await spontaneous labor. Cesarean section is rarely indicated for medical complications of pregnancy. It is used prophylactically in the setting of an intracranial lesion such as an arteriovenous malformation or aneurysm, for which concerns include rupture as well

as deteriorating maternal status or coagulopathy with an unripe cervix. The judicious use of induction of labor for maternal and fetal indications may be warranted for the medically unstable patient at term after her medical status is optimized. In cases of maternal or fetal compromise, decisions on delivery are based on gestational age and maternal medical stability.

For the truly unstable gravida, resuscitation of the mother is an absolute prerequisite for resuscitation of the fetus, as the fetus is completely dependent on the mother for oxygenation and perfusion. Delivery when the mother is acidotic, whether from sepsis or diabetic ketoacidosis, leads only to two sick patients, whereas correction of metabolic disturbances often leads to a better maternal and neonatal outcome. A sign of effective ventilation in a critically ill patient is the lack of contractions or fetal heart rate decelerations, because maternal hypoxia leads to both and to the necessity of delivery in a critically ill mother for the sake of her fetus. Avoidance of labor in the critically ill mother until she is medically stabilized can be crucial, because the physiologic changes that occur during labor, delivery, and the postpartum period can be dramatic. With each contraction, there is an increase in the amount of blood flow that returns to the heart, as well as changes in heart rate that are related to pain and anxiety. These normal changes are well tolerated by the healthy woman but may compromise the patient with a fixed ejection fraction. Tachycardia limits diastolic filling, and therefore a lack of anesthesia may further compromise cardiac output. Valsalva maneuvers decrease the return of blood to the heart, and both systemic and pulmonary perfusion can therefore have a profound effect on cardiac output and oxygenation. Thus, the use of forceps and vacuum has been proposed in patients with cardiac disease to avoid the shift in blood volume and its effect on cardiac output. The avoidance of labor and elective cesarean delivery to "control" of factors of labor only leads to increases in blood loss and risk of infection. Consultation with anesthesiologists is critical for the delivery of these patients. Epidural anesthesia has been shown to neutralize many of the cardiovascular changes seen in labor, which are probably related more to the effect of pain than to the process of labor.

After delivery, the expected shift in fluids and blood volume from the uteroplacental circulation to the maternal circulation in the first 48 hours place women with cardiovascular disease and heart failure at increased risk for heart failure and arrhythmias. Therefore, cardiac monitoring should be continued for at least 24 hours after delivery.

Close collaboration of specialists in maternal-fetal medicine and subspecialties can only improve the outcomes of these high-risk pregnancies. It allows for the understanding of the physiologic changes of pregnancy and how they affect both the mother and her fetus in the normal and compromised state, and it enables the incorporation of advances in medical technology into their care.

References

1. Briggs GG, Freeman RK, Yaffe SJ: Drugs in Pregnancy and Lactation: A Reference Guide to Fetal and Neonatal Risk, 6th ed. Baltimore, Williams & Wilkins, 2001.
2. Institute of Medicine, Food and Nutrition Board, Committee on Nutritional Status During Pregnancy and Nutrition: Nutrition

During Pregnancy and Lactation: An Implementation Guide. Washington, D.C., National Academy Press, 1992.

3. Worthington-Roberts B, Williams SR: Nutrition in Pregnancy and Lactation, 5th ed. Dubuque, Ia, WCB/McGraw-Hill, 1997.

4. March of Dimes website, *www.modimes.org.*

5. Mills JL: Malformations in infants of diabetic mothers. Teratology 1982;25:385-394.

6. Reece EA, Homko CJ, Wu YK, Wiznitzer A: The role of free radicals and membrane lipids in diabetes-induced congenital malformations. J Soc Gynecol Invest 1998;5:178-187.

7. Reece EA, Homko CJ: Why do diabetic women deliver malformed infants? Clin Obstet Gynecol 2000;43:32-45.

8. Miller E, Hare JW, Cloherty JP, et al: Elevated maternal hemoglobin A$_{1c}$ in early pregnancy and major congenital anomalies in infants of diabetic mothers. N Engl J Med 1981;304:1331-1334.

9. Lucas MJ, Leveno KJ, Williams ML, et al: Early pregnancy glycosylated hemoglobin, severity of diabetes, and fetal malformations. Am J Obstet Gynecol 1989;161:426-431.

10. Fuhrmann K, Reiher H, Semmler K, et al: Prevention of congenital malformations in infants of insulin-dependent diabetic mothers. Diabetes Care 1983;6:219-223.

11. Cousins L: The California Diabetes and Pregnancy Programme. A statewide collaborative programme for the pre-conception and prenatal care of diabetic women. Baillieres Clin Obstet Gynaecol 1991;5:443-449.

12. Diabetes Control and Complications Research Group: Pregnancy outcomes in the Diabetes Control and Complications Trial. Am J Obstet Gynecol 1996;174:1343-1353.

13. Elixhauser A, Weschler JM, Kitzmiller JL, et al: Cost-benefit analysis of preconception care for women with established diabetes mellitus. Diabetes Care 1993;16:1146-1157.

14. Platt LD, Koch R, Azen C, et al: Maternal phenylketonuria collaborative study, obstetric aspects and outcomes: The first 6 years. Am J Obstet Gynecol 1992;166:1150-1160.

15. Holmes LB, Harvey EA, Coull BA, et al: The teratogenicity of anticonvulsant drugs. N Engl J Med 2001;344:1132-1138.

16. Monson RR, Rosenberg L, Hartz SC, et al: Diphenylhydantoin and selected congenital malformations. N Engl J Med 1973;289:1045-1049.

17. Nulman I, Scolnik D, Chitayat D, et al: Findings in children exposed in utero to phenytoin and carbamazepine monotherapy: Independent effects of epilepsy and medications. Am J Med Genet 1997;68:18-24.

18. Azarbayjani F, Danielsson BR: Pharmacologically induced embryonic dysrhythmia and episodes of hypoxia followed by reoxygenation: A common teratogenic mechanism for antiepileptic drugs? Teratology 1998;57:117-126.

19. Jones KL, Lacro RV, Johnson KA, et al: Pattern of malformation in the children of women treated with carbamazepine during pregnancy. N Engl J Med 1989;320:1661-1666.

20. Matalon S, Schechtman S, Goldzweig G, et al: The teratogenic effect of carbamazepine: A meta-analysis of 1255 exposures. Reprod Toxicol 2002;16:9-17.

21. Clayton-Smith J, Donnai D: Fetal valproate syndrome. J Med Genet 1995;32:724-727.

22. Dansky LV, Andermann E, Rosenblatt D, et al: Anticonvulsants, folate levels, and pregnancy outcome: A prospective study. Ann Neurol 1987;21:176-182.

23. Finnell RH, Buehler BA, Kerr BM, et al: Clinical and experimental studies linking oxidative metabolism to phenytoin-induced teratogenesis. Neurology 1992;42(4, Suppl 5):25-31.

24. Buehler BA, Bick D, Delimont D: Prenatal prediction of risk of the fetal hydantoin syndrome. N Engl J Med 1993;329:1660-1661.

25. Samren EB, van Duijn CM, Koch S, et al: Maternal use of antiepileptic drugs and the risk of major congenital malformations: A joint European prospective study of human teratogenesis associated with maternal epilepsy. Epilepsia 1997;38:981-990.

26. Warburton D, Kinney A: Chromosomal differences in susceptibility to meiotic aneuploidy. Environ Mol Mutagen 1996;28:237-247.

27. Delvaux I, van Tongerloo A, Messiaen L, et al: Carrier screening for cystic fibrosis in a prenatal setting. Genet Test 2001;5:117-125.

28. Old J, Petrou M, Varnavides L, et al: Accuracy of prenatal diagnosis for haemoglobin disorders in the UK: 25 years' experience. Prenat Diagn 2000;20:986-991.

29. Kaback MM: Screening and prevention in Tay-Sachs disease: Origins, update, and impact. Adv Genet 2001;44:253-265.

30. Whitten CF, Whitten-Shurney W: Sickle cell. Clin Perinatol 2001;28:435-448.

31. Cuckle H: Biochemical screening for Down syndrome. Eur J Obstet Gynecol Reprod Biol 2000;92:97-101.

32. Cusick W, Rodis JF, Vintzileos AM, et al: Predicting pregnancy outcome from the degree of maternal serum alpha-fetoprotein elevation. J Reprod Med 1996;41:327-332.

33. Nadel AS, Norton ME, Wilkins-Haug L: Cost-effectiveness of strategies used in the evaluation of pregnancies complicated by elevated maternal serum alpha-fetoprotein levels. Obstet Gynecol 1997;89 (5, Pt 1):660-665.

34. van Rijn M, van der Schouw YT, Hagenaars AM, et al: Adverse obstetric outcome in low- and high-risk pregnancies: Predictive value of maternal serum screening. Obstet Gynecol 1999;94:929-934.

35. Cheng EY, Luthy DA, Zebelman AM, et al: A prospective evaluation of a second-trimester screening test for fetal Down syndrome using maternal serum alpha-fetoprotein, hCG, and unconjugated estriol. Obstet Gynecol 1993;81:72-77.

36. MacDonald ML, Wagner RM, Slotnick RN: Sensitivity and specificity of screening for Down syndrome with alpha-fetoprotein, hCG, unconjugated estriol, and maternal age. Obstet Gynecol 1991;77:63-68.

37. Spencer K: Accuracy of Down syndrome risks produced in a first-trimester screening programme incorporating fetal nuchal translucency thickness and maternal serum biochemistry. Prenat Diagn 2002;22:244-246.

38. Lennon CA, Gray DL: Sensitivity and specificity of ultrasound for the detection of neural tube and ventral wall defects in a high-risk population. Obstet Gynecol 1999;94:562-566.

39. Watson WJ, Chescheir NC, Katz VL, et al: The role of ultrasound in evaluation of patients with elevated maternal serum alpha-fetoprotein: A review. Obstet Gynecol 1991;78:123-128.

40. Barisic I, Clementi M, Hausler M, et al: Evaluation of prenatal ultrasound diagnosis of fetal abdominal wall defects by 19 European registries. Ultrasound Obstet Gynecol 2001;18:309-316.

41. Crane JP, LeFevre ML, Winborn RC, et al: A randomized trial of prenatal ultrasonographic screening: Impact on the detection, management, and outcome of anomalous fetuses. The RADIUS Study Group. Am J Obstet Gynecol 1994;171:392-399.

42. Goncalves LF, Romero R: A critical appraisal of the RADIUS study. Fetus 1993;3:7-18.

43. Bakketeig LS, Eik-Nes SH, Jacobsen G, et al: Randomized controlled trial of ultrasonographic screening in pregnancy. JAMA 1984;2:207-211.

44. Shirley IM, Bottomley F, Robinson VP: Routine radiographer screening for fetal abnormalities by ultrasound in an unselected low risk population. Br J Radiol 1992;65:565-569.

45. Chitty LS, Hunt GH, Moore J, et al: Effectiveness of routine ultrasonography in detecting fetal structural abnormalities in a low risk population. BMJ 1991;303:1165-1169.

46. Magriples U, Copel JA: Accurate detection of anomalies by routine ultrasonography in an indigent clinic population. Am J Obstet Gynecol 1998;179:978-981.

47. Bahado-Singh RO, Mendilcioglu I, Copel JA: Ultrasound markers of fetal Down syndrome. JAMA 2001;285:2857-2858.

48. Brambati B: Chorionic villus sampling. Curr Opin Obstet Gynecol 1995;7:109-116.

49. Sutcharitchan P, Embury SH: Advances in molecular diagnosis of inherited hemoglobin disorders. Curr Opin Hematol 1996;3:131-138.

50. Froster UG, Jackson L: Limb defects and chorionic villus sampling: Results from an international registry, 1992-94. Lancet 1996;347: 489-494.

51. Grover CM, Thulliez P, Remmington JS, et al: Rapid prenatal diagnosis of congenital toxoplasma infection by using polymerase chain reaction and amniotic fluid. J Clin Microbiol 1990;28:2297-2301.

52. Lynch L, Daffos F, Emanuel D, et al: Prenatal diagnosis of fetal cytomegalovirus infection. Am J Obstet Gynecol 1991;165:714-718.

53. Wen LZ, Xing W, Liu LQ, et al: Cytomegalovirus infection in pregnancy. Int J Gynaecol Obstet 2002;79:111-116.

54. Feldman B, Aviram-Goldring A, Evans MI: Interphase FISH for prenatal diagnosis of common aneuploidies. Methods Mol Biol 2002;204:219-241.

55. Field NT, Gilbert WM: Current status of amniotic fluid tests of fetal maturity. Clin Obstet Gynecol 1997;40:366-386.

56. Moise KJ: Management of rhesus alloimmunization in pregnancy. Obstet Gynecol 2002;100:600-611.

57. Liley AW: Foetal transfusion in haemolytic disease. Bibl Gynaecol 1966;38:146-157.

58. Daffos F, Capella-Pavlovsky M, Forestier F: Fetal blood sampling via the umbilical cord using a needle guided by ultrasound. Prenat Diagn 1983;3:271-277.

59. Hickok DE, Mills M: Percutaneous umbilical blood sampling: Results from a multicenter collaborative registry. The Western Collaborative Perinatal Group. Am J Obstet Gynecol 1992;166:1614-1617.

60. Manning FA: IUGR: Etiology, pathophysiology, diagnosis and treatment. In Manning FA (ed): Fetal Medicine: Principles and Practice. E. Norwalk, Conn, Appleton & Lange, 1995, pp 307-386.

61. Manning FA, Platt LD, Sipos L: Antepartum fetal evaluation: Development of a fetal biophysical profile. Am J Obstet Gynecol 1980;136:787-795.

62. Manning FA, Baskett TF, Morrison I, et al: Fetal biophysical profile scoring: A prospective study in 1,184 high-risk patients. Am J Obstet Gynecol 1981;140:289-294.

63. Manning FA, Morrison I, Lange IR, et al: Fetal assessment based on fetal biophysical profile scoring: Experience in 12,620 referred high-risk pregnancies. I: Perinatal mortality by frequency and etiology. Am J Obstet Gynecol 1985;151:343-350.

64. Arduini D, Rizzo G, Romanini C, et al: Fetal blood flow velocity waveforms as predictors of growth retardation. Obstet Gynecol 1987;70:7-10.

65. Brar HS, Platt LD: Reverse end-diastolic flow velocity on umbilical artery velocimetry in high-risk pregnancies: An ominous finding with adverse pregnancy outcome. Am J Obstet Gynecol 1988;159:559-561.

66. Bahado-Singh RO, Kovanci E, Jeffres A, et al: The Doppler cerebro-placental ratio and perinatal outcome in intrauterine growth restriction. Am J Obstet Gynecol 1999;180:750-756.

67. Galan HL, Ferrazzi E, Hobbins JC: Intrauterine growth restriction (IUGR): Biometric and Doppler assessment. Prenat Diagn 2002;22:331-337.

68. Sterne G, Shields LE, Dubinsky TJ: Abnormal fetal cerebral and umbilical Doppler measurements in fetuses with intrauterine growth restriction predicts the severity of perinatal morbidity. J Clin Ultrasound 2001;29:146-151.

69. Mari G, Detti L, Oz U, et al: Accurate prediction of fetal hemoglobin by Doppler ultrasonography. Obstet Gynecol 2002;99:589-593.

70. Zimmerman R, Carpenter RJ Jr, Durig P, Mari G: Longitudinal measurement of peak systolic velocity in the fetal middle cerebral artery for monitoring pregnancies complicated by red cell alloimmunisation: A prospective multicentre trial with intention-to-treat. BJOG 2002;109:746-752.

71. Mari G, Deter RL, Carpenter RL, et al: Noninvasive diagnosis by Doppler ultrasonography of fetal anemia due to maternal red-cell alloimmunization. Collaborative Group for Doppler Assessment of the Blood Velocity in Anemic Fetuses. N Engl J Med 2000;6:342:9-14.

72. Main DM, Gabbe SG: Risk scoring for preterm labor: Where do we go from here? Am J Obstet Gynecol 1987;157:789-793.

73. Goldenberg RL, Davis RO, Copper RL, et al: The Alabama preterm birth prevention project. Obstet Gynecol 1990;75:933-939.

74. Grimes D, Schulz K: Randomized clinical trials of home uterine activity monitoring: A review and critique. Obstet Gynecol 1992;79:137-142.

75. Iams J, Johnson F, O'Shaughnessy R: A prospective random trial of home uterine activity monitoring in pregnancies at increased risk of preterm labor, Part II. Am J Obstet Gynecol 1988;159:595-603.

76. American College of Obstetricians and Gynecologists (ACOG): Assessment of Risk Factors for Preterm Birth. Practice Bulletin #31. Washington, D.C., ACOG, October 2001.

77. Goldenberg RL, Mercer BM, Iams JD, et al: The preterm prediction study: Patterns of cervicovaginal fetal fibronectin as predictors of spontaneous preterm delivery. National Institute of Child Health and Human Development Maternal-Fetal Medicine Units Network. Am J Obstet Gynecol 1997;177:8-12.

78. Goldenberg RL, Klebanoff M, Carey JC, et al: Vaginal fetal fibronectin measurements from 8 to 22 weeks' gestation and subsequent spontaneous preterm birth. Am J Obstet Gynecol 2000;183:469-475.

79. Iams JD, Goldenberg RL, Mercer BM, et al: The preterm prediction study: Can low-risk women destined for spontaneous preterm birth be identified? Am J Obstet Gynecol 2001;184:652-655.

80. Goldenberg RL, Iams JD, Das A, et al: The Preterm Prediction Study: Sequential cervical length and fetal fibronectin testing for the prediction of spontaneous preterm birth. National Institute of Child Health and Human Development Maternal-Fetal Medicine Units Network. Am J Obstet Gynecol 2000;182:636-643.

81. Gomez R, Romero R, Edwin SS, et al: Pathogenesis of preterm labor and preterm premature rupture of membranes associated with intra-amniotic infection. Infect Dis Clin North Am 1997;11:135-176.

82. Romero R, Gomez R, Ghezzi F, et al: A fetal systemic inflammatory response is followed by the spontaneous onset of preterm parturition. Am J Obstet Gynecol 1998;179:186-193.

83. Caritis S, Toig G, Heddinger L, Ashmead G: A double-blind study comparing ritodrine and terbutaline in the treatment of preterm labor. Am J Obstet Gynecol 1984;150:7-14.

84. Canadian Preterm Labor Investigators Group: Treatment of preterm labor with the beta-agonist ritodrine. N Engl J Med 1992;327:308-312.

85. Effect of corticosteroids for fetal maturation on perinatal outcomes. NIH Consensus Statement 1994;12:1-24.

86. Committee on Obstetric Practice: ACOG committee opinion: Antenatal corticosteroid therapy for fetal maturation. Obstet Gynecol 2002;99(5, Pt 1):871-873.

87. Fontenot T, Lewis DF: Tocolytic therapy with preterm premature rupture of membranes. Clin Perinatol 2001;28:787-796, vi.

88. Mercer BM, Miodovnik M, Thurnau GR, et al: Antibiotic therapy for reduction of infant morbidity after preterm premature rupture of the membranes. JAMA 1997;278:989-995.

89. Ferguson J, Hensleigh P, Kredenster D: Adjunctive use of magnesium sulfate with ritodrine for preterm labor tocolysis. Am J Obstet Gynecol 1984;148:166-171.

90. Hollander D, Nagey D, Pupkin M: Magnesium sulfate and ritodrine hydrochloride: A randomized comparison. Am J Obstet Gynecol 1987;156:631-637.

91. Niebyl JR, Blake DA, White RD, et al: The inhibition of premature labor with indomethacin. Am J Obstet Gynecol 1980;136:1014-1019.

92. Moise KJ, Huhta JC, Sharif DS, et al: Indomethacin in the treatment of premature labor: Effects on the fetal ductus arteriosus. N Engl J Med 1988;319:327-331.

93. Niebyl J, Witter F: Neonatal outcome after indomethacin treatment for preterm labor. Am J Obstet Gynecol 1986;155:747-749.

94. Ferguson J, Dyson D, Holbrook R, et al: Cardiovascular and metabolic effects associated with nifedipine and ritodrine tocolysis. Am J Obstet Gynecol 1989;161:788-795.

DIABETES AND PREGNANCY

Anne B. Kenshole

The changes in the maternal milieu that characterize the diabetic state can have profound effects on the growth and development of the fetus, increasing the risk of perinatal morbidity and mortality, as well as having adverse effects that can persist throughout adult life. Physiologic adaptations induced by pregnancy can unmask latent maternal diabetes or result in transient worsening of preexisting vascular compromise.

OVERVIEW OF CARBOHYDRATE METABOLISM

The body requires a constant source of energy, and this is provided mainly by glucose. On entering a cell, glucose may undergo oxidative (i.e., glycolysis) or nonoxidative metabolism, chiefly glycogen synthesis. Therefore, the regulation of plasma glucose levels and the entry of glucose into cells are of critical importance.

The Postprandial Phase

After the ingestion of carbohydrates, plasma glucose concentrations begin to rise. This change is detected by the islets of the endocrine pancreas, which contain specialized insulin-secreting cells (β cells). In response, insulin secretion increases rapidly, and circulating plasma insulin concentrations rise. Insulin interacts with its receptor in hepatocytes and peripheral tissues, such as skeletal muscle and adipocytes. In muscle and, to a lesser extent, in fat, insulin promotes cellular glucose uptake, removing glucose from the systemic circulation. The synthesis of glycogen, a storage form of glucose, is also promoted in myocytes. Muscle amino acid uptake is triggered, with a simultaneous inhibition of proteolysis. Insulin also inhibits lipolysis in adipocytes and secondarily decreases the release of free fatty acids. In the liver, insulin promotes the storage of excess glucose as glycogen while simultaneously decreasing both glycogenolysis (the breakdown of glycogen) and gluconeogenesis (the production of new glucose).

The Postabsorptive Phase

Four to 6 hours after meal ingestion, when circulating glucose concentrations have fallen to baseline, insulin levels also decline to basal levels. Thus, glucose and amino acid uptake by muscle is reduced. Glucose uptake by fat is also attenuated. Meanwhile, and as a direct result of the decreased circulating concentration of insulin, the liver is transformed from an organ of net glucose disposal to one of net glucose production, in an attempt to support ambient glucose concentrations. Initially, this occurs primarily through glycogenolysis. As glycogen stores decrease, gluconeogenesis contributes a greater proportion to overall hepatic glucose production. This occurs via the conversion of lactate, amino acids (primarily alanine), and, to a lesser extent, glycerol.

The Fasting Phase

Twelve hours or more after a meal, glycogen stores are further depleted, and gluconeogenesis becomes the prime source of circulating glucose. Because amino acids are a major substrate of this new glucose production, gluconeogenesis requires net protein catabolism. In addition, the simultaneous breakdown of fat plays a key metabolic role at this time. The low circulating insulin concentrations allow lipolysis to proceed unabated, providing glycerol to the liver for gluconeogenesis, as well as free fatty acids for conversion to ketone bodies. The latter may be oxidized for energy by certain tissues. Although ketone bodies, chiefly acetoacetate and β-hydroxybutyrate, accumulate, metabolic acidosis does not typically result, because the ketone bodies are rapidly cleared by the kidneys and their systemic levels remain low.

The cycle is initiated once again with food ingestion, indicated by a rise in glucose and amino acid concentrations, which leads to another prompt increase in insulin secretion, followed by the movement of glucose and amino acids into cells and, once again, suppression of hepatic glucose output.

In summary, in the fed state, insulin serves both as an anabolic factor and as an anticatabolic factor. It enhances the supply of energy to cells in the form of glucose, enabling ongoing metabolism, growth, and development. It simultaneously inhibits the breakdown of fat and protein stores while attenuating the production of glucose from the liver. Conversely, during periods of fasting, it is the relative absence of insulin that allows for endogenous glucose production, primarily from the liver, in addition to catabolism of muscle and fat stores to meet the body's continuous requirements for energy.

METABOLIC CHANGES DURING NORMAL PREGNANCY

In pregnancy, important changes occur in carbohydrate, lipid, and ketone body and amino acid metabolism that serve to enhance nutrient supply to the fetus. A progressive state of insulin resistance is induced, resulting in a 2.5-fold to threefold increase in insulin secretion by term.[1,2] Fasting plasma glucose (FPG) levels decline during the third trimester, reflecting the increasing demand for glucose with accelerating fetal growth. Postprandial glucose levels are slightly higher than in the nonpregnant state. During the first and second trimesters, the pregnant woman is in an anabolic state; her fat deposits increase as a result of hyperphagia and enhanced lipogenesis. A catabolic state characterizes the third trimester, with enhanced lipolytic activity in adipose tissue, which results in increased plasma levels of free fatty acids and glycerol and a consequent increased production of triglycerides. Glycerol becomes the preferred gluconeogenetic substrate; other more essential substrates such as amino acids are saved for the fetus. Maternal triglycerides do not cross the placenta but are hydrolyzed, releasing fatty acids to the fetus. The enhanced ketogenesis that occurs during fasting in late pregnancy permits the easy transfer of ketones to the fetus, in whom they are used as fuels for oxidative metabolism as well as lipogenic substrates.

In the postprandial phase, resistance to the cellular actions of insulin dominates, most notably at the level of skeletal muscle, in which insulin allows glucose entry into cells, thus lowering plasma glucose concentrations. This has been demonstrated definitively through the glucose "clamp" technique. In such studies, a pharmacologic amount of insulin is administered to subjects, and glucose uptake (or "disposal") into peripheral tissues is determined by the amount of exogenous dextrose necessary to maintain glucose concentrations in the normal range. Such investigations have demonstrated a 50% to 70% decline in insulin sensitivity by the third trimester, in comparison with that in nonpregnant control subjects. The effect of insulin on the liver, in which it attenuates endogenous glucose production, may also be decreased during pregnancy. Although human placental lactogen, cortisol, and a placental growth

hormone (GH) variant make major contributions to the insulin resistance of pregnancy, tumor necrosis factor α has been shown to be the most significant independent predictor of insulin sensitivity.[3] Elevated leptin levels further contribute to progressive insulin resistance.[4]

Placental GH behaves similarly to native GH, a known counterregulatory hormone. The secretion of native pituitary GH is actually suppressed because of placental secretion of the GH variant, which itself stimulates insulin-like growth factor 1 (IGF-1) production by the liver and peripheral tissues.

Elevated estrogen, progesterone, and prolactin concentrations also decrease insulin sensitivity during pregnancy; insulin sensitivity is further affected by increasing caloric intake, body weight, and adiposity, together with a decrease in physical activity. Other hormones known to affect insulin secretion or action include glucagon and catecholamines, but their secretion is not known to be altered by pregnancy.

Carbohydrate Metabolism in Pregnancy

As a result of diminishing maternal sensitivity to insulin, pregnancy is characterized by increased circulating insulin, because, in health, the maternal β cells compensate for the added demand by enhanced insulin secretion. The teleologic explanation for the insulin resistance of pregnancy is not clear. Some authorities have speculated that the small increases in circulating glucose concentrations enable nutrient flux from mother to fetus, allowing for the fetus' growth and development. Insulin resistance may also promote the accumulation of adipose tissue, a mechanism that allows for maternal caloric storage.

In the fasting state, two important changes occur in maternal carbohydrate metabolism. First, the FPG level declines. The reason for this phenomenon is not fully apparent, inasmuch as the caloric demand of the fetus in early pregnancy is too small to serve as a nutritional "drain" on the mother. Early findings indicate that a decrease in hepatic gluconeogenesis, primarily from decreased amino acid substrate availability, is responsible. This could result from the impact of placental hormones on amino acid release from skeletal muscle. With the progression of pregnancy, however, the shunting of actual calories to the fetus may play a greater role in the relative maternal fasting hypoglycemia of pregnancy. In a study of pregnant women during the second trimester, no change in either basal glucose turnover or gluconeogenesis was found. This suggests that the decline in maternal FPG concentrations does indeed result from utilization by the growing fetus, whose development is probably fueled by the increase in maternal postprandial plasma glucose levels.[5] During fasting, a generalized enhancement of fat catabolism is additionally observed, a direct result of the lipolytic effect of pregnancy, which has been attributed to the effects of placental GH variant.[6] This results in increased circulating concentrations of free fatty acids, providing greater substrate to the liver for ketone body production. The mild fasting hypoglycemia is associated with a compensatory decrease in insulin levels, which allows for further enhancement of ketone production. The effects of

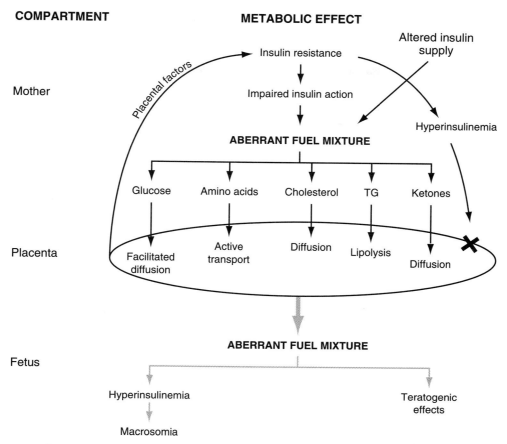

COMPARTMENT   **METABOLIC EFFECT**

Figure 2–1. Diagrammatic representation of changes in the maternal metabolic environment during the pregnancy of a diabetic patient and their effects on the placenta and fetus. TG, triglycerides. (Adapted from Hod M, Rabinerson D, Peled Y: Gestational diabetes mellitus: Is it a clinical entity? Diabetes Rev 1995;3:604.)

the maternal metabolic environment on the fetus are shown in Figure 2-1.

In summary, pregnancy is characterized by accelerated starvation during fasting, when glucose levels fall and fat breakdown is augmented, followed by a state of facilitated anabolism after feeding, which enhances nutrient supply to the fetus.

MATERNAL-FETAL INTERACTIONS AND INTERMEDIARY METABOLISM

The growth of the fetus during the 9 months of gestation is an impressive biologic feat of energy efficiency, involving the transport of a massive amount and assortment of nutrients from the mother to the fetus. This fetal demand represents a significant metabolic obligation on the part of the mother, requiring maternal nutrient storage. Very little is understood about the maternal provision for the nutritional demands of the developing embryo in early gestation. Later in gestation, however, the placenta serves as a conduit for most of the important nutrients. Carbohydrates, in the form of glucose, traverse the placental circulation through a process of facilitated transport via insulin-dependent placental glucose transporters.[7] Ambient fetal glucose concentrations are known to be 20 to 40 mg/dL lower than

simultaneous maternal levels. Thus, the placenta, which is insulin-independent, may act as a partial inhibitor of glucose transport. Active transport of amino acids across the placenta also occurs and is, in part, concentration dependent.[8] Free fatty acids pass freely, although the actual transport mechanisms are not well understood; concentrations are generally higher in the mother than in the fetus. Triglycerides do not cross the placenta, being hydrolyzed to free fatty acids and glycerol within the placenta.[9] Ketone bodies such as acetoacetate and β–hydroxybutyrate are freely diffusible across the placenta, and fetal and maternal concentrations are equal. Glucose supports the energy requirement of the fetus; amino acids are incorporated into proteins, and free fatty acids are re-esterified into fats by fetal tissues. However, access of the principal hormones that govern maternal intermediary metabolism, including that of insulin, is blocked by the placenta. Instead, from the 11th week of gestation onwards, fetal metabolism is controlled by insulin derived from the fetal pancreas.

In the setting of suboptimally controlled diabetes, elevated fetal glucose levels stimulate fetal insulin secretion. This provides one explanation for the excessive fetal growth, or macrosomia, that is the hallmark of the diabetic pregnancy.

In summary, nutrient supply flows essentially freely from the mother to the fetus, whereas the endocrine systems that control the metabolic fate of these nutrients remain separate. During pregnancy in the diabetic patient, higher-than-normal maternal concentrations of glucose and free fatty acids provide increased anabolic substrate for the fetus, giving rise to a series of metabolic changes that result in abnormally increased fetal growth. Therefore, an important goal in managing the diabetic pregnancy is to maintain maternal glucose concentration as close to normal as possible throughout the entire pregnancy.

OVERVIEW OF DIABETES

Diagnosis

The diagnosis of diabetes is made when the FPG concentration is 126 mg/dL or higher, or when any ambient levels are over 200 mg/dL, in conjunction with typical symptoms, such as polyuria, polydipsia, and weight loss. Alternatively, the diagnosis may be made after a standard oral glucose tolerance test (OGTT) with a 75-g glucose load.[10] The OGTT is not performed routinely, because the diagnosis is usually determined easily from one of the other two methods. The glycosylated hemoglobin A_{1c} (HbA_{1c}) is usually, but not invariably, elevated in these situations; however, the test for HbA_{1c} is specific but insensitive and is therefore not widely accepted as a way of establishing the diagnosis.

Classification

Type 1 Diabetes

The term *diabetes* indicates solely the presence of chronic hyperglycemia (Table 2–1). The underlying causes, however, may be quite disparate in pathophysiologic terms. Type 1 diabetes mellitus, formerly referred to as *insulin-dependent diabetes mellitus* or *juvenile-onset diabetes mellitus,* generally occurs in individuals younger than 40 years, usually younger than 30. Clinically, the onset is typically abrupt and obvious, with marked hyperglycemia developing over several days to weeks, usually in association with weight loss, fatigue, polyuria, and polydipsia and often with blurring of vision and, ultimately, volume contraction. The presence of ketoacidosis indicates absolute deficiency of insulin, which results in both hyperglycemia and unrestrained lipolysis. In this setting, increased circulating concentrations of free fatty acids provide substrate to the liver for the production of both new glucose and ketone bodies. Because renal ketone clearance is decreased as a result of volume contraction, circulating ketone concentrations rise, leading to an anion gap metabolic acidosis. If uncorrected, the dehydration and acid-base disturbance lead to further

electrolyte abnormalities, cardiac dysrhythmias, hemodynamic collapse, and, ultimately, death.

In contrast to patients with type 2 diabetes, individuals with type 1 diabetes are often lean.

The etiologic pathogenesis of this disease remains incompletely understood, although it ultimately results from autoimmune destruction of pancreatic islets, which involves both genetic and environmental factors. Although pancreatic islet destruction may occur over a period of years, the clinical manifestations of type 1 diabetes develop rapidly when a critical number of islet cells have failed. Several autoantibodies, such as those directed against glutamic acid decarboxylase (an enzyme within the β cells) and insulin itself, can be detected early in the course of the disease.

Type 2 Diabetes

Type 2 diabetes mellitus, previously termed *non–insulin-dependent diabetes mellitus,* is in many ways an entirely separate disorder. The autoimmune markers of type 1 diabetes are typically absent. Although relative pancreatic insufficiency is, by definition, present in all individuals with type 2 diabetes, the first and perhaps primary disorder in most is peripheral insulin resistance, primarily at the level of skeletal muscle. These two pathophysiologic defects, in combination with augmented hepatic glucose production, which similarly results from the tandem of decreased pancreatic insulin supply and hepatocyte resistance to insulin action, form what has been described as the "triumvirate" of type 2 diabetes[11] (Fig. 2–2).

The natural history of type 2 diabetes begins with a period of insulin resistance with preserved, indeed augmented, insulin secretion. As occurs in normal pregnancy, this insensitivity to insulin action in peripheral tissues is compensated by enhanced pancreatic insulin production, leading to elevated circulating insulin concentrations. Thus, the plasma glucose level remains normal. As the disease progresses, pancreatic islet cell function begins to falter and is no longer able to meet demands for increased insulin secretion. As a result, relative insulin insufficiency and hyperglycemia develop, first manifested in the postprandial setting, whereas fasting glucose levels are usually preserved until late in the course of the disease. Insulin levels at this

TABLE 2–1   Classification of Diabetes Mellitus

Type 1 diabetes mellitus
Type 2 diabetes mellitus
Diabetes resulting from another disease process (secondary diabetes)
Gestational diabetes mellitus

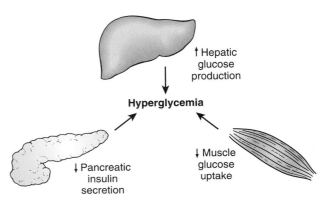

Figure 2–2. Major pathophysiologic contributions to hyperglycemia in type 2 diabetes.

point may actually still be higher than those measured in control subjects. In contrast to patients with type 1 diabetes, typical patients with type 2 diabetes have traditionally been middle-aged or older at presentation; however, type 2 diabetes is now being increasingly recognized among overweight children and young adults with a family history of type 2 diabetes or in ethnic groups with high rates of diabetes. Of individuals with type 2 diabetes, 80% are overweight or obese with excess adipose accumulation within the abdomen, in the so-called "android" pattern, which is a marker of the insulin-resistant state. Insulin secretion persists to some extent in most affected patients; thus, ketoacidosis is rare. Because of renal glucose clearance, plasma glucose elevations plateau in the range of 250 to 350 mg/dL, in the absence of a superimposed deterioration in renal function or marked dehydration. In many patients with type 2 diabetes, a group of other clinical findings is also commonly encountered, including abdominal adiposity, hypertension, dyslipidemia, microalbuminuria and increased risk of premature cardiovascular disease. This constellation of findings is referred to as the *insulin resistance syndrome*, the *metabolic syndrome*, or "syndrome X."[12]

Some cases of diabetes mellitus are difficult to categorize because affected patients have features of both type 1 and type 2. Lean individuals who appear to have type 2 are increasingly recognized to have progressive β cell failure, a manifestation of slowly developing type 1. Several new forms of diabetes have been described. One is known as *maturity-onset diabetes of the young*. Affected individuals present with diabetes during childhood or their teens. Although they may initially experience severe hyperglycemia, sometimes even with ketoacidosis, later they are often able to maintain normal blood glucose levels with oral agents alone. One subtype of maturity-onset diabetes of the young has been associated with an abnormality in pancreatic glucorecognition—that is, the ability of the islet cells to "sense" ambient glycemia—which is related to a defect in the gene coding for the enzyme glucokinase.

Other forms of diabetes include gestational diabetes mellitus (GDM), which is first detected during pregnancy. As later discussed, GDM is being increasingly recognized as little more than a manifestation of type 2 diabetes that is condensed into a shorter timeframe.[13] Secondary diabetes mellitus (Table 2–2) is diabetes for which the origin is attributed to a separate disease process. This is further subdivided into diabetes originating from diseases of the endocrine pancreas (pancreatitis, cystic fibrosis, thalassemia, or hemochromatosis), other endocrinopathies (hyperthyroidism, Cushing's syndrome, acromegaly, and pheochromocytoma), and a number of genetic syndromes. Secondary diabetes is uncommon in general and is rare in pregnant women.

THE MANAGEMENT OF DIABETES

Most people with type 1 diabetes are now on a regimen of two, three, or four injections of insulin each day; insulin pumps are gaining ever-increasing acceptance, because of the enhanced quality of life that they offer, as well as improved glycemic control. Frequent measurement of capillary glucose levels with a hand-held meter is a vital component of successful control, as is educating each affected patient to use a combination of estimating the amount of carbohydrates ingested at each meal or snack, coupled with adjustments in individual insulin doses to accommodate for the postprandial glycemic excursions that are predicted. Additional adjustments in food and insulin have to be made to reduce the likelihood of exercise-induced hypoglycemia. Although such intensive management can result in HbA_{1c} levels in the normal or near-normal range, high and sustained motivation is required on the part of the patient and his or her caregivers. Such tight control increases the likelihood of more frequent and more severe hypoglycemia.

Several insulin types are available, each with their own pharmacokinetic profile involving unique onset, peak, and duration of action (Table 2–3). Patients with the best control are usually on individualized programs involving multiple injections of mixtures of various insulin types. A comprehensive diabetic management program also involves intensive education, a well-balanced meal plan, and the judicious use of exercise.

In contrast, type 2 diabetes is often initially treated with a combination of diet, emphasizing caloric restriction, and exercise, with the goal of weight loss of 5% to 10% of the weight at presentation. These steps, however, are commonly inadequate by themselves for attaining desirable glucose control. Thus, most patients soon require oral hypoglycemic agents, often a combination of two or more that have different mechanisms of action. Metformin or one of the thiazolidinediones are effective in combating the insulin resistance that typifies impaired glucose tolerance or early type 2 diabetes, whereas the

---

TABLE 2–2   Disorders Associated with Secondary Diabetes

Genetic defects in β cell function (e.g., maturity-onset diabetes of the young)
Genetic defects in insulin action (e.g., leprechaunism)
Exocrine pancreatic diseases (e.g., pancreatitis, cystic fibrosis)
Other endocrinopathies (e.g., Cushing's syndrome, acromegaly, pheochromocytoma)
Drug/chemical-induced (e.g., glucocorticoids, pentamidine)
Infections (e.g., congenital rubella, cytomegalovirus)
Uncommon forms of immune-mediated diabetes (e.g., "stiff-man" syndrome)
Other genetic syndromes (e.g., Klinefelter's, Prader-Willi, Laurence-Moon-Biedl syndromes; myotonic dystrophy)

TABLE 2–3   Pharmacokinetics of Human Insulin

Insulin Type	Time Course of Action		
	Onset	Peak	Duration
Rapid acting: Lispro Insulin, Aspart	10-15 min	1-2 hr	3-4 hr
Short acting: Regular Intermediate acting	0.5-1 hr	2-5 hr	5-8 hr
NPH	2-4 hr	6-10 hr	16-24 hr
Lente	3-4 hr	6-12 hr	16-24 hr
Long acting: Ultralente	6-10 hr	18 hr	24-30 hr
Glargine	90 min	None	24 hr

secretagogues are chiefly of value in lean patients with type 2 diabetes or in combination therapy when HbA_{1c} levels remain unacceptably elevated (Table 2–4). Of particular interest is that none of these medications is currently approved for use in pregnancy; therefore, they should be used with caution in women of childbearing age, unless adequate contraception is being practiced. An increasing number of women with the polycystic ovary syndrome with or without associated impaired glucose tolerance and type 2 diabetes are taking metformin to enhance ovulation.

Metformin, a biguanide, works mainly by suppressing hepatic glucose output. It also has a modest effect on peripheral glucose uptake. Beneficial effects on peripheral insulin sensitivity have also been measured, although, as with the sulfonylureas, it has been difficult to discern whether this is a primary or secondary effect. Use of metformin may result in diarrhea, but this usually abates with continued use and slow dosage titration. It has also been associated in rare cases with lactic acidosis, usually in patients already predisposed, such as those with renal failure, hepatic dysfunction, or ethanol abuse. The α-glucosidase inhibitors (e.g., acarbose) are not targeted at a specific lesion of diabetes but impair intestinal carbohydrate absorption by inhibiting the action of an enzyme in the small intestinal brush border. This attenuates the postprandial glucose excursion. Acarbose ingestion frequently leads to gastrointestinal distress, especially flatulence, as may be expected from a drug that increases carbohydrate load to the distal intestine. The thiazolidinediones act mainly by enhancing uptake of glucose at the peripheral level, together with a modest reduction in hepatic glucose output. They are increasingly used, in combination with metformin or in an "insulin-sparing" strategy, together with one or more daily injections of insulin. The safety of the thiazolidinediones in pregnancy has not been established.

The meglitinides (e.g., repaglinide) are chemically dissimilar to sulfonylureas but also increase pancreatic insulin secretion.

It should be reiterated that, despite the advent of new antidiabetic pharmacologic agents, mainstays of therapy continue to be diet, exercise, and attainment of ideal body weight. Concurrent treatment of associated conditions—specifically, other cardiovascular risk factors, such as obesity, hyperlipidemia, and hypertension—is also imperative.

Diabetic Complications

Diabetes-related complications include those resulting from microvascular and macrovascular disease. Microvascular complications primarily involve the kidneys (nephropathy), the eyes (retinopathy), and the peripheral nerves (neuropathy), although the pathogenesis of neuropathy is probably a combination of mechanical disruption of the myelin sheath and microcirculatory impairment. Macrovascular complications involve the coronary arteries, the cerebral circulation, and the vascular supply to the lower extremities, which may result in myocardial infarction, stroke, and peripheral vascular disease, respectively.

Diabetic Nephropathy

Diabetic nephropathy begins with a period of glomerular hyperfiltration, leading to intraglomerular hypertension. After a variable period of years, glomerular injury develops, and, eventually, glomerular scarring and loss occur. Abnormal protein excretion progresses from microalbuminuria (20 to 300 mg/day) to macroalbuminuria (>300 mg/day) and sometimes to frank nephrotic syndrome levels (protein excretion >3.5 g/day). The glomerular filtration rate eventually declines and azotemia results, ultimately necessitating renal replacement therapy, either dialysis or organ transplantation. Diabetes is the second most common cause of renal failure in North America. Treatment with angiotensin-converting enzyme inhibitors has been shown to delay the progression to end-stage renal failure and is routinely prescribed to patients with diabetes once microalbuminuria is detected. Angiotensin-converting enzyme inhibitors are teratogenic, however, and although there is general agreement that they should not be used in the second and third trimesters, uncertainty persists as to whether they should be discontinued in preparation for pregnancy.

Diabetic Retinopathy

The retinal microvasculature is also frequently involved in long-standing diabetes. Background diabetic retinopathy is manifested clinically by the detection of hard exudates, microaneurysms, and minor hemorrhages. This condition is not usually associated with visual loss but is a marker for the future development of more significant disease. Preproliferative retinopathy is manifested by the presence of cotton-wool spots, which are indicative of retinal infarctions. Such ischemia of the retina eventually provides an angiogenic stimulus, although the new blood vessels that form are frequently abnormal in both appearance and structure. In proliferative retinopathy, blood vessel fragility predisposes to significant retinal and vitreous hemorrhage. Edema of the retina may also occur. Involvement of the macula results in visual loss. Studies have confirmed a beneficial effect on sight preservation with laser photocoagulation in the setting of both macular edema and proliferative diabetic retinopathy.

TABLE 2–4	Primary Mechanisms of Action of Oral Agents for Type 2 Diabetes			
Class of Drug	↑ Pancreatic Insulin Secretion	↓ Hepatic Glucose Production	↑ Peripheral Glucose Utilization	↓ Gut Carbohydrate Absorption
Sulfonylureas/meglitinides	X			
Biguanides	X	X	X	
Thiazolidinediones		X	X	
α-Glucosidase inhibitors				X

Diabetic Neuropathy

Diabetic neuropathy has protean manifestations. The most common form is somatosensory peripheral neuropathy. This results in sensory loss in a stocking-glove distribution, often in association with paraesthesias or dysesthesias. Acute mononeuropathies may also occur; either cranial or peripheral nerves or even entire spinal nerve roots may be affected. Autonomic neuropathy, although less common, may have a more significant impact on the patient's quality of life, and multiple organs may be affected. In the gastrointestinal tract, diabetic gastroparesis and diabetic diarrhea lead to significant disability. Involvement of the urinary tract may result in atonic bladder, urinary retention, a predisposition to urinary tract infections, and overflow incontinence. In men, erectile dysfunction results from autonomic neuropathy, vascular disease, or both. Cardiovascular involvement may manifest with orthostatic hypotension. Unawareness of hypoglycemia constitutes a hazard to the patient and to society in general and necessitates targeting blood glucose to higher levels than usual. To date, no treatment, other than improvement in glycemic control, has been shown to delay or reverse the neuropathic complications of diabetes. However, several therapeutic modalities can be directed at symptom amelioration. Specific treatment regimens can help control the various manifestations of autonomic dysfunction.

The diabetic complication that causes the most morbidity and premature death is atherosclerotic disease of the large vessels. Patients with diabetes are at a twofold to fourfold higher risk of both stroke and myocardial infarction than is the general population. The risk is even higher in women than in men. Coronary artery disease, which is often asymptomatic, is a hazard for women with type 1 and type 2 diabetes who are still in their reproductive years. Because of lower extremity vascular occlusions, diabetes is the leading cause of nontraumatic amputations in North America. The accelerated aggressive atherosclerosis that characterizes diabetes has multiple causes, including coexisting hypertension and dyslipidemia. The role of hyperglycemia in the development and progression of atherosclerosis remains uncertain.

The Relationship between Glycemic Control and Complications

The role of hyperglycemia in the development and progression of microvascular complications was confirmed in 1993 with the publication of the Diabetes Control and Complications Trial (DCCT),[14] a large multicenter, randomized, prospective trial comparing conventional with intensive glycemic control. In this study, approximately 1400 patients with type 1 diabetes were randomly assigned to receive either conventional or intensive insulin regimens. The patients in the first group (control subjects) were administered one or two insulin injections daily and met with the investigators every 3 to 4 months. The goal was to maintain an asymptomatic state but not to achieve any specific degree of glycemic control. The latter group (intensively treated subjects) took injections three to four times per day or used an insulin pump, and these subjects met with the study team monthly, with even more frequent telephone consultation. Their glycemic control was targeted to approach normal levels. The therapeutic dichotomy resulted in and was able to maintain an absolute HbA_{1c} difference of approximately 2% between the two groups (9% for conventional therapy vs. 7% for intensive). After 9 years, significant differences in the rates of the development of diabetes complications were observed, with 56% to 76% decreases in the appearance or progression of retinopathy, microalbuminuria, and peripheral nerve dysfunction. Despite these encouraging findings, intensive glucose control is not without its risks: Subjects randomly assigned to this group experienced three times as many severe hypoglycemic episodes as those who were assigned to a conventional regimen. On the basis of this study, however, most type 1 diabetes patients should be considered for tight glycemic control with the target goals as set forth by the American Diabetes Association (ADA) (Table 2-5).

The largest prospective study of type 2 diabetes is the United Kingdom Prospective Diabetes Study.[15] This large and complex study confirmed that the major risk was macrovascular disease, especially coronary artery disease; however, there was no statistically significant correlation with glycemic control. Metformin monotherapy reduced the rate of cardiovascular outcomes in obese patients. Several studies, including the United Kingdom Prospective Diabetes Study, have confirmed the importance of tight blood pressure control in patients with type 2 diabetes. The drugs or the class of drug used may be less important than maintaining target levels.

DIABETES AND PREGNANCY

Before the discovery of insulin in 1922, girls with diabetes frequently did not survive to childbearing age. In those who did, diabetes during pregnancy was associated with high maternal and infant mortality rates, both approaching 50%[16]; stillbirths were the primary causes of perinatal deaths. Insulin resulted in a miraculous reduction in the maternal mortality rate, although perinatal losses were not substantially reduced. Women with more advanced and severe disease finally had the opportunity to become pregnant safely. Since 1970, much has been learned about the important relationship between maternal glycemic control before and during pregnancy and fetal outcomes. The perinatal mortality rate has simultaneously improved as an intensive approach to the diabetic pregnancy has become standard. In the 1960s, for example, the perinatal mortality rate in the pregnancies of women with type 1 was approximately 250 per 1000 live births. By the 1980s,

TABLE 2–5 Glycemic Goals for Adults with Diabetes	
Criterion	**Goal**
Hemoglobin A_{1c} (%)	<7.0%
Preprandial plasma glucose	90-150 mg/dL
Postprandial plasma glucose	<180 mg/dL

From American Diabetes Association: 2004 Clinical practice recommendations. Diabetes Care 2004;27(Suppl 1).

the rate had fallen more than 90%, to 20 per 1000. Indeed, a true shift in the therapeutic paradigm had occurred.

Whereas the primary goal in the diabetic pregnancy used to be maternal and fetal survival, today's chief concern is to approximate the clinical outcomes of nondiabetic pregnancies, particularly with regard to maternal health and the rates of congenital anomalies, fetal macrosomia, and perinatal complications.

Despite ongoing advances in the field, diabetes during pregnancy, particularly when it is poorly controlled, continues to be associated with several significant threats to the health of both the mother and her children. Most studies in developed countries continue to report a 5% to 8% congenital anomaly rate, which is responsible for 50% of the perinatal mortality observed.[17] Outcomes of diabetic pregnancies in developing regions remain much worse.[18]

Risk to both the fetus and the mother in the diabetic pregnancy is associated with the degree of glycemic control, the coexistence of cardiovascular or renal complications, and other factors, such as maternal obesity and hypertensive disorders. An essential concept that has developed from years of epidemiologic observation is the differential effect of diabetic control just before conception and during the first 7 weeks of gestation, when organogenesis is occurring, in comparison with that during the second and third trimesters. Glycemic control during the early phase affects primarily the risk of fetal congenital malformations, whereas maternal outcomes, the risk of fetal macrosomia (and its attendant obstetric complications), and much of the risk of neonatal complications are influenced by management in the latter phase.

Classification

The White classification of diabetic pregnancy is of historic significance.[19] It is featured in Table 2-6. Although it remains in widespread use, it may not be fully applicable to modern diabetic management, because its primary focus is on the duration of maternal diabetes, which is no longer a prime determinant of maternal and fetal outcome. In addition, the White classification did not account for a degree of glycemic control before or during the pregnancy. A simpler classification is now used in many centers (Table 2-7). This schema places the diabetes primarily in the context of the pregnancy (i.e., as a preexisting

condition) or one that was acquired during pregnancy. In addition, practical emphasis is placed on the maternal complications that are known to influence or to be influenced by the progress of the pregnancy (particularly retinopathy, renal disease, and cardiovascular disease). Type 1 or type 2 diabetes that existed before the pregnancy is termed *pregestational diabetes*. Diabetes that is diagnosed during the pregnancy is termed *gestational diabetes*. This terminology does not distinguish between the important subset of women with previously unrecognized type 2 diabetes and women with "true" gestational diabetes in whom carbohydrate intolerance of varying degrees is induced by the insulin resistance that characterizes the latter half of pregnancy.

Pregestational Diabetes

Fertility and Contraceptive Options

In diabetic women with reasonable glycemic control, fertility is well maintained.[20] Only in women with very poorly controlled diabetes, often in the setting of a major eating disorder, does a form of hypothalamic amenorrhea that results in infertility occur. Women with the polycystic ovary syndrome and hyperandrogenism are at increased risk for impaired glucose tolerance or type 2 diabetes and have impaired fertility. However, women with type 1 diabetes with onset at an early age and duration of diabetes of 20 years or more can achieve successful pregnancies. As a result, pregnancy is a common event in diabetic women of childbearing age. Therefore, it is important for physicians caring for women with diabetes to assist them in planning each pregnancy: if necessary, delaying conception until glycemic control has been optimized and vascular complications stabilized. Preventing unwanted pregnancies is crucial. This is particularly true in patients with preexisting complications, which may worsen during pregnancy, or when control is inadequate. Thus, appropriate birth control counseling should be offered to all diabetic women of reproductive ability. The continuous use of a reliable and acceptable form of contraception is the primary concern. Oral contraceptives are the preferred method for most women with diabetes. The low-dose preparations now used have minimal effects on carbohydrate and lipid metabolism. Previous concerns that intrauterine devices might predispose

TABLE 2-6   White Classification of Diabetes in Pregnancy

Class	Description
A	Abnormal glucose tolerance test result (asymptomatic; normal glucose levels achieved with diet only)
B	Adult-onset diabetes (age ≥20 years) and short disease duration (<10 years)
C	Youth-onset diabetes (ages 10-19 years) or relatively long disease duration (10-19 years)
D	Childhood onset (age <10 years), very long disease duration (≥20 years), or evidence of background retinopathy
E	Any diabetes with evidence of vascular disease in the pelvis (diagnosed by plain radiograph)
F	Any diabetes with the presence of renal disease
R	Any diabetes with the presence of proliferative retinopathy
RF	Any diabetes with both renal disease and proliferative retinopathy
G	Any diabetes with a history of multiple failures during pregnancy
H	Any diabetes with atherosclerotic heart disease
T	Any diabetes after renal transplantation

From Hare JW: Gestational diabetes and the White classification. Diabetes Care 1980;3:394.

TABLE 2–7   Alternative Classification of Diabetes in Pregnancy

Pregestational Diabetes ("Overt" Diabetes)
1. Type 1 diabetes
   a. Complicated by retinopathy
   b. Complicated by nephropathy
   c. Complicated by coronary artery disease
2. Type 2 diabetes
   a. Complicated by retinopathy
   b. Complicated by nephropathy
   c. Complicated by coronary artery disease

Pregnancy-Related or Gestational Diabetes
1. Diet-controlled
2. Insulin-requiring

the woman with diabetes to an increased risk of infection have abated. Periodic intramuscular injection of depot formulations of progesterone is another reasonable option because of its effectiveness, especially in patients in whom compliance or appropriate follow-up cannot be secured. Surgical sterilization should be offered to any woman who chooses, for any reason, not to become pregnant.

Epidemiology

Pregestational diabetes includes both type 1 and type 2 (Fig. 2–3). In North America, 2 to 4 per 1000 pregnancies involves a woman with type 1 diabetes. In these women, neither early age at onset nor longer duration of diabetes is now thought to be predictive of adverse perinatal or

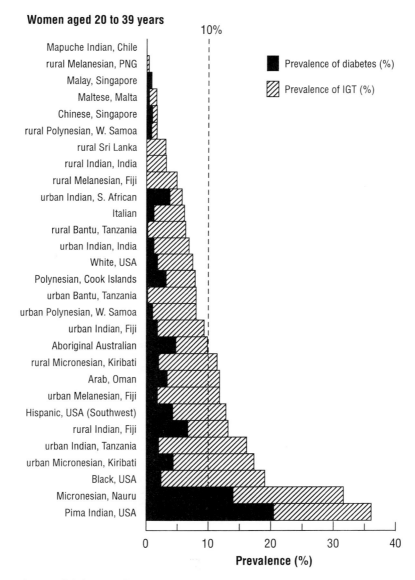

Figure 2–3. Worldwide prevalences of diabetes mellitus and impaired glucose tolerance (IGT) in women from the ages of 20 to 39. PNG, Papua New Guinea. (From World Health Organization Ad Hoc Diabetes Reporting Group: Diabetes and impaired glucose tolerance in women aged 20-39 years. World Health Stat Q 1992;45:324.)

maternal outcomes. On the other hand, the presence of vascular complications affecting one or more systems has significant implications for both mother and child. This situation was previously perceived as uncommon; however, current data suggest that approximately 1% of pregnancies in unselected populations involve women with type 2 diabetes, but the prevalence is considerably higher, ranging from 3% to 6%, among aboriginal women. A population-based survey carried out in the United States in 1995 found that type 2 diabetes accounted for 65% of pregestational diabetic pregnancies that year, in comparison with only 26% in 1980. The patterns of adverse fetal and maternal outcome are the same in type 2 and type 1 diabetes. Major congenital anomalies were detected in 4.4% of infants born to women with a diagnosis of pregestational type 2 diabetes, which is similar to the rate of 4.6% in infants of women with previously unrecognized type 2 diabetes, the diagnosis being confirmed by glucose tolerance testing 6 weeks post partum. Among women with type 1 in that study, major congenital anomalies were found in 5.9% of infants.[21] Type 2 also confers an increased risk of maternal morbidity and perinatal mortality. In a Japanese study,[22] nonproliferative retinopathy was found in 28% and proliferative retinopathy in 4.3% of gravidas with type 2; 1.4% had nephropathy. The perinatal mortality rate was four times higher among infants of mothers with type 2 diabetes than in those of mothers with type 1 in a New Zealand study.[23] Congenital malformations accounted for only 2% of the perinatal deaths.

Furthermore, there was a sevenfold increase in the rate of late fetal death among the infants of women with type 2 diabetes. Potential confounding factors included the older age and greater incidence of obesity of the women with type 2 diabetes who also presented for management later in pregnancy. Many women with type 2 diabetes, as well as their caregivers, perceive type 2 diabetes as having less significance with regard to pregnancy and are therefore less likely to plan their pregnancies. There is clearly a need to educate all women with pregestational diabetes mellitus as well as health professionals about the importance of prepregnancy planning and meticulous management throughout pregnancy.

Fetal Implications

The abnormal metabolic milieu of the diabetic pregnancy can have deleterious effects on the fetus at all stages of gestation (Fig. 2–4). Thus, the diabetic pregnancy is associated with multiple potential complications for the fetus and neonate, which directly or indirectly result from the maternal metabolic derangements. Although the risk of pregnancy-related complications in pregestational diabetic pregnancies has definitively been shown to be decreased[24] with improved glycemic control, the other metabolic derangements that characterize the diabetic pregnancy contribute to the increased perinatal morbidity and mortality that are still encountered.

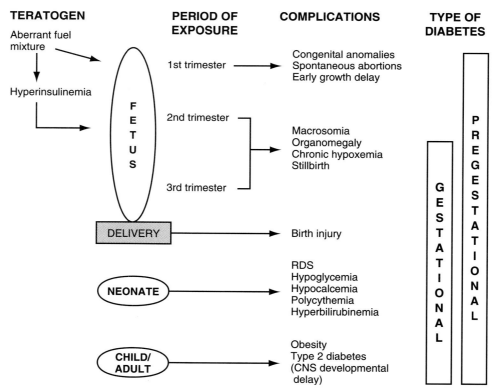

Figure 2–4. Diagrammatic representation of the multiple deleterious effects of the pregnancy of a diabetic patient on the children, during the various periods of fetal and postnatal life. CNS, central nervous system; RDS, respiratory distress syndrome. (Adapted from Hod M, Rabinerson D, Peled Y: Gestational diabetes mellitus: Is it a clinical entity? Diabetes Rev 1995;3:605.)

Congenital Anomalies

The reported incidence of malformations continues to be between two and four times the expected frequency, with a positive correlation between periconceptional glycosylated hemoglobin levels and malformation rates. Diabetic embryopathy, however, is multifactorial. Abnormalities in levels of arachidonic acid and myoinositol levels, generation of excess oxygen free radicals, lipid peroxidation, somatomedin inhibitors, mitochondrial damage, and activation of apoptotic pathways have been implicated.[25] Nevertheless, obtaining the best day-to-day blood glucose levels and the lowest glycosylated hemoglobin measurement that can be safely achieved in all women with pregestational diabetes should be a standard of care. During the periconception period, achieving average fasting capillary glucose concentrations of 70 to 130 mg/dL and a glycosylated hemoglobin measurement less than four standard deviations above normal minimizes the risk of glycemia-related congenital anomalies.[26]

A wide variety of anomalies have been described, most involving the cardiac, neural, skeletal, gastrointestinal, and genitourinary structures (Table 2-8). The most common include ventricular and atrial septal defects; transposition of the great vessels; caudal regression syndrome and other neural tube defects; gastrointestinal atresias; and urinary tract malformations, such as renal agenesis, cystic kidney, and duplex ureter.

In a seminal study in 1983, Fuhrmann and colleagues reported a 5.5% congenital malformation rate among 420 infants born to women with type 1 diabetes, in comparison with 1.4% in a nondiabetic control group.[27] Greene and associates assessed outcomes in 303 pregnant women with type 1 diabetes.[28] The incidence of major malformations was 3.0% in the group with first trimester HbA$_1$ values of 9.3% or less, whereas it was 40% with HbA$_1$ levels above 14.4%; this comparison yielded a risk ratio of 13. Note was made, however, of a broad range of control over which the risks were not substantially elevated (Fig. 2-5). Miller and colleagues also found a significantly higher incidence of major congenital anomalies in the infants of women with elevated HbA$_{1c}$ values.[29] In this study, 13% of 116 women with type 1 diabetes delivered infants with

TABLE 2-8   Congenital Malformations Found More Frequently in Infants of Mothers with Pregestational Diabetes

Cardiac
   Transposition of the great vessels
   Atrial septal defect
   Ventricular septal defect
Spinal/central nervous system
   Spina bifida
   Anencephaly
   Hydrocephalus
Gastrointestinal
   Anal/rectal atresia
Genitourinary
   Renal agenesis
   Cystic kidney
   Ureteral duplex
Other
   Caudal regression syndrome
   Situs inversus

From Kucera J: Rate and type of congenital anomalies among offspring of diabetic women. J Reprod Med 1971;7:61-70.

major congenital anomalies. The mean initial HbA$_1$ level was significantly higher in the group with major anomalies (9.6% vs. 8.4%), and there was no relationship to the White classification. When the study population was divided into women with glycohemoglobin values higher than 8.5% and those with values less than 8.5%, a significant difference in the malformation rate was seen: Of the children, 22% in the poorly controlled group and 3% in the well-controlled group were affected. Ylinen and colleagues measured HbA$_1$ at the end of the 15th week of gestation in 142 type 1 diabetic pregnancies.[30] The HbA$_1$ level was 9.5% in women with pregnancies complicated by fetal malformations, significantly higher than that in unaffected pregnancies (8%). In addition, malformations occurred in 35% of pregnancies in women with HbA$_1$ levels at 10% or more, in 13% of those with HbA$_1$ levels between 8% and 9.9%, and in only 5% of those with levels below 8%.

That factors other than maternal glycemic control contribute to fetal anomalies was also suggested by the Diabetes in Early Pregnancy (DIEP) study, analyzed by

HEMOGLOBIN A$_1$ LEVELS AND DIABETIC PREGNANCY RISK

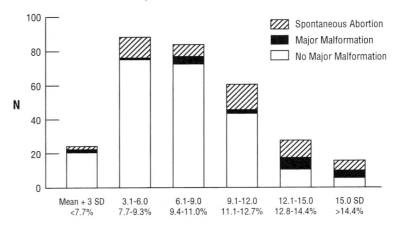

Figure 2–5. Major malformations and spontaneous abortions according to first trimester hemoglobin A$_1$ (HbA$_1$) levels in 303 pregnancies of women with insulin-requiring diabetes. (From Greene M, Hare JW, Cloherty JP, et al: First-trimester hemoglobin A$_1$ risk for major malformation and spontaneous abortion in diabetic pregnancy. Teratology 1989;39:227. Reprinted by permission of John Wiley & Sons, Inc.)

Mills and colleagues.[31] They found no relationship between increased malformation rates in infants of diabetic mothers and glycemic control during the period of organogenesis. In this study, 347 diabetic and 389 control women were enrolled within 21 days of conception. An additional 279 diabetic women entered the study after 21 days. Major malformations occurred in the infants of 4.9% of the early-entry diabetic women, 9% of the late-entry diabetic women, and 2.1% of the control group. The differences were statistically significant between the early-entry diabetic group and the control subjects, as well as between the early- and late-entry diabetic subjects. In early-entry subjects, mean blood glucose and HbA_1 levels during the early first trimester were not significantly higher than in the women whose infants were malformed. Early glycemic data were not available in the late-entry diabetic women. Thus, the failure to find a correlation between glycemic control and malformation rate may lie in the fact that the early-entry patients were generally well controlled. Thus, any differences may have eluded detection because of the statistical design of the trial. Indeed, virtually all the early-entry study subjects would have been included in the "well-controlled" group of Miller and colleagues. Together, the data of Miller and Mills and their respective associates appear to conclude that poor maternal glycemic control explains some but not all of the propensity toward fetal malformations in the pregestational diabetic pregnancy.

Similarly, patient education and initiating intensive management before conception have been demonstrated to significantly decrease but not normalize the risk of congenital malformations.[32]

In Fuhrmann and associates' study, a subgroup of 125 women began intensive treatment before conception; only one malformation (0.8%) occurred in this group.[27] Steel and colleagues compared the gestational outcomes of 143 women with type 1 diabetes who had attended a preconception clinic with the outcomes of 96 diabetic women who did not receive specific pregestational care.[33] The preconception care recipients had lower HbA_1 levels in the first trimester (8.4% vs. 10.5%) and a higher incidence of hypoglycemia (27% vs. 8%) but fewer infants with congenital anomalies (1% vs. 10%). Kitzmiller and coworkers recruited 84 women with type 1 diabetes for intensive preconception care, and their outcomes were compared with those of 110 women who were already pregnant when referred to the investigators at 6 to 30 weeks of pregnancy.[34] Only one major anomaly (1.2%) occurred among the infants in the preconception care recipients, in comparison with 12 (10.9%) of 110 in the postconception group. Transient hypoglycemia during embryogenesis was experienced by 60% of women in the preconception group. This was not associated with detectable sequelae in the children. In the DCCT, 270 pregnancies occurred during 9 years among the more than 1400 patients with type 1 diabetes. In the patients who received conventional treatment, the mean level of HbA_{1c} fell from 8.1% to 6.6% during the pregnancies. In the intensively managed group, the corresponding data were 7.4% and 6.6%. Nine congenital malformations occurred: eight in the control group, whose treatment was generally not intensified until after the discovery of pregnancy,

and only one in the intensively managed group. The small numbers involved resulted in borderline statistical significance.

Early intensive diabetes management not only is advantageous for maternal and fetal health but also has been shown to be cost effective. A financial analysis of the California Early Diabetes and Pregnancy Program concluded that $5 was ultimately saved for every dollar spent by the program, which served to improve the diabetic management of women with type 1 diabetes in the preconception phase.[35]

Early Pregnancy Loss

The risk of spontaneous abortions in diabetic pregnancies is increased according to some but not all reports.[36,37] As in the case of fetal malformations, maternal HbA_{1c} levels at the end of the first trimester are positively correlated with this risk. A nonlinear relationship appears to exist between the spectrum of glycemic control and pregnancy loss: Risks are much higher with the highest HbA_{1c} percentiles.

In one uncontrolled observational study of 132 pregnancies in 91 women with type 1 diabetes, the spontaneous abortion rate was 30%, the incidence peaking between the 10th and 12th gestational weeks. This is more than twice the frequency reported in the literature from normal pregnancies. This group of patients was, however, generally treated suboptimally by modern standards during the preconception phase. Higher abortion rates were associated with more advanced White classification, but relationship with glycemic control was not assessed.

In the outcomes study of 303 pregnant women with type 1 diabetes by Greene and colleagues,[28] spontaneous abortions occurred in 12.4% of women with first trimester HbA_1 levels of 9.3% or less but in 37.5% of those with HbA_1 levels above 14.4%, which yielded a risk ratio of 3. As with congenital anomalies, there was a broad range of control over which the risks were not substantially elevated (see Fig. 2–5).

In the DIEP study,[24] the incidence of spontaneous abortion in 386 women with generally well-controlled type 1 diabetes pregnancies (16.1%) was not substantially different from that in a normal control group of 432 women (16.2%). In the diabetic women who did have spontaneous abortions, however, higher fasting and postprandial glucose levels in the first trimester were detected, in compared with those whose pregnancies continued to term. The authors calculated that in the subgroup of women with poor first trimester control, an increase of 1 standard deviation in HbA_{1c} above the normal range was associated with an increase of 3 % in the rate of pregnancy loss (Fig. 2–6).

Studies continue to show that the incidence of both congenital anomalies and pregnancy loss depends only in part on the degree of preconception care received by the diabetic woman and the level of glycemic control achieved.[36-40] Of the 270 pregnancies in the DCCT, rates of spontaneous abortion were not significantly different between the intensively and conventionally treated groups (10.4% vs. 13.3%).[41]

The exact explanation for the association of diabetes with fetal loss is unclear but presumably involves several

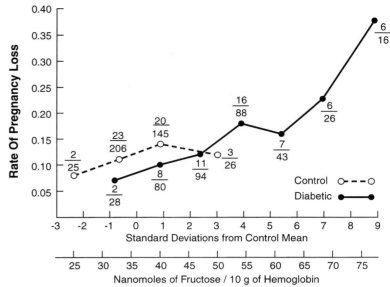

Figure 2–6. Rate of pregnancy loss by mean first trimester hemoglobin A₁ (HbA₁) in 375 women with type 1 diabetes and 402 subjects in the control group, from the Diabetes in Early Pregnancy (DIEP) study. The number of pregnancy losses (numerator) and the total number of women at each level of HbA₁ (denominator) are shown. (From Mills J, Simpson JL, Driscoll SG, et al: Incidence of spontaneous abortion among normal women and insulin-dependent diabetic women whose pregnancies were identified within 21 days of conception. N Engl J Med 1988;319:1620.)

factors working in concert. These factors may include hyperosmolality; ketosis; disruption of glycolysis; DNA glycosylation; inhibitors of various growth factors, such as IGF-1; arachidonic acid deficiency; the generation of oxygen radicals; altered myoinositol metabolism; cell membrane lipid peroxidation[42]; and decreased prostaglandin concentrations.[43]

Macrosomia

Suboptimal glycemic control spurs fetal growth during the second and third trimesters, as excess nutrients (glucose, amino acids, and free fatty acids) are delivered to the fetus. Excess glucose from the maternal circulation stimulates insulin production by fetal β cells, leading to increased anabolic processes, including the deposition of stored calories as fetal fat. Endocrine secretion by the fetal pancreas begins by the 11th gestational week, and it is after this that fetal macrosomia may first be detected by ultrasonography. The increase in fetal body fat occurs in the insulin-dependent tissues, such as the liver, intraabdominal, and thigh adipose stores.[44] Macrosomia may occur in the presence of adequate maternal glycemic control, which indicates that fetal hyperinsulinemia induced by hyperglycemia is only one of several factors that lead to macrosomia.[45] Nevertheless, several groups have convincingly demonstrated that the best predictor of fetal size is maternal postprandial plasma glucose concentrations during the third trimester. This relationship is stronger than that between fetal size and either maternal fasting glucose or HbA₁c level. These data support the accepted position that strict control should be maintained throughout the entire pregnancy. Macrosomia is variously defined as a weight of 4000 or 4500 g, and this may in part explain the wide range in the incidence of macrosomia, from 8% to 43%, noted in type 1 pregnancies.

Late Fetal Demise

Stillbirth rates in pregestational diabetic pregnancies continue to be reported with a frequency of 0% to 4%,[29,46,47] which is a marked improvement in comparison with previous eras. This has presumably resulted from an overall improvement in medical and obstetric care in addition to more sophisticated methods of monitoring fetal well-being. The risk rises as term approaches; therefore, in many centers, induction of delivery at 38 weeks of gestation is standard. The exact reasons for fetal demise are unclear but may be related to maternal diabetic ketoacidosis, fetal acidosis, or placental insufficiency resulting from underlying vasculopathy. Placental insufficiency is thought to be the cause of the increased rate of sudden intrauterine demise that is seen with macrosomic fetuses or in women with type 1 diabetes of long duration, even in the absence of overt vascular complication.

A progressive decline in perinatal death rates has been achieved. Most large series report a neonatal mortality rate in the 5% range; 50% of deaths are attributed to congenital malformations that are incompatible with life. The respiratory distress syndrome, which was previously a major cause of neonatal demise, is encountered less often, in part because of the widespread use of amniocentesis for assessment of fetal lung maturity as well as surfactant treatment of the neonate.

Neonatal Morbid Conditions Associated with Diabetic Pregnancies

Other than fetal loss, congenital malformations and macrosomia, the infant of the diabetic mother is at risk for several other morbid conditions. These include neonatal hypoglycemia, hypocalcemia, hyperbilirubinemia, polycythemia/hyperviscosity, and self-limiting asymmetrical septal hypertrophy. Maternal glycemic control during the latter weeks of gestation and during labor affects the likelihood of each of these adverse outcomes,[48] with the exception of septal hypertrophy, which occurs unpredictably and is unrelated to glycemic control.[49]

Neonatal Hypoglycemia

Currently defined as a serum glucose level of less than 35 to 40 mg/dL at term during the first 12 hours of life, neonatal hypoglycemia has been observed in 30% to 50% of the children of diabetic mothers, depending on the value used. Approximately one fourth of infants born to diabetic mothers experience early hypoglycemia.[50] Neonatal blood glucose levels normally decrease after birth into the range of 50 to 60 mg/dL, although this is not usually associated with any symptoms. Glucose values even lower than 50 mg/dL are also usually well tolerated.[51] However, when glucose concentrations drop below 30 mg/dL, symptoms such as lethargy, failure to feed, and seizures may become apparent. Neonatal hypoglycemia in the children of diabetic mothers is caused in part by fetal β cell hyperplasia, with resultant fetal hyperinsulinism. In addition, simultaneously immature gluconeogenic enzymes and a discontinuation of the maternal nutrient supply play a role. Inappropriately elevated fetal insulin levels at this time also impede the required mobilization of fat stores to provide both ketone bodies and glycerol substrate for neonatal gluconeogenesis. A sluggish rise in neonatal pancreatic glucagon secretion slows lipolysis, further inhibiting hepatic glucose production.

Whether hypoglycemia in neonates is truly deleterious is not well understood.[52] Hypoglycemia may, however, have worse implications for premature infants. Hypoglycemia typically occurs in these infants 1 to 3 hours after delivery and usually resolves during the first day after birth. Strict maternal glycemic control in late pregnancy and during labor and delivery has been shown to reduce the incidence of this complication.

Neonatal Hypocalcemia

Infants of diabetic mothers are also at risk for hypocalcemia during the first few days after birth. Prematurity and birth asphyxia may be contributing factors. In full-term infants from diabetic pregnancies, early sluggishness in parathyroid function has been described. Maternal and consequently neonatal hypomagnesemia leads to physiologic neonatal hypoparathyroidism, resulting from decreases in both secretion and action of parathyroid hormone. Hypomagnesemia occurs in pregnant women with poorly controlled diabetes, primarily because of excess renal losses. Transient neonatal hypocalcemia occurs in approximately 7% of diabetic births. As expected, decreased risk is noted with strict maternal glycemic control.[53]

Polycythemia

An increased incidence of neonatal polycythemia has also been reported; it is probably caused by fetal anoxia secondary to placental insufficiency or the effects of fetal hyperinsulinism, which stimulates fetal erythropoietin production. Increased levels of maternal HgbA$_{1c}$, which binds tightly to oxygen, thereby reducing placental oxygen transfer, provides another explanation. In some cases, a hyperviscosity syndrome may supervene. Affected infants have a plethoric appearance, and venous hematocrits may climb above 60%. Intravascular sludging with tissue anoxia may result, leading to right-sided heart failure, cerebral nervous system dysfunction, and renal vein thrombosis. In one series, the incidence was 7% in gestational diabetes and 11% in pregestational diabetes, but polycythemia was not seen at all in nondiabetic subjects.[48]

Neonatal Hyperbilirubinemia

Neonatal hyperbilirubinemia may follow 20% to 25% of diabetic pregnancies and also appears to be proportional to maternal glucose levels during gestation. The cause is directly related to prematurity, a generalized immaturity of hepatic bilirubin conjugation enzymes, increased red blood cell breakdown, and frequently accompanying neonatal polycythemia.

Respiratory Distress Syndrome

There is an intrinsic risk of respiratory distress syndrome in the infants of diabetic pregnancies, because of physiologic pulmonary immaturity, which predisposes them to hyaline membrane disease. This disease is thought to result from decreased synthesis of surfactant, as a result of fetal hyperglycemia or fetal hyperinsulinism. The risk of respiratory distress syndrome is increased when poor maternal glycemic control has been present and in premature infants. Because of a drop in the rate of prematurity in most diabetic pregnancies, the risk of respiratory distress syndrome has fallen to less than 5%.[54] Antenatal prediction of fetal lung maturity is possible by assessing the lecithin/sphingomyelin ratio or the concentration of phosphatidylglycerol concentration in amniotic fluid.

Birth Asphyxia and Injury

The infants of diabetic mothers have a higher incidence of birth asphyxia, to which they are predisposed because of macrosomia, especially the asymmetrical macrosomia that is common in all types of diabetic pregnancy. A difference of 2.6 cm in the ultrasonographically determined abdominal and biparietal diameters has been shown to be predictive of shoulder dystocia with its attendant risks of brachial plexus and anoxic injury.[55] Cord blood leptin levels have been noted to be significantly higher in infants asymmetrically large for gestational age than in infants of similar weight but symmetrical growth. Other birth injuries and complications include shoulder dystocia,[56,57] brachial plexus injury (Erb's palsy),[58] fractures of the clavicle and humerus, cerebral injury, and increased requirements for forceps delivery or cesarean section. Optimal glycemic control reduces but does not normalize the risk for these adverse outcomes.

Future Development

Neurodevelopmental consequences of maternal type 1 diabetes mellitus were studied by Sells and colleagues in

109 infants of diabetic mothers and compared with outcomes in 90 control infants.[59] The results showed that mothers with insulin-dependent diabetes who maintain good control during pregnancy can expect to have infants who are neurodevelopmentally normal. In those whose diabetes is suboptimally controlled, however, subtle cognitive deficiencies have been described. The risk of future type 1 diabetes in the children of mothers with type 1 diabetes is 1.3%. (The risk for those with fathers with type 1 diabetes is 6%.) There is an apparent greater genetic predisposition in type 2 diabetes, the risk being approximately 15% with one affected parent and as high as 60% to 75% when both parents are affected.[60]

Maternal Considerations

Glycemic Control

In patients with pregestational diabetes, the progressive insulin resistance of pregnancy results in increased insulin requirements, typically twofold to threefold the prepregnancy dose, particularly during the second half of pregnancy. In one study of 237 pregnancies in women with type 1 diabetes, the mean absolute increase in insulin dose was 52 U a day, although individual variation was wide. The increase in insulin was directly related to maternal weight gain in the second trimester.[61] The previously described normal swings in blood glucose from hypoglycemia to postprandial hyperglycemia present further challenges to the maintenance of good glycemic control.

Women with type 1 diabetes are particularly susceptible to increased frequency and severity of hypoglycemia, particularly during the first half of pregnancy. Rosenn and associates performed a series of hyperinsulinemic hypoglycemic clamp studies in a group of 17 women with type 1 diabetes before pregnancy and during the second and third trimesters.[62] The diabetic women demonstrated decreased epinephrine, cortisol, and glucagon responses to hypoglycemia in comparison with their own prepregnancy baseline responses and with those of a control group of 10 healthy women. The GH response during pregnancy was decreased in both groups in comparison with prepregnancy levels. These data may explain the increased propensity of hypoglycemia in pregnant women with type 1 diabetes. During an insulin-induced controlled fall in plasma glucose levels in another study, pregnant women with type 1 diabetes demonstrated failure to increase both their glucagon and epinephrine levels, in comparison with nonpregnant control subjects. In addition, the plasma glucose level, necessary to prompt release of both epinephrine and GH, was 5 to 10 mg/dL lower than in the control group. The authors concluded that the frequency of hypoglycemia in intensively treated pregnant women with diabetes may result, in part, from impairment of counterregulatory hormonal responses.[63]

Severe hypoglycemia does indeed occur frequently during tightly controlled diabetic pregnancies, as demonstrated by Kimmerle and colleagues, who recorded episodes of severe hypoglycemia (defined as impairment of consciousness necessitating intravenous glucose or glucagon) in 85 pregnancies in 77 women with type 1 diabetes.[64] Overall, 94 episodes of severe hypoglycemia occurred in 35 pregnancies. Of these, 80% occurred before the 20th gestational week (median, at the 12th week), and 77% occurred during sleep. Despite this, however, no permanent maternal sequelae were seen, and fetal outcomes were favorable, with no perinatal mortality or congenital anomalies. There persists concern, however, that frequent and/or major maternal hypoglycemia may have deleterious effects on the long-term neuropsychologic development of these infants.[65]

Hellmuth and colleagues found an incidence of 37% of nocturnal hypoglycemia during the first trimester.[66] The best predictive value was a blood glucose level below 108 mg/dL at 2300 hours, which resulted in a risk of nocturnal hypoglycemia of 71%, whereas the chance of avoiding nocturnal hypoglycemia was 83% if the before-bedtime blood glucose level was 108 mg/dL or higher.

It is clearly necessary to individualize treatment goals in the diabetic pregnancy, weighing both the risks and benefits to the mother and the fetus, so that an optimal balance between good glycemic control and the risks of hypoglycemia can be achieved.[67]

The tendency toward ketosis that is observed in normal pregnancy is also accentuated in the diabetic patient. Indeed, omission of insulin injections or the development of a superimposed infection may result in diabetic ketoacidosis more rapidly than would normally occur in the nonpregnant situation. Ketoacidosis develops rapidly and subtly in pregnancy with lower plasma glucose levels than otherwise found. In one third of episodes, glucose levels at presentation were lower than 200 mg/dL.[68] In spite of aggressive management, ketoacidosis still has grave consequences for the fetus, who is intolerant of acidemia, with resulting fetal distress and potential for intrauterine death.

Inadequate caloric ingestion may also manifest itself as low-grade ketonuria and can be avoided by increasing caloric intake to prevent potential deleterious effects to the fetus.[69,70]

Obstetric Complications

Hypertensive Disorders

Hypertensive disorders as a whole occur more frequently in diabetic pregnancies; the risk of eclampsia or preeclampsia is threefold to fourfold higher than in normal pregnancies. In a detailed review, preeclampsia rates ranged from 9% to 66% in patients with type 1 diabetes.[71] The rate increased with increasing severity of diabetes by the White classification; the highest rate was reported in women with pregravid diabetic nephropathy. The relationship between glycemic control and preeclampsia was explored by Hiilesmaa and associates.[72] The adjusted odds ratios for preeclampsia were 1.6 for each 1% increment in the glycosylated hemoglobin value at 4 to 14 (median 7) weeks of gestation and 0.6 (0.5 to 0.8) for each 1% decrement achieved during the first half of pregnancy. Changes in glycemic control during the second half of pregnancy did not significantly alter the risk of preeclampsia. Women with underlying renal dysfunction are particularly at risk. In the case of pregestational diabetes, possible explanations for this phenomenon include underlying vasculopathy, decreased glomerular filtration rate, and the well-recognized sodium retentive properties of insulin itself. In gestational diabetes, underlying activation of the sympathetic nervous system and abnormalities of renal salt handling presumably contribute, along with the effects of insulin, if administered. The incidence of pregnancy-induced hypertension (including preeclampsia) in pregestational diabetes is approximately 15%, or two to four times higher than in control pregnancies.[71] In more advanced diabetes, according to the White classification, the incidence is approximately 30%. Hypertensive disorders are also more frequent when glycemic control is poor.

Preterm Labor

Preterm labor complicates approximately 10% to 30% of pregestational diabetic pregnancies,[73] and this rate also increases with worsening severity of disease, elevated plasma glucose levels, and the presence of urogenital infections.

Polyhydramnios

An overall incidence of polyhydramnios of 16% in all diabetic pregnancies, with comparatively higher rates in patients with pregestational diabetes, has been noted. A pathophysiologic explanation for this phenomenon is not clear, although increased fetal urinary flow and altered osmolality of amniotic fluids have been raised as possibilities.

Pyelonephritis

The incidence of pyelonephritis in diabetic pregnancies is reported to be 4%. This may result from the combination of altered immune function in the patient with poorly controlled diabetes and an increased incidence of incomplete bladder emptying secondary to diabetic neuropathy. One study[74] has shown a positive correlation with fasting blood glucose levels. Screening and treatment of asymptomatic bacteriuria may reduce the incidence of urinary tract infections during pregnancy.

Cesarean Section

The rate of cesarean section for diabetic mothers is at least twofold higher than for their nondiabetic counterparts because of a combination of an increased incidence of preeclampsia and macrosomia, together with worsening of preexisting maternal retinal and renal compromise.

Diabetic Complications and Pregnancy

The potential for development of retinal and renal compromise is influenced by several factors, including genetic predisposition, the duration of diabetes, and glycemic control. Typically, type 1 manifests at puberty; therefore, because it has typically been present 10 to 15 years by the time pregnancy ensues, microvascular complications are not uncommon. Although macrovascular disease in women of reproductive age is uncommon, women with diabetes are at risk, especially those who smoke and are hypertensive.

Diabetic Retinopathy

The incidence of diabetic retinopathy is closely associated with the duration of diabetes, as well as with the degree of

previous glycemic control. The actual mechanisms by which glycemia adversely affects the retinal vasculature are not well understood but are probably multifactorial. An increasingly important role is being ascribed to various local growth factors, such as vascular endothelial growth factor and IGF-1. Of note, maternal concentrations of both of these factors increase during pregnancy, which may in part provide a pathophysiologic basis for the worsening of diabetic retinopathy that is often encountered during pregnancy.

As a general rule, background retinopathy rarely worsens or progresses to proliferative retinopathy during pregnancy.[75,76] In a cross-sectional study of 1358 women with type 1 diabetes, retinopathy was less common in parous women, even when the data were adjusted for glycemic control.[77] Thus, there is no epidemiologic proof that pregnancy promotes persistent acceleration of early microvascular complications. On the other hand, established proliferative retinopathy may worsen during pregnancy. To assess the influence of pregnancy on the progression of diabetic retinopathy, a prospective cohort of 155 women with type 1 diabetes in the DIEP study[76] (Fig. 2-7) was monitored from the preconception period to 1 month post partum. Of subjects with no proliferative retinopathy at baseline, only 10% experienced progression. If minimal, mild, or moderate-to-severe nonproliferative retinopathy was seen at baseline, the risk of progression was 21%, 19%, and 55%, respectively. Of patients with moderate to severe nonproliferative retinopathy, 29% progressed to proliferative disease, whereas only 6% of those with mild retinopathy did so. Predictors of progression were initial HbA_{1c} levels and the degree to which plasma glucose levels were lowered. Rapid improvement in control is recognized to exacerbate

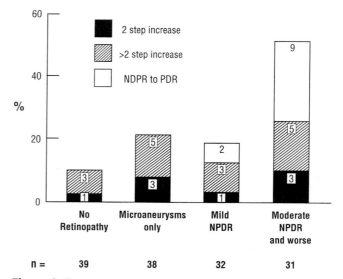

Figure 2–7. Progression rates of diabetic retinopathy during pregnancy, stratified by baseline retinopathy. More severe preconception retinopathy is associated with a greater chance of progression during pregnancy. NPDR, nonproliferative diabetic retinopathy; PDR, proliferative diabetic retinopathy. (From Chew E, Mills JL, Metzger BE, et al: Metabolic control and progression of retinopathy: The Diabetes in Early Pregnancy Study. Diabetes Care 1995;18:633.)

retinopathy; this finding provides further justification for optimizing glycemic control before conception. Therefore, patients with moderate to severe nonproliferative diabetic retinopathy must be monitored closely, particularly if their diabetes was suboptimally controlled during the preconception period. Another study demonstrated that diabetic women are at increased risk for retinopathy progression if they develop hypertension during pregnancy.[78] Pregnancy-induced accentuation of retinal changes generally remits by 6 months post partum. In general, it appears that pregnancy does not alter the long-term course of diabetic retinopathy.

Most authorities recommend that laser photocoagulation therapy be provided before conception to women with proliferative retinal changes. Preconception evaluation by an ophthalmologist experienced in the management of retinal diseases is recommended if diabetes has been present for more than 5 years. During pregnancy, follow-up evaluations should be performed periodically, usually every trimester but more frequently if any changes are observed or in patients at high risk.

Diabetic Nephropathy

Diabetic nephropathy affects 30% to 40% of people with type 1 diabetes. Genetic susceptibility and glycemic control are contributing factors. Patients present initially with an increase in the glomerular filtration rate and with microalbuminuria and rising blood pressure levels 5 to 15 years after diagnosis; progression to overt proteinuria, declining glomerular filtration rate, and accelerating hypertension ultimately result in end-stage renal failure. Microalbuminuria is unlikely to develop de novo during pregnancy, but preconception microalbuminuria tends to increase and is associated with an increased risk of pregnancy-induced hypertension and preeclampsia.[79] Early nephropathy does not appear to progress during pregnancy, whereas women with more advanced renal compromise may experience significant and progressive deterioration in renal function as pregnancy progresses.

The hyperfiltration of pregnancy increases intraglomerular pressure. With the superimposed effect of associated hypertensive disorders, further impairment of renal function may result. Studies to date have included small numbers of women with relatively short postpartum follow-up, and results concerning the risk of accelerated progression of nephropathy during and after pregnancy have conflicted.[80-82]

Perinatal outcome is adversely affected by the development of deteriorating renal function during pregnancy; adverse effects include smallness for gestational age, prematurity, stillbirth, and increased risk for maternal hypertensive disorders.[83]

Neuropathy

By itself, diabetic neuropathy is not a contraindication to pregnancy. However, women with debilitating, painful dysesthesias who, as a result, require analgesic medication may present an unquantifiable risk to their fetuses. In addition, those affected by autonomic dysfunction, such as orthostatic hypotension and delayed gastric emptying (gastroparesis), may find pregnancy particularly difficult, because both blood pressure and gastric emptying decline in most normal pregnancies.

Macrovascular Disease

Pregnancy in women with diabetes and coronary artery disease is extremely risky. Active and significant macrovascular disease may pose a strong contraindication to pregnancy in the diabetic woman.[84,85] For example, a woman with ongoing cardiac ischemia necessarily runs the risk of decompensation during pregnancy, in view of the superimposed demands placed on the heart.

It is prudent to make the patient aware of the serious maternal risk and to recommend a permanent method of sterilization. Myocardial infarction or ischemic cardiac event are probably underreported; 20 cases of such events before, during, or shortly after pregnancy were reported in the literature between 1953 and 1998. Among cases of infarction during pregnancy or in the puerperium, seven mothers and seven infants died, whereas in the seven cases in which the myocardial event occurred before pregnancy, all of the mothers and infants survived. The better outcomes reported since 1980 may reflect improved care or reporting bias of unexpectedly successful outcomes despite preexisting coronary artery disease. The increased cardiac output during pregnancy and, in particular, the immediate 60% to 80% increase in cardiac output that occurs in the immediate postpartum period leaves the woman at risk for pulmonary edema and further myocardial damage. It appears that those diabetic women at risk for or with evidence of coronary disease should undergo exercise testing, preferably with nuclear myocardial perfusion imaging, before conception. If significant coronary insufficiency is documented, revascularization should be contemplated before pregnancy is considered.[86] However, there exist several case reports of successful pregnancies in women after recent revascularization procedures.

Management of Diabetes

The theme of modern glycemic management during the diabetic pregnancy is to approximate the nondiabetic state: that is, to maintain blood glucose levels as close to normal as possible. Such care necessarily requires the cooperative efforts of a clinical team that includes the obstetrician, internist, diabetologist, diabetes educator, and neonatologist.[87,88] This intensive approach necessarily involves an extraordinary commitment on the part of both the patient and the health care team, but the potential benefits to both the mother and the infant are immeasurable. For the patient, effective self-management includes careful attention to dietary intake, regular physical exercise, and frequent monitoring of capillary glucose levels with a home monitor whose accuracy has been demonstrated. Most patients taking insulin require multiple injections per day. The clinical team managing the pregnancy must be responsible for providing patient education, guidance, and counseling. Frequent follow-up, ideally in a specialized multidisciplinary clinic to optimize efficiency and enhance cross-disciplinary decision making, is recommended. Regular telephone contact further enhances compliance and appropriate insulin adjustments. Consultation with appropriate subspecialists, such as an ophthalmologist, is arranged as indicated.

Preconception Counseling and Assessment

As described, it is now well recognized that glucose control before conception and during early gestation (first 6 to 8 weeks) is the primary determinant of the risk for various congenital anomalies and early fetal loss. The degree of glycemic control during the second and third trimesters of pregnancy is correlated with the degree of fetal macrosomia, late fetal demise, and several neonatal complications, as well as with maternal complications, such as hypertensive disorders. It is therefore imperative that all women with pregestational diabetes attain strict glycemic control (if not already achieved during the preconception phase) as soon as possible upon the discovery of pregnancy. A brief hospitalization to speedily determine the most effective regimen is sometimes desirable.

Ideally, prepregnancy management should be initiated 3 to 6 months before intended conception. The shorter time is usually adequate for the women with diabetes of brief duration and reasonable control. In this situation, the goal is to obtain a glycosylated hemoglobin level in the normal range. Typically, diabetes of long duration becomes progressively more difficult to control because patients are less able to perceive hypoglycemia. Allowing 6 months to try different insulin regimens, including, in some cases, initiating use of an insulin pump, helps ensure that conception occurs with the best glycemic control that is attainable. Under these circumstances, a glycosylated hemoglobin level of 8% may be an acceptable target; this has not been shown to be associated with a significantly increased risk of congenital anomaly.[26] This is also the time to consider laser therapy for any women with preproliferative retinopathy. When angiotensin-converting enzyme inhibitors are being used to control hypertension or protein excretion in the urine, they should be continued until conception has occurred. Autoimmune thyroid dysfunction is common and may be subtle. The thyroid-stimulating hormone and thyroid peroxidase autoantibodies should be checked in all women with type 1 diabetes.[89] An association has been noted between high levels of autoantibodies and higher glycosylated hemoglobin levels in early pregnancy. Screening for asymptomatic bacteriuria should be considered. Diabetic women with recurrent urinary tract infections should undergo urologic workup before conception.

Treatment options for women with diabetes during pregnancy who require insulin therapy include a variety of insulin combinations. The most common protocols utilize mixtures of intermediate insulin, such as neutral protamine Hagedorn (NPH) or Lente with short-acting insulin (Regular Insulin). The time course of action for the currently available insulin types is described in Table 2–3. The peak effect of NPH and Lente is 6 to 10 hours after injection, with a duration of action of 18 to 24 hours. Regular Insulin peaks at 2 to 4 hours, and the duration of action is 6 to 8 hours. Ultralente generally has a modest peak, with an effectiveness that lasts 24 to 36 hours. Insulin glargine

is a long-acting "peakless" insulin. Two rapid-acting analogs, insulin lispro and insulin aspart (Novo Rapid) are available. Both have an alteration in the amino acid sequence in the β chain of the insulin molecule. These new structures inhibit the tendency of conventional Regular Insulin to form hexamers, which delays its absorption. The onset of action of both analogs occurs within 10 to 15 minutes, and their action peaks within 1 to 2 hours. These analogs provide better postprandial control and diminish the tendency for hypoglycemia before the next meal. Their pharmacokinetic profile appears to make them ideal for use during pregnancy, in view of the marked insulin resistance that occurs and leads to significant postprandial hyperglycemia; however, neither insulin lispro nor insulin aspart[90] is yet approved for use during pregnancy in North America.

Continuous subcutaneous insulin infusion via an insulin pump offers the type 1 diabetic patient the opportunity for the most intensive glycemic control. Insulin pump therapy can be initiated during pregnancy without transient disturbance in glycemic control.[91]

The computerized pump provides a continuous basal rate of insulin, which may change according to the hour of the day, meeting the basal metabolic demands of the body. In addition, intermittent and variable boluses of insulin are given before meals, to offset the anticipated glycemic excursions that are expected to follow nutrient ingestion. It should be realized that the actual modality of insulin administration in the patient with type 1 diabetes is, by itself, not critical. Of much more importance is the degree of glycemic control achieved. Indeed, the regimen must be individualized for each patient, and creative programs are sometimes necessary: for example, to accommodate shift work.

From the preconception phase onward, fasting blood glucose levels should be maintained between 90 and 105 mg/dL, with 2-hour postprandial readings less than 140 mg/dL (Table 2–9). Constant glucose monitoring systems that continually plot blood glucose levels over a 72-hour period are useful in detecting nocturnal hypoglycemia or demonstrating a progressive overnight rise in glucose levels (the dawn phenomenon). An insulin pump with a programmable progressive increase in basal insulin delivery through the night is the most effective way of combating the dawn phenomenon.

Otherwise, a suboptimally controlled (i.e., high) blood glucose level before breakfast is addressed by increases of 5% to 10% in the dose of the intermediate insulin injected during the previous evening. If the glucose level after breakfast (or that before lunch) is not controlled, a dose

TABLE 2–9 Glycemic Goals for Intensive Management of Diabetes during Pregnancy

Criterion	Goal (mg/dL)	
	Preconception and First Trimester	**Second Trimester**
Preprandial glucose level	70-100	60-90
Postprandial glucose level at 2 hr	<140	<120

of short- or rapid-acting insulin is administered before breakfast. Suboptimal control before supper can be corrected by increases in the intermediate insulin dose administered at breakfast, whereas hyperglycemia after supper (or at bedtime) can be corrected by increases in the dose of short- or rapid-acting insulin before supper. Changes in insulin dosage should generally be made at no more frequent intervals than every 3 to 4 days, so that *trends* in glycemia and not isolated glucose aberrations are addressed. Variations in caloric content, activity level, and especially emotional stress may affect glucose readings substantially. Therefore, appropriate dosage adjustments must take these variables into account. To ensure proper glycemic control, capillary blood glucose readings should be checked four to six times per day throughout pregnancy in all pregestational diabetic patients, if insulin is required. A pattern of blood glucose readings before breakfast and 2 hours after meals with occasional monitoring of premeal and 3:00 A.M. values is useful in monitoring the impact of the changes in diet, exercise, and insulin requirements that pregnancy involves. The preprandial capillary blood glucose determinations are of particular value if the dosage of the short- or rapid-acting insulin is varied from one meal to another on the basis of a "sliding scale." Proactive insulin adjustments, based on the expected level of activity before the next meal, allow for flexibility in mealtimes and food choices in addition to enhancing control. Patients may additionally modulate their dose on the basis of their caloric intake (carbohydrate counting), as well as taking into account their anticipated postprandial activity level. In most cases, an adjustment of ±2 to ±4 U of the short- or rapid-acting insulin is required. Postprandial glycemic excursions may be particularly difficult to control in pregnancy; therefore, significant increases in short- or rapid-acting insulin, beyond the usual proportions that are more in keeping with successful regimens outside pregnancy, are often required. Self-adjustment of insulin doses by the patient is encouraged; alternatively, adjustments in the dose of insulin can be made either in the physician's office or through frequent telephone contact.

As previously discussed, the hormonal milieu of pregnancy results in both impaired insulin action and enhanced lipolysis. As a consequence, ketoacidosis may occur both more frequently and at a lower plasma glucose concentration during pregnancy than in the nonpregnant state. All efforts should be made to avoid this development, because of possible deleterious fetal effects from maternal ketone bodies, which have ready access to the fetal circulation. Although the rates of ketoacidosis in pregnancy continue to fall, it is nevertheless of grave consequence to the fetus, with a fetal death rate of 10%.[69] In one study, the neurodevelopment in children of diabetic pregnancies appeared to be correlated negatively with maternal β-hydroxybutyrate levels in the third trimester.[71] In general, if the blood glucose level is high and ketones are present, the patient requires more insulin. If ketones are present but the glucose level is normal, the patient requires extra calories, particularly before bedtime. The detection of small amounts of ketone in an overnight urine sample, in association with a fasting blood glucose level that is higher than usual, may indicate undetected nocturnal hypoglycemia.

Formal nutritional evaluation should be encouraged in any pregnant woman with diabetes. The diet should offer 30 to 35 kcal/kg, consisting of three meals and a bedtime snack, comprising 50% to 60% carbohydrates and less than 30% fat, with adequate amounts of dietary fiber. Further carbohydrate restriction to 40% of total calories may decrease postprandial glucose surges.

A total average weight gain of 25 to 30 pounds is endorsed by the ADA's committee on maternal nutrition. A weight gain of 15 to 25 pounds is acceptable in overweight women. This can be achieved by limiting daily intake to 20 to 25 kcal/kg.

A regular exercise program should also be considered, because physical activity has been shown to improve insulin sensitivity and glucose levels in both pregnant and nonpregnant diabetic patients. Exercise during pregnancy is both safe and desirable for those with diabetes.[91a,92]

Once conception has occurred, office visits should be scheduled as often as necessary to maintain desirable control throughout the pregnancy, particularly during the last trimester when insulin resistance increases and when most of the insulin dosage adjustments are required. As an index of recent glycemic control, HbA_{1c} levels are measured at least every trimester to corroborate the results of capillary glucose monitoring. Some clinicians use fructosamine concentrations, in lieu of HbA_{1c}, the former representing the degree of glycemic control over a shorter period of 2 to 3 weeks, as opposed to the 2 to 3 months reflected by the HbA_{1c}.[93]

Blood pressure and urinary albumin excretion should be monitored closely, in view both of the increased frequency of hypertensive disorders, including preeclampsia, that accompany diabetic pregnancy, and of the possibility of the deterioration in renal function linked to the diabetes itself. Routine laboratory assessment of renal function should also be performed, particularly in patients with preexisting renal disease. A retinal evaluation should occur every trimester in those without known eye disease and every 1 to 2 months in those with established retinopathy. If visual symptoms develop, an immediate assessment is necessary.

Obstetric Management

First Trimester

Because of the increased risk of preterm delivery, accurate dates must be established in diabetic pregnancies. Ultrasound evaluation should therefore be performed during the late first trimester, before macrosomia becomes established, because macrosomia makes exact dating by size more difficult. However, some investigators have observed a slight growth delay early in diabetic pregnancies, which makes it difficult to date properly by size alone. The usual prenatal tests should also be provided, as for nondiabetic women.

Second and Third Trimesters

As previously discussed, the adverse influence of maternal hyperglycemia on the fetus changes from one of a potential teratogen to one of a potent stimulator of in utero growth. Thus, high maternal glucose levels are associated with macrosomia and its attendant obstetric complications.

Maintaining strict blood glucose control helps attenuate this excessive growth. Ideally, the FPG is maintained below 90 mg/dL, and postprandial blood glucose levels are maintained below 120 mg/dL (see Table 2-9); however, targets have to be individualized especially in women subject to hypoglycemia unawareness, by day or by night. When these levels are achieved, HbA_{1c} is usually maintained within the normal range.

During this time, office visits should occur every 2 to 3 weeks initially, then every 2 weeks, and eventually weekly in the third trimester, depending on the degree of glycemic control achieved, the presence of concomitant diseases, and the woman's experience with previous pregnancies. This schedule not only facilitates proper glycemic control but also allows for the detection of obstetric and medical complications.

As in nondiabetic pregnancies, α-fetoprotein concentrations for the detection of neural tube defects should be measured between the 16th and 21st weeks. Falsely low values in diabetic subjects have been reported by some investigators, especially if glycemic control is poor. Most of the evidence, however, indicates that it remains a reliable test for most patients, especially when used in conjunction with ultrasonography.

Induction of Fetal Lung Maturation

Betamethasone is routinely given to enhance fetal lung maturation whenever premature delivery is likely. The significant insulin resistance that is induced often results in hyperglycemia that persists for up to 5 days after the second of two daily injections. Ketoacidosis has been described. Using an algorithm by which the usual insulin dose was increased by 27% on the first day after betamethasone administration, followed by 45%, 40%, 31%, and 11% on succeeding days, one group of investigators achieved near-normal glycemia throughout the period of treatment.[94] Using an insulin infusion facilitates glycemic management in the presence of such rapidly changing insulin sensitivity.

Antepartum Fetal Surveillance

Antenatal fetal monitoring for signs of compromise in the diabetic pregnancy is performed through various methods, including fetal heart rate testing (nonstress test or contraction stress test) and the biophysical profile score. The preference of test varies from one center to another, and tests are often used in conjunction. The use of fetal vessel Doppler flow velocimetry has been promoted by some centers but has not gained widespread acceptance. Fetal assessments should be performed biweekly, beginning some time between the 26th and 36th gestational weeks, depending on the glycemic control achieved by the mother, the progress of the pregnancy to date, and the underlying risk category of the pregnancy. During the late second trimester and throughout the third trimester, hydramnios, macrosomia, and other fetal abnormalities can be detected by periodic serial ultrasound examinations. Results of antepartum testing should be interpreted cautiously, however, because the test results may not always be concordant with the actual condition of the pregnancy in the diabetic patient.

The nonstress test is the preferred method for assessment of fetal well-being during diabetic pregnancies.

Generally initiated at 32 weeks in women without vascular compromise, testing is started earlier in the presence of maternal hypertension or suspected fetal growth delay. Twice-weekly nonstress tests should be considered if the risk of fetal compromise is high because of macrosomia or intrauterine growth restriction, because intrauterine death has been described within 1 week of a reactive nonstress test. The use of the fetal biophysical profile enables evaluation of amniotic fluid in addition to four parameters of fetal well-being. A score of 8 or more out of 10 is predictive of a reassuring tracing during labor and of normal Apgar scores. In the type 1 diabetes, progressively rising insulin requirements may plateau, generally between 34 to 36 weeks. A muted rise in insulin requirements and early plateauing may be seen in women with long-standing diabetes or vascular compromise, heralding placental insufficiency. A physiologic decline in insulin requirements in late pregnancy may occur in conjunction with placental maturation; however, a rapid decline in insulin requirement—20% or more over a 7-day period—mandates increased fetal surveillance because it suggests placental insufficiency.

The Timing and Route of Delivery

The timing of delivery in the diabetic pregnancy continues to be a controversial issue and is determined by obstetric and medical considerations. The possibility of fetal demise in a potentially hostile uterine environment needs to be weighed against the risk of potential prematurity. Antepartum fetal lung maturation assessment and placental function testing now allow for a more educated determination of the appropriate delivery date. Fetuses that appear most threatened according to such physiologic test results and most likely to survive ex utero can be delivered by induction or cesarean section. In general, women whose pregnancies have been complicated by poor glycemic control or who have other high-risk characteristics should be delivered once fetal lung maturation is secured. However, if the pregnancy has been otherwise uncomplicated with good glycemic control and normal fetal growth, there is little inherent reason to alter the natural course of the pregnancy. In this situation, routine vaginal delivery should be planned. If the fetal growth curve suggests that prolonging gestation beyond 38 weeks is likely to result in a macrosomic infant, induction of labor at that time should be considered. Some authorities still recommend elective induction between 36 and 38 weeks because of the increased potential for stillbirth in late pregnancy.[95] Whenever delivery before 38 weeks is contemplated, a lecithin/sphingomyelin ratio of 2.0 or more and the presence of phosphatidylglycerol are proof of fetal lung maturity. Respiratory distress syndrome is rarely seen in the infant of the diabetic mother in the presence of these values. Although vaginal delivery is the goal, rates of cesarean sections in diabetic pregnancies remain high because of a combination of concern about the association between macrosomia and shoulder dystocia, especially when the estimated fetal weight is 4500 g or higher. Coexisting preeclampsia (the rate of which is increased in multiparous as well as nulliparous type 1 diabetic pregnancies), the potential for fetal compromise that is evident when control is suboptimal, and the presence of maternal vascular complications further contribute to the twofold to threefold increase in cesarean section rates that continue to be recorded. The cost-benefit ratio of elective cesarean section for suspected macrosomia in diabetic pregnancies is a matter of ongoing debate.[96]

Labor and Delivery

It is important to maintain maternal glucose levels within the normal range to prevent stimulation of the fetal pancreas during labor and to minimize the risk of fetal hypoglycemia. Women with type 1 diabetes without endogenous insulin require a constant supply of exogenous insulin. A continuous insulin infusion is the best way to maintain blood glucose levels within target: that is, between 60 and 120 mg/dL. During insulin infusion, capillary glucose monitoring should be performed every 1 to 2 hours and the insulin drip adjusted to maintain glucose levels within target. If labor is prolonged, a 5% dextrose in water solution should be infused together with the insulin. Alternatively, if intravenous insulin is not used, Regular Insulin or an analog can be administered every 3 to 6 hours subcutaneously according to a sliding scale so as to maintain the desired blood glucose concentrations. This regimen usually results in greater lability in glycemic control.

Postpartum Care

The superimposed insulin resistance of pregnancy rapidly resolves after delivery, often with complete normalization of the blood glucose levels in patients with type 2 diabetes. Patients with type 1 diabetes may experience a "honeymoon" period during which no insulin is required for hours, occasionally for a day or more. This is attributed to increased insulin sensitivity resulting from suppression of pituitary GH. Capillary blood glucose levels are measured every 4 hours, and insulin is initiated when a level of 180 mg/dL is found. Because enhanced insulin sensitivity may persist for several days and hypoglycemia should be avoided, doses equivalent to or somewhat less than prepregnancy requirements are appropriate. During the puerperium, the combination of discomfort and the initiation of breast feeding, together with the abrupt alteration in the maternal hormonal milieu, results in lability of blood glucose levels, necessitating more liberal glycemic targets than usual. Because major or frequent hypoglycemia is undesirable in a woman caring for a newborn infant, temporary blood glucose goals may be set at 80 to 150 mg/dL.

Insulin should be discontinued at delivery in the woman with type 2 diabetes. Blood glucose levels are then monitored every 6 hours. If significant hyperglycemia occurs, insulin is used in preference to oral agents during lactation.

Breast-feeding is encouraged in all women but is generally associated with greater difficulty in maintaining good glycemic control.[97]

The incidence of postpartum thyroiditis is increased in women with type 1 diabetes; approximately 25% of such women are affected, a threefold increase over that observed in the nondiabetic population.[98] Therefore, women with type 1 diabetes should be vigilantly monitored post partum for any sign or symptoms of either thyrotoxicosis or hypothyroidism.

Gestational Diabetes Mellitus

GDM continues to be one of the most controversial issues in fetal maternal medicine. Because of changing and sometimes conflicting recommendations for universal or selective screening, disagreement also persists about the appropriate diagnostic criteria for the glucose tolerance test by which the diagnosis is made and, ultimately, by uncertainty about the significance of modest elevation of maternal glucose levels in pregnancy for the woman and her offspring. Current recommendations concerning diagnosis and management should be regarded as tentative pending the result of prospective studies that have sufficient power to resolve these important issues.

Definition

Currently defined as carbohydrate intolerance of varying severity with onset or first recognition during pregnancy, GDM encompasses three different conditions: (1) "true" gestational diabetes, which develops in the later half of the pregnancy as a result of the altered hormonal milieu; (2) previously unrecognized type 2 diabetes, which is discovered as result of screening; and (3) the uncommon case in which the first manifestation of type 1 diabetes occurs when a woman is pregnant. The implications for the woman and her children, both with regard to pregnancy outcome and in the long term, are different in each situation and account for some of the continuing uncertainties and conflicting findings that exist in the literature on GDM. The incidence of type 2 diabetes masquerading as GDM reflects the prevalence in the population being studied; for example, in one study, 46% of women were reclassified as having type 2 diabetes on postpartum glucose tolerance testing.

Risk Factors (Table 2-10)

In a large survey of almost 15,000 pregnancies, of which nearly 5% were complicated by GDM, multivariate analysis showed an increased risk in mothers with older maternal ages, those with a family history of diabetes, those who smoked, those with increased body mass index (BMI) (especially those who gained weight early in adulthood), and those who were nonwhite.[99] In a smaller survey of more than 1100 women of whom 7% had GDM, increased risk was encountered in women older than 30 years, those

---

TABLE 2-10   Risk Factors for Pregnancy-Related Diabetes Mellitus

Age >30 years
Obesity
Insulin resistance
Polycystic ovary syndrome
History of pregnancy-related diabetes mellitus during previous pregnancy
History of large-for-gestational-age infant during previous pregnancy
Family history of type 2 diabetes (first-degree relative)
Ethnicity (Native Americans; African Americans; Hispanic Americans, and Asian Americans; Pacific Islanders)

with a family history of diabetes in a first-degree relative, and those with a BMI greater than 30 kg/m². [100] However, the incidence of GDM in women even without known definable risk factors in this study remained considerable, at almost 5%. As observed in type 2 diabetes, central fat distribution appears to serve as an independent risk factor for GDM. [101] The polycystic ovary syndrome is another risk factor, which appears to be independent of BMI, [102] particularly in those with pregestational hyperinsulinemia. [103]

A woman with a history of a pregnancy complicated by GDM is likely to experience a recurrence during future pregnancies. Recurrence rates of between 20% and 50% have been reported and are doubled among women who require insulin during the earlier pregnancy. [104] During the second pregnancy, a higher dosage of insulin is often required. Women who develop GDM again during subsequent pregnancies have a higher BMI (especially if BMI is 35 kg/m² or greater), higher plasma glucose concentrations during OGTT, and a higher incidence of neonates who are large for gestational age during the index pregnancy. Early recurrent GDM (i.e., that detected before 24 weeks) occurs in 5% of women with prior GDM and often indicates previously undetected type 2 diabetes. [13] It is interesting that delivery of a child with macrosomia (weighing >4000 g), despite no abnormalities on OGTT, increases the risk of GDM in future pregnancies threefold.

In addition to the risk of glucose intolerance in subsequent pregnancies, women with a history of GDM represent a group at high risk for the future development of type 2 diabetes. [105] Rates reflect the prevalence of type 2 diabetes in the population studied. The annual incidence ranges from a low of 0.5% per year to a high of 7.5%. [106] Up to 50% may develop diabetes 5 years after delivery. Having delivered a macrosomic child increases the risk of future diabetes sixfold, despite no abnormalities detectable by OGTT. Therefore, all these individuals require continuing surveillance of their carbohydrate metabolism after delivery.

Many authorities believe that GDM and type 2 diabetes mellitus are usually nothing more than different stages of the same general disease process. The evidence for this is based on similar epidemiologic characteristics, similar comorbid features, and a shared pathogenesis. [13]

Pathogenesis

Like type 2 diabetes, GDM is marked by a variable combination of decreased insulin action resulting from peripheral insulin resistance and relatively decreased insulin secretion. The severity of the hyperglycemia correlates with the degree of these impairments. It is therefore logical to consider GDM as a prodrome of type 2 diabetes that is unmasked by pregnancy. As in type 2 diabetes, the underlying insulin resistance, although not initially clinically apparent, may have been present for years. Initially, this is compensated for by increased pancreatic insulin production, which results in normal glucose uptake by peripheral tissues and suppression of hepatic glucose output. With the superimposed insulin resistance of pregnancy (especially during the second half), further augmentation of insulin production may not be possible or adequate. The result is decreased peripheral glucose

uptake, increased hepatic glucose output, and, as a result, increased circulating plasma glucose concentrations. As in type 2 diabetes, this is first apparent postprandially and subsequently appears in the fasting state.

Diagnosis

Oral Glucose Tolerance Test

The American College of Obstetrics and Gynecology recommends universal screening; that is, all pregnant women should be screened for GDM between the 24th and 28th weeks. The ADA recommends selective screening, thus avoiding the need to screen gravidas at low risk. To be considered at low risk, a woman must be younger than 25 years, be of normal body weight, have no family history of diabetes, and not be a member of an ethnic or racial group with a high prevalence of diabetes. The U.S. Preventive Services Task Force [107] concluded that the evidence is insufficient to recommend or warn against routine screening for gestational diabetes and that better quality evidence is needed to determine whether the benefits of screening for GDM outweigh the harm. Until such evidence is available, clinicians may reasonably choose either not to screen at all or to screen only women at increased risk for GDM. The Task Force found insufficient evidence that screening for GDM substantially reduces important adverse health outcomes for mothers or their infants (for example, cesarean delivery, birth injury, or neonatal morbidity or mortality). Screening produces frequent false-positive results, and the diagnosis of GDM may be associated with other adverse outcomes, such as negatively affecting a women's perception of her health, but data are limited. In 2002 the Canadian Society of Obstetricians and Gynecologists revised their guidelines for screening and concluded that a single approach to testing for GDM cannot be recommended at the present because there is not enough evidence-based data proving the beneficial effect of a large-scale screening program. Until a large perspective randomized control trial shows a clear clinical benefit for screening and consequently treating GDM, recommendations will necessarily be based on consensus or expert opinion. Currently, the clinician therefore has the options of universal or selective screening; the option of not screening for GDM is also considered acceptable. [108]

Early screening in pregnancy is, however, recommended for any woman with underlying risk factors for type 2 diabetes, including those with previously known impaired glucose tolerance, with obesity, with hypertension or hyperlipidemia, or with the polycystic ovary syndrome; those who are members of at-risk ethnic groups (women of African, Hispanic, Asian and Aboriginal origin); and those with a family history of type 2 diabetes.

In the United States, most centers currently use the diagnostic recommendations and criteria of the National Diabetes Data Group (NDDG) (Table 2–11). This consists of a two-step process, initially a screen consisting of a 50-g oral glucose challenge (the glucose challenge test), which can be performed at any time during the day without regard to meal ingestion. Patients with a 1-hour plasma glucose value of 140 mg/dL or higher should be further evaluated with the more formal and rigorous 3-hour

OGTT unless the screen value is higher than 180 mg/dL, which is predictive of an abnormal result. For the OGTT, the patient should fast at least 8 hours but no more than 14 hours. In addition, her diet during the 3 previous days should have unrestricted carbohydrate intake. The patient is administered 100 g of glucose orally, with venous blood sampled at baseline and hourly for 3 hours while continuing the fast. The woman should remain seated and refrain from smoking. The diagnosis of GDM is made when two values or more surpass the following four thresholds for plasma glucose concentrations: 105 mg/dL (5.8 mmol/L) for fasting; 190 mg/dL (10.6 mmol/L) at 1 hour; 165 mg/dL (9.2 mmol/L) at 2 hours; and 145 mg/dL (8.1 mmol/L) at 3 hours. These thresholds are based on the O'Sullivan criteria but are extrapolated to plasma determinations from the original whole blood readings. At some centers, the more stringent criteria of Carpenter and Coustan (see Table 2–11) are used: ≥95 mg/dL (5.3 mmol/L) for fasting; ≥180 mg/dL (10 mmol/L) at 1 hour; ≥155 mg/dL (8.6 mmol/L) at 2 hours; and ≥140 mg/dL (7.8 mmol/L) at 3 hours. These values were adapted from the NDDG, on the basis of a more recent plasma glucose reagent methodology, and are recommended by the ADA. The NDDG criteria have continued to be accepted by the Second through Fourth International Workshop Conferences on Gestational Diabetes Mellitus between 1985 and 1998.

Women with one abnormal value in the 3-hour OGTT should undergo repeat testing. The incidence of neonatal macrosomia in infants of women with such "borderline" results has been reported to be as high as 20%.[109] In addition, one group has shown a decreased gestational morbidity rate if glucose-"intolerant" women (as defined by a positive result of a 50-g glucose challenge test but a negative result of a 100-g glucose tolerance test) are placed on an aggressive nutritional protocol. The incidence of macrosomia in this group decreased from 18% to 7%, and the cesarean section rate dropped from 30% to 20%.[110]

There is no distinct relationship between the absolute plasma glucose values during the oral glucose challenge or OGTT and the risk of macrosomia in women with either glucose intolerance of pregnancy or frank gestational diabetes. In women with GDM, however, average fasting and postprandial glucose concentrations are higher in those with macrosomic newborns than in those with nonmacrosomic newborns.[111]

The World Health Organization (WHO) supports the 2-hour 75-gram OGTT for detecting GDM (see Table 2–11). The criteria are the same as those for assessing glucose tolerance in nonpregnant adults, with the important modification that impaired glucose tolerance (2-hour plasma glucose level >7.8 mmol/L [140 mg/dL]) be treated in pregnancy as diabetes. In one comparison of the NDDG and WHO diagnostic methods, the prevalence of GDM in the same 709 women proved significantly different. GDM was diagnosed in only 1.4% of women by the NDDG criteria but in 15.7% through WHO parameters. In all the women with abnormal NDDG tests, GDM was additionally detected with the WHO 75-g OGTT. Notably, of the 14 women with macrosomic infants, six had abnormal WHO test results, although only three received abnormal diagnoses by NDDG criteria. These findings suggest that the WHO criteria are better at predicting gestational morbidity than the more cumbersome schema of the NDDG.[112] The Fourth International Workshop-Conference on GDM modified its prior recommendation, aligning them with the recommendations of Carpenter and Coustan (see Table 2–11).

Obviously, there is considerable controversy regarding whether to screen women for GDM and, if so, the most appropriate way. As in all tests that serve to screen for or diagnose disease, enhanced sensitivity usually results in lowered specificity. It is clear that random glucose measurements have both poor sensitivity and specificity, rendering them inadequate for assessing abnormal glucose tolerance in pregnancy.[113] Some authorities have argued, however, that a fasting blood glucose determination may be a more effective and efficient screen than the glucose challenge, because in some series only 15% of women with positive challenges are found to be truly diabetic on the basis of the 3-hour test.[114] Others have encouraged the utilization of generally higher glycemic criteria. For instance, no effects on neonatal morbidity, mortality, or birth trauma were observed in a study that relaxed the WHO criteria of diagnosing GDM, using a 2-hour plasma glucose level of 9 mmol/L (162 mg/dL) instead of the usual 7.8 mmol/L (140 mg/dL). Women in whom GDM

TABLE 2–11   Criteria for an Abnormal Result of an Oral Glucose Tolerance Test for the Diagnosis of Gestational Diabetes Mellitus*

	Criteria		
Time	National Diabetes Data Group (100 g) (≥2 Abnormal Results)	Carpenter and Coustan (100 g) (≥2 Abnormal Results)	World Health Organization (75 g) (>1 Abnormal Result)
0-hour fasting	≥105 mg/dL (5.8 mmol/L)	≥95 mg/dL (5.3 mmol/L)	≥140 mg/dL (7.8 mmol/L)[†]
1-hour fasting	≥190 mg/dL (10.6 mmol/L)	≥180 mg/dL (10.0 mmol/L)	—
2-hour fasting	≥165 mg/dL (9.2 mmol/L)	≥155 mg/dL (8.6 mmol/L)	≥200 mg/dL (7.8 mmol/L)
3-hour fasting	≥145 mg/dL (8.1 mmol/L)	≥140 mg/dL (7.8 mmol/L)	—

Data from the National Diabetes Data Group: Classification and diagnosis of diabetes mellitus and other categories of glucose intolerance. Diabetes 1979;18:1039; Carpenter MW, Coustan DR: Criteria screening tests for gestational diabetes. Am J Obstet Gynecol 1982;144:768; and World Health Organization: Diabetes mellitus: Report of a WHO Study Group [Tech. Rep. Ser. No. 727]. Geneva, World Health Organization, 1985.
*All results based on venous plasma determinations.
†If fasting result is <140 mg/dL and the 2-hour result is 140-199 mg/dL, the diagnosis is "impaired glucose tolerance," and, during pregnancy, the patient should be treated in the same aggressive manner as if she had frank "diabetes."

would have been diagnosed according to standard criteria gave birth to children who were heavier than average.[115] Some authorities advocate using different thresholds for various ethnic groups, on the basis of the variable reliability of the screening criteria in individual populations. For instance, in one study, 27% of white patients failed the 50-g glucose challenge, whereas the corresponding failure rates in black, Asian, and Filipino patients were 18%, 41%, and 31%, respectively. When the women with "glucose challenge failures" in these groups were subjected to the formal 3-hour OGTT, the GDM rates were 17%, 43%, 12%, and 12%, respectively. It therefore appears that the predictive value of the glucose challenge varies substantially by ethnicity.[116]

Other Tests

Because the renal glucose threshold decreases during normal gestation, glycosuria is common during pregnancy. Therefore, there is no role for urine glucose screening to diagnose diabetes during pregnancy. HbA_{1c} is a poorly sensitive test for diagnosing GDM, in part because of the length of time necessary to increase the percentage of glycosylation of the hemoglobin molecule. In addition, because this test represents an average ambient glucose concentration, the initial postprandial glucose elevations that occur may not result in a significant HbA_{1c} increase over the normal range. For these reasons, HbA_{1c} cannot be used as a screening tool for GDM.

Complications

A few studies have found an increased risk for fetal malformations in pregnancies complicated by GDM.[117] Because organogenesis is complete by 7 weeks of gestation, it is surmised that pregestational diabetes existed but was detected only during pregnancy.

Macrosomia is the main adverse outcome in GDM. The incidence of fetal macrosomia, defined as a birth weight of more than 4000 g, varies from 10% to 20%, and that of fetuses large for gestational age (>90th percentile) is 15% to 35%.[118] Postprandial hypoglycemia seems to be most predictive of the development of fetal macrosomia.[119] The risk of shoulder dystocia rises with the weight of the infant and may approach 50% in infants who weigh 4500 grams or more in GDM, a twofold to threefold increase.[120]

For this reason, elective cesarean section may be considered when the estimated fetal weight exceeds 4 to $4\frac{1}{2}$ kg in these infants; however, prenatal estimation of weight in infants large for gestational age is of limited accuracy, and the cost-benefit ratio of elective induction or routine cesarean delivery for suspected macrosomia is a matter of debate.[96]

A pilot study has raised important questions about the value of diagnosing and treating GDM. No difference in birth weight, rates of macrosomia, operative delivery, or neonatal metabolic disorders was found in a study of 300 women with gestational diabetes randomly assigned to be managed by strict glycemic control and tertiary level obstetric care in comparison with women who underwent twice-weekly blood glucose measurement and received routine obstetric care.[121] Wen and associates compared fetal and maternal outcome in two regions of Ontario

that have contrasting policies on prenatal screening. Prenatal glucose screening was discontinued in 1989 in the metropolitan Hamilton area, whereas it was continued in most of the rest of the province. No difference was found in any outcome measure, including macrosomia and cesarean section rates, in the screened and the unscreened populations.[122]

Some investigators have found an increased perinatal mortality rate among the infants of mothers with GDM. In one previous large survey of more than 116,000 pregnancies, GDM was associated with an increased risk of perinatal death, with an adjusted odds ratio of 1.5. Infants of women with GDM that was diagnosed only retrospectively had an even higher rate of perinatal mortality (odds of 2:3).[123] No subsequent study has combined current obstetric and medical practice with sufficient power to detect any small increase in perinatal mortality rate that might occur.

Although the infants of mothers with any form of diabetes during pregnancy have been shown to be at increased future risk for the development of obesity and type 2 diabetes, at this time manipulation of the intrauterine metabolic milieu has not been shown to be preventative. Conversely, aggressive control of maternal hyperglycemia has been shown to increase the risk of intrauterine growth restriction, which is now recognized as a risk factor for cardiovascular disease in adult life.[124]

Risk of Hypertensive Disorder

Whether the risk of preeclampsia is increased in women with GDM is debatable. Data supporting both viewpoints exist, mostly from retrospective or case-control studies. Most studies have found that women with GDM who develop pregnancy-related hypertension tend to be older and heavier and to exhibit more marked insulin resistance and hyperinsulinemia.

Diabetic Management

Traditional management was with dietary restriction and exercise with the addition of insulin in women with blood glucose levels that exceeded target levels. The effects of primary dietary therapy in women with gestational diabetes on fetal growth and neonatal outcomes were evaluated by the Cochrane Library in 2001.[125] Four studies involving 612 women were included. The trials were small and of variable quality. No differences were detected between primary dietary therapy and no primary dietary therapy for birth weights exceeding 4000 g (odds ratio, 0.78; 95% confidence interval, 0.4521 to 1.35) or cesarean deliveries (odds ratio, 0.97; 95% confidence interval, 0.6521 to 1.44). It was concluded that there was not enough evidence to evaluate the use of primary dietary therapy for women who showed impaired glucose metabolism during pregnancy. Traditionally, however, a diet consisting of 30 to 32 kcal/kg/day is recommended for nonobese women with GDM. In obese women, further restriction may be warranted, as low as 25 kcal/kg per day.[126] The effectiveness and safety of markedly hypocaloric diets are unproven during pregnancy. The diet should be initially individualized in consultation with a nutritionist familiar with the unique requirements during pregnancy. In general, the dietary program should consist of 50% to 60% of complex carbohydrates, less than 30% fat, and adequate fiber (25 g/1000 kcal). Further decreases in carbohydrate intake may prevent postprandial hyperglycemia, and simple sugars should generally be avoided. Daily caloric intake should be divided as equally as possible among three meals and one or two snacks. Specifically, inclusion of a bedtime snack is important for preventing fasting ketosis. Regular and graduated physical exercise is considered an important component of any program and has generally been shown to be safe and effective in women with GDM. Treatment goals are to maintain preprandial glucose levels below 90 mg/dL and 2-hour postprandial levels below 120 mg/dL.

Insulin Use in Gestational Diabetes Mellitus

The use of insulin in GDM continues to be one of the most important but unresolved issues. To date, no large randomized trial in unselected populations has adequately addressed the level of maternal glycemia that warrants its use, the optimal insulin regimen that should be employed or, most important, the target blood glucose levels that will favorably affect fetal and maternal outcomes. The impact of insulin use in GDM has been addressed by the United States Preventive Services Task Force.[107] The Task Force found that although insulin therapy does decrease the incidence of fetal macrosomia in women with more severe degrees of hyperglycemia, the magnitude of any effect on maternal and neonatal health outcomes is not clear. The evidence is insufficient to determine the magnitude of health benefit for any treatment among the numerous women with GDM and milder degrees of hyperglycemia.

Insulin therapy is recommended by some authorities for patients who are unable to maintain the FPG at or below 105 mg/dL or their 2-hour postprandial glucose levels at or below 120 mg/dL. Others recommend using the 1-hour postprandial glucose reading of less than 140 mg/dL as a threshold for the initiation of insulin therapy.[127] Unlike type 1 diabetes, type 2 diabetes can often be managed with one or two daily injections alone, sometimes consisting of solely intermediate-acting insulin. Consistent glycemic targets are more commonly achieved through the use of a mixture of insulins with both short and intermediate durations of action, usually NPH and Regular Insulin, administered before breakfast and the evening meal. In other patients, however, more aggressive regimens as previously described may be necessary. Insulin requirements typically rise throughout the third trimester, including the final 2 weeks, during which time the dose required may increase more than 25%.

The use of oral hypoglycemic agents in pregnancy is currently being reevaluated. In a pilot study[127] in which women with gestational diabetes were treated with glyburide, no adverse maternal or fetal outcomes were evident. In women with the polycystic ovary syndrome, metformin therapy throughout pregnancy may protect against the development of gestational diabetes[128]; in one study, its use appeared to be safe.[129]

The woman with GDM should perform home glucose monitoring, initially three or four times per day, both before and after meals, in order to assess for the need for insulin therapy. Those in whom GDM is managed with diet alone and is stabilized may reduce their monitoring to twice daily, being sure that at least some of these checks are performed postprandially. Assessment of urine ketones is also helpful. If insulin treatment is initiated, the goal should be to normalize glucose concentrations; however, despite maintaining this target, excess fetal growth may nonetheless occur, inasmuch as many factors other than glycemia determine fetal growth.

Maintenance of appropriate weight gain should be monitored. Fearing the need for insulin, some women may inadvisably restrict their caloric intake. The detection of persistent overnight ketonuria should prompt a review of carbohydrate and total energy intake.

Obstetric Management

There is no agreed-upon protocol for antepartum testing in women with GDM. Most centers begin routine testing on these patients in the early third trimester, especially if glucose control has been suboptimal or if insulin is required. A rational program consists of daily recording of fetal movement counts beginning at week 36 and weekly nonstress or biophysical profile testing beginning at weeks 32 to 36. Periodic ultrasonography is also useful for assessing amniotic fluid volume and fetal growth.

Timing and Route of Delivery

In general, gestation can proceed to term, followed by vaginal delivery; however, if macrosomia is suspected, induction of labor at or after 38 weeks may be considered, or elective cesarean section may be recommended if the estimated fetal weight is 4500 g or more.

Labor and Delivery

At the time of delivery, medical management of the insulin-requiring women with GDM is less complex than for those with type 1 diabetes; however, maintenance of normal maternal glucose levels continues to be necessary to prevent fetal hyperinsulinism and minimize the risk of neonatal hypoglycemia. Depending on the prelabor degree of hyperglycemia and the total daily dose of insulin, the woman with GDM who requires insulin during pregnancy may require little to no insulin during labor, because of her fasting status and high energy requirements at this time. Capillary glucose determinations should be performed every 2 hours during labor, and glucose levels should be maintained between 60 and 120 mg/dL. Small doses of short-acting insulin can be administered subcutaneously when the glucose levels climb above this threshold, or, preferably, an insulin infusion drip can be used, as discussed in the section on pregestational diabetes. It is advisable in most cases to avoid intermediate-acting insulin at this time. If labor begins shortly after the administration of intermediate insulin, capillary blood glucose should be monitored closely and intravenous dextrose solution should be provided.

A "labeling effect" induced by the diagnosis of GDM was noted in the Toronto Tri-Hospital program.[130] In this large study, women with GDM who received "usual care" had infants with macrosomia rates comparable with those of infants of nondiabetics but were significantly more likely to be delivered by cesarean section.

Postpartum Care

After delivery, plasma glucose levels normalize in most women. Capillary glucose determinations should initially be performed two to four times per day. If persistent hyperglycemia is noted, undiagnosed pregestational diabetes may have actually been present. In women whose blood glucose levels normalize after delivery, a follow-up FPG test should be performed 4 to 6 weeks postpartum. Some authorities recommend that a 75-g OGTT be performed at that time, with subsequent referral if abnormalities are detected. Women with GDM have up to a 50% risk of developing type 2 diabetes within 5 to 10 years of delivery. Therefore, ongoing monitoring is indicated, and annual fasting blood glucose determinations suffice for this. This is an ideal opportunity for ongoing nutritional assessment, and counseling is geared at weight maintenance, the judicious use of exercise, and other lifestyle modifications. In addition, appropriate family planning should be considered, including provision of contraception.

References

1. Catalano P, Tyzbir E, Roman N, et al: Longitudinal changes in insulin release and insulin resistance in non-obese pregnant women. Am J Obstet Gynecol 1991;165:1667.
2. Buchanan T, Metzger B, Freinkel N, Bergman R: Insulin sensitivity and B-cell responsiveness to glucose during late pregnancy in lean and moderately obese women with normal glucose tolerance of mild gestational diabetes. Am J Obstet Gynecol 1990;162:1008.
3. Kirwan JP, Hauguel-De Mouzon S, Lepereq J, et al: TNF-alpha is a predictor of insulin resistance in human pregnancy. Diabetes 2002;51:2207.
4. Vitoratos N, Salamelekis E, Kassanos D, et al: Maternal plasma leptin levels and their relationship to insulin and glucose in gestation-onset diabetes. Gynecol Obstet Invest 2001;51:17.
5. Chiasson J, el Achkar G, Ducros F, et al: Glucose turnover and gluconeogenesis during pregnancy in women with and without insulin-dependent diabetes mellitus. Clin Invest Med 1997;20:140.
6. Freinkel N: The Banting lecture 1980: Of pregnancy and progeny. Diabetes 1990;13:209.
7. Thorens B, Charron M, Lodish H: Molecular physiology of glucose transporters. Diabetes Care 1990;13:209.
8. Holzman I, Lemons J, Meschia G, Battaglia F: Uterine uptake of amino acids and placental glutamine-glutamate balance in the pregnant ewe. J Dev Physiol 1979;1:137.
9. Bonnet B, Brunzell J, Gown A, Knopp R: Metabolism of very-low-density lipoprotein triglyceride by human placental cells: The role of lipoprotein lipase. Metabolism 1992;41:596.
10. American Diabetes Association: Screening for type 2 diabetes. Diabetes Care 2003;26:S21.
11. Defronzo R: Lilly Lecture 1987. The triumvirate: beta cell, muscle, liver: A collusion responsible for NIDDM. Diabetes 1988;37:667.
12. Reaven G: Banting Lecture 1998. Role of insulin resistance in human disease. Diabetes 1988;37:1595.
13. Pendergrass M, Fazoni E, DeFronzo R: Non–insulin-dependent diabetes mellitus and gestational diabetes mellitus: Same disease another name? Diabetes Rev 1995;3:566.
14. DCCT Research Group: The effect of intensive treatment to diabetes on the development and progression of long-term complications in insulin-dependent diabetes mellitus. N Engl J Med 1993;329:977.
15. Intensive blood glucose control with sulphonylureas or insulin compared with conventional treatment and risk of complications in type 2 diabetes (UKPDS 33). UK Prospective Diabetes Study (UKPDS) Group. Lancet 1998;352:837.
16. Gabbe S: A story of two miracles: Impact of the discovery of insulin on pregnancy in women with diabetes mellitus. Obstet Gynecol 1992;79:295.
17. Weintrob N, Karp M, Hod M: Short- and long-range complications in offspring of diabetic mothers. J Diabetes Complications 1996;10:294.
18. al-Dabbous I, Owa J, Nasserallah Z, al-Qurash I: Perinatal morbidity and mortality in offspring of diabetic mothers in Qatif, Saudi Arabia. Eur J Obstet Gynecol Reprod Biol 1996;65:165.
19. White P: Pregnancy complicating diabetes. Am J Med 1949;7:609.
20. Kjaer K, Hagen C, Sando S, Eshoj O: Infertility and pregnancy outcome in an unselected group of women with insulin-dependent diabetes mellitus. Am J Obstet Gynecol 1992;166:1412.
21. Farrell T, Neale L, Cundy T: Congenital anomalies in the offspring of women with type 1, type 2 and gestational diabetes. Diabet Med 2002;19:322.
22. Omori Y, Minei S, Testuo T, et al: Current status of pregnancy in diabetic women: A comparison of pregnancy in IDDM and NIDDM mothers. Diabetes Res Clin Pract 1994;24(Suppl S):273.
23. Cundy T, Gamble G, Townend K, et al: Perinatal mortality in type 2 diabetes mellitus. Diabet Med 2000;17:33.
24. Mills J, Simpson J, Driscoll S, et al: Incidence of spontaneous abortion among normal women and insulin-dependent diabetic women whose pregnancies were identified within 21 days of conception. N Engl J Med 1988;319:1617.
25. Reece E, Homko C, Wu Y: Multifactorial basis of the syndrome of diabetic embryopathy. Teratology 1997;54:171.
26. Ray JG, O'Brien TE, Chan W: Preconception care and the risk of congenital anomalies in the offspring of women with diabetes mellitus: A meta-analysis. Q J Med 2001;94:435.
27. Fuhrmann K, Reiher H, Semmler K, et al: Prevention of congenital malformations in infants of diabetic mothers. Diabetes Care 1983;83:173.
28. Greene M, Hare J, Cloherty J, et al: First-trimester hemoglobin A$_1$ and risk for major malformation and spontaneous abortion in diabetic pregnancy. Teratology 1989;39:225.
29. Miller E, Hare J, Cloherty J, et al: Elevated maternal hemoglobin A$_{1c}$ in early pregnancy and major congenital anomalies in infants of diabetic mothers. N Engl J Med 1981;304:1331.
30. Ylinen K, Qula P, Stenman U-H, et al: Risk of minor and major malformations in diabetics with high haemoglobin A$_{1c}$ values in early pregnancy. BMJ 1984;289:345.
31. Mills J, Knopp R, Simpson J, et al: Lack of relation of increased malformation rates in infants of diabetic mothers to glycemic control during organogenesis. N Engl J Med 1988;318:671.
32. Willhoite M, Bennert HJ, Palomaki G, et al: The impact of preconception counseling on pregnancy outcomes. The experience of the Maine Diabetes in Pregnancy Program. Diabetes Care 1993;16:450.
33. Steel J, Johnstone F, Hepburn D, Smith A: Can prepregnancy care of diabetic women reduce the risk of anomalous babies? BMJ 1990;301:1070.
34. Kitzmiller J, Gavin L, Gin G, et al: Preconception care of diabetes: Glycemic control prevents congenital malformations. JAMA 1991;265:731.
35. Scheffler R, Feuchtbaum L, Phibbs C: Prevention: The cost-effectiveness of the California Diabetes and Pregnancy Program. Am J Public Health 1992;82:168.
36. Rosenn B, Miodovnik M, Combs CA, et al: Glycemic thresholds for spontaneous abortion and congenital malformations in insulin dependent diabetes mellitus. Obstet Gynaecol 1994;84:515.
37. Lorenzen T, Pociot F, Johannesen J, et al: A population-based survey of frequencies of self-reported spontaneous and induced abortions in Danish women with type 1 diabetes mellitus. Danish IDDM Epidemiology and Genetics Group. Diabet Med 1999; 16:472.
38. Chia Y, Chua S, Thai A, et al: Congenital abnormalities and pregestational diabetes mellitus in pregnancy. Singapore Med J 1996; 37:380.
39. Albert T, Landon M, Wheller J, et al: Prenatal detection of fetal anomalies in pregnancies complicated by insulin-dependent diabetes mellitus. Am J Obstet Gynecol 1996;174:1424.
40. Hawthorne G, Robson S, Ryall E, et al: Prospective population based survey of outcome of pregnancy in diabetic women: Results of the Northern Diabetic Pregnancy Audit. BMJ 1994;315:279.
41. Pregnancy outcomes in the Diabetes Control and Complications Trial. Am J Obstet Gynecol 1996;174:1343.
42. Carone D, Loverro G, Greco P, et al: Lipid peroxidation products and antioxidant enzymes in red blood cells during normal and diabetic pregnancy. Eur J Obstet Gynecol Reprod Biol 1993; 51:103.
43. Schoenfeld A, Erman A, Wurchaizer S, et al: Yolk sac concentration of prostaglandin E$_2$ in diabetic pregnancy. Prostaglandin 1995; 50:121.

44. Kehl R, Krew M, Thomas A, Catalano P: Fetal growth and body composition in infants of women with diabetes mellitus during pregnancy. J Matern Fetal Med 1996;5:273.

45. Combs C, Gunderson E, Kitzmiller J, et al: Relationship of fetal macrosomia to maternal postprandial glucose control during pregnancy. Diabetes Care 1992;15:1251.

46. Gestation and Diabetes in France Study Group: Multicenter survey of diabetic pregnancy in France. Diabetes Care 1991;14:994.

47. Roberts A, Pattison N: Pregnancy in women with diabetes mellitus. Twenty years experience: 1968-1987. N Z Med J 1990;103:211.

48. Kuo P, Lin C, Chen Y, Chen H: The effect of third-trimester glycemic control on maternal and perinatal morbidities in pregestational diabetes mellitus. J Formosan Med Assoc 1992;91:237.

49. Sheehan PQ, Rowland TW, Shah BL, et al: Maternal diabetic control and hypertrophic cardiomyopathy in infants of diabetic mothers. Clin Pediatr (Phila) 1986;25:266.

50. Ogata E: Perinatal morbidity in offspring of diabetic mothers. Diabetes Rev 1995;3:652.

51. Tanzer F, Yazar N, Yazar H, Icagasioglu D: Blood glucose levels and hypoglycaemia in full term neonates during the first 48 hours of life. J Trop Pediatr 1997;43:58.

52. Silverman B, Rizzo T, Green O, et al: Long-term prospective evaluation of offspring of diabetic mothers. Diabetes 1991;40:121.

53. DeMarini S, Mimouni F, Tsang R, et al: Impact of metabolic control of diabetes during pregnancy on neonatal hypocalcemia: A randomized study. Obstet Gynecol 1994;83:918.

54. Kjos S, Walther F, Montoro M, et al: Prevalence and etiology of respiratory distress in infants of diabetic mothers: Predictive value. Am J Obstet Gynecol 1990;163:898.

55. Cohen B, Penning S, Major C, et al: Sonographic prediction of shoulder dystocia in infants of diabetic mothers. Obstet Gynecol 1996;88:10.

56. Nocon J, McKenzie D, Thomas L, Hansell R: Shoulder dystocia: An analysis of risks and obstetric maneuvers. Am J Obstet Gynecol 1993;168:1732.

57. Yeo G, Lim Y, Yeong C, Tan T: An analysis of risk factors for the prediction of shoulder dystocia in 16,471 consecutive births. Ann Acad Med Singapore 1995;24:836.

58. Lewis D, Raymond R, Perkins M, et al: Recurrence rate of shoulder dystocia and neonatal morbidity and mortality. Am J Obstet Gynecol 1995;172:1369.

59. Sells C, Robinson N, Brown Z, Knopp R: Long-term developmental follow-up of infants of diabetic mothers. J Pediatr 1994;125:S9.

60. Hagay Z, Reece E: Diabetes mellitus in pregnancy and periconceptional genetic counseling. Am J Perinatol 1992;9:87.

61. Steel J, Johnstone F, Hume R, Mao J: Insulin requirements during pregnancy in women with type 1 diabetes. Obstet Gynecol 1994;83:253.

62. Rosenn B, Miodovnik M, Khoury J, Siddiqi T: Counterregulatory hormonal responses to hypoglycemia during pregnancy. Obstet Gynecol 1996;87:568.

63. Diamond M, Reece E, Caprio S, et al: Impairment of counterregulatory hormone responses to hypoglycemia in pregnant women with insulin-dependent diabetes mellitus. Am J Obstet Gynecol 1992;166:707.

64. Kimmerle R, Heinemann L, Delecki A, Berger M: Severe hypoglycemia incidence and predisposing factors in 85 pregnancies of type 1 diabetic women. Diabetes Care 1992;15:1034.

65. ter Braak EW, Evers I, Willem Erkelens D, Visser GH: Maternal hypoglycemia during pregnancy in type 1 diabetes: maternal and fetal consequences. Diabetes Metab Res Rev 2002;18:96.

66. Hellmuth E, Damm P, Molstea-Pedersen L, et al: Prevalence of nocturnal hypoglycemia in first trimester of pregnancy in patients with insulin-treated diabetes mellitus. Acta Obstet Gynecol Scand 2000;79:958.

67. Rosenn B, Siddiqi T, Miodovnik M: Normalization of blood glucose in insulin-dependent diabetic pregnancies and the risks of hypoglycemia: A therapeutic dilemma. Obstet Gynecol Surv 1995;50:56.

68. Cullen M, Reece E, Homko C, et al: The changing presentations of diabetic ketoacidosis during pregnancy. Am J Perinatol 1996;13:449.

69. Montoro M, Myers V, Mestman J, et al: Outcome of pregnancy in diabetic ketoacidosis. Am J Perinatol 1993;10:1.

70. Rizzo A, Dooley S, Metzger B, et al: Prenatal and perinatal influences on long-term psychomotor development in offspring of diabetic mothers. Am J Obstet Gynecol 1995;173:1753.

71. Sibai B: Risk factors, pregnancy complications and prevention of hypertensive disorders in women with pregravid diabetes mellitus. J Matern Fetal Med 2000;9:62.

72. Hiilesmaa V, Suhonen L, Terano K: Glycemic control is associated with preeclampsia but not with pregnancy-induced hypertension in women with type 1 diabetes mellitus. Diabetologia 2000;43:1534.

73. Hanson U, Persson B: Outcome of pregnancies complicated by type 1 insulin dependent diabetes in Sweden. Am J Perinatol 1993;4:330.

74. Rosenn B, Miodovnik M, Combs C, et al: Poor glycemic control and antepartum obstetric complications in women with insulin-dependent diabetes. Int J Gynaecol Obstet 1993;43:21.

75. Klein B, Moss S, Klein R: Effect of pregnancy on progression of diabetic retinopathy. Diabetes Care 1990;13:34.

76. Chew E, Mills J, Metzger B, et al: Metabolic control and progression of retinopathy. The Diabetes in Early Pregnancy Study. National Institute of Child Health and Human Development Diabetes in Early Pregnancy Study. Diabetes Care 1995;18:631.

77. Chaturvedi N, Stephenson J, Fuller J: The relationship between pregnancy and long-term maternal complications in the EURODIABIDDM complication study. Diabetic Med 1995; 12:494.

78. Rosenn B, Miodovnik M, Kranias G, et al: Progression of diabetic retinopathy in pregnancy: Association with hypertension in pregnancy. Am J Obstet Gynecol 1992;166:1214.

79. Ekbom P, Damm P, Feldt-Rasmussen B, et al: Pregnancy outcome in type 1 diabetic women with microalbuminuria. Diabetes Care 2001;24:1739.

80. Purdy L, Hantsch C, Molitch M, et al: Effect of pregnancy on renal function in patients with moderate to severe diabetic renal insufficiency. Diabetes Care 1996;19:1067.

81. MacKie A, Doddridge MC, Gamsu HR, et al: Outcome of pregnancy in patients with insulin dependent diabetes mellitus and nephropathy with moderate renal impairment. Diabetes Med. 1996;13:96.

82. Miodovnik M, Rosenn B, Khoury J, et al: Does pregnancy increase the risk for development and progression of diabetic nephropathy? Am J Obstet Gynecol 1996;174:1180.

83. Biesenbach G, Stoger H, Zazgornik J: Influence of pregnancy on progression of diabetic nephropathy and subsequent requirement of renal replacement therapy in female type 1 diabetic patients with impaired renal function. Nephrol Dial Transplant 1992;7:105.

84. Rosenn B, Miodovnik H: Medical complications of diabetes mellitus in pregnancy. Clin Obstet Gynecol 2000;43:17.

85. Pombar X, Strassner H, Fenner P: Pregnancy in a woman with class H diabetes mellitus and previous coronary artery bypass graft: A case report and review of the literature. Obstet Gynecol 1995; 85:825.

86. Gordon M, Landon M, Boyle J, et al: Coronary artery disease in insulin-dependent diabetes mellitus of pregnancy (class H): A review of the literature. Obstet Gynecol Surv 1996;51:437.

87. Bailey B, Caldwell M: A team approach to managing pre-existing diabetes complicated by pregnancy. Diabetes Educator 1996;22:111.

88. Jovanovic-Peterson L, Peterson C: Pregnancy in the diabetic woman. Guidelines for a successful outcome. Endocrinol Metab Clin North Am 1992;21:433.

89. Fernandez-Soto L, Gonzales A, Lobon J, et al: Thyroid peroxidase autoantibodies predict poor metabolic control and need for thyroid treatment in pregnant IDDM women. Diabetes Care 1997;20:1524.

90. Buchbinder A, Miodovnik M, Khoury J, et al: Is the use of insulin lispro safe in pregnancy? J Matern Fetal Neonatal Med 2002;11:232.

91. Gabbe S, Holing E, Temple P: Benefits, risks, costs and patient satisfaction associated with insulin pump therapy for the pregnancy complicated by type 1 diabetes mellitus. Am Obstet Gynecol 2000;182:1283.

91a. Jovanovic-Peterson L, Peterson C: Exercise and the nutritional management of diabetes during pregnancy. Obstet Gynecol Clin North Am 1996;23:75.

92. Bung P, Bung C, Artal R, et al: Therapeutic exercise for insulin-requiring gestational diabetics: Effects on the fetus—results of a randomized prospective longitudinal study. J Perinat Med 1993;21:125.

93. Hughes P, Agarwal M, Newman P, Morrison J: An evaluation of fructosamine estimation in screening for gestational diabetes mellitus. Diabet Med 1995;12:708.

94. Mathiesen ER, Christensen AB, Hellmuth E, et al: Insulin dose during glucocorticoid treatment for fetal lung maturation in diabetic pregnancy: Test of an algorithm. Acta Obstet Gynecol Scand 2002;81:835.

95. Steel J, Johnstone F: Guidelines for the management of IDDM in pregnancy. Drugs 1996;52:60.

96. Rouse D, Goldenberg R, Cliver S: The effectiveness and costs of elective delivery for fetal macrosomia diagnosed by ultrasound. JAMA 1996;276:1480.

97. Gagne M, Leff E, Jefferis S: The breast-feeding experience of women with type 1 diabetes. Health Care Women 1992;13:249.

98. Alvarez-Marfany M, Roman S, Drexler A, et al: Long-term prospective study of postpartum thyroid dysfunction in women with insulin dependent diabetes mellitus. J Clin Endocrinol Metab 1994;79:10.

99. Solomon C, Willett W, Carey V, et al: A prospective study of pregravid determinants of gestational diabetes mellitus. JAMA 1997;278:1078.

100. Moses R: The recurrence rate of gestational diabetes in subsequent pregnancies. Diabetes Care 1996;19:1348.

101. Branchtein L, Schmidt M, Mengue S, et al: Waist circumference and waist-to-hip ratio are related to gestational glucose tolerance. Diabetes Care 1997;20:509.

102. Urman B, Sarac E, Dogan L, Gurgan T: Pregnancy in infertile PCOD patients. Complications and outcome. J Reprod Med 1997;42:501.

103. Lanzone A, Caruso A, Di Simone N, et al: Polycystic ovary disease. A risk factor for gestational diabetes? J Reprod Med 1995;40:312.

104. Wein P, Dong Z, Beischer N, Sheedy M: Factors predictive of recurrent gestational diabetes diagnosed before 24 weeks' gestation. Am J Perinatol 1995;12:352.

105. Stowers J, Sutherland H, Kerridge EF: Long range implications for the mother. The Aberdeen experience. Diabetes 1985;34(Suppl 2):106.

106. O'Sullivan J: Diabetes mellitus after GDM. Diabetes 1991;40(Suppl 2):131.

107. Screening for gestational diabetes: A summary of the evidence for the U.S. Preventive Services Task Force. Obstet Gynecol 2003;101:380-392.

108. Berger H, Crane J, Farine D, et al: Screening for gestational diabetes mellitus. J Obstet Gynaecol Can 2002;24:894.

109. Kaufman R, McBride P, Amankwah K, Huffman D: The effect of minor degrees of glucose intolerance on the incidence of neonatal macrosomia. Obstet Gynecol 1992;80:97.

110. Jovanovic-Peterson L, Bevier W, Peterson C: The Santa Barbara County Health Care Services program: Birth weight change concomitant with screening for and treatment of glucose-intolerance of pregnancy: A potential cost-effective intervention? Am J Perinatol 1997;14:221.

111. Verman A, Mitchell B, Demianczuk N, et al: Relationship between plasma glucose levels in glucose-intolerant women and newborn macrosomia. J Matern Fetal Med 1997;6:187.

112. Deerochanawong C, Putiyanun C, Wongsuryrat M, et al: Comparison of National Diabetes Data Group and World Health Organization criteria for detecting gestational diabetes mellitus. Diabetologia 1996;39:1070.

113. Mathai M, Thomas T, Kuruvila S, Jairaj P: Random plasma glucose and the glucose challenge test in pregnancy. Natl Med J India 1994;7:160.

114. Sacks D, Greenspoon J, Fotheringham N: Could the fasting plasma glucose assay be used to screen for gestational diabetes? J Reprod Med 1992;37:907.

115. Nord E, Hanson U, Persson B: Blood glucose limits in the diagnosis of impaired glucose tolerance during pregnancy: Relation to morbidity. Acta Obstet Gynecol Scand 1995;74:589.

116. Nahum G, Huffaker B: Racial differences in oral glucose screening test results: Establishing race-specific criteria for abnormality in pregnancy. Obstet Gynecol 1993;81:517.

117. Hawthorne G, Snodgrass A, Tunbridge M: Outcome of diabetic pregnancy and glucose intolerance in pregnancy: An audit of fetal loss in Newcastle General Hospital 1977-1990. Diabetes Res Clin Pract 1994;25:183.

118. Langer O: Is normal glycemia the correct threshold to prevent complications in the pregnant diabetic patient? Diabetes Rev 1996;4:2.

119. Deveciana M, Major C, Morgan M, et al: Postprandial versus preprandial blood glucose monitoring in women with GDM requiring insulin therapy. N Engl J Med 1995;333:1237.

120. Langer O, Berkus H, Huff R, et al: Shoulder dystocia: Should the fetus weighing ≥4000 grams be delivered by cesarean section? Am J Obstet Gynecol 1991;165:831.

121. Garner P, Okun N, Keely E, et al: A randomized control trial of strict glycemic control and tertiary level obstetrical care versus routine obstetric care in the management of gestational diabetes: A pilot study. Am J Obstet Gynecol 1997;177:190.

122. Wen SW, Liu S, Kramer MS, et al: Impact of prenatal glucose screening on the diagnosis of gestational diabetes and on pregnancy outcome. Am J Epidemiol 2000;152:1009.

123. Beischer N, Wein P, Sheedy M, et al: Identification and treatment of women with hyperglycemia diagnosed during pregnancy can significantly reduce perimortality rates. Aust N Z Obstet Gynecol 1996;36:239.

124. Ong KK, Dunger DB: Perinatal growth failure: The road to obesity, insulin resistance and cardiovascular disease in adults. Best Pract Res Clin Endocrinol Metab 2002;16:191.

125. Walkinshaw SA: Dietary regulation for "gestational diabetes." Cochrane Database Syst Rev 2000;(2):CD000070.

126. American Diabetes Association: Gestational diabetes mellitus. Diabetes Care 2003;26:S103.

127. Langer O: When diet fails: Insulin and oral hypoglycemic agents as alternative for the management of gestational diabetes mellitus. J Matern Fetal Neonatal Med 2002;11:218.

128. Glueck CJ, Wang P, Koboyashi S, et al: Metformin therapy throughout pregnancy reduces the development of gestational diabetes in women with polycystic ovary syndrome. Fertil Steril 2002;77:520.

129. Glueck CJ, Wang P, Goldenberg N, Sieve-Smith L: Pregnancy outcomes among women with polycystic ovary syndrome treated with metformin. Hum Reprod 2002;17:2858.

130. Naylor C, Sermer M, Chen E, et al: Cesarean delivery in relation to birth weight and gestational glucose intolerance: Pathophysiology or practice style? JAMA 1996;275:1165.

HYPERTENSIVE DISORDERS IN PREGNANCY

Phyllis August

Hypertension is one of the most common medical complications of pregnancy and affects both maternal and fetal health, sometimes with life-threatening consequences. Hypertensive disorders are important causes of premature delivery, intrauterine growth restriction, and intrauterine fetal death. Maternal complications include those attributable to excessive increases in blood pressure, such as stroke, acute cardiac decompensation, and acute renal failure. Hypertensive disorders in pregnancy remain one of the leading causes of maternal death worldwide, accounting for 10% to 20% of maternal deaths worldwide.[1,2] A large epidemiologic survey of hospital discharges reported that the rate of maternal mortality from hypertensive disorders in pregnancy is 1.4 per 100,000 deliveries.[3]

Because ensuring the well-being of the mother does not always ensure the most favorable fetal outcome, clinical management is challenging, and decisions regarding the timing of delivery have profound lifelong effects on both the mother and the child. Although many, if not most, patients with hypertensive disorders in pregnancy are managed by obstetricians and specialists in perinatology, the internist is often involved, particularly when hypertension is severe and necessitates multidrug therapy or when additional medical disorders, such as renal disease or preexisting hypertensive conditions, are present. A thorough understanding of the diagnostic categories, clinical manifestations, pathophysiology, and treatment of hypertension helps maximize the chances of favorable outcome for both the mother and the fetus. A comprehensive review of these issues is presented in this chapter.

PHYSIOLOGIC ADAPTATIONS IN NORMAL PREGNANCY

Some of the important physiologic changes in pregnancy that are relevant to cardiovascular and renal function are reviewed, to provide a foundation for the discussion of hypertensive disorders.

Cardiac and Hemodynamic Alterations

Normal pregnancy is characterized by generalized vasodilation so marked that, despite increases in cardiac output and plasma volume in the range of 40%, mean arterial pressure decreases approximately 10 mm Hg.[4,5] The decrement in blood pressure is apparent in the first trimester, reaching a nadir by midpregnancy.[4] Blood pressure then increases gradually, approaching prepregnancy values at term, but may transiently increase to values slightly above the individual's nonpregnant level during the puerperium. Women with preexisting or chronic hypertension also manifest such decrements, which may be as great as 15 to 20 mm Hg.[6]

The control of blood pressure in normal pregnancy, including the influence of pressor systems (autonomic nerves and catecholamines, renin-angiotensin, vasopressin), baroreceptor function, endothelial cell function, and volume-mediated changes, has been evaluated only sporadically. Furthermore, results of animal studies are frequently contradictory, in part because of differences among species. Thus, there is a critical need to explain normal vascular physiology in pregnancy if the additional alterations in blood pressure regulation in hypertensive women are to be understood.

The primary features of blood pressure regulation during pregnancy are vasodilation and lower blood pressure, both of which have been documented to occur in women by as early as 6 weeks into the pregnancy.[7] There is evidence, mainly from animal models, that basal and stimulated nitric oxide increases in pregnancy and may account for these effects.[8] The basis for the increased nitric oxide is not known; however, steroid hormones, including estrogen and progesterone, may play a role.[9] Other potential mediators of vasodilation include prostacyclin[10]; relaxin,[11] a protein secreted by the corpus luteum during pregnancy; calcitonin gene–related peptide,[12] a vasoactive peptide produced by neural tissue; vascular endothelial growth factor (VEGF)[13]; angiotensin1-7,[14]; and adrenomedullin,[15] a potent vasodilatory peptide with plasma levels that increase during pregnancy.

Data are conflicting as to whether the autonomic nervous system is more active in the control of blood pressure during pregnancy. Different investigators have used different protocols and measurements to ascertain autonomic function, which is one reason for disparate results. A summary of noninvasive tests of autonomic cardiovascular function in pregnancy concluded that there appears to be decreased baroreceptor sensitivity in normal pregnant women, in comparison with nonpregnant women.[16] Pregnancy is also associated with diminished bradycardic response to orthostatic stress, increased tachycardia ratio in response to the Valsalva maneuver, and less change in systolic blood pressure in response to cold exposure.[17,18] Investigators have utilized the microneurographic technique to measure muscle sympathetic nerve activity and have reported increased activity in normal pregnancy, particularly in late pregnancy.[19] The impact of these alterations on blood pressure regulation during pregnancy is not clear.

The renin-angiotensin system is markedly stimulated during normal pregnancy.[5] Normotensive gravidas demonstrate an exaggerated hypotensive response to angiotensin-converting enzyme inhibition, in comparison with nonpregnant women, which suggests that this system is stimulated to help maintain normal blood pressure.[20]

Primary vasodilation and lower blood pressure would be expected to be accompanied by increased cardiac output and increased blood volume, both of which are features of normal pregnancy. Although varying results with regard to the extent and timing of these changes have been reported, one review suggested that the increase in cardiac output occurs early in the first trimester, with a further rise in the second trimester, followed by variable changes in the third trimester that are dependent on individual patient variables.[21] Chapman and colleagues performed elegant longitudinal studies of renal and hemodynamic parameters in normal pregnant women and demonstrated that plasma and blood volume increased significantly from the nonpregnant state at 6 weeks, reaching maximal levels at week 36 of pregnancy.[7]

Renal Changes

Profound alterations in renal hemodynamics, including increases in glomerular filtration rate and renal blood flow of approximately 50%, occur in normal pregnancy.[22] Micropuncture studies of single-nephron glomerular filtration rate in pregnant rats indicate that the increase in glomerular filtration rate is caused by increased glomerular plasma flow, which, in turn, is a result of renal vasodilatation.[23] Experimental evidence supports a role of nitric oxide and other vasodilators, including relaxin (mentioned previously), in mediating the renal vasodilation in normal pregnancy.[11,24,25] In addition to the alterations in renal hemodynamics, many other renal adaptations to pregnancy have been reported, including increased uric acid clearance, alterations in plasma osmolality, increased urinary excretion of calcium, and increased glucosuria and aminoaciduria.[26]

Endocrine Changes

The endocrine adaptations to pregnancy are the most dramatic physiologic adjustments that occur. The fetus, the placenta, and the maternal ovary and adrenal gland participate in the production of large amounts of estradiol-17β, estriol, progesterone, aldosterone, deoxycorticosterone, human placental lactogen, and human chorionic gonadotropin, as well as other pregnancy-specific peptide hormones and prostaglandins. Although considerable progress has been made in the understanding of the synthesis and metabolism of these substances, less is known regarding the precise ways in which these hormones maintain a normal pregnancy. Both estrogen and progesterone have vascular, renal, and hemodynamic effects; therefore, it is quite likely that these hormones interact with other regulatory systems in the control of blood pressure during pregnancy.[27-29] For example, elevated levels of estrogens during pregnancy are, in part, responsible for the elevations in renin substrate. Progesterone is natriuretic and appears to inhibit the renal tubular effect of aldosterone. There is also evidence that sex hormones modulate vascular responses in pregnancy by altering production of local vasodilators such as nitric oxide and calcitonin gene–related peptide.[9,12]

CLASSIFICATION OF HYPERTENSIVE DISORDERS IN PREGNANCY

Accurate diagnosis of hypertension in pregnancy is of utmost importance, because preeclampsia is associated with adverse maternal and fetal outcome if not recognized early. Critical interventions, such as decisions regarding the timing of delivery, are often based on clinical impressions of the disease responsible for the hypertension; thus, appropriate diagnosis may have significant implications for the future health of the fetus.

Many classification schemes of the hypertensive disorders in pregnancy have been used; this has resulted in confusion for both clinician and investigator. The classification scheme that has been in widespread use in the United States, and has proved to be clinically useful, is the 1972 recommendation of the Committee on Terminology of the American College of Obstetricians and Gynecologists (Table 3–1).[30] This classification scheme has also been endorsed by the National High Blood Pressure Education Program.[31] Four categories of hypertension in pregnancy are recognized: (1) preeclampsia-eclampsia, a syndrome occurring only in pregnancy and the puerperium and defined by the new onset of hypertension (systolic blood pressure of >140 mm Hg or diastolic blood pressure of >90 mm Hg) accompanied by new onset proteinuria, defined as 300 mg or more per 24 hours (eclampsia is the convulsive form); (2) chronic hypertension, which is hypertension that preceded pregnancy and is due to essential or secondary hypertension; (3) chronic hypertension with superimposed preeclampsia; (4) and gestational hypertension, which is high blood pressure appearing first after midpregnancy, and is distinguished from preeclampsia by the absence of proteinuria. This category is broad, and includes women who later develop diagnostic criteria for

TABLE 3–1   Classification of Hypertension in Pregnancy

Disorder	Description
Preeclampsia-eclampsia	Multisystem disorder that usually manifests in the latter half of first pregnancy, characterized by hypertension, proteinuria, thrombocytopenia, mild renal dysfunction, and, on occasion, abnormal results of liver function tests
Chronic hypertension	Hypertension that precedes pregnancy and that may represent essential hypertension or any form of secondary hypertension (e.g., renal disease, renovascular hypertension, pheochromocytoma, hyperaldosteronism)
Chronic hypertension with superimposed preeclampsia	The development of worsening hypertension, new-onset proteinuria, hyperuricemia, or thrombocytopenia in the latter half of pregnancy in a woman with chronic hypertension
Gestational hypertension	Hypertension detected after midpregnancy; no proteinuria
	If blood pressure returns to normal by 12 weeks after delivery, then diagnosis is transient hypertension
	If hypertension persists, then diagnosis is chronic hypertension

Modified from Report of the National High Blood Pressure Education Working Group on Hypertension in Pregnancy. Am J Obstet Gynecol 2000;183:S1-S22.

preeclampsia, as well as women with chronic hypertension in whom blood pressure decreased in early pregnancy, masking the true diagnosis. Gestational hypertension which resolves postpartum, and which was not in retrospect preeclampsia, is more likely to occur in women who develop essential hypertension later in life.

In clinical practice, overdiagnosis of preeclampsia may result in closer surveillance and possibly better outcomes. Underdiagnosis poses maternal as well as fetal risks. Thus, it may be prudent to consider a woman with gestational hypertension to be *at risk* for preeclampsia. It is also worth emphasizing that even when rigorous clinical diagnostic criteria are applied, there is a fairly high rate of error. Correlations between clinical diagnosis and renal histologic features have demonstrated that as many as 20% of primigravid women with a clinical diagnosis of preeclampsia have underlying renal disease or hypertensive nephrosclerosis.[32]

PREECLAMPSIA-ECLAMPSIA

This disorder is unique to pregnancy and is a clinical syndrome that affects both the mother and the fetus. Alterations in the placental circulation leading to reduced placental perfusion are an important aspect of the pathophysiologic mechanisms of the preeclamptic syndrome (see later discussion). These alterations in placental circulation probably occur early in the second trimester, whereas the maternal manifestations of the disease are not apparent until much later in pregnancy, most often near term. The most common and well-known maternal clinical features are hypertension, proteinuria, and edema. Other manifestations include coagulation disorders, particularly thrombocytopenia, and liver dysfunction.

Epidemiology

Preeclampsia is more common in nulliparous women, the incidence in such women ranging from 2% to 10% in different populations.[33-36] Risk factors in addition to nulliparity include positive family history; multiple gestations; presence of underlying chronic hypertension, renal disease, or diabetes; obesity; hydatidiform mole; extremes of reproductive age; and second- or early third-trimester preeclampsia in a previous pregnancy (Table 3–2). Three of the four major features of the metabolic syndrome (insulin resistance/glucose intolerance, obesity, hypertension) are risk factors for preeclampsia.[37,38] Dyslipidemia (low levels of high-density lipoproteins, hypertriglyceridemia, hypercholesterolemia) has been reported to increase the risk for preeclampsia in some but not all studies.[38] Although preeclampsia is usually a disease of first pregnancy, the risk of recurrence is higher in the second pregnancy of affected women than in women who have had a normal first pregnancy. Careful follow-up studies performed before 1960 in Scotland reported a risk of recurrent preeclampsia of 3.4% in second pregnancies of women who had preeclampsia with their first pregnancies.[39] The risk of recurrent hypertension without proteinuria was even higher, approaching 25%. More recent investigations suggest that if preeclampsia occurred early in the first pregnancy (in the second trimester), then the risk of recurrence may be as high as 60%.[40] In one report of women who had the HELLP (hemolysis, elevated liver enzymes, and low platelet count) syndrome before 28 weeks' pregnancy, the recurrence rate of preeclampsia in subsequent pregnancies was 55%.[41] The recurrence rate of HELLP syndrome was only 6%. Interestingly, if there is a change in paternity, the risk of preeclampsia in multiparas is almost as high as it is for the first pregnancy.[42] Prior spontaneous or elective abortion is protective against subsequent preeclampsia only among women who conceive again with the same partner.[43]

TABLE 3–2   Risk Factors for Preeclampsia

Nulliparity
Positive family history
Multiple gestations
Chronic hypertension
Renal disease
Diabetes
Obesity
Hydatidiform mole
Extremes of reproductive age
History of early (second trimester) preeclampsia in first pregnancy

The incidence of eclampsia has declined since the 1920s largely because of the greater availability of prenatal care. According to data from the United States, the United Kingdom, and New Zealand, the incidence of eclampsia is between 0.5 and 0.8 per 1000 pregnancies.[36]

The long-term prognosis of women with preeclampsia is a matter that has been debated over the years. Chesley monitored 267 women who survived eclampsia in a first pregnancy and reported that the prevalence of later hypertension was not different from that in age- and race-matched controls.[44] There was, however, a significant increase in the prevalence of chronic hypertension among women who had eclampsia as multiparas, and, interestingly, women who never had preeclampsia or eclampsia had lower rates of later hypertension than did the general population. There have been few, if any, subsequent longitudinal studies of women who had preeclampsia in pregnancy; however, it has been observed that some women with preeclampsia have certain risk factors that are associated with cardiovascular disease, such as hyperlipidemia, obesity, and glucose intolerance.[38] This raises the question of whether women who had preeclampsia in pregnancy are at increased risk for coronary or other cardiac disease as they get older. One case-control study of women with prior preeclampsia evaluated hormonal profiles approximately 17 years after delivery. In comparison with controls, women with prior preeclampsia had elevated serum testosterone levels, which the authors speculated might be associated with increased vascular morbidity.[45] A retrospective cohort study of more than 3000 women from Aberdeen, Scotland, reported that women with hypertensive diseases in pregnancy are at greater risk for hypertension and stroke, and less so for ischemic heart disease, later in life.[46] This study did not report the parity of the cases of hypertension in pregnancy. In summary, preeclamptic pregnancy is more clearly associated with later hypertensive disease than with other cardiovascular disease. Women with recurrent preeclampsia or hypertensive pregnancy appear to be at greater risk, as do those who develop either condition as multiparas. Because there is overlap between risk factors for preeclampsia and those for cardiovascular disease, it is not known whether preeclampsia that occurs solely in the first pregnancy without recurrence is an independent risk factor for cardiovascular disease.

Diagnosis

The classic features of preeclampsia are hypertension in association with proteinuria. Previous definitions included edema; however, this sign is nonspecific and may be present in gravidas with normal blood pressure. The disease occurs after 20 weeks, most often in nulliparas, and the diagnosis is more easily made when women have well-documented normotension in early pregnancy. The criterion for the diagnosis of hypertension is a blood pressure of 140/90 mm Hg or higher after the 20th week of pregnancy. Previous criteria considered increments in blood pressure (30 mm Hg for systolic pressure, 15 mm Hg for diastolic pressure) to be diagnostic of hypertension in pregnancy; however, consensus groups have concluded that these criteria are also too nonspecific and may lead to classifying as many as 25% of

pregnant woman as hypertensive.[31] Nevertheless, it should be appreciated that many young women have midpregnancy blood pressures as low as 90/60 mm Hg. Thus, significant increases in blood pressure (from 90/60 to 120/80 mm Hg) should be monitored closely, although they may not signify the development of preeclampsia. Failure to appreciate that seemingly "normal levels" of blood pressure can be abnormal is one reason why the diagnosis of preeclampsia may be missed in its early stages.

Hypertension is but one of many manifestations of preeclampsia, and focusing on this clinical feature alone may lead to erroneous approaches to therapy that unduly emphasize lowering the blood pressure. Other features of preeclampsia include cerebral symptoms, such as headache and visual disturbances; epigastric or right upper quadrant pain with nausea or vomiting; thrombocytopenia; and abnormal liver enzyme levels. Nevertheless, blood pressure is measured at every antepartum visit. Thus, it is not surprising that hypertension has been the focus of many investigations regarding pathophysiologic processes and therapy in preeclampsia. Also, most maternal deaths attributed to preeclampsia occur in the setting of uncontrolled hypertension and ensuing intracerebral hemorrhage.

The hypertension associated with preeclampsia may be widely variable from moment to moment,[47] and two observers measuring blood pressure successively may obtain very different readings. Preeclampsia hypertension is also characterized by alterations in the normal circadian rhythm of blood pressure; therefore, in women with this disease, blood pressure may not decrease during the night. This has been demonstrated with ambulatory blood pressure monitoring, and it has also been shown that alterations in circadian blood pressure variability are present as early as the first trimester in women who later develop preeclampsia.[48]

Proteinuria is one of the classic laboratory features of preeclampsia; although it frequently appears late in the course, its presence greatly bolsters the diagnosis. The criterion for abnormal urinary protein excretion in pregnancy is 0.3 g or more in a 24-hour specimen, or greater than 1+ in a random urine specimen. The amount of protein excreted by preeclamptic patients might vary greatly, ranging from barely abnormal to frankly nephrotic amounts.

Edema frequently accompanies normal pregnancy; therefore, its presence alone is not useful in diagnosing preeclampsia, and its absence does not eliminate the diagnosis. For example, sudden and rapid weight gain often precedes overt manifestations of the disease. On the other hand, severe disease can occur even in the absence of edema ("dry" preeclampsia).

Laboratory tests are very helpful both in verifying and establishing a diagnosis and in assessing the severity of preeclampsia. For this reason, it is helpful to establish baseline data in patients at high risk (e.g., chronic hypertensive patients, diabetic patients, and women with multiple pregnancies or strong family histories of preeclampsia). The standard tests recommended for the evaluation of preeclampsia are summarized in Table 3–3. A number of other biochemical abnormalities occur in preeclampsia, and some may be useful in predicting gravidas at risk. Indeed, the importance of early prediction in managing

TABLE 3–3   Laboratory Evaluation of Women Who Develop Hypertension after Midpregnancy

Test	Rationale
Hemoglobin and hematocrit	Hemoconcentration supports diagnosis of preeclampsia and is an indicator of severity; values may be decreased, however, if hemolysis accompanies the disease
Blood smear	Signs of microangiopathic hemolytic anemia (e.g., schistocytes) favor diagnosis of preeclampsia and may be present when blood pressure is only mildly elevated
Platelet count	Decreased levels suggest severe preeclampsia
Urinalysis	If qualitative dipstick result is 1+ or greater, a quantitative measurement of protein excretion should be done. Hypertensive gravidas with proteinuria should be considered to have preeclampsia (pure or superimposed) until proved otherwise
Serum creatinine level	Most cases of preeclampsia are associated with only mild elevations in creatinine; rising levels, especially when associated with oliguria, suggest severe preeclampsia
Serum uric acid level	Increased levels aid in the differential diagnosis of preeclampsia and may reflect disease severity
Serum aspartate aminotransferase Alanine aminotransferase	Abnormal values suggest severe preeclampsia and hepatic involvement
Lactic acid dehydrogenase	Elevated levels are associated with hemolysis and hepatic involvement and suggest severe preeclampsia
Serum albumin	Values may be decreased even in the absence of heavy proteinuria, and this decrease may result from "capillary leak" or hepatic involvement in preeclampsia

this disorder underscores the continued "quest" to identify laboratory abnormalities present before clinical manifestations of the disease, and identification of such predictors should also help clinicians understand the pathogenesis. Some of the tests that have been investigated and found to be potentially useful as predictors of preeclampsia are those of urinary calcium excretion, urinary kallikrein excretion, plasma fibronectin levels, antithrombin III levels, and ambulatory blood pressure monitoring; however, none are sufficiently sensitive or specific to be recommended for routine use in clinical practice (reviewed by Friedman and Lindheimer[49]).

Preeclampsia is characterized by the unpredictable nature of its clinical course. Women with mildly elevated blood pressure and even minimal proteinuria can rapidly progress to eclampsia, the convulsive form of the disorder. Thus, all cases should be considered potentially dangerous, regardless of whether they are classified as "mild" or "severe." However, certain signs are particularly ominous: systolic blood pressure of 160 mm Hg or more or diastolic blood pressure of 110 mm Hg or more; nephrotic range proteinuria; significant azotemia (serum creatinine >1.2 mg/dL); platelet count less than 100,000/mm³ or evidence of microangiopathic hemolytic anemia; elevated hepatic enzymes; headache or other cerebral or visual disturbances; epigastric pain; and pulmonary edema.

A variant of the classic form of preeclampsia is the HELLP syndrome.[50] As mentioned previously, this acronym refers to the specific laboratory abnormalities that characterize this manifestation of preeclampsia: *h*emolysis, *e*levated *l*iver function test results, and *l*ow *p*latelet count. The clinical significance of this syndrome is that it is associated with a particularly adverse maternal and fetal prognosis.[51] Most obstetricians consider the development of the HELLP syndrome to be an urgent indication for delivery, because the laboratory abnormalities can reach life-threatening levels with profound thrombocytopenia and extremely elevated levels of hepatic enzymes. A rare complication of preeclampsia is hepatic rupture, in which subcapsular hepatic bleeding occurs. This complication is probably more commonly preceded by the laboratory features of HELLP syndrome. At present, it is not known

why some women with preeclampsia develop HELLP syndrome, whereas others develop the more classic manifestations. Different maternal susceptibility genes may be responsible, and this is clearly an area worthy of further study. HELLP syndrome may represent a more severe form of generalized maternal endothelial cell dysfunction/damage, in comparison with other cases of preeclampsia. Indeed, the features of HELLP syndrome are very similar and sometimes difficult to distinguish from those of other microangiopathic syndromes that may develop in late pregnancy, such as hemolytic-uremic syndrome and thrombotic thrombocytopenic purpura. These latter disorders are characterized by vascular endothelial cell damage, elicited by unknown antigens or toxic substances. Distinction of these disorders from HELLP syndrome is important because treatment of HELLP syndrome is urgent delivery, and treatment of hemolytic-uremic syndrome or thrombotic thrombocytopenic purpura may require plasma infusion or plasmapheresis.[52]

The diagnosis of preeclampsia may be straightforward when a nulliparous woman develops the sudden onset of significant hypertension in association with proteinuria and edema. Making an accurate diagnosis becomes more challenging when only some of the features are present. Finally, a correct diagnosis is usually achieved through a careful analysis of patient risk factors, of gestational age of the fetus at delivery, and of changes in blood pressure in comparison with early pregnancy and through the recognition that some of the laboratory abnormalities can be quite subtle and must be evaluated in the context of normal values for pregnant women. When a woman has newly diagnosed hypertension in the latter part of pregnancy and ambiguous laboratory test results, the safest course is to assume that the diagnosis is preeclampsia. Thus, appropriate maternal and fetal surveillance can be instituted.

Pathophysiology

Preeclampsia is a syndrome with both maternal and fetal manifestations. Current evidence suggests that abnormalities in placental adaptation to the maternal spiral arteries that supply blood to the developing fetoplacental unit are among the earliest changes responsible for the disease.[53] These abnormalities in placental function are present in the early second trimester; thus, they precede, and probably directly cause, the multisystemic maternal disorder.[54-56] Maternal susceptibility factors are also important in the pathophysiologic processes of preeclampsia, inasmuch as reduced placental perfusion in association with fetal growth restriction may occur in pregnancies of women who do not develop preeclampsia. Considerable progress has been made in the understanding of some of the cellular and biochemical abnormalities that might contribute to the placental disease. The maternal syndrome has also been well characterized. However, the cause of preeclampsia remains elusive, as does the mechanism whereby placental vascular abnormalities can result in a systemic, albeit temporary, disease in the mother. What follows is a review of some of the important features of the pathophysiology of the preeclamptic syndrome, beginning with the evidence for a genetic component, followed by a discussion of both fetal and placental as well as maternal manifestations.

Genetics of Preeclampsia

Family studies have shown that genetic factors play a role in preeclampsia; however, the precise pattern of inheritance is unknown. Several models of inheritance have been suggested, including a maternal dominant gene model with reduced penetrance, a maternal-fetal gene model, or a maternal and fetal gene interaction model (reviewed by Lachmeijer et al.[57]). In addition, mitochondrial inheritance and genomic imprinting, as well as environmental factors, may also contribute to the expression of the disease.[57] Difficulties in defining a strict phenotype of preeclampsia, the variability of expression of the syndrome, and the fact that the disease is sex-limited and is expressed only during pregnancy have made genetic studies difficult. Lachmeijer and colleagues exhaustively reviewed studies of the various candidate genes and genomewide scans performed as of 2002.[57] Despite extensive research, the molecular genetic basis of preeclampsia remains unclear, although there are some promising data that suggest that the 2p13 locus may be important with regard to maternal susceptibility.

The Placenta

The placenta is considered to be of central pathogenetic importance in preeclampsia.[56,58] This is because delivery is the most successful, if not the only definitive, cure of this disease. Also, preeclampsia is more likely to occur in women with hydatidiform moles (a rapidly growing placenta but no fetus) as well as in those with multiple pregnancies (increased placental mass). In addition, there are several animal models, whose manifestations mimic certain features of preeclampsia in humans, which have been produced by creating transient or chronic uterine ischemia.[59]

Normal placentation, it appears, involves the transformation of the branches of the maternal uterine arteries—the spiral arteries—from thick-walled, muscular arteries into sacklike flaccid vessels that permit delivery of greater volumes of blood to the uteroplacental unit. This transformation involves invasion of the spiral artery walls by invasive cytotrophoblast cells of the placenta. These cells migrate in a retrograde manner involving first the decidual and then the myometrial segments of the arteries, causing considerable disruption at all layers of the vessel wall (Fig. 3–1).[53-55,60,61] The mechanisms involved in this complex process are only beginning to be elucidated; they involve alterations in the expression of adhesion molecules, proteinase, and proteinase inhibitor in such a way that the cytotrophoblast cells acquire an invasive phenotype. This process whereby cytotrophoblast cells invade maternal blood vessels and assume an endothelial phenotype has been described as *cytotrophoblast pseudovasculogenesis* and is believed to be stimulated in part by the hypoxic milieu of the developing placenta.[62,63]

In women destined to develop preeclampsia, the extent of interstitial invasion by cytotrophoblasts is variable but frequently shallow. Endovascular invasion is incomplete; it may occur in the decidual but not the myometrial segments of the artery; and in some vessels, the process does not occur at all.[53-55,64-66] The arteries, therefore, remain thick walled and muscular, the diameters in the myometrial segments being half those measured during normal pregnancy. It has been reported that in preeclampsia, the invading cytotrophoblasts fail to properly express adhesion receptors that are necessary for normal remodeling of the maternal spiral arteries.[64,65] This failure of cytotrophoblast invasion of the spiral arteries is considered to be the morphologic basis for decreased placental perfusion in preeclampsia. It has been suggested that the basis for these abnormalities may be dysregulated immunologic interaction between mother and fetus.

Another placental lesion described in preeclampsia is called *acute atherosis* and is characterized by accumulation of fat-laden macrophages and perinuclear cell infiltrates. This lesion is believed to occur only in arteries that have not been invaded by trophoblast cells. Of interest is a study of 400 placentas from preeclamptic women, in which vascular lesions in the placenta correlated with severity of clinical disease.[67]

Preeclampsia is also associated with a greater degree of placental infarction than is seen in normal pregnancy. However, the placenta has considerable physiologic reserve, which explains why some patients experience fetal loss or their infants are growth restricted, whereas most preeclamptic patients deliver infants whose weights are normal for their gestational age. Nevertheless, preeclampsia is associated with an increased incidence of intrauterine growth restriction and fetal death. In view of the abnormalities described earlier, it is not surprising that the fetus would be affected by this disease. What remains an enigma is the mechanism whereby the placental changes lead to the maternal syndrome that develops in late pregnancy.

Immunologic Mechanisms

An intriguing area of ongoing investigation that addresses the link between the placental and maternal disease involves the nature of the immune response at the maternal-placental interface and how alterations in this response might lead to preeclampsia. There are several unique aspects of the immune response in pregnancy that appear to play a role in normal placental development. In comparison with other circulating cells in the body, trophoblast cells do not

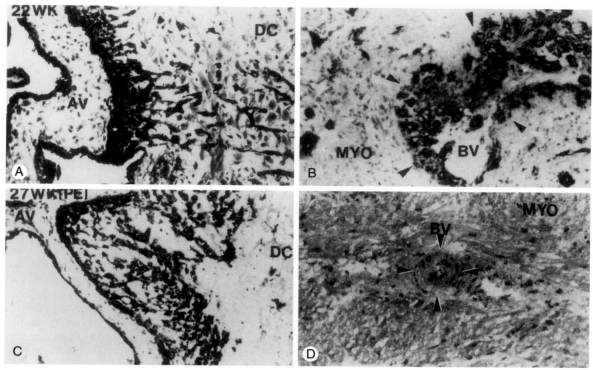

Figure 3–1. Placental bed biopsy specimens from normal and preeclamptic pregnancy, demonstrating the migrations of cytotrophoblasts throughout the decidua and myometrium. Anchoring villus formation and cytotrophoblast invasion in normal (**A, B**) and preeclamptic (**C, D**) pregnancy. During the second trimester, cytotrophoblasts with elongated shape emanate (**A**) from anchoring villus (AV) columns and are found throughout the decidua (DC) and (**B**) from the adjacent third of the myometrium (MYO) and lining the blood vessels (BV). In preeclampsia, cytotrophoblasts retain their connections with the cell columns and fail to invade the decidua and myometrium (**C**). There is no evidence of cytotrophoblast invasion of the blood vessels, which remain uniformly constricted (**D**). *Arrowheads* mark perimeters of blood vessels. (From Zhou Y, Damsky CH, Chiu K, et al: Preeclampsia is associated with abnormal expression of adhesion molecules by invasive cytotrophoblasts. J Clin Invest 1993;91:950, by copyright permission of the American Society for Clinical Investigation.)

express the classic human leukocyte antigen (HLA) antigens; rather, they express a nonclassical antigen, HLA-G, which may have an important role in protecting the placenta from the deleterious effects of a local maternal immune response.[68] Several reports suggest that placental tissue from preeclamptic pregnancies express less, or different, HLA-G, and researchers postulate that this may result in a breakdown in maternal tolerance to the immunologically foreign placenta.[69] There are also reports of increased levels of inflammatory cytokines such as tumor necrosis factor α and interleukin-2 in placental tissue as well as in serum from preeclamptic women.[70-73] It is hypothesized that these factors may be involved in the initiation of a systemic immune-mediated illness in the mother.

The observation that preeclampsia occurs primarily in nulliparous women, whose subsequent pregnancies tend to be uncomplicated thereafter unless there is a change in paternity, has been cited as support for alterations in immune response as a factor in the pathogenesis of preeclampsia.[74] Epidemiologic reports also indicate that the prevalence of preeclampsia is decreased in women who received heterologous blood transfusions, practiced oral sex, or had a long period of cohabitation that preceded an established pregnancy, which suggests that prior exposure

to paternal antigens might be protective.[75] It has also been observed that certain pathologic changes in the placental vasculature resemble those of allograft rejection. Furthermore, increased T cell, natural killer cell, and neutrophil activation are reported in preeclampsia.[75]

Pathophysiology of the Maternal Manifestations of Preeclampsia

The maternal syndrome of preeclampsia is characterized by vasoconstriction, in association with evidence for vascular endothelial cell dysfunction and activation of the coagulation system. There are reduced blood flow and relative ischemia in the kidneys, liver, brain, and placenta as a consequence of generalized vasoconstriction. In many humoral and autacoid systems, there are simultaneous perturbations that are related to volume and blood pressure control as well as to clotting. However, it is often difficult to determine whether changes described represent cause or effect.

Blood Pressure in Preeclampsia

Preeclamptic women do not develop frank hypertension until late pregnancy, but vasoconstrictor influences may be present considerably earlier. For instance, alterations in vascular reactivity may already be present by week 20 of pregnancy, and both longitudinal and epidemiologic surveys suggest that women destined to develop preeclampsia have slightly higher "normal" blood pressure (e.g., diastolic levels >70 mm Hg) as early as the second trimester.[76,77] These findings have been confirmed with ambulatory blood pressure monitoring.[78]

As mentioned, blood pressure in preeclampsia is characteristically labile. Pressor responses to several peptides and amines (e.g., norepinephrine and angiotensin) are exaggerated.[79] The hypertension of preeclampsia resolves post partum, usually within the first few days; but normalization may take 2 to 4 weeks in severe cases.[80] The precise mechanisms of preeclamptic hypertension are obscure. Investigations of the various pressor systems and locally acting peptides are briefly summarized as follows.

During normal pregnancy, the renin-angiotensin system is stimulated, probably in response to vasodilation and lower blood pressure.[81] In contrast, in women with preeclampsia, plasma renin activity, plasma aldosterone concentration, urinary aldosterone excretion, and angiotensin II levels are suppressed, although often not to prepregnancy levels. There is evidence that the renin-angiotensin system is stimulated early in pregnancy in women who later develop preeclampsia and that the developing vasoconstriction and hypertension turn off renin secretion. As renin levels decrease, the sensitivity to angiotensin II increases, often well before the clinical signs of preeclampsia.[82] This loss of the normal refractoriness to angiotensin II has been used as a screening test to identify gravidas in midpregnancy who are at risk for the development of preeclampsia.

Although plasma norepinephrine levels are unaltered in preeclampsia, there is increased pressor sensitivity to this catecholamine in preeclampsia. Noninvasive studies of autonomic cardiovascular function have not revealed any clearcut differences between normal pregnant and preeclamptic women.[83] However, electromyoneurographic studies of skeletal muscle have demonstrated higher sympathetic nerve activity in preeclampsia, which resolves post partum.[19]

Alterations in eicosanoid metabolism occur in normal pregnancy, and further changes accompany preeclampsia. Most research in this area relates to effects of pregnancy on prostacyclin (prostaglandin I_2 [PGI_2]) and thromboxane A_2 (TXA_2) production, both of which are products of cyclooxygenase metabolism of arachidonic acid. There exists evidence that prostaglandin formation is increased in normal human pregnancy, particularly vasodilatory prostanoids (mostly PGI_2) produced principally by vascular endothelial cells.[84] Longitudinal studies of the urinary metabolite of PGI_2, 2,3-dinor-6-keto prostaglandin $F_{1\alpha}$, have demonstrated that this substance increases in the first trimester, the increments are sustained through term,[85] and decreases in PGI_2 are detectable early in the second trimester in women who later develop preeclampsia. A prospective study of prostaglandin metabolites in pregnancy demonstrated that reductions in PGI_2, but not TXA_2, occur months before the clinical onset of preeclampsia.[86]

The literature is substantial, suggesting that alterations in prostaglandin metabolism underlie the pathogenesis of preeclampsia.[84-90] Manifestations such as increments in vascular reactivity and blood pressure, as well as

intravascular coagulation, have been proposed to be caused by an imbalance between PGI_2 and TXA_2 synthesis, resulting in a relative or absolute PGI_2 deficiency.[87] Reduced PGI_2 production has been reported in various tissues and body fluids from preeclamptic women in comparison with normotensive controls. These findings are consistent with the growing evidence that preeclampsia is characterized by generalized vascular endothelial cell dysfunction (see later discussion), which leads to diminished production of PGI_2, as well as of other vasodilatory endothelial cell products.

In spite of the large body of evidence supporting a role for alterations in prostaglandin metabolism in preeclampsia, it is important to emphasize that these substances are difficult to measure, and caution is advised in interpretation of results. Furthermore, these substances act locally; thus, measurements from peripheral blood may not reflect local effects. Nevertheless, the notion that preeclampsia is characterized by a relative deficiency of PGI_2 (with preservation of or increased TXA_2 production) has been the basis of several large and costly multicenter randomized trials designed to evaluate the ability of low-dose aspirin (which inhibits platelet TXA_2 generation but spares vascular PGI_2 production) to prevent preeclampsia. Most of these trials did not demonstrate a beneficial effect of aspirin on pregnancy outcome.

Endothelial Cell Function and Preeclampsia

Increased knowledge of the role of the vascular endothelial cells in the modulation of adjacent vascular smooth muscle contractile activity, as well as in coagulation and regulation of blood flow, has led to the appreciation of the significance of alterations in endothelial cell function in the pathophysiologic mechanisms of preeclampsia, as well as other chronic cardiovascular conditions, such as atherosclerosis and essential hypertension. Endothelial cells, which have receptors for numerous vasodilators and constrictors, produce hormones, autacoids, and mitogenic cytokines, including PGI_2, nitric oxide, and endothelin. The pathophysiologic changes of preeclampsia, particularly those present before clinically apparent disease, support the hypothesis that altered endothelial function contributes to many of the changes observed in the preeclamptic syndrome.[91] Women with preeclampsia manifest increased circulating markers of endothelial activation (von Willibrand factor, cellular fibronectin, thrombomodulin, endothelin, vascular cell adhesion molecule).[56] Preeclamptic blood vessels demonstrate reduced endothelial mediated vasodilation in vitro,[56] and in vivo studies have shown that flow mediated (endothelium-dependent) dilatation is impaired in women with previous preeclampsia.[92] Most recently, plasma concentrations of asymmetric dimethylarginine, the endogenous inhibitor of endothelial nitric oxide synthase, has been shown to be elevated in women with evidence of abnormal endothelial function before the development of preeclampsia.[93]

There are numerous reports of a hypertensive syndrome produced by inhibiting nitric oxide synthase in various experimental models of pregnancy, with some features similar to human preeclampsia.[94-96] Results from women with preeclampsia are conflicting, with reports of increased as well as decreased serum and urinary metabolites of nitric oxide in preeclampsia.[97-99]

Endothelins represent another vasoactive endothelial cell product postulated to play a role in preeclampsia.[100-104] In this regard, circulating levels of endothelin-1 are generally (but not universally) reported to be increased in this disorder, but it is unclear whether such levels have pathogenic significance or are a byproduct of endothelial damage.

The evidence for endothelial cell dysfunction in the pathogenesis of the maternal manifestations of preeclampsia is strong; however, its cause remains obscure (Fig. 3–2). Postulated to be of pathogenic significance are circulating factors, of placental origin, that are toxic to endothelial cells.[105,106] Indeed, sera from women destined to develop or manifest preeclampsia are cytotoxic to endothelial cells or cause endothelial cell activation in vitro (assessed by nitric oxide and PGI_2 generation).[106] Sera from preeclamptic patients are also mitogenic and increase messenger RNA for, as well as production of, the platelet-derived growth factor α in culture.[107] There is also a growing body of evidence implicating increased lipid peroxides as well as byproducts of increased oxidative stress, possibly released by the placenta in response to hypoxia or ischemia, in the genesis of endothelial cell damage in preeclampsia.[56,108-111] Another placenta-derived substance that may play an important role in the maternal manifestations of preeclampsia is soluble fms-like tyrosine kinase 1 (sFlt1), which is a variant of the VEGF receptor and acts as an antagonist of VEGF.[112] Maynard and colleagues demonstrated that this substance is elevated in women with preeclampsia, disappears after delivery, and is associated with decreased levels of free VEGF and endothelial dysfunction.[112] Administration of sFlt1 to pregnant rats induces hypertension, proteinuria, and glomerular endotheliosis. Experiments of conditional knockout of VEGF also demonstrate that mice with reduced VEGF develop the classic renal lesion of preeclampsia, glomerular endotheliosis.[113] There are other potential placenta-derived substances that have been suggested as mediators of maternal endothelial cell damage, including leptin and tumor necrosis factor α.[114,115]

Metabolic Disturbances in Preeclampsia

Hyperinsulinemia, obesity, glucose intolerance, hypertension, and dyslipidemia (e.g., increased triglyceride levels, reduced levels of high-density lipoproteins) are associated with cardiovascular disease, including essential hypertension. Insulin resistance and hyperinsulinemia (mediated by hormonal changes) are also characteristic of normal pregnancy and are maximal in the third trimester.[38] Several laboratories have reported exaggerated metabolic disturbances in patients with preeclampsia, including hypertriglyceridemia, increased levels of free fatty acids, decreased levels of lipoprotein a, increased insulin levels, and glucose intolerance.[116-121] These observations are intriguing, particularly because they may be related to the evidence for increased oxidative stress in preeclampsia (lipid abnormalities may result in increased oxidative stress), as well as to the recognition that obesity is a significant risk factor for preeclampsia. However, it remains uncertain whether these factors are pathogenic in hypertensive pregnancy or whether they may be markers of the disease process.

Cardiac Function in Preeclampsia

Data conflict with regard to the effect of preeclampsia on the heart. This reflects the failure of most investigators to define precisely their study populations, which frequently include women with chronic hypertension and renal disease. Also, many reports describe term and/or intrapartum events, the gravidas receiving a variety of medications (e.g., magnesium sulfate or antihypertensive agents) as well as intravenous solutions of variable solute content. Moreover, preeclampsia is an evolving disorder, and hemodynamics may change as the disease progresses. Thus, it is not surprising that the cardiac output of preeclamptic patients has been described as decreased, increased, and unchanged.

Wallenburg and colleagues[122-124] studied nulliparous gravidas who developed third trimester hypertension and proteinuria, before any therapeutic intervention. They measured cardiac output and vascular resistance with pulmonary artery catheters and found cardiac output to be decreased in women with preeclampsia in comparison with controls. Peripheral vascular resistance was increased, and pulmonary capillary wedge pressure was low normal. Lang and associates[125] used echocardiography and confirmed the decrements in cardiac output and increments in peripheral vascular resistance in preeclampsia. A study of eclamptic women also demonstrated similar changes in hemodynamics.[126]

In contrast are the results of Cotton and colleagues[127] who, using invasive hemodynamic monitoring, reported variable changes in cardiac output; many patients had increased values. Perhaps the most controversial findings are those of Easterling and colleagues,[128] who performed

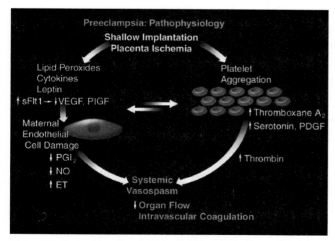

Figure 3–2. In this schema of the pathogenesis of preeclampsia, decreased uteroplacental blood flow resulting in placental ischemia is hypothesized to lead to maternal disease (systemic vasospasm, decreased organ flow, and intravascular coagulation) by causing the release of toxic substances that mediate generalized endothelial cell damage and platelet aggregation. Damaged endothelial cells may produce fewer vasodilatory substances (prostacyclin [PGI_2], nitric oxide [NO]) and release mitogenic factors (platelet-derived growth factor [PDGF]). Platelet aggregation, a consequence of endothelial damage, in turn leads to increased thromboxane A_2. Platelet aggregation and endothelial damage aggravate placental ischemia. ET, endothelin; PlGF, placental growth factor; SFlt1, soluble fms-like tyrosine kinase 1; VEGF, vascular endothelial growth factor.

serial echocardiographic studies throughout their patients' pregnancies and observed that a small group of women who eventually developed preeclampsia had strikingly increased cardiac outputs and decreased peripheral vascular resistance throughout pregnancy; some patients "crossed over" by developing increased peripheral vascular resistance and decreased cardiac output when disease became severe. These results are intriguing in that the pathophysiologic development of preeclampsia seems to follow that described in certain forms of essential hypertension, but the latter has a time course of years, whereas preeclampsia develops over months.

Plasma volume and red blood cell mass are increased in normal pregnancy, although the decrease in blood pressure in association with stimulation of the renin-angiotensin system suggests that the increase in volume is secondary to vasodilation and is perceived as normal. Plasma volume in preeclamptic women has been measured with Evans blue dye, and most investigators report that the volume is decreased.[17,66,123-127] Again, the decrease in plasma volume may be secondary to vasoconstriction and hypertension, although there are some reports that decreases in plasma volume may precede hypertension.[33,79,129,130] These latter reports have led to the use of volume expansion therapy in combination with vasodilator drugs in the treatment of preeclampsia. The suppression of the renin-angiotensin system in preeclampsia suggests that the decrease in plasma volume is secondary to vasoconstriction and a "smaller" intravascular compartment. Finally, the decrease in intravascular volume, often associated with hypoalbuminemia and hemoconcentration, may relate to a "leaky" vasculature that accompanies preeclampsia.

Renal Changes

The renal lesion that is characteristic of preeclampsia is termed *glomerular endotheliosis*.[79,131-133] The glomeruli are enlarged and swollen but not hypercellular, primarily because of hypertrophy of the intracapillary cells (mainly endothelial but mesangial as well), which encroach on the capillary lumina, giving the appearance of a bloodless glomerulus. The changes vary, depending on the severity of the lesion, but are widespread. Thrombosis and fibrin-like material, as well as foam cells, may be present, and epithelial crescents have been described in rare instances. Ultrastructural examination reveals extensive swelling and vacuolization primarily of endothelial cells and, to a lesser extent, of the mesangial cells. The basement membrane is usually not thickened, and foot processes are usually well preserved, even when severe proteinuria is present. Localized lesions resembling those of focal and segmental glomerulosclerosis are present in about 20% of women with preeclampsia. The significance of this finding is not clear; some authorities consider it to be a sequela of preeclampsia, a form of secondary focal and segmental glomerulosclerosis, whereas others consider that it may be a manifestation of preexisting subclinical nephrosclerosis.

Both glomerular filtration rate and renal blood flow decrease in preeclampsia, the former more so than the latter, leading to a decrease in filtration fraction.[79] The decrement is usually modest (25%) even when morphologic changes are pronounced. In rare cases, renal insufficiency may be severe, and acute tubular or cortical necrosis has been linked to preeclampsia, especially when marked coagulopathy is present.[134] Fractional urate clearances decrease, often before overt disease, with hyperuricemia being an important feature of preeclampsia. Abnormal proteinuria, another hallmark of the disease, may appear late in the clinical course and tends to be nonselective.

Sodium excretion is impaired in preeclampsia, documented best by studies of the renal excretory ability after acute saline infusion.[135] The genesis of this defect remains poorly understood, because it occurs in the presence of decreased intravascular volume but increased interstitial space and atrial natriuretic factor levels, as well as suppression of the renin-angiotensin system.

Renal handling of calcium is also abnormal in preeclampsia.[136] Gravidas are normally hypercalciuric, perhaps because of increases in glomerular filtration rate, as well as increases in 1,25-dihydroxyvitamin D_3, which results in an "absorptive hypercalciuria."[137] Preeclampsia, however, is characterized by marked reduction in the fractional excretion of calcium, leading to striking hypocalciuria. Alterations in calcium regulatory hormones, including reduced plasma levels of 1,25-dihydroxyvitamin D_3 and increased parathyroid hormone, are also present.[138] Thus the hypocalciuria may be caused by increased distal tubular calcium reabsorption, or, alternatively, there may be enhanced proximal tubular reabsorption, as seen with sodium.

Coagulation Abnormalities

Preeclampsia is associated with activation of the coagulation cascade, leading at times to frank evidence of disseminated intravascular coagulation.[139] There are many reports documenting increased consumption of various clotting components, including factor VII, as well as decreases in inhibitors of coagulation such as antithrombin III. Decrements in antithrombin III have been reported to occur before overt disease.[140] An increased incidence of resistance to activated protein C has also been reported in women with preeclampsia.[141] There is some evidence that fibrinolytic activity is reduced, which may relate to fibrin deposits in kidney and placenta, but the fibrinolytic system in general has not been well studied in preeclampsia.

Alterations in platelet number and function are recognized features of preeclampsia.[139,142-146] There are variable reports of whether platelet counts change in normal pregnancy and in which direction, but some investigators have noted decreases that they ascribed to increased platelet activation in comparison to the nonpregnant state. In this setting, preeclamptic women experience further declines, which are often apparent before other signs or symptoms of the disease. At times, thrombocytopenia becomes severe, and even life-threatening, especially when it is part of the HELLP variant described previously.

The exact mechanisms responsible for thrombocytopenia are unclear. Increased platelet activation has been observed, as well as enhanced aggregation and destruction, which appear to result from endothelial damage. Platelet activation may lead to increased generation of TXA_2, which may, in turn, increase vasoconstriction and platelet aggregation. Increased release of platelet products such as serotonin may also contribute to enhanced vasoconstriction, and pharmacologic agents that inhibit serotonin have been used successfully in the treatment of preeclampsia.[147,148]

Hepatic Changes

Liver dysfunction accompanying preeclampsia may range from mild enzyme abnormalities to the ominous HELLP syndrome, with markedly elevated transaminase levels and even subcapsular bleeding or hepatic rupture. In general, liver involvement is a sign of more severe disease and is associated with lower platelet counts, more severe proteinuria, and more maternal complications.[149] Histologic findings include periportal hemorrhages, ischemic lesions, and fibrin deposition. They are well described in the classic autopsy studies of Sheehan and Lynch[150] and are consistent with both endothelial damage and activation of the coagulation system. There are several clinical and laboratory similarities between the rare complication termed *acute fatty liver of pregnancy* and preeclampsia, and evidence of hepatocyte fat deposition has been observed in liver biopsy specimens obtained from preeclamptic patients.[151] The liver abnormalities associated with preeclampsia usually resolve within the first postpartum week, whereas the liver damage associated with acute fatty liver of pregnancy tends to be more severe and may even lead to hepatic failure, which is exceedingly rare in preeclampsia.

Central Nervous System Manifestations

Eclampsia, the convulsive phase of preeclampsia, is the most common central nervous system complication of hypertension, and most maternal deaths attributable to hypertension occur in women with eclampsia. Additional clinical mani-festations include headache, visual disturbances, blurred vision, scotomata, and, in rare cases, cortical blindness. On occasion, focal neurologic signs may develop, which should prompt radiologic investigation, because subdural hematoma is a complication, albeit rare, of preeclampsia.[152]

Pathologic specimens reveal varying degrees of hemorrhages and petechiae, vasculopathy with vessel wall damage and fibrinoid necrosis (possibly related to chronic hypertension), ischemic brain damage, and microinfarctions.[153] There is some controversy regarding whether cerebral edema is a feature of eclampsia or whether it is a postmortem phenomenon. The cause of the hemorrhage is debated; possibilities include vasospasm and ischemia, infiltration of the vascular wall with fibrinoid material leading to focal edema, thrombosis, and rupture. Studies involving transcranial Doppler analysis of the cerebral circulation have documented increases in cerebral blood flow velocity, which have been interpreted as consistent with cerebral vasospasm in women with preeclampsia and eclampsia.[154-156] The role of elevated blood pressure in the pathogenesis of the cerebral manifestations of preeclampsia remains disputed. The mechanisms for the convulsion are not known, and the role of hypertension in eclamptic seizures is also controversial.

Eclamptic patients have been evaluated with computed tomography and magnetic resonance imaging.[157,158] Some studies have yielded relatively normal results, and others describe a variety of abnormalities, most of which are usually transient. Lesions consistent with cerebral edema and hemorrhage, as well as hypodense areas believed to represent localized edema induced perhaps by hypoxia, have been described in the computed tomographic scans.[159] Hemorrhage and edema have also been documented by magnetic resonance imaging, and of interest are reports of changes in the posterior hemispheres or in the vascular watershed areas, findings consistent with global ischemia induced by vasospasm.[157,159] In rare cases, hemorrhages may be major and associated with permanent neurologic sequelae. The predominance of posterior lesions may explain the increased incidence of visual disturbances in preeclampsia-eclampsia. CT or MRI evidence of cerebral edema are in contrast to those of some autopsy studies. One possible explanation might be the greater use of intravenous fluids to treat preeclampsia, especially when oliguria is present. Cerebral edema observed on computed tomography may be a consequence of excess administration of fluids in patients with low oncotic pressure resulting from hypoalbuminemia. In addition, reversible, predominantly posterior leukoencephaolopathy may develop in patients with eclampsia.[160] The findings on neuroimaging are characteristic of subcortical edema without infarction.

Prevention and Treatment

The cause or causes of preeclampsia remain unknown; thus, treatment remains empirical. The principles of treatment have changed little since the early 1970s, despite advances in understanding its pathophysiologic mechanisms. Outcomes are improving primarily because of early recognition of the disease, close maternal and fetal surveillance, seizure prophylaxis, judicious use of antihypertensive therapy, and timely delivery. The ultimate goal of therapy is prevention, which, unfortunately, remains elusive.

Prevention

Many strategies to prevent preeclampsia have been attempted over the years, including sodium restriction, diuretics, high-protein diets, and antihypertensive medication, and all have been unsuccessful. Since 1990, considerable resources have been allocated toward determining whether either low-dose aspirin or calcium supplementation is an effective preventive strategy.

Several small studies conducted in the mid-1980s suggested that low-dose aspirin (50 to 150 mg/day) administered early in pregnancy may prevent preeclampsia (reviewed in several sources[161-165]). It was hypothesized that such therapy reversed the imbalances between PGI_2 and TXA_2 that may be responsible for some of the manifestations of this disease. Since 1993, several large trials have been completed, and most have not demonstrated a beneficial effect of aspirin for the prevention of preeclampsia. In a National Institutes of Health (NIH)–sponsored randomized, placebo-controlled trial of 3135 healthy nulliparous women, 4.6% of the aspirin recipients and 6.3% of the placebo recipients developed preeclampsia; the difference was barely significant.[166] There was a slight increase in placental abruption in the group taking aspirin. A larger trial conducted largely in the United Kingdom (the Collaborative Low-dose

Aspirin Study in Pregnancy [CLASP]) of 9309 women at slightly increased risk failed to demonstrate any decrease in the incidence of preeclampsia in the treated group.[167] In this study, there was no increase in placental abruption in the aspirin-treated patients. Several subsequent large trials in Brazil, Barbados, Jamaica, and the United States, with a total of more than 13,000 women at moderate or high risk, found no significant differences in the incidence of preeclampsia, fetal growth restriction, preterm births, or adverse outcomes in women receiving aspirin and in controls. A summary of all large trials conducted suggests that aspirin treatment will prevent the occurrence of early onset preeclampsia in approximately 15% of women at risk and reduced fetal growth restriction by 18%.[165] A systematic review of 14 trials that included more than 12,000 women showed a small but significant benefit of aspirin therapy in reducing perinatal death (odds ratio, 0.79) and preeclampsia (odds ratio, 0.86), and an increase of 215 g in mean birth weight. Aspirin therapy is safe and not associated with increased risk of bleeding or placental abruption.[165]

It appears that aspirin may be beneficial only in women at high risk. In the NIH trial, a benefit was observed in women with higher blood pressures at recruitment. In the CLASP trial, there was a reduction in the incidence of early-onset preeclampsia in treated women. Furthermore, the issue of compliance has been raised, and reanalysis of results of the NIH trial based on circulating TXA_2 levels and of pill counts suggest that aspirin may, in fact, reduce the incidence of preeclampsia and result in improved fetal outcome.[168] An additional concern regarding the CLASP trial is that the therapy may have been initiated (up to 26 weeks) too late for the aspirin to be beneficial or that perhaps the dose was too low (60 mg/day).

It has been suggested that the women enrolled in the earlier trials were at too low a risk to detect a significant benefit of aspirin; however, a multicenter trial of women with high-risk pregnancies (because of chronic hypertension, diabetes, multiple pregnancy) did not demonstrate a reduced incidence of preeclampsia in the treated group.[169] The current data do not support the prophylactic use of low-dose aspirin in pregnant women at low or medium risk for preeclampsia or in women with mild chronic hypertension. However, low-dose aspirin may be effective in a defined group of predominantly parous women at high risk, not only in preventing preeclampsia but also in reducing its severity.

Another preventive strategy that has received considerable attention is calcium supplementation. Low calcium intake has been implicated in the pathogenesis of preeclampsia,[170] and a trial of 1094 nulliparous pregnant women,[171] as well as a metaanalysis,[172] suggested that calcium supplementation with 2 g of calcium carbonate daily can prevent preeclampsia. Again, a large NIH multicenter randomized clinical trial of 4589 women failed to support these earlier findings.[173] However, subsequent trials conducted outside the United States have continued to demonstrate a beneficial effect of calcium supplementation for the prevention of preeclampsia.[174,175] A possible explanation for the discrepancy in these results is the dietary calcium intake in these populations. In the NIH trial, both the placebo and treatment recipients had baseline calcium intake of more than 1000 g/day. In contrast, in the trials in which calcium has been beneficial, the calcium intake in the population was well below the recommended dietary allowance for pregnancy. Thus, calcium supplementation may be beneficial in women with low calcium intake but may not be necessary if calcium intake is adequate.

Oxidative stress is currently a plausible hypothesis for the mechanism of endothelial injury in preeclampsia. A study of 283 women considered to be at increased risk of preeclampsia because of abnormal uterine artery Doppler waveforms at 18 to 22 weeks participated in a randomized clinical trial; treated women received 1000 mg vitamin C daily and 400 IU vitamin E, in comparison with placebo.[176] This study demonstrated a significant benefit of antioxidant therapy in reducing the incidence of preeclampsia. Currently, two large trials of antioxidant therapy in prevention of preeclampsia are in progress in the United States and the United Kingdom.

Other approaches to prevention, including fish oil, diuretics, sodium restriction, and magnesium, have not been successful.[177,178] Nevertheless, although prevention of preeclampsia is usually not possible, avoidance of severe complications may be accomplished by early recognition of the disease before such complications develop. If early signs of severe disease are detected, hospitalization should be strongly considered to enable close monitoring of the patient. If preeclampsia is detected early, bed rest and close monitoring of maternal and fetal condition may enable prolongation of pregnancy in some cases.

Treatment

The ultimate goal of treating a patient with preeclampsia is delivery of a mature, healthy infant without compromising maternal health. When preeclampsia is mild and develops close to term, the perinatal death rate and the rates of preterm delivery, fetal growth restriction, and placental abruption are similar to those of normotensive pregnancies. When the disease manifests near term and fetal maturity is certain, the definitive treatment is delivery. In contrast, both perinatal and maternal morbidity are increased when the disease is severe, particularly when disease develops in the second trimester, and the fetus is still quite immature. In such cases, decisions regarding timing of delivery are difficult.

Antepartum Management of Preeclampsia before 37 Weeks

The standard approach to treatment of preeclampsia includes bed rest in the hospital with daily maternal and fetal surveillance.[179] Investigators have questioned whether hospitalization or bed rest is necessary for women with mild preeclampsia and mild hypertension. In the absence of definitive data from randomized clinical trials, reduced activity and modified bed rest is a safe strategy. Hospitalization is preferred in cases when optimum, close outpatient follow-up is not possible. Further evaluation of these approaches with randomized clinical trials is warranted.

Adequate maternal surveillance should include regular assessment for signs of severe disease.[180] This includes evaluation of symptoms that may precede eclampsia (headache, visual changes, altered mentation, right upper quadrant pain, epigastric pain) and close monitoring of blood pressure. Laboratory tests are an important aspect of maternal surveillance, as they detect progression of disease. Routine laboratory tests recommended for women with suspected or diagnosed preeclampsia include measurements of 24-hour urine protein, serum creatinine, serum uric acid, platelets, and liver enzymes. The frequency with which these tests should be performed depends on the initial findings and the severity of the disease.

Fetal testing is also indicated in women with preeclampsia, because nonreassuring fetal heart rate patterns or poor growth may be an indication for delivery, even if the maternal condition is stable. Routine fetal monitoring includes daily fetal movement counts, nonstress testing, and biophysical profile. These tests should be performed at the time of diagnosis and then one to two times weekly until delivery. Ultrasound evaluation of fetal weight and amniotic fluid volume are also recommended. Some authorities recommend Doppler flow velocimetry for detection of increased umbilical artery impedance.

If signs of severe disease are present (i.e., persistent hypertension with diastolic blood pressures higher than 110 mm Hg, abnormal results of liver function tests, low platelet count, oliguria, or deteriorating renal function), then delivery is recommended if pregnancy has reached 34 weeks.[31] Indications for delivery regardless of gestational age of the fetus include imminent eclampsia, multiorgan dysfunction, severe fetal growth restriction, placental abruption, or nonreassuring results of fetal testing. Conservative management in such cases may not be associated with improved fetal outcome and may, in fact, result in serious maternal morbidity.

In some situations, however, postponing delivery may be appropriate. A woman may develop preeclampsia far before term with only mild to moderate hypertension and no signs of deteriorating renal or hepatic function or coagulopathy. In some cases, valuable time may be gained for the fetus by temporizing. In some cases, it may be necessary to administer antihypertensive therapy to maintain maternal blood pressure in a safe range. Such women should be treated in the hospital, where it is easier to monitor progression of the maternal disease and to intercede rapidly when complications arise. Also, hospitalization enables frequent antepartum testing to diagnose fetal jeopardy. The decision to continue the pregnancy can then

be made on a day-to-day basis. Indeed, one report of a conservative approach to women in whom preeclampsia developed between 24 and 27 weeks suggested that such an approach resulted in improved perinatal survival.[180] It must be emphasized, however, that conservative treatment of early preeclampsia is appropriate only when aggressive monitoring of maternal and fetal status is possible.

Antihypertensive Therapy

The role of antihypertensive therapy (Table 3–4) in the management of preeclampsia is controversial. The basis for this controversy is that it is still uncertain whether the uteroplacental circulation is autoregulated; and thus the impact of lowering maternal blood pressure on placental perfusion is of great concern, especially because diminished uteroplacental blood flow usually is already present in preeclampsia. Lowering maternal blood pressure does not cure or reverse preeclampsia, and it may not benefit the fetus. Nevertheless, maternal health is of utmost importance; thus lowering blood pressure is indicated when maternal cerebrovascular or cardiovascular safety is at risk.

There is disagreement about which level of blood pressure should be treated. Many women with preeclampsia have previously been normotensive, so that blood pressure levels that would normally be tolerated in individuals with chronic hypertension cause symptoms in women with acute preeclampsia. For women in the peripartum period, many physicians, including myself, would begin antihypertensive therapy when the diastolic blood pressure approaches 100 mm Hg. Blood pressure should not be aggressively lowered, because this may cause fetal heart rate decelerations. This recommendation is not based on data from controlled clinical trials, however it is supported by consensus-based guidelines.[31] If delivery is expected within 24 to 48 hours, parenteral agents are usually advisable. If temporization for more than 48 hours is anticipated, then an oral agent is preferable.

The drug most commonly used in management of hypertension in the peripartum period is intravenous hydralazine, a drug that most obstetric staff know well and one with a long history of safe and effective use in women with preeclampsia.[181,182] In addition to the well-known side effects of tachycardia, headache, tremulousness, nausea, and vomiting, some reports suggest that

TABLE 3–4 Drug Treatment of Peripartum Hypertension Caused by Preeclampsia

Drug	Dose and Route	Onset of Action	Adverse Effects	Comments
Hydralazine	5 mg IV or IM, then 5-10 mg every 20-40 min	IV: 10 min IM: 10-30 min	Headache, flushing, tachycardia, nausea	Extensive experience in this setting; well-documented safety and efficacy
Labetalol	20 mg IV, then 20-80 mg every 20-30 min, up to 300 mg	5-10 min	Flushing, headache, vomiting, tingling of scalp	—
Nifedipine	5-10 mg PO; repeat in 30 min if necessary; sublingual route not recommended	10-15 min	Flushing, headache, tachycardia, nausea, inhibition of labor	May cause abrupt drop in blood pressure; may cause hypotension if magnesium sulfate is used
Diazoxide	30-50 mg IV every 15 min	2-5 min	Inhibition of labor, hyperglycemia, fluid retention	Should be used only in refractory cases; may cause hypotension

IM, intramuscularly; IV, intravenously; PO, per os (orally).

hydralazine administered in the setting of severe volume contraction may cause rapid and excessive decrements in blood pressure and may provoke oliguria as well as fetal heart rate decelerations.[183,184] Therefore, treatment should commence with 5-mg doses, followed by 5- to 10-mg increases every 20 to 30 minutes. Parenteral labetalol has been administered to women with preeclampsia with favorable results.[185-188] This drug is a combined α and β blocker, and studies suggest that uteroplacental blood flow is maintained after parenteral use.[187,188]

Several features of calcium channel blockers make them attractive agents for controlling hypertension in women with preeclampsia. These drugs have a rapid onset of action, rarely cause hypotension, and are relatively free of serious adverse effects. Moreover, calcium channel blockers have been demonstrated to reduce cerebral vasospasm (measured by transcranial Doppler waveforms) in women with preeclampsia.[189] The use of calcium channel blockers in pregnancy has been investigated in several, largely uncontrolled studies. The results demonstrate that these agents are effective in controlling blood pressure[190,191]; however, caution is warranted because a few anecdotal reports suggest that the interaction of magnesium sulfate and calcium channel blockers has led to precipitous drops in blood pressure and even neuromuscular blockade.[192]

Finally, in an occasional patient, severe hypertension is resistant to the antihypertensive agents previously discussed; such a patient may require diazoxide or sodium nitroprusside. The latter drug has been associated with cyanide poisoning of sheep fetuses (albeit with large doses); however, when necessary, the mother's health should be considered first.

Anticonvulsant Therapy

Magnesium sulfate has been the drug of choice (in the United States) for the prevention of convulsions in women with preeclampsia, and for the treatment of eclampsia.[179] Although in the past, critics have claimed that this drug is ineffective because it is not an established anticonvulsant, two large clinical trials demonstrated the superiority of magnesium sulfate compared with either phenytoin or diazepam.[193,194] Two randomized, placebo-controlled trials demonstrated that magnesium sulfate is superior to placebo for prevention of convulsions in women with severe preeclampsia.[195-197] One trial enrolled more than 10,000 women with preeclampsia in 33 countries, many in developing nations.[197] Magnesium reduced the rate of eclampsia in the entire group (0.8% versus 1.9%; relative risk, 0.42; 95% confidence interval, 0.29 to 0.60); however, in the 1560 women in developed Western nations, the rates of eclampsia were 0.5% in the treated groups and 0.8% in the placebo groups (relative risk, 0.67; 95% confidence interval, 0.19 to 2.37).

Hemodynamic Monitoring

In occasional severe or complicated cases, invasive hemodynamic monitoring may be useful, particularly when refractory oliguria, pulmonary edema, or refractory hypertension is present.[198] It must be stressed that these circumstances are extremely rare; and if experienced personnel are not available for catheter insertion and maintenance, then the risks may outweigh the benefits.

Postpartum Hypertension

Hypertension associated with preeclampsia may resolve in the first postpartum week, although in more severe cases, blood pressure may continue to rise after delivery and the hypertension may persist for 2 to 4 weeks post partum.[199,200] Ferrazzani and colleagues[200] stressed that the time required for the blood pressure to normalize post partum correlates both with laboratory markers indicative of renal impairment and with early delivery. Of interest, blood pressure in normotensive women is higher during the first 5 postpartum days,[201] and it has been proposed that this may relate to the shifting of fluid from the interstitial space to the intravascular compartment that occurs in the immediate puerperium. No large clinical treatment trials have focused solely on hypertension in the immediate puerperium. This is unfortunate, because severe hypertension in the setting of resolving vasospasm may interfere with cerebral autoregulation, resulting in seizures or cerebrovascular accidents. Thus, in the absence of more definitive data, I recommend that systolic blood pressure levels of 150 mm Hg or higher and diastolic levels of 100 mm Hg or higher be treated in the puerperium. Women with postpartum hypertension should not receive bromocriptine, because of anecdotal reports that such therapy paradoxically exacerbates the hypertensive syndrome and may cause cerebrovascular accidents.[202]

Hypertension may first be diagnosed in the postpartum period. When this occurs, the differential diagnosis includes postpartum preeclampsia or eclampsia, unrecognized chronic hypertension that was masked by pregnancy, and, in rare cases, microangiopathic syndromes such as hemolytic-uremic syndrome or thrombotic thrombocytopenic purpura.

Postpartum preeclampsia or eclampsia is uncommon, and in some cases, careful scrutiny of antepartum records reveals evidence of preeclampsia before delivery. However, there are instances of well-documented normotensive deliveries in which hypertension in association with laboratory features of preeclampsia has appeared late in the first postpartum week or afterward. Late postpartum eclampsia has also been observed, the seizures occurring after the first postpartum week.[203-205] The pathogenesis of these phenomena is poorly understood and certainly is at odds with the traditional concept of preeclampsia-eclampsia as disorders observed only during pregnancy or the immediate puerperium, caused by abnormalities in placental development. There are no standard protocols for the management of these late postpartum syndromes. Some authorities use the traditional approach of parenteral magnesium sulfate, whereas others concerned about previously subclinical epilepsy use phenytoin. In most instances, the disease resolves within 48 to 72 hours.

Hypertension appearing de novo in the puerperium without laboratory abnormalities suggestive of preeclampsia probably represents undiagnosed chronic hypertension. In some cases the blood pressure had normalized during pregnancy as a response to the physiologic vasodilation that accompanies pregnancy. In most cases the underlying disorder is essential hypertension; however, secondary causes should be considered when there are unusual features such as severe hypertension, hypokalemia, or symptoms suggestive of pheochromocytoma.

CHRONIC HYPERTENSION DURING PREGNANCY

The incidence of preexisting or chronic hypertension in pregnant women has not been quantified exactly. According to current estimates of the prevalence of hypertensive disorders during pregnancy, chronic hypertension probably complicates 2% to 5% of pregnancies. Also, because preeclampsia or gestational hypertension in multiparous women may be unrecognized chronic hypertension, the incidence may be higher. Finally, in certain parts of the world, particularly industrialized urban areas, many women postpone childbearing; thus, the incidence of preexisting hypertension complicating pregnancy is more common.

Chronic hypertension complicating pregnancy is diagnosed by high blood pressure known to predate conception. Most women with chronic hypertension have essential (also called primary) hypertension, but as many as 10% may have underlying renal or endocrine disorders (i.e., secondary hypertension).

Diagnosis

When hypertension has been clearly documented before conception, the diagnosis of chronic hypertension in pregnancy is straightforward. It is also the most likely diagnosis when hypertension is present before 20 weeks of pregnancy, although isolated, rare cases of preeclampsia before this time have been reported, particularly in the presence of hydatidiform mole.

Difficulties arise when pregnant women with stage 1 and even stage 2 hypertension present initially in the second trimester, after having experienced the pregnancy-associated "physiologic" decrease in blood pressure. These women have been presumed to be normotensive and are later erroneously diagnosed with preeclampsia if blood pressure rises in the third trimester. In such cases, a diagnosis of either hypertension of pregnancy or chronic hypertension is most likely when the increased blood pressure is not accompanied by proteinuria and when other classic laboratory abnormalities consistent with preeclampsia are absent. It may not be possible to distinguish between gestational hypertension and chronic hypertension until post partum. Women with gestational hypertension become normotensive in the postpartum period (although not necessarily immediately), whereas those with chronic hypertension remain hypertensive and in some cases become more hypertensive as the levels of the vasodilatory hormones of pregnancy decrease. Because women with gestational hypertension may be at increased risk of essential hypertension and may even be considered to have "latent essential hypertension," such women, who have been normotensive before pregnancy, on occasion develop sustained hypertension after delivery.

Because 15% to 25% of women with chronic hypertension develop *superimposed* preeclampsia, it may be impossible to diagnose chronic hypertension in this setting until well after delivery. In other instances, women with well-documented hypertension before conception demonstrate normal blood pressures throughout their entire pregnancy, only to return to prepregnancy hypertensive levels post partum.

Clinical Impact of Chronic Hypertension During Pregnancy

Although there is little doubt that perinatal morbidity and mortality are increased among women with chronic hypertension who develop superimposed preeclampsia in comparison with hypertensive pregnant women with uncomplicated preexisting essential hypertension,[206] the maternal and fetal risks of pregnancies in this latter group are less clear. Some women experience accelerated hypertension during pregnancy, with resultant target organ damage (e.g., to the heart, brain, and kidneys), although this is extremely uncommon in the absence of preeclampsia. One exception may be the case of the rare women with severe hypertension (stage 3 or 4) before conception, many of whom have underlying renal disease or secondary hypertension.

Placental abruption may be associated with life-threatening maternal hemorrhage, and the risk of abruption is increased threefold in women with chronic hypertension.[207] Some women with secondary forms of hypertension, such as from chronic renal disease and collagen disorders, may suffer from irreversible deterioration in renal function. In the case of systemic lupus erythematosus, there may be multiorgan system morbidity, regardless of the development of superimposed preeclampsia. Finally, although the expectation is that pregnancies in women with uncomplicated chronic hypertension will be successful, these women are more likely to be hospitalized for hypertension and to undergo cesarean delivery.[208]

As discussed, underlying hypertension is a recognized risk factor for preeclampsia.[209] The National High Blood Pressure Education Program Working Group Report definition of superimposed preeclampsia is as follows: a significant increase in blood pressure (30 mm Hg for systolic pressure, 15 mm Hg for diastolic pressure) in association with new-onset proteinuria (≥300 mg/day) and hyperuricemia or features of HELLP syndrome occurring after midpregnancy.[31] According to these criteria, the incidence of superimposed preeclampsia in women with chronic hypertension is between 20% and 25%.[208-211]

Effects of Chronic Hypertension on Fetal Outcome

The rate of perinatal mortality is higher in pregnancies accompanied by chronic hypertension, and these excess losses are caused primarily by superimposed preeclampsia. The relative risk of perinatal death has been reported to be 3.6 in women with superimposed preeclampsia in comparison with those with uncomplicated chronic hypertension.[208] The incidence of perinatal death is also significantly higher in the latter group than in normotensive controls (relative risk, 2.3). The risk of preterm delivery is increased by fourfold in women with chronic hypertension, largely because of indicated preterm delivery. Data confirm an incidence of preterm delivery of 33%

in women with chronic hypertension. Fetal growth restriction is also more common with chronic hypertension, especially when superimposed preeclampsia develops.

An unquantified risk to fetal well-being is exposure in utero to antihypertensive medications. Metaanalyses suggest that lowering blood pressure with antihypertensive medication may contribute to fetal growth restriction.[212] Careful clinical trials evaluating maternal outcomes as well as long-term outcomes of exposed offspring have been conducted with a limited number of agents, primarily methyldopa.[213] Because of its proven safety, this drug remains the drug of choice for hypertension during pregnancy, although nifedipine and labetolol are also widely used as first line agents.

Secondary Hypertension

These forms of hypertension are quite rare in comparison with essential hypertension and account for 2% to 5% of cases of hypertension diagnosed and treated at specialized centers. In routine care groups, however, their numbers are lower. The most common causes are renal disease, renovascular hypertension, aldosteronism, Cushing's syndrome, and pheochromocytoma. The prevalence of secondary hypertension in women of childbearing age has not been determined. Of importance, the prognosis may be better when a diagnosis of secondary hypertension is made before conception, because most forms of secondary hypertension are associated with increased maternal and fetal morbidity and mortality, and some cases may be cured with surgery.

Renal Disease

A detailed discussion of renal disease and pregnancy is presented in Chapter 13. There are, however, several points to emphasize regarding the management of hypertension associated with intrinsic renal disease. Kidney disease is the most common cause of secondary hypertension and may result from anatomic or congenital abnormalities, glomerulonephritis, diabetes, systemic lupus erythematosus, or interstitial nephritis.

All young women with newly diagnosed hypertension should be screened for intrinsic renal disease, with blood tests for renal function and urinalysis for detection of proteinuria or red blood cells. Those with a strong family history of renal disease should be screened with ultrasonography for polycystic kidney disease. This autosomal dominant disorder often manifests as hypertension in the third and fourth decades. When renal disease is detected, regardless of its cause, these women should be counseled in regard to increased maternal and fetal risks with impaired renal function (preconception serum creatinine level ≥1.4 mg/dL) or poorly controlled hypertension.

Pregnant women with renal disease should be managed by a multidisciplinary team of obstetricians and nephrologists. This is particularly appropriate for renal transplant recipients, in whom concerns regarding immunosuppression and risk of infection and rejection necessitate coordinated specialty care. Therapy for hypertension is similar to that in gravidas with essential hypertension, although

many nephrologists treat hypertension more aggressively during pregnancy when there is underlying renal disease.

Renovascular Hypertension

This entity refers to hypertension caused by anatomic lesions of the renal arteries. The narrowing of the lumen leads to diminished blood flow to one or both kidneys, with resultant renal ischemia, stimulation of the renin-angiotensin system, and ensuing hypertension. Renovascular hypertension in women of childbearing age is usually caused by fibromuscular dysplasia, a nonatherosclerotic, noninflammatory vascular-occlusive disease.[214]

Knowledge of renovascular hypertension in pregnancy is based on a handful of case reports and a few limited series of patients totaling approximately 25 cases. Many of the patients manifested early and severe preeclampsia and poor pregnancy outcomes.[215-219] One retrospective comparison of pregnancy outcomes in four patients with known renovascular hypertension matched to 20 women with essential hypertension demonstrated that those with renovascular hypertension were younger (25 versus 36 years) and had higher blood pressure levels during pregnancy.[220] All four women with renovascular hypertension developed superimposed preeclampsia, in contrast to 30% of those with essential hypertension.

Of interest are sporadic cases of early pregnancy detection of renovascular hypertension, and successful revascularization during midpregnancy, with good pregnancy outcome.[218,219] Hennessy and colleagues also documented the experiences of two women whose pregnancies, when they had untreated renovascular hypertension, were complicated by severe preeclampsia. Both underwent successful angioplasty post partum, and their subsequent pregnancies were normal.[220] In view of the dramatic clinical improvement that usually follows revascularization, as well as the anecdotal experience described earlier, it seems justified to rule out renovascular hypertension before conception in young women with clinical features suggestive of this condition. Pregnant women with renovascular hypertension who have not undergone revascularization are at considerable risk, especially for superimposed preeclampsia and fetal complications. Temporizing therapy with angiotensin-converting enzyme inhibitors or angiotensin II receptor-blocking agents is precluded for use in pregnancy because of the dangers that these agents post to the fetus, but treatment of hypertension with other drugs that suppress renin secretion is possible. Those most likely to be effective are methyldopa and β-adrenergic receptor blockers.

Primary Aldosteronism

This form of hypertension results from increased secretion of aldosterone and may be caused by a solitary adrenal adenoma (Conn's syndrome) or bilateral adrenal hyperplasia. There is also a variant, labeled *nodular hyperplasia,* that is characterized by enlargement of the adrenal glands, which contain one or more adenomas that secrete most of the aldosterone.

Several cases of aldosteronism have been reported in pregnancy.[221-231] Some of these have been complicated by considerable morbidity, including severe hypertension, hypokalemia, preeclampsia, and poor fetal outcome, but there are also cases in which hypertension and hypokalemia have been ameliorated during pregnancy.[226,231] It is hypothesized that such improvement, when it occurs, is a consequence of the high levels of progesterone that antagonize the actions of aldosterone.[226]

Primary aldosteronism is difficult to diagnose in pregnant women because of the marked alterations in the renin-angiotensin-aldosterone system that occur in normal pregnancy. Both renin and aldosterone production are markedly increased; urine aldosterone excretion is fivefold increased over that commonly observed in nonpregnant patients with primary aldosteronism. Moreover, mild hypokalemia is not unusual in the course of a normal pregnancy. Greater degrees of hypokalemia (≤ 3 mEq/L), however, are unusual and should be investigated.

Treatment of aldosteronism diagnosed during pregnancy is controversial.[228-231] If blood pressure improves spontaneously or is easily controlled with antihypertensive drugs, then it is reasonable to postpone surgical intervention until post partum. Spironolactone, reported to cause virilization in female rodent fetuses exposed in utero, should be avoided.[232] Calcium channel blockers have been reported to be beneficial in nonpregnant patients with aldosteronism[233]; thus, I would prescribe these latter agents, especially if methyldopa proved ineffective. However, when faced with severe hypertension resistant to therapy and marked hypokalemia (≤ 2.8 mEq/L) or any level of hypokalemia necessitating very large replacement doses, it may be prudent to consider surgery. During pregnancy, magnetic resonance imaging is preferable to computed tomography because ionizing radiation is not used in the former. Adrenal vein sampling has not been reported in pregnancy and is unadvisable because this procedure must be done with fluoroscopically guided catheter placement. Thus, documentation of a unilateral adenoma during pregnancy may be suboptimal, which is one reason why surgery may be indicated for treatment failure alone. In this regard, there are several reports of surgical removal of adenomas during the second trimester, followed by favorable maternal and fetal outcomes.[224,228,229,231]

Pheochromocytoma

More than 100 cases of pheochromocytoma manifesting during pregnancy or in the immediate puerperium have been reported, and both maternal and fetal morbidity and mortality rates are extremely high when the presence of the tumor is unknown before delivery.[234-243] There are also cases of unsuspected pheochromocytoma manifesting as myocardial infarction in pregnant women.[239,240] Other serious complications include cardiac arrhythmias, shock, pulmonary edema, cerebral hemorrhage, and hemorrhaging into the tumor.[241] In several instances, the presenting signs and symptoms—late pregnancy accelerated hypertension, proteinuria, and seizures—were indistinguishable from those of preeclampsia or eclampsia.[242] In fact, there is a suggestion that the clinical manifestations may be more dramatic as pregnancy progresses because the enlarged uterus is more likely to compress the tumor.

Surgical removal is the therapy of choice when a pheochromocytoma is diagnosed in the initial two trimesters, although successful medical management throughout the entire pregnancy has been reported.[225] Preoperative management includes α blockade with either phenoxybenzamine[237,238] or combinations of α and β blockers. Placental transfer of phenoxybenzamine has been reported and may lead to perinatal depression and hypotension in newborns.[243] Labetalol, an α and β blocker, has also been used successfully during pregnancy.[236]

The approach to treatment in the third trimester is more variable and includes combined cesarean delivery and tumor resection, tumor resection followed by delivery, and delivery followed by tumor resection at a later date. Once the predicted chance of fetal survival is high, I prefer the combined procedure of cesarean delivery and immediate tumor resection.[237,242]

Cushing's Syndrome

This disease, too, is quite rare in pregnant hypertensive women, possibly because patients with Cushing's syndrome have a variety of menstrual irregularities.[244] Also, the syndrome may be difficult to diagnose because the hormonal alterations of normal pregnancy mimic those of the disease.[245] Of importance, Cushing's syndrome is associated with excessive maternal morbidity; hypertension, superimposed preeclampsia, diabetes, and congestive heart failure are the most common complications. There is also a high incidence of preterm delivery, growth restriction, and fetal death. Management includes surgical resection of the tumor during the first trimester and surgery after delivery in the third trimester, whereas therapeutic approaches in the second trimester are more complex. In this case, the risks of surgery must be weighed against the risks of medication to treat hypercortisolism.[245]

Principles of Management of Chronic Hypertension in Pregnancy

The treatment goals for chronic hypertension in pregnant women are different from the goals of treatment of hypertension in nonpregnant patients. In the latter, the primary concern is prevention of long-term cardiovascular morbidity and mortality. Blood pressure control is essential, and the report of the Joint National Committee on Prevention, Detection, Evaluation, and Treatment of High Blood Pressure[246] recommended maintaining systolic levels between 120 and 135 mm Hg and diastolic levels between 75 and 85 mm Hg. Management also includes aggressive attention to modifying other cardiovascular risk factors, such as blood lipid and glucose levels, body weight, and smoking. Some of these concerns are relevant during pregnancy (e.g., smoking, blood glucose), but others are not (weight loss, aerobic exercise).

Preconception Counseling

Management ideally begins before conception and includes ruling out and treating secondary causes of hypertension. Women in whom hypertension is known to have been present for 5 years or more require careful evaluation for evidence of target organ damage (i.e., left ventricular hypertrophy, retinopathy, and azotemia). Pregnant women 35 years of age or older, particularly those with chronic illnesses, should be screened for occult coronary disease, and this is particularly important in women with type I diabetes with evidence of vascular complications. Ideally, adjustment of medications should also precede conception, and, of course, drugs with known deleterious fetal effects (especially angiotensin-converting enzyme inhibitors and angiotensin II receptor antagonists) should be discontinued. Risks posed by pregnancy are best discussed and less emotionally evaluated before conception. For example, women with stages 1 and 2 hypertension should be informed of the high likelihood of a favorable outcome but should still be told of the risks of superimposed preeclampsia and the fetal complications associated with this disorder. This is also the best time to emphasize the importance of compliance and that frequent office or clinic visits increase the likelihood of detecting preeclampsia and other complications well before they become life-threatening to the mother or the fetus. Women with young children and those in the workforce should be informed of the possibility that lifestyle adjustments will be necessary, especially if complications develop. This allows them to plan ahead for increased support both at home and at work. Finally, early planning, including the assembling of a multidisciplinary team consisting of the obstetrician and internists, optimizes the chances of a successful outcome in hypertensive women with other medical complications (e.g., renal transplant recipients, those with diabetic nephropathy, those with systemic lupus erythematosus).

Nonpharmacologic Management

Pregnant hypertensive women, in contrast to their non-pregnant counterparts, are not advised to exercise vigorously, although careful studies of the effects of aerobic exercise on pregnancy outcome have not been performed. However, moderate exercise such as a walking program three to five times a week is acceptable. The major concern regarding vigorous exertion is that women with chronic hypertension are at risk for preeclampsia, a condition characterized by decreased uteroplacental blood flow, and such exercise may compromise blood flow even further.

Excessive weight gain, of course, is not advisable, but again, in contrast to therapy in nonpregnant populations, obese women should not be advised to lose weight during pregnancy. Dietary adjustments in pregnant women with chronic hypertension have not been extensively investigated. Salt restriction, an important component of management in nonpregnant populations, is less important in pregnancy, in which extremely low sodium intakes (≤2 g/day) may even jeopardize the physiologic plasma volume expansion that normally occurs. However, in women with "salt-sensitive" hypertension successfully managed with a low-sodium diet before conception, it is reasonable to continue such diets during pregnancy, limiting restriction to between 60 and 80 mEq/day. Increased dietary calcium intake (i.e., more than the recommended 1200 mg/day)

may be beneficial in nonpregnant hypertensive patients, but data pertaining to pregnancy are inconclusive. In this regard, metaanalyses of small trials of the efficacy of supplementation to prevent preeclampsia in normotensive women were encouraging, whereas a large, carefully conducted, randomized, placebo-controlled trial failed to detect any beneficial actions of added calcium in normotensive primiparous women. Other dietary approaches such as supplementation with magnesium or with fish oil have been investigated in normotensive pregnant women, with negative results, but have not been studied in women with chronic hypertension.[247]

Pharmacologic Management

Guidelines for antihypertensive therapy during pregnancy (Table 3–5) are less clear than those for nonpregnant hypertensive women. For the latter, compelling data from large population studies document the benefits of lowering blood pressure with medication, even in women with only mild hypertension.[246] During pregnancy, however, although maternal safety remains the primary concern, there is also a desire to minimize exposure of the fetus to drugs, given their unknown long-term effects on growth and development. A systematic review of clinical trials of hypertension found only 13 randomized clinical trials in which antihypertensive therapy was compared with either no treatment or placebo in women with chronic hypertension.[248] The most commonly used drug, methyldopa, was given to only a little more than 200 subjects. Six trials showed no reduction in perinatal mortality with antihypertensive treatment, whereas three reported a trend toward lower perinatal mortality with treatment. A debatable issue is whether lowering blood pressure prevents superimposed preeclampsia, but there is little or no convincing evidence to support this contention.[248,249] Thus, it is permissible to tolerate higher blood pressure levels during pregnancy that do not harm in the short term while limiting use of antihypertensive drugs. In this regard, most pregnant women with chronic hypertension have only mild or very moderate elevations in blood pressure and require little or no medication at all. However, "appropriate" or "tolerable" levels of blood pressure during pregnancy for these patients seem to have been set empirically, and multicenter clinical trials are needed to support or reject such practices.

I recommend the guidelines of the National High Blood Pressure Education Program Working Group Report on High Blood Pressure in Pregnancy,[31] in which antihypertensive drug treatment is begun only when maternal blood pressure reaches diastolic levels of 100 mm Hg or more. There are, however, exceptions, including parenchymal renal disease and evidence of target organ damage (e.g., retinopathy and cardiac hypertrophy), in which case therapy is recommended once levels are 90 mm Hg or more.

The argument of whether to treat becomes more debatable in regard to fetal well-being. Some evidence suggests fetal benefits when mild to moderate hypertension is treated with antihypertensive drugs during pregnancy.[250] For instance, in one frequently cited trial, treatment with methyldopa was associated with a reduction in perinatal

TABLE 3–5   Antihypertensive Therapy for Chronic Hypertension in Pregnancy

Drug	Dose	Additional Comments
Methyldopa	500-3000 mg in 2-4 divided doses	Considered drug of choice because of extensive experience and well-documented maternal and fetal safety
Hydralazine	50-300 mg in 2-4 divided doses	Extensive experience; few adverse effects; may cause tachycardia
Labetalol	200-1200 mg in 2-3 divided doses	Similar in efficacy to methyldopa, less experience Other β blockers have been reported to be associated with smaller infants when used early in pregnancy; sporadic cases of liver toxicity
β Blockers	Variable	Possibility of fetal bradycardia, lower birth weight (when used early in pregnancy)
Calcium channel blockers	Variable	Accumulating data support maternal and fetal safety; may cause lower extremity edema; may inhibit labor; may interact with magnesium sulfate
α Blockers	Variable	No data for use in pregnancy
Clonidine	0.1-0.8 mg in 2-4 divided doses	Limited data
Thiazide diuretics	Variable	May be associated with diminished volume expansion in pregnancy; may be necessary, in lower doses, in salt-sensitive hypertensive patients
Angiotensin-converting enzyme inhibitors	Variable	Contraindicated in pregnancy: causes neonatal anuric renal failure, neonatal death, fetal loss in animals
Angiotensin receptor antagonists	Variable	No data in pregnancy; contraindicated in view of data with angiotensin-converting enzyme inhibitors

mortality, primarily midtrimester loss,[251] but a similar benefit was not evident in another large trial.[252]

In summary, the unknown but potential hazards of antihypertensive treatment during pregnancy are sufficient reasons for withholding drug treatment when hypertension is mild (diastolic levels of 90 to 99 mm Hg), particularly during the initial trimester. As noted, many affected patients experience a physiologic decrease in blood pressure that on occasion reaches normotensive levels. Patients whose diastolic levels are 100 mm Hg or more, however, should be treated, whereas evidence of renal disease or end-organ damage necessitates initiation of treatment at lower levels (≥90 mm Hg).

Specific Antihypertensive Agents

Evaluation of most antihypertensive agents during pregnancy has been sporadic, and there are almost no follow-up data with regard to the children exposed to the drug in utero. In fact, the only antihypertensive agent for which creditable follow-up exists is methyldopa.[213] No adverse effects were documented with the use of this agent, which is one reason why it is considered one of the safest drugs for use during pregnancy. Methyldopa is usually prescribed alone, but on occasion the direct-acting vasodilator hydralazine has been added to the regimen; this drug, too, has a long history of use in pregnancy and appears safe.[253] A brief summary regarding other groups of antihypertensive agents follows.

β-Adrenoreceptor blockers have been used extensively to lower blood pressure in pregnancy.[254] Most reports are of women enrolled as patients relatively late in pregnancy, in the second or third trimesters. The preponderance of data attests to the overall safety of β-blockers; however, when treatment is begun early in pregnancy, the birth weight may be lower, an observation supported by a recent metaanalysis of 29 trials that included 2500 women.[254]

Labetalol, a combined β- and α-adrenergic blocker, has been used widely in pregnancy, with periodic claims of its superiority to other agents. In comparative trials with methyldopa, it appears to have similar efficacy and similar incidence of maternal side effects,[255,256] but when it is compared with placebo, significant fetal benefits have not been demonstrated.[257] Thus, I use it as a second-line antihypertensive agent in the treatment of gravidas with chronic hypertension.

There are limited trials of the efficacy of calcium channel blockers in pregnant women; many of these trials have been uncontrolled.[257-260] One concern about prescribing these agents relates to the high incidence of superimposed preeclampsia in chronic hypertensive patients, a complication that mandates immediate initiation of parenteral magnesium therapy.[261] The potential interactions between magnesium and calcium channel blockers have been discussed.

Angiotensin-converting enzyme inhibitors are contraindicated in pregnancy because of their association with fetopathy and neonatal renal failure and death.[262-265] These observations have led to similar rejection of the use of angiotensin II receptor antagonists in pregnancy. One case report of a woman exposed to losartan during midpregnancy reported oligohydramnios, pulmonary hypoplasia, hypoplastic skull bones, and ultimate intrauterine demise at 31 weeks.[266]

There is only limited experience with α blockers in pregnancy. Because of their efficacy in controlling the signs and symptoms of pheochromocytoma, they are indicated in the medical management of this condition. The use of diuretics in pregnancy has been controversial, mainly because of concern that saluretic therapy interferes with the physiologic volume expansion of normal pregnancy (although proof of this is limited). The National High Blood Pressure Education Program Working Group on High Blood Pressure in Pregnancy condemned using diuretics in preeclampsia but noted that they need not be discontinued if the woman was receiving these drugs before conception.[31] Because most pregnant patients have only mild or moderate hypertension, it is safe to discontinue diuretic therapy, especially in view of the physiologic declines in pressure during the initial trimesters. I do, however, prescribe these drugs to women in whom hypertension appears refractory to the first-line medication because of salt sensitivity.

Antihypertensive Medications and Lactation

Studies of the possible effects of antihypertensive agents on breast-feeding infants are limited. In general, drugs that are bound to plasma proteins are not transferred to breast milk.[267] Lipid-soluble drugs may achieve higher concentrations than may water-soluble drugs.[268] Methyldopa is considered safe, and preliminary data suggest that the levels in breast milk are low. Several β blockers are concentrated in breast milk; atenolol and metoprolol are concentrated in high levels, and propranolol and labetalol, in very low levels.[269] Captopril levels in breast milk have been reported to be low; however, in view of the adverse effects of angiotensin-converting enzyme inhibitors on neonatal renal function, I do not recommend these agents to lactating women. There are only limited reports of calcium channel blockers and their transfer into breast milk; however, no adverse effects have been reported.[270,271] A systematic review of excretion of antihypertensive medication into human breast milk suggested that drugs with high protein binding were less likely to be excreted in breast milk.[272] Finally, although the concentration of diuretics in breast milk is usually low, these agents may reduce the quantity of milk production and interfere with the ability to breast-feed successfully.[268]

References

1. Chang J, Elam-Evans LD, Berg CJ, et al: Pregnancy-related mortality surveillance—United States, 1991-1999. MMWR Surveill Summ 2003;52(2):1.
2. Rajaram P, Agrawal A, Swain S: Determinants of maternal mortality: A hospitality based study from south India. Indian J Matern Child Health 1995;6:7.
3. Zhang J, Meikle S, Trumble A: Severe maternal morbidity associated with hypertensive disorders in pregnancy in the United States. Hypertens Pregnancy 2003:22:203.
4. Bader ME, Bader RA: Cardiovascular hemodynamics in pregnancy and labor. Clin Obstet Gynecol 1968;11:924.
5. Wilson M, Morganti AA, Zervoudakis I, et al: Blood pressure, the renin-aldosterone system and sex steroids throughout normal pregnancy. Am J Med 1980;68:97.
6. August P, Lenz T, Ales KL, et al: Longitudinal study of the renin-angiotensin-aldosterone system in hypertensive pregnant women: Deviations related to development of superimposed pre-eclampsia. Am J Obstet Gynecol 1990;163:1612.
7. Chapman AB, Abraham WT, Zamudio S, et al: Temporal relationships between hormonal and hemodynamic changes in early human pregnancy. Kidney Int 1998;54:2056.
8. Deng A, Engels K, Baylis C: Impact of nitric oxide deficiency on blood pressure and glomerular hemodynamic adaptations to pregnancy in the rat. Kidney Int 1996;50:1121.
9. Liao QP, Buhimschi IA, Saade G, et al: Regulation of vascular adaptation during pregnancy and post-partum: Effects of nitric oxide inhibition and steroid hormones. Hum Reprod 1996;11:2777.
10. Goeschen K, Henkel E, Behrens O: Plasma prostacyclin and thromboxane concentrations in 160 normotensive, hypertensive and preeclamptic patients during pregnancy, delivery and the postpartum period. J Perinat Med 1993;21:481.
11. Novak J, Danielson LA, Kerchner LJ, et al: Relaxin is essential for renal vasodilation during pregnancy in conscious rats. J Clin Invest 2001;107:1469.
12. Gangula PRR, Zhao H, Supowit S, et al: Pregnancy and steroid hormones enhance the vasodilation responses to CRGP in rats. Am J Physiol 1999;276:H284.
13. Ni Y, May V, Braas K, Osol G: Pregnancy augments uteroplacental vascular endothelial growth factor gene expression and vasodilator effects. Am J Physiol 1997;273:H938.
14. Howard RB, Husain A: Rat ovarian angiotensin II receptors, renin, and angiotensin I–converting enzyme during pregnancy and the postpartum period. Biol Reprod 1992;47:925.
15. Jerat S, Morrish DW, Davidge ST, Kaufman S: Effect of adrenomedullin on placental arteries in normal and preeclamptic pregnancies. Hypertension 2001;37:227.
16. Rang S, Wolf H, Montfrans GA, Karemaker JM: Non-invasive assessment of autonomic cardiovascular control in normal human pregnancy and pregnancy-associated hypertensive disorders: A review. J Hypertens 2002;20:2111.
17. Lucini D, Strappazzon P, Vecchia LD, et al: Cardiac autonomic adjustments to normal human pregnancy: Insight from spectral analysis of R-R interval and systolic arterial pressure variability. J Hypertens 1999;12:1899.
18. Blake MJ, Martin A, Manktelow BN, et al: Changes in baroreceptor sensitivity for heart rate during normotensive pregnancy and the puerperium. Clin Sci 2000;98:259.
19. Greenwood JP, Scott EM, Stoker JB, et al: Sympathetic neural mechanisms in normal and hypertensive pregnancy in humans. Circulation 2001;104:2200.
20. August P, Muller FB, Sealey JE, Edersehim TG: The stimulated renin-angiotensin system in pregnancy maintains blood pressure. Lancet 1995;345:896.
21. van Oppen ACC, Stigter RH, Bruinse HW: Cardiac output in normal pregnancy: A critical review. Obstet Gynecol 1996;87:310.
22. Davison JM, Dunlop M: Renal hemodynamics and tubular function in normal human pregnancy. Kidney Int 1980;18:152.
23. Baylis C: Effect of early pregnancy on glomerular filtration rate and plasma volume in the rat. Renal Physiol 1980;2:333.
24. Danielson LA, Conrad DP: Acute blockade of nitric oxide synthase inhibits renal vasodilatation and hyperfiltration during pregnancy in chronically instrumented conscious rats. J Clin Invest 1995;96:482.
25. Cadnapaphornchai MA, Ohara M, Morris KG, et al: Chronic NOS inhibition reverses systemic vasodilation and glomerular hyperfiltration in pregnancy. Am J Physiol Renal Physiol 2001;280:F592.
26. Conrad KP, Lindheimer MK: Renal and cardiovascular alterations. In Lindheimer MD, Roberts JM, Cunningham FG (eds): Chelsey's Hypertensive Disorders in Pregnancy, 2nd ed. Stamford, Conn, Appleton & Lange, 1999, pp 2263-2326.
27. Veille JC, Morton MJ, Burry K, et al: Estradiol and hemodynamics during ovulation induction. J Clin Endocrinol Metab 1986;63:721.
28. Berl T, Better OS: Renal effects of prolactin, estrogen, estrogen and progesterone. In Brenner BM, Stein JH (eds): Hormonal Function and the Kidney. New York, Churchill Livingstone, 1979, pp 194-214.
29. Oparil S, Ehrlich EN, Lindheimer MD: Effect of progesterone on renal sodium handling in man: relation to aldosterone excretion and plasma renin activity. Clin Sci Mol Med 1975;49:139.
30. Hughes EC (ed): Obstetric-Gynecologic Terminology. Philadelphia, FA Davis, 1972, pp 422-423.
31. Report of the National High Blood Pressure Education Program Working Group on High Blood Pressure in Pregnancy. Am J Obstet Gynecol 2000;183:S1.
32. Fisher KA, Luger A, Spargo BH, et al: Hypertension in pregnancy: Clinical-pathological correlations and remote prognosis. Medicine 1981;60:267.
33. Chesley LC: Hypertensive Disorders in Pregnancy. New York, Appleton-Century-Crofts, 1978.
34. Moutquin JM, Rainville C, Giroux L, et al: A prospective study of blood pressure in pregnancy: Prediction of pre-eclampsia. Am J Obstet Gynecol 1985;151:191.
35. Saftlas AF, Olson DR, Franks AL, et al: Epidemiology of preeclampsia and eclampsia in the United States, 1979-1986. Am J Obstet Gynecol 1990;163:460.
36. Ness RB, Roberts JM: Epidemiology of hypertension. In Lindheimer MD, Roberts JM, Cunningham FG (eds): Chelsey's Hypertensive Disorders in Pregnancy, 2nd ed. Stamford, Conn, Appleton & Lange, 1999, pp 43-67.

37. Sibai BM, Ewell M, Levine RJ, et al: Risk factors associated with preeclampsia in healthy nulliparous women. The Calcium for Preeclampsia Prevention (CPEP) Study Group. Am J Obstet Gynecol 1997;177:1003.

38. Seely EW, Solomon CG: Insulin resistance and its potential role in pregnancy-induced hypertension. J Clin Endocrinol Metab 2003;88:2393.

39. MacGillivray I: Some observations on the incidence of pre-eclampsia. J Obstet Gynaecol Br Emp 1958;65:536.

40. Sibai BM, Mercer B, Sarinoglu C: Severe preeclampsia in the second trimester: Recurrence risk and long-term prognosis. Am J Obstet Gynecol 1991;165:1408.

41. Chames MC, Haddad B, Barton JR, et al: Subsequent pregnancy outcome in women with a history of HELLP syndrome at < or = 28 weeks of gestation. Am J Obstet Gynecol 2003;188:1504.

42. Trupin LS, Simon LP, Eskenazi B: Change in paternity: A risk factor for pre-eclampsia in multiparas. Epidemiology 1996;7:240.

43. Saftlas AF, Levine RJ, Klebanoff MA, et al: Abortion, changed paternity, and risk of preeclampsia in nulliparous women. Am J Epidemiol 2003;157:1108.

44. Chesley LC: Hypertension in pregnancy: Definitions, familial factor and remote prognosis. Kidney Int 1980;18:234.

45. Laivouri H, Kaaja R, Rutanen EM, et al: Evidence of high circulating testosterone in women with prior pre-eclampsia. J Clin Endocrinol Metab 1998;83:344.

46. Wilson BJ, Watson MS, Prescott GJ, et al: Hypertensive diseases of pregnancy and risk of hypertension and stroke in later life: Results from cohort study. BMJ 2003;326:845.

47. Ekholm EMK, Tahvanainen KUO, Metsala T: Heart rate and blood pressure variabilities are increased in pregnancy-induced hypertension. Am J Obstet Gynecol 1997;177:1208.

48. Ayala DE, Hermida RC, Mojon A, et al: Circadian blood pressure variability in healthy and complicated pregnancies. Hypertension 1997;30:603.

49. Friedman SA, Lindheimer MD: Prediction and differential diagnosis. In Lindheimer MD, Roberts JM, Cunningham FG (eds): Chesley's Hypertensive Disorders in Pregnancy, 2nd ed. Stamford, Conn, Appleton & Lange, 1999, pp 201-229.

50. Weinstein L: Syndrome of hemolysis, elevated liver enzymes, and low platelet count: A severe consequence of hypertension in pregnancy. Am J Obstet Gynecol 1982;142:159.

51. Sibai MB, Ramadan MK, Usta I, et al: Maternal morbidity and mortality in 442 pregnancies with hemolysis, elevated liver enzymes, and low platelets (HELLP syndrome). Am J Obstet Gynecol 1993;169:1000.

52. Sibai BM, Kustermann L, Velasco J: Current understanding of severe preeclampsia, pregnancy-associated hemolytic uremic syndrome, thrombotic thrombocytopenic purpura, hemolysis, elevated liver enzymes, and low platelet syndrome, and postpartum acute renal failure: Different clinical syndromes or just different names? Curr Opin Nephrol Hypertens 1994;3:436.

53. Robertson WB, Brosens I, Dixon G: Maternal uterine vascular lesions in the hypertensive complications of pregnancy. In Lindheimer MD, Katz AI, Zuspan FP (eds): Hypertension in Pregnancy. New York, John Wiley, 1976, pp 115-129.

54. Fox H: The placenta in pregnancy hypertension. In Rubin PC (ed): Handbook of Hypertension, vol 10: Hypertension in Pregnancy. New York, Elsevier, 1988, pp 16-37.

55. Pijnenborg R: Trophoblast invasion and placentation in the human: Morphological aspects. Trophoblast Res 1990;4:33.

56. Roberts JM, Lain KY: Recent insights into the pathogenesis of preeclampsia. Placenta 2002;23:359.

57. Lachmeijer AMA, Dekker G, Pals G, et al: Searching for preeclampsia genes: The current position. Eur J Obstet Gynecol 2002;105:94.

58. Lyall F, Myatt L: The role of the placenta in preeclampsia—a workshop report. Placenta 2002;23:S142.

59. Podjarny E, Baylis C, Losonczy G: Animal models of preeclampsia. Semin Perinatol 1999;23:2.

60. Zhou Y, Fisher SJ, Janatpour M, et al: Human cytotrophoblasts adopt a vascular phenotype as they differentiate: A strategy for successful endovascular invasion? J Clin Invest 1997;99:2139.

61. Norwitz ER, Schust DJ, Fisher SJ: Implantation and the survival of early pregnancy. N Engl J Med 2001;345:1400-1408.

62. Damsky CH, Fisher SJ: Trophoblast pseudo-vasculogenesis: Faking it with endothelial adhesion receptors. Curr Opin Cell Biol 1998;10:660.

63. Fisher SJ: The placenta dilemma. Semin Reprod Med 2000;18:321.

64. Zhou Y, Damsky CH, Chiu K, et al: Pre-eclampsia is associated with abnormal expression of adhesion molecules by invasive cytotrophoblasts. J Clin Invest 1993;91:950.

65. Zhou Y, Damsky CH, Fisher SJ: Pre-eclampsia is associated with failure of human cytotrophoblast to mimic a vascular adhesion phenotype: One cause of defective endovascular invasion in this syndrome? J Clin Invest 1997;99:2152.

66. Brosens JJ, Pijnenborg R, Brosens IA: The myometrial junctional zone spiral arteries in normal and abnormal pregnancies: A review of the literature. Am J Obstet Gynecol 2002;187:1416.

67. Ghidini A, Salafia CM, Pezzullo JC: Placental vascular lesions and likelihood of diagnosis of pre-eclampsia. Obstet Gynecol 1997;90:542.

68. Kovats S, Librach C, Fisch P, et al: Expression and possible function of the HLA-G chain in human cytotrophoblasts. Science 1990;248:220.

69. Main E, Chiang M, Colbern G: Nulliparous preeclampsia (PE) is associated with placental expression of a variant allele of the new histocompatibility gene: HLA-G. Am J Obstet Gynecol 1994;170:289.

70. Hamai Y, Fujii T, Yamashita T, et al: Evidence for an elevation in serum interleukin-2 and tumor necrosis factor–alpha levels before the clinical manifestations of preeclampsia. Am J Reprod Immunol 1997;38:89.

71. Hamai Y, Fujii T, Yamashita T, et al: Pathogenetic implication of interleukin-2 expressed in pre-eclamptic decidual tissues: A possible mechanism of deranged vasculature of the placenta associated with pre-eclampsia. Am J Reprod Immunol 1997;38:83.

72. Conrad KP, Benyo DF: Placental cytokines and the pathogenesis of preeclampsia. Am J Reprod Immunol 1997;37:240.

73. Wang Y, Walsh SW: TNF alpha concentrations and mRNA expression are increased in preeclamptic placentas. J Reprod Immunol 1996;32:157.

74. Beer AE: Possible immunologic bases of preeclampsia/eclampsia. Semin Perinatol 1978;2:39.

75. Taylor RN: Review: Immunology of pre-eclampsia. Am J Reprod Immunol 1997;37:79.

76. Fallis N, Langford HG: Relationship of second trimester blood pressure to toxemia of pregnancy. Am J Obstet Gynecol 1967;87:123.

77. Page EW, Christianson R: The impact of mean arterial pressure in the middle trimester upon the outcome of pregnancy. Am J Obstet Gynecol 1976;125:740.

78. Kyle PM, Clark SJ, Buckley D, et al: Second trimester ambulatory blood pressure in nulliparous pregnancy: A useful screening test for preeclampsia? Br J Obstet Gynaecol 1993;100:914.

79. Lindheimer MD, Katz AI: Renal physiology and disease in pregnancy. In Seldin DW, Giebisch G (eds): The Kidney: Physiology and Pathophysiology, 2nd ed. New York, Raven Press, 1992, pp 3371-3431.

80. Ferrazzani S, Caruso A, De Carolis S, et al: The duration of hypertension in puerperium of preeclamptic women relates to fetal growth, renal impairment and week of delivery. Am J Obstet Gynecol 1994;171:506.

81. August P, Sealey JE: The renin-angiotensin system in normal and hypertensive pregnancy and in ovarian function. In Laragh JH, Brenner BM (eds): Hypertension: Pathophysiology, Diagnosis, and Management. New York, Raven Press, 1990, pp 1761-1778.

82. Gant NF, Daley GL, Chand S, et al: A study of angiotensin II pressor response throughout primigravid pregnancy. J Clin Invest 1973;51:2682.

83. Greenwood JP, Scott EM, Walker JJ: The magnitude of sympathetic hyperactivity in pregnancy induced hypertension and preeclampsia. Am J Hypertens 2003;16:194.

84. Fitzgerald DJ, FitzGerald GA: Eicosanoids in the pathogenesis of pre-eclampsia. In Laragh J, Brenner BM (eds): Hypertension: Pathophysiology, Diagnosis, and Management. New York, Raven Press, 1990, pp 1789-1807.

85. Fitzgerald DJ, Entmann SS, Mulloy K, FitzGerald GA: Decreased prostacyclin biosynthesis preceding the clinical manifestations of pregnancy-induced hypertension. Circulation 1987;75:956.

86. Mills JL, Dersimonian R, Raymond E, et al: Prostacyclin and thromboxane changes predating clinical onset of preeclampsia. A multicenter prospective study. JAMA 1999;282:356.

87. Walsh SW: Pre-eclampsia: An imbalance in placental prostacyclin and thromboxane production. Am J Obstet Gynecol 1985;152:335.

88. Fitzgerald DJ, Rocki W, Murray R, et al: Thromboxane A_2 synthesis in pregnancy-induced hypertension. Lancet 1990;1:751.

89. Walsh SW, Behr MJ, Allen NJ: Placental prostacyclin production in normal and toxemic pregnancies. Am J Obstet Gynecol 1985;151:110.

90. Catella F, Lawson JA, Fitzgerald DJ, Fitzgerald GA: Endogenous biosynthesis of arachidonic acid epoxids in humans: Increased formation in pregnancy-induced hypertension. Proc Natl Acad Sci U S A 1990;87:5893.

91. Roberts JM, Taylor RN, Musci TJ, et al: Pre-eclampsia: An endothelial cell disorder. Am J Obstet Gynecol 1989;161:1200.

92. Chambers JC, Fusi L, Makil IS, et al: Association of maternal endothelial dysfunction with preeclampsia. JAMA 2001;285:1607.

93. Savvidou MD, Hingorani AD, Tsikas D, et al: Endothelial dysfunction and raised plasma concentrations of asymmetric dimethylarginine in pregnant women who subsequently develop preeclampsia. Lancet 2003;361:1511.

94. Baylis C, Beinder E, Suto T, August P: Recent insights into the roles of nitric oxide and renin-angiotensin in the pathophysiology of preeclampsia pregnancy. Semin Nephrol 1998;18:208.

95. Baylis C, Engels K: Adverse interactions between pregnancy and a new model of systemic hypertension produced by chronic blockade of endothelial derived relaxing factor. Clin Exp Hypertens B 1992;11:117.

96. Molnar M, Suto T, Toth T, Hertelendy F: Prolonged blockage of NO synthesis in gravid rats produces sustained hypertension, proteinuria, thrombocytopenia, and IUGR. Am J Obstet Gynecol 1994;170:1458.

97. Seligman SP, Abramson SB, Young BK, Buyon JP: The role of nitric oxide (NO) in the pathogenesis of preeclampsia. Am J Obstet Gynecol 1994;170:290.

98. Begum S, Yamasaki M, Michizuki M: Urinary levels of nitric oxide metabolites in normal pregnancy and preeclampsia. J Obstet Gynaecol Res 1996;22:551.

99. Silver RK, Kupferminc MJ, Russell TL, et al: Evaluation of nitric oxide as a mediator of severe pre-eclampsia. Am J Obstet Gynecol 1996;175:1013.

100. Taylor RN, Varma M, Teng NN, et al: Women with preeclampsia have higher plasma endothelin levels than women with normal pregnancies. J Clin Endocrinol Metab 1990;71:1675.

101. Nova A, Sibai BM, Barton JR, et al: Maternal plasma level of endothelin is increased in pre-eclampsia. Am J Obstet Gynecol 1991;165:724.

102. Clark BA, Halvorson L, Sachs B, Epstein FH: Plasma endothelin levels in preeclampsia: Elevation and correlation with uric acid levels and renal impairment. Am J Obstet Gynecol 1992;166:962.

103. Schiff E, Ben-Baruch G, Peleg E, et al: Immunoreactive circulating endothelin-1 in normal and hypertensive pregnancies. Am J Obstet Gynecol 1992;166:624.

104. Benigni A, Orisio S, Gaspari F, et al: Evidence against a pathogenetic role for endothelin in pre-eclampsia. Br J Obstet Gynaecol 1992;99:798.

105. Roberts JM, Edep ME, Goldfein A, Taylor RN: Sera from preeclamptic women specifically activate human umbilical vein endothelial cells in vitro: Morphological and biochemical evidence. Am J Reprod Immunol 1992;27:101.

106. Davidge ST, Signorella AP, Hubel CA, et al: Distinct factors in plasma of preeclamptic women increase endothelial nitric oxide or prostacyclin. Hypertension 1996;28:758.

107. Taylor RN, Casal DC, Jones L, et al: Selective effects of preeclamptic sera on human endothelial cell procoagulant protein expression. Am J Obstet Gynecol 1991;165:1705.

108. Hubel CA, Roberts JM, Taylor RN, et al: Lipid peroxidation in pregnancy: New perspectives on preeclampsia. Am J Obstet Gynecol 1989;161:1025.

109. Barden A, Beilin LJ, Ritchie J, et al: Plasma and urinary 8-isoprostane as an indicator of lipid peroxidation in preeclampsia and normal pregnancy. Clin Sci 1996;91:711.

110. Poranen AK, Ekblad U, Uotila P, Ahotupa M: Lipid peroxidation and antioxidants in normal and preeclamptic pregnancies. Placenta 1996;17:401.

111. Serdar Z, Gur E, Develioglyu O, et al: Placental and decidual lipid peroxidation and antioxidant defenses in preeclampsia. Lipid peroxidation in preeclampsia. Pathophysiology 2002;9:21-25.

112. Maynard SE, Min JY, Merchan J, et al: Excess placental soluble fms-like tyrosine kinase 1 (sFLt1) may contribute to endothelial dysfunction hypertension, and proteinuria in preeclampsia. J Clin Invest 2003;111:649.

113. Eremina V, Sood M, Haigh J, et al: Glomerular-specific alterations of VEGF-A expression lead to distinct congenital and acquired renal diseases. J Clin Invest 2003;111:707.

114. Sagawa N, Yra S, ItohH, et al: Role of leptin in pregnancy—a review. Placenta 2002;23:S80.

115. Serin IS, Ozcelik B, Basbug M, et al: Predictive value of tumor necrosis factor alpha (TNF-alpha) in preeclampsia. Eur J Obstet Gynecol Reprod Biol 2002;100:143.

116. Sattar N, Bendomir A, Berry C, et al: Lipoprotein subfraction concentrations in preeclampsia: Pathogenic parallels to atherosclerosis. Obstet Gynecol 1997;89:403.

117. Murai JT, Muzykanskiy E, Taylor RN: Maternal and fetal modulators of lipid metabolism correlate with the development of pre-eclampsia. Metabolism 1997;46:963.

118. Lorentzen B, Birkeland KI, Endresen JM, Henriksen T: Glucose intolerance in women with pre-eclampsia. Acta Obstet Gynecol Scand 1998;77:22.

119. Wang J, Mimuro S, Lahoud R, et al: Elevated levels of lipoprotein A in women with pre-eclampsia. Am J Obstet Gynecol 1998;178:146.

120. Long PA, Abell DA, Beischer NA: Importance of abnormal glucose tolerance (hypoglycemia and hyperglycemia) in the etiology of preeclampsia. Lancet 1977;1:923.

121. Solomon CG, Graves SW, Greene MF, Seely EW: Glucose intolerance as predictor of hypertension in pregnancy. Hypertension 1994;23:717.

122. Groenendijk R, Wallenburg HCS: Hemodynamic measurements in preeclampsia: Preliminary observations. Am J Obstet Gynecol 1984;150:232.

123. Wallenburg HCS: Hemodynamics in hypertensive pregnancy. In Rubin PC (ed): Handbook of Hypertension, vol 10: Hypertension in Pregnancy. New York, Elsevier, 1988, pp 66-101.

124. Visser W, Wallenburg HCS: Central hemodynamic observations in untreated preeclamptic patients. Hypertension 1991;17:1072.

125. Lang RM, Pridjian G, Feldman T, et al: Alterations in left ventricular mechanics in pregnancy induced hypertension (pre-eclampsia): Increased afterload or cardiomyopathy? Am Heart J 1991;121:1768.

126. Hankins GDV, Wendel DG, Cunningham FG, Leveno KJ: Longitudinal evaluation of hemodynamic changes in eclampsia. Am J Obstet Gynecol 1984;150:506.

127. Cotton DB, Longmire S, Jones MM, et al: Cardiovascular alterations in severe pregnancy-induced hypertension. Am J Obstet Gynecol 1988;158:523.

128. Easterling TR, Benedetti TJ, Schmucker RC, Millard SP: Maternal hemodynamics in normal and preeclamptic pregnancies: A longitudinal study. Obstet Gynecol 1990;76:1061.

129. Gallery EDM, Hunyor SN, György AZ: Plasma volume contraction: A significant factor in both pregnancy-associated hypertension (pre-eclampsia) and chronic hypertension in pregnancy. Q J Med 1979;48:593.

130. Brown MA, Zammit VC, Mitar DM: Extracellular fluid volumes in pregnancy-induced hypertension. J Hypertens 1992;10:61.

131. Gaber LW, Spargo BH, Lindheimer MD: The nephropathy of pre-eclampsia-eclampsia. In Tisher CC, Brenner BM (eds): Renal Pathology, 2nd ed. Philadelphia, JB Lippincott, 1994, pp 419-441.

132. Fisher KA, Luger A, Spargo BH, Lindheimer MD: Hypertension in pregnancy: Clinical-pathological correlations and remote prognosis. Medicine 1981;60:267.

133. Packham DK, Mathews DC, Fairley KF, et al: Morphometric analysis of pre-eclampsia in women biopsied in pregnancy and postpartum. Kidney Int 1988;34:704.

134. Pertuiset N, Grünfeld J-P: Acute renal failure in pregnancy. Baillieres Clin Obstet Gynaecol 1994;8:333.

135. Brown MA, Gallery EDM, Ross MR, Esber RP: Sodium excretion in normal and hypertensive pregnancy: A prospective study. Am J Obstet Gynecol 1988;159:297.

136. August-Taufield P, Ales K, Resnick L, et al: Hypocalciuria in preeclampsia. N Engl J Med 1987;316:715.

137. Gertner JM, Coustan DR, Kliger AS, et al: Pregnancy as a state of physiologic absorptive hypercalciuria. Am J Med 1986;81:451.

138. August P, Marcaccio B, Gertner JM, et al: Abnormal 1,25 dihydroxyvitamin D metabolism in preeclampsia. Am J Obstet Gynecol 1992;4:1295.
139. Weiner CP: Clotting alterations associated with the pre-eclampsia/eclampsia syndrome. In Rubin PC (ed): Handbook of Hypertension, vol 10: Hypertension in Pregnancy. New York, Elsevier, 1988, pp 241-257.
140. Weiner CP, Brandt J: Plasma antithrombin III activity: An aid in the diagnosis of preeclampsia-eclampsia. Am J Obstet Gynecol 1982;142:275.
141. Lindoff C, Ingemarsson I, Martinsson G, et al: Pre-eclampsia is associated with a reduced response to activated protein C. Am J Obstet Gynecol 1997;176:457.
142. Redman CWG, Bonnar J, Beilin L: Early platelet consumption in pre-eclampsia. BMJ 1978;1:467.
143. Stubbs TM, Lazarchick J, Van Dorsten P, et al: Evidence of accelerated platelet production and consumption in nonthrombocytopenic pre-clampsia. Am J Obstet Gynecol 1986;155:263.
144. Ballegeer VC, Spitz B, De Baene LA, et al: Platelet activation and vascular damage in gestational hypertension. Am J Obstet Gynecol 1992;166:629.
145. Norris LA, Gleeson N, Sheppard BL, Bonnar J: Whole blood platelet aggregation in moderate and severe pre-eclampsia. Br J Obstet Gynaecol 1993;100:684.
146. Konijnenberg A, Stokkers EW, van der Post JA, et al: Extensive platelet activation in preeclampsia compared with normal pregnancy: Enhanced expression of cell adhesion molecules. Am J Obstet Gynecol 1997;176:461.
147. Weiner CP: The role of serotonin in the genesis of hypertension in pre-eclampsia. Am J Obstet Gynecol 1987;156:885.
148. Steyn DW, Odendaal HJ: Randomised controlled trial of ketanserin and aspirin in prevention of pre-eclampsia. Lancet 1997;350:1267.
149. Girling JC, Dow E, Smith JH: Liver function tests in pre-eclampsia: Importance of comparison with a reference range derived for normal pregnancy. Br J Obstet Gynaecol 1997;104:246.
150. Sheehan HL, Lynch JB: Pathology of Toxaemia of Pregnancy. London, Churchill Livingstone, 1973.
151. Barton JR, Riely CA, Adamec TA, et al: Hepatic histopathologic condition does not correlate with laboratory abnormalities in HELLP syndrome. Am J Obstet Gynecol 1992;167:1538.
152. Giannina G, Smith D, Belfort MA, Moise KJ: Atraumatic subdural hematoma associated with pre-eclampsia. J Matern Fetal Med 1997;6:93.
153. Richards A, Graham D, Bullock R: Clinicopathological study of neurological complications due to hypertensive disorders of pregnancy. J Neurol Neurosurg Psychiat 1988;51:421.
154. Ohno Y, Kawai M, Wakahara Y, et al: Transcranial assessment of maternal cerebral blood flow velocity in patients with pre-eclampsia. Acta Obstet Gynecol Scand 1997;76:928.
155. Riskin-Mashiah S, Belfort MA, Saade GR, Herd JA: Transcranial Doppler measurement of cerebral velocity indices as a predictor of preeclampsia. Am J Obstet Gynecol 2002;187:1667.
156. Qureshi AI, Frankel MR, Ottenlips JR, Stern BJ: Cerebral hemodynamics in preeclampsia and eclampsia. Arch Neurol 1996;53:1226.
157. Dahmus MA, Barton JR, Sibai BM: Cerebral imaging in eclampsia: Magnetic resonance imaging versus computed tomography. Am J Obstet Gynecol 1992;167:935.
158. Moodley J, Bobat SM, Hoffman J, Bill PLA: Electroencephalogram and computerised cerebral tomography findings in eclampsia. Br J Obstet Gynaecol 1993;100:984.
159. Drislane FW, Wang AM: Multifocal cerebral hemorrhage in eclampsia and severe preeclampsia. J Neurol 1997;244:194.
160. Hinchey J, Chaves C, Appignani B, et al: A reversible posterior leukoenphalopathy syndrome. N Engl J Med 1996;334:494.
161. Imperiale TF, Stollenwerk-Petrulis A: A meta-analysis of low-dose aspirin for the prevention of pregnancy induced hypertensive disease. JAMA 1991;226:261.
162. Collins R: Antiplatelet agents for IUGR and pre-eclampsia. In Enkin M, Keirse MJ, Renfrew M, Neilson JP (eds): Pregnancy and Childbirth Module. Cochrane Database of Systemic Reviews, Review No. 04000, May 4, 1994.
163. Dekker G, Sibai B. Primary, secondary, and tertiary prevention of pre-eclampsia. Lancet 2001;357:209.
164. Duley L, Henderson-Smart D, Knight M, King J: Antiplatelet drugs for prevention of pre-eclampsia and its consequences: Systematic review. BMJ 2001;322:329-333.
165. Coomarasamy A, Honest H, Papaioannou S, et al: Aspirin for prevention of preeclampsia in women with historical risk factors: a systematic review. Obstet Gynecol. 2003 Jun;101(6):1319-32.
166. Sibai BM, Caritis SN, Thom E, et al, and the National Institutes of Child Health and Human Development Network of Maternal-Fetal Medicine Units: Prevention of preeclampsia with low-dose aspirin in healthy nulliparous women. N Engl J Med 329:1213, 1993.
167. CLASP: A randomised trial of low-dose aspirin for the prevention and treatment of pre-eclampsia among 9364 women. CLASP (Collaborative Low-dose Aspirin Study in Pregnancy) Collaborative Group. Lancet 1994;343:619.
168. Hauth JC, Goldenberg RL, Parker CR, et al: Maternal serum thromboxane B_2 reduction versus pregnancy outcome in a low-dose aspirin trial. Am J Obstet Gynecol 1995;173:575.
169. Caritis S, Sibai B, Hauth J, et al, and The National Institutes of Child Health and Human Development Network of Maternal-Fetal Medicine Units: Low-dose aspirin to prevent preeclampsia in women at high risk. N Engl J Med 1998;338:701.
170. Belizan JM, Villar J: The relationship between calcium intake and edema-, proteinuria-, and hypertension-gestosis: An hypothesis. Am J Clin Nutr 1980;33:2202.
171. Belizan J, Villar J, Gonzalez L, et al: Calcium supplementation to prevent hypertensive disorders of pregnancy. N Engl J Med 1991;325:1399.
172. Bucher HC, Guyatt GH, Cook RJ, et al: Effect of calcium supplementation on pregnancy-induced hypertension and preeclampsia: A meta-analysis of randomized controlled trials. JAMA 1996;275:1113.
173. Levine RJ, Hauth JC, Curet LB, et al: Trial of calcium to prevent preeclampsia. N Engl J Med 1997;337:69.
174. Lopez-Jaramillo P, Delgado F, Jacome P, et al: Calcium supplementation and the risk of preeclampsia in Ecuadorian pregnant teenagers. Obstet Gynecol 1997;90:162.
175. Purwar M, Kulkarni H, Motghare V, Dhole S: Calcium supplementation and prevention of pregnancy induced hypertension. J Obstet Gynecol Res 1996;22:425.
176. Chappell LC, Seed PT, Briley AL, et al: Effect of antioxidants on the occurrence of preeclampsia in women at increased risk: A randomized trial. Lancet 1999;354:810.
177. Onwude JL, Lillford RJ, Hjartardottir H, et al: A randomized double blind placebo controlled trial of fish oil in high risk pregnancy. Br J Obstet Gynaecol 1995;102:95.
178. Sibai BM, Villar MA, Bray E: Magnesium supplementation during pregnancy: A double-blind randomized controlled clinical trial. Am J Obstet Gynecol 1989;161:115.
179. Pritchard JA, Cunningham FG, Pritchard FA: The Parkland Memorial Hospital protocol for treatment of eclampsia: Evaluation of 245 cases. Am J Obstet Gynecol 1984;148:951.
180. Sibai BM, Akl S, Fairlie F, Morett M: A protocol for managing severe preeclampsia in the second trimester. Am J Obstet Gynecol 1990;163:733.
181. Paterson-Brown S, Robson SC, Redfern N, et al: Hydralazine boluses for the treatment of severe hypertension in pre-eclampsia. Br J Obstet Gynaecol 1994;101:409.
182. Belfort M, Uys P, Dommisse J, et al: Hemodynamic changes in gestational proteinuric hypertension: The effects of rapid volume expansion and vasodilator therapy. Br J Obstet Gynaecol 1989;96:634.
183. Vink GJ, Moodley JH, Philpott RH: Effect of dihydralazine on the fetus in the treatment of maternal hypertension. Obstet Gynecol 1980;55:519.
184. Walker JJ, Greer I, Calder AA: Treatment of acute pregnancy-related hypertension: Labetalol and hydralazine compared. Postgrad Med J 1983;59:168.
185. Davey DA, Dommisse J, Garden A: Intravenous labetalol and intravenous dihydralazine in pregnancy. In Riley A, Symonds EM (eds): The Investigation of Labetalol in the Management of Hypertension in Pregnancy. Amsterdam, Excerpta Medica, 1982, pp 51-61.
186. Ashe RG, Moodley J, Richards AM, et al: Comparison of labetalol and dihydralazine in hypertensive emergencies of pregnancy. S Afr Med J 1987;71:354.

187. Lunell NO, Nylund L, Lewander R, et al: Acute effect of antihypertensive drug, labetalol, on uteroplacental blood flow. Br J Obstet Gynaecol 1982;89:640.

188. Jouppiila P, Kirkinen P, Koivula A, et al: Labetalol does not alter the placental and fetal blood flow or maternal prostanoids in preeclampsia. Br J Obstet Gynaecol 1986;93:543.

189. Belfort MA, Saade GR, Moise KJ, et al: Nimodipine in the management of preeclampsia: Maternal and fetal effects. Am J Obstet Gynecol 1994;172:1652.

190. Sibai BM, Barton JR, Akl S, et al: A randomized prospective comparison of nifedipine and bed rest versus bed rest alone in the management of preeclampsia remote from term. Am J Obstet Gynecol 1989;879:167.

191. Fenakel K, Fenakel G, Appelman Z, et al: Nifedipine in the treatment of severe preeclampsia. Obstet Gynecol 1991;77:331.

192. Snyder SW, Cardwell MS: Neuromuscular blockade with magnesium sulfate and nifedipine. Am J Obstet Gynecol 1989;161:35.

193. Which anticonvulsant for women with eclampsia? Evidence from the Collaborative Eclampsia Trial. Lancet 345:1455, 1995.

194. Lucas MJ, Leveno KJ, Cunningham FG: A comparison of magnesium sulfate with phenytoin for the prevention of eclampsia. N Engl J Med 1995;333:201.

195. Duley L, Gulmezoglu AM, Henderson-Smart DJ: Magnesium sulphate and other anticonvulsants for women with pre-eclampsia. Cochrane Database Syst Rev 2003;(2):CD000025.

196. Livingston JC, Livingston LW, Ramsey R, et al: Magnesium sulfate in women with mild preeclampsia: A randomized controlled trial. Obstet Gynecol 2003;101:217-220.

197. Magpie Trial Collaboration Group: Do women with pre-eclampsia, and their babies, benefit from magnesium sulphate? The Magpie Trial: A randomised placebo-controlled trial. Lancet 2002;359:1877.

198. Fox DB, Troiano NH, Graves CR: Use of the pulmonary artery catheter in severe preeclampsia: A review. Obstet Gynecol Surv 1996;51:684.

199. Walters BNJ, Walters T: Hypertension in the puerperium [Letter]. Lancet 1987;2:330.

200. Ferrazzani S, Caruso A, De Carolis S, et al: The duration of hypertension in puerperium of preeclamptic women relates to fetal growth, renal impairment and week of delivery. Am J Obstet Gynecol 1994;171:506.

201. Walters BNJ, Thompson ME, de Swiet M: Blood pressure in the puerperium. Clin Sci 1986;71:589.

202. Makdassi R, De Cagny B, Lobjoie E, et al: Convulsions, hypertension crisis and acute renal failure in postpartum: Role of bromocriptine? Nephron 1996;72:732.

203. Lubarsky SL, Barton JR, Friedman SA, et al: Late postpartum eclampsia revisited. Obstet Gynecol 1994;83:502.

204. Brady WJ, De Behnke DJ, Carter CT: Postpartum toxemia: Hypertension, edema, proteinuria and unresponsiveness in an unknown female. J Emerg Med 1995;13:643.

205. Chames MC, Livingston JC, Ivester TS, et al: Late postpartum eclampsia: A preventable disease? Am J Obstet Gynecol 2002;186:1174.

206. Dunlop JCH: Chronic hypertension and perinatal mortality. Proc R Soc Med 1966;59:838.

207. Ananth CV, Savitz DA, Williams MA: Placental abruption and its association with hypertension and prolonged rupture of membranes: A methodologic review and meta-analysis. Obstet Gynecol 1996;88:309.

208. Rey E, Couturier A: The prognosis of pregnancy in women with chronic hypertension. Am J Obstet Gynecol 1994;171:410.

209. Sibai BM, Lindheimer M, Hauth J, et al: Risk factors for preeclampsia, abruptio placentae, and adverse neonatal outcomes among women with chronic hypertension. National Institute of Child Health and Human Development Network of Maternal-Fetal Medicine Units. N Engl J Med 1998;339:667.

210. Mabie WC, Pernoll ML, Biswas MK: Chronic hypertension in pregnancy. Obstet Gynecol 1986;67:197.

211. Sibai BM, Abdella TN, Anderson GD: Pregnancy in 211 patients with mild chronic hypertension. Obstet Gynecol 1983;61:571.

212. von Dadelszen P, Ornstein MP, Bull SB, et al: Fall in mean arterial pressure and fetal growth restriction in pregnancy hypertension: A meta-analysis. Lancet 2000;355:87.

213. Ounsted M, Cockburn J, Moar VA, Redman CWG: Maternal hypertension with superimposed pre-eclampsia: Effects on child development at 7$\frac{1}{2}$ years. Br J Obstet Gynaecol 1983;90:644.

214. Stanley JC: Arterial fibrodysplasia. In Novick AC, Scoble J, Hamilton G (eds): Renal Vascular Disease. London, WB Saunders, 1996, pp 21-35.

215. Hotchkiss RL, Nettles JB, Wells DE: Renovascular hypertension in pregnancy. South Med J 1971;64:1256.

216. Koskela O, Kaski P: Renal angiography in the follow-up examination of toxemia of late pregnancy. Acta Obstet Gynecol Scand 1971;50:41.

217. Roach CJ: Renovascular hypertension in pregnancy. Obstet Gynecol 1973;42:856.

218. McCarron DA, Keller FS, Lundquist G, Kirk PE: Transluminal angioplasty for renovascular hypertension complicated by pregnancy. Arch Intern Med 1982;142:1727.

219. Easterling TR, Brateng D, Goldman ML, et al: Renovascular hypertension during pregnancy. Obstet Gynecol 1991;78:921.

220. Hennessy A, Helseth G, August P: Renovascular hypertension in pregnancy. Increased incidence of severe pre-eclampsia. J Am Soc Nephrol 1997;8:316A.

221. Crane MG, Andes JP, Harris JJ, et al: Primary aldosteronism in pregnancy. Obstet Gynecol 1964;23:200.

222. Neerhof MG, Shlossman PA, Poll DS, et al: Idiopathic aldosteronism in pregnancy. Obstet Gynecol 1991;78:489.

223. Gordon RD, Fishman LM, Liddle GW: Plasma renin activity and aldosterone secretion in a pregnant woman with primary aldosteronism. J Clin Endocrinol Metab 1967;27:385.

224. Lotgering FK, Derkx FMH, Wallenburg HCS: Primary hyperaldosteronism in pregnancy. Am J Obstet Gynecol 1986;155:986.

225. Colton R, Perez GO, Fishman LM: Primary aldosteronism in pregnancy. Am J Obstet Gynecol 1984;150:892.

226. Biglieri EG, Slaton PE: Pregnancy and primary aldosteronism. J Clin Endocrinol Metab 1976;27:1628.

227. Merrill RH, Dombrowski RA, MacKenna JM: Primary hyperaldosteronism during pregnancy. Am J Obstet Gynecol 1984;150:786.

228. Solomon CG, Thiet MP, Moore F, Seely EW: Primary hyperaldosteronism in pregnancy: A case report. J Reprod Med 1996;41:255.

229. Aboud E, Deswiet M, Gordon H: Primary aldosteronism in pregnancy—should it be treated surgically? Irish J Med Sci 1995;164:279.

230. Webb JC, Bayliss P: Pregnancy complicated by primary aldosteronism. South Med J 1997;90:243.

231. Baron F, Sprauve ME, Huddleston JF, Fisher AJ: Diagnosis and surgical treatment of primary aldosteronism in pregnancy: A case report. Obstet Gynecol 1995;86:644.

232. Hecker A, Hasan SH, Neumann F: Disturbances in sexual differentiation of rat foetuses following spironolactone treatment. Acta Endocrinol 1980;95:540.

233. Nadler JL, Hsueh W, Horton R: Therapeutic effect of calcium channel blockade in primary aldosteronism. J Clin Endocrinol Metab 1985;60:896.

234. Leak D, Carroll JJ, Robinson DC, Ashworth EJ: Management of pheochromocytoma during pregnancy. Obstet Gynecol Surv 1977;32:583.

235. Schenker JG, Chowers I: Pheochromocytoma and pregnancy: Review of 89 cases. Obstet Gynecol Surv 1971;26:739.

236. Lyons CW, Colmorgen GH: Medical management of pheochromocytoma in pregnancy. Obstet Gynecol 1988;72:450.

237. Burgiss GE: Alpha blockade and surgical intervention of pheochromocytoma in pregnancy. Obstet Gynecol 1979;53:266.

238. Stenstrom G, Swolin K: Pheochromocytoma in pregnancy: Experience of treatment with phenoxybenzamine in three patients. Acta Obstet Gynecol Scand 1985;64:357.

239. Jessurun CR, Adam K, Mosie KJ, Wilansky S: Pheochromocytoma-induced myocardial infarction in pregnancy: A case report and literature review. Texas Heart Institute J 1993;20:120.

240. Hamada S, Hinokio K, Naka O, et al: Myocardial infarction as a complication of pheochromocytoma in a pregnant woman. South Eur J Obstet Gynecol Reprod Biol 1996;70:197.

241. Lie JT, Olney BA, Spittel JA: Perioperative hypertensive crisis and hemorrhagic diathesis: Fatal complication of clinically unsuspected pheochromocytoma. Am Heart J 1980;100:716.

242. Freier DT, Thompson NW: Pheochromocytoma and pregnancy: The epitome of high risk. Surgery 1993;114:1148.

243. Santeiro ML, Stromquist C, Qyble L: Phenoxybenzamine placental transfer during the third trimester. Ann Pharmacother 1996;30:1249.

244. Buescher MA, McClamrock HD, Adashi EY: Cushing syndrome in pregnancy. Obstet Gynecol 1992;79:130.

245. Van der Spuy ZM, Jacobs HS: Management of endocrine disorders and pregnancy. II: Pituitary, ovarian and adrenal disease. Postgrad Med J 1984;60:312.

246. The Sixth Report of the Joint National Committee on Prevention, Detection, Evaluation, and Treatment of High Blood Pressure. Arch Intern Med 1997;157:2413.

247. Lindheimer MD: Pre-eclampsia-eclampsia: Preventable? Have disputes on its treatment been resolved? Curr Opin Nephrol Hypertens 1996;5:452.

248. Ferrer RL, Sibai BM, Mulrow CD, et al: Management of mild chronic hypertension during pregnancy: A review. Obstet Gynecol 2000;96:849.

249. Redman CWG: Controlled trials of antihypertensive drugs in pregnancy. Am J Kidney Dis 1991;17:149.

250. Fletcher AE, Bulpitt CJ: A review of clinical trials in pregnancy. In Rubin PC (ed): Handbook of Hypertension, vol 10: Hypertension in Pregnancy. New York, Elsevier, 1988, pp 186-201.

251. Redman CWG, Beilin LJ, Bonnar J: Treatment of hypertension in pregnancy with methyldopa: Blood pressure control and side effects. Br J Obstet Gynaecol 1977;84:419.

252. Gallery EDM, Ross MR, Gyory AZ: Antihypertensive treatment in pregnancy: Analysis of different responses to oxprenolol and methyldopa. BMJ 1985;29:563.

253. Hogstedt S, Lindeberg S, Axwlsson O, et al: A prospective controlled trial of metoprolol-hydralazine treatment in hypertension during pregnancy. Acta Obstet Gynecol Scand 1985;64:505.

254. Magee LA, Duley L: Oral beta-blockers for mild to moderate hypertension during pregnancy. Cochrane Database Syst Rev 2003;(3):CD002863.

255. Plouin PF, Breart G, Maillard F, et al: Comparison of antihypertensive efficacy and perinatal safety of labetalol and methyldopa in the treatment of hypertension in pregnancy: A randomized controlled trial. Br J Obstet Gynaecol 1988;95:868.

256. Symonds EM, Lamming GD, Jadoul F, Broughton-Pipkin F: Clinical and biochemical aspects of the use of labetalol in the treatment of hypertension in pregnancy: Comparison with methyldopa. In Riley A, Symonds M (eds): The Investigation of Labetalol in the Management of Hypertension in Pregnancy. Amsterdam, Excerpta Medica, 1982, pp 62-76.

257. Sibai BM, Gonzalez AR, Mabie WC, Moretti M: A comparison of labetalol plus hospitalization versus hospitalization alone in the management of preeclampsia remote from term. Obstet Gynecol 1987;70:323.

258. Lindberg B, Lindeberg S, Marsal K, Andersson KE: Calcium channel blockade (isradipine) in treatment of hypertension in pregnancy: A randomized placebo-controlled study. Am J Obstet Gynecol 1995;173:872.

259. Jannet D, Carbonne B, Sebban E, Milliez J: Nicardipine versus metoprolol in the treatment of hypertension during pregnancy: A randomized comparative trial. Obstet Gynecol 1994;84:354.

260. Magee LA, Schick B, Donnenfeld AE, et al: The safety of calcium channel blockers in human pregnancy: A prospective multicenter cohort study. Am J Obstet Gynecol 1996;174:823.

261. Waisman GD, Mayorga LM, Camera MI, et al: Magnesium plus nifedipine: Potentiation of hypotensive effect in preeclampsia? Am J Obstet Gynecol 1988;159:308.

262. Rosa FW, Bosco LA, Graham CF, et al: Neonatal anuria with maternal angiotensin-converting enzyme inhibition. Obstet Gynecol 1989;74:371.

263. Hanssens M, Keirse MJ, Vankelecom F, Van Assche FA: Fetal and neonatal effects of treatment with angiotensin-converting enzyme inhibitors in pregnancy. Obstet Gynecol 1991;78:128.

264. Pryde PG, Sedman AB, Nugent CE: Angiotensin converting enzyme inhibitor fetopathy. J Am Soc Nephrol 1993;3:1575.

265. Postmarketing surveillance for angiotensin-converting enzyme inhibitor use during the first trimester of pregnancy—United States, Canada, and Israel, 1987-1995. MMWR Morbid Mortal Wkly Rep 1997;46:240.

266. Saji H, Yamanaka Y, Hagiwara A, Ijiri R: Losartan and fetal toxic effects. Lancet 2001;357:363.

267. Committee on Drugs: The transfer of drugs and other chemicals into human milk. Pediatrics 1994;93:137.

268. White WB: Management of hypertension during lactation. Hypertension 1984;6:297.

269. Atkinson H, Begg EJ: Concentrations of beta-blocking drugs in human milk. J Pediatr 1990;116:156.

270. Ehrenkranz RA, Ackerman BA, Hulse JD: Nifedipine transfer into human milk. J Pediatr 1989;114:478.

271. Anderson P, Bondesson U, Mattiasson I, et al: Verapamil and norverapamil in plasma and breast milk during breast feeding. Eur J Clin Pharmacol 1987;31:625.

272. Beardmore KS, Morris JM, Gallery ED: Excretion of antihypertensive medication into human breast milk: A systematic review. Hypertens Pregnancy 2002;21:85.

4

HEMATOLOGIC ASPECTS OF PREGNANCY

Thomas P. Duffy

Pregnancy elicits a reorientation of physiologic priorities of the woman's body to help ensure optimal development of the maturing fetus. Specific alterations occur in the hematologic system during pregnancy as the mother provides the nutrients for fetal hematopoiesis and her body prepares for the hemostatic challenge of childbirth. In the nonpregnant state, iron flow is primarily in the direction of cells engaging in hemoglobin synthesis. This vector is altered during pregnancy; the trophoblastic cells of the placenta become the major target for iron delivery.[1] The iron needs of the fetus take precedence over those of the mother, permitting the attainment in an infant of a normal hemoglobin level even while iron deficiency develops in the mother.[2]

As pregnancy evolves, there is also an accommodation in the hemostatic defenses of the mother to anticipate the separation of the placenta from the uterine wall. An increase in the levels of several coagulation factors occurs with a concomitant reduction in fibrinolytic activity[3]; a new, specific plasminogen activator inhibitor is produced by the placenta.[4] These alterations combine to create a "hypercoagulable" state[5] that persists for several weeks after the delivery of the infant. Coagulation abnormalities, in the setting of venous stasis caused by the enlarging uterus, explain the expectant mother's predisposition to thrombosis. The hypercoagulable state, although posing a risk to the mother, is advantageous in the setting of pregnancy but may pose a threat when combined with thrombophilic disorders.

The hematologic system significantly affects and is affected by the course of pregnancy. The approach to recognition and management of hematologic problems during this state requires a reorientation and expansion of the physician's focus to include the fetus and its specific needs. Any therapeutic decisions must be examined for their dual effects on both the mother and the fetus. It is only with this combined focus that the hematologic care of the pregnant woman will be properly served.[6]

ANEMIA DURING PREGNANCY

The red blood cell (RBC), an elegant example of structure matching function, is essentially a mass of hemoglobin contained within an easily deformable and permeable membrane. The excess surface area–volume ratio of the membrane contributes to the biconcave shape of the RBC and confers upon the RBC a plasticity that allows it to pass through the microvasculature of the body. This pliable structure endows the RBC with its essential role in the delivery of oxygen to tissues, allowing RBCs with the diameter of 7 μm to filter easily through capillaries as small as 0.5 μm in diameter.

Hemoglobin production occurs within the marrow in maturing RBCs; heme synthesis, taking place in and around cellular mitochondria, is matched to globin chain synthesis in a 1:1 ratio and takes place within the cytoplasm of the cell. Cell division continues until an optimal hemoglobin level exists in the developing RBC. The end product of marrow erythropoiesis, an enucleated cell, is then released from the marrow and still contains some remnants of a polyribosomal network. This reticulum network can be detected with supravital stains, permitting the enumeration of the daily output of reticulocytes, or young RBCs, produced by the marrow. Under steady-state conditions, RBC survival is approximately 100 days in circulation, which accounts for the normal reticulocyte count of 1% to 1.5%. Senescent RBCs are removed by the spleen, whose reticuloendothelial network recognizes a "senescent" antigen, which appear on RBCs as they age.[7,8]

The mass of RBCs in the peripheral blood is maintained within optimal boundaries by a humoral feedback mechanism that responds to oxygen tension of RBCs that perfuse the kidney. Erythropoietin, a glycoprotein with a molecular weight of 55,000 kD, is secreted by renal peritubular interstitial cells that respond to the redox state of heme molecules in the circulating blood.[9] With a decrease in hematocrit of oxygen tension, erythropoietin secretion rises with stimulation of the marrow and increases the production and release of RBCs. Erythropoietin acts on a population of erythropoietin-responsive cells derived from a common precursor pool of multipotential stem cells within the marrow. Stem cell deficiency, which occurs in aplastic or hypoplastic anemias, results in anemia, accompanied by varying degrees of leukopenia and thrombocytopenia. This triad of cytopenias or pancytopenia may also have its origin in any maturation defect of the stem cell, as occurs either in megaloblastic anemias[10] or with overactivity of the spleen, which occurs in hypersplenic states.

Under normal conditions, the hematocrit of a woman is 42% ± 5%, and her hemoglobin measures 12.5 to 15 g/dL. As pregnancy advances, physiologic hydremia or hemodilution occurs with an expansion in the RBC and plasma volumes. The condition is referred to as *hemodilution* because the plasma volume expansion of 50% outdistances a 30% increase in RBC mass during the first two trimesters. The drop in hematocrit to approximately 30% and in hemoglobin to 10.5 to 11 g/dL represents a "physiologic" anemia that favors the fetus by enhancing perfusion of the placenta and anticipates the blood loss that attends normal childbirth.[11] As opposed to this "physiologic" anemia of pregnancy, the true anemias of pregnancy represent a real reduction in the RBC mass and not a dilution of the RBC mass (Table 4-1). These anemias most frequently originate from production defects secondary to iron or folate deficiency[12]; a few anemias during pregnancy, such as hemolytic or aplastic anemia, have other causes.[13] Anemia is not an uncommon complication of pregnancy, as either a component of a primary, underlying hematologic condition or as a secondary complication of pregnancy. Its frequency is heavily influenced by the socioeconomic circumstances of the mother, because nutrition and prenatal care most commonly determine the overall incidence of these complications.[2] Pregnancy, with its increased demands on the mother, often unmasks a borderline nutritional state, resulting in new anemia or worsening of antecedent anemias.

GENERAL APPROACH TO THE ANEMIC PATIENT

Recognition of anemia during pregnancy requires awareness of the reduced levels associated with the physiologic hydremia of pregnancy. Established guidelines demonstrate that a hemoglobin level below 10.5 g/dL in any trimester constitutes anemia for this state. Evaluation for the cause of anemia initially focuses on two measurements: (1) the reticulocyte count and (2) the mean corpuscular volume (MCV) of the RBC.[14] The reticulocyte count requires a supravital staining of the peripheral smear; it is not a value that is generated from an electronic counter. The normal reticulocyte count is 1% to 2.5%.

If the feedback erythropoietin circuit of the body is intact, the development of anemia should cause a compensatory reticulocytosis. Failure to mount an appropriate reticulocyte response in the presence of anemia indicates that the marrow is a source of anemia; during pregnancy, these hyporegenerative anemias are usually caused by nutritional deficiencies, such as iron or folate deficiency. An inadequate reticulocyte response also accompanies erythropoietin-deficient erythropoiesis, the cause of anemia that accompanies progressive renal failure. A low reticulocyte count generally points to the marrow or erythropoietin deficiency as the source of anemia and, if peripheral blood studies such as iron, folate, and erythropoietin measurements do not provide an answer, a bone marrow examination is indicated to determine the cause of the anemia.

When RBC survival is shortened, such as with hemolysis or bleeding, the resultant anemia leads to heightened erythropoietin stimulation of the marrow and an increase in reticulocytes. An elevated reticulocyte count is the hallmark of hypergenerative anemias, conditions whose causes exist outside the marrow. Bleeding must be ruled out. Examination of the peripheral smear for RBC morphologic changes, immunologic Coombs' testing, and hemoglobin electrophoresis are some of the means of investigating the cause of hemolytic anemias associated with an elevated reticulocyte count. The latter count is important in the crucial implication of the marrow or the extramarrow environment in the causation of anemia, and thus its measurement is critical in any patient in whom anemia is discovered.

Use of the MCV of RBCs is a second method of identifying the source of anemia, although it is less helpful in pregnancy than in the nonpregnant state. This relative lack of utility is based on the frequency of mixed or combined nutritional abnormalities as causes of anemia during pregnancy. Iron deficiency, with its attendant reduction in RBC size, may be masked by folate deficiency and its creation of macrocytic RBCs. The MCV in such patients may be normal, although an RBC sizing index, which provides a plot of RBC size, uncovers different cell populations in a combined deficiency.[15]

Another deterrent to the use of MCV is the fact that all anemias are initially normocytic because the original RBC pool is only slowly diluted by the entry of abnormal cells. Nonetheless, a low MCV (<80 fL) indicates iron deficiency, and a high MCV (>95 fL) is attributable to folate deficiency until proven otherwise.

The reticulocyte count and MCV measurement narrow the possible causes of anemia and dictate the further tests necessary to refine the diagnosis. Previous hematologic values in the prepregnancy state and documentation of any familial hematologic conditions may help with the recognition that the hematologic condition antedated the pregnancy. Such patients may have an exaggerated but

---

TABLE 4-1   Anemia during Pregnancy

True anemia versus physiologic anemia or hydremia of pregnancy (Hb <10.5 g/dL)

Elevated reticulocyte count indicates blood loss or hemolysis

Low or absent reticulocyte count indicates marrow failure, usually iron or folate deficiency

Low MCV (<80 fL) indicates iron deficiency anemia; confirmed with serum ferritin measurement

High MCV (>95 fL) indicates folate deficiency; confirmed with RBC folate measurement

Normal MCV (80-95 fL) indicates possible combined deficiency; investigated with RBC sizing index

Hb, hemoglobin; MCV, mean corpuscular volume; RBC, red blood cell.

tolerable decrease in hemoglobin during pregnancy, a phenomenon that is most common in the hemoglobinopathy states.

IMPACT OF ANEMIA ON THE FETUS AND THE MOTHER

The fetus is a remarkably successful "parasite" of the mother, and nowhere is this more evident than in the hematologic system. Iron is delivered to the fetus against a concentration gradient, which helps guarantee a normal hemoglobin in the fetus. Placental hypertrophy accompanies maternal anemia, and increased oxygen extraction by the fetus further compensates for any decrease in hemoglobin.[16,17] It is therefore not surprising that modest anemia (8.5 to 10.5 g/dL) in the mother poses little threat to the fetus and that the literature is controversial regarding the degree of risk that any anemia poses for the fetus or mother.[18] There is only minimal evidence that iron deficiency in the mother is associated with decreased fertility,[19] whereas folate deficiency leads to an increased risk of spontaneous abortion.[20]

Modest anemias, with a hemoglobin level higher than 8.5 g/dL, do not necessitate transfusion but nonetheless merit investigation and correction whenever possible.[6] These anemias may be a "sickness index" of the body, calling attention to an overlooked disorder or deficiency. Correction of the anemia also optimizes the hematologic environment in which the fetus is developing and maturing.

More severe anemias (hemoglobin level <8.5 g/dL) in the last 4 weeks of pregnancy are considered grounds for transfusion, especially to anticipate any hemorrhage that might complicate childbirth.

NUTRITIONAL DEFICIENCY ANEMIAS

Iron Deficiency Anemia

The iron needs of the body for hemoglobin synthesis are provided for by a coordinated system of conservation and recycling of this essential element.[21] RBCs, after a life cycle of 100 to 120 days, are removed from peripheral blood by splenic reticuloendothelial cells; their hemoglobin is degraded, and the iron core reenters a pool that becomes available for new hemoglobin synthesis. Daily RBC production requires approximately 30 to 35 mg of iron per day, of which all but 1 to 2 mg is derived from the recycling of storage pool iron (Table 4–2). This 1 to 2 mg is the daily loss of iron from the body. The storage pool exists as either ferritin, with iron molecules housed in a protein shell, or hemosiderin, a more complicated and larger iron molecule composed of lipids, carbohydrates, and protein. A man has approximately 1000 mg of iron in this pool, whereas a woman has only 300 to 500 mg of iron in storage. The difference is attributed to iron losses incurred with menstruation. Adolescents of either gender frequently have little iron storage because of the needs of their expanded blood pool and the inadequate amounts of iron in their diets.

TABLE 4–2   Temporal Sequence in the Development of Iron Deficiency Anemia

Mobilization of marrow stores of iron; fall in serum ferritin (<15 pmol/L)
Fall in serum iron; elevation in iron-binding capacity with transferrin saturation (<15%)
Anemia, initially normochromic, normocytic
Anemia, hypochromic, microcytic

Only 1 to 2 mg of iron needs be absorbed daily to correct for daily losses and to supplement the storage iron that is recycled for hemoglobin synthesis. The normal American diet contains approximately 15 mg of iron per day; thus, only 10% to 15% of ingested iron must be absorbed each day. As a consequence of pregnancy, which results in the expansion of the mother's blood pool and fetal iron needs, stored iron and absorbed iron may be inadequate for the increased needs of pregnancy. Iron supplementation for expectant mothers has become standard because of these increased needs in addition to the borderline iron stores of expectant young mothers.[2]

The hallmark of advanced iron deficiency is a hypochromic microcytic anemia (MCV< 80), but this condition is only the terminus in a stepwise decline in total body iron. When a deficiency first occurs, iron is initially mobilized from the storage depots of reticuloendothelial cells and parenchymal liver cells. Ferritin levels in the peripheral blood parallel levels of stored iron, and radioimmunoassay for this iron complex allows quantitation of iron stores. After all iron has been mobilized from storage, levels of the iron transport protein, transferrin, increase. This combination leads to a low-percentage saturation of transferrin; saturation levels of less than 15% are the marker for iron-deficient erythropoiesis.

Anemia, initially normochromic and normocytic, finally supervenes. Such a result occurs only after the conserved stores of iron have been depleted and when serum iron levels are inadequate to fulfill the needs for hemoglobin synthesis.

Diagnosis

Florid iron deficiency is easily recognized from its hypochromic, microcytic blood picture, but earlier stages in the deficiency may be more muted. Even in non–iron-deficient expectant mothers, a low level of serum iron and an elevated level of transferrin are present. These parameters of pseudo–iron deficiency represent how the alterations in iron flow during pregnancy favor the needs of the fetus. However, ferritin levels remain a reliable gauge of iron stores and are the preferred means of evaluating iron needs during pregnancy.[22] A ferritin level of 80 pmol/L in midpregnancy (20 weeks) indicates that iron stores are adequate for supporting the needs of pregnancy and that supplemental iron is not necessary[23]; a ferritin level of less than 12 pmol/L indicates that iron deficiency is present and must be corrected.[24] Caution must be used in the interpretation of ferritin levels because this protein is an acute-phase reactant; low levels may be falsely elevated when inflammation or infection complicate iron deficiency anemia. In this case, ferritin levels of less than 60 to 100 pmol/L are considered indicative of iron deficiency. The measurement of serum transferrin receptor levels is another method of identifying iron deficiency in the setting of inflammation or infection.[25]

Treatment

Iron replacement or supplementation is easily achieved in most patients with oral administration of ferrous sulfate or gluconate tablets.[26] These tablets are better absorbed on an empty stomach, but gastrointestinal intolerance is frequent with this practice; ingestion of iron with meals is better tolerated, and this may be the preferred regimen, although absorption is lessened. Gradual introduction of medication (from one to three tablets daily) also improves tolerance and patient compliance. Iron may cause constipation in some patients and thus may limit its use, unless attention to elimination accompanies its prescription.

Some patients who do not tolerate iron tablets can be given an iron solution, which is best taken through a straw to avoid staining the teeth. If oral iron is not tolerated and iron replacement is necessary, intramuscular or intravenous administration of iron as ferric gluconate is possible.[27] This preparation has replaced iron dextran as the preferred parenteral iron preparation because of its greater safety, proved in comparison trials of the two agents. Its administration carries a very small risk of acute anaphylaxis, and it is thus necessary to employ caution with its use. Intravenous iron administration allows iron replacement in patients with inflammatory bowel disease and also allows a more rapid repletion than is possible with oral iron.[28]

Impact of Iron Deficiency on the Fetus and Mother

Although there is controversy regarding the contribution of anemia to complications in pregnancy, iron deficiency anemia has been definitively implicated as increasing the risk of low birth weight, prematurity, and perinatal mortality. Iron deficiency anemia during pregnancy results in an increased threefold risk of low birth weight and a twofold risk of preterm delivery.[29] Iron deficiency anemia is also associated with large placental weight and a high ratio of placental weight to birth weight.[30] The implications of this discordance are important, because these placental alterations are known predictors of adult hypertension, which appears to originate in fetal life.[17]

The specific deficiency of iron may result in a generalized nutritional deficiency because of the association of pica with iron deficiency. Pica, which is a bizarre craving for oral ingestion of foodstuff or other unusual substances,[31] may lead to the consumption of large amounts of materials such as clay (geophagia),[32] starch (amylophagia), or ice (pagophagia).[33,34] Not only may these materials substitute for other nutritious calories but they can exaggerate iron deficiency by complexing iron within the gut. The effects of ingestion of baking powder have even been confused with eclampsia.[35] Recognition of pica allows detection of iron deficiency, and correction of the latter can resolve the former.

Folic Acid Deficiency in Pregnancy

Folic acid is an essential cofactor in the conversion of uridine to thymidine in nucleic acid synthesis within all cells. A deficiency of folic acid results in megaloblastic hematopoiesis, with a macrocytic anemia frequently accompanied by varying degrees of leukopenia and thrombocytopenia.[36] However, macrocytic RBC indices for recognition of a megaloblastic process may be misleading during pregnancy because of a concomitant iron-deficient microcytic process. Even in the absence of macrocytic indices, an excellent marker of a megaloblastic process is hypersegmentation of polymorphonuclear cells in the peripheral blood. This abnormality should be sought in any anemic pregnant patient, because its presence indicates folate or vitamin B_{12} deficiency unless proven otherwise. Vitamin B_{12} deficiency is not a strong concern during pregnancy; deficiency of this vitamin is usually associated with sterility, and large stores of this vitamin in the body are not outstripped by the demands of pregnancy. A rare report of neurologic impairment in a newborn born to a mother subsisting on a restricted vegetarian diet has been attributed to a vitamin B_{12}-deficient state.[37] Discovery of a megaloblastic process during pregnancy remains equated with folate deficiency unless the dietary history dictates consideration of vitamin B_{12} deficiency.

Folate stores within the body are limited. The increased cellular demands for this vitamin—which provides for the expanding maternal and fetal blood pools and for the enlargement of the uterus and placenta—may outstrip the available supply. Folate deficiency is more frequent with twin pregnancies and with multiparity, the latter being associated with repeated states of negative folate balance. Reduced oral intake secondary to hyperemesis gravidarum is a common prologue to folate deficiency. Alcohol consumption, which interferes with folate metabolism, may worsen the deficiency. Cigarette smoking also reduces the availability of folate.

Diagnosis

The diagnosis of folate deficiency is simple once the entity (of folate deficiency) is considered as contributing to anemia. Hypersegmentation of polymorphonuclear cells, macrocytic indices, large ovalocytes, leukopenia, and thrombocytopenia are the classic effects of the disorder. Marked elevation of lactose dehydrogenase (LDH) is a serum marker of the extreme degree of ineffective intramedullary hematopoiesis that a megaloblastic process represents. The macrocytic character of anemia, as manifested by the MCV, may be lost when there is a combined folate and iron deficiency; a dimorphic RBC population on the peripheral smear is the clue to this double nutritional jeopardy. Folate-responsive aplastic anemia has also been reported during pregnancy.[10]

Confirmation of the diagnosis requires measurement of RBC folate levels, determined by radioimmunoassay. Serum levels of the vitamin are not diagnostic and should not be used as a basis of the diagnosis. Other biochemical assays are available to demonstrate folate deficiency (e.g., formiminoglutamic acid test), but they are unnecessary for diagnosing folate deficiency.

Treatment

In view of the marginal stores of folate within the body and the increased demands for this vitamin during pregnancy, folate supplementation has become a standard component of prenatal care[39]; supplementation of folate is also recommended antenatally for its role in preventing neural tube defects. Most prenatal vitamins contain 1 mg of folate, an amount that is adequate for fulfilling the escalated folate needs of pregnancy; higher amounts are required for hemolytic disorders, such as sickle disease or thalassemia, in which a 5-mg daily supplement is indicated. In addition to its ease of administration and freedom from any side effects, supplements can eliminate any contribution of folate deficiency to anemia during pregnancy.[12]

Impact of Folate Deficiency on the Fetus and Mother

Folate deficiency, as a cause of maternal anemia, is associated with premature birth, although its role in this pathologic process is not as well known as that of iron deficiency.[20] Folate deficiency has also been implicated in the genesis of neural tube defects and in cleft palate development.[38] The fetus is usually spared the development of anemia because folate, like iron, is transferred against a concentration gradient to a dense accumulation of folate receptors on the placenta. The fetus effectively drains the mother of available folate, which is an additional example of the fetus as a successful "parasite" of the mother.

HEMOGLOBINOPATHIES IN PREGNANCY

Significant shortening of RBC survival occurs secondary to alterations in structure (sickle hemoglobin) or quantity (thalassemia) of hemoglobin chains.[40] These are inherited disorders, which in their most severe forms are associated with hemolytic anemia as well as progressive multiorgan failure. Repeated sickling crises result in widespread microvascular blockade with obliteration of normal perfusion and function of several organs, including the spleen, the lungs,[41] and the kidneys.[42] Iron overload, the aftermath of years of ineffective erythropoiesis and transfusional support in thalassemia, damages the heart, liver, and endocrine system. Therefore, patients with hemoglobinopathies enter pregnancy at increased risk of morbidity and mortality secondary to the combination of underlying anemia and multiorgan dysfunction.[43] Successful management of these pregnancies requires attention to hematologic needs and negative consequences of organ dysfunction, both of which are often exaggerated by the demands of pregnancy.

Sickle Hemoglobinopathy

Sickle hemoglobin differs from the normal hemoglobin by only a single amino acid substitution, valine for glutamic acid, in the β chain of the hemoglobin molecule. The homozygous form of the disease, SS ($\alpha_2\beta_2^s$), results in an RBC hemoglobin pool that is almost completely sickle hemoglobin; the heterozygous form of the disease, AS ($\alpha_2\beta_1\beta^s$), has approximately 60% to 70% normal hemoglobin and 30% to 40% sickle hemoglobin. SS disease, associated with a lifelong severe hemolytic anemia (hematocrit ~20% to 25%), is punctuated by repeated painful crises caused by logjam formation by sickled cells in the microvasculature. The major factor precipating sickling of RBCs is hypoxemia, with worsening of the process by acidosis and hypertonicity. The crisis frequently involves the long bones with necrosis of the marrow, but no organ is safe from the assault of sickling. SS patients are functionally asplenic from birth and undergo anatomic autosplenectomy by adolescence; the absence of the spleen greatly contributes to the markedly increased incidence and severity of infection in the patient. The kidneys participate in a similar phenomenon, with a functional dismantling of the medullary countercurrent mechanism from birth, followed by an anatomic papillectomy in early adolescence. The handicap is mirrored in an inability to concentrate urine, a significant disability when fluid retention is necessary to buffer the fluid losses associated with fever.

The greatest threat to the affected patient is acute chest syndrome, in which a pulmonary infiltrate with fever, which leads to hypoxemia, hypertonicity, and acidosis, recreates in vivo the conditions that induce sickling in vitro. These infiltrates, formerly believed to be mainly infectious in origin, are now thought to arise more frequently from in situ sickling or embolized necrotic marrow from sickled bones. Monitoring of oxygen saturation in such patients is mandatory, with maintenance of the oxygen saturation at greater than 85 mm Hg to prevent sickling; oxygen saturation below this level necessitates exchange transfusion to prevent a lethal outcome. SS patients experience all of these complications to a varying degree, and other interacting hemoglobinopathies (hemoglobin S–thalassemia, SC) participate in the same spectrum of complications but often to a lesser intensity. In this regard, SC hemoglobinopathy may have a silent clinical course even with a close-to-normal hematocrit; this hemoglobinopathy may initially present with an episode of severe pulmonary thrombosis in the peripartum period.

Patients heterozygous for the sickle cell gene are only slightly affected by the amino acid substitution. Such patients are not anemic; the heterozygous state does not result in a hemolytic process. However, a concentrating defect occurs in their kidneys, and their urine is isosthenuric from birth. Renal papillary necrosis, sometimes accompanied by hematuria, results in scarred kidneys. This alteration is associated with an increased risk of pyelonephritis that may occur during pregnancy and complicate its course. Asymptomatic bacteriuria should be identified and treated aggressively in this group.

The chemotherapeutic agent hydroxyurea is now frequently administered to patients with sickle cell disease for its demonstrated role in assuaging the clinical severity of the disorder. Its use is not recommended during pregnancy, and such patients, both female and male, should be counseled about the risks involving conception while the drug is taken.[44]

Diagnosis

The diagnosis of these hemoglobinopathies is sought with hemoglobin electrophoresis. In the homozygous form (SS), almost all hemoglobin is sickle hemoglobin, with a small amount of A_2 and fetal hemoglobin; larger amounts of fetal hemoglobin indicate a sickle cell–thalassemic state whose clinical severity is close to that of the homozygous state. Heterozygous sickle trait (AS) is identified by its larger percentage of normal hemoglobin and its mainly asymptomatic course.

Anemia with reticulocytosis is usually present, although patients with SC hemoglobin may have a close-to-normal hematocrit. Sickle cells may or may not be evident on the peripheral smear, although a sickle preparation (RBCs exposed to a reducing agent, such as sodium metabisulfite) induces the sickling phenomenon; target cells are usually evident in all these conditions except in sickle trait, in which the smear is normal.

Splenomegaly in any adult with sickle hemoglobin is excellent evidence that an interacting hemoglobinopathy (e.g., hemoglobin S–thalassemia) is present; patients with SS disease have undergone autosplenectomy by adulthood as a universal accompaniment of their disease.

Hemoglobin electrophoresis should be a part of all prenatal evaluations in black patients. Recognition of the hemoglobinopathy is important because of the special threat that pregnancy poses to this group. Identification of the asymptomatic heterozygous state is also important because of its implication for the fetus if the father is a heterozygote or has an interacting hemoglobinopathy. Prenatal diagnosis is possible with chorionic villous biopsy or amniocentesis to obtain material for DNA analysis.[45,46]

Treatment

Controversy has persisted with regard to the role of prophylactic transfusions in the management of pregnant patients with sickle cell disease.[47] The previously documented excessive morbidity and mortality rates for both the mother and fetus in sickle cell pregnancy has now been reduced as a result of better general management of pregnancy, without the need for prophylactic transfusion.[48,49] By not undergoing transfusions routinely, these patients are not exposed to the multiple risks of alloimmunization, viral infections, and iron overload. However, the nonuse of transfusions imposes a serious responsibility on the physician to closely monitor any pregnancy and anticipate the many threats that it presents to the mother and fetus. Cardiac iron disease may be unmasked with the development of eclampsia or even with the demands of a normal pregnancy. Any serious complication such as acute chest syndrome, stroke, or papillary necrosis necessitates intervention with exchange transfusions; more painful crises should also be handled in the same manner.

The objective of transfusions in the patient with sickle cell disease is not simply to elevate the hemoglobin to the 10 g/dL range but to simultaneously reduce the percentage of sickle hemoglobin. This is best accomplished by an exchange transfusion of 2 U out and 3 to 4 U in. With this maneuver, the sickle hemoglobin percentage usually falls to approximately 40%, the desired end point of the exchange. Serial determinations of the percentage of sickle hemoglobin and hematocrit then dictate further need for transfusion throughout the remainder of the pregnancy.[50]

Cesarean section is not necessary and is not indicated for delivery unless there are special obstetric needs; patients need to undergo exchange before this surgical procedure and before receiving any general anesthesia. Epidural anesthesia is well tolerated, with close attention to avoiding hypotension or hypoxemia; anatomic positioning is also important for reducing the uterine compression of the inferior vena cava.

Patients with sickle cell disease are in special need of increased folate supplementation. Folic acid, 5 mg/day, should be prescribed because of the ongoing RBC needs. Some sickle cell patients also need iron supplementation; this need can be identified if the ferritin level is less than 80 to 120 pmol/L during pregnancy. Of note, the incidence of pica appears significantly increased in sickle cell patients and may compromise iron availability for hemoglobin synthesis.

Thalassemia

The thalassemias represent a diverse spectrum of hematologic disorders, all of which share some alteration in the modulation of globin chain synthesis.[51,52] A multiplicity of genetic alterations is translated into clinical pictures that range from death in utero (hydrops fetalis) to a benign state with α- and β-thalassemia trait. The conditions are named according to the chain in which synthesis is diminished or absent; this defect in globin chain synthesis results in defective hemoglobin synthesis, the cause of hypochromia and microcytosis. The more important complication of the unbalanced globin chain synthesis, however, is the accumulation of free globin chains that are not linked to their partners to form the normal hemoglobin tetramer. These chains damage the developing RBCs by oxidative injury, resulting in chronic hemolysis and, ultimately, in iron overload. Patients with severe thalassemia require transfusional support to maintain an adequate RBC count; this iron infusion, in the form of RBCs, supplements the iron accumulation that accompanies thalassemic lesions.[53]

There are major, intermediate, and minor variations of thalassemia; these categories are defined by their clinical severity, corresponding to the number of gene deletions creating the abnormalities. In homozygous β-thalassemia, both β chain messages are missing, and severe anemia and secondary organ damage constitute the clinical course of the disease. In β-thalassemia intermedia, both β chains may be missing, but the lesion is modified because there is a parallel reduction in the α-chains as a result of an inherited defect at the α locus. Patients in this group may be modestly anemic but not in need of transfusion. β-Thalassemia trait is caused by the lack of only one locus of the globin genes and results in microcytosis without any significant anemia. Its major significance is its confusion with iron deficiency anemia and the inappropriate iron therapy that is frequently administered to such patients.

Diagnosis

Thalassemia must be suspected in the ethnic groups from which its name is derived. Thalassemia or Mediterranean anemia predominantly affects blacks and individuals of Italian or Greek descent; different genetic alterations are responsible for the disorder in different groups. Variant thalassemias are now being recognized frequently in immigrant groups from Asia.

Microcytosis, target cells, and splenomegaly are features of these anemias. Definitive categorization of the type of thalassemia may be possible with hemoglobin electrophoresis, in which elevations in A_2 or fetal hemoglobin levels represent the compensation for decreased levels of A hemoglobin.

Some variants are not identifiable on electrophoresis, and study of α and β chain synthesis is required; DNA probes are available to identify many of the genetic alterations that are causal in thalassemia. Prenatal diagnosis of some variants of thalassemia is possible with these probes.[54,55]

Impact on the Fetus and Mother

Thalassemia major is infrequently an obstetric problem, because the associated iron overload usually results in failure of pubertal growth and delayed sexual development.[56] Affected patients are often infertile and anovulatory, manifesting hypogonadotropic hypogonadism as a result of hemosiderin deposition in the hypothalamus and pituitary gland. There have been approximately 40 reported pregnancies in this group, with a high incidence of fetal loss.[57,58]

Pregnancy may precipitate cardiac failure in this iron overload state; affected patients need close cardiovascular monitoring and maintenance of the hemoglobin at a level of 10 g/dL. Thalassemia intermedia and thalassemia minor are no impediments to pregnancy, but they necessitate extra folate supplementation.[59] In the presence of adequate ferritin levels (80 to 120 pmol/L), iron administration is not necessary in these groups.

HEMOLYTIC DISEASE OF THE NEWBORN

Hemolytic disease of the newborn occurs after alloimmunization of a mother against paternally derived fetal antigens, usually of the Rh subgroup; the sensitization arises because fetomaternal bleeding frequently occurs during pregnancy, especially at the time of delivery. The exposure that causes sensitization may escape detection because of the absence of prenatal care or because immunization occurs during a miscarried or aborted pregnancy. Routine administration at 28 weeks' gestation of $Rh_O(D)$ immune globulin (300 mg intramuscularly) to an Rh-negative mother when the father is Rh-positive, or when the father's Rh status is unknown, effectively suppresses Rh immunization. This intervention has become an accepted standard of obstetric care.[60,61] Prevention of sensitization is imperative because no therapy is successful in suppressing active Rh immunization once it has begun. In that situation,

all subsequent pregnancies with Rh-positive infants are complicated by increasing sensitization and antibody response. Administration of high-dose intravenous immune globulins has not proved to significantly ameliorate severe erythroblastosis fetalis.[62] The incidence of hemolytic disease of the newborn has dramatically declined, a phenomenon attributable largely to Rh immune globulin administration.[63,64]

Once sensitization of the Rh-negative mother has occurred, all subsequent pregnancies need serial monitoring to recognize the presence of antibodies and to determine their levels. Identification of pregnant women at risk requires documentation of their ABO and Rh types and a screen for antibodies with an indirect Coombs test; the Coombs test detects antibodies in a woman's serum whose targets are not only the Rh locus but also other minor group RBC antigens such as Kell, Duffy, and others that may also cause fetal hemolysis. An antibody titer of less than 1:16 is not associated with any problems for the fetus, but the mother still needs monitoring at 2- to 4-week intervals beginning at 16 to 18 weeks of pregnancy. If the father is heterozygous at the Rh locus, a fetal blood sample to determine the blood type may obviate the need for further monitoring if the fetus is found to be Rh-negative. Umbilical vein blood sampling is possible before the 27-week interval, when amniocentesis becomes a means of determining the impact of the immune reaction directed against the fetal RBCs. [65-67]

Diagnosis

Amniocentesis, performed under ultrasound guidance, enables sampling of amniotic fluid to determine its content of bilirubin as an index of the severity of fetal hemolysis.[68] Spectrophotometric measurement of the deviation in optical density at 450 nm (Liley's index) is a reliable reflection of the degree of hemolysis threatening the infant's survival. Amniocentesis and ultrasound monitoring of fetal development are usually adequate to deal with the problems of Rh and most other RBC sensitizations. Kell sensitization is not mirrored in the amniotic fluid analysis, because the severity of anemia does not correlate with the optical density measurements; a more invasive, more direct assessment with fetal blood sampling is indicated in this situation and whenever any question arises in the course of more standard monitoring.[69]

Impact of Hemolytic Disease of the Newborn on the Fetus and Mother

The immediate and major threat of maternal sensitization is the potential for a degree of hemolysis in the fetus that leads to hydrops fetalis. Severe anemia may result in high-output cardiac failure with marked fluid retention; extreme hepatic and splenic hematopoiesis is associated with portal hypertension as a second cause of the hydrops state. Affected infants can still be salvaged by direct intravascular transfusions, whose results are better than those of the previous modality of intraperitoneal administration of the blood to correct the anemia. Such interventions require the skills of obstetricians who care for women at high risk; they must explain the need for specialized medical care in these circumstances.

Another, more delayed threat of Rh immunization is central nervous system damage, kernicterus, that follows exposure of the fetal brain to hyperbilirubinemia. Identification of infants at risk anticipates this danger after birth and allows early intervention with phototherapy or exchange transfusion before any damage has occurred.

The problems generated by Rh and other minor group incompatibilities do not usually arise with ABO incompatibility. The reason for the relative innocence of this form of maternal-fetal incompatibility is the almost immediate destruction of the potential sensitizer, the fetal RBCs. Large amounts of the alloantibody are present, and they destroy the intruding foreign RBCs. A second reason for the benignity of ABO incompatibility is the generation of immunoglobulin M antibodies in response to this sensitization. These, in contrast with the immunoglobulin G antibodies of Rh sensitization, cannot cross the placental barrier and cannot create the problems of fetal hemolysis.

APLASTIC ANEMIA

Bone marrow hypoplasia or aplasia is the hematopoietic lesion responsible for aplastic anemia. Numerous insults to the marrow, including infection, drugs or toxins, and humoral and cell-mediated immune mechanisms may produce this condition, which results in varying degrees of pancytopenia in the peripheral blood. Because aplastic anemia in some pregnant patients remits with termination or completion of the pregnancy and sometimes recurs in subsequent pregnancies, a cause-and-effect relationship between aplasia and pregnancy is strongly suspected. Management of the condition has been dictated by this association; termination of pregnancy is offered when severe aplasia complicates the early stages of pregnancy. In the later stages, blood component support with RBCs and platelets may be necessary; spontaneous delivery is preferred. There is no evidence of any transmission of the condition to the fetus.[70-72]

Constitutional aplastic anemia or Fanconi's anemia may not be clinically recognized until a woman is in her childbearing years. The implications of this diagnosis are the same as those of acquired aplastic anemia.[73,74]

In rare cases, acquired aplastic marrow states respond to steroid therapy, and limited experience with antilymphocyte globulin has demonstrated its safety in pregnancy.[70] The role of growth factors in pregnancy is not yet fully established, although granulocyte colony–stimulating factor has been administered to pregnant women with agranulocytosis without any apparent harm to the fetus.[75] Aplasia that persists after pregnancy may necessitate bone marrow transplantation for its permanent cure.[76]

PURE RED BLOOD CELL APLASIA

Pure RBC aplasia may appear in an acute form when parvovirus specifically infects marrow erythroblasts; this aplasia presents its greatest threat to those individuals suffering from a chronic hemolytic process. The supervention of an RBC production defect upon a hemolytic anemia seriously compounds the problem of an already shortened RBC survival. Serologic evidence (e.g., immunoglobulin M) of active parvovirus infection or measurement of the viral load establishes the cause of aplasia and enables use of intravenous immune globulin to successfully treat the condition. Immune globulin preparations contain antiparvovirus antibodies, which explains their efficacy in this infection-mediated aplasia.[77]

Parvovirus B19 infection during pregnancy infrequently leads to an adverse outcome: miscarriage or hydrops fetalis. The likelihood of a healthy outcome in this case is very high; the risk is most significant if the infection occurs during the second trimester. No significant protection or vaccine yet exists for protection against the infection, although 40% to 60% of women in their childbearing years possess parvovirus B19 antibodies and are therefore immune from a recurrence of the infection. The Centers for Disease Control and Prevention recommend that infected pregnant women be informed of the risks of such infections and that they make their personal decisions regarding the pregnancy after proper education and counseling.[78,79]

Pure RBC aplasia, like aplastic anemia, may also complicate pregnancy and recur with subsequent pregnancies.[80] A high correlation of this marrow condition with thymomas has been shown, and both cellular and humoral immunologic mechanisms have been demonstrated to play a role.[81]

PAROXYSMAL NOCTURNAL HEMOGLOBINURIA

Paroxysmal nocturnal hemoglobinuria (PNH) receives its descriptive title from the complement-mediated lysis of RBCs that occurs when sleep-associated hypoventilation causes a slight fall in pH as a result of increasing carbon dioxide pressure; this alteration in pH activates complement that attacks the complement-sensitive RBCs present in patients with PNH. This sensitivity of PNH cells is part of a larger defect in several membrane-based molecules; a particular deficiency of so-called decay accelerating factor results in prolonged and excessive complement activity on these cells, with their premature destruction.[82,83]

A sugar water or acid-hemolysis test was used to diagnose this condition in the past; flow cytometry now identifies the involved cell population on the basis of missing cell membrane markers.

Hemolysis with anemia draws attention to PNH, but of greater importance, especially during pregnancy, is the threat of thrombosis.[84,85] PNH constitutes a hypercoagulable state, in which platelets participate in membrane defects that frequently result in thrombosis.[86] The threat of this complication has led many clinicians to recommend termination of pregnancy in patients with PNH, although some such pregnancies have been successful.[87]

Intravascular hemolysis often results in iron deficiency because of iron loss from the kidneys in the form of hemoglobin. Iron must be administered cautiously and slowly, because young RBCs in this disorder are more likely to participate in hemolysis. Transfusions of RBCs need to be ABO specific and administered through a filter, because any leukoagglutinin reaction may activate complement and lead to hemolysis.[88]

MYELOPROLIFERATIVE DISORDERS

All the myeloproliferative disorders are stem cell disorders characterized by panhyperplasia of marrow elements with increased production of peripheral blood elements. Polycythemia vera (PCV), essential thrombocythemia (ET), chronic myelogenous leukemia (CML), and myeloid metaplasia constitute these disorders, although myeloid metaplasia is rarely seen in women of childbearing age. When pregnancy occurs in a patient with a myeloproliferative disorder, there are distinct complications that are unique to each of the subgroups.

Polycythemia Vera

In PCV, erythrocytosis is the major lesion, although leukocytosis and thrombocytosis are also present in varying degrees. Thrombosis is a major complication of PCV, and infarction of the placenta is a documented result of the elevated cytocrit (percentage volume of cells per sample).[89] Phlebotomy is an effective method of managing PCV. Special care is given to keep the hematocrit in the 30% range, because higher hematocrits are associated with increased rates of fetal loss.[90] Other means of depressing the marrow are available with the use of chemotherapy or biologic agents (interferon), but these agents are not as attractive as phlebotomy for use during pregnancy. Interferon alfa does control PCV and appears free of mutagenic effects upon the fetus[91]; its use is still not recommended for treatment of PCV during pregnancy unless phlebotomy proves unsuccessful.

Essential Thrombocythemia

ET is a myeloproliferative disorder characterized by platelet counts that usually exceed 1 million/μL. Thrombosis is a major threat in this disorder, although, paradoxically, some of these patients experience a bleeding tendency.[92] Pregnant patients with ET have an increased risk of first trimester abortion.[93] Administration of aspirin in some patients has enabled such pregnancies to proceed without thrombosis; its administration must be used with caution in ET patients in whom bleeding, rather than thrombosis, is the expression of the defect. The quandary is resolved by some clinicians with the administration of aspirin only to patients with ET who demonstrate a normal bleeding time.

Plateletpheresis is an acute, short-term method of reducing the platelet count in ET; this may be indicated when a thrombotic event occurs or when a patient needs preparation for immediate surgery. Chemotherapy with hydroxyurea (Hydrea) lowers the platelet count, but its use is not recommended during pregnancy. Interferon treatment in an ET patient before pregnancy has enabled an event-free pregnancy during which thrombocytosis did

not recur. This treatment has also been used during pregnancy to successfully reduce the platelet count without adverse effects on the fetus.[94] A new agent, anagrelide HCl, has a specific platelet-lowering effect through its action on the megakaryocyte, but its safety during pregnancy has not been determined.[95]

Chronic Myelogenous Leukemia

CML may appear during pregnancy, usually as an asymptomatic elevation in the white blood cell count. This leukocytosis may be mistaken for the benign increase in white blood cells that sometimes accompanies pregnancy. The distinction is important because of the prognosis for a patient with CML and the question of desirability of continuing the pregnancy in the presence of this condition. The diagnosis of CML is made simple because of the presence of a characteristic chromosomal marker in 90% to 95% of patients with CML. This 9;22 translocation, the Philadelphia chromosome, is an acquired defect, and the condition is not transmitted to the fetus. A molecular probe for the *bcr-c-abl* fusion gene is now available and is more sensitive than the identification of the Philadelphia chromosome in CML on the basis of morphology.

If pregnancy is allowed to proceed in a woman with CML, leukapheresis is a proven method of controlling any massive increase in granulocyte mass.[96] Chemotherapy has been given during the second and third trimesters of pregnancy without adverse effects upon the fetus.[97] Interferon has also been used successfully to manage CML during pregnancy.[91] Imatinib mesylate (Gleevec) is now front-line therapy for CML, but it is not recommended for use during pregnancy. An opportunity to provide a solution for the disorder in the mother should not be overlooked; transplantation of a child's marrow to a mother has been successfully performed. Stem cells collected from cord blood may enable marrow transplantation if human leukocyte antigens are an appropriate match. This potential donor source may simplify the process of performing such transplantation in the future, because transplantation is still the only cure for CML that is currently available.[98]

HEMATOLOGIC MALIGNANCIES

Lymphomas, especially Hodgkin's disease, are not uncommon in women of childbearing age and may first occur during pregnancy. Unfortunately, their presence may be overlooked because of the understandable reluctance of physicians to use radiographs during this period. Symptoms such as sweating, pruritus, and back pain may all be attributed to the pregnant state, further lessening the likelihood of these diagnoses during pregnancy. The result is progression of the tumor to a more advanced and potentially incurable stage.

Discovery of lymphoma during the first trimester is an indication for abortion if chemotherapy is necessary to treat the malignancy; later in pregnancy, either chemotherapy or deferral of treatment until after delivery is an option in these cases.[99] The choice of chemotherapy is affected by the patient's desire for future children. Doxorubicin (Adriamycin)–bleomycin-vinblastine-dacarbazine (ABVD) regimens are preferred over mechlorethamine–vincristine (Oncovin)–procarbazine-prednisone (MOPP) regimens in Hodgkin's disease because of the lesser incidence of sterility with use of ABVD.[97]

Acute leukemia occurring during pregnancy[100] raises the same considerations that arise with lymphoma. The options are actually less limited because of the greater seriousness of the diagnosis of leukemia and its likelihood of a lethal outcome even with aggressive therapy. Elective termination of pregnancy is advisable if this is acceptable to the patient. Chemotherapy can be deferred for only a brief time. Successful delivery of healthy infants has occurred when acute leukemia has been treated with cytarabine and anthracycline-based regimens in the second and third trimesters.[101]

Treatment of acute promyelocytic leukemia with all-*trans*-retinoic acid during pregnancy has induced remission without any adverse consequences for the fetus.[102]

PLATELET DISORDERS

Platelets are small, granulated particles that arise by demarcation from the cytoplasm of megakaryocytes within the marrow. During their 8- to 10-day survival in the peripheral blood, platelets participate in endothelial maintenance and in formation of platelet plugs at the site of vessel breaks or ruptures. Petechial lesions are the characteristic lesions in thrombocytopenic states and are the end result of RBC extravasation outside the defective endothelial barriers. A normal platelet count is in the range of 200,000/μL to 400,000/μL, a number well in excess of the 10,000/μL to 20,000/μL platelet count below which spontaneous bleeding may occur. Platelet number is not, however, the only determinant of this facet of hemostasis; qualitative disruptions in platelet function may result in bleeding even with a normal platelet count. A prolonged bleeding time is the means of demonstrating this cause of a bruising or bleeding tendency in an individual without thrombocytopenia. The converse situation also exists: Low platelet counts may be associated with normal bleeding times, especially when enhanced peripheral consumption of platelets is accompanied by the release of young, hemostatically more effective platelets from the marrow.

There are strict parallels between erythropoiesis and thrombopoiesis: Both manifest a humoral feedback system that maintains peripheral counts within specific limits. Thrombopoiesis is slightly more complicated than erythropoiesis, because there are both specific megakaryocyte stimulatory factors and thrombopoietins that determine platelet number.[103] The oxygen-sensing device within the kidneys that causes erythropoietin release is well defined; its counterpart in thrombopoiesis is not known, although there is a suggestion that the endothelium or platelet components (platelet factor 4) may perform this function. The spleen also plays a larger role in platelet than in RBC physiology, although it is the major graveyard for senescent forms of both elements. Under normal circumstances, approximately one third of the platelet mass is in residence within the spleen. Even larger numbers are

sequestered as the spleen enlarges, which explains the contribution of splenomegaly of any cause to the development of thrombocytopenia (Table 4–3).

The approach to the patient with thrombocytopenia parallels the approach to anemia, although there is no widely available test comparable with the RBC reticulocyte count that enumerates daily platelet production. In place of the reticulocyte count, a cruder index capitalizes on the larger size of young platelets. A mean platelet volume can be measured with electronic counters, and a shift to a large size is considered evidence of a stimulated, turned-on marrow.

Flow quantitation of platelet RNA content has been developed to improve this semiquantitative sizing index but is not yet generally available.[104]

With significant thrombocytopenia (confirmed by examination of the peripheral smear), a bone marrow aspiration may be necessary to evaluate megakaryocytopoiesis and thrombopoiesis. Conditions as varied as aplastic anemia, leukemia, megaloblastic processes, or amegakaryocytic states may be discovered on marrow examination. Timidity in performing the study is inappropriate in thrombocytopenic states, because bleeding rarely complicates the procedure, and the information obtained is often valuable in determining the cause of thrombocytopenia.

Peripheral consumption of platelets usually has an immunologic basis or is caused by participation in pathologic clotting or endothelial interaction. In contrast with RBCs, in which bleeding results in anemia, this same challenge of bleeding is usually associated with thrombocytosis; bleeding is not an acceptable explanation for thrombocytopenia unless massive blood loss has occurred, followed by replacement with packed RBCs. Excess consumption of platelets commonly accompanies many disorders in pregnancy, with the real possibility that platelet consumption is a primary contribution to the pathophysiologic mechanisms of these disorders.[105] Platelet alterations are important not only for their role in normal hemostasis and the threat of bleeding but also because thrombocytopenia may be an early indication of serious complications in pregnancy.

Idiopathic Thrombocytopenic Purpura

Several incitants leading to immune sensitization of platelets are known; drugs and viral infections are the leading

---

TABLE 4–3   Causes of Thrombocytopenia during Pregnancy

Marrow lesion (aplasia, leukemia, etc.)
Accelerated consumption of platelets with normal coagulation
   parameters
     Splenomegaly
     Immune thrombocytopenia (antiplatelet antibodies)
     Thrombotic thrombocytopenia purpura
     Eclampsia
Accelerated consumption of platelets with abnormal coagulation
   parameters
     Disseminated intravascular coagulation
     HELLP syndrome

causes, and perturbed immune function as a component of collagen vascular and lymphoproliferative disorders may play a role.[105a] During pregnancy, these common causes of idiopathic thrombocytopenic purpura (ITP) must be supplemented by consideration of pregnancy itself as the immune sensitizer leading to thrombocytopenia. The initial appearance of thrombocytopenia during pregnancy and its disappearance after pregnancy makes a cause-and-effect relationship likely, although the basis of the sensitization is not established.[106]

Thrombocytopenia carries a special threat during pregnancy because of the pathophysiology of ITP and its potential for concomitant sensitization of the fetus. Accelerated platelet destruction in ITP is secondary to the presence of antibodies, usually of the immunoglobulin G subclass, which have specific platelet membrane antigens as their target.[107] Platelets coated with antibody are removed by the reticuloendothelial cells of the body, predominantly within the spleen. Antibodies of the immunoglobulin G subclass are able to traverse the placenta with the potential for sensitization of fetal and maternal platelets. Thrombocytopenia within the fetus is surrounded by the additional fears of bleeding during a vaginal delivery, although some clinicians believe that this threat is overrated[108]; trauma to the brain may occur as the infant's cranium is remodeled in passage through the vaginal vault. Documentation of thrombocytopenia in the fetus of a woman with ITP may affect the decision regarding the mode of delivery to anticipate and to prevent this threat of a vaginal delivery; cesarean section is recommended by many (but not all) clinicians to avoid this complication when significant fetal thrombocytopenia is present. There is growing advocacy for allowing a vaginal delivery even in the face of fetal thrombocytopenia; this position would obviate the need and risks of umbilical blood sampling.

ITP during pregnancy is, therefore, a multifaceted problem that influences the course of pregnancy and perhaps the choice of the mode of delivery. The complex decisions that surround the management of such patients make the correct diagnosis of ITP essential to anticipate these problems.[109,110] Monitoring of the infant's platelet count is essential because of the potential transmission of ITP to fetuses of mothers with ITP.

Diagnosis

Immune thrombocytopenia, like autoimmune hemolytic anemia, can be documented by analyzing the patient's serum for the presence of antibodies against the imputed antigens.[111] The indirect assay, a Western blot test, is a specific test for ITP and identifies antibodies that usually have the membrane glycoproteins IIB-IIIA and IB/IX as their target.[112,113] The direct assay, using platelet immunofluorescence, demonstrates the presence of immunoglobulins on the patient's own platelets. This assay, although a very sensitive test for ITP, is very nonspecific, because most thrombocytopenic states are characterized by elevated immunoglobulin levels on the platelet surface.[110]

Unfortunately, the presence or absence of platelet antibodies does not correlate in a 1:1 ratio with the presence or absence of thrombocytopenia in the infant; in fact, no feature of immune thrombocytopenia is a reliable predictor of the fetal platelet count.[114] The risk of severe fetal thrombocytopenia is low in infants born to mothers with no history of ITP before pregnancy or with absence of circulating antibodies in those with such a prior history of the condition.[115] However, the 20% to 40% incidence of fetal thrombocytopenia and its associated risk of cranial bleeding in 1% to 3% of such infants has resulted in the recommendation for determining fetal platelet counts before delivery. Such samples are obtained either by percutaneous umbilical blood sampling (PUBS) before the onset of labor or by fetal scalp vein sampling once the baby's head has descended within reach of a lancet.[116] A fetal platelet count of greater than $50,000/\mu L$ is considered an adequate level to permit a vaginal delivery[117] but many obstetricians favor a vaginal delivery irregardless of the platelet count.

Fears regarding fetal thrombocytopenia are not warranted when new-onset maternal thrombocytopenia of greater than $100,000/\mu L$ occurs during pregnancy. This so-called gestational thrombocytopenia[118] carries no threat of significant platelet lowering in the fetus, making it unnecessary to obtain fetal platelet counts.[119] However, the cause of maternal thrombocytopenia should still be determined, because it may be a clue to other conditions that need to be recognized. Thrombocytopenia is often a harbinger of eclampsia and may accompany anticardiolipin antibodies during pregnancy.[120-122]

Treatment

Treatment of ITP[123] during pregnancy is usually restricted to mothers with platelet counts less than 30-50,000/μL. Steroids at a dosage of 1 mg/kg of oral prednisone are initiated with tapering as soon as possible to a dose that maintains the platelet count in the 30-50,000/μL range. The 30-50,000/μL level is not a strict indication for initiating steroids, because many clinicians use steroids only in those patients who have symptomatic bruising or bleeding and in asymptomatic thrombocytopenic patients with a bleeding time greater than 20 minutes.[124] This spares a majority of such patients the many threatening side effects of steroids during pregnancy. Steroids are frequently administered in the 2 to 3 weeks before delivery because of a suggestion that their administration favorably affects the infant's platelet count. This practice has also come into question because of doubt regarding transplacental passage of the steroids.[125]

Intravenous immune globulins have become an excellent, albeit expensive, substitute for steroids in the treatment of ITP.[126,127] An initial course of 1 g/kg/day for 2 days usually elevates the platelet count for approximately 2 to 3 weeks. Punctuation of this effect can be achieved by repeat infusions of smaller amounts (400 mg/kg at 3 to 4 week intervals). This treatment does not appear to affect the fetal count in either direction and allows the patient to escape the hypertensive, diabetogenic threat of steroids. Its use should probably be governed by the same indications as the use of steroids in this condition; platelet number is not the determinant but rather evidence for platelet functional deficiency with a prolonged bleeding time or actual bruising and bleeding.

Splenectomy is a very effective method of reversing thrombocytopenia in ITP states. This intervention is only an option in midpregnancy, because the risk of spontaneous abortion is too great with its performance in early or late pregnancy. If steroid or immune globulin treatment has failed in early pregnancy, splenectomy is best performed in the early part of the second trimester; laparoscopic splenectomy has reduced the morbidity of this procedure, permitting its use when indicated during pregnancy.[128] Platelet transfusions are not more than a very transient option, because they are rapidly destroyed and also create a risk of alloimmunization. Platelet transfusions may be used for acute emergencies (central nervous system bleeding, major gastrointestinal bleeding) while awaiting the impact of steroids or immunoglobulins on the bleeding episode. Fortunately, steroid or immune globulin therapy are all that are usually necessary to manage the condition.

Eclampsia

Eclampsia and preeclampsia are obstetric conditions with major hematologic manifestations that serve not only as markers of these diseases but are also of pathologic significance as their cause.[129,130] Although the specific etiology of eclampsia and preeclampsia is unknown, platelet-endothelial activation is an omnipresent phenomenon in the hypertensive disorders of pregnancy.[131] In addition to altered angiotensin II sensitivity, platelet consumption and activation are anticipators in early pregnancy of this third-trimester disorder.[122] Multiple hematologic alterations also accompany the condition, with some evidence of disseminated intravascular coagulation (DIC) (see section on Disseminated Intravascular Coagulation) in addition to primary platelet endothelial interactions. Antithrombin III deficiency,[132] reduced protein C and S, and elevation of fibrin split products (FSP)[133] are the findings that support a consumptive pattern in the disorder.

Platelet consumption and indices of endothelial activation, however, outdistance the evidence for DIC, supporting platelet-endothelial interaction as the major derangement in eclampsia. Epidemiologic and laboratory studies suggest that immune mechanisms underlie the endothelial damage; antivascular endothelial antibodies,[134] complement activation,[135] and antiphospholipid antibodies have all been identified in various series of eclamptic patients.[136] Altered endothelial reactivity is manifested by reduced prostacyclin-thromboxane ratio favoring vasoconstriction.[137] Elevated circulating endothelin levels have also been demonstrated in eclamptic patients, further exaggerating the problems in the vessel wall.[138] The past brief enthusiasm for the use of aspirin to reduce the incidence of eclampsia has been dampened by studies demonstrating its lack of effectiveness; the blanket recommendation for universal use of aspirin in pregnancy is no longer advisable. Its use is restricted to those cases in which there is a history of eclampsia or the identification of a risk for eclampsia on the basis of abnormal angiotensin II testing.[139-142] Even in these candidates for aspirin use, some clinicians would delay its introduction until the 13th week of pregnancy because of fear of teratogenicity with its use during the first trimester.

Thrombocytopenia in eclampsia has its major risks in placental disruption and fetal loss. Antiplatelet antibodies are not present, thus eliminating any fear of immune thrombocytopenia in the fetus. Management of eclampsia usually consists of delivery of the infant when this is possible based on its maturation.[143] Platelet support is appropriate when the count is less than 50,000 or at higher platelet levels if any evidence of increased bleeding or bruising exists.

The hematologic lesion in eclampsia is not restricted to the platelet; striking abnormalities may occur in the RBC line as a result of increased sheer stress to the RBC membranes within the microvasculature. This traumatic hemolysis creates a characteristic morphologic picture with helmet cells, schistocytes, and microspherocytes on the peripheral smear; serum LDH levels are elevated secondary to the intravascular rupture of RBCs, the same mechanism that is responsible for the release of free hemoglobin and its saturation of its binding protein, haptoglobin.[144]

HELLP Syndrome

Eclampsia, with hemolysis and thrombocytopenia, may be complicated by hepatic decompensation in addition to its more common involvement of the kidney and central nervous system.[145] Recognition of HELLP (hemolysis with elevated liver enzymes and low platelets) syndrome is important, because this form of toxemia may be free of the usual renal or hypertensive clues to the diagnosis.[146] This syndrome also creates its own particular morbidity because hepatic failure is associated with decreased synthesis of numerous clotting factors.[147] Because management of the HELLP syndrome is the same as management of eclampsia (i.e., delivery of the infant), these patients need more aggressive coagulation resuscitation. Platelets and fresh frozen plasma (3 to 4 U every 6 to 8 hours) are administered according to the degree of coagulopathy and fluid balance of the patient. Severe depletion of fibrinogen should be managed with infusions of cryoprecipitate (10 U), with levels monitored to maintain the fibrinogen level greater than 150 mg/dL.

Thrombotic Thrombocytopenic Purpura

Eclampsia, with its multisystem organ involvement, closely resembles another platelet endothelial disorder, thrombotic thrombocytopenic purpura (TTP).[106,148] The resemblance is troublesome because of the differing therapeutic implication of each condition; eclampsia is managed with delivery of the infant, whereas TTP is treated with plasmapheresis and plasma infusions. The confusion with eclampsia is understandable, because of the pentad of TTP (thrombocytopenia, hemolytic anemia, fever, and renal and central nervous system involvement), fever is the only facet that is not a feature of eclampsia;

10% to 25% of TTP cases occur during pregnancy. The confusion of eclampsia with TTP[149] during pregnancy has led to the recommendation that the clinical picture of TTP or eclampsia during pregnancy calls for delivery of the infant, as in eclampsia. When this picture occurs earlier in pregnancy, before the third trimester, the case is managed as TTP, with plasmapheresis and/or plasma infusions.[150] LDH levels and platelet counts are monitored as markers of response to therapy. Platelet infusions are avoided in TTP because of the fear of fueling the process of thrombosis; plasmapheresis should be performed before any necessary infusion of platelets.

Thrombotic thrombocytopenic purpura is not a distinct clinical entity with a single known cause. It is more properly considered a syndrome, often occurring after a bout of diarrhea with enterotoxin-producing *Escherichia coli* or *Shigella* species. The role of von-Willebrand factor–cleaving protease deficiency as an inherited or acquired disorder is now established in TTP.[151] Measurement of this cleaving factor is becoming more available, and thus the clinical diagnosis and management may become less problematic. The syndrome may not manifest itself until the postpartum period, at which time plasmapheresis and plasma infusions are the indicated therapy. The hemolytic-uremic syndrome is also a microangiopathic process in which the major manifestations are renal failure, thrombocytopenia, and hemolytic anemia. Renal support is usually the major intervention; plasmapheresis and plasma infusions are reserved for progressive disease.[152]

Other Thrombocytopenic and Platelet Functional Deficiency States in Pregnancy

Inherited forms of thrombocytopenia may be associated with a lifelong bruising tendency or become manifest or recognized during pregnancy.[153] Bernard-Soulier syndrome is a thrombocytopenic state compounded by a deficiency of platelet glycoprotein Ib; its seriousness derives from the absence of this glycoprotein receptor for von Willebrand factor (vWF).[154,155] A subtype (IIb) of von Willebrand disease (vWD) may also be associated with thrombocytopenia, in which the platelet deficiency is exaggerated during pregnancy. An abnormal vWF is manufactured in this condition, which accelerates platelet consumption; thrombocytopenia worsens during pregnancy because of the physiologic increase in vWF that accompanies this state.[156] Hermansky-Pudlak syndrome is characterized by oculocutaneous albinism and a storage-pool defect of the platelets, which leads to a hemorrhagic diathesis.[157]

Management of these conditions involves administration of platelets.[158] This approach is also appropriate when a qualitative platelet abnormality exists, even in the presence of a normal platelet count. Normalization of the bleeding time is the desired end point of such intervention. Desmopressin (DDAVP) administration may also correct the bleeding tendency in these disorders. Type IIb vWD necessitates management as discussed in the treatment of vWD (see section on von Willebrand disease).

COAGULOPATHIES IN PREGNANCY

von Willebrand Disease

The most common coagulopathy that creates problems during pregnancy is vWD, a disorder that results from a deficiency of a plasma factor that acts as a bridging molecule between platelets and endothelium.[159] Its most characteristic clinical feature is a prolonged bleeding time, which accompanies the soft tissue and mucous membrane bleeding that complicates the disorder. The standard screening coagulation assay is the partial thromboplastin time (PTT), which may or may not be prolonged, depending on the severity of the factor deficiency. There is much variability in the several subtypes of the disorder, which is attributable to molecular lesions that affect the production or assembly of this large, multimeric adhesive glycoprotein.

vWF is synthesized and stored within endothelial cells and megakaryocytes. Deficient factor levels can be boosted with varying success in the several subtypes after the intravenous administration of DDAVP. This intervention can be repeated at 12-hour intervals, but the effect is usually lost after one or two repetitions. For patients who fail to respond to DDAVP (frequently those with type III vWD), correction of the deficiency is possible with administration of factor VIII concentrates containing significant amounts of vWF. These concentrates are now more free than they formerly were of viral contamination, eliminating the need for use of fresh-frozen plasma or cryoprecipitate as a source of vWF.

During pregnancy, these interventions may not be necessary, because there is usually a pregnancy-related rise in vWF that allows a vaginal delivery without major risk of bleeding. Postdelivery bleeding may necessitate intervention with DDAVP or concentrates as the vWF level returns to the nonpregnant, deficient levels.

Type IIb vWD is associated with thrombocytopenia, which worsens as pregnancy progresses.[156] The defect in this subgroup is an abnormal vWF that causes accelerated platelet clearance. As the levels of vWF increase with advancing pregnancy, a parallel reduction in platelet number occurs. This interaction in type IIb vWD has led to the recommendation that affected patients not receive DDAVP for treatment of their disorder, because endothelial release of the abnormal factor exaggerates the thrombocytopenia. Factor VIII concentrates containing vWF can be used to correct the bleeding tendency when necessary in this subtype.[160]

Congenital Coagulation Abnormalities

A coagulopathy that may prolong the PTT and may initially manifest during pregnancy is factor XI deficiency.[161] This condition occurs most commonly in Ashkenazi Jewish individuals and may first become clinically significant during the hemostatic challenge of childbirth. Affected patients can be managed with infusion of fresh-frozen plasma during childbirth, because only 25% of normal factor XI levels is necessary for hemostasis. Small amounts of fresh-frozen plasma usually suffice to manage this problem.

A rarer coagulopathy, factor XIII deficiency, has implications for pregnancy beyond those of bleeding.[162,163] This factor is necessary for crosslinking of fibrin monomers and stabilization of the fibrin clot. Factor XIII–deficient individuals experience poor wound healing, recurrent miscarriage, and delayed bleeding after trauma. Routine coagulation screening with prothrombin time and PTT does not identify deficiency of this factor; a urea solubility test is necessary to recognize the unstable fibrin clot present in factor XIII deficiency. Fresh-frozen plasma corrects the deficiency; its administration has allowed normal pregnancy and delivery to occur.

Other coagulopathies, including factor VII deficiency, factor IX deficiency, and dysfibrinogenemias, may complicate pregnancy.[164] Factor VII deficiency causes a prolonged prothrombin time without any abnormality in the PTT; it can be managed in the peripartum period with infusions of factor VII concentrates.[165] Factor IX, an even rarer deficiency in women, can be treated with the same concentrates.[166] Dysfibrinogenemias may cause bleeding or thrombosis; if bleeding is a problem, cryoprecipitate is a solution to the problem.

Coagulopathies not only are a threat in and around delivery but also may complicate procedures and local anesthesia. Invasive procedures need coverage with the missing components to avoid excessive bleeding complications. Affected patients pose particular problems during pregnancy and should be managed in close association with a hematologist.[167,168]

Disseminated Intravascular Coagulation

DIC is caused by activation of the coagulation cascade within the intravascular space. This pathologic sequence results in a combined threat of thrombosis and bleeding, the former attributable to thrombin activation and the latter to incorporation and consumption of the body's hemostatic factors within thrombi. The process is a dynamic one; its clinical features are determined by the inciting cause, the speed of the process, and the ability of the host to regenerate the clotting factors that are consumed. Fleeting DIC often accompanies saline-induced abortions, with no clinical consequences, whereas life-threatening bleeding may be the aftermath of abruptio placentae or amniotic fluid embolism.[169]

The speed of the process has led to the distinguishing of DIC states in pregnancy into two categories of "slow" and "fast."[170] "Slow" DIC occurs with fetal death, in which the precipitant of the clotting cascade is thought to be the release of tissue factors from the decomposing fetus into maternal circulation. This consumption of coagulation factors may result in spontaneous delivery of a dead fetus.[171] "Fast" DIC has several possible causes in the pregnant woman, including amniotic fluid embolism, abruptio placentae, and clostridial sepsis. All of these significant complications may result in a major bleeding diathesis because of the rapid depletion of clotting factors as amniotic fluid or endotoxin tips off the cascade.[172]

Amniotic fluid embolism is the most threatening of these obstetric emergencies because the consumption coagulopathy is accompanied by cardiopulmonary collapse.[173]

This condition occurs most commonly in the setting of prolonged and difficult labor in a multiparous woman; it is heralded by the development of shock, hypoxemia, and generalized bleeding.[174] The diagnosis can be confirmed by demonstrating amniotic fluid components in blood obtained from the pulmonary vascular circuit.[175] Monoclonal antibodies against these components are now available to make a more sensitive diagnosis of this condition.[176] Cardiopulmonary support, steroids, and correction of the coagulopathy constitute its management in preparation for delivery of the infant.[177] Platelets, fresh-frozen plasma, and cryoprecipitate may all be necessary to correct the global deficiency created by the consumptive process.

Abruptio placentae is associated with the same threat of DIC, and its management entails a similar correction of any coagulopathy before delivery of the infant.[178] Pain and bleeding are the usual hallmarks of abruptio placentae, although some patients may present in shock without pain, which thus diverts attention from this cause of an obstetric emergency.[179] Abruptio placentae has now assumed a more prominent profile because of its causal relationship to cocaine abuse; the latter may hinder recognition of the entity because it alters the patient's perception of pain.[180]

Severe DIC accompanies clostridial sepsis as a complication of abortions.[181] *Clostridium welchii* organisms release lecithinase, which causes massive intravascular hemolysis that can destroy virtually all circulating RBCs. Unfortunately, even with the most aggressive intervention with antibiotics and blood component support, few patients survive this catastrophe.

Administration of heparin to halt DIC is not dictated in these consumption coagulopathies. Correction of the clotting defects, circulatory support, and delivery of the infant are recommended interventions. The recommendations for management of slow DIC with fetal death are the same: induction and delivery under blood component support. The administration of heparin has successfully allowed one twin to survive DIC caused by the other twin's death in utero.[182] This finding may be important in the management of fetal death caused by selective reduction in fetal number in a multiple pregnancy.

Acquired Inhibitors of Coagulation

Pregnancy is one of the conditions associated with the spontaneous appearance of circulating inhibitors, usually directed against factor VIII.[183] The laboratory evidence for the abnormality is the presence of a prolonged PTT that is not corrected with a mixing experiment. It is an acquired abnormality, because it occurs in women with no history of hemophilia or bleeding. If the titer of the antibody is low, infusions of factor VIII concentrate may overwhelm the inhibitor acutely but with the risk of escalating the inhibitor titer. Porcine factor VIII may be used to elude the antibody effects, but sensitization to this factor also occurs. Intravenous immune globulins have successfully eliminated the antibody in some patients. If the titer remains high and bleeding is a problem, infusions of vitamin K–dependent factor concentrate can bypass the inhibitor and prevent or halt bleeding. Concentrates of factor VIII inhibitor bypassing activity also produce the same effect. A recombinant activated factor VII is now available to correct for the presence of the inhibitor and has become the treatment of choice for this problem.

References

1. Okuyana T, Tawada T, Furuya H, Villee CA: The role of transferrin and ferritin in the fetal-maternal-placental unit. Am J Obstet Gynecol 1995;152:344.

2. Schwartz WJ III, Thurnau GR: Iron deficiency anemia in pregnancy. Clin Obstet Gynecol 1995;38:443.

3. Ballegeer V, Mombaerts P, Declerk PJ, et al: Fibrinogen response to venous occlusion and fibrin fragment D-dimer levels in normal and complicated pregnancy. Thromb Haemost 1987;58:1032.

4. Lecander I, Astedt B: Isolation of a new specific plasminogen activator inhibitor from pregnancy plasma. Br J Haematol 1986;62:221.

5. Roberts D, Schwartz RS: Clotting and hemorrhage in the placenta—a delicate balance. N Engl J Med 2002;347:57.

6. Williams MD, Wheby MS: Anemia in pregnancy. Med Clin North Am 1992;76:631.

7. Clark MR, Shohet SB: Red cell senescence. Clin Haematol 1985;14:223.

8. Magnani M, DeFlora A (eds): Red Blood Cell Aging. New York, Plenum Press, 1991.

9. Harstad TW, Mason RA, Cox SM: Serum erythropoietin quantitation in pregnancy using an enzyme-linked immunoassay. Am J Perinatol 1992;9:233.

10. Solano FX, Couricell RB: Folate deficiency presenting as pancytopenia in pregnancy. Am J Obstet Gynecol 1986;154:1117.

11. Hytten F: Blood volume changes in normal pregnancy. Clin Haematol 1985;14:601.

12. Horn E: Iron and folate supplements during pregnancy. BMJ 1988;297:1325.

13. van Besien K, Tricot G, Golichowski A, et al: Pregnancy-associated aplastic anemia. Eur J Haematol 1991;47:253.

14. Berliner N, Duffy T, Abelson H: Approach to the adult and child with anemia. In Hoffman R, Benz E, Shattil S, et al (eds): Hematology: Basic Principles and Practice, 2nd ed. New York, Churchill Livingstone, 1995, pp 468-483.

15. Thompson WG: Red cell distribution width in alcohol abuse and iron deficiency anemia [Letter]. JAMA 1992;267:1071.

16. Delpapa EH, Edelstone DI, Milley JR, et al: Effects of chronic maternal anemia on systemic and uteroplacental oxygenation in near term pregnant sheep. Am J Obstet Gynecol 1992;166:1007.

17. Godfrey KM, Redman CW, Barker DJ, et al: The effect of maternal anemia and iron deficiency on the ratio of fetal weight to placental weight. Br J Obstet Gynaecol 1991;98:886.

18. Klebanoff MA, Shiono PH, Berendes HW, et al: Facts and artifacts about anemia and pre-term delivery. JAMA 1989;162:511.

19. Rushton DH, Ramsay ID, Gilkes JJ, et al: Ferritin and fertility [Letter]. Lancet 1991;337:1554.

20. Pietrzik K, Prinz R, Reusch K, et al: Folate status and pregnancy outcomes. Ann N Y Acad Sci 1992;669:371.

21. Duffy TP: Iron deficiency. In Spivak J, Eichner E (eds): The Fundamentals of Clinical Hematology, 3rd ed. Baltimore, Johns Hopkins University Press, 1993, pp 17-26.

22. Foulkes J, Goldie DJ: The use of ferritin to assess the need for iron supplements in pregnancy. J Obstet Gynecol 1982;3:11.

23. Guldholt IS, Trolle BG, Hvidman LE: Iron supplementation during pregnancy. Acta Obstet Gynecol Scand 1991;70:9.

24. Romslo I, Haram K, Sagen V, et al: Iron requirements in normal pregnancy as assessed by serum ferritin, serum transferring saturation and erythrocyte protoporphyrin determinations. Br J Obstet Gynaecol 1988;90:101.

25. Punnonen K, Irjala K, Rajamaki A: Serum transferring receptor and its ratio to serum ferritin in the diagnosis of iron deficiency. Blood 1997;89:1052.

26. Vogt C: Iron requirements of pregnancy. Clin Issues Perinat Womens Health Nurs 1991;2:364.

27. Faich G, Strobos J: Sodium ferric gluconate complex in sucrose: Safer intravenous iron therapy than iron dextrans. Am J Kidney Dis 1999;33:464.

28. Bayoumeu F, Subiran-Buisset C, Baka NE, et al: Iron therapy in iron deficiency anemia in pregnancy: Intravenous route versus oral route. Am J Obstet Gynecol 2002;186:518.

29. Scholl TO, Hediger ML, Fischer RL, et al: Anemia vs. iron deficiency: Increased risk of pre-term delivery in a prospective study. Am J Clin Nutr 1992;55:985.

30. Steer P: The effect of maternal anaemia and iron deficiency on the ratio of fetal weight to placental weight. Br J Obstet Gynaecol 1992;99:271.

31. Crosby WH: Pica: A compulsion caused by iron deficiency. Br J Haematol 1976;34:341.

32. Woywodt A, Kiss A: Geophagia: The history of earth-eating. J R Soc Med 2002;95:143.

33. Horner RD, Lackey J, Kolasa K, et al: Pica practices of pregnant women. J Am Diet Assoc 1991;91:34.

34. Smulian JC, Motiwala S, Sigman RK: Pica in a rural obstetric population. South Med J 1995;88:1236.

35. Barton JR, Riely CA, Sibai BM: Baking powder pica mimicking pre-eclampsia. Am J Obstet Gynecol 1992;167:98.

36. Campbell BA: Megaloblastic anemia in pregnancy [Review]. Clin Obstet Gynecol 1995;38:455.

37. Higginbottom MC, Sweetman L, Nyhan ML: A syndrome of methylmalonic aciduria, homocystinuria, megaloblastic anemia and neurologic abnormalities in a vitamin B_{12} deficient breast-fed infant of a strict vegetarian. N Engl J Med 1978;299:17.

38. March of Dimes: Folic acid supplementation and prevention of birth defects. J Nutr 2002;132:2356S.

39. Ali SA, Economides DL: Folic acid supplementation. Obstet Gynecol 2000;12:507.

40. Bunn H, Forget B: Hemoglobin—Molecular, Genetic, and Clinical Aspects. Philadelphia, WB Saunders, 1986.

41. VanEnk A, Vicshers G, Jansen W, et al: Maternal death due to sickle cell chronic lung disease. Br J Obstet Gynaecol 1992;99:162.

42. Sarjeant G: Sickle Cell Disease. New York, Oxford University Press, 1992.

43. Perry KG Jr, Morrison JC: The diagnosis and management of hemoglobinopathies during pregnancy. Semin Perinatol 1990;14:90.

44. Oklene-Frempoing K, Smith-Whitley K: Use of hydroxyurea in children with sickle cell disease. Semin Hematol 1977;34:30.

45. Day NS, Tadin M, Christiano AM, et al: Rapid prenatal diagnosis of sickle cell diseases using oligonucleotide ligation assay coupled with laser-induced capillary fluorescence detection. Prenat Diagn 2002;22:686.

46. Phillips OP, Elias S: Prenatal diagnosis of hematologic disorders. Clin Obstet Gynecol 1995;38:558.

47. Smith JA, Espeland M, Bellevue R, et al: Pregnancy in sickle cell disease: Experience of the cooperative study of sickle cell disease. Obstet Gynecol 1996;87:199.

48. Koshy M, Burd L, Wallace D, et al: Prophylactic red cell transfusions in pregnant patients with sickle cell disease. N Engl J Med 1988;319:1447.

49. Sun PM, Wilburn W, Raynor BD, Jamieson D: Sickle cell disease in pregnancy: Twenty years of experience at Grady Memorial Hospital, Atlanta, Georgia. Am J Obstet Gynecol 2001;184:1127.

50. Danielson CF: The role of red blood cell exchange transfusion in the treatment and prevention of complications of sickle cell disease. Ther Apher 2002;6:24.

51. Higgs DR, Wood WG, Jarman AP, et al: The alpha-thalassemias. Ann N Y Acad Sci 1990;612:15.

52. Kazazian HH Jr, Dowling LE, Boehm CD, et al: Gene defects in beta-thalassemia and their prenatal diagnosis. Ann N Y Acad Sci 1990;612:1.

53. VanderWeyden MB, Foug H, Hallam LI, et al: Red cell ferritin and iron overload in heterozygous beta-thalassemia. Am J Hematol 1989;30:201.

54. Cao A, Saba L, Galanello R, Rosatelli M: Molecular diagnosis and carrier screening for beta thalassemia. JAMA 1997;278:1273.

55. Fischel-Ghodsian N: Prenatal diagnosis of hemoglobinopathies. Clin Perinatol 1990;17:811.

56. Kilpatrick SJ, Laros RK: Thalassemia in pregnancy. Clin Obstet Gynecol 1995;38:485.

57. Kumar RM, Rizk DE, Khuranna A: Beta-thalassemia major and successful pregnancy. J Reprod Med 1997;42:294.

58. Mordel N, Birkenfeld A, Goldfarb AN, et al: Successful full-term pregnancy in homozygous beta-thalassemia major. Obstet Gynecol 1989;73:837.

59. Leung CF, Lao TT, Chang AM: Effect of folate supplement on pregnant women with beta-thalassemia minor. Eur J Obstet Gynecol Reprod Biol 1989;33:209.

60. Anonymous: Rh_O(D) immune globulin IV for prevention of Rh isoimmunization and for treatment of ITP. Med Lett Drugs Ther 1996;38:6.

61. Bowman JM: Antenatal suppression of Rh alloimmunization. Clin Obstet Gynecol 1991;34:296.

62. Chitkara U, Bussel J, Alvarez N, et al: High-dose intravenous gamma globulin: Does it have a role in the treatment of severe erythroblastosis fetalis? Obstet Gynecol 1990;76:703.

63. Hadley AG: Laboratory assays for predicting the severity of haemolytic disease of the fetus and newborn. Transpl Immunol 2002;10:191.

64. Tannirandorn Y, Rodeck CH: Management of immune hemolytic disease in the fetus. Blood Rev 1991;5:1.

65. Management of isoimmunization in pregnancy. ACOG Technical Bulletin number 148—October 1990. Int J Gynaecol Obstet 1992;37:57.

66. Gollin YG, Copel JA: Management of the Rh-sensitized mother. Clin Perinatol 1995;22:545.

67. Stockman, J: Overview of the state of the art of Rh disease: History, current clinical management and recent progress. J Pediatr Hematol Oncol 2001;23:554.

68. Stetyn DW, Pattinson RC, Odendaal HJ: Amniocentesis—still important in the management of severe rhesus incompatibility. S Afr Med J 1992;82:321.

69. Kanhai HH: Management of severe red cell immunization in pregnancy. Eur J Obstet Gynecol Reprod Biol 1991;42:S90.

70. Aitchison RG, Marsh JC, Hows JM, et al: Pregnancy associated aplastic anemia: A report of 5 cases and review of current management. Br J Haematol 1989;73:541.

71. Pajor A, Kelemen E, Szakacs Z, Lehoczky D: Pregnancy in idiopathic aplastic anemia (report of 10 patients). Eur J Obstet Gynecol Reprod Biol 1992;45:19.

72. Tichelli A, Socie G, Marsh J, Barge R, et al: Outcome of pregnancy and disease course among women with aplastic anemia treated with immunosuppression. Ann Intern Med 2002;137:164.

73. Alter BP, Frissora CL, Halperin DS, et al: Fanconi's anemia and pregnancy. Br J Haematol 1991;77:410.

74. Alter BP, Kumar M, Lockhart LL, et al: Pregnancy in bone marrow failure syndromes: Diamond-Blackfan anaemia and Shwachman-Diamond syndrome. Br J Haematol 1999;107:49.

75. Fujiwaki R, Hata T, Hata K, et al: Effective treatment of drug-induced agranulocytosis using recombinant human granulocyte colony stimulating factor in pregnancy. Gynecol Obstet Invest 1995;40:276.

76. Ball SE: The modern management of severe aplastic anemia. Br J Haematol 2000;110:41.

77. Young N: Hematologic and hematopoietic consequences of B19 parvovirus infection. Semin Hematol 1988;25:159.

78. Brown KE, Young NS: Human parvovirus B19: Pathogenesis of disease. In Anderson LJ, Young NS (eds): Monographs in Virology, vol 20: Human Parvovirus B19. Basel, Switzerland, Karger, 1997, pp 105-119.

79. Nunoue T, Kusuhara K, Hara T: Human fetal infection with parvovirus B19 maternal infection time in gestation, viral persistence and fetal prognosis. Pediatr Infect Dis J 2002;21:1133.

80. Banavali SD, Parikh PM, Charak BS, et al: Corticosteroid-responsive pure red cell aplasia in rheumatoid arthritis and its association with pregnancy. Am J Hematol 1989;31:58.

81. Fisch P, Handgretinger R, Schaefer HE: Pure red cell aplasia. Br J Haematol 2000;111:1010.

82. Rosse WF: Paroxysmal nocturnal hemoglobinuria and decay-accelerating factor. Annu Rev Med 1990;41:431.

83. Schultz DR: Erythrocyte membrane protein deficiencies in paroxysmal nocturnal hemoglobinuria. Am J Med 1989;87:22.

84. Solal-Celigney P, Tertian G, Fernandez H, et al: Pregnancy and paroxysmal nocturnal hemoglobinuria. Arch Intern Med 1988;148:593.

85. Ray JG, Burrows RF, Gusberg JS: PNH and the risk of venous thrombosis: Review and recommendations for management of the pregnant and nonpregnant patient. Haemostasis 2000;30:103.

86. Sholar PW: The continuing problem of thrombosis in paroxysmal nocturnal hemoglobinuria. N Y State J Med 1992;92:88.

87. Imai A, Takagi H, Kawabata I, et al: Successful pregnancy in a patient with paroxysmal nocturnal hemoglobinuria. Arch Gynecol Obstet 1989;246:121.

88. Sirchia G, Zanell A: Transfusion of PNH patients. Transfusion 1990;30:479.

89. Ferfusen JE II, Ueland K, Aronson W: Polycythemia rubra vera and pregnancy. Obstet Gynecol 1983;62:16S.

90. Spivak JL: The optimal management of PCV. Br J Haematol 2002;116:243.

91. Baer MR, Ozer H, Foon KA: Interferon-alpha therapy during pregnancy in chronic myelogenous leukemia and hairy cell leukemia. Br J Haematol 1992;81:167.

92. Griesshammer M, Heimpel H, Pearson TC: Essential thrombocythemia and pregnancy. Leuk Lymphoma 1996;22(Suppl 1):57.

93. Wright CA, Tefferi A: A single institutional experience with 43 pregnancies in essential thrombocythemia [Review]. Eur J Haematol 2001;66:152.

94. Delage R, Demers C, Cantin G, Roy J: Treatment of essential thrombocythemia during pregnancy with interferon-alpha. Obstet Gynecol 1996;87:814.

95. Tefferi A, Solberg LA, Silverstein MN: A clinical update in polycythemia vera and essential thrombocythemia. Am J Med 2000;109:141.

96. Fitzgerald D, Rowe JM, Heal J: Leukapheresis for control of chronic myelogenous leukemia during pregnancy. Am J Hematol 1986;22:213.

97. Doll DC, Ringenberg QS, Yarbro JW: Antineoplastic agents and pregnancy. Semin Oncol 1989;16:337.

98. Newton I, Charbord P, Schaal JD, et al: Toward cord blood banking: Density separation and cryopreservation of cord blood progenitors. Exp Hematol 1993;21:671.

99. Ward F, Weiss R: Lymphoma and pregnancy. Semin Oncol 1989;16:397.

100. Pejovic T, Schwartz P: Leukemia. Clin Obstet Gynecol 2002;45:866.

101. Caligiuri M, Mayer R: Pregnancy and leukemia. Semin Oncol 1989;16:388.

102. Incerpi MH, Miller DA, Posen R, Byrne J: All-trans-retinoic acid for treatment of acute promyelocytic leukemia in pregnancy. Obstet Gynecol 1997;89:826.

103. Gewirtz AM: Megarkaryocytopoiesis: The state of the art. Thromb Haemost 1995;74:204.

104. Rinder HM, Munz UJ, Ault KA, et al: Reticulated platelets in the evaluation of thrombopoietic disorders. Arch Pathol Lab Med 1993;117:606.

105. Romero R, Mazor M, Lockwood CJ, et al: Clinical significance, prevalence and natural history of thrombocytopenia in pregnancy induced hypertension. Am J Perinatol 1989;6:32.

105a. Kelton JG: ITP complicating pregnancy [Review]. Blood 2002;16:43.

106. McCrae K, Cines D: Thrombotic microangiopathy during pregnancy. Semin Hematol 1997;34:148.

107. Kunicki T, Newman P: The molecular immunology of human platelet proteins. Blood 1992;80:1386.

108. Crowther MA, Burrows RF, Ginsberg J, Kelton JG: Thrombocytopenia in pregnancy: Diagnosis, pathogenesis and management. Blood Rev 1996;10:8.

109. George JN, Woolf SH, Raskob GE, et al: Idiopathic thrombocytopenic purpura: A practice guideline developed by explicit methods for the American Society of Hematology. Blood 1996;88:3.

110. Kelton JG, Powers PJ, Carter CJ: A prospective study of the usefulness of the measurement of platelet-associated IgG for the diagnosis of idiopathic thrombocytopenic purpura. Blood 1982;60:1050.

111. Beardsley DS: Platelet autoantigens: Identification and characterization using immunoblotting. Blut 1989;59:47.

112. Berchtold P, Wenger M: Autoantibodies against platelet glycoproteins in autoimmune thrombocytopenic purpura: Their clinical significance and response to treatment. Blood 1993;81:1246.

113. Keifel V, Santoso S, Kaufmann E, et al: Autoantibodies against platelet glycoprotein Ib/IX: A frequent finding in autoimmune thrombocytopenic purpura. Br J Haematol 1991;79:256.

114. Burrows RF: Platelet disorders in pregnancy. Curr Opin Obstet Gynecol 2001;13:115.

115. Samuels P, Bussel JB, Braitman LE, et al: Estimation of the risk of thrombocytopenia in the offspring of pregnant women with presumed thrombocytopenia. N Engl J Med 1990;323:229.

116. Garmel SH, Craigo SD, Morin LM, et al: The role of percutaneous umbilical blood sampling in the management of immune thrombocytopenic purpura. Prenat Diagn 1995;15:439.

117. Dan U, Barkai G, David B, et al: Management of labor in patients with idiopathic thrombocytopenic purpura. Gynecol Obstet Invest 1989;27:193.

118. Aster RH: "Gestational" thrombocytopenia: A plea for conservative management. N Engl J Med 1990;323:264.

119. Copplestone JA: Asymptomatic thrombocytopenia developing during pregnancy (gestational thrombocytopenia): A clinical study. Q J Med 1992;8:593.

120. Eisenberg GM: Antiphospholipid syndrome: The reality and implications. Hosp Prac 1992;27:119.

121. Minakami H, Yamada H, Suzuki S: Gestational thrombocytopenia and pregnancy-induced antithrombin deficiency: Progenitors to the development of the HELLP syndrome and acute fatty liver of pregnancy. Semin Thromb Hemost 2002;28:515.

122. Redman CW: Platelets and the beginning of pre-eclampsia. N Engl J Med 1990;323:478.

123. British Committee for Standards in Haematology General Haematology Task Force: Guidelines for the investigation and management of idiopathic thrombocytopenic purpura in adults, children and in pregnancy. Br J Haematol 2003;120:574.

124. Ballem PJ, Buskard N, Wittmann BK, et al: ITP in pregnancy: Use of the bleeding time as an indicator for treatment. Blut 1989;59:131.

125. Christiaens GC, Neiuwenhuis HK, von Dem Borne AE, et al: Idiopathic thrombocytopenic purpura in pregnancy: A randomized trial on the effect of antenatal low dose corticosteroids on neonatal platelet count. Br J Obstet Gynaecol 1990;97:893.

126. Gibson J, Laird PP, Joshua DE, et al: Very high dose intravenous gammaglobulin in thrombocytopenia of pregnancy. Aust N Z J Med 1989;19:151.

127. Godeau B, Lesage S, Divine M, et al: Treatment of adult chronic autoimmune thrombocytopenic purpura with repeated high dose intravenous immunoglobulin. Blood 1993;82:1415.

128. Anglin BV, Rutherford C, Ramus R, et al: Immune thrombocytopenic purpura during pregnancy: Laparoscopic treatment. JSLS 2001;5:63.

129. Leduc L, Wheeler JM, Kirshon B, et al: Coagulation profile in severe pre-eclampsia. Obstet Gynecol 1992;79:14.

130. Weiner CP: Preclampsia-eclampsia syndrome and coagulation. Clin Perinatol 1991;18:713.

131. Saleh AA, Bottoms SF, Farag AM, et al: Markers for endothelial injury, clotting and platelet activation in pre-eclamsia. Arch Gynecol Obstet 1992;251:105.

132. Weiner CP: The mechanism of reduced antithrombin III activity in women with pre-eclampsia. Obstet Gynecol 1988;72:847.

133. Gaffney PJ, Creighton LJ, Callus M: Monoclonal antibodies to crosslinked fibrin degradation products: Evaluation in a variety of clinical conditions. Br J Haematol 1988;68:91.

134. Rappaport VJ, Hirata G, Yap HK, et al: Antivascular endothelial cell antibodies in severe eclampsia. Am J Obstet Gynecol 1990;162:138.

135. Haeger M, Unander M, Bengtsson A: Complement activation in relation to development of pre-eclampsia. Obstet Gynecol 1991;78:46.

136. Sibai BM: Immunologic aspects of pre-eclampsia. Clin Obstet Gynecol 1991;34:27.

137. Walsh S: Pre-eclampsia: An imbalance in placental prostacyclin and thromboxane production. Am J Obstet Gynecol 1985;152:335.

138. Schiff S, Ben-Baruch G, Peleg E, et al: Immunoreactive circulating endothelin-1 in normal and hypertensive pregnancies. Am J Obstet Gynecol 1992;166:624.

139. CLASP: A randomised study of low-dose aspirin for the prevention and treatment of pre-eclampsia among 9364 pregnant women. CLASP (Collaborative Low-dose Aspirin Study in Pregnancy) Collaborative Group. Lancet 1994;343:619.

140. Schiff S, Peleg E, Goldenberg M, et al: The use of aspirin to prevent pregnancy-induced hypertension and lower the ratio of thromboxane A_2 to prostacyclin in relative high-risk pregnancies. N Engl J Med 1989;321:351.

141. Subtil D, Goeusse P, Puech F, et al: Aspirin (100 mg) used for prevention of pre-eclampsia in nulliparous women: The Essai Regional Aspirine Mere-Enfant study (Part 1). BJOG 2003; 110:475.

142. Sureau C: Prevention of perinatal consequences of pre-eclampsia with low-dose aspirin: Results of the Epreda trial. The Epreda Trial Study Group. Eur J Obstet Gynecol Reprod Biol 1991;41:71.

143. Dildy GA III, Cotton DB: Management of severe pre-eclampsia and eclampsia. Crit Care Clin 1991;7:829.

144. Schrocksnadel H, Sitte B, Stekel-Berger G, et al: Hemolysis in hypertensive disorders of pregnancy. Gynecol Obstet Invest 1992;34:211.

145. Dotsch J, Hohmann M, Kuhl PG: Neonatal morbidity and mortality associated with maternal hemolysis elevated liver enzymes and low platelet syndrome. Eur J Pediatr 1997;156:389.

146. Fairlie F, Sibai B: HELLP syndrome. In Greer IA, Turpie AG, Forbes CD (eds): Haemostasis and Thrombosis in Obstetrics and Gynecology. London, Chapman & Hall, 1992, p 203.

147. DeBoer K, Buller H, Ten Cate J, et al: Coagulation studies in the syndrome of haemolysis, elevated liver enzymes and low platelets. Br J Obstet Gynaecol 1991;98:42.

148. Weiner CP: Thrombotic microangiopathy in pregnancy and postpartum period. Semin Hematol 1987;24:119.

149. Schwartz M, Brenner W: The obfuscation of eclampsia by thrombotic thrombocytopenic purpura. Am J Obstet Gynecol 1978;131:18.

150. Rozdinski E, Hertenstein B, Schmeiser T, et al: Thrombotic thrombocytopenic purpura in early pregnancy with maternal and fetal survival. Ann Hematol 1992;64:245.

151. George JN, Sadler JE, Lämmle B: Platelets: Thrombotic thrombocytopenic purpura. Hematology (Am Soc Hematol Educ Program) 2002;(1):315-334.

152. McMinn JR, George JN: Evaluation of women with clinically suspected thrombotic thrombocytopenic purpura–hemolytic uremic syndrome during pregnancy. J Clin Apheresis 2001;16:202.

153. Fausset B, Silver R: Congenital disorders of platelet function. Clin Obstet Gynecol 1999;42:390.

154. Peng TC, Kickler TS, Bell WR, et al: Obstetric complications in a patient with Bernard-Soulier syndrome. Am J Obstet Gynecol 1991;165:425.

155. Saade G, Homsi R, Seoud M: Bernard-Soulier syndrome in pregnancy: A report of four pregnancies in one patient and review of the literature. Eur J Obstet Gynecol Reprod Biol 1991;40:149.

156. Rick ME, Williams SB, Sacher RA, et al: Thrombocytopenia associated with pregnancy in a patient with type IIB von Willebrand's disease. Blood 1987;69:786.

157. Wax JR, Rosengren S, Spector E, et al: DNA diagnosis and management of Hermansky-Pudlak syndrome in pregnancy. Am J Perinatol 2001;18:159.

158. Edozian LC, Jip J, Mayers FN: Platelet storage pool deficiency in pregnancy. Br J Clin Pract 1995;49:220.

159. Chediak JR, Alban GM, Maxey B: von Willebrand's disease and pregnancy: Management during delivery and outcome of offspring. Am J Obstet Gynecol 1986;155:618.

160. Nishino M, Nishino S, Sugimoto M, et al: Changes in factor VIII binding capacity of von Willebrand factor and factor VIII coagulant activity in two patients with type 2B von Willebrand disease after hemostatic treatment and during pregnancy. Int J Haematol 1996;64:127.

161. Steinberg MH, Saletaris S, Funt M, et al: Management of factor XI deficiency in gynecologic and obstetric patients. Obstet Gynecol 1986;68:130.

162. Boda Z, Pfliegler G, Muszbek L, et al: Congenital factor XIII deficiency with multiple benign breast tumors and successful pregnancy with substitutive therapy. Haemostasis 1989;19:348.

163. Egbring R, Kroniger A, Seitz R: Factor XIII deficiency: Pathogenic mechanism and clinical significance [Review]. Semin Thromb Hemost 1996;22:419.

164. Rigby FB, Nolan TE: Inherited disorders of coagulation in pregnancy. Clin Obstet Gynecol 1995;38:497.

165. Robertson LE, Wasserstrum N, Bazez E, et al: Hereditary factor VII deficiency in pregnancy: Peripartum treatment with factor VII concentrate. Am J Hematol 1992;40:38.

166. Guy GP, Baxi LV, Hurlet-Jensen A, et al: An unusual complication in a gravida with factor IX deficiency. Obstet Gynecol 1992;80:502.

167. Greer IA, Lowe GD, Walker JJ, et al: Hemorrhagic problems in obstetrics and gynecology in patients with congenital coagulopathies. Br J Obstet Gynaecol 1991;98:909.

168. Lusher, JM: Screening and diagnosis of coagulation disorders. Am J Obstet Gynecol 1996;175:778.

169. Richey ME, Gilstrap LC III, Ramin SM: Management of disseminated intravascular coagulopathy. Clin Obstet Gynecol 1995;38:514.
170. Weiner CP: The obstetric patient and disseminated intravascular coagulation. Clin Perinatol 1986;13:705.
171. Romero R, Copel JA, Hobbins JC, et al: Intrauterine fetal demise and hemostatic failure: The fetal death syndrome. Clin Obstet Gynecol 1985;28:24.
172. Lockwood CJ, Bach R, Guha A, et al: Amniotic fluid containing tissue factor: A potent initiator of coagulation. Am J Obstet Gynecol 1991;165:1335.
173. Tuffnell, DJ: Amniotic fluid embolism. Curr Opin Obstet Gynecol 2003;15:119.
174. Masson RG: Amniotic fluid embolism. Clin Chest Med 1992; 13:657.
175. Clark SL: Amniotic fluid embolism. Crit Care Clin 1991;7:877.
176. Kobayashi H, Ohi H, Terao T: A simple, noninvasive, sensitive method of diagnosis of amniotic fluid embolism by monoclonal TKH-2 that recognizes NeuAC alpha 2-6 GalNAC. Am J Obstet Gynecol 1993;168:848.

177. Hardin L, Fox LS, O'Quinn AG: Amniotic fluid embolism. South Med J 1991;84:1046.
178. Twaalfhoven FC, van Roosmalen J, Briet E, et al: Conservative management of placental abruption complicated by severe clotting disorders. Eur J Obstet Gynecol Reprod Biol 1992; 46:25.
179. Mechem CC, Knopp RK, Feldman D: Painless abruptio placentae associated with disseminated intravascular coagulation and syncope. Ann Emerg Med 1992;21:833.
180. Fleming AD: Abruptio placentae. Crit Care Clin 1991;7:865.
181. Pritchard J, Whalley PJ: Abortion complicated by *Clostridium perfringens* infection. Am J Obstet Gynecol 1971;111:484.
182. Romero R, Duffy TP, Berkowitz R, et al: Prolongation of a preterm pregnancy complicated by death of a single twin in utero and disseminated intravascular coagulation. N Engl J Med 1984; 310:772.
183. Staikowsky F, Blanchin I, Pineat-Vincent F, et al: Inhibitors of factor VIII C and pregnancy: Review of the literature. J Gynecol Obstet Biol Reprod (Paris) 1991;20:817.

5

VENOUS THROMBOEMBOLISM DURING PREGNANCY*

Peter McPhedran

The commonest form of thrombosis that occurs during pregnancy involves veins of the calf, thigh, and pelvis. The most important aspect of such lower extremity and pelvic venous thrombosis is that on occasion, during pregnancy and post partum, it leads to pulmonary embolism (PE), which is a major threat to the life of a pregnant woman. Surveys in England and the United States rank PE as the first or second most frequent cause of death during and after pregnancy.[1-3] Many of these deaths can be prevented. In England, the number of maternal deaths from PE has declined since treatment with anticoagulants came into wide use.[4,5] The same decrease in mortality appears to have taken place in the U.S.[6] However, anticoagulants themselves are dangerous to the pregnant woman and the fetus. In addition, women who have experienced venous thrombosis in pregnancy are sometimes left with chronic pain and swelling of their legs.[7,8]

Humans are equipped with a complex hemostatic system consisting of tissue-derived clotting activators, blood platelets, and proenzyme clotting factors, which are activated when blood vessels are injured or cut. A system of natural anticoagulants and fibrinolytic agents works to limit clotting and dissolve thrombi (Fig. 5–1). *Thrombosis,* or obstruction of a blood vessel by platelets and fibrin, can be blood preserving and lifesaving. However, it is often undesirable, causing ischemia and infarction of limbs and vital organs (if the thrombus is in an artery) or swelling and pain, usually in lower extremities and sometimes in association with pulmonary embolization with or without infarction (if the thrombus is in a major vein).

Virchow's formulation of the three causes of thrombosis was offered in the mid-19th century and is still accepted.[14] Thrombosis was (and is) thought to be the consequence of (1) alterations in the vessel wall, (2) slowing of blood flow (or *stasis*), and (3) changes in blood components. Alterations in the vessel wall take the form of damage to the clot-inhibiting endothelial surface, which exposes thrombogenic substances within the vessel wall, such as collagen and basement membrane. Trauma to the vessel wall occurs most obviously during delivery, whether vaginal or operative. Blood flow from leg and pelvic veins is slowed during pregnancy by pressure on iliac veins by the gravid uterus. Changes in blood components during normal pregnancy include moderate to marked increases in certain clotting factors and decreases in some components of the natural anticoagulant and fibrinolytic systems (Table 5–1).[10] Some of these changes are mild and/or inconsistent; others, such as the increases in fibrinogen and factor VIII and the decrease in protein S, are dramatic and consistent. Although it is unclear whether any single one or combination of these physiologic changes in blood components actually causes thrombosis in pregnancy,† it is interesting that the changes overlap with those brought about by birth control pills, which, like pregnancy, are believed to cause an increased risk of thrombosis.[15,16] Patient-specific abnormalities of the hemostatic and fibrinolytic systems, congenital and acquired, that sometimes cause hypercoagulable states in nonpregnant individuals, also cause an increase in the risk of venous thromboembolism (VTE) during pregnancy (Table 5–2). Some of these disorders also cause various complications of pregnancy believed to result from placental thrombosis. Patients with these disorders are considered to be at high risk for thrombosis

---

*Venous thromboembolism (VTE) during pregnancy has many parallels with VTE in nonpregnant individuals. The differences are emphasized. Various aspects of thrombosis in pregnancy have been well summarized in several secondary sources, including the version of this chapter in the third edition of this volume and in original papers in the clinical literature.[9-13] I have consulted these secondary sources and journal articles while composing the present chapter, and I refer to both types of sources.

†For example, it has not been shown that patients with especially large increases in fibrinogen are more prone to VTE during pregnancy. Nor has it been shown that patients who have had VTE have particularly high fibrinogen levels.

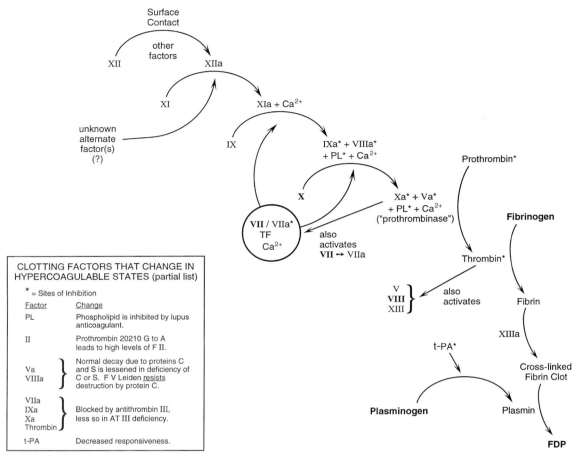

Figure 5–1. An outline of blood clotting showing components altered in hereditary and acquired hypercoagulable states. Some clotting factors that increase in pregnancy are shown in boldface. FDP, fibrin degradation product; PL, phospholipid; t-PA, tissue plasminogen activator; TF, tissue factor.

during pregnancy and are potential candidates for prophylactic anticoagulants (further described in the section on treatment).

INCIDENCE

Some frequencies of deep venous thrombosis (DVT), PE, and fatal PE during pregnancy and post partum, according to various authors, are presented in Table 5–3. This table emphasizes sources in which positive diagnoses were confirmed by imaging and emphasizes current studies. There have been many useful presentations of such data in which the diagnoses of VTE, DVT, and PE rested on *clinical* diagnoses; many of these are presented in Table 5–2 in the previous edition of this book.[17] The more current data presented here in Table 5–3 indicates that the frequency of VTE in pregnancy and the puerperium in Western (and some other) populations is about 1 per 1000 deliveries. About two thirds of these events manifest as DVTs and one third as PEs. VTE events are scattered throughout pregnancy and the puerperium.[18] The incidence of all VTE events may be higher post partum, and that of PE is indeed higher.[15,18,19] The rate of mortality from PE remains about 1 per 100,000 pregnancies, according to several sources

(see Table 5–3). Because current VTE incidence data are supported by confirmatory imaging tests, they may be accepted as more reliable but minimum estimates. Current rates are lower than those previously given, sometimes one tenth of previous rates. This could be interpreted as a correction of past clinical overdiagnoses or as representing an improvement in care. Also, rates of VTE in Western nations may not reveal much about rates in Asia or Africa, where genetic causes of thrombophilia common in Western nations are rare and standards of medical care may be different.

MANIFESTATIONS AND DIAGNOSIS

Patients with VTE disease in pregnancy may present with symptoms of DVT or symptoms of PE after an asymptomatic DVT.[20] It is often said and written that the *clinical* methods of detecting VTE are insensitive and inadequate, and this is relevant especially in pregnancy, in which some dyspnea and edema are normal. However, without suspicion raised by clinical evaluation, patients do not undergo ultrasonography or ventilation-perfusion (V/Q) scans, and the condition often goes undiagnosed.

Characteristic symptoms of DVT include pain, swelling, tenderness, warmth, and color change that occur

TABLE 5–1 Some Clotting and Fibrinolytic Factor Changes during Pregnancy (All Revert Post Partum)

Factors	Comment	Reference
Increased		
Fibrinogen	Marked increase	122, 123
Factor VII	—	123, 124
Factor VIII	Marked increase	122, 123
von Willebrand antigen	—	122, 123
Factor X	—	122, 123
PAI-1	Placental	127–129
PAI-2	Endothelial; marked increase	127, 129, 130
Plasminogen	Increase in these reflects decreased fibrinolysis	71, 122, 124
Antiplasmin		71, 122, 124
FDP	Fibrinolysis is not totally shut down	71, 123, 131
D-Dimer		70, 72, 127, 132–134
Heparin "resistance"	Composite of fibrinogen, factor VIII, and unknown substance	135
Decreased		
APC resistance ratio*	Lower but usually still in normal range	136, 137
Factor XI	—	122
"Fibrinolysis"	Overall	55, 71, 128
t-PA, t-PA release	Lower levels and blunting of normal increase after venous occlusion	70, 135
Protein S	Functional or free	136, 138–141
Platelets	At term	142
PT and PTT	Shortening reflects increased clotting factors	143, 144

There are other pertinent references on hemostatic changes in pregnancy.[125, 145-148]
*A *lower* APC resistance ratio means *increased* resistance to the action of activated protein C.
APC, activated protein C; FDP, fibrin degradation product; PAI, plasminogen activator inhibitor; PT, prothrombin time; PTT, partial thromboplastin time; t-PA, tissue plasminogen activator.

in the leg, especially in the left leg of the pregnant woman. Risk of PE is associated with popliteal, femoral, or iliac phlebitis; thus, thigh swelling is an especially important sign. However, 20% to 30% of patients with calf phlebitis also have or develop iliac or femoral phlebitis.[21] Regardless of which part of the leg is swollen or tender, the first diagnostic move should be to perform a sensitive test for upper leg vein thrombosis. Traditionally, this was usually done with contrast venography and later by impedance plethysmography (IPG)[22]; the current method is ultrasonography with vein compression and Doppler flow analysis. Venography shows the entire venous system (calf to iliac vessels) and is the only currently available, reliable method for detecting DVTs in the calf.‡ However, the dye used in venography may itself cause phlebitis, and the added benefit of seeing the iliac vessels must be given up to avoid radiation exposure to the fetus. IPG and, now, ultrasonography are the most sensitive techniques for detecting DVTs in the thigh; therefore, these techniques have been most frequently used. If iliac

‡Iodine 131–labeled fibrinogen was used in a sensitive test for new thrombi in leg veins but was never usable in pregnant women; it is now unavailable.

vessels *must* be visualized (e.g., if there is a strong suspicion of DVT but a negative finding on thigh vessel ultrasonography), abdominal computed tomography (CT), with its attendant radiation hazard, or magnetic resonance imaging (MRI) appears to be the technique of choice.[23-27]

It is sometimes difficult, but important, to proceed with urgent, aggressive imaging evaluation if VTE is suspected in a pregnant women. If a Doppler ultrasound imaging study demonstrates new upper leg vein thrombosis, immediate heparin or low-molecular-weight heparin anticoagulation is required. In the past, a study showing only calf vein thrombosis might have been an indication for serial IPG[22,28] or ultrasound studies every second or third day for 1 to 2 weeks to monitor for the development of higher venous thrombosis; meanwhile, symptomatic treatment, such as analgesics, warm soaks, and elevation, was applied. Many, perhaps most, providers would now recommend anticoagulation in patients with evidence of a DVT restricted to the calf. Anticoagulation in patients with calf DVT has apparently become more common as outpatient use of both low-molecular-weight heparin (LMWH) and regular heparin has gained broader acceptance.

Probably the most common presenting *symptom* in a patient with PE is dyspnea.[25,29] The physical examination may reveal tachycardia, tachypnea, and perhaps a few rales or wheezes. At this point in the examination, in urgent visit settings, pulse oximetry would be performed and might show low oxygen saturation (<92%). One leg, usually the left, may be swollen and, less commonly, warm and tender if the patient has an associated DVT. Arterial blood gas measurements are likely to show low partial pressure of oxygen (<85 mm Hg), low partial pressure of carbon dioxide, and low oxygen saturation. Routine chest radiographs may show avascular areas in the lung fields or other abnormalities but do not show pneumonia or congestive heart failure. (In this situation, the chest radiograph is as important for what it does *not* show as for what it does show.) If there is pulmonary infarction (about 10% of PEs), hemoptysis, pleuritic chest pain, and a pleural friction rub or signs of effusion may be found. Routine laboratory tests may reveal elevated levels of lactic dehydrogenase and bilirubin, and chest radiography may reveal atelectasis or pleural-based opacity or a pleural effusion. If the PE is large or massive, the patient presents with severe dyspnea, hypoxia, and hypotension. Examination may reveal cyanosis, jugular venous distention, a right ventricular heave (lower left sternal border), and a loud and widely split pulmonic second sound. Even the routine chest radiograph may show an absence (cutoff) of large vessels beyond the hilar region on one side. In such a large PE, the electrocardiogram may show right axis shift with S_1, Q_3, and T_3 changes and P pulmonale; echocardiographic studies may show right ventricular strain with elevated pulmonary pressures.

However, some PEs are asymptomatic and can be found only by pulmonary vascular imaging studies, which, again, are especially likely to be positive among patients who have iliac, femoral, or popliteal vein thrombosis.

Some of the more routine and seemingly tangential examinations and tests performed on a dyspneic pregnant woman may be helpful in preventing a mistaken diagnosis of PE. Symptoms of high fever accompanied by

TABLE 5–2   Putative Risks of Venous Thromboembolism (VTE) during Pregnancy from Clinical Risk Factors and Known Thrombophilias*

Clinical Factors	Frequency of Cause	Risk of VTE	Need for Prophylaxis in Pregnancy†	Need for Prolonged Anticoagulation after Event
Obesity, older age, multiparity, operative delivery	Common	+	No	Unknown
History of VTE				
Spontaneous	Uncommon	+++	Yes	Yes
Provoked (e.g., trauma)	Uncommon	+	No	No
Thrombophilias (TPs)				
Deficiency				
Antithrombin III	Rare	+++	Yes	Yes
Protein C	Rare	++	Possibly	Yes
Protein S	Rare	++	Possibly	Yes
Factor V Leiden	Common	+	No	No
APCR decrease without factor V Leiden	Common	+	No	No
Prothrombin mutation	Common	+	No	No
Hyperhomocystinemia	Common	+	No (folate Rx)	Not if homocysteine is corrected
Multiple TPs in the same person (or TPs and clinical factors)	Uncommon	+++	Yes	Possibly
Elevated factor VIII, IX, or XI	Common	+	No	Unknown
Antiphospholipid syndrome	Common	+	No	No

*This table is based on a topic well covered by Kearon et al.[149] and by Rosene-Montella and Barbour[150] (Table 8).
†In the absence of a history of thrombosis.
APCR, activated protein C resistance; VTE, venous thromboembolism.
+, slight; ++, moderate; +++, high.

leukocytosis, left shift (increased band neutrophils), and purulent and bloody sputum may correlate with pneumonia on chest radiograph. A chest film may reveal unexpected signs of pneumothorax or congestive heart failure.

The most important noninvasive diagnostic study for PE in any dyspneic, tachypneic patient is a radioisotopic lung V/Q scan. This technique entails locating one or more ventilated areas of lung that are nonperfused (a V/Q "mismatch"), together with a chest film free of infiltrate in the nonperfused area. Such a result is a "high-probability" scan and is sufficient to support the decision to anticoagulate. A less conclusive V/Q scan in a patient

TABLE 5–3   Some Estimates of the Frequency of Venous Thromboembolism during Pregnancy and Post Partum

Events/Denominators	Rate	Type of Assessment	Time of Study	Year of Report	Reference (Location)
Venous Thromboembolism					
Pregnancies	0.5-3.0	Radiographic	—	1997	18
Deliveries (268,525)	1/1627 or 0.6/1000	Doppler studies, V/Q scans, etc. (all clinically diagnosed and confirmed)	1978-1996	1999	151 (United States)
Pregnancies ≥24 wk (395,335)	0.85/1000	Objective confirmation	1988-1997	2001	152 (London)
Deliveries (39,757)	1.25/1000	Doppler venography	1986-1998	2002	153 (Saudi Arabia)
Deep Venous Thrombosis					
Pregnancies	0.7%	Plethysmography	—	1979	154, 155 (Sweden)
Cesarean sections (169)	1.8%	Venography	—	1983	154, 155 (Sweden)
Antepartum	1/10,000	Venography	—	1986	156
Postpartum (15,000 deliveries)	6/10,000	Confirmation of clinical diagnosis	—	1986	156
Pregnancies (63,300 over 11 years)	1.2/1000	Ultrasonography	—	1998	157 (Denmark)
Pulmonary Embolism					
Pregnancies	1/750	"Lung scan," angiography	—	1967	154 (Sweden)
Fatal Pulmonary Embolism					
Vaginal deliveries	1/100,000	Public health statistics	—	1981	1
Cesarean section	7/100,000	Public health statistics	—	1981	1
Pregnancies	1.3/100,000	Public health statistics	1985-1993	1998	5 (United Kingdom)
	2.1/100,000	Public health statistics	1994-1996	1998	5 (United Kingdom)
Deliveries	1.2/100,000	Public health statistics	Not given	2002	158 (Singapore)

V/Q, ventilation-perfusion.

clinically suspected of PE might lead to pulmonary angiography (a more invasive but more sensitive and specific test), in which, again, a large nonperfused segment of lung is sought. An alternative, perhaps preferable, study for the patient with an equivocal V/Q lung scan is ultrasonography of veins in the thigh. This study is less invasive and, if the result is positive, is equal justification for anticoagulation. CT of the chest—"helical" or "spiral" CT—has been used instead of V/Q scans with perhaps less sensitivity but good specificity; sensitivity is said to be improving. Also, patients with large venous thrombi always have ongoing fibrinolysis, which can be detected by tests for fibrin degradation products, or the D-dimer. Nonpregnant patients being evaluated for VTE may be permitted to bypass the special imaging studies if the D-dimer test result is negative and the clinical point score is not too high.[30] However, a negative D-dimer test is less likely to aid in the exclusion of VTE in pregnancy, inasmuch as there is often an increase in D-dimer in normal pregnancy (see Table 5-1). Also, pregnancy often causes false positivity

of the clinical criteria for VTE, and the D-dimer–point score algorithm has not yet been tested in this setting. Physicians are hesitant about exposing the fetus to any roentgen rays, but confirming or excluding a diagnosis of DVT or PE may save the patient's and her baby's lives.

TREATMENT

Patients with documented new or acute popliteal, femoral, or iliac venous thrombosis or PE require immediate parenteral anticoagulation with regular or unfractionated heparin or one of its low-molecular-weight derivatives (Tables 5-4 and 5-5). The purpose of this treatment is to prevent a PE in the patient with iliofemoral thrombosis and to prevent reembolization in the patient who has already had a PE. The body's own fibrinolytic system is expected to dissolve most clots already present. If regular heparin is used, anticoagulation is often initiated with a bolus of 80 U/kg, followed by continuous intravenous

TABLE 5–4 Anticoagulant Treatment of Venous Thromboembolism (VTE) during Pregnancy

	Heparin*	LMWH	Warfarin (Avoid in First Trimester)
Mechanism of action	Activates antithrombin III to bind rapidly to thrombin, factor Xa, and other serine protease factors	Action primarily against factor Xa	Prevents completion of synthesis of vitamin K–dependent clotting factors (II, VII, IX, X)
Anticoagulant program (treatment levels)	Start with IV heparin infusion: about 80 U/kg bolus then 18 U/kg/hr adjusted by PTT or heparin assay	Start with 1 mg/kg q12h, assay anti–factor Xa	Start with heparin infusion as described in "Heparin" column; start warfarin 5 mg/day concurrently or up to a week later
	Maintenance dosage is about 10,000-20,000 U SC q12h, push to PTT 1.5-2 × control PTT or to heparin assay level of 0.5-0.8 U/mL 4 hr after dose	Maintenance dosage is the same dosage adjusted to heparin level (same target)	Maintenance is usually 2-10 mg PO daily, or enough to push INR to 2-3
Duration	From diagnosis of VTE to 6-8 weeks post partum; withheld during labor, resumed or replaced by warfarin, warfarin post partum	Same as for heparin	From diagnosis of VTE or 12 weeks of pregnancy, whichever is later, until 36 weeks of pregnancy (heparin is used before, if necessary, and after)
Advantages†			
Prevention of recurrent VTE disease	Effective	Effective	Effective
Convenience day to day	Self-injection	Self-injection	Pill
Convenience and safety of delivery	Easy to discontinue, or reverse with protamine	Longer time to dissipate; no sure antidote (protamine is partially effective)	A little harder to discontinue or reverse; reverse with vitamin K or plasma if necessary
Effect on breast milk	None	None	None or insignificant
Disadvantages†			
Bleeding risk	Present	Present	Present
Fetal loss in comparison to normal pregnancy	Normal or increased	Probably the same as heparin	Increased
Issue with epidurals	Yes (but heparin is easiest to reverse and confirm)	Yes	Yes
Embryopathy	No	No	Characteristic
Fetal anticoagulation	No, does not cross placenta	No	Yes; crosses placenta
Osteoporosis	Occasional, can be severe	Rare	Not seen
Thrombocytopenia and thrombosis	A potential issue (low platelets in 3%-5% of patients taking heparin)	Less common	No
Cost	Drug is cheap; monitoring is costly over time	Drug is very costly	Drug is cheap; monitoring is costly over time

*Heparin or low-molecular-weight heparin (LMWH) is currently preferred in most situations; warfarin may be preferable in patients with artificial heart valves.
†See also Table 5-5.
INR, international normalized ratio; IV, intravenously; PO, per os (orally); PTT, partial thromboplastin time; SC, subcutaneously.

TABLE 5–5   Some Published Information on Low-Molecular-Weight Heparin (LMWH) Use in Pregnancy

Year Published	No. of Patients (Pregnancies)	Indications	LMWH Dosage	Target Levels: Anti–Factor Xa	Intent	Outcome for Fetus	Reference
1992	6 (6)	DVTs, SVTs, PEs, most current	Enoxaparin, 40 mg, 1-2 times/day	—	Follows UH treatment	5 delivered successfully; 1 died	159
1992	11 (17)	VTED postpartum, or on OCPs; SABs; protein C deficiency (1), protein S deficiency (1)	Dalteparin, 2500-7500 U total, divided doses	0.1- to 0.25 U/mL trough	Prophylactic	15 delivered successfully; 2 fetal deaths	160
1994	24 (27)	VTED risk	Dalteparin, 2500-7500 U, split in 1-2 doses/day	0.2-0.6 U/mL, achieved 2-6 hr after dose	Prophylactic	24 delivered successfully; 3 SABs	161
1994	16 (18)	VTED or thrombophilia or lupus	Enoxaparin, 20-40 mg once/day	Checked; no target	Prophylactic	14 delivered successfully; 4 SABs	162
1996	7 (7)	History of VTED and thrombophilia	Nadroparin, 2000-4000 U/day	Checked; no target	Prophylactic	7 delivered successfully	163
1996	2 (2)	Starr Edwards mitral valves	Nadroparin, 0.1 mL/10 kg b.i.d.	0.6-0.7 U/mL	Prophylactic (treatment doses)	Both delivered successfully	164
1997	18 (18)	DVT this pregnancy, 6 thrombophilic	Nadroparin, 6150 U/day	—	Intermediate	17 FTNDs, 1 SAB	165
1997	32 (34)	VTED in this or previous pregnancy plus 11 with APS, 6 with protein S deficiency, 2 with protein C deficiency	Dalteparin, 5000 U, 1-2 times/day ± ASA	Trough: 0.15-0.2 U/mL Peak (+2 hr): 0.4-0.6 U/mL	Treatment	27 successful deliveries, 7 infant deaths	166
1999	486 (literature and multicenter review)	Previous VTE or APS; previous fetal loss; or (a few) current issues	Nadroparin, enoxaparin, dalteparin, reviparin, tinzaparin Low to high dose	Various	Various	Women with comorbid conditions, such as APS, had 13.4% adverse fetal outcomes; those without, comorbidity, 3.1%	102
1998	4	Treatment of DVTs and PEs	Enoxaparin, dosage of 1 mg/kg q12h decreased to q12h at labor onset	0.4-1.0 U/mL after 3 hr Mean peak: 0.67 U/mL	Treatment	Good	167
1999	728 (40 paper reviews)	Thrombo-prophylaxis	Dalteparin, enoxaparin, certoparin, nadroparin, other "-parins" Low to high	Various; 0.1-1.6 U/mL	VTE prevention	Generally safe and effective No randomized studies	168
2000	50 (57)	Thrombo-prophylaxis or treatment	Enoxaparin at 40 mg/day	Observed mean: 0.235 U/mL	Prevention or treatment	Safe and effective for mothers except for 2 bleeds post partum	169

APS, antiphospholipid syndrome; ASA, acetylsalicylic acid; DVT, deep venous thrombosis; FTND, full-term normal delivery; OCP, oral contraceptive pill; PE, pulmonary embolism; SAB, spontaneous abortion; SVT, superficial venous thrombosis; UH, unfractionated heparin; VTED, venous thromboembolic disease.

infusion at 18 U/kg/hour. Some physicians would choose lower loading and maintenance dose formulas for pregnant patients and adjust the dose upward if necessary. Heparin effect is monitored by partial thromboplastin time (PTT), and the patient's PTT is usually pushed to 1.5 to 2 times the control level. PTT is measured before (as a baseline) and then 2 to 6 hours after heparin is started, and measurement is repeated one to several times during the first day to ensure that the patient is well anticoagulated.[31,32] Any recurrences of PE tend to be early but are largely prevented by good anticoagulation.

Some authors recommend the use of heparin assays instead of the PTT for monitoring anticoagulation during pregnancy, reporting that the PTT is relatively insensitive to the effect of heparin (i.e., there is heparin resistance), especially late in pregnancy. This resistance to the effect of heparin probably occurs because increased levels of factor VIII and fibrinogen in the plasma of pregnant women oppose the heparin anticoagulant effect,[33-35] if not necessarily the antithrombotic effect. A heparin assay (anti–factor Xa) is more cumbersome; thus, most patients are monitored by the PTT when it responds to reasonable doses of heparin. However, the use of the heparin assay does seem appropriate when the amount of heparin required to get a patient's PTT to more than 1.5 times control is much more than 18 U/kg/hour.

In nonpregnant individuals with VTE, a transition is made to oral anticoagulation with warfarin, which is begun simultaneously with heparin or up to several days after its initiation; the switch is usually complete after 4 days to a week of concomitant heparin and warfarin administration. The transition is sometimes delayed in very ill patients, because physicians have most confidence in the protective effect of heparin in acute situations. On the other hand, physicians may hasten the switch because of fear of heparin-induced thrombocytopenia (HIT) and its especial risk of thrombosis (HITT). HIT and HITT complications are said to occur in up to 5% and 0.5% of therapeutically heparinized patients, respectively, after at least 4 days of exposure to heparin. However, there have been few reports of HIT or HITT in pregnancy.[36] Warfarin, once initiated, is regulated by prothrombin time, expressed as an international normalized ratio; the target ratio is 2.5 in nonpregnant patients with VTE. Warfarin is then usually continued 3 to 6 months.

In a pregnant patient who needs continuing anticoagulation, warfarin was recommended for use after the period of greatest risk for congenital anomalies, the 6th to 12th weeks of gestation,[37,38] to be continued until 36 weeks, when a switch back to heparin was suggested to decrease the risk of bleeding at delivery, because heparin dosing can conveniently be reduced or withheld at the time of delivery.[39] An alternative and now preferable protocol[40,41] is to continue heparin after an initial 3- to 7-day infusion as an every-12-hour subcutaneous injection, with the 6-hour PTT pushed to 1.5 to 2 times the control level (see Table 5–4). Heparin dosing is usually withheld when the patient goes into labor but is resumed 6 to 12 hours after delivery to cover the initiation of oral anticoagulants. Heparin and warfarin are then restarted, with warfarin to be continued for 6 to 8 weeks post partum.

Heparin is still a reasonable choice for the treatment of VTE during pregnancy. However, LMWH is now often preferred. (For PE, intravenous heparin is still preferred.) Most local experience with LMWH is with enoxaparin. It can be started as acute therapy for a DVT, the standard dose being 1 mg/kg every 12 hours. Monitoring is perhaps less necessary than with heparin but still recommended

in pregnancy. Target levels for treatment of VTE are about 0.5 to 0.8 U of heparin per milliliter of plasma, 4 hours after a dose of heparin, and the test (heparin level or anti–factor Xa) may be repeated intermittently during pregnancy. Advantages of LMWH include a more consistent response at standard dosing, lower frequencies of HIT and HITT, and less osteoporosis.[42-45] LMWH can also be used in various prophylactic modes: The typical prophylactic dosage for enoxaparin is 30 mg subcutaneously every 12 hours or 40 mg subcutaneously once a day (see Table 5–5 for representative dosages from the literature). A major downside is cost, which is high for LMWH.

One likely exception to the general preference for heparins, standard heparin or LMWH, for VTE treatment and prophylaxis during pregnancy involves women with artificial/prosthetic heart valves. The use of heparin and LMWH in these patients seems to be complicated by a higher risk of thromboembolism originating on the prosthetic valve than is found in patients taking warfarin.[46] This topic is discussed in Chapter 6.

For the pregnant patient who presents with a large PE, is hypoxic and hypotensive, and exhibits right ventricular strain on echocardiography, treatment should probably begin with a fibrinolytic agent, such as streptokinase, urokinase, tissue plasminogen activator (t-PA), or, if fibrinolytics are contraindicated, surgical embolectomy.[47] The postpartum state is a contraindication to fibrinolytic agents, as are any recent surgery and any serious bleeding tendency. Most of the clinical experience is with streptokinase, and the success rate is high. Success is defined here as a high rate of maternal and fetal survival among reported cases.[48] However, streptokinase does not work for a patient who has had a recent streptococcal infection. Streptokinase dosing is 250,000 U infused over 30 minutes, followed by an infusion of 100,000 U/hour for 12 to 36 hours. Urokinase is given as a 4400-U/kg initial bolus, followed by 4400 U/kg/hour, usually for 12 hours. The possibility of a therapeutic response to these two agents is supported by development of a "lytic state" (marked prolongation of the thrombin time and a fall in the fibrinogen level after several hours).[47] Availability of these two fibrinolytic agents may be an issue. t-PA has also been used to treat large VTE events. Its advantage relates to its stronger action against fibrin in clot than against fibrinogen and circulating clotting factors. A dose that has been used is 100 mg intravenously over 2 hours. However, there appears to be little experience with this agent against VTEs in pregnancy.[49] If any fibrinolytic agent is used, full-dose heparin is instituted after the period of therapeutic fibrinolysis.

ANTICOAGULANT PROPHYLAXIS IN PREGNANT WOMEN AT SPECIAL RISK OF VENOUS THROMBOEMBOLISM

Patients who are hypercoagulable, especially those who tend to develop venous clots, are often referred for investigation by hematologists. There is an evolving set of risk factors for venous thrombosis: demographic characteristics, other clinical characteristics, and blood changes, genetic and acquired. The blood changes are often referred to as *hypercoagulable* or *thrombophilic* states (see Table 5–2).[50-53] The workup, at least for hematologists, has become somewhat standardized, although it is full of pitfalls (Table 5–6). Several of the tests yield misleading results if done in, for example, patients taking anticoagulants, those with liver disease, or even those with acute thrombosis.

Hypercoagulable states may contribute to VTE that appears "spontaneous": that is, without any obvious provocative stimuli. Such stimuli include recent trauma, a recent economy class plane flight, and a period of increased risk, such as pregnancy. However, inherited thrombophilias also do contribute to *provoked* thrombosis. Patients who experience clotting as a result of these thrombophilias are relatively young and often have positive family histories of venous thrombosis. Levels of risk assigned to different thrombophilias should determine the recommended intensity of prophylactic anticoagulation. However, these estimates vary among different authorities.

The clearest candidates for prophylactic anticoagulation are women with a history of VTE during a previous pregnancy[54,55] or outside of pregnancy, especially if the VTE was spontaneous or unprovoked, is recurrent, or is associated with a positive family history.[18] Patients with other clinical risk factors for VTE listed in Table 5–2 also deserve consideration for prophylaxis, as do patients with some of the blood abnormalities listed. Numeric estimates of the clinical risks of thrombosis in patients with genetic/hereditary and acquired thrombophilias are offered in the literature. Most or all of these estimates are based on retrospective studies of risks in patients with VTE found to have thrombophilia or in studies of their relatives. In studies of relatives of such patients, VTE frequency in relatives affected by the thrombophilia is compared with that in relatives unaffected by the thrombophilia.[56,57] Unfortunately, estimates of risk made by different authors seem to vary widely; for example, the risk of VTE for a pregnant woman with antithrombin III (AT III) deficiency and no VTE history is given as 40%[58] and 4%.[59]

However, useful principles do emerge from this literature. A personal or perhaps family history of spontaneous VTE (i.e., not provoked by such things as trauma or birth control pills) in the patient with a thrombophilia does imply a relatively high risk of recurrence. AT III deficiency and perhaps proteins C and S deficiencies confer higher risks for future VTEs than does factor V Leiden or the prothrombin mutation. Combinations of two or more genetic thrombophilias confer relatively high risk, as does a genetic thrombophilia in a patient with one or more clinical risk factors.

As mentioned previously, patients with clinical or blood abnormalities conferring increased risk of venous thrombosis are often considered for prophylactic anticoagulation with heparin or a LMWH. Dose intensity varies from 5000 U of regular heparin every 12 hours to full therapeutic levels, often 20,000 units every 12 hours. If enoxaparin is used, the range is from 40 mg once a day, or 30 mg twice a day, to therapeutic doses of 1 mg/kg twice a day, or 1.5 mg/kg once a day, with initial and/or occasional monitoring by heparin assay. Heparin or LMWH therapy is usually withheld during labor and delivery and is then resumed briefly post partum as a "bridge" to warfarin. Warfarin is started after delivery and then continued for 6 to 8 weeks post partum.[60] LMWHs, such as enoxaparin or dalteparin, are now widely used at prophylactic or therapeutic dosages instead of treatment with regular heparin. LMWHs, again, have higher bioavailability, a more predictable effect, and a longer half-life (sometimes being given once a day) and carry less risk of HIT and HITT. They also, however, have less of a track record in this situation and are much more expensive.

TABLE 5–6   Testing for Venous Hypercoagulability

Condition (Specimen*)	Test Type	Interference	Other Conditions Affecting Test Results
Antithrombin III deficiency (blue)	Functional or immunologic	Heparin lowers	Liver disease, acute thrombosis
Protein C deficiency (blue)	Functional or immunologic	Warfarin lowers	Liver disease, acute thrombosis
Protein S deficiency (blue)	Functional or immunologic	Warfarin lowers	Liver disease, acute thrombosis
Factor V Leiden (purple)	Gene amplification	No	Any contamination with other blood
APCR screen for factor V Leiden (blue)	Coagulation	Heparin may affect	None
Prothrombin mutation (purple)	Gene amplification	No	Contamination
Hyperhomocystinemia (green)	Fluorescence polarization immunoassay	No	Vitamin deficiencies and/or treatment of them
Elevated factors VIII, IX, XI (blue)	Coagulation	No	Inflammatory state
Antiphospholipid syndrome			
Partial thromboplastin time (blue)	Coagulation	Heparin and warfarin	Liver disease
Russell's venom viper clotting time (blue)	Coagulation	Heparin and warfarin (and low-molecular-weight heparin)	Liver disease
Anticardiolipin antibody (red)	ELISA (immunologic)	No	None

*Blue, citrate anticoagulated; purple, ethylenediaminetetraacetic acid anticoagulated; green, heparinized; red, no anticoagulant
APCR, activated protein C resistance; ELISA, enzyme-linked immunosorbent assay.

The mere presence of factor V Leiden[61] or even deficiency of one of the natural anticoagulants may or may not imply risk of thrombosis during pregnancy. Families differ, probably because of undetected thrombophilic cofactors. However, many pregnant women who are known to have heterozygous or homozygous factor V Leiden or a deficiency of AT III, protein C, or protein S have a personal or family history of thrombophilia; otherwise, the tests would not have been done. The medical history is likely to include episodes of VTE in a person who may not have clinical risk factors other than current pregnancy. Such episodes may have occurred repeatedly. They are likely to have occurred in relatives, because factor V Leiden, the prothrombin mutation, and the natural anticoagulant deficiencies are inherited in a dominant manner, in which the pattern of thrombophilia follows the pattern of the deficiencies in affected families.[62] As noted previously, it has been recommended that patients with natural anticoagulant deficiency, especially AT III deficiency, undergo anticoagulation during pregnancy.[60,63] The risk of VTE in women with factor V Leiden appears to be lower than in those with deficiency of AT III, protein C, or protein S.[64-66] However, some families with deficiencies of natural anticoagulants do not have thrombophilia. This variability in clinical manifestations among affected families was established early in families with protein C deficiency.[67] The question of what to do for a pregnant woman known to have such a deficiency, with no personal or family history of VTE, is still generally unresolved. More prospective data are needed.

The treatment for the nonpregnant patient with factor V Leiden or natural anticoagulant deficiency who experiences thrombosis, especially unprovoked or recurrent thrombosis, is long-term oral anticoagulation; however, as noted, pregnancy is probably an indication for using subcutaneous heparin or LMWH instead.

OTHER ABNORMALITIES

Other, less common abnormalities of plasma proteins implying hypercoagulability have been identified and may cause VTE, but their overall importance and their roles in pregnancy are still to be determined. Some abnormalities cause problems with the normal process of fibrinolysis; some unusual fibrinogens (dysfibrinogenemias) result in the formation of fibrin clots that are not easily lysed by a normal plasminogen-plasmin system.[68] A few of these conditions have been associated with increased VTE disease in pregnancy. Plasminogen can be congenitally reduced in amount or can be dysfunctional. Endogenous t-PA levels normally increase in a vein upstream of an occlusion (tourniquet or thrombus). In some people, t-PA is unresponsive to such stimulation, and this unresponsiveness has been associated with hypercoagulable states. Alternatively, natural t-PA inhibitor can be present in excess, which has also been associated with thrombosis.[69] Abnormalities of both t-PA and t-PA inhibitor are reported to be the rule during pregnancy.[70-72] However, to date there seems to be no special correlation between thrombosis and extreme values of t-PA and t-PA inhibitor during pregnancy.

OTHER TYPES OF THROMBOTIC DISEASE DURING PREGNANCY

Antiphospholipid Syndrome: Thrombosis and Obstetric Complications

A relatively common acquired hypercoagulable state, the antiphospholipid syndrome (APS), involves venous or arterial thrombosis; recurrent miscarriage, probably caused by placental thrombosis[73]; and, in some patients, livedo reticularis and thrombocytopenia—all in association with antibody to phospholipid-binding proteins (usually referred to simply as *antiphospholipid antibodies*).[74] The presence of lupus anticoagulant (LAC) or anticardiolipin antibodies, confirmed by laboratory study, completes the syndrome (Table 5-7). If LAC is present, as it is in 75% of patients with APS, it usually prolongs the PTT.[75,76] Anticardiolipin antibodies are also present in 75% of patients with APS. Many patients with APS have both LAC and anticardiolipin antibodies.

APS was originally identified among patients with systemic lupus erythematosus. It was also noted early among psychotic patients taking high-dose phenothiazine drugs[77] and, later, among patients with a variety of chronic infections, including human immunodeficiency virus and acquired immunodeficiency syndrome (AIDS). Some patients with APS/LAC appear to be less susceptible to hypercoagulable states than do others; it has been noted that LAC caused by infection (e.g., AIDS) does not cause thrombophilia.[78]

Laboratory tests that can identify APS are listed in Table 5-7. An active hospital clinical laboratory generates many sets of coagulation test results (e.g., prothrombin

---

TABLE 5-7   Laboratory Test Results Likely to be Abnormal in Patients with Antiphospholipid Syndrome

Tests for Lupus Anticoagulant (LAC)*
APTT: sensitivity varies with the partial thromboplastin activator
    If prolonged, it shortens with increasing phospholipid (PL) added to PTT mixture
    If mixed with normal plasma APTT is still markedly prolonged ("positive mixing study")
Russell's viper venom time
    A snake venom that clots by activating factor X; the test is sensitive to anti-PL activity of LAC

Tests for Anticardiolipin Antibody
ELISA for IgG and IgM antibodies
Varieties:
    IgG is often clinically important, especially in high titer
    IgM is sometimes important
    IgA is uncertain
    β_2-glycoprotein 1

Other Test Results that May Be Abnormal in Antiphospholipid Syndrome
Platelets (low)
Antinuclear antibodies
Venereal Disease Research Laboratory

*Those favored at Yale University.
APTT, activated partial thromboplastin time; ELISA, enzyme-linked immunoassay; IgG and IgM, immunoglobulins G and M; PL, phospholipid; PTT, partial thromboplastin time.

time, PTT) that include an isolated prolongation of the PTT. If the unexpected prolongation of a patient's PTT is not caused by heparin treatment or heparin contamination of the patient's blood sample, LAC is a likely cause (although not all PTT activators are equally sensitive to LACs[79]). In a hospital setting, heparin must always be excluded. When an isolated prolonged PTT is evaluated, polybrene is added to the patient's plasma; the PTT is shortened if the prolongation is caused by heparin, and then extra phospholipid is added, which will shorten the PTT if the prolongation is caused by LAC. Next, a "mixing study," a 1 + 1 mixture of the patient's plasma and normal plasma, is performed, followed by a 1-hour 37°F incubation and a repeated measurement of the PTT of the mixture. The result of the mixing study is considered positive for a circulating anticoagulant: LAC, or perhaps antibody to factor VIII, if the PTT of this mixture is still prolonged. If the patient is not a "bleeder" according to the history, LAC is more likely to be present. Any other clotting test sensitive to the antiphospholipid effect of LAC will also be prolonged, and Russell's viper venom clotting time (RVVCT) is sensitive and relatively convenient for this purpose. This snake venom is able to cause clotting by activating factor X; the RVVCT detects LAC because the test is sensitive, like the PTT, to the antiphospholipid effect of LAC. Patients with antiphospholipid syndrome may have abnormalities in one or more of these tests. It is often hard to be sure whether a patient really has APS from the test results. Results of one or two of these tests may be positive, the others negative. There are many borderline situations.

LAC is an acquired defect that often causes VTE or arterial thrombosis; about one third of patients with LAC are found to have arterial or venous thromboembolism. LAC is always on the list of hypercoagulable states to be sought in nonpregnant patients with thrombosis, including, for example, young people with unexplained strokes. In pregnancy, the association of LAC and APS with fetal loss has overshadowed their association with thrombosis. This dual role of LAC may have also led investigators to wonder whether other blood abnormalities that cause thrombosis would also cause complications of pregnancy (see later discussion). Although LAC is likely to be found in a woman with a history of multiple miscarriages, it was shown not to be at increased frequency among women with a single miscarriage.[80] However, pregnant women with LAC and a history of thrombosis or miscarriage, or a high titer of anticardiolipin antibody, appear to have a high risk of pregnancy loss.[81]

Treatment and prophylaxis of LAC effects in pregnancy has involved trials of corticosteroids, aspirin, and either heparin or LMWH anticoagulation. The combination of steroids and aspirin increased the success rate of pregnancies in LAC patients but was associated with a high rate of preeclampsia.[82] Although the best form of treatment is still uncertain, treated patients seem to do better than untreated patients.[83] The best current policy for an antiphospholipid antibody–positive patient who has a history of miscarriage is probably to treat with aspirin, with or without heparin or LMWH, and definitely to use heparin or LMWH therapy if the patient has a history of thrombosis.[75,84]

The association of APS and LAC with both thrombosis and miscarriage, which was first widely noted and studied in the 1980s, initiated a series of investigations that demonstrated that other hypercoagulable states are an important and perhaps leading cause of a number of complications of pregnancy.[4,85-89] Because the list of hypercoagulable states has lengthened since 1980, and especially since 1995, higher percentages of patients with complications of pregnancy, now the majority, are noted to be affected by one or another of the known hypercoagulable states. Although most of these data are retrospective—for example, the frequency of factor V Leiden in women who have had miscarriages is compared with the frequency of this thrombophilia in controls who have not had miscarriages—there have also been prospective treatment trials of patients with thrombophilias in which complications of pregnancy are apparently decreased in women who undergo prophylactic anticoagulation. These studies are still evolving.

The list of hypercoagulable states associated with complications of pregnancy is presented in Table 5–2, under the heading "Thrombophilias." Complications of pregnancy evaluated in relation to these thrombophilias have included miscarriage, intrauterine fetal death, preeclampsia, abruptio placentae, and intrauterine growth retardation.[90]

Homocystinuria/Homocystinemia

Homocystinuria is an autosomal recessive deficiency of cystathionine β-synthase that leads to elevated plasma levels of homocysteine and methionine in the blood and urine. Homocysteine, if elevated, appears to be responsible for vascular damage, both arterial and venous. Patients homozygous for this condition may suffer from mental retardation, seizures, lens dislocation, osteoporosis, and thromboembolism.[91,92] A high rate of pregnancy loss was reported in Mudd and colleagues' survey, but this study involved many miscarriages in a minority of women with homocystinuria.[91] Prophylaxis against VTE might not be necessary unless the patient herself had a history of VTE or miscarriage, although Walters and de Swiet recommended low-dose aspirin therapy during pregnancy, dextran during labor, and heparin post partum.[92] A few thrombotic episodes have been diagnosed in women with homocystinuria during and after pregnancy but not enough to state that the thrombotic tendency is excessive in comparison with unaffected women.[93,94] In addition to patients homozygous for cystathionine β-synthase deficiency, many patients with the more common but lesser degrees of homocystinemia resulting from a variety of causes are at increased risk for venous and arterial disease. Patients with methylene tetrahydrofolate reductase deficiency and patients with vitamin B_{12} or folate deficiencies also develop hyperhomocystinemia. In pursuit of this diagnosis, patients may undergo loading with methionine, a homocysteine precursor, to bring out a tendency for hyperhomocystinemia, but this would not be done during pregnancy. It is important to detect hyperhomocystinemia because the abnormality is dangerous, but it can usually be corrected by treatment with folic acid, pyridoxine, and vitamin B$_{12}$.[95,96] In some patients with tendencies for elevated homocysteine, the condition is probably not discovered during pregnancy, even if homocysteine levels are checked, because of the requirement to treat all pregnant women with folic acid to protect against neural tube defects. Nonetheless, homocysteine levels are worth checking in a pregnant woman with VTE, because hyperhomocystinemia, although dangerous, often responds to treatment. Correction of hyperhomocystinemia may require large doses of folate or a combination of folate with vitamins B$_6$ and B$_{12}$. There have been rare reports of patients who have required the active form of folic acid as leucovorin or folinic acid to reverse the elevated homocysteine levels, but leucovorin or folinic acid seems not to have been administered in pregnancy.[97]

Septic Pelvic Thrombophlebitis

Septic pelvic thrombophlebitis manifests post partum and clinically resembles endometritis that fails to clear with antibiotic treatment. Presenting signs are persistent fever, abdominal pain, and tenderness. Septic pulmonary emboli may constitute a complication and are associated with positive blood cultures.[98,99] The preceding event may be a cesarean section,[100] and the phlebitis may originate in or be confined to ovarian veins.[101,102] The diagnosis can be established by ultrasonography, pelvic CT, pelvic MRI, and, at times, by laparoscopy.[103] A positive venogram may demonstrate iliac vein thrombosis. The condition is dangerous, and a risk of death exists despite antibiotics. Once the diagnosis is confirmed, some authorities would add heparin anticoagulation to the antibiotic coverage[104]; this should eliminate the febrile state that persisted with antibiotic treatment. The value of adding heparin to the treatment regimen has been challenged by a randomized, controlled study in which treatment with antibiotics plus heparin is compared with antibiotic treatment alone. Duration of fever was no different in heparinized patients.[105] Whether the risk of fatal PE is lessened by the addition of heparin is still undetermined.

Rates of septic pelvic phlebitis and ovarian vein thrombosis have been reported; pelvic phlebitis was identified after 1 per 3000 deliveries (but 1 per 800 cesarean sections) at Parkland Hospital.[105] Ovarian vein thrombosis (with the septic pelvic thrombophlebitis syndrome) was estimated to occur in between 1 per 500 and 1 per 2000 deliveries in an Israeli population.[106] Of 22 patients in whom this condition was detected in the study from Israel, 11 also had a thrombophilia (factor V Leiden, protein S deficiency, or homozygosity for methylene tetrahydrofolate reductase C677T).

Cerebral Venous Thrombosis

Cerebral venous thrombosis, a rare and previously hard-to-diagnose critical event, manifests, usually post partum, with fever, headache, vomiting, seizures, obtundation, and hemiplegia or other localizing signs. Papilledema is frequent. The incidence in the United States has been found to be about 11 per 100,000 deliveries.[107]

The differential diagnosis is broad, including strokes and eclampsia. The diagnosis can be made from angiography, CT, or MRI. Treatment includes dexamethasone and antiseizure medications (if indicated) and administration of anticoagulants, if the patient fails to improve on steroids and if intracerebral hemorrhage has been ruled out.[108-110] Cerebral venous thrombosis has been associated with factor V Leiden in a series and with deficiencies of AT III, protein S, APS, and Behçet's syndrome in case reports.[111-116]

Thrombosis in Patients Undergoing Ovarian Stimulation

Ovarian stimulation for the purpose of in vitro fertilization has occasionally resulted in venous or arterial thrombosis, sometimes during an ensuing pregnancy. Ovarian stimulation results in acquired activated protein C resistance, thought to be caused by increased estrogen levels.[117] The thrombotic tendency has been attributed to ovarian hyperstimulation syndrome, with the combination of hemoconcentration and hyperestrogenism, but thrombosis has sometimes occurred in the absence of this syndrome.[118] Venous thromboses have occurred at unusual sites, including internal jugular vein. The prevalence of these thromboses is unknown, but there have been numerous case reports.[118,119] Individual cases have occurred in patients with factor V Leiden and AT III deficiency.[120,121]

CONCLUSIONS

Venous thromboembolic disease includes a set of dangerous conditions whose incidence is increased during pregnancy and that are even more common during the early postpartum period. Modes of presentation and methods of diagnosis resemble those in nonpregnant individuals, with the following exceptions: (1) The development of some leg edema and dyspnea, important clues to VTE in nonpregnant individuals, may be a normal accompaniment of pregnancy; (2) venous compression by the uterus affects the noninvasive imaging tests (venous ultrasonography and IPG) that detect popliteal, femoral, and iliac venous occlusion; (3) roentgen and gamma radiation in diagnostic tests must be used judiciously, only as necessary, to minimize fetal exposure; and (4) chronic anticoagulation entails special hazards to the fetus (especially warfarin embryopathy). Whereas the reward for successful treatment of thromboembolic disease in pregnancy is great, failure to detect and treat various types of thromboembolic disease in these patients sometimes has catastrophic results.

There is an evolving literature on the blood causes—genetic and acquired—of hypercoagulability. It now appears that many of the 8 to 14 blood changes that tend to cause venous thrombosis in the general population also affect pregnancy. These conditions often lead to VTE in pregnancy but are also responsible for many known obstetric complications.

Treatment of VTE has been improved by the addition of LMWH to the therapeutic armamentarium. These agents are currently particularly useful in prophylaxis of VTE. They may also be helpful in preventing diverse complications of pregnancy in patients with hypercoagulable states.

References

1. Bonnar J: Venous thromboembolism and pregnancy. Clin Obstet Gynaecol 1981;8:455.
2. Kaunitz AW, Hughes JM, Grimes DA, et al: Causes of maternal mortality in the United States. Obstet Gynecol 1985;65:605.
3. Sachs BP, Brown DAJ, Driscoll SG, et al: Maternal mortality in Massachusetts. Trends and prevention. N Engl J Med 1987;316:667.
4. Bonnar J: Epidemiology of venous thromboembolism in pregnancy and the puerperium. In Greer IA, Turpie AGG, Forbes CD (eds): Haemostasis and Thrombosis. London, Chapman & Hall, 1992, p 260.
5. Department of Health: Why Mothers Die. Report on Confidential Enquiries into Maternal Deaths in the United Kingdom 1994-1996. London, The Stationery Office, 1998, pp 20-38.
6. Moore JG, OLeary JA, Johnson PM: The changing impact of pulmonary thromboembolism in obstetrics. Am J Obstet Gynecol 1967;97:507.
7. Bergqvist D, Bergqvist A, Lundhagen A, Matsch T: Long term outcome of patients with venous thromboembolism during pregnancy. In Greer IA, Turpie AGG, Forbes CD (eds): Haemostasis and Thrombosis. London, Chapman & Hall, 1992, p 349.
8. Sandison AJP, Panayiotopoulos YP, Taylor PR: Venous thromboembolism during pregnancy [Letter]. N Engl J Med 1996;335:1846.
9. de Swiet M: Thromboembolism. In de Swiet M (ed): Medical Disorders in Obstetric Practice. Oxford, UK, Blackwell Scientific, 2002, pp 97-124.
10. Forbes CD, Greer IA: Physiology of haemostasis and the effect of pregnancy. In Greer IA, Turpie AGG, Forbes CE (eds): Haemostasis and Thrombosis. London, Chapman & Hall, 1992, pp 15, 16.
11. LeClerc JR: The diagnosis of venous thromboembolism during pregnancy and the postpartum period. In Greer IA, Turpie AGG, Forbes CD (eds): Haemostasis and Thrombosis. London, Chapman & Hall, 1992, p 267-303.
12. LeClerc JR, Hirsh J: Venous thromboembolic disorders. In Burrow GN, Ferris TF (eds): Medical Complications during Pregnancy, 3rd ed. Philadelphia, WB Saunders, 1988, pp 204-223.
13. Schmidt GA, Hall JB: Pulmonary disease. In Barron WM, Lindheimer MD (eds): Medical Disorders During Pregnancy. St. Louis, CV Mosby, 2000, pp 217-228.
14. Virchow R: Phlogose und Thrombose in Gefasssystem. In Virchow R (ed): Gesamelte Abhandlungen Zur Wissenschaflichen Medecin. Frankfurt, Von Medinger Sohn, 1856, pp 458-636.
15. Drill VA, Calhoun DW: Oral contraceptives and thromboembolic disease. JAMA 1968;206:77.
16. Wessler S, Gitel S: Thrombotic complications of oral contraceptives. In Colman RW, Hirsh J, Marder VJ, Salzman EW (eds): Hemostasis and Thrombosis. Philadelphia, JB Lippincott, 1987, p 1159.
17. Burrow G, Duffy TP (eds): Medical Complications of Pregnancy, 5th ed. Philadelphia, WB Saunders, 1999, p 100.
18. Barbour LA: Current concepts of anticoagulant therapy in pregnancy. Obstet Gynecol Clin North Am 1997;24:499.
19. Carter C, Gent M, LeClerc JR: The epidemiology of venous thrombosis. In Colman RW, Hirsh J, Marder VJ, Salzman EW (eds): Hemostasis and Thrombosis. Philadelphia, JB Lippincott, 1982, p 1190.
20. Witlin AG, Mattar FM, Saade GR, et al: Presentation of venous thromboembolism during pregnancy. Am J Obstet Gynecol 1999;181:1118.
21. Lagerstedt CI, Olsson CG, Fagher BO, et al: Need for long term anticoagulant treatment in symptomatic calf vein thrombosis. Lancet 1985;2:515.
22. Hull RD, Hirsh J, Carter C, et al: Diagnostic efficacy of impedance plethysmography for clinically suspected deep-vein thrombosis. Ann Intern Med 1985;102:21.
23. Anderson DR, Lensing AW, Wells PS, et al: Limitations of impedance plethysmography in the diagnosis of clinically suspected deep vein thrombosis. Ann Intern Med 1993;118:25.
24. Kearon C, Julian JA, Newman TE, Gusberg JS, et al: Noninvasive diagnosis of deep vein thrombosis. Ann Intern Med 1998;128:663.
25. Rutherford SE, Phelan JP: Deep venous thrombosis and pulmonary embolus. In Clark SL, Cotton DB, Hankins GDV, Phelan JP (eds): Critical Care Obstetrics. Boston, Blackwell, 1991, pp 150, 155-8, 159.
26. Spritzer CE: Magnetic resonance imaging of deep venous thrombosis in pregnant women with leg edema. Obstet Gynecol 1995;85:603.
27. Wheeler HB, Anderson FA Jr: Impedance plethysmography and DVT diagnosis [Letter]. Ann Intern Med 1993;119:246.
28. Tollefsen DM: Disorders of hemostasis. In Dunagan WC, Ridner ML (eds): Manual of Medical Therapeutics. Boston, Little, Brown, 1989, p 337.
29. Rosenow EC III, Osmundson PJ, Brown ML: Pulmonary embolism. Mayo Clin Proc 1981;56:161.
30. Wells PS, Anderson DR, Rodger M, et al: Derivation of a simple clinical model to categorize patients' probability of pulmonary embolism: Increasing the models' utility with the simpliRED D-dimer. Thromb Haemost 2000;83:416.
31. Brill-Edwards P, Ginsberg JS, Johnston M, Hirsh J: Establishing a therapeutic range for heparin therapy. Ann Intern Med 1993;119:104.
32. Hirsh J: Anticoagulants in venous thromboembolism. Clin Haematol 1990;3:691.
33. Chunilal SD, Young E, Johnston MA, et al: The APTT response of pregnant plasma to unfractionated heparin. Thromb Haemost 2002;87:92.
34. Edson JR, Krivit W, White JG: Kaolin partial thromboplastin time: High levels of procoagulants producing short clotting times or masking deficiencies of other procoagulants or low concentrations of anticoagulant. J Lab Clin Med 1967;70:463.
35. Poller L: Laboratory control of anticoagulant therapy. Semin Thromb Hemost 1986;12:13.
36. Greinacher A, Eckhardt T, Mussmann J, et al: Pregnancy complicated by heparin associated thrombocytopenia. Thromb Res 1993;71:123.
37. Hall JAG, Pauli RM, Wilson KM: Maternal and fetal sequelae of anticoagulation during pregnancy. Am J Med 1980;68:122.
38. Iturbe-Alessio I, Fonseca MC, Mutchinik O, et al: Risks of anticoagulant therapy in pregnant women with artificial heart valves. N Engl J Med 1986;315:390.
39. Duffy T: Hematologic aspects of pregnancy. In Hoffman R, Benz EJ, Shattil SJ, et al (eds): Hematology: Basic Principles and Practice. New York, Churchill Livingstone, 1991, p 1709.
40. Ginsberg JS: Fetal abnormalities and anticoagulants. In Greer IA, Turpie AGG, Forbes CD (eds): Haemostasis and Thrombosis. London, Chapman & Hall, 1992, p 361.
41. Ginsberg JS, Hirsh J: Use of anticoagulants during pregnancy. Chest 1989;95(Suppl):156S.
42. Dahlman TC: Osteoporotic fractures and the recurrence of thromboembolism during pregnancy and the puerperium in 184 women undergoing thromboprophylaxis with heparin. Am J Obstet Gynecol 1993;168:1265.
43. de Swiet M, Dorrington-Ward P, Fidler J, et al: Prolonged heparin therapy in pregnancy causes bone demineralization (heparin induced osteopenia). BJOG 1983;90:1129.
44. Griffiths HT, Liu DTY: Severe heparin osteoporosis in pregnancy. Postgrad Med J 1984;60:424.
45. Wise PH, Hall AJ: Heparin induced osteopenia in pregnancy. BMJ 1980;281:110.
46. Chan WS, Anand S, Ginsberg JG: Anticoagulation of pregnant women with mechanical heart valves. Arch Intern Med 2000;160:191.
47. Loscalzo J: Fibrinolytic therapy. In Beutler E, Lichtman MA, Coller BS, et al (eds): Williams Hematology, 6th ed. New York, McGraw-Hill, 2001, pp 1803-1811.
48. Turrentine MA, Braems G, Ramirez MA: Use of thrombolytics for the treatment of thromboembolic disease during pregnancy. Obstet Gynecol Surv 1995;50:534.
49. Grand A, Ghadban W, Perret SP, et al: Ilio-femoral thrombosis treated with tissue plasminogen activator in a pregnant woman. Ann Cardiol Angeiol (Paris) 1996;45:517.

50. Morrison AE, Walker IO, Black WP: Protein C deficiency presenting as deep venous thrombosis in pregnancy. Case report. BJOG 1988;95:1077.

51. Seligsohn U, Lubetsy A: Medical progress: Genetic susceptibility to venous thrombosis. N Engl J Med 2001;344:1222.

52. Vogel J, de Moerloose PA, Bounameaux H: Protein C deficiency and pregnancy: A case report. Obstet Gynecol 1989;73:455.

53. Winter JH, Fenech H, Ridler W, et al: Familial antithrombin III deficiency. Q J Med 1982;204:373.

54. Gallus AS: Anticoagulants in the prevention and treatment of thromboembolic problems in pregnancy including cardiac problems. In Greer IA, Turpie AGG, Forbes CD (eds): Haemostasis and Thrombosis. London, Chapman & Hall, 1992, pp 334-335.

55. Stamm H: Die thromboembolischen Erkrankungen. Fortschr Geb Gynakol 1969;39:8.

56. Friedrich PW, Sanson BJ, Simioni P, et al: Frequency of pregnancy-related venous thromboembolism in anticoagulant factor deficient women. Ann Intern Med 1996;125:955.

57. Trauscht-Van Horn JJ, Capeless EL, Easterling TR, Bovill EG: Pregnancy loss and thrombosis with protein C deficiency. Am J Obstet Gynecol 1992;167:968.

58. McColl MD, Walker ID, Freer IA: The role of inherited thrombophilia in venous thromboembolism associated with pregnancy. BJOG 1999;106:756.

59. Gerhardt A, Scharf RE, Zotz RB: Effect of hemostatic risk factors on the individual probability of thrombosis during pregnancy and the puerperium. Thromb Haemost 2003;90:77.

60. Toglia MR, Weg JG: Venous thromboembolism during pregnancy. N Engl J Med 1996;335:108.

61. Bokarewa MI, Bremme K, Blomback M: Arg^{506}-Gln mutation in factor V and risk of thrombosis during pregnancy. Br J Haematol 1996;92:473.

62. Thaler E, Lechner K: Antithrombin III deficiency and thromboembolism. Clin Haematol 1981;10:369.

63. De Stefano V, Leone G, DeCarolis S, et al: Management of pregnancy in women with antithrombin III congenital defect: Report of four cases. Thromb Haemost 1988;59:193.

64. Dizon-Townson D, Nelson LM, Jang H, et al: The incidence of factor V Leiden mutation in an obstetric population and its relationship to deep vein thrombosis. Am J Obstet Gynecol 1997;176:883.

65. Hallak M, Sanderowicz J, Cassel A, et al: Activated protein C resistance (factor V Leiden) associated with thrombosis in pregnancy. Am J Obstet Gynecol 1997;176:889.

66. Pabinger I, Schneider B: Thrombotic risk in hereditary antithrombin III, protein C, or protein S deficiency. Gesellschaft fur Thrombose—und Hamostaseforschung (GTH) Study Group on Natural Inhibitors. Arterioscler Thromb Vasc Biol 1996;16:742.

67. Miletich J, Sherman L, Broze G Jr: Absence of thrombosis in subjects with heterozygous protein C deficiency. N Engl J Med 1987;317:991.

68. Haverkate F, Samama M: Familial dysfibrinogenemia and thrombophilia. Thromb Haemost 1995;73:151.

69. Nilsson IM, Ljungner H, Tengborn L: Two different mechanisms in patients with venous thrombosis and defective fibrinolysis. BMJ 1985;18:1453.

70. Ballegeer V, Mombarts P, Declerk PJ, et al: Fibrinolytic response to venous occlusion and fibrin fragment D-dimer levels in normal and complicated pregnancy. Thromb Haemost 1987;58:1030.

71. Bonnar J, McNicol GP, Douglas AS: Fibrinolytic enzyme system and pregnancy. BMJ 1969;3:387.

72. Woodfield DG, Cole SK, Allan AGE, et al: Serum fibrin degradation products throughout normal pregnancy. BMJ 1968;4:665.

73. Many A, Pauzner R, Carp M: Treatment of patients with antiphospholipid antibodies during pregnancy. Am J Reprod Immunol 1992;28:216.

74. Lubbe WF, Butler WS: Acquired defects of coagulation—the lupus anticoagulant. In Greer IA, Turpie AGG, Forbes CD (eds): Haemostasis and Thrombosis. London, Chapman & Hall, 1992, p 392.

75. Hunt BJ, Khamashta MA: Management of the Hughes syndrome. Clin Exp Rheumatol 1996;14:115.

76. Malm J, Laurell M, Dahlback B, et al: Changes in the plasma levels of vitamin K dependent protein C and S and of C4b-binding protein during pregnancy and oral contraception. Br J Haematol 1988;68:437.

77. Gastineau DA, Kazimer KJ, Nichols WL, et al: Lupus anticoagulant: An analysis of clinical and laboratory features of 219 cases. Am J Hematol 1985;19:265.

78. Triplett DA, Brandt JT, Musgrave KA, Orr CA: The relationship between lupus anticoagulants and antibodies to phospholipid. JAMA 1988;259:550.

79. Mannucci PM, Canciani MT, Mari D, et al: The varied sensitivity of partial thromboplastin and prothrombin time reagents in the demonstration of the lupus like anticoagulant. Scand J Haematol 1979;22:423.

80. Infante-Rivard C, David H, Gauthier R, Rivard GE: Lupus anticoagulants, anticardiolipin antibodies, and fetal loss. A case control study. N Engl J Med 1991;325:1063.

81. Finazzi G, Brancaccio V, Moia M, et al: Natural history and risk factor for thrombosis in 360 patients with antiphospholipid antibodies: a four-year prospective study from the Italian Registry. Am J Med 1996;100:530.

82. Lubbe WF, Walker EB: Chorea gravidarum associated with circulating lupus anticoagulant: Successful outcome of pregnancy with prednisone and aspirin therapy. BJOG 1983;90:487.

83. Reece AE, Gabrielli, Cullen MF, et al: Recurrent adverse pregnancy outcome and antiphospholipid antibodies. Am J Obstet Gynecol 1990;163:162.

84. Lima F, Khamashta MA, Buchanan NMM, et al: A study of 60 pregnancies with the antiphospholipid syndrome. Clin Exp Rheumatol 1996;14:131.

85. Brenner B, Mandel H, Lanir N, et al: Activated protein C resistance can be associated with recurrent fetal loss. Br J Haematol 1997;97:551.

86. Kupferminc MJ, Eldor A, Steinman N, et al: Increased frequency of genetic thrombophilia in women with complications of pregnancy. N Engl J Med 1999;341:384.

87. Preston FE, Rosendaal FR, Walker ID, et al: Increased fetal loss in women with heritable thrombophilia. Lancet 1996;348:1734.

88. Rai R, Regan L, Hadley E, et al: Second trimester pregnancy loss is associated with activated protein C resistance. Br J Haematol 1996;92:489.

89. Therakan T, Baxi LV, Diuguid D: Protein S deficiency in pregnancy: A case report. Am J Obstet Gynecol 1993;168:141.

90. Brenner B: Thrombophilia and pregnancy. Clin Adv Hematol Oncol 2003;1:351.

91. Mudd SH, Skovby F, Levy HL, et al: The natural history of homocystinuria due to cystathionine β-synthase deficiency. Am J Hum Genet 1985;37:1.

92. Walters B, de Swiet M: Bone disease, disease of the parathyroid glands, and some other metabolic disorders. In de Swiet M (ed): Medical Disorders in Obstetric Practice. Oxford, UK, Blackwell Scientific, 1989, p 713.

93. Constantine G, Green A: Untreated homocystinuria: A maternal death in a woman with four pregnancies. BJOG 1987;94:803.

94. Lamon JM, Lenke RR, Levy HL, et al: Selected metabolic diseases. In Schulman JD, Simpson JL (eds): Genetic Diseases in Pregnancy. New York, Academic Press, 1981, pp 6-8.

95. Den Heijer M, Koster T, Blom HJ, et al: Hyperhomocysteinemia as a risk factor for deep vein thrombosis. N Engl J Med 1996;334:759.

96. Peng F, Triplett D, Barna L, Morrical D: Pulmonary embolism and premature labor in a patient with both factor V Leiden mutation and methylenetetrahydrofolate reductase gene C677T mutation. Thromb Res 1996;83:243.

97. Franken DG, Boers GHJ, Blom HJ, et al: Treatment of mild hyperhomocysteinemia in vascular disease patients. Arterioscler Thromb 1994;14:465.

98. McElin TW, LaPata RE, Westenfelder GO, et al: Postpartum ovarian vein thrombosis and microaerophilic streptococcal sepsis. Obstet Gynecol 1970;35:632.

99. Witlin A, Sibai BM: Postpartum ovarian vein thrombosis after vaginal delivery: A report of 11 cases. Obstet Gynecol 1995;85: 7757.

100. Malkamy H: Heparin therapy in postcesarean septic pelvic thrombophlebitis. Int J Gynaecol Obstet 1980;17:564.

101. Salomon O, Apter S, Shahan D, et al: Risk factors associated with postpartum ovarian vein thrombosis. Thromb Haemost 1999;82:1015.

102. Sanson B-J, Lensing AWA, Prins MH, et al: Safety of low molecular weight heparin in pregnancy: A systematic review. Thromb Haemost 1999;81:668.

103. Bahnson RR, Wendel EF, Vogelzang RL: Renal vein thrombosis following puerperal ovarian vein thrombophlebitis. Am J Obstet Gynecol 1985;152:290.

104. Weiner CP: Diagnosis and management of thromboembolic disease during pregnancy. Clin Obstet Gynecol 1985;28:107.

105. Brown CE, Stettler RW, Twickler D, et al: Puerperal septic pelvic thrombophlebitis: Incidence and response to heparin therapy. Am J Obstet Gynecol 1999;181:143.

106. Salomon D, Apter S, Shaham D, et al: Risk factors associated with postpartum ovarian vein thrombosis. Thromb Haemost 1999;82:1015.

107. Lanska DJ, Kryscio RJ: Risk factors for peripartum and postpartum stroke and intracranial venous thrombosis. Stroke 2000;31:1274.

108. Bousser MG, Chiras J, Bories J, et al: Cerebral venous thrombosis—a review of 38 cases. Stroke 1985;16:199.

109. Halpern JP, Morris JGL, Driscoll GL: Anticoagulants and cerebral venous thrombosis. Aust N Z J Med 1984;14:643.

110. Wiebers DO, Whisnant JP: The incidence of stroke among pregnant women in Rochester Minnesota 1955 through 1979. JAMA 1985;254:3055.

111. Arunkalaivanan AS, Barrington JW: Late puerperal sagittal sinus thrombosis associated with primary antiphospholipid antibody syndrome. J Obstet Gynecol 2002;22:682.

112. Burneo JG, Elias SB, Barkley GL: Cerebral venous thrombosis due to protein S deficiency in pregnancy. Lancet 2002;359:892.

113. Galan HL, McDowell AB, Johnson PR, et al: Puerperal cerebral venous thrombosis associated with decreased free protein S. J Reprod Med 1995;40:859.

114. Gokcil Z, Odabasi Z, Vural O, et al: Cerebral venous thrombosis in pregnancy: The role of protein S deficiency. Acta Neurol Belg 1998;98:36.

115. Martinelli I, Landi G, Merati G, et al: Factor V gene mutation is a risk factor for cerebral venous thrombosis. Thromb Haemost 1996;75:373.

116. Wechsler B, Genereau T, Biousse V, et al: Pregnancy complicated by cerebral venous thrombosis in Behçet's disease. Am J Obstet Gynecol 1995;173:1627.

117. Curvers J, Nap AW, Thomasson MC, et al: Effect of in-vitro fertilization treatment and subsequent pregnancy on the protein C pathway. Br J Haematol 2001;115:400.

118. Aurousseau MH, Samama MU, Belhassen A, et al: Risk of thromboembolism in relation to an in-vitro fertilization programme: Three case reports. Hum Reprod 1995;10:94.

119. Hignett M, Spence JE, Claman P: Internal jugular vein thrombosis: A late complication of ovarian hyperstimulation syndrome despite mini-dose heparin prophylaxis. Hum Reprod 1995;10:3121.

120. Ellis MH, Nun IB, Rathaus V, et al: Internal jugular vein thrombosis in patients with ovarian hyperstimulation syndrome. Fertil Steril 1998;69:140.

121. Kligman I, Noyes N, Benadiva CA, Rosenwaks Z: Massive deep vein thrombosis in a patient with antithrombin III deficiency in a patient undergoing ovarian stimulation for in vitro fertilization. Fertil Steril 1995;63:673.

122. Hellgren M, Blomback M: Studies on blood coagulation and fibrinolysis in pregnancy, during delivery and in the puerperium. I: Normal condition. Gynecol Obstet Invest 1981;12:141.

123. Stirling Y, Woolf I, North WRS, et al: Haemostasis in normal pregnancy. Thromb Haemost 1984;52:176.

124. Beller FK, Ebert C: The coagulation and fibrinolytic enzyme system in normal pregnancy and the puerperium. Eur J Obstet Gynaecol Reprod Biol 1982;13:177.

125. Inglis TCM, Stuart J, George AJ, et al: Haemostatic and rheological changes in normal pregnancy and pre-eclampsia. Br J Haematol 1982;50:461.

126. Scholtes MCW, Gerretsen G, Haak HL: The factor VIII ratio in normal and pathological pregnancies. Eur J Obstet Gynaecol Reprod Biol 1983;16:89.

127. Bellart J, Gilabert R, Fontcuberta J, et al: Fibrinolysis changes in normal pregnancy. J Prenat Med 1997;25:368.

128. Lecander I, Astedt B: Isolation of a new specific plasminogen activator inhibitor from pregnancy plasma. Br J Haematol 1986;62:221.

129. Nilsson IM, Felding P, Lecander I, et al: Different types of plasminogen activator inhibitors in plasma and platelets in pregnant women. Br J Haematol 1986;62:215.

130. Booth N, Reith A, Bennalt B, et al: A plasminogen activator inhibitor (PAI-2) circulates in two molecular forms in pregnancy. Thromb Haemost 1988;59:77.

131. Thorburn J, Drummond MM, Whigham KA, et al: Blood viscosity and haemostatic factors in late pregnancy, pre-eclampsia, and fetal growth retardation. BJOG 1982;89:117.

132. Bellart J, Gilabert R, Miralles RM, et al: Endothelial cell markers and fibrinopeptide A to D-dimer ratio as a measure of coagulation and fibrinolysis balance in normal pregnancy. Gynecol Obstet Invest 1998;46:17.

133. Chabloz O, Reber G, Boehlen F, et al: TAFI antigen and D-dimer levels during normal pregnancy and at delivery. Br J Haematol 2001;115:150.

134. Francalanci L, Comeglio P, Alessandro-Liotta A, et al: D-dimer plasma levels during normal pregnancy measured by specific ELISA. Int J Clin Lab Res 1997;27:65.

135. Choi JW, Pai SH: Tissue plasminogen activator levels change with plasma fibrinogen concentrations during pregnancy. Ann Hematol 2002;81:611.

136. Clark P, Brennand J, Conkie JA, et al: Activated protein C sensitivity, protein C, protein S and coagulation in normal pregnancy. Thromb Haemost 1998;79:1166.

137. Kjellberg U, Andersson NE, Rosen S, et al: APC resistance and other hemostatic variables during pregnancy and the puerperium. Thromb Haemost 1999;81:527.

138. Alving BM, Comp PC: Recent advances in understanding clotting and evaluating patients with recurrent thrombosis. Am J Obstet Gynecol 1992;167:1184.

139. Comp PC, Thurman GR, Welsh J et al: Functional and immunologic protein S levels are decreased during pregnancy. Blood 1986;68:881.

140. Lefkowitz JB, Clark SH, Barbour LA: Comparison of protein S functional and antigenic assays in normal pregnancy. Am J Obstet Gynecol 1996;175:657.

141. Oruc S, Saruc M, Koyuncu, et al: Changes in the plasma activities of protein C and S during pregnancy. Aust N Z J Obstet Gynaecol 2000;40:448.

142. Boehlen F, Hohlfeld P, Extermann P, et al: Platelet count at term in pregnancy: A reappraisal of the threshold. Obstet Gynecol 2000;95:29.

143. Cerneca F, Ricci G, Simeone R, et al: Coagulation and fibrinolysis changes in pregnancy. Increased levels of procoagulants and reduced levels of inhibitors during pregnancy induce a reactive fibrinolysis. Eur J Obstet Gynaecol Reprod Biol 1997;73:31.

144. Shimano S, Kurosu T, Hayama K, et al: Differences of IgG and IgM antibodies to phospholipids and APTT among non-pregnant and pregnant women. J Obstet Gynecol Res 1998;24:299.

145. Hayashi M, Inoue T, Hoshimoto K, et al: The levels of five markers of hemostasis and endothelial status at different stages of normotensive pregnancy. Acta Obstet Gynecol Scand 2002;81:208.

146. Mannucci PM, Vigano S, Bottasso B, et al: Protein C antigen during pregnancy, delivery, and the puerperium. Thromb Haemostas 1984;52:217.

147. Persson BL, Steinberg P, Holmberg L, et al: Transaminating enzymes in maternal plasma and placenta in human pregnancies complicated by intrauterine growth retardation. J Dev Physiol 1980;2:37.

148. Weiner CP, Brandt J: Plasma antithrombin III activity in normal pregnancy. Obstet Gynecol 1980;56:601.

149. Kearon C, Crowther M, Hirsh J: Management of patients with hereditary hypercoagulable disorders. Annu Rev Med 2000;51:169.

150. Rosene-Montella K, Barbour LA: Thromboembolic disease and hypercoagulable states. In Lee RV, Rosene-Montella K, Barbour LA, et al (eds): Medical Care of the Pregnant Patient. Philadelphia, American College of Physicians, 2000, pp 423-448.

151. Gherman RB, Goodwin TM, Leung B, et al: Incidence, clinical characteristics, and timing of objectively diagnosed venous thromboembolism during pregnancy. Obstet Gynecol 1999;94:730.

152. Simpson EL, Lawrenson RA, Nightingale AL, Farmer RD: Venous thromboembolism in pregnancy and the puerperium: Incidence and additional risk factors from a London perinatal database. BJOG 2001;108:56.

153. Soomro RM, Bucur IJ, Noorani S: Cumulative incidence of venous thromboembolism during pregnancy and puerperium: A hospital based study. Angiology 2002;53:429.

154. Bergqvist A, Bergqvist D, Hallbrook T: Acute deep venous thrombosis after caesarian section. Acta Obstet Gynecol Scand 1979;58:473.
155. Bergqvist A, Bergqvist D, Hallbrook T: Deep venous thrombosis during pregnancy. Acta Obstet Gynecol Scand 1983;62:443.
156. Kierkegaard A: Incidence and diagnosis of deep vein thrombosis associated with pregnancy. Acta Obstet Gynecol Scand 1983;62:239.
157. Andersen BS, Steffensen FH, Sorensen HT, et al: The cumulative incidence of venous thrombosis during pregnancy and puerperium—an 11-year Danish population based study of 63,300 pregnancies. Acta Obstet Gynecol Scand 1998;77:170.
158. Tan JY: Thrombophilia in pregnancy. Ann Acad Med Singapore 2002;31:328.
159. Gillis S, Shushan A, Eldor A: Use of low molecular weight heparin for prophylaxis and treatment of thromboembolism in pregnancy. Int J Gynaecol Obstet 1992;39:297.
160. Melissari E, Parker CJ, Wilson HV, et al: Use of low molecular weight heparin in pregnancy. Thromb Hemost 1992;68:652.
161. Rasmussen C, Wadt J, Jacobsen B: Thromboembolic prophylaxis with low molecular weight heparin during pregnancy. Int J Gynaecol Obstet 1994;47:121.
162. Sturridge F, de Swiet M, Letsky E: The use of low molecular weight heparin for thromboprophylaxis in pregnancy. BJOG 1994;101:69.
163. Boda Z, Laszlo P, Rejto L, et al: LMWH vs thromboprophylaxis during the whole period of pregnancy [Letter]. Thromb Haemost 1996;76:124.
164. Lee LH, Liauw PCY, Ng ASH: Low molecular weight heparin for thromboprophylaxis during pregnancy in two patients with mechanical mitral valve replacement. Thromb Haemost 1996;76:628.
165. Daskalaskis G, Antsaklis A, Papageorgion I, Michalas S: Thrombosis prophylaxis after treatment during pregnancy. Eur J Obstet Gynaecol 1997;74:165.
166. Hunt BJ, Doughty HA, Majumdar G, et al: Thromboprophylaxis with low molecular weight heparin (Fragmin) in high risk pregnancies. Thromb Haemost 1997;77:39.
167. Thomson AJ, Walker ID, Greer IA: Low molecular weight heparin for immediate management of thromboembolic disease in pregnancy. Lancet 1998;352:1904.
168. Ensom MH, Stephenson MD: Low molecular weight heparins in pregnancy. Pharmacotherapy 1999;19:1013.
169. Ellison J, Walker ID, Green IA: Antenatal use of enoxaparin for prevention and treatment of thromboembolism in pregnancy. Int J Gynaecol Obstet 2000;107:1116.

PREGNANCY AND CARDIOVASCULAR DISEASE

John F. Setaro and Teresa Caulin-Glaser

GENERAL CONSIDERATIONS

Cardiovascular disease in women affects 1% of all pregnancies, and it remains the major cause of nonobstetric maternal mortality in the United States.[1] Despite key advances in the diagnosis and management of circulatory diseases in pregnancy since 1980, this field continues to pose great challenges as three broad trends converge. First, successful treatment of congenital heart disease has created a new population of clinically complex patients who are able to reach childbearing age. Second, there is an increasing trend toward pregnancies in older women who are susceptible to heart diseases acquired in adulthood. Third, immigration from underdeveloped nations has reacquainted Western medicine with a cohort of young childbearing patients who have rheumatic heart disease.

Although maternal death during pregnancy in women with cardiovascular disease is uncommon, pregnant women are at significant risk for complications, including congestive heart failure, arrhythmias, and stroke.[2] Even in the context of comprehensive prenatal care, pregnancy in women with cardiovascular disease is associated with significant cardiac and neonatal consequences. Independent predictors of maternal cardiac complications include cyanosis, poor functional class, left ventricular outflow obstruction, arrhythmias, left ventricular systolic dysfunction, and prior cardiac events.[2]

Pregnancy is associated with major alterations in circulatory physiology. These changes, which occur throughout pregnancy, are necessary for the healthy growth and development of the fetus. The pregnant woman is in a hyperdynamic and volume-overloaded state as a result of these physiologic transformations, which increases demand on the cardiovascular system. In normal women, the cardiac reserve is sufficient to accommodate an increase in workload. However, women with underlying cardiovascular disease may already be compromised hemodynamically or at least marginally compensated; with the additional hemodynamic burden of pregnancy, there may be significant risk to the mother, the fetus, or both. Poor functional status and cyanosis are linked strongly to maternal and fetal complications. Therefore, pregnancy may exacerbate the underlying disease, increasing the risk of morbidity and mortality.

In the Western world, delayed childbearing has emerged as a risk factor for maternal morbidity and mortality, as well as a greater incidence of genetic abnormalities in the fetus. Women older than 35 years have a maternal death rate five times higher than that in women younger than 34 years. Parity tends to increase with age and both magnify the degree of risk. A woman aged 35 years or older who is also a primigravida has a 20-fold greater risk than does a woman who is 34 years of age or younger and multiparous. There is a need for redefinition of preconception/early pregnancy risk stratification in the older woman to include full and careful cardiovascular risk assessment.[3-7] The rate of mortality from cardiovascular events is reported to be higher than that from abortion, genital sepsis, and hemorrhage (Fig. 6–1).[8] Women older than 40 years are at enhanced risk for more frequent antepartum complications, need for cesarean section, preeclampsia, and placenta previa.[3] Age alone is a major risk factor for maternal death.[9] Advanced maternal age implies increased vulnerability to diseases known to complicate pregnancy, such as diabetes mellitus and hypertension. Infants of women with gestational hypertension and chronic hypertension tend to have worse perinatal outcomes, such as low birth weight, preterm birth, diseases of prematurity, and death, than do infants of normotensive women.[10] The presence of cardiovascular risk factors such as smoking, hyperlipidemia, obesity, and sedentary lifestyle may amplify the risk of morbidity and mortality in both mothers and infants when childbearing is delayed. Maternal smoking during pregnancy is associated with premature birth, decreased head circumference, stillbirth, intrauterine growth restriction, and neonatal death.[11] Obesity during pregnancy heightens tendencies for hypertension and cardiac dysfunction. In comparison with women of normal weight, there is a significant increase in pregnancy-induced hypertension in obese patients.

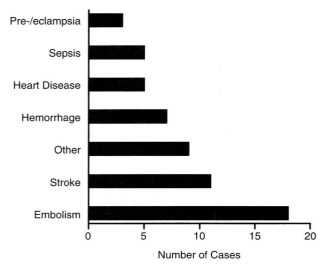

Figure 6–1. Maternal deaths, direct and indirect, in Sweden, 1980-1988 (N = 59). (From Hogberg U, Innala E, Sandstrom A, et al: Maternal mortality in Sweden, 1980-1988. Obstet Gynecol 84:240-244, 1994. Reprinted with permission from the American College of Obstetricians and Gynecologists.)

When pregnancy is considered, weight management should be addressed in women older than 40 years, as well as in those with congenital cardiac disorders.[12]

Management of the patient with a complex medical profile ideally begins before pregnancy with clear delineation of the cardiac abnormality, the safety of pregnancy to the mother and the fetus, and the advisability of becoming pregnant (Table 6–1). Comprehensive evaluation and management of patients best serves this objective. The team of caregivers should clearly understand the cardiovascular disease process as well as the physiologic changes anticipated as pregnancy progresses. This team optimally includes the general obstetrician, a specialist in

TABLE 6–1 High-Risk Factors for Maternal and/or Fetal Morbidity and Mortality

Cyanotic heart disease
Eisenmenger's syndrome and/or severe pulmonary hypertension
Severe aortic stenosis
Mitral regurgitation or aortic regurgitation with NYHA class III or
    IV symptoms
Valve disease resulting in severe pulmonary hypertension
    (pulmonary pressure >75% of systemic pressure)
Valve disease with severe left ventricular dysfunction
    (left ventricular ejection fraction < .40)
Mechanical prosthetic valve necessitating warfarin therapy
Aortic regurgitation or aortic involvement in
    Marfan's syndrome
Aortic coarctation with valvular involvement
Left ventricular dysfunction with NYHA class III or
    IV symptoms

Adapted from Guidlines for the management of patients with valvular heart disease. J Am Coll Cardiol 1998;32:1486-1588.
NYHA, New York Heart Association.

Maternal-Fetal Medicine, a cardiologist, and an anesthesiologist. Pregnancy-related morbidity and mortality for the mother and the fetus should be clearly and frankly addressed with the patient. The requirements during the pregnancy for the safe and healthy delivery of both mother and fetus should be outlined. These elements may have implications for diet, activity, medication, or intervention/surgery. In addition, patients with congenital cardiovascular abnormalities need genetic counseling for discussion of possible transmission of their conditions to the fetus. In general, there may be a 5% to 10% inheritance risk for the fetus, in the absence of other additional risk factors or syndromes. Fetal echocardiography should be performed at 18 to 20 weeks of gestation.[13]

HEMODYNAMIC ALTERATIONS IN NORMAL PREGNANCY

Pregnancy is associated with physiologic changes that increase the hemodynamic burden on the cardiovascular system. The care team must understand that these changes place pregnant women with cardiovascular disease at risk for complications during the pregnancy, labor, and the puerperium.

The arterial blood pressure of the pregnant woman is influenced by position. Brachial artery pressure varies from sitting to lying in the lateral recumbent supine position. The arterial pressure is lowest at midpregnancy. Diastolic blood pressure decreases to a greater extent than does systolic pressure. The upper extremity venous pressure remains unchanged during pregnancy, but blood flow in the lower extremities is impaired except when the patient is in the lateral recumbent position. This finding is most notable during the third trimester and is attributed to occlusion of the pelvic veins and of the inferior vena cava by the uterus. The consequence of this impedance to blood flow is the development of dependent edema and varicose veins.[14,15]

Normal pregnancy is not associated with significant changes in the electrocardiogram (ECG). There may be a sinus tachycardia, and the electrical axis deviates to the left because of the altered position of the heart. The diaphragm is elevated with increased uterine size and displaces the heart upward to the left with a slight rotation on the long axis. On chest radiographs, the cardiac silhouette appears larger than in the nonpregnant state because of the development of hemodynamically insignificant pericardial effusions.[16]

Auscultation of the heart may also elicit altered findings during pregnancy. In a study of 50 normal pregnant women undergoing phonocardiography at different stages of pregnancy, a systolic flow murmur was demonstrated in more than 90% of the women.[17] The majority of murmurs disappeared after delivery. However, a systolic murmur graded as greater than II/VI warrants further evaluation. The investigators also documented an increase in intensity and widened splitting of the first heart sound, because of increased contractility, and the presence of a third heart sound. A fourth heart sound is not normal. An increase in blood flow in the mammary vessels in late pregnancy may result in a continuous murmur over the breasts, often termed a *mammary souffle.*

Cardiac output measured in the lateral recumbent position increases by 30% to 50% with pregnancy.[18,19] Augmentation of cardiac output is a result of an increase in stroke volume and heart rate. Heart rate levels at term are 10% to 20% higher than those observed before pregnancy. The heart rate continues to rise throughout pregnancy. The stroke volume returns to prepregnancy levels by the end of pregnancy. Falling systemic vascular resistance and blood pressure also influence the cardiac output. The systolic blood pressure decreases slightly, whereas there is a more significant decline in the diastolic pressure. Blood pressure returns to prepregnancy levels at approximately 20 weeks of pregnancy. The systemic vascular resistance falls during the first and early second trimesters and slowly returns to prepregnancy levels after delivery. The rise in cardiac output commences in the first trimester and continues during the second and third trimesters.[20,21] The maximization of cardiac output when measured in the lateral recumbent position is most notable during the last trimester, when the gravid uterus in the supine position impedes venous return to the heart (Fig. 6–2). Studies have shown a reduction in cardiac output by 0.6 L per minute in the supine position.[22,23] It is uncommon for significant hypotension and bradycardia to develop because of position, but these may be relieved if the woman assumes the lateral recumbent position.

The initiation of labor promotes additional changes in the cardiovascular system. The sympathetic nervous system is stimulated by pain and anxiety, leading to a further increase in cardiac output of approximately 10% to 15%. Each contraction of the uterus forces an autotransfusion of 300 to 500 mL of blood into the central venous system. The total augmented cardiac output is therefore nearly 50% higher than that observed during the pregnancy.[24,25] Cardiac output is also affected by any type of anesthesia used during the delivery. Epidural anesthesia is associated with an increase of only 40% in cardiac output, and general anesthesia, which is rarely recommended, with an augmentation of only 25%.[25,26] In the postpartum period, there are further increases in cardiac output because of decreased colloid osmotic pressure, maternal blood volume redistribution, and the decompression of the central venous system with delivery of the fetus and placenta. The cardiac output can increase to 80% of the value before vaginal delivery. The increase is somewhat less with cesarean section: approximately 50%.[27] A report of more than 500 pregnant women with cardiovascular disease documented 10 maternal deaths, 8 of which occurred during the puerperium.[28] Such findings emphasize the importance of close observation and management after delivery.

In pregnancy, there is an increase in blood volume and ventricular volume (Fig. 6–3). There is, however, significant individual variation in the observed volume expansion, ranging from 40% to 45% of the prepregnancy volume state.[29-31] The degree of expansion is quite variable. Maternal blood volume begins to rise at 6 weeks of pregnancy and reaches a maximum by the end of the second trimester. During pregnancy, both water and sodium are retained.

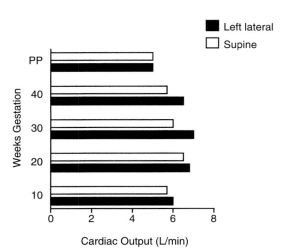

Figure 6–2. Cardiac output measured in the left lateral and supine position during uncomplicated pregnancies. pp, post partum. (Data from Capeless EL, Clapp JF: Cardiovascular changes in early phases of pregnancy. Am J Obstet Gynecol 1989;161:1449; Ueland K, Hansen JM: Maternal cardiovascular dynamics. 2: Posture and uterine contractions. Am J Obstet Gynecol 1969;103:1; and Robson SC, Hunter S, Boys RJ, Dunlop W: Serial study of factors influencing changes in cardiac output during human pregnancy. Am J Physiol 1989;256:H1060.)

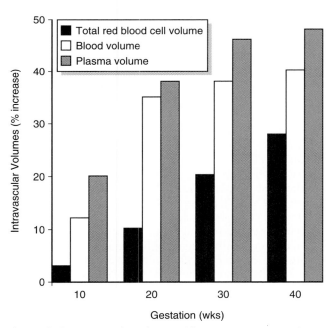

Figure 6–3. Intravascular volumes with pregnancy. At term there is a 50% increase in plasma volume and a 25% increase in total red cell volume, resulting in a 40% increase in total blood volume. (Data from Whittaker PG, MacPhail S, Lind T: Serial hematologic changes and pregnancy outcome. Obstet Gynecol 1996;88:33; Pritchard JA: Changes in the blood volume during pregnancy and delivery. Anesthesiology 1965;26:393; and Chesley LC: Plasma and red cell volumes during pregnancy. Am J Obstet Gynecol 1972;112:440.)

Total body water has the potential to increase by 6 to 8 L in association with the retention of 500 to 900 mEq of sodium. This fluid exists primarily in the extracellular space.[32,33] The amplification in blood volume is caused by an increase in red blood cells and plasma. Plasma volume increases to a much greater extent than does the total red blood cell volume. Plasma volume increases in singleton and twin pregnancies by 50% and 70%, respectively. Red blood cell volume increases by approximately 33% at the end of pregnancy.[34] Greater erythrocyte production results in erythroid hyperplasia with a mildly elevated reticulocyte count during pregnancy.[35] Despite this increase in erythropoiesis, the erythrocyte concentration and the hematocrit decrease during pregnancy in the setting of an even greater increase in plasma volume. A relative anemia results, with hemoglobin levels in the range of 11 to 13 mg/dL. A hemoglobin level below 11 mg/dL in the latter stages of pregnancy should be considered not a normal volume-related finding but rather a signal of iron deficiency.[36] Iron demands of pregnancy are not fully met from iron absorbed from the diet and mobilized from body stores. Several studies have supported the use of iron supplementation during pregnancy, proven to elevate hemoglobin concentration and to improve oxygen-carrying capacity of blood.[37,38] The enlargement in total volume peaks during the third trimester and declines minimally until delivery. The changes in blood volume are regulated by hormonal fluxes associated with pregnancy. Rising placental estrogen is associated with sodium retention via the renin-angiotensin-aldosterone system, thereby increasing plasma volume. Augmented progesterone, prolactin, and placenta somatomammotropin release are associated with the increase in erythropoiesis.[39]

Related to blood volume expansion is a minimal increase in left ventricular end-diastolic volume, as assessed echocardiographically by Katz and colleagues.[40] This study revealed that both left ventricular wall mass and end-diastolic dimension increases with pregnancy. The change in stroke volume was found to be directly proportional to end-diastolic volume. The stroke volume rises by 20% to 25%, with the ejection fraction remaining constant. Therefore, cardiac changes occur during pregnancy to adjust to the new hemodynamic demands of the mother and fetus. Myocardial mass increases by approximately 10% to 15%, and remodeling occurs. Several echocardiographic studies disclose that normal pregnancy is associated with a reversible fall in contractility. Left ventricular hypertrophy and atrophy occur and are linked to changes in the hemodynamic load associated with pregnancy.[41] Other investigators have shown that these changes are not cumulative with multiparity, which implies that the cardiovascular system is capable of adapting to multiple episodes of volume overload during pregnancies without permanent structural or functional alterations.[42] Multiple pregnancies are associated with higher cardiac output as a result of an increase in inotropy.[43] The increased demand resulting from augmented heart rate and inotropy suggests a decrease in cardiac reserve.

Clark and colleagues[44] reported right-sided heart catheterization data, collected during the third trimester and repeated 11 to 13 weeks post partum in 10 women, thus illustrating the following normal pregnancy-related hemodynamic parameters. There was a 43% increase in cardiac output, a 17% increase in heart rate, a 21% decrease in systemic vascular resistance, and a 34% decrease in pulmonary vascular resistance (Table 6-2). There was no change in the mean arterial pressure, pulmonary capillary wedge pressure, central venous pressure, or left ventricular stroke work index.

At delivery and during the postpartum period in the normal patient, large quantities of fluid are rapidly mobilized, with a consequent major diuresis. In the patient who has cardiovascular disease, such a fluid load may pose a significant challenge. It is imperative that all caregivers of women with cardiovascular disease appreciate the risk for the development of cardiac failure at all stages of pregnancy, labor, delivery, and the puerperium.

ROLE OF MATERNAL EXERCISE

Several studies have addressed the effects of exercise during pregnancy on maternal and fetal outcome, spontaneous abortion, birth weight, and labor. Overall, pregnancy is not a contraindication to exercise.[45,46] The American College of Obstetricians and Gynecologists suggests that women who have participated in aerobic exercise before becoming pregnant may continue to exercise during pregnancy.[47] A woman's overall health, in regard to both obstetric and medical risks, should be evaluated before an exercise program is prescribed. Each activity should be reviewed individually for its potential risk. Sports with a high risk of abdominal trauma should be avoided.[47] For the inactive woman, the recommended exercise would be walking. Several investigators have documented fetal bradycardia in association with maximal maternal exercise (heart rate >180 beats/minute) but not with submaximal exercise (heart rate <150 beats/minute).[48] Clapp, however, showed an improved metabolic efficiency with exercise in conditioned walking. For women without heart disease, the recommendation is to walk or participate in aerobic exercise for up to 30 minutes per day.[49] These investigators proved that aerobic exercise at 50% to 85% of maximum capacity had diverse beneficial effects: decrease in the length of labor, fewer cesarean sections, and decreased fetal distress, without an increase in spontaneous abortions. The investigators did note a decrease in fetal birth weight secondary to a decrease in fat mass, a finding of uncertain relevance.[49-52]

TABLE 6-2 Hemodynamic Changes with Pregnancy*	
Cardiac output	↑ 43%
Systemic vascular resistance	↓ 21%
Pulmonary vascular resistance	↓ 34%
Heart rate	↑ 17%
Stroke index	↑ 17%
Mean arterial pressure	↓ 4%
Osmotic pressure	↓ 14%

Adapted from Clark SL, Cotton DB, Lee W, et al: Central hemodynamic assessment of normal term pregnancy. Am J Obstet Gynecol 1989;161:1439.
*Central hemodynamic changes in 10 normal pregnant women between 35 and 38 weeks of pregnancy. Measurements were performed in patients in the lateral position.
↑, increased; ↓, decreased.

Fetal growth has actually been shown to increase in moderately trained women in comparison with well-trained women. During exercise, there may be a small increase in fetal heart rate (5 to 25 beats per minute), possibly related to stimulation from the maternal vasoactive hormones, training-induced uterine contractions, or, less likely, a reduction in oxygen delivery.[53] Women who have underlying cardiovascular disease, hypertension, multiple pregnancies, or complications during pregnancy should not initiate new exercise programs during the pregnancy.

CARDIOVASCULAR DIAGNOSIS

Normal pregnant women experience many symptoms that can be suggestive of heart disease. Shortness of breath, palpitations, fatigue, and peripheral edema all may appear during normal pregnancy. Although the diagnosis of cardiovascular disease may be known before conception, the hemodynamic changes associated with the pregnancy often catalyze the first symptoms and signs. Table 6–3 lists symptoms and physical findings that may signal the presence of cardiovascular disease.[54] Documenting the history and physical examination during pregnancy may be difficult, and further diagnostic testing is typically indicated to determine the presence or severity of cardiovascular disease. Most diagnostic tests are safe and noninvasive. In general, radiographic and radionuclide studies are avoided, especially during the first trimester.

Chest radiography is occasionally indicated for the evaluation of both cardiac size and pulmonary vessels. Fetal radiation exposure is extremely small (0.07 mrad) and is below the level of acceptable risk for any gestational age.[55] Lead apron shielding should be used with all studies, although internal scatter renders this method only partly preventive. Electrocardiography is associated with nonspecific ST segment alterations as well as a 15-degree leftward axis deviation in a normal pregnancy. Increased premature ventricular and atrial contractions are commonly noted.

TABLE 6–3   Indicators of Cardiovascular Disease with Pregnancy

Signs
Digital clubbing
Cyanosis
Persistent jugular venous distention
Systolic murmur equal to or greater than grade 3/6
Cardiomegaly
Pulmonary hypertension indicated by increased P_2 and left parasternal lift
Persistent arrhythmia
Diastolic murmur
Persistent splitting of S_2

Symptoms
Chest pain with exertion or stress
Syncope
Hemoptysis
Progressive orthopnea
Progressive dyspnea
Paroxysmal nocturnal dyspnea

Reports have also suggested that inferior ST segment depression is relatively frequent during pregnancy.[56] If significant arrhythmia is suspected, Holter or event monitoring is recommended.

Echocardiography is a widely used and safe procedure during pregnancy. It provides both structural and functional information about the heart. However, it is not indicated unless cardiovascular disease or abnormalities are suspected. The study should be performed and interpreted only by well-trained specialists because normal pregnancy-induced changes such as increased left atrial size, physiologic pericardial effusions, or tricuspid regurgitation may be misinterpreted as abnormal.[57]

Cardiac catheterization, because of radiation and contrast exposure, is avoided if possible during pregnancy. There are situations, however, in which the benefits of the procedure outweigh the risks.

Radionuclide examinations are not recommended in pregnant women. Studies have demonstrated that some isotopes, even those bound to albumin, can cross the placenta and reach the fetal circulation.[58]

DISEASES OF THE MYOCARDIUM

Dilated Cardiomyopathy

The manifestation of cardiomyopathy during pregnancy is reflected in signs and symptoms of congestive heart failure. Symptoms include chest discomfort, dyspnea, paroxysmal nocturnal dyspnea, and cough.[59] Echocardiography is useful for demonstrating chamber enlargement and depressed ventricular function. The cause of cardiomyopathy may be myocarditis, toxins, or idiopathic.[60,61] In severe cases manifested by advanced clinical heart failure, maternal outcomes may be quite poor.[62,63]

Treatment consists of limitation in activity and sodium intake during pregnancy. Anemia, infection, and fever all magnify the physiologic effects of left ventricular dysfunction and should be treated vigorously. Reasonable measures include careful use of diuretics, while monitoring closely for hypokalemia, as well as the initiation of digoxin for inotropic support and hydralazine as an afterload-reducing agent. Anticoagulation therapy with heparin may be indicated if left ventricular dysfunction is severe. The use of angiotensin-converting enzyme inhibitors or angiotensin receptor blockers should be avoided. The prognosis of idiopathic cardiomyopathy is poor; definitive therapy for patients with end-stage heart failure is cardiac transplantation.[64,65]

Peripartum Cardiomyopathy

Peripartum cardiomyopathy is a rare disorder of unknown origin that is seen in late pregnancy or in the early puerperium, technically defined as the last month of pregnancy and the first five months post partum. Estimates of incidence vary from 1 in 1300 to 1 in 15,000 pregnancies.[66] Diagnosis is confined to a narrow time period and requires echocardiographic evidence of left ventricular systolic dysfunction.[67] The mortality rate associated with the disease in the United States is reported to be 25% to 50%.[68] Deaths from peripartum cardiomyopathy are caused by progressive congestive heart failure, arrhythmias, and thromboembolic events. The disease was first described in 1849 but was not well characterized until the early 1970s, when diagnostic criteria were developed by Demakis and colleagues.[66] According to epidemiologic studies, the disease occurs most frequently in multiparous women, in women older than 30 years, and in black women. In addition, it is associated with a history of hypertension, preeclampsia, cesarean section, and multiple pregnancies.[69]

Investigations suggest that the development of cardiomyopathy during the gestational period is associated with a greater frequency of disease regression. Fifty percent of affected patients are reported to regain normal cardiac function 6 to 12 months after the diagnosis. A report by Witlin and colleagues, however, demonstrated a much worse prognosis: 92.9% of patients had persistent or progressive disease.[70] Most studies suggest that improvement in and recovery of cardiac function should occur within 6 months of diagnosis. Patients who recover left ventricular function have a markedly improved survival rate.[71] Women with persistent left ventricular dysfunction are at high risk for additional morbidity and mortality with subsequent pregnancies.[72] The risk with repeated pregnancy in women who had peripartum cardiomyopathy but who regained left ventricular function remains controversial. However, a study of subsequent pregnancies in women who had peripartum cardiomyopathy with later normalization of left ventricular function showed an average 20% decrease in left ventricular function in 21% of the women with subsequent pregnancies. In addition, 21% of the women developed symptoms of heart failure. In 25% of the women who had persistent left ventricular dysfunction caused by peripartum cardiomyopathy, subsequent pregnancies were associated with an additional decrease of more than 20% in systolic function. Symptoms of heart failure occurred in 44% of the women, and the mortality rate was 19%.[73]

A small series describes a good outlook for subsequent pregnancies in patients whose left ventricular contractility improved after peripartum cardiomyopathy.[74] Treatment should be the same as described for dilated cardiomyopathy. Heart transplantation has been performed and prognosis has thereby improved; however, there is a higher frequency of rejection than in other cardiac transplant recipients. Immunosuppressive therapy has been used successfully in only a small number of patients.[75,76]

Hypertrophic Cardiomyopathy

Cardiomyopathies that are characterized as hypertrophic may have various causes. The optimal management and prognosis for many of these conditions are unclear. Hypovolemia or increased left ventricular contractility may increase outflow obstruction and must be avoided during pregnancy. Arrhythmias are frequently a complication of these disorders, and β-adrenergic blocker therapy may be beneficial. The use of spinal and epidural anesthetics is associated with vasodilation and should be avoided during labor and delivery.

RHYTHM DISORDERS

Palpitations, presyncope, and dizziness are frequent symptoms during pregnancy and often lead to referral for cardiac evaluation. Reports are conflicting as to whether there is an increase in incidence of arrhythmia with pregnancy or whether patients are more closely monitored and rhythm disturbances are therefore diagnosed more frequently.[77] Enhanced sympathetic nervous system activity in pregnancy has been proposed by some investigators as a cause of increased incidence of arrhythmia.

Most arrhythmias are not associated with structural heart disease and should be evaluated and managed in the same manner as in the nonpregnant patient. The rhythm should first be evaluated by electrocardiography because this may provide an indication of the underlying cause of the patient's symptoms, such as long QT syndrome. The woman's hemodynamic status should direct the therapy, with reversible causes being corrected if possible. When arrhythmias are well tolerated and patients are minimally symptomatic, a conservative approach is recommended. When arrhythmias cause debilitating symptoms or hemodynamic compromise, therapy is indicated. No antiarrhythmic drug is completely safe during pregnancy; however, many are well tolerated and can be given with relatively low risk to mother and fetus. If possible, drug therapy should be avoided during the first trimester. Compounds with the most extensive history of safe use should be the first-line agents.[78] Electrical cardioversion is not contraindicated in the pregnant woman, nor is the use of intravenous antiarrhythmic medications.

Bradyarrhythmias

Bradycardia may have several causes, some of which are reversible. Drugs, including β-adrenergic blockers or nondihydropyridine calcium channel blockers, and metabolic abnormalities, including hypoxia, acidosis, and hyperkalemia, may be causative and can be corrected. Sinus node dysfunction and atrioventricular block, including complete heart block, may cause bradycardia. Therapy is required only in symptomatic patients. Labor and delivery can be associated with syncope in women with atrioventricular block and may necessitate temporary pacing. If necessary, permanent pacemakers can be inserted safely during pregnancy. Women who have undergone prior pacemaker placement are able to have successful pregnancies.[79]

Tachyarrhythmias

Sinus tachycardia, with heart rates faster than 100 beats/minute, must be evaluated. The causes include dehydration, fever, anemia, infection, drugs, anxiety, and pain. The underlying cause should be corrected; pharmacologic therapy is not usually warranted.

Paroxysmal supraventricular tachycardia may indicate the presence of dual or accessory pathways in the heart that allow a reentrant tachycardia. The baseline ECG should be carefully evaluated for short PR intervals and delta waves, which suggest Wolff-Parkinson-White syndrome (preexcitation).[80] Therapy for these rhythms may include digoxin, β-adrenergic blockers, calcium channel blockers, or adenosine. Adenosine is generally safe to use in pregnancy and is the drug of choice for acute termination of a supraventricular tachycardia. The use of these drugs has been tolerated without any significant compromise to the fetus.[81]

Atrial fibrillation or flutter is usually a marker for an underlying structural or metabolic abnormality. Rate control is achieved acutely with intravenous verapamil, diltiazem, or β blockers. The use of a calcium channel blocker or digitalis for rate control with paroxysmal episodes is appropriate. Persistent atrial fibrillation, even in the absence of structural heart disease, is still associated with a risk for thromboembolic events, and anticoagulation with heparin or at least aspirin is indicated. Atrial fibrillation in patients who have mitral stenosis should be treated with digoxin and heparin during pregnancy.

Ventricular tachycardia in the pregnant woman warrants evaluation for underlying structural or metabolic causes.[82] Immediate therapy parallels that in the nonpregnant state. If the patient is hemodynamically stable, intravenous lidocaine or procainamide may be used initially. If the woman is not hemodynamically stable, synchronized DC cardioversion is indicated. β Blocker therapy has been used effectively to treat these patients, which suggests that a hyperadrenergic state may precipitate the rhythm. The use of an implantable cardioverter-defibrillator should be considered in women with life-threatening ventricular arrhythmias. Pregnancy does not increase the complications related to implantable cardioverter-defibrillators or result in an increase in the number of discharges.[83]

Long QT syndrome may be acquired or congenital. Affected patients are at risk for syncope, recurrent ventricular tachycardia, and sudden cardiac death. The drugs associated with an acquired long QT interval, including class IA antiarrhythmic medications and tricyclic amines, should be discontinued. Antihistamines such as astemizole and terfenadine are no longer available. In congenital long QT syndrome, β-adrenergic blocker therapy should be initiated. Recurrent ventricular tachycardia warrants an electrophysiologic consultation. Congenital long QT syndrome can be transmitted genetically to offspring.

Ventricular fibrillation requires full cardiopulmonary resuscitation procedures with nonsynchronized DC cardioversion at 360 J.[84]

CONGENITAL HEART DISEASE

One percent of all pregnancies in the United States are complicated by maternal cardiovascular disease. Increasing numbers of women with congenital heart disease are surviving to adulthood because of advances in medical and cardiovascular surgical techniques. As a result, pregnancies in patients with complex cardiovascular anomalies are occurring more frequently. A report by Mendelson and Lang suggested three groups of congenital heart disease: (1) left-to-right shunts associated with volume overload, such as atrial and ventricular septal defects, patent ductus arteriosus, and anomalous pulmonary venous return; (2) right-to-left shunts that result in cyanosis, such as tetralogy of Fallot and Eisenmenger's syndrome; and (3) anomalies associated with pressure overload, such as aortic stenosis, pulmonary stenosis, coarctation of the aorta, and hypertrophic subaortic stenosis.[81]

Whereas the risk for a congenital cardiac malformation in an infant of a normal mother is 0.8% to 1.0%, it is significantly higher when genetically determined anomalies have affected a family member or when the pregnant woman has congenital heart disease. Fetal echocardiographic screening in women with congenital heart disease should be performed to confirm or rule out fetal congenital heart disease and to assess for a malformation or arrhythmia.[85]

Left-to-Right Shunts

Most affected women have undergone surgical repair before pregnancy; however, some residual defect may remain, or the defect may have been previously undiagnosed.

The degree of shunting is determined by the resistances of the pulmonary and systemic vascular systems, both of which decrease during pregnancy; therefore, pregnancy itself does not significantly alter the degree of shunting.[86] If pulmonary vascular disease has developed, a decrease in left-to-right shunting may occur. If a large shunt is present, then ventricular arrhythmias, ventricular dysfunction, and progression of pulmonary hypertension can be present. Women with acyanotic congenital lesions, in the absence of pulmonary hypertension, generally tolerate pregnancy, labor, and delivery.

Atrial Septal Defect

Seventy percent of atrial septal defects in women are ostium secundum defects; many affected patients are asymptomatic. These women may develop symptoms for the first time during pregnancy after the development of pulmonary hypertension and atrial arrhythmias.

The physical examination is significant for persistent splitting of the second heart sound in association with a systolic ejection murmur. Chest radiographic examination may demonstrate increased pulmonary blood flow. Electrocardiographic findings are significant for a right bundle branch block with a right axis deviation (left axis deviation with ostium primum defects). Echocardiography with Doppler analysis verifies the diagnosis, as well as associated lesions and pulmonary pressures.

Pregnancy is well tolerated in the absence of complications such as pulmonary hypertension. No reports to date suggest that surgical repair before pregnancy improves rates of maternal morbidity and mortality. Antibiotic prophylaxis is usually not necessary because endocarditis is rare. Up to 85% of affected women have uncomplicated deliveries, but a 15% fetal loss rate is associated with this condition. The defect is inherited in 5% to 10% of offspring of a parent with an atrial septal defect.[87]

Ventricular Septal Defect

This is the most common cardiac anomaly. Most ventricular septal defects close spontaneously or are detected and repaired during childhood. Pregnancy is well tolerated if pulmonary hypertension is absent.

Physical examination is significant for a holosystolic murmur that may be associated with a thrill at the left sternal border. Echocardiography with Doppler analysis verifies the diagnosis, as well as associated lesions and pulmonary pressures.

When the defect is unrepaired, endocarditis may occur, and prophylaxis with antibiotics is necessary. This condition is associated with maternal mortality if pulmonary hypertension is present. The fetal loss rate is 25%, and this defect is inherited in 5% to 8% of offspring of a parent with this condition.[87]

Patent Ductus Arteriosus

This lesion is usually repaired in childhood. Unrepaired lesions in adulthood are usually asymptomatic. The physiologic consequences of the lesion are related to its size. This defect is usually well tolerated during pregnancy in the absence of pulmonary hypertension.

Physical examination is significant for a wide pulse pressure and a machinery-like murmur that is harsh and continuous, best heard at the upper left sternal border and under the left clavicle. The ECG usually demonstrates left ventricular hypertrophy. Echocardiography with Doppler analysis confirms the diagnosis, as well as associated lesions and pulmonary pressures.

Endocarditis is common with this lesion, and therefore antibiotic prophylaxis is recommended. The fetal loss rate is estimated at 5% to 7% with this defect, and the lesion is inherited in 4% to 5% of cases.[87]

Right-to-Left Shunts

Right-to-left shunting can occur with any lesion when obstruction to right ventricular outflow exists or when pulmonary vascular resistance exceeds the systemic vascular resistance. Hypoxemic disorders are linked to intrauterine growth restriction, premature delivery, and fetal demise. Whittemore and colleagues reported a 35% fetal loss rate in women with cyanotic congenital cardiovascular disease.[88] Hypoxemia associated with polycythemia and hematocrit greater than 65% correlates with almost universal fetal wastage.[89] Maternal morbidity and mortality rates for these defects range from 10% to 50%. A paper describing 96 pregnancies in 44 women with cyanotic heart defects reported maternal cardiac events in 32%, including one death; prematurity in 37%; and low birth weight among live births in 43%.[90] Successful surgical correction before pregnancy improves the outcome for both the mother and offspring.[91]

Tetralogy of Fallot

This lesion is the most common cause of right-to-left shunting of blood past the pulmonary bed with the subsequent development of cyanosis. Tetralogy of Fallot consists of ventricular septal defect, pulmonary valve stenosis, right ventricular hypertrophy, and an overriding aorta. During pregnancy, the peripheral vascular resistance

decreases with an increase in shunting and worsening of cyanosis. Surgical correction of the defect should be performed before pregnancy if possible.[92] The risk of complications in pregnancy is generally low in women who have experienced successful correction. However, late sequelae of corrective surgery can increase the complication rate associated with pregnancy. These sequelae include residual shunt, arrhythmia, pulmonary valve regurgitation, pulmonary artery hypertension, and left ventricular dysfunction. It is critical to review all prior surgical repair reports and perform a comprehensive cardiovascular evaluation in patients who have undergone a corrective surgical procedure.

The physical examination findings are significant for digital clubbing and cyanosis. Chest radiographs and ECGs demonstrate right ventricular hypertrophy. Echocardiography with Doppler analysis substantiates the diagnosis, as well as associated lesions.

There is an increased risk of maternal and fetal morbidity and mortality when tetralogy of Fallot is present. If pregnancy occurs, venous return and systemic vascular resistance must be maintained to preserve pulmonary blood flow. In one series, 5 of 16 patients with corrected tetralogy of Fallot experienced a deterioration in cardiac functional class during pregnancy; three of the five experienced progression of pulmonary valve regurgitation.[93] Vaginal delivery is recommended unless there is an indication for cesarean section, and the use of epidural anesthetics should be avoided if possible.[94]

Transmissibility of the defect from parent to offspring was examined in a large collaborative study.[95] The authors found cardiac defects with significantly greater frequency in the children of affected women than in children of affected men. The authors measured a 3% incidence of inheritance overall, with a 2% incidence in siblings and a 0.3% incidence in second- and third-degree relatives, which suggests a polygenic disorder with a small number of interacting genes.[95] Genetic counseling and analysis before conception allow patients with the tetralogy to know whether the 22q11 deletion syndrome is present; if it is absent, the risk of fetal defects is low.[96]

Eisenmenger's Syndrome

In this syndrome, right-to-left shunting in any cardiac lesion arises as a result of the development of pulmonary hypertension.[97] The vasodilation associated with pregnancy increases the degree of right-to-left shunting, resulting in worsening cyanosis.

Physical examination findings are significant for digital clubbing and cyanosis. Chest radiographs and ECGs demonstrate right ventricular hypertrophy. Echocardiography with Doppler analysis substantiates the diagnosis, defines related lesions, and estimates pulmonary pressures.

It has been reported that the maternal and fetal mortality rates associated with this condition are 30% to 50%.[98] Women with this syndrome should be discouraged from becoming pregnant. Management during labor and delivery is very difficult. Venous return and right ventricular filling must be maintained, and blood loss and the use of epidural anesthetics should be avoided. The cause of death is usually right ventricular failure associated with cardiogenic shock.

Transposition of the Great Vessels

The original surgical approaches to transposition of the great vessels focused on redirecting atrial flow patterns (Mustard and Senning procedures) and resulted in complications in adulthood such as sinus node dysfunction, atrial arrhythmias, and systolic dysfunction. The complications among 43 pregnancies in 31 women with this type of surgical repair included a 14% incidence of congestive heart failure and arrhythmias, as well as one death. The sequelae of the current corrective surgical approach, the arterial switch procedure, has not been evaluated on a large scale, inasmuch as very few of these patients have not yet reached childbearing age.[99] In a large prospective, multicenter study of pregnancy in congenital heart disease, a small subset (four women) had undergone the arterial switch procedure for transposition of the great vessels.[93] One patient experienced a decline in functional class; however, all four completed normal pregnancies.

Fontan Repair

The Fontan procedure routes systemic venous return directly to the lungs and is performed for conditions in which there is a single ventricular pumping chamber. Affected women are at elevated risk for cardiovascular complications during pregnancy. There is increased hemodynamic load on the right atrium and the single ventricular chamber; a 2% maternal mortality has been reported.[100] Progressive venous congestion, ventricular failure, atrial clot formation, and rhythm disturbances are frequently witnessed complications in the pregnant patient who has undergone a Fontan repair. A high rate of miscarriage may be related to extreme congestion of the intrauterine veins.[96] Nonetheless, successful pregnancies have been reported in the current literature.[101]

Pressure Overload

Pressure overload results from obstructive lesions that may reflect isolated congenital lesions or a part of a more complex congenital defect. Aortic and pulmonary stenosis is discussed in the section on rheumatic and valvular heart disease. Coarctation of the aorta and idiopathic hypertrophic subaortic stenosis are also typified by pressure overload.

Coarctation of the Aorta

This is an uncommon defect, and it sometimes appears as part of a constellation of other congenital findings such as bicuspid aortic valve and cerebral artery aneurysms. The defect is usually situated at the level of the subclavian artery.

Physical examination findings include brachial hypertension, with upper and lower extremity pulse discrepancy and, over the back, audible bruits caused by collateral blood flow. Chest radiographs are notable for rib notching. Echocardiography with Doppler analysis establishes the diagnosis and serves to define associated lesions.

Most studies report that maternal morbidity and mortality rates are increased with this defect.[102] However, a preliminary study reported improved outcomes with no maternal deaths and one fetal death in women with coarctation of the aorta.[103] Current recommendations remain that corrective surgery should be performed before pregnancy whenever possible, although there are numerous reports of successful pregnancies with careful management.[104,105] The major complications are hypertension, congestive heart failure, endocarditis, and rupture of the aorta. Treatment of high blood pressure is usually required.[54,105,106] Management of hypertension can be difficult during pregnancy because control of upper body blood pressure may lead to hypotension below the coarctation site, thereby compromising the fetus. Prophylactic antibiotics are necessary because of the high risk of endocarditis. The risk of aortic rupture is highest in the third trimester, during labor and delivery, and early in the puerperium. In addition, women who have undergone repair in childhood are at risk of aortic rupture because of the development of aneurysms at the site of repair. The rate of fetal loss is approximately 10% with this defect. Offspring have a 2% incidence of inheriting the defect, as well as a 6% incidence of other congenital cardiac diseases,[54,105] although other authors suggest a higher risk.[107]

Idiopathic Hypertrophic Subaortic Stenosis

This autosomal dominant trait is associated with chest pain, syncope, dyspnea, arrhythmias, and sudden cardiac death. It can appear in the company of other disorders, such as Friedreich's ataxia, Turner's syndrome, neurofibromatosis, and pheochromocytoma. Symptoms become clinically manifest in the second or third decade of life and may be first appreciated during pregnancy.

Physical examination findings are notable for a dynamic systolic ejection murmur, best heard at the base, and a rapidly rising carotid pulse. The murmur of mitral regurgitation may also be present. The diagnosis is confirmed by echocardiography with Doppler analysis.

Outflow obstruction may be increased because of the normal fall in peripheral vascular resistance with pregnancy, in combination with a decrease in venous return from compression of the inferior vena cava by the gravid uterus, and because of blood loss associated with delivery.[108,109] Complex arrhythmias may develop and lead to sudden cardiac death.[110,111] A contemporary series described two maternal deaths in 199 cases of live births in a cohort of 91 affected women. Both patients had high-risk characteristics and had been advised against pregnancy: One had a resting left ventricular outflow gradient of greater than 100 mm Hg, and the other had a strong family history of sudden cardiac death.[111]

Management is directed toward avoidance of hypotension and tachycardia because both can diminish left ventricular diastolic filling and increase outflow obstruction. Recommendations should include limitation of stress and strenuous activity, which increase the force of myocardial contraction and thus magnify the ventricular outflow obstruction. Blood volume and venous return must be maintained during pregnancy and especially during labor and delivery. β-Blocking agents should be used if indicated. Conventional advice has favored avoidance of the use of epidural anesthetics, although a published series reported few complications and generally favorable outcomes.[112] Antibiotic prophylaxis should be provided at delivery.

Marfan's Syndrome

This autosomal dominant trait disorder results from a genetic abnormality of the fibrillin gene. Connective tissue weakness leads to the following cardiovascular abnormalities: dilatation of the aortic wall and root, aortic valve regurgitation, and mitral valve prolapse.[113] Affected patients who become pregnant are at risk of potential catastrophic aortic dissection.[114]

On physical examination, cardiovascular findings include evidence of mitral or aortic regurgitation by auscultation. Chest radiographic findings may demonstrate enlargement of the ascending aorta. Echocardiography allows aortic root measurement as well as assessment of related cardiac defects.

Although reports on the rate of maternal morbidity and mortality with pregnancy are conflicting, there is general agreement that women with dilation of the aorta or other cardiovascular manifestations are at risk for life-threatening cardiovascular complications.[115,116] One report found an association among aortic dimension larger than 4.0 cm, progression of aortic dilation, and decreased cardiac function as risk factors during pregnancy in women with Marfan's syndrome. Pregnancy should be discouraged in these individuals. Maternal activity should be limited, and prophylactic β-adrenergic blocker therapy should be applied during pregnancy. Ideal monitoring includes blood pressure analysis and serial echocardiographic studies. If there is progressive aortic root dilation or if the aortic root diameter equals 5.5 cm, necessary surgical repair can be carried out during pregnancy with good outcomes.[114] Acute dissection of the ascending aorta during pregnancy is a surgical emergency; dissections distal to the subclavian artery merit medical management. Cesarean section is advised in patients with Marfan's syndrome and aortic root involvement.[117] Normal vaginal deliveries have been accomplished in patients with Marfan's syndrome who do not have demonstrable cardiovascular abnormalities.[114] Successful pregnancies have been described in patients with Marfan's syndrome who have undergone surgical replacement of aortic root and arch.[118]

Related syndromes include Ehlers-Danlos syndrome type IV, in which connective tissue fragility may lead to aortic dissection and excessive bleeding post partum, and non-Marfan familial syndromes of aortic enlargement and dissection. Careful monitoring and medical management is essential for the success of pregnancies in these high-risk patients.[96]

Ebstein's Anomaly

In Ebstein's anomaly, the tricuspid valve is dysplastic and displaced into the right ventricle. If the defect is mild and no cyanosis exists, pregnancy is usually well tolerated.[119]

Pregnancy in patients who have a more severe Ebstein anomaly may be attended by complications such as tricuspid regurgitation, right ventricular dysfunction, right ventricular outflow obstruction with right-to-left shunting, and cyanosis. This anomaly is also associated with Wolff-Parkinson-White preexcitation syndrome, with heightened risk of arrhythmias.

RHEUMATIC, VALVULAR, AND PERICARDIAL DISORDERS

Rheumatic heart disease in women of childbearing age has declined in prevalence in most of the United States; however, it is still a major source of maternal morbidity throughout many regions in the underdeveloped world. As immigration to industrialized nations increases, clinicians in the developed societies will encounter patients with rheumatic heart disease more frequently. Other types of congenital and acquired valvular abnormalities necessitate careful management in the pregnant patient as well.

Rheumatic Fever

Acute rheumatic fever is rare in the United States. However, it continues to be a foremost health concern worldwide, particularly in areas of socioeconomic disadvantage and limited access to antibiotics for streptococcal infection treatment. Bouts of rheumatic fever tend to recur during pregnancy, and vulnerable patients should be maintained on antibiotic prophylaxis.[120] Sydenham's chorea is known to reappear during pregnancy and is termed *chorea gravidarum*.

Arthralgias, chest discomfort, fever, subcutaneous nodules, erythema marginatum, and chorea, with culture or serologic findings of streptococcal infection, mark the acute manifestation of rheumatic fever. Cardiac involvement may encompass pericarditis, myocarditis, valvulitis, endocarditis, and conduction system abnormalities. Examination reveals a pericardial friction rub; an apical systolic murmur with an apical mid-diastolic (Carey-Coombs) murmur, signaling mitral involvement; a diastolic murmur of aortic regurgitation at the lower left sternal border; and signs of pulmonary congestion. Tricuspid valvulitis may be discovered, usually in the context of mitral and aortic valve findings.

Therapy consists of antibiotics (penicillin), as well as measures to relieve congestive heart failure, pain, and inflammation.

Mitral Stenosis

Congenital mitral stenosis is a rare entity. The most frequent cause of obstructive mitral valve disease is rheumatic disease; mitral stenosis is the most commonly seen rheumatic valvular lesion in pregnancy. The diagnosis of significant mitral stenosis exerts an important prognostic influence on maternal course. In a large study, complications were predicted by (1) the presence of left-sided obstructive disease, such as mitral stenosis, aortic valve stenosis, and hypertrophic subaortic stenosis; (2) the presence of cyanosis or poor New York Heart Association functional class; (3) the presence of myocardial dysfunction; (4) previous occurrence of arrhythmia; and (5) a prior cardiac event.[121] Patients who possessed none, one, or more than one of these characteristics at the start of pregnancy experienced a cardiac complication rate of 3%, 30%, and 66%, respectively (Fig. 6–4). A larger multicenter study subsequently validated the importance of these five risk factors: maternal complication rates were 3%, 27%, and 62%, respectively, for the same groups.[2] Another series of pregnant patients with valve disease confirmed that the most adverse outcomes were observed in women who had significant mitral or aortic valve obstructive disease.[122]

A multicenter evaluation of neonatal outcomes addressed prematurity, intrauterine growth restriction, cerebral hemorrhage, respiratory distress syndrome, and death as end points.[123] Adverse outcomes were forecast by maternal cardiac risk factors such as abnormal functional capacity or cyanosis and left-sided valve obstruction. Yet neonatal outcomes were significantly worsened by the presence of noncardiac risk factors such as smoking, use of anticoagulant drugs throughout pregnancy, multiple pregnancy, and maternal age older than 35 or younger than 20 years (Fig. 6–5).[123] This report was particularly notable as the first demonstration of a significant interaction between cardiac and noncardiac risk factors in the clinical course of pregnant women who have congenital heart disorders.

Twenty-five percent of patients with mitral stenosis experience their first symptoms, including cough, fatigue,

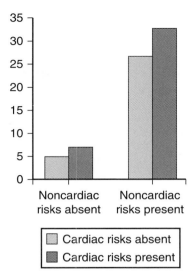

Figure 6–5. Neonatal adverse event rate, based on presence of maternal cardiac risk factors (poor functional capacity/cyanosis, left-sided obstructive lesion) versus noncardiac maternal risks factors (smoking, use of anticoagulant drugs throughout pregnancy, multiple pregnancy, and maternal age older than 35 or younger than 20 years). (Adapted from Siu SC, Colman JM, Sorensen S, et al. Adverse neonatal and cardiac outcomes are more common in pregnant women with cardiac disease. Circulation 2002;105:2179.)

dyspnea, orthopnea, or hemoptysis, during pregnancy. The physical examination reveals an accentuated first heart sound, and an opening snap may be present. A new diastolic apical rumbling murmur is suspicious and can be verified with echocardiography.

In pregnancy, the pathophysiologic mechanism of mitral stenosis is founded upon several important changes that take place after the 20th week: namely, the increase in heart rate and the rise in plasma volume and cardiac output. These natural alterations combine with mitral valve obstruction to reduce the diastolic filling time of the left ventricle, which can produce a doubling of the pressure gradient across the mitral valve. Forward cardiac output may decline, and in severely affected patients, there is a rise in the pulmonary capillary wedge pressure, leading to symptomatic pulmonary congestion. Elevated pulmonary pressures may engender right ventricular enlargement, hepatomegaly, ascites, jugular venous distention, and peripheral edema.

Left atrial enlargement predisposes to clot formation and systemic thromboembolization, as well as atrial fibrillation, which itself can provoke pulmonary edema. Sinus tachycardia at the time of labor may cause pulmonary edema as well. Volume shifts in pregnancy can have diverse effects in mitral stenosis. The rise in central volume in the setting of obstructed inflow to the left ventricle during contractions in labor and immediately post partum as the uterus rapidly shrinks can swiftly lead to pulmonary edema. At the same time, the presence of the valvular obstruction requires adequate filling pressures, or preload, in order to maintain cardiac output; thus, hypovolemia or reduced venous return is equally deleterious.

Labor itself causes an increase of 8 to 10 mm Hg in pulmonary capillary wedge pressure.[124] Marked intravascular

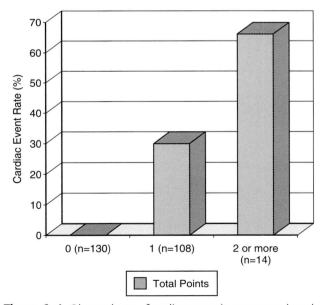

Figure 6–4. Observed rate of cardiac events in pregnancy, based on total number of points in risk factor evaluation. One point was given for each of the following: left-sided obstructive disease, cyanosis or poor New York Heart Association functional class, myocardial dysfunction, prior arrhythmia, and prior cardiac event. (Adapted from Siu CS, Sermer M, Harrison DA, et al: Risk and predictors for pregnancy-related complications in women with heart disease. Circulation 1997;96:2789.)

volume shifts in the first 24 hours after delivery may cause extreme circulatory instability in the postpartum interval (Fig. 6–6).

Pregnant patients with mitral stenosis who are in New York Heart Association functional class I or II have a favorable outlook with regard to mortality, although one series reported a 35% morbidity rate, including pulmonary edema, arrhythmia, and fetal or neonatal adverse events.[125] Whether these patients would benefit from preventive medical or transcatheter interventions is not yet defined. Patients with class III symptoms may be given digoxin and placed on bed rest after the 20th week. Class IV symptoms or the presence of atrial fibrillation portends an adverse maternal and fetal outcome. Limitation in activity, fatigue, and anxiety, with treatment for anemia and infection, are appropriate for all patients with mitral stenosis. Rheumatic fever prophylaxis[120] and antibiotic prophylaxis during labor and delivery are recommended, although some authors advise deferring peripartum antibiotic treatment unless active pelvic infection is present.[8,126] Anticoagulant agents should be given to patients with a history of systemic embolization, and atrial fibrillation should be addressed with digoxin or β-adrenergic blockers. Hospitalization is recommended for patients with pulmonary congestion, particularly in the presence of significant arrhythmias that necessitate pharmacologic or electrical cardioversion. In a series of 1000 pregnant women with cardiac disease collected over 10 years, the complication rate for those with rheumatic heart disease was 21.4%.[127] Heart failure, arrhythmia, thromboembolism, and endocarditis were described.[127]

If congestive heart failure is resistant to medical treatment during pregnancy, a mechanical approach to mitral stenosis involving balloon valvuloplasty or valve replacement

has been successful.[8,128-132] Subsequent childhood development after maternal mitral balloon valvuloplasty is normal.[133]

Mitral Regurgitation and Mitral Valve Prolapse

In contrast to left-sided obstructive lesions such as mitral stenosis, left-sided valve regurgitation is relatively well tolerated in pregnancy. Decreased systemic vascular resistance reduces arterial impedance to the ejection of blood from the left ventricle, favoring forward rather than regurgitant flow and mimicking the beneficial actions of afterload-reducing pharmacotherapy. Elevated heart rates in pregnancy reduce diastolic filling time, thereby moderating potentially excessive preload volume.

Causes of mitral valve regurgitation in women of childbearing age include rheumatic disease, rupture of the chordae tendineae, annular dilatation caused by cardiomyopathic ventricular dilation, prior bacterial endocarditis, and, in rare cases, myxomatous changes. Symptoms include dyspnea and fatigue, with the finding of a holosystolic murmur at the cardiac apex, often radiating to the axilla. Pulmonary congestion and right-sided heart failure may predominate in advanced cases. Left atrial enlargement predisposes to atrial fibrillation. The diagnosis of mitral regurgitation can be confirmed by echocardiography. Treatment consists of sodium restriction, diuretics, and digoxin in patients with heart failure. Afterload-reducing agents such as hydralazine may be useful, and antibiotic prophylaxis with delivery should be considered.

Mitral valve prolapse exists in 2% to 10% of young women but generally does not affect pregnancy.[134] Physical findings, such as the midsystolic click, often disappear with pregnancy-induced cardiac geometric changes that compensate for the redundancy of valve tissue. In rare cases, patients experience chest discomfort or rhythm disturbances and should be managed with reassurance. Therapy with β-adrenergic blockers can be employed if patients are highly symptomatic. If a murmur is audible, antibiotic prophylaxis should be administered at the time of delivery.

Aortic Stenosis

This left-sided obstructive lesion may be congenital or rheumatic in origin and is relatively uncommon in pregnancy. If aortic stenosis is severe (with a valve area of less than 1.0 cm^2), pregnancy imposes a major risk on mother and fetus. Mild to moderate aortic stenosis may be tolerated in pregnancy with careful management.[135] Earlier studies defined mortality rates up to 17%,[136] and more recent data have confirmed left-sided obstructive disease as a principal maternal risk factor.[121] Surgical treatment before pregnancy improves outcomes in severe cases.[121] Termination of pregnancy in patients with aortic stenosis carries a reported high maternal mortality rate, probably based on hypovolemia occurring during the procedure. Hypovolemia is disadvantageous in severe aortic stenosis, in which a hypertrophied and obstructed left ventricle

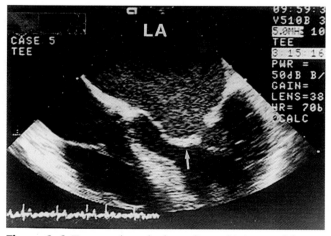

Figure 6–6. Transesophageal echocardiographic image of rheumatic mitral valve stenosis (*arrow*), enlargement of the left atrium (LA), and spontaneous echocardiographic contrast in the left atrium, probably representing microthrombi in a 36-year-old woman of West Indian ancestry. The patient presented with transient ischemic neurologic attack, atrial fibrillation, and heart failure at 30 weeks of pregnancy. She had previously undergone closed surgical commissurotomy with subsequent recurrence of stenosis. (Courtesy of Eugene Parent, MD, Section of Cardiovascular Medicine, Department of Internal Medicine, Yale University School of Medicine.)

depends on adequate venous return (i.e., preload) for appropriate filling.

Dyspnea with exertion, chest discomfort, and presyncope are the cardinal symptoms of aortic stenosis and may appear in the second or third trimester. Physical evidence includes delayed carotid upstrokes and a harsh crescendo-decrescendo murmur radiating from the right upper sternal border to the neck. The presence of a fourth heart sound and a single second heart sound indicate severe obstruction, which can be verified with echocardiography. In pregnant patients with aortic stenosis, activity should be limited and diuretic treatment for pulmonary congestion used with great caution. In rare cases, balloon valvuloplasty as a palliative measure may be considered before delivery.[137,138] Antibiotic prophylaxis during labor and delivery is advised.

Aortic Regurgitation

Similar to mitral regurgitation, this left-sided regurgitant abnormality is well tolerated in pregnancy. The natural decrease in systemic vascular resistance reduces afterload, thereby favoring forward rather than regurgitant flow. Causes include rheumatic disease, congenital bicuspid valve, and endocarditis. Aortic root dilation, as in Marfan's syndrome, should also be considered.

Dyspnea and fatigue occur commonly, and physical findings include a rapidly collapsing peripheral pulse and a blowing diastolic murmur at the left lower sternal border. If the regurgitation is rheumatic in origin, mitral valve murmurs may be heard as well. In advanced stages, pulmonary congestion or peripheral edema can be found. Echocardiography is useful in substantiating the diagnosis of aortic regurgitation and identifying aortic root enlargement or endocarditic lesions.

Therapy for aortic regurgitation in pregnancy consists of limiting activity and prescribing digoxin and diuretics when pulmonary congestion is present. Afterload-reducing agents have been used to stabilize the progression of aortic regurgitation in nonpregnant subjects; therefore, it is reasonable to consider hydralazine, or perhaps nifedipine, for pregnant women who have moderate to severe disease. Antibiotic prophylaxis during delivery is advisable.

Pulmonic Stenosis and Regurgitation

Pulmonic stenosis is uncommon, usually congenital in origin. Symptoms include dyspnea, chest discomfort, and syncope. Physical data include right ventricular lift, systolic murmur heard at the left sternal border that lessens with inspiration, and pulmonary ejection click. Pulmonic stenosis is generally well tolerated during pregnancy, although correction of the lesion before pregnancy is desirable. Balloon valvuloplasty is a rational option in severely affected pregnant patients.

Isolated pulmonic valvular regurgitation is very unusual and is typically well tolerated in pregnancy. More common is pulmonic regurgitation secondary to pulmonary hypertension. In this case, it is the primary condition that creates an adverse prognosis.

Tricuspid Stenosis and Regurgitation

Tricuspid valve stenosis is a rare lesion, usually rheumatic in origin and is almost always linked to left-sided rheumatic valve abnormalities. A successful balloon tricuspid valvuloplasty in pregnancy has been described.[139]

Tricuspid regurgitation during pregnancy may be physiologic.[140] Severe tricuspid regurgitation is often a structural consequence of endocarditis or a functional result of pulmonary hypertension. Jugular venous elevation, liver enlargement, and a holosystolic murmur at the left lower sternal border that increases with inspiration may be present. Antibiotic prophylaxis during delivery is recommended.

Endocarditis and Antibiotic Prophylaxis

Unexplained fever, fatigue, and malaise in a pregnant woman with structural heart disease should raise the prospect of endocarditis. Physical examination findings, blood culture results, and echocardiographic evaluation allow early antibiotic treatment to prevent the need for urgent valve replacement.

Prophylaxis against recurrent rheumatic fever with penicillin should be given to susceptible patients.[120] The general question of antibiotic prophylaxis during delivery for women with congenital or valvular heart disease has been debated. In one study of 519 pregnancies in women with rheumatic valvular or congenital heart disease, no antibiotic prophylaxis was given during delivery. The authors reported that no patient developed endocarditis.[8] Moreover, there is no evidence from any prospective controlled trial to suggest that antibiotic prophylaxis is effective in preventing endocarditis in any setting.[126] Current American Heart Association guidelines do not recommend prophylaxis during normal delivery unless active pelvic infection is diagnosed. Prophylaxis is optional for patients who have prosthetic valves, complex cyanotic congenital disease, or surgically created systemic-to-pulmonary shunts.[126]

These guidelines have sparked much discussion. In view of the unpredictable nature of peripartum events and the severe consequences of endocarditis, some authors proposed prophylaxis for all patients with congenital and valve disease, except in cases of isolated secundum type atrial septal defects or ligation of a persistent ductus arteriosus 6 months or more earlier.[141] One review supported the role of physician discretion in this area.[124] We concur with the objections to these guidelines and favor antibiotic prophylaxis as a prudent, low-risk, and clinically logical strategy for the time of delivery and the immediate postpartum interval.

Prophylaxis consists of 2.0 g of intramuscular or intravenous ampicillin, plus intravenous gentamicin, 1.5 mg/kg, not to exceed 120 mg, within 30 minutes of initiating of the procedure or delivery, and then 1.0 g of intramuscular or intravenous ampicillin 6 hours later. For penicillin-allergic patients, vancomycin, 1.0 g, is given intravenously over 1 to 2 hours, along with intramuscular or intravenous gentamicin, 1.5 mg/kg, not to exceed 120 mg. Completion of dosing 30 minutes before beginning the procedure is advised.[126]

Pericardial Diseases

Pericarditis is unusual in pregnancy, although an asymptomatic pericardial effusion is relatively common, often an incidental finding. These silent fluid collections are typically mild or moderate in size, although they can be large.[142] In one series, they were found late in pregnancy, and all had resolved 2 months post partum.[142] A published report described an incidence of pericardial effusion of 42% in normal pregnant women and identified no correlation between the presence of fluid and hematologic, serum protein, or albumin status.[143] In this study left ventricular function was normal in all cases, excluding congestive heart failure or cardiomyopathy as a cause of the effusion.[143] Asymptomatic effusion occurs more frequently in primigravidas and becomes more common as pregnancy advances; effusions were seen in 15%, 19%, and 44% of patients in the first, second, and third trimesters, respectively.[144] Two papers identified effusions as more common in patients who had gained more weight in pregnancy,[142,144] leading one author to hypothesize silent effusions as the product of salt and water retention.[142]

Autoimmune disorders such as lupus erythematosus, malignancy, tuberculosis, and post–viral inflammation status can cause pericardial symptoms and hemodynamic compromise if an effusion leads to cardiac tamponade.[145-148] Dyspnea, fatigue, tachycardia, hypotension with paradoxical pulse, distended neck veins, and distant heart tones suggest pericardial tamponade. Echocardiography can confirm tamponade by identifying right-sided chamber collapse in diastole. In treatment of pregnant patients, surgical pericardiectomy[149] and ultrasonographically guided needle aspiration with catheter drainage have been reported (Fig. 6–7).[150]

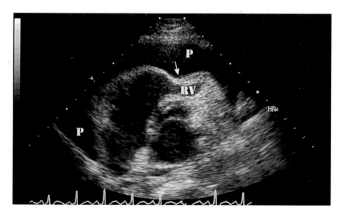

Figure 6–7. Transthoracic echocardiographic image of pericardial effusion (P) with tamponade in a primiparous 31-year-old woman at 26 weeks of pregnancy, who presented with dyspnea, neck vein distention, and peripheral congestion 10 weeks after a self-limited upper respiratory virus-type syndrome. *Arrow* indicates region of right ventricular (RV) collapse in diastole. Symptoms and findings resolved after ultrasonographically guided needle aspiration and catheter drainage of the effusion. (Courtesy of Nassir Azimi, MD, Section of Cardiovascular Medicine, Department of Internal Medicine, Yale University School of Medicine.)

PROSTHETIC VALVES AND CARDIAC SURGERY

Significant clinical issues exist regarding (1) choice of valve prosthesis in women of childbearing potential, (2) management of anticoagulation in pregnant women who have mechanical heart valves, and (3) the prospect of heart surgery during pregnancy. In general, the presence of a prosthetic heart valve is considered a relative contraindication to pregnancy because of maternal risks of death, heart failure, thromboemboli, hemorrhage, rhythm disturbances, and bacterial endocarditis. Nevertheless, many patients choose to become pregnant, and there is much controversy regarding optimal management in this area.

Choice of Valve in Women of Childbearing Potential

When feasible, mechanical correction of a moderate to severe valve abnormality should be accomplished before conception,[121] particularly when New York Heart Association class III or class IV symptoms exist. There are advantages as well as disadvantages to the placement of either bioprosthetic (tissue) or mechanical (metallic) valves. A bioprosthesis has low thrombogenic potential, and thus there is no need for anticoagulation in pregnancy. However, a bioprosthesis has a limited natural life, often necessitating a second open-heart surgical procedure for replacement within 10 to 15 years, a significant drawback for young women who must survive the morbidity and mortality risks of repeated surgery while still raising young children.[151] Moreover, the conventional view holds that pregnancy may accelerate the deterioration of tissue valves[152,153]; however, current data are contradictory.[154] Authors of large series have observed that pregnancy does not accelerate structural deterioration or reduce lifespan of bioprosthetic valves.[155] A mechanical prosthesis has the definite advantage of durability, and certain valve types have maintained structural and functional integrity for 25 years or more after implantation. However, anticoagulant agents must be given, particularly in the hypercoagulable pregnant state,[156] to avoid potentially catastrophic valve thrombosis. In pregnant women, there is a greater thrombotic risk for mechanical versus bioprostheses.[155] Some women require anticoagulation independently of valve type, and thus selection of a mechanical valve that necessitates anticoagulation may be reasonable. A parallel indication for anticoagulation is the presence of noncardiac thrombophlebitic or embolic disease, atrial fibrillation, rheumatic mitral valve disease, left atrial enlargement, or cardiac chamber thrombus.

Percutaneous, or transcatheter, balloon valvuloplasty may represent a temporizing alternative. This procedure may enable a patient to complete her pregnancy without having to confront the complications of severe valvular stenosis or the risks of anticoagulation. Definitive surgical replacement can then be performed when childbearing is concluded. Balloon valvuloplasty has excellent long-term benefits in congenital pulmonic stenosis and rheumatic mitral stenosis. Aortic valvuloplasty is useful in selected situations such as congenital noncalcific valve disease, although the 6-month rate of recurrent stenosis is greater than 50% when calcific lesions, often present in rheumatic aortic valve disease, are approached with balloon valvuloplasty, which thereby limits its utility. In a recent case, however, aortic valvuloplasty was performed successfully in the 20th week of pregnancy to relieve left-sided heart failure caused by a transvalvular gradient of 120 mm Hg, with subsequent delivery of a healthy newborn at term by cesarean section.[93]

Anticoagulation and the Prosthetic Valve

The management of anticoagulation in pregnant patients who have mechanical prosthetic cardiac valves or significant thromboembolic disorders is subject to controversy, with considerable geographic variations in practice worldwide.[157-160] Overall, the rate of maternal mortality attributable to mechanical valve thrombosis in pregnancy is 1% to 4%.[161] Warfarin is favored for reliable prosthetic valve thromboprophylaxis, although its use during the first trimester creates risk of embryopathy, particularly in the 6th to 12th weeks. Fetal hemorrhage, loss, and malformations have been described with the use of warfarin in the first trimester.[162] Teratogenic effects may be found in up to 25% of exposures; they include nasal hypoplasia, optic atrophy, radiographic bone stippling, saddle-nose deformity, frontal bossing, short stature, cataracts, and mental retardation.[163] However, other series suggest high rates of normal pregnancies and deliveries with the use of warfarin throughout, with heparin introduced only at term.[157,160,164-166] In one report, no warfarin embryopathy was found in 58 patients when daily doses of 5 mg or less were used.[167]

Because of the risk of embryopathy, the practice in the United States is to substitute the use of subcutaneous unfractionated heparin in place of warfarin. The large and highly charged heparin molecule does not cross the placental barrier. However, protection against potentially devastating valve thrombosis may not be complete,[168-171] even when anticoagulation is optimized with the use of a subcutaneous heparin infusion pump.[172] One series reported that first trimester subcutaneous heparin in a three-times-daily dose (partial thromboplastin time 1.5 to 2.5 times that of control values) was not effective in preventing valve thrombosis, nor was the frequency of fetal loss much improved over warfarin therapy.[173] One large review showed that, in comparison with warfarin, heparin use in the first trimester doubled maternal thromboembolism and death risk to 9.2% and 4.2%, respectively.[124,161] Citing a lower incidence of embryopathy in newer series as well as reports of valve thrombosis on heparin, several international authors have suggested that warfarin be used exclusively until term.[160,169,174] Heparin therapy may have other adverse effects as well, including thrombocytopenia, osteoporosis, and fetal intracranial microhemorrhage.

Noting that most valve thromboses on heparin occurred in early-generation ball-and-cage or tilting-disk mechanical valves in the thrombus-prone mitral position, Elkayam proposed a system of risk stratification to be used until prospective randomized trials are conducted and results are available.[175] Elkayam advised a full discussion of fetal embryopathic risks versus maternal thrombotic risks with the patient and her family. Elkayam then advised that women who have first-generation mitral valves should either use warfarin until term or enter the hospital for intravenous heparin therapy during the organogenetic 6th through 12th weeks. Other authors have advised intravenous heparin as well[176]; however, we view this approach as inconvenient, costly, and perhaps providing no greater benefit than full-dose subcutaneous heparin with partial thromboplastin time maintained at 2.0 to 3.0 times the control value.

Less controversial is Elkayam's advice that women who have first-generation aortic valves or who possess less thrombogenic second-generation bileaflet valves in either position may be treated with full-dose subcutaneous heparin on a three-times-daily basis during the 6th to 12th weeks. Again, close monitoring is essential, with frequently evaluated midinterval partial thromboplastin times adjusted to 2.0 to 3.0 times the control values.[175] Other guidelines favor the addition of low-dose aspirin as an antithrombotic supplement to warfarin or heparin.[177,178] Educating prospective parents as to the risks and benefits of alternative anticoagulation strategies is essential.[124]

Low-molecular-weight heparin (LMWH) administered subcutaneously has been proposed for use in pregnant patients with mechanical valves. However, current data are mixed[178,179]: One manufacturer advised against its use in pregnancy because of uncontrolled small series reports of valve thrombosis and teratogenicity.[180] Because LMWH does not traverse the placental barrier, the plausibility of teratogenicity has been questioned.[156,181] Although standard weight-based dosing for LMWH represents an advantage over frequent anticoagulation monitoring for conventional unfractionated heparin, it is possible that pregnant women may metabolize the compound differently in comparison with nonpregnant patients, which would thus invalidate weight-based dosing schemes and explain reported episodes of valve thrombosis. To address this problem, it may be useful to evaluate levels of antifactor Xa (antibody to activated factor X) to ensure proper dosing.[181] However, in a series evaluating 69 pregnancies in women at high risk for thromboembolism, there were neither prenatal thrombotic episodes nor instances of thrombocytopenia with a daily dose of 40 mg, although the question of bone demineralization was raised in treated patients.[182] Other small series suggest benign outcomes with LMWH.[183] Further studies in a controlled setting are required before LMWH can be recommended with confidence for valve thromboprophylaxis in the organogenetic phase of gestation.

At term, the warfarin-related hemorrhagic risk is significant. Heparin is then substituted because of its short-acting properties. Heparin can be suspended during parturition and resumed several hours later. Some authors advise cesarean section to avoid fetal hemorrhage associated with normal delivery if warfarin is present as labor commences, although it is simpler to reverse anticoagulation temporarily with fresh-frozen plasma. Warfarin may be continued during lactation without risk to the infant,[141] and heparin does not enter breast milk.

The use of other antithrombotic compounds has initiated interest. Low-dose aspirin (50 to 100 mg daily) may reduce the risk of pregnancy-induced hypertension in some groups[184] and is not linked to adverse effects in offspring, such as hemorrhage or premature closure of the ductus arteriosus that is based on prostaglandin inhibition.[185] A randomized placebo-controlled evaluation of 60 mg of aspirin daily, intended to prevent preeclampsia in patients at high risk, showed no adverse fetal or maternal effect in the active therapy group.[186] Aspirin may enhance the antithrombotic effect of subcutaneous heparin in pregnancy.[175] Dipyridamole therapy can cause fetal loss.[164] There are no reports of sulfinpyrazone use in pregnancy, and clopidogrel and ticlopidine have been given on an anecdotal basis. Case studies suggest that thrombolytic agents such as tissue plasminogen activator (t-PA) for myocardial infarction[187] and urokinase for prosthetic valve thrombosis[175] may be employed during pregnancy, although such measures must be reserved for life-threatening scenarios because of possible increased risk of placental abruption.

Surgical and Transcatheter Cardiac Procedures

Surgical or transcatheter (percutaneous or interventional) cardiac corrective procedures may be needed in extreme circumstances such as refractory heart failure or cardiogenic shock caused by severe valve disease, myocardial infarction or unstable angina.[8,121,188,189] Maternal risks are no greater than in the nonpregnant patients; however, fetal risks include teratogenicity in the first trimester, and fetal loss associated with cardiopulmonary bypass is frequent, probably linked to changes in placental blood flow.[190] Cardiopulmonary bypass is associated with fetal bradycardia, measured by continuous fetal monitoring, and is corrected by increasing the blood flow rate from the bypass pump.[141,191] Nonpulsatile blood flow to the placenta during cardiopulmonary bypass may be harmful.[192] Ideal management includes maintenance of normothermia, use of the left lateral decubitus position after the second trimester, and increasing pump flow to equal the physiologic maternal cardiac output that is commensurate with the stage of pregnancy.[190] Under these methods, fetal losses are reduced to fewer than 15% with benign maternal outcomes.[188,190] Combined cardiac surgery and cesarean section has been described in third trimester patients.

Severe mitral or aortic valve stenosis may be approached by transcatheter balloon valvuloplasty as an alternative to open surgical treatment and cardiopulmonary bypass.[128-132,137,138,193,194] Although often employed as a temporizing measure in pregnancy, long-term results are generally favorable for mitral disease.[128] Appropriate candidates include those who do not have major mitral regurgitation or excessive calcification of valve structures. Fetal risks from ionizing radiation suggest the use of lead shielding, or, more advantageous, transesophageal echocardiographic guidance (Fig. 6–8).[164]

Severe unstable cases of ischemic heart disease may warrant coronary bypass surgery. This operation has been accomplished in pregnancy with favorable maternal and fetal outcomes by using standard cardiopulmonary bypass techniques.[195] In cases of a single left internal

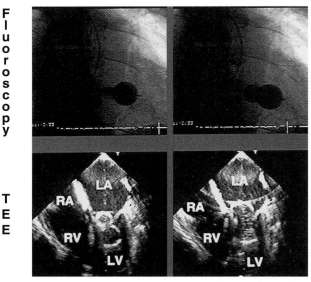

Figure 6–8. Transcatheter mitral balloon valvuloplasty with the Inoue device by fluoroscopy with companion transesophageal echocardiographic images. At left, half-inflated balloon with partial relief of mitral valve stenosis. At right, full opening of balloon and valve. LA, left atrium; LV, left ventricle; RA, right atrium; RV, right ventricle. (Courtesy of John Lasala, MD, PhD, Cardiac Catheterization Laboratory, Barnes Hospital–Washington University of St. Louis.)

mammary graft to an anterior vessel, the operation has been performed successfully on a warm beating heart without fetal risks of cardiopulmonary bypass (off-pump procedure).[196,197]

Although there are no reports of cardiac transplantation during pregnancy, a number of patients have become pregnant after transplantation. Significant issues include need for immunosuppression, accelerated atherosclerosis, and hemodynamic maladaptation related to cardiac denervation in patients and the clinician's inability to conduct fluoroscopically guided surveillance cardiac biopsies.[198] Adverse outcomes included an elevated incidence of maternal hypertension, preeclampsia, prematurity, and low birth weight.[199,200]

Despite the risks of ionizing radiation, transcatheter coronary balloon angioplasty[201,202] and intracoronary stent placement[197] have been accomplished with benign maternal and fetal results.[203] The presence of a cardiac pacemaker or an automatic implantable cardioverter-defibrillator has not been associated with increased device-related complications.[204] Cardioverter-defibrillator placement during pregnancy has been reported.[205]

CORONARY, PERIPHERAL VASCULAR, AND LIPID DISORDERS

With increasing maternal age, the obstetric population is vulnerable to acquired coronary and peripheral vascular atherosclerotic disorders that may affect the course of pregnancy.[9] Nonatherosclerotic arterial diseases such as fibromuscular dysplasia, vasospastic disorders, Takayasu's arteritis, and late sequelae of Kawasaki's disease also may be seen in pregnancy. Venous thrombotic disorders in pregnancy present diagnostic and therapeutic challenges.

Atherosclerotic Risk Factors and Hyperlipidemia

Risk factors for atherosclerotic coronary artery disease in women of childbearing age, as in the general population, include family history, advancing age, hypertension, hyperlipidemia, diabetes mellitus, cigarette smoking, oral contraceptive use, obesity, and physical inactivity. Hyperlipidemia, diabetes, and obesity are more prevalent with increasing age.[6,206] Normal pregnancy represents an up-regulation in the inflammatory cascade.[207] There may be characteristics shared with nonpregnant subjects in whom a similar up-regulation reflects a pre-atherosclerotic state. Vascular response to the metabolic stress of pregnancy may be predictive of future atherosclerotic events in women.[207] The use of oral contraceptive agents is discouraged in high risk women older than 35 years, particularly if they are smokers or have hypertension.[208] Oral contraceptives may be linked to coronary artery disease through their thrombogenic, hyperlipidemic, and hypertensive effects. Smoking cessation is required for maternal health reasons and for reducing the risk of fetal and neonatal complications.[209,210]

As in the case of hypertension, hyperlipidemia is often difficult to treat because most lipid-modifying drugs are unsuitable for use in pregnant patients. Physiologic changes in lipid metabolism in pregnancy are founded upon the stimulatory actions of estrogen, insulin, and lipoprotein lipase, allowing metabolic adaptation that favors the conservation of glucose and energy for the fetus. Enhanced adipose tissue lipolysis promotes a rise in available triglyceride substrates. Lipoprotein lipase activity decreases, leading to slower triglyceride clearance.[211] Hypertriglyceridemia is the principal finding in maternal hyperlipidemia. In the normal pregnancy, a modest rise in total serum cholesterol is observed as well, along with a fall in the beneficial high-density lipoprotein cholesterol concentration; the reason for the latter is not clear.[212] Diabetes mellitus and alcoholism can cause secondary lipid disorders. Severe hyperlipidemia can be associated with hypoxemia and fetal growth restriction.[213] Myocardial infarction during pregnancy was observed in a young woman with elevated levels of the atherogenic lipoprotein Lp_a.[214]

Pregnancy is challenging for patients who have preexisting hyperlipidemia, and multiple pregnancies may increase coronary risk in some patients, although there are no definite conclusions for the general population.[215] Dietary counseling is the standard approach for maternal hyperlipidemia. Drugs that alter hepatic metabolism, such as gemfibrozil, niacin in pharmacologic doses, and 3-hydroxy-3-methylglutaryl–coenzyme A (HMG-CoA) reductase inhibitors of the lovastatin class, should be avoided. Cholesterol-lowering bile acid sequestrants such as colestipol, cholestyramine, and colesevelam are not absorbed systemically and therefore are safe in women of childbearing age. However, the tendency of bile acid sequestrants to raise serum triglyceride levels is a drawback in hyperlipidemic

pregnant patients. In extreme situations of genetically based gestational hypertriglyceridemia, serum values may reach 5000 mg/dL, resulting in pancreatitis. The clinical presentation is noteworthy for abdominal pain, eruptive xanthomas, and lipemia retinalis. Serum may appear grossly lipemic. For such patients, extracorporeal lipid elimination with plasma exchange apheresis has been used.[211]

Coronary Artery Disease and Myocardial Infarction

Angina pectoris and myocardial infarction are relatively rare in pregnancy.[216,217] Myocardial infarction complicates fewer than 1 in 10,000 pregnancies[217]; nevertheless, maternal mortality averages 20%. Multigravid patients are more likely to experience myocardial infarction, and cardiac events tend to occur in the third trimester and peripartum intervals. Important causes include atherosclerosis[187]; thrombus related to the hypercoagulable gravid state; embolism; spontaneous dissection[197,218] linked to arterial wall structural changes in pregnancy, such as smooth muscle proliferation and reduced collagen synthesis[217,219]; inflammatory syndromes[220]; and spasm with structurally normal coronary vessels.[221] Other causes include Kawasaki's disease with aneurysmal coronary dilation, connective tissue disorders,[222] the use of ergot derivatives and oxytocin, and pheochromocytoma.[223,224] Anterior infarction is noted most frequently, and the majority of angiographic and pathologic studies do not reveal atherosclerosis.[216,217] Myocardial infarction is associated with pregnancy-induced hypertension and eclampsia. Vasoconstrictive stimuli may serve as the link connecting these entities.[217]

The diagnosis of coronary artery disease may be difficult because of a low index of suspicion and nonspecific electrocardiographic ST segment and T wave changes found in normal pregnant women, in particular at the time of cesarean section with regional anesthesia.[225,226] Low-level exercise treadmill studies may be useful for documenting coronary artery disease, and echocardiography is safe and accurate in defining regions of ischemia or infarction. At the time of labor and the early postpartum interval, blood levels of creatine kinase with positive MB isoenzymes can be elevated. Although this elevation simulates that observed during a myocardial infarction, these enzymes are believed to arise from the uterus and placenta.[227] Cardiac troponin level measurements may be useful, however, because unlike creatine kinase, troponin levels normally do not become elevated in pregnancy and delivery.[228] Radionuclide scintigraphy and catheterization with angiography carry radiation risks to the fetus and should be avoided.

Therapy for symptomatic coronary artery disease consists of low-dose aspirin, β-adrenergic blockers, nitrates, and heparin. Careful observation and management are essential during the physiologically stressful time of labor and delivery.[229] For women who have coronary artery disease or who have sustained a myocardial infarction, there is no clear advantage of cesarean over vaginal delivery or vice versa. The former averts prolonged and stressful labor, whereas the latter avoids surgical, anesthetic, and postoperative risks.[217,229] The left lateral decubitus position maximizes cardiac output and should relieve pain and anxiety quickly. Oxygen is administered, and myocardial oxygen consumption minimized through pharmacologic regulation of elevated pulse or blood pressure. Oxytocin and ergot derivatives can promote arterial spasm and should be avoided. Invasive hemodynamic monitoring is useful in cases of ongoing myocardial ischemia, congestive heart failure, or hemodynamic instability.

For acute myocardial infarction in pregnancy, thrombolytic therapy with t-PA has been reported as safe and effective.[177,216] A large molecule with a very short half-life, t-PA does not cross the placental barrier to a significant degree. Because of the risk of hemorrhage, t-PA should not be given near the time of delivery. Low-dose aspirin, heparin, judicious doses of nitrates, oxygen, and β-adrenergic blockers may be employed. Cardiac catheterization with transcatheter therapeutic intervention requires ionizing radiation for fluoroscopy and should be deferred unless medically refractory symptoms or hemodynamic instability occurs. Intra-aortic balloon pump counterpulsation techniques have been used in myocardial infarction during pregnancy when shock is present.[230] Percutaneous coronary balloon angioplasty, intracoronary stent placement, and surgical myocardial revascularization with or without cardiopulmonary bypass pump have been conducted successfully in pregnant patients.[195-197,201,202] A radial artery versus femoral artery approach to angiography and angioplasty can offer advantages in the pregnant woman by reducing fetal radiation exposure.[231] A case report describes the successful use of immunosuppressive therapy for myocardial infarction with multiple sites of spontaneous coronary dissection.[220] In patients who experienced an earlier myocardial infarction, subsequent normal pregnancies have been reported.[209]

Peripheral Vascular Diseases

Chronic disorders of the arterial system may complicate pregnancy, or new syndromes may appear with pregnancy. Arterial changes observed in pregnancy include heightened vascular fragility. A tendency toward maternal cerebrovascular accidents has been defined.[106] Aortic dissection, most commonly associated with Marfan's syndrome or coarctation of the aorta, may be more frequent in pregnancy. Transesophageal echocardiography furnishes an accurate diagnosis without exposure to ionizing radiation. Drug treatment emphasizes reduction in vascular shear forces, as in nonpregnant patients, through modification of the rate of rise in aortic pressure.[141] β-Adrenergic blockade, combined with afterload reducing agents such as hydralazine, satisfies this objective in the pregnant patient. To limit sharp rises in blood pressure associated with labor, cesarean section may be preferred.

Nonatherosclerotic arterial diseases such as fibromuscular dysplasia, vasospastic disorders, late sequelae of Kawasaki's disease, and Takayasu's arteritis may complicate pregnancy.[232,233] Fibromuscular dysplasia and Takayasu's arteritis are observed mainly in young women. In particular, Takayasu's arteritis or pulseless disease may pose challenges in managing the pregnant patient. There are maternal complications in half of all pregnancies in patients who

have Takayasu's arteritis. In addition to the aorta, multiple central and peripheral arterial distributions may have occlusive disease (Fig. 6–9). Hypertension and heart failure may be prominent, although peripheral indirect blood pressure measurements can underestimate central arterial pressure.[234] Because of blood pressure elevations with uterine contraction, cesarean section is preferred if hypertension or congestive heart failure proves refractory to medical management.[141] However, with careful hemodynamic monitoring and pharmacologic management, vaginal delivery may be considered.[234] Glucocorticoid treatment appears to bring benefit only in the acute phase of the disease.

Venous thrombophlebitis is often seen in pregnancy. The capacitance of the venous network increases in the gravid state, with consequent higher venous pressure and associated distention. Flow may decrease, thereby producing stasis, thrombosis, and embolization. Establishing the diagnosis may be difficult because edema and tenderness are often natural findings in pregnancy. Doppler ultrasonography can identify venous occlusion without the use of ionizing radiation, although contrast venography is helpful when the diagnosis is in doubt.[235] Because of warfarin-related embryopathy, the preferred anticoagulant is heparin, and if there is a prior history of thromboembolic disease, prophylactic anticoagulation should be given in the third trimester, when recurrence rates are highest. After delivery, computed tomography with radiocontrast can be used to identify iliac or pelvic thromboses.

CARDIOVASCULAR MEDICATIONS IN PREGNANCY AND LACTATION

During pregnancy, if serious cardiovascular or hypertensive conditions necessitate pharmacotherapy, agents

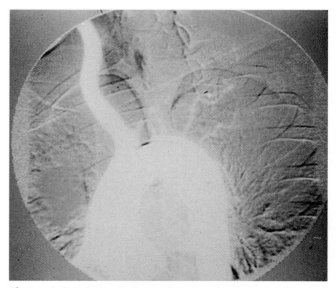

Figure 6–9. Takayasu's disease: Aortography demonstrating occlusion of left carotid and bilateral subclavian arteries in a severely hypertensive pregnant woman of Asian Indian ancestry. The right carotid artery is the sole major aortic arch branch that remains patent.

should be prescribed in the lowest effective dosage. Cardiovascular drugs traverse the placental barrier with varying levels of ease. For the fetus, the point of maximum drug sensitivity is the period of organogenesis occurring in the first trimester.

In pregnancy, there is a wide spectrum of clinical and investigative experience with drugs that affect the circulation. The range of data spans the extensive and reassuring experience with methyldopa and digoxin, the limited but often promising findings associated with β-adrenergic blockers and calcium channel blockers, the limited but clearly unfavorable findings relating to angiotensin converting enzyme inhibitors, and the minimal information concerning minoxidil and sotalol. Ethical objections make drug study in pregnancy very difficult, and observations derived from animal models may not apply to humans.

The use of cardiovascular drugs in lactating women has become a significant issue because of the intersection of two trends: the rising popularity of breast-feeding and the greater number of women bearing children at older ages when medication is prescribed for essential hypertension or other circulatory conditions.[236] In mothers who are breast-feeding, drug passage into milk is influenced principally by the concentration gradient between plasma and milk. The agent's lipid solubility, extent of ionization, protein-binding capacity, and pH of the breast milk all play subsidiary roles. As a result of the lower pH of milk than of plasma, weak acids such as diuretics appear in lower concentration in milk than in plasma. Conversely, weak bases such as β-adrenergic blockers are measured in greater concentration in breast milk than in plasma. Milk concentration may equal plasma concentration for certain drugs, but because of partial absorption and extensive distribution of drug in the neonate, there may be no measurable clinical toxicity. Digoxin and β-adrenergic blockers are generally regarded as safe in lactation, although well-conducted human studies have been limited. Drugs that appear in the lowest concentration in breast milk are typically considered most desirable.[237] Careful clinical observation should be maintained when children are breast-feeding while the mother is receiving any cardiovascular compound.

α-Adrenergic Blockers

Experience with α-adrenergic blockers has been limited, and these compounds have been combined with β-adrenergic blockers in severe hypertensive cases without adverse neonatal effects.[237] There are no reports of the use of these agents in lactating mothers.

α Agonists

Methyldopa has been employed and studied extensively, and it is considered a safe first-line drug for hypertensive pregnant patients.[237] Children of mothers who received methyldopa had no demonstrable abnormalities on evaluation after the seventh year of life.[238] The α agonist clonidine was compared with methyldopa in a randomized controlled manner, and both agents were proved safe

in pregnancy.[239] Although both methyldopa and clonidine appear in breast milk, no consequences in the newborn have been noted for either drug.[236,240]

Angiotensin-Converting Enzyme Inhibitors and Receptor Blockers

Angiotensin-converting enzyme inhibitors such as captopril, enalapril, lisinopril, fosinopril, quinapril, benazepril, trandolapril, perindopril, and others cross the placenta rapidly[241,242] and are associated with fetal loss, oligohydramnios, low birth weight, cranial ossification abnormalities, and neonatal renal failure. The angiotensin-converting enzyme inhibitors are therefore not recommended in pregnancy.[243,244] This advice extends to the related class of angiotensin II receptor blockers, such as losartan, valsartan, irbesartan, candesartan, telmisartan, eprosartan, and olmesartan.[245] Captopril concentration in breast milk is extremely low.[246]

Antiarrhythmic Agents

Quinidine passes the placental barrier but is generally viewed as safe in pregnancy. Fetal thrombocytopenia and ototoxicity have been reported in association with therapeutic doses, and toxic doses may induce premature labor or fetal loss. Quinidine appears in modest concentration in breast milk. The quantity absorbed by the infant is unlikely to pose clinical issues,[141,247] unless the child is premature, in which case hepatic accumulation of quinidine may be observed.[248] There has been less clinical experience with procainamide. Although this compound crosses the placenta, no adverse effects have been reported. Disopyramide has been employed in rare cases for heart rhythm indications. No ill effects on the fetus have been recognized, although stimulation of uterine contractions is cited as a side effect.[249] The breast milk concentration of disopyramide approximates that of maternal plasma, although the drug is unmeasurable in the breast-feeding infant. Lidocaine has been used in obstetric settings as an anesthetic rather than an antiarrhythmic agent. Elevated maternal blood levels pose a risk of reversible fetal or neonatal central nervous system depression, apnea, hypotonia, seizure, and bradycardia. Bretylium is not preferred because it has been linked with abnormal uteroplacental perfusion.

Mexiletine has been the subject of few reports, with no teratogenic or long-term complications noted, although bradycardia and hypoglycemia have been witnessed acutely.[250] Mexiletine is excreted in a high ratio of breast milk concentration to plasma concentration,[251,252] although ingestion by the infant may produce drug levels well below the therapeutic range.[247] Flecainide has been given safely and successfully in treating fetal tachycardia and maternal ventricular tachycardia; however, there is a paucity of overall experience.[253,254] Propafenone crosses the placenta, and published experience is quite sparse.[255] Phenytoin is undesirable in light of reports of increased risks of congenital cardiac anomalies, cleft palate, mental retardation, and craniofacial malformations.[256]

Sotalol use in pregnancy has not been adequately evaluated. This agent crosses the placenta and appears in high concentration in breast milk.[257] Amiodarone is typically used only in refractory rhythm disturbances. This compound traverses the placental barrier, and some case reports have been favorable; however, congenital hypothyroidism, goiter, prematurity, hypotonia, and bradycardia haven been described.[258,259] Amiodarone is secreted in significant concentration in breast milk and probably should be avoided in this setting. Adenosine as therapy for maternal tachyarrhythmias is safe.[260,261] Ibutilide is not recommended for gestational use because of teratogenic and embryocidal effects in experimental models. Breast milk concentrations of this drug have not been analyzed.

Anticoagulant and Antiplatelet Compounds

Clinical experience and advice regarding warfarin, unfractionated heparin and LMWH, thrombolytic agents, aspirin, dipyridamole, sulfinpyrazone, ticlopidine, and clopidogrel have been presented in the foregoing section on anticoagulation and prosthetic valves in pregnancy.

β-Adrenergic Blockers and Combined α-β Blockers

β-Adrenergic blockers are well tolerated late in pregnancy, but fetal growth restriction has been reported when they are used early in pregnancy. Postnatal growth, however, is unaffected.[262] Fetal bradycardia and neonatal hypoglycemia, apnea, and hyperbilirubinemia have been observed. Atenolol, metoprolol, and propranolol have been used extensively.[237,255,263] $β_2$-Adrenergic receptor stimulation promotes uterine muscular relaxation. Therefore, selective $β_1$-adrenergic blockers such as atenolol or metoprolol are preferred in order to avoid the uterine stimulation that is often seen when nonselective agents such as propranolol block $β_2$-adrenergic receptors.

Combined α- and β-adrenergic blocking agents such as labetalol are well tolerated and useful in hypertensive pregnant patients.[264] Despite reduced maternal blood pressure, uteroplacental blood flow is not diminished when labetalol is used.[265] In an animal model, the use of labetalol had no adverse effect on fetal heart rate, blood pressure, or acid-base status.[266] Long-term follow-up concerning use of labetalol during pregnancy in humans is limited.[267]

As weak bases, β-adrenergic blockers appear in greater concentration in breast milk than in plasma. On the basis of protein-binding properties, hydrophilic β-adrenergic blockers such as atenolol are observed in greater concentrations in milk than are lipophilic agents such as propranolol; thus, use of the latter has a theoretical advantage.[237] The breast-feeding newborn may experience side effects of bradycardia and somnolence.[263]

Calcium Channel Blockers

Experience is limited, but there is accumulating evidence favoring the safety of this class of cardiovascular agents in pregnancy. Calcium channel blockers, also known as calcium antagonists or calcium entry blockers, can be divided into four groups: the dihydropyridine (nifedipine), papaverine (verapamil), benzothiazepine (diltiazem), and tetralol (mibefradil) subclasses. In an animal model, there was a low incidence of fetal cardiovascular malformations with exposure to these four subclasses.[268] A prospective multicenter study observed no increased risk of teratogenicity in infants exposed to calcium channel blockers during the first trimester.[269]

Nifedipine has been used to treat severe essential hypertension and hypertensive emergencies in pregnancy.[270] In one series, nifedipine lowered maternal blood pressure without adverse impact on umbilical artery blood flow-velocity waveforms.[271] Sublingual administration has been associated with sudden hypotension and cerebral ischemia in the general medical population and thus should be avoided in pregnancy to prevent uteroplacental hypoperfusion. Prematurity and low birth weights have been reported in association with the use of nifedipine during pregnancy. The drug may cause uterine relaxation and therefore has been employed as a tocolytic agent. In an animal model, the dihydropyridine calcium channel blocker nicardipine did not adversely affect fetal heart rate, blood pressure, or acid-base status.[266] Nifedipine has been evaluated favorably for use in lactating mothers,[272] and the similar dihydropyridine agent nimodipine is secreted minimally in breast milk.[273]

Verapamil has been used to regulate maternal and fetal tachycardias, severe gestational hypertension, and premature labor. At the onset of full-term labor, this agent should not be administered, so as to avoid dysfunctional labor or postpartum hemorrhage secondary to lack of uterine muscular tone. Use of verapamil in lactating women is probably benign.[272]

Few reports describe use of the benzothiazepine compound diltiazem in pregnancy. Diltiazem is probably acceptable in lactation.[272] The tetralol subclass of calcium channel blockers, including the agent mibefradil, has not been fully evaluated for use in pregnancy or lactation. Because of concerns regarding medication interactions, mibefradil is not available for clinical use at present. Congenital anomalies in the form of aortic arch branching variants were discovered in animal fetuses after gestational exposure to mibefradil.[268]

Diuretics

Diuretics are generally not favored in pregnancy because of their propensity to decrease maternal blood volume, thereby jeopardizing fetal nutrition, oxygenation, and growth. Hypokalemia, hyponatremia, and thrombocytopenia have been reported in neonates. Loop agents should be carefully titrated. Previously hypertensive patients taking diuretics who become pregnant may benefit from a change to another blood pressure–lowering agent. However, some authorities advocate continuing diuretics if blood pressure regulation is optimal with diuretic use in the sodium-sensitive subject.[267] If a potassium-conserving agent is needed, safety data for amiloride are favorable.[274] Spironolactone harbors antiandrogen activity and may feminize male fetuses.[275] Diuretics may suppress milk production in lactation and are not recommended.[237]

Inotropic and Pressor Agents

Cardiac glycosides such as digoxin cross the placenta, and the resulting plasma concentration in the fetus equals that of the mother without consequence. Digoxin has been employed widely for treatment of maternal and fetal heart failure and supraventricular tachyarrhythmias. In pregnancy, digoxin has an increased volume of distribution and augmented renal clearance. Relatively high doses may be needed to achieve the desired therapeutic effect. Serum levels may be difficult to interpret because of a gestational increase in the concentration of physiologic digoxin-like substances. The use of digoxin in lactating mothers is safe.

Intravenous inotropic and pressor agents such as dopamine, dobutamine, amrinone, milrinone, epinephrine, and norepinephrine pose hazards by suppressing placental blood flow and provoking uterine contractions.[276] Such agents should be used with extreme caution and are recommended for life-threatening situations only.[277] Ephedrine probably represents a better alternative pressor in pregnancy, although most experience with this agent lies in treatment of hypotension caused by hypovolemia, or vasodilation induced by spinal anesthesia, rather than cardiogenic shock.[276,278]

Nitrates and Vasodilators

Nitrate preparations are safe for use in pregnancy, although they are not ideal antihypertensive agents, in view of their primary venodilatory role. On the basis of vascular relaxation, nitrates assist in the therapy of preeclampsia or intrauterine fetal growth restriction.[279-281] Patients treated with nitroglycerin must be observed for hypotension to avoid serious consequences to the fetus.[282] The use of nitrates in lactating women has not been widely reported.

Hydralazine is safe and effective for both blood pressure control and afterload reduction indications in pregnancy. As an arterial dilator, it provides a complementary mechanism of action when used as an adjunct to β-adrenergic blockers. Rare reports link hydralazine with neonatal thrombocytopenia.

Sodium nitroprusside should be avoided in pregnancy because the metabolites thiocyanate and cyanide are potentially toxic. Fetal cyanide poisoning has been produced in animal models. The use of minoxidil, the most potent oral vasodilating antihypertensive agent, has not been tested in pregnancy or lactation.

Statins and Other Lipid-Modifying Drugs

HMG-CoA reductase inhibitors (statins) of the lovastatin class should be avoided in pregnancy, in light of animal toxicity studies demonstrating increased rates of malformations.[262] However, inadvertent first trimester exposure to statins was not accompanied by increased adverse events in humans.[283] Statins are secreted in breast milk.

Niacin (nicotinic acid) carries no risk in pregnancy when used as a vitamin supplement in physiologic doses. Pharmacologic lipid-lowering doses of niacin have not been assessed in pregnancy. Bile acid sequestrants (resins), such as colestipol, cholestyramine, and colesevelam, are not systemically absorbed and thus are safe. Fibrates, such as gemfibrozil and fenofibrate, may be harmful, inasmuch as malformations have appeared in animal models. Although ezetimibe acts in the intestine, it is absorbed and metabolized in the liver and is not recommended for use during pregancy.

CARDIAC EFFECTS OF OBSTETRIC DRUGS

Obstetric medications can have a major impact on circulatory function. Tocolytic agents and uterine stimulants are surveyed as follows.

Tocolytic Compounds

Drugs administered to suppress premature uterine contractions may stimulate the heart. Terbutaline, a β-adrenergic agonist, causes uterine relaxation through activation of β_2 receptors. Terbutaline, isoxsuprine, salbutamol, and ritodrine (the latter no longer marketed in the United States) may provoke tachycardia with hemodynamic decompensation in patients who have structural heart disease, particularly left-sided obstructive lesions, myocardial ischemia, or rapid rhythm disorders. Heightened myocardial contractility generated by β-adrenergic tocolytic agents can magnify outflow obstruction in patients who have hypertrophic subaortic stenosis. In such instances, nifedipine is preferred.

Adverse cardiac effects of terbutaline in pregnancy include chest discomfort, dyspnea, irregular pulse, electrocardiographic changes, or pulmonary edema.[284] In one series, tocolytic use was the most common cause of pulmonary edema in pregnancy.[285] Several effects may account for pulmonary edema, including elevated heart rate and cardiac output, myocardial dysfunction related to prolonged catecholamine exposure, increased capillary permeability, and associated excess fluid administration.[235,276] This condition responds to cessation of terbutaline therapy and the institution of oxygen and diuretics.

Uterine Stimulants

Prostaglandins and oxytocin may have cardiovascular consequences when given to induce labor. As vasodilators, prostaglandins are well tolerated in volume overload states. They are not advisable for use for hypertrophic subaortic stenosis because of the hazard of worsened outflow obstruction with hypotension. Oxytocin is favored in this setting.[141] Reactive hypertension and volume retention may accompany the use of oxytocin, and this agent should be given carefully if heart disease has been diagnosed.

MANAGEMENT DURING SURGERY, LABOR, AND DELIVERY

Physiologic stress of labor, delivery, cesarean section, or other surgical operations during pregnancy may be intolerable in the woman who has cardiac disease. Patients are particularly prone to complications in the immediate postpartum interval as vena caval compression is relieved and heavy blood volume is reinjected into the maternal circulation from the uterus. Left-sided heart filling pressure, stroke volume, and cardiac output all rise, increasing the risk of pulmonary congestion in the patient who has depressed ventricular function or left-sided obstructive pathologic processes.

Method of Anesthesia

Epidural or neuraxial anesthesia may blunt the hemodynamic changes associated with vaginal delivery, but it does not modify the rise in cardiac output that accompanies uterine contractions.[141] Because of the potential for hypotension and reduced cardiac filling pressures with epidural anesthesia, this technique should be avoided or used with great caution in patients who have right-sided heart lesions with major preload dependence, such as Eisenmenger's syndrome, tetralogy of Fallot, or complex cyanotic congenital heart disease.[286] Moreover, in patients with these diagnoses and in those who have Ebstein's anomaly, the systemic vasodilation associated with epidural anesthesia can exacerbate right-to-left shunting and lead to greater cyanosis. Preload-dependent left-sided obstructive lesions such as hypertrophic subaortic stenosis and aortic valve stenosis suggest the need for great caution if epidural anestesia is used. Patients who have mitral valve stenosis may tolerate epidural anesthesia quite well because the generalized vasodilation can improve their pulmonary congestion, particularly in the postpartum interval of enhanced circulating volume.

Alternatives to standard neuraxial or epidural anesthesia include inhalation analgesia, pudendal nerve block, intrathecal opiate treatment, and systemic parenteral analgesia. Nalbuphine (Nubain) is useful in this setting because it produces less respiratory depression than do other opiates, because of its strong narcotic antagonist characteristics. General anesthesia usually is not required.

Perioperative and Peripartum Management in the Complex Patient

Cesarean section may limit the stress of vaginal delivery in patients who have heart disease. This method avoids prolonged labor with hemodynamically destabilizing contractions.[286] However, cesarean section entails the major surgery, blood loss, and the possibility of stress associated with endotracheal intubation and extubation if general anesthesia is required.[141] If vaginal delivery is selected for patients with cardiac disease, elective low or outlet forceps delivery may shorten the second stage of labor. Placing the patient in the left lateral decubitus position prevents hypotension[287] and may be especially effective when epidural anesthesia is given. To protect against hypertension with contractions, cesarean section is advised for patients with Marfan's syndrome or aortic dissection. In most other categories of maternal heart disease, vaginal delivery is feasible if invasive pulmonary artery and arterial pressure monitoring are feasible. In a large series of women with congenital heart lesions, 79% were able to deliver vaginally with careful monitoring.[93] Invasive monitoring can prevent extreme fluctuations in hemodynamics and may guide fluid, diuretic, vasodilator, or pressor therapy.[234,276] These suggestions apply as well to patients undergoing nonobstetric surgical procedures while pregnant. Rapid echocardiographic assessment of high-risk cardiac patients is valuable, particularly at delivery, and can be complemented by invasive methods to generate a full hemodynamic profile.[288]

FUTURE DIRECTIONS

Technologic innovations and advances in scientific understanding have contributed to the welcome progress in the field of cardiovascular disease in pregnancy. Evolving diagnostic and management techniques now enable improved outcomes in affected mothers and offspring. However, three risk-prone groups are joining the childbearing population: (1) adults who have undergone surgical correction of complex congenital heart disease, (2) patients who become pregnant after 40 years of age and who are thus vulnerable to acquired cardiovascular disorders, and (3) women immigrating from areas where rheumatic heart disease is still endemic in young people.

The future may bring greater understanding of how cardiac and noncardiac risk factors interact to alter maternal and neonatal outcomes. Further insights will be gained into the origin of peripartum cardiomyopathy. Prospective trials may illustrate benefits of preventive pharmacotherapy in patients who have heart valve disease. Criteria for selecting artificial valves in young women will be refined. Randomized studies may clarify the contested issues of optimal anticoagulation in pregnancy and the value of peripartum antibiotic prophylaxis in women with structural heart disease. The scope of safe drug use in pregnancy will expand slowly because of the challenges involved in human testing. Finally, progress in genetic inquiry will allow better estimation of the transmissibility of congenital heart lesions from mother to infant.

References

1. Rochat RW, Koonin LM, Atrash HK, et al, and the Maternal Mortality Collaborative: Maternal mortality in the United States: Report from the Maternal Mortality Collaborative. Obstet Gynecol 1996;72:91.
2. Siu SC, Sermer M, Colman JM, et al: Prospective multicenter study of pregnancy outcomes in women with heart disease. Circulation 2001;104:515.
3. Seoud MA, Nassar AH, Usta IM, et al: Impact of advanced maternal age on pregnancy outcome. Am J Perinatol 2002;19:1.
4. Syverson CG, Shavkin W, Atrash HK, et al: Pregnancy-related mortality in New York City, 1980-1984. Am J Obstet Gynecol 1991;164:603.

5. Dorfman SF: Maternal mortality in New York City 1981-1983. Obstet Gynecol 1990;76:317.
6. Hansen JP: Older maternal age in pregnancy outcome: A review of the literature. Obstet Gynecol Surv 1986;41:726.
7. Buehler JW, Kaunitz AM, Hogue CJ, et al: Maternal mortality in women aged 35 years and older: United States. JAMA 1986;255:53.
8. Mc Faul PB, Dornan JC, Lamki H, Boyle D: Pregnancy complicated by maternal heart disease: A review of 519 women. Br J Obstet Gynaecol 1988;95:861.
9. Hogberg U, Innala E, Sandstrom A: Maternal mortality in Sweden, 1980-1988. Obstet Gynecol 1994;84:240.
10. Ray JG, Burrows RF, Burrows EA, Vermeulen MJ: McMaster outcome study of hypertension in pregnancy. Early Hum Dev 2001;64:129.
11. Kallen K: The impact of maternal smoking during pregnancy on delivery outcome. Eur J Public Health 2001;11:329.
12. Tomoda S, Tamura T, Sudo Y, Ogita S: Effects of obesity on pregnant women: Maternal hemodynamic change. Am J Perinatol 1996;13:73.
13. Callan NA, Maggio M, Steger S et al: Fetal echocardiography: indications for referral, prenatal diagnosis, and outcomes. Am J Perinatol 1991;8:390.
14. McLennan CE: Antecubital and femoral venous pressure in normal and toxemic pregnancy. Am J Obstet Gynecol 1943;45:568.
15. Wright HP, Osborn SB, Edmunds DG: Changes in rate of flow of venous blood in the leg during pregnancy, measured with radioactive sodium. Surg Gynecol Obstet 1950;90:480.
16. Enein M, Zina AA, Kassem M, El-Tabbakh G: Echocardiography of the pericardium in pregnancy. Obstet Gynecol 1987;69:851.
17. Cutforth R, MacDonald CB: Heart sounds and murmurs in pregnancy. Am Heart J 1966;71:741.
18. Mabie WC, DiSessa TG, Crocker LG, et al: A longitudinal study of cardiac output in normal human pregnancy. Am J Obstet Gynecol 1994;170:849.
19. Duvekot JJ, Cheriex EC, Pieters FAA, et al: Early pregnancy changes in hemodynamics and volume homeostasis are consecutive adjustments triggered by a primary fall in systemic vascular tone. Am J Obstet Gynecol 1993;169:1382.
20. Easterling TR, Benedetti TJ, Schmucker BC, Millard SP: Maternal hemodynamics in normal and preeclamptic pregnancies: A longitudinal study. Obstet Gynecol 1990;76:1061.
21. Capeless EL, Clapp JF: Cardiovascular changes in early phases of pregnancy. Am J Obstet Gynecol 1989;161:1449.
22. Ueland K, Hansen JM: Maternal cardiovascular dynamics. 2: Posture and uterine contractions. Am J Obstet Gynecol 1969;103:1.
23. Robson SC, Hunter S, Boys RJ, Dunlop W: Serial study of factors influencing changes in cardiac output during human pregnancy. Am J Physiol 1989;256:H1060.
24. Ueland K, Metcalfe J: Circulatory changes in pregnancy. Clin Obstet Gynecol 1975;18:41.
25. Robson SC, Dunlop W, Boys RJ, Hunter S: Cardiac output during labor. BMJ 1987;295:1169.
26. Mc Anulty JH: Anesthesia during pregnancy in the patient with heart disease. In Bonica JJ, McDonald JS (eds): Principles and Practice of Obstetric Analgesia and Anesthesia, 2nd ed. Baltimore, Lippincott, Williams & Wilkins, 1995, pp 1013-1039.
27. James C, Banner T, Caton D: Cardiac output in women undergoing cesarean section with epidural or general anesthesia. Am J Obstet Gynecol 1989;160:1178.
28. Etheridge MJ, Pepperell RJ: Heart disease and pregnancy at the Royal Women's Hospital. Med J Aust 1977;2:227.
29. Whittaker PG, MacPhail S, Lind T: Serial hematologic changes and pregnancy outcome. Obstet Gynecol 1996;88:33.
30. Pritchard JA: Changes in the blood volume during pregnancy and delivery. Anesthesiology 1965;26:393.
31. Chesley LC: Plasma and red cell volumes during pregnancy. Am J Obstet Gynecol 1972;112:440.
32. Lindheimer MC, Katz AL: Sodium and diuretics in pregnancy. N Engl J Med 1973;299:891.
33. Lindheimer MC, Richardson DA, Ehrlich EN, Katz AI: Potassium homeostasis in pregnancy. J Reprod Med 1987;32:517.
34. Pritchard JA, Adams RH: Erythrocyte production and destruction during pregnancy. Am J Obstet Gynecol 1960;79:750.
35. Widness JA, Clemons GK, Garcia JF, Schwartz R: Plasma immunoreactivity erythropoietin in normal women studied

sequentially during and after pregnancy. Am J Obstet Gynecol 1984;149:646.
36. Huisman A, Aarnoudse JG, Heuvelmans JHA, et al: Whole blood viscosity during normal pregnancy. Br J Obstet Gynaecol 1987;94:1143.
37. Chisholm M: A controlled clinical trial of prophylactic folic acid and iron in pregnancy. J Obstet Gynaecol Br Commonw 1966;73:191.
28. Kaneshige E: Serum ferritin as an assessment of iron stores and other hematologic parameters during pregnancy. Obstet Gynecol 1981;57:238.
39. Longo L: Maternal blood volume and cardiac output during pregnancy: A hypothesis of endocrinologic control. Am J Physiol 1983;245:721.
40. Katz R, Karliner JS, Resnick R: Effects of a natural volume overload state (pregnancy) on left ventricular performance in normal human subjects. Circulation 1978;58:434.
41. Mone SM, Sanders SP, Colan SD: Control mechanisms for physiological hypertrophy of pregnancy. Circulation 1996;15:667.
42. Sadaniantz A, Saint Laurent L, Parisi AF: Long-term effects of multiple pregnancies on cardiac dimensions and systolic and diastolic function. Am J Obstet Gynecol 1996;174:1061.
43. Veille JC, Morton MJ, Burry KJ: Maternal cardiovascular adaptations to twin pregnancy. Am J Obstet Gynecol 1985;153:261.
44. Clark SL, Cotton DB, Lee W, et al: Central hemodynamic assessment of normal term pregnancy. Am J Obstet Gynecol 1989;61:1439.
45. Hauth JC, Gilstrap LC III, Widmer K: Fetal heart rate reactivity before and after maternal jogging during the third trimester. Am J Obstet Gynecol 1982;142:545.
46. Carpenter MW, Sady SP, Hoegsberg B, et al: Fetal heart rate response to maternal exertion. JAMA 1988;259:3006.
47. Committee on Obstetric Practice: Exercise during pregnancy and the postpartum period. Number 267, January 2002. American College of Obstetricians and Gynecologists. Int J Gynaecol Obstet 2002;77:79.
48. Watson MJ, Katz VL, Hackney AC, et al: Fetal responses to maximal swimming and cycling exercise during pregnancy. Obstet Gynecol 1991;77:382.
49. Clapp JF: Oxygen consumption during treadmill exercise before, during, and after pregnancy. Am J Obstet Gynecol 1989;161:1458.
50. Clapp JF, Capeless EL: Neonatal morphometrics after endurance exercise during pregnancy. Am J Obstet Gynecol 1990;163:1805.
51. Clapp JF, Little KD: The interaction between regular exercise and selected aspects of women's health. Am J Obstet Gynecol 1995;173:2.
52. Clapp JF: The course of labor after endurance exercise during pregnancy. Am J Obstet Gynecol 1990;163:1799,
53. Riemann MK, Kanstrup Hansen IL: Effects on the foetus of exercise in pregnancy. Scand J Med Sci Sports 2000;10:12.
54. Metcalfe J, McAnulty JH, Ueland K (eds): Burwell and Metcalf's Heart Disease and Pregnancy, 2nd ed. Boston, Little, Brown, 1986.
55. Brent RL: The effect of embryonic and fetal exposure to x-ray, microwaves, and ultrasound: Counseling the pregnant and non-pregnant patient about these risks. Semin Oncol 1989;16:347.
56. Carruth JE, Mivis SB, Brogan DR, Wenger NK: The electrocardiogram in normal pregnancy. Chest 1981;102:1075.
57. Limacher MC, Ware JA, O'Meara ME, et al: Tricuspid regurgitation during pregnancy: Two-dimensional and pulsed Doppler echocardiographic observations. Am J Cardiol 1985;55:1059.
58. Mettler FA, Guiberteau MJ: Essentials of Nuclear Medicine Imaging. Philadelphia, WB Saunders, 1991.
59. Veille JC: Peripartum cardiomyopathies: A review. Am J Obstet Gynecol 1984;148:806.
60. Sanderson JE, Olsen EGJ, Gatie D: Peripartum heart disease: An endomyocardial biopsy study. Br Heart J 1986;56:285.
61. Cunningham FG, Pritchard JA, Hankins GDV, et al: Idiopathic cardiomyopathy or compounding cardiovascular vents. Obstet Gynecol 1986;67:157.
62. Yacoub A, Martel MJ: Pregnancy with primary dilated cardiomyopathy. Obstet Gynecol 2002;99:928.
63. Koželj M, Novak-Antolic Ž, Noc M, Antolic G: Idiopathic dilated cardiomyopathy in pregnancy. Acta Obstet Gynecol Scand 2003;82:389.
64. Cunningham FG: Peripartum cardiomyopathy. Contemp Obstet Gynecol 1995;40:98.

65. Lee W, Cotton DB: Peripartum cardiomyopathy: Current concepts and clinical management. Clin Obstet Gynecol 1989;32:54.

66. Demakis JG, Rahimtoola SH, Sutton GC, et al: Natural course of peripartum cardiomyopathy. Circulation 1971;44:1053.

67. Pearson GD, Veille JC, Rahimtoola S, et al: Peripartum cardiomyopathy: National Heart, Lung, and Blood Institute and Office of Rare Diseases workshop recommendations and review. JAMA 2000;283:1183.

68. Elkayam U, Ostrzega EL, Shotan A: Peripartum cardiomyopathy. In Gleicher N (ed): Principles and Practice of Medical Therapy in Pregnancy, 2nd ed. E. Norwalk, Conn, Appleton & Lange, 1992.

69. O'Connell JB, Costanzo-Nordin MR, Subramanian R, et al: Peripartum cardiomyopathy: Clinical, hemodynamic, histologic and prognostic characteristics. J Am Coll Cardiol 1986;8:52.

70. Witlin AG, Mabie WC, Sibai BM: Peripartum cardiomyopathy: An ominous diagnosis. Am J Ostet Gynecol 1997;176:182.

71. Carvalho A, Brandao A, Martinez EE, et al: Prognosis in peripartum cardiomyopathy. Am J Cardiol 1989;64:540.

72. Lampert MB, Weinert L, Hibbard J, et al: Contractile reserve in patients with peripartum cardiomyopathy and recovered left ventricular function. Am J Obstet Gynecol 1997;176:189.

73. Elkayam U, Tummala PP, Rao K, et al: Maternal and fetal outcomes of subsequent pregnancies in women with peripartum cardiomyopathy. N Engl J Med 2001;344:1567.

74. Avila WS, De Carvalho MEC, Tschaen CK, et al: Pregnancy and peripartum cardiomyopathy: A comparative and prospective study. Arq Bras Cardiol 2002;79:489.

75. Futterman LG, Lemberg L: Peripartum cardiomyopathy: An ominous complication of pregnancy. Am J Crit Care 2000;9:362.

76. Bozkurt B, Villanueva FS, Holubkov R, et al: Intravenous immune globulin in the therapy of peripartum cardiomyopathy. J Am Coll Cardiol 1999;34:177.

77. Rotmensch HH, Rotmensch S, Elkayam U: Management of cardiac arrhythmias during pregnancy: Current concepts. Drugs 1987;33:623.

78. Joglar JA, Page RL: Treatment of cardiac arrhythmias during pregnancy: Safety considerations. Drug Saf 1999;20:85.

79. Jaffe R, Gruber A, Feigin M, et al: Pregnancy with an artificial pacemaker. Obstet Gynecol Surv 1987;42:137.

80. Widerhorn J, Widerhorn ALM, Rahimtoola SH, Elkayam U: WPW syndrome during pregnancy: Increased incidence after supraventricular arrhythmias. Am Heart J 1992;123:796.

81. Mendelson MA, Lang RM: Pregnancy and heart disease. In Baron WM, Lindheimer MD (eds): Medical Disorders during Pregnancy, 2nd ed. St. Louis, Mosby–Year Book, 1995, p 129.

82. Brodsky M, Doria R, Allen B, et al: New onset ventricular tachycardia during pregnancy. Am Heart J 1992;123:933.

83. Natale A, Davidson T, Geiger MJ, Newby K: Implantable cardioverter-defibrillators and pregnancy: A safe combination. Circulation 1997;96:2808.

84. Lee RV, Rodgers BD, White LM, Harvey RC: Cardiopulmonary resuscitation of pregnant women. Am J Med 1986;81:311.

85. Oberhansli I, Extermann P, Jaggi E, et al: Fetal echocardiography in pregnancies of women with congenital heart disease—clinical utility and limitations. Thorac Cardiovasc Surg 2000;48:323.

86. Metcalfe J, Ueland K: Maternal cardiovascular adjustments to pregnancy. Prog Cardiovasc Dis 1974;16:363.

87. Morris CD, Menashe VD: Evidence for maternal transmission of congenital heart defects. Circulation 1993;88(Suppl I):98.

88. Whittemore R, Hobbins JC, Engle MA: Pregnancy and its outcome in women with and without surgical treatment of congenital heart disease. Am J Cardiol 1982;50:641.

89. Shime J, Mocarski EJM, Hasting D, et al: Congenital heart disease in pregnancy: Short- and long-term implications. Am J Obstet Gynecol 1987;156:313.

90. Presbitero P, Somerville J, Stone S, et al: Pregnancy in cyanotic congential heart disease. Outcome of mother and fetus. Circulation 1994;89:2673.

91. Singh H, Bolton PJ, Oakley CM: Pregnancy after surgical correction of tetralogy of Fallot. BMJ 1982;285:168.

92. Morris CD, Menashe VD: 25 year mortality after surgical repair of congenital heart defect in childhood: A population-based cohort study. JAMA 1991;266:3447.

93. Kaemmerer H, Bauer U, Stein JI, et al: Pregnancy in congenital cardiac disease: An increasing challenge for cardiologists and obstetricians—a prospective multicenter study. Z Kardiol 2003;92:16.

94. Patton DE, Lee W, Cotton DB, et al: Cyanotic maternal heart disease in pregnancy. Obstet Gynecol Surv 1990;45:594.

95. Burn J, Brennan P, Little J, et al: Recurrence risks in offspring of adults with major heart defects: Results from first cohort of British collaborative study. Lancet 1998;351:311.

96. Task Force on the Management of Cardiovascular Diseases during Pregnancy of the European Society of Cardiology: Expert consensus document on management of cardiovascular diseases during pregnancy. Eur Heart J 2003;24:761.

97. Nugent EW, Planter WH, Edwards JE, Williams WH: The pathology, abnormal physiology, clinical recognition, and medical and surgical treatment of congenital heart disease. In Hurst JW, Schlant RC, Rackley CE, et al (eds): The Heart, 7th ed. New York, McGraw-Hill, 1990, p 655.

98. Gleicher N, Midwall J, Hochberger D, Jaffin H: Eisenmenger's syndrome and pregnancy. Obstet Gynecol Surv 1979;34:721.

99. Genoni M, Jenni R, Hoerstrup SP, et al: Pregnancy after atrial repair for transposition of the great arteries. Heart 1999;81:276.

100. Canobbio M, Mair D, Van Der Velde M, et al: Pregnancy outcomes after the Fontan repair. J Am Coll Cardiol 1996;28:763.

101. Hoare JV, Radford D: Pregnancy after Fontan repair of complex congenital heart disease. Austral N Z J Obstet Gynecol 2001;41:464.

102. McAnulty JH, Metcalfe J, Ueland K: Heart disease in pregnancy. In Hurst JW, Schlant RC, Rackley CE, et al (eds): The Heart, 7th ed. New York, McGraw-Hill, 1990, p 1465.

103. Connolly H, Ammash NM, Warnes C: Pregnancy in women with coarctation of the aorta. J Am Coll Cardiol 1996;27:43A.

104. Sherer DM: Coarctation of the descending thoracic aorta diagnosed during pregnancy. Obstet Gynecol 2002;100:1094.

105. Beauchesne LM, Connolly HM, Ammash NM, Warnes CA: Coarctation of the aorta: Outcome of pregnancy. J Am Coll Cardiol 2001;38:1728.

106. Barrett JM, Vanhooydonk JD, Bochm FH: Pregnancy related rupture of arterial aneurysms. Obstet Gynecol Surv 1982;37:557.

107. Whittemore R, Wells JA, Castellsague X: A second-generation study of 427 probands with congenital heart defects and their 837 children. J Am Coll Cardiol 1994;23:1459.

108. Kolibash AJ, Ruis DE, Lewis RP: Idiopathic hypertrophic subaortic stenosis in pregnancy. Ann Intern Med 1975;82:791.

109. Oakley GD, McGarry K, Limb DG, Oakley CM: Management of pregnancy in patients with hypertrophic cardiomyopathy. BMJ 1979;1:1749.

110. Shah DM, Sunderji SG: Hypertrophic cardiomyopathy and pregnancy: Report of a maternal mortality and review of literature. Obstet Gynecol Surv 1985;40:444.

111. Autore C, Conte MR, Piccininno M, et al: Risk associated with pregnancy in hypertrophic cardiomyopathy. J Am Coll Cardiol 2002;40:1864.

112. Thaman R, Varnava A, Hamid MS, et al: Pregnancy related complications in women with hypertrophic cardiomyopathy. Heart 2003;89:752.

113. Pyeritz RE, McKusick VA: The Marfan syndrome: Diagnosis and management. N Engl J Med 1979;300:772.

114. Elkayam U, Ostrzega E, Shotan A, Mehra A: Cardiovascular problems in pregnant women with the Marfan syndrome. Ann Intern Med 1995;123:117.

115. Mor-Yosef S, Younis J, Granat M, et al: Marfan's syndrome in pregnancy. Obstet Gynecol Surv 1988;43:382.

116. Murdoch JL, Walker BA, Helpern BL, et al: Life expectancy and causes of death in the Marfan syndrome. N Engl J Med 1972;298:804.

117. Lind J, Wallenburg HC: The Marfan syndrome and pregnancy: A retrospective study in a Dutch population. Eur J Obstet Gynecol Reprod Biol 2001;98:28.

118. Williams A, Child A, Rowntree J, et al: Marfan's syndrome: Successful pregnancy after aortic root and arch replacement. Br J Obstet Gynaecol 2002;109:1187.

119. Waickman LA, Skorton DJ, Varner MW, et al: Ebstein's anomaly and pregnancy. Am J Cardiol 1984;53:357.

120. Dajani AS, Bisno AL, Durack DT, et al: Prevention of rheumatic fever. Circulation 1988;78:1082.

121. Siu CS, Sermer M, Harrison DA, et al: Risk and predictors for pregnancy-related complications in women with heart disease. Circulation 1997;96:2789.

122. Hameed A, Karaalp IS, Tummala PP, et al: The effect of valvular heart disease on maternal and fetal outcome of pregnancy. J Am Coll Cardiol 2001;37:893.

123. Siu SC, Colman JM, Sorensen S, et al: Adverse neonatal and cardiac outcomes are more common in pregnant women with cardiac disease. Circulation 2002;105:2179.

124. Reimold SC, Rutherford JD: Valvular heart disease in pregnancy. N Engl J Med 2003;349:52.

125. Silversides CK, Colman JM, Sermer M, Siu SC: Cardiac risk in pregnant women with rheumatic mitral stenosis. Am J Cardiol 2003;91:1382.

126. Dajani AS, Taubert KA, Wilson W, et al: Prevention of bacterial endocarditis: Recommendations by the American Heart Association. JAMA 1997;277:1794.

127. Avila WS, Rossi EG, Ramires JAF, et al: Pregnancy in patients with heart disease: Experience with 1,000 cases. Clin Cardiol 2003;26:135.

128. Patel JJ, Mitha AS, Hassen F, et al: Percutaneous balloon mitral valvotomy in pregnant patients with tight pliable mitral stenosis. Am Heart J 1993;125:1106.

129. Saleh MH, El-Fiky AA, Fahmy M, et al: Use of biplane transesophageal echocardiography as the only imaging technique for percutaneous balloon mitral commissurotomy. Am J Cardiol 1996;78:103.

130. Farhat MB, Ayari M, Maatouk F, et al: Percutaneous balloon versus closed and open mitral commissurotomy. Seven year followup results of a randomized trial. Circulation 1998;97:245.

131. DeSouza JA, Martinez EE, Ambrose JA, et al: Percutaneous balloon mitral valvuloplasty in comparison with open mitral valve commissurotomy for mitral stenosis during pregnancy. J Am Coll Cardiol 2001;37:900.

132. Nercolini DC, da Rocha Loures Bueno R, Eduardo Guérios E, et al: Percutaneous mitral balloon valvuloplasty in pregnant women with mitral stenosis. Catheter Cardiovasc Interv 2002;57:318.

133. Kinsara AJ, Ismail O, Fawzi ME: Effect of balloon mitral valvuloplasty during pregnancy on childhood development. Cardiology 2002;97:155.

134. Rayburn WF: Mitral valve prolapse and pregnancy. In Elkayam U, Gleicher N (eds): Cardiac Problems in Pregnancy: Diagnosis and Management of Maternal and Fetal Disease, 2nd ed. New York, Alan R. Liss, 1990, p 181.

135. Silversides CK, Colman JM, Sermer M, et al: Early and intermediate-term outcomes of pregnancy with congenital aortic stenosis. Am J Cardiol 2003;91:1386.

136. Easterling TR, Chadwick HS, Otto CM, Benedetti TJ: Aortic stenosis in pregnancy. Obstet Gynecol 1988;72:113.

137. Banning AP, Pearson JF, Hall RJC: Role of balloon dilatation of the aortic valve in pregnant patients with aortic stenosis. Br Heart J 1993;70:544.

138. Lao TT, Adelman AG, Sermer M, Colman JM: Balloon valvuloplasty for congenital aortic stenosis in pregnancy. Br J Obstet Gynaecol 1993;100:1141.

139. Gamra H, Betbout F, Ayari M, et al: Recurrent miscarriages as an indication for percutaneous tricuspid valvuloplasty during pregnancy. Cathet Cardiovasc Diagn 1997;40:283.

140. Campos O, Andrade JL, Bocanegra J, et al: Physiologic multivalvular regurgitation during pregnancy: A longitudinal Doppler echocardiographic study. Int J Cardiol 1993;40:265.

141. Elkayam U: Pregnancy and cardiovascular disease. In Braunwald E (ed): The Heart: A Textbook of Cardiovascular Medicine (5th ed.). Philadelphia, WB Saunders, 1997, p 1846.

142. Haïat R, Halphen, C, Clément F, Michelon B: Silent pericardial effusion in late pregnancy. Chest 1981;79:171.

143. Enein M, Zina AAA, Kassem M, El-Tabbakh G: Echocardiography of the pericardium in pregnancy. Obstet Gynecol 1987;69:851.

144. Abduljabbar HSO, Marzouki KMH, Zawawi TF, Khan AS: Pericardial effusion in normal pregnant women. Acta Obstet Gynecol Scand 1991;70:291.

145. Averbuch M, Bojko, A, Levo Y: Cardiac tamponade in the early postpartum period as the presenting and predominant manifestation of systemic lupus erythematosus. J Rheumatol 1986;13:1444.

146. Khabele D, Chasen S: Cardiac tamponade as an unusual presentation of advanced breast cancer in pregnancy. J Reprod Med 1999;44:989.

147. Mecacci F, LaTorre P, Paretti E, et al: Acute pericarditis in pregnancy. Report of a case. Minerva Ginecol 2000;52:259.

148. Hagley MT, Shaub TF: Acute pericarditis with a symptomatic pericardial effusion complicating pregnancy: A case report. J Reprod Med 1993;38:813.

149. Richardson PM, LeRoux BT, Rogers NM, Gotsman GS: Pericardiectomy in pregnancy. Thorax 1970;25:627.

150. Azimi N, Selter J, Abbott JD, et al: A pregnant woman with pericardial tamponade. Case report and review of the literature. Angiology 2004 (in press).

151. Bloomfield P: Choice of heart valve prosthesis. BMJ 2002;87:583.

152. Badduke BR, Jamieson WRE, Miyagishima RT, et al: Pregnancy and childbearing in a population with biologic valvular prostheses. J Thorac Cardiovasc Surg 1991;102:179.

153. Jamieson WRE, Janusz MT, Miyagishima RT, et al: Carpentier-Edwards standard porcine bioprostheses—primary tissue failure (structural valve deterioration) by age groups. Ann Thorac Surg 1988;46:155.

154. Jamieson WRE, Miller DC, Akins CW, et al: Pregnancy and bioprostheses: Influence on structural valve deterioration. Ann Thorac Surg 1995;60(Suppl):S282.

155. North RA, Sadler L, Stewart AW, et al: Long-term survival and valve-related complications in young women with cardiac valve replacements. Circulation 1999;99:2669.

156. Greer IA: Exploring the role of low-molecular weight heparins in pregnancy. Semin Thromb Hemost 2002;28(Suppl 3):25.

157. Mayosi B, Commerford PJ, Levetan BN: Anticoagulation for prosthetic valves during pregnancy [Letter]. Clin Cardiol 1996;19:921.

158. Conti CR: Anticoagulation for mechanical valve prostheses during pregnancy. Clin Cardiol 2003;26:303.

159. Evans W, Laifer SA, McNanley TJ, Ruzycky A: Management of thromboembolic disease associated with pregnancy. J Matern Fetal Med 1997;6:21.

160. Al-Lawati AA, Venkitraman M, Al-Delaime, Valliathu J: Pregnancy and mechanical heart valve replacement: Dilemma of anticoagulation. Eur J Cardiothorac Surg 2002;22:223.

161. Chan WS, Anand S, Ginsberg JS: Anticoagulation of pregnant women with mechanical heart valves. A systematic review of the literature. Arch Intern Med 2000;160:191.

162. Ayhan A, Yapar EG, Yuce K, et al: Pregnancy and its complications after cardiac valve replacement. Int J Gynaecol Obstet 1991;35:117.

163. Hall JG, Pauli RM, Wilson KM: Maternal and fetal sequelae of anticoagulation during pregnancy. Am J Med 1980;69:122.

164. Sareli P, England MJ, Berk MR, et al: Maternal and fetal sequelae of anticoagulation during pregnancy in patients with mechanical heart valve prostheses. Am J Cardiol 1989;63:1462.

165. John S, Ravikumar E, Jairaj PS, et al: Valve replacement in the young patient with rheumatic heart disease. Review of a twenty year experience. J Thorac Cardiovasc Surg 1990;99:631.

166. Cotrufo M, DeFeo M, DeSanto LS, et al: Risk of warfarin during pregnancy with mechanical valve prosthesis. Obstet Gynecol 2002;99:35.

167. Vitale N, DeFeo M, DeSanto LS, et al: Dose-dependent fetal complications of warfarin in pregnant women with mechanical heart valves. J Am Coll Cardiol 1999;33:1637.

168. Iturbe-Alessio I, Fonseca M, Mutchinik O, et al: Risks of anticoagulation therapy in pregnant women with heart valves. N Engl J Med 1986;315:1390.

169. Hanania G, Thomas D, Michel PL, et al: Pregnancy and prosthetic heart valves: A French cooperative retrospective study of 155 cases. Eur Heart J 1994;15:1651.

170. Lecuru F, Desnos M, Taurelle R: Anticoagulant therapy in pregnancy: Report of 54 cases. Acta Obstet Gynecol Scand 1996;75:217.

171. Siu SC, Colman JM: Heart disease and pregnancy. Heart 2001;85:710.

172. Watson WJ, Freeman J, O'Brien C, Benson M: Embolic stroke in a pregnant patient with a mechanical heart valve on optimal heparin therapy. Am J Perinatol 1996;13:371.

173. Salazar E, Izaguirre R, Verdejo J, Mutchinik O: Failure of adjusted doses of subcutaneous heparin to prevent thromboembolic phenomena in pregnant patients with mechanical cardiac valve prostheses. J Am Coll Cardiol 1996;27:1698.

174. Oakley CM: Valvular disease in pregnancy. Curr Opin Cardiol 1996;11:159.

175. Elkayam U: Anticoagulation in pregnant women with prosthetic heart valves: A double jeopardy. J Am Coll Cardiol 1996;27:1704.

176. Hung L, Rahimtoola SH: Prosthetic heart valves and pregnancy. Circulation 2003;107:1240.

177. Bonow RO, Carabello B, DeLeon AC, et al: Guidelines for the management of patients with valvular heart disease: Executive summary. A report of the American Collage of Cardiology/American Heart Association task force on practice guidelines. Circulation 1998;98:1949.

178. Lupton M, Oteng-Ntim E, Ayida G, Steer PJ: Cardiac disease in pregnancy. Curr Opin Obstet Gynecol 2002;14:137.

179. Rowan JA, McCowan MLE, Raudkivi PJ, North RA: Enoxaparin treatment in women with mechanical heart valves during pregnancy. Am J Obstet Gynecol 2001;185:633.

180. Lovenox Injection [package insert]. Bridgewater, N.J., Aventis Pharmaceuticals, 2002.

181. Ginsberg JS, Chan WS, Bates SM, Kaatz S: Anticoagulation of pregnant women with mechanical heart valves. Arch Intern Med 2003;163:694.

182. Nelson-Piercy C, Letsky EA, de Swiet M: Low-molecular-weight heparin for obstetric thromboprophylaxis: Experience of sixty-nine pregnancies in sixty-one women at high risk. Am J Obstet Gynecol 1997;176:1062.

183. Shapira Y, Sagie A, Battler A: Low-molecular-weight heparin for the treatment of patients with mechanical heart valves. Clin Cardiol 2002;25:323.

184. Sibai BM, Caritis SN, Thom E, et al: Prevention of pre-eclampsia with low dose aspirin in healthy nulliparous pregnant women. N Engl J Med 1993;329:1213.

185. DiSessa TG, Moretti ML, Khoury A, et al: Cardiac function in fetuses and newborns exposed to low-dose aspirin during pregnancy. Am J Obstet Gynecol 1994;171:892.

186. Caritis S, Sibai B, Hauth J, et al: Low-dose aspirin to prevent preeclampsia in pregnant women. N Engl J Med 1998;338:701.

187. Schumacher B, Belfort MA, Card RJ: Successful treatment of acute myocardial infarction during pregnancy with tissue plasminogen activator. Am J Obstet Gynecol 1997;176:716.

188. Rossouw GJ, Knott-Craig CJ, Barnard PM, et al: Intracardiac operation in seven pregnant women. Ann Thorac Surg 1993;55:1172.

189. Alessandrini F, Lapenna E, Nasso G, et al: Successful thrombectomy for thrombosis of aortic composite valve graft in pregnancy. Ann Thorac Surg 2003;75:1317.

190. Pomini F, Mercogliano D, Cavaletti C, et al: Cardiopulmonary bypass in pregnancy. Ann Thorac Surg 1996;61:259.

191. Levy DL, Warriner RA, Burgess GE: Fetal response to cardiopulmonary bypass. Obstet Gynecol 1980;56:112.

192. Khandelwal M, Rasanen J, Ludormirski A, et al: Evaluation of fetal and uterine hemodynamics during maternal cardiopulmonary bypass. Obstet Gynecol 1996;88:667.

193. Onderoglu L, Tuncer ZS, Oto A, Durukan T: Balloon valvuloplasty during pregnancy. Int J Gynaecol Obstet 1995;49:181.

194. Yaryura RA, Carpenter RJ, Duncan JM, Wilansky S: Management of mitral valve stenosis in pregnancy: Case presentation and review of the literature. J Heart Valve Dis 1996;5:16.

195. Garry D, Leikin E, Fleisher AG, Tejani N: Acute myocardial infarction in pregnancy with subsequent medical and surgical management. Obstet Gynecol 1996;87:802.

196. Silberman S, Fink D, Berko RS, et al: Coronary artery bypass surgery during pregnancy. Eur J Cardiothorac Surg 1996;10:925.

197. Klutstein MW, Tzivoni D, Bitran D, et al: Treatment of spontaneous coronary artery dissection: Report of three cases. Cathet Cardiovasc Diagn 1997;40:372.

198. Laifer SA, Yeagley CJ, Armitage JM: Pregnancy after cardiac transplantation. Am J Perinatol 1994;11:217.

199. Scott JR, Wagoner LE, Olsen SL, et al: Pregnancy in heart transplant recipients. Management and outcome. Obstet Gynecol 1993;82:324.

200. Branch KR, Wagoner LE, McGrory CH, et al: Risks of subsequent pregnancies on mother and newborn in female heart transplant recipients. J Heart Lung Transplant 1998;17:698.

201. Ascarelli MH, Grider AR, Hsu HW: Acute myocardial infarction during pregnancy managed with immediate percutaneous transluminal coronary angioplasty. Obstet Gynecol 1996;88:655.

202. Eickman FM: Acute coronary artery angioplasty during pregnancy. Cathet Cardiovasc Diagn 1996;38:369.

203. Cayenne S, Manzoor N, Conard A, et al: Cardiac procedures during pregnancy. An interesting case and review. Cardiovasc Rev Rep 2000;21:145.

204. Natale A, Davidson T, Geiger MJ, Newby K: Implantable cardioverter-defibrillators and pregnancy: A safe combination? Circulation 1997;96:2808.

205. Olufolabi AJ, Charlton GA, Allen SA, et al: Use of implantable cardioverter defibrillator and anti-arrhythmic agents in a parturient. Br J Anaesth 2002;89:652.

206. Gordon MC, Landon MB, Boyle J, et al: Coronary artery disease in insulin-dependent diabetes mellitus of pregnancy (class H): A review of the literature. Obstet Gynecol Surv 1996;51:437.

207. Sattar N, Greer IA: Pregnancy complications and maternal cardiovascular risk: Opportunities for intervention and screening? BMJ 2002;325:157.

208. Chasan-Taber L, Stampfer MJ: Epidemiology of oral contraceptives and cardiovascular disease. Ann Intern Med 1998;128:467.

209. Velasco JG, Requena A, Gonzalez A: Pregnancy after myocardial infarction. Int J Gynaecol Obstet 1994;47:291.

210. Medical-care expenditures attributable to cigarette smoking during pregnancy—United States, 1995. MMWR Morb Mortal Wkly Rep 1997;46:1048.

211. Swoboda K, Derfler K, Koppensteiner R, et al: Extracorporeal lipid elimination for treatment of gestational hyperlipidemic pancreatitis. Gastroenterology 1993;104:1527.

212. Lewis CE, Funkhouser E, Raczynski JM, et al: Adverse effect of pregnancy on high density lipoprotein (HDL) cholesterol in young adult women: The CARDIA Study. Coronary Artery Risk Development in Young Adults. Am J Epidemiol 1996;144:247.

213. Economides DL, Crook D, Nicolaides KH: Hypertriglyceridemia and hypoxemia in small-for-gestational-age fetuses. Am J Obstet Gynecol 1990;162:382.

214. Ulm MR, Obwegeser R, Ploeckinger B, et al: A case of myocardial infarction complicating pregnancy—a role for prostacyclin synthesis stimulating plasma factor and lipoprotein (a)? Thromb Res 1996;83:237.

215. Salameh WA, Mastrogiannis DS: Maternal hyperlipidemia in pregnancy. Clin Obstet Gynecol 1994;37:66.

216. Badui E, Enciso R: Acute myocardial infarction during pregnancy and puerperium: A review. Angiology 1996;47:739.

217. Roth A, Elkayam U: Acute myocardial infarction associated with pregnancy. Ann Intern Med 1996;125:751.

218. Esinler I, Yigit N, Ayhan A, et al: Coronary dissection during pregnancy. Acta Obstet Gynecol Scand 2003;82:194.

219. Dhawan R, Singh G, Fesniak H: Spontaneous coronary artery dissection: The clinical spectrum. Angiology 2002;53:89.

220. Koller PT, Cliffe CM, Ridley DJ: Immunosuppressive therapy for peripartum-type spontaneous coronary artery dissection: Case report and review. Clin Cardiol 1998;21:40.

221. Fujito T, Inoue T, Mizoguchi K, et al: Acute myocardial infarction during pregnancy. Cardiology 1996;87:361.

222. Athanassiou AM, Turrentine MA: Myocardial infarction and coronary artery dissection during pregnancy associated with type IV Ehlers-Danlos syndrome. Am J Perinatol 1996;13:181.

223. Hamada S, Hinokio K, Naka O, et al: Myocardial infarction as a complication of pheochromocytoma in a pregnant patient. Eur J Obstet Gynecol Reprod Biol 1996;70:197.

224. Satani O, Katsuragi M, Hano T, et al: Pheochromocytoma-related myocardial damage following delivery. Hypertens Res 1996;19:291.

225. Camann W, Trunfio GV, Kluger R, Steinbrook RA: Automated ST-segment analysis during cesarean delivery: Effects of ECG filtering modality. J Clin Anesth 1996;8:564.

226. Eisenach JC, Tuttle R, Stein A: Is ST segment depression of the electrocardiogram during cesarean section merely due to cardiac sympathetic block? Anesth Analg 1994;78:287.

227. Abramov Y, Abramov D, Abrahamov A, et al: Elevation of serum creatine phosphokinase and its MB isoenzyme during normal labor and early puerperium. Acta Obstet Gynecol Scand 1996;75:255.

228. Shade GH, Ross G, Bever FN, et al: Troponin I in the diagnosis of acute myocardial infarction in pregnancy labor, and postpartum. Am J Obstet Gynecol 2002;187:1719.

229. Cohen WR, Steinman T, Patsner B, et al: Acute myocardial infarction in a pregnant woman at term. JAMA 1983;250:2179.

230. Allen JN, Wewers MD: Acute myocardial infarction with cardiogenic shock during pregnancy: Treatment with intra-aortic balloon counterpulsation. Crit Care Med 1990;18:888.

231. Sharma GL, Loubeyre C, Morice MC: Safety and feasibility of the radial approach for primary angioplasty in acute myocardial infarction during pregnancy. J Invasive Cardiol 2002;14:359.

232. Ishikawa A, Matsura S: Occlusive thromboaortopathy (Takayasu's disease) and pregnancy. Am J Cardiol 1982;50:1293.

233. Wong VCW, Wang RYC, Tse TF: Pregnancy and Takayasu's arteritis. Am J Med 1983;75:597.

234. Winn HW, Setaro JF, Mazor M, et al: Severe Takayasu's arteritis in pregnancy: The role of central hemodynamic monitoring. Am J Obstet Gynecol 1988;159:1135.

235. Rizk NW, Kalassian KG, Gilligan T, et al: Obstetric complications in pulmonary and critical care medicine. Chest 1996;110:791.

236. White WB: Management of hypertension during lactation. Hypertension 1984;6:297.

237. White WB: Cardiovascular therapy during pregnancy and lactation. In Messerli FH (ed): Cardiovascular Drug Therapy (2nd ed.). Philadelphia, WB Saunders, 1996, pp 269-279.

238. Cockburn J, Moar VA, Ounsted N, et al: Final report of the study on hypertension during pregnancy. The effects of specific treatment on the growth and development of the children. Lancet 1982;2:647.

239. Horvath JS, Phippard A, Korda A, et al: Clonidine hydrochloride: A safe and effective antihypertensive agent in pregnancy. Obstet Gynecol 1985;66:634.

240. White WB, Andreoli JW, Cohn RD: Alpha-methyldopa disposition in mothers with hypertension and in their breast-fed infants. Clin Pharmacol Ther 1985;4:387.

241. Ducsay CA, Umezaki H, Kaushal KM, et al: Pharmacokinetic and fetal cardiovascular effects of enalaprilat administration to maternal rhesus macaques. Am J Obstet Gynecol 1996;175:50.

242. Reisenberger K, Egarter C, Sternberger B, et al: Placental passage of angiotensin-converting enzyme inhibitors. Am J Obstet Gynecol 1996;174:1450.

243. Shotan A, Widerhorn J, Hurst A, Elkayam U: Risks of angiotensin converting enzyme inhibition during pregnancy: Experimental and clinical evidence, potential mechanisms, and recommendations for use. Am J Med 1994;96:451.

244. Postmarketing surveillance for angiotensin-converting enzyme inhibitor use during the first trimester of pregnancy—United States, Canada, and Israel, 1987-1995. MMWR Morb Mortal Wkly Rep 1997;46:240.

245. Saji H, Yamanaka M, Hagiwara A, Ijiri R: Losartan and fetal toxic effects. Lancet 2001;357:363.

246. Devlin RG, Fleiss PM: Captopril in human blood and breast milk. J Clin Pharmacol 1981;21:110.

247. Mitani GM, Steinberg I, Lien E, et al: The pharmacokinetics of antiarrhythmic agents in pregnancy and lactation. Clin Pharmacokinet 1987;12:253.

248. Hill LM, Malkasian GD: The use of quinidine sulfate throughout pregnancy. Obstet Gynecol 1979;54:366.

249. Leonard RF, Braun TE, Levy AM: Initiation of uterine contractions by disopyramide during pregnancy. N Engl J Med 1978;299:84.

250. Timmis AD, Jackson G, Holt DW: Mexiletine for control of ventricular dysrhythmias in pregnancy. Lancet 1980;2:647.

251. Lewis AM, Patel L, Johnston A, et al: Mexiletine in human blood and breast milk. Postgrad Med J 1981;57:546.

252. Lownes HE, Ives TJ: Mexiletine use in pregnancy and lactation. Am J Obstet Gynecol 1987;157:446.

253. Allan LD, Chita SK, Sharland GK, et al: Flecainide in the treatment of fetal tachycardias. Br Heart J 1991;65:46.

254. Connaughton M, Jenkins BS: Successful use of flecainide to treat new onset maternal ventricular tachycardia in pregnancy. Br Heart J 1994;72:297.

255. Cox JL, Gardner M: Treatment of cardiac arrhythmias during pregnancy. Prog Cardiovasc Dis 1993;36:137.

256. Joglar JA, Page RL: Treatment of cardiac arrhythmias during pregnancy. Safety considerations. Drug Saf 1999;20:85.

257. Hackett LP, Wojnar-Horton RE, Dusci LJ, et al: Excretion of sotalol in breast milk. Br J Clin Pharmacol 1990;29:277.

258. Matsumura LK, Born D, Kunii IS, et al: Outcome of thyroid function in newborns from mothers treated with amiodarone. Thyroid 1992;2:279.

259. Valensise H, Civitella C, Garzetti GG, Romanini C: Amiodarone treatment in pregnancy for dilated cardiomyopathy with ventricular malignant extrasystole and normal maternal and neonatal outcome. Prenat Diagn 1992;12:705.

260. Podolsky SM, Varon J: Adenosine use during pregnancy. Ann Emerg Med 1991;20:1027.

261. Elkayam U, Goodwin TM: Adenosine therapy for supraventricular tachycardia during pregnancy. Am J Cardiol 1995;75:521.

262. James PR: Cardiovascular disease. Best Pract Res Clin Obstet Gynecol 2001;15:903.

263. Frishman WH, Chesner M: Beta-adrenergic blockers in pregnancy. Am Heart J 1988;115:147.

264. Michael CA: The evaluation of labetalol in the treatment of hypertension complicating pregnancy. Br J Clin Pharmacol 1982; 13(Suppl 1):127.

265. Nylund L, Lunell NO, Lewander R, et al: Labetalol for the treatment of hypertension in pregnancy. Pharmacokinetics and effects on the utero-placental blood flow. Acta Obstet Gynecol Scand 1984;118(Suppl):71.

266. Sakamoto H, Misumi K, Matsuda Y, Ikenoue T: Effects of antihypertensive drugs on maternal and fetal hemodynamics and uterine blood flow in pregnant goats—comparison of nicardipine and labetalol. J Vet Med Sci 1996;58:515.

267. Cunningham FG, Lindheimer MD: Hypertension in pregnancy. N Engl J Med 1992;326:927.

268. Scott WJ, Resnick E, Hummler H, et al: Cardiovascular alterations in rat fetuses exposed to calcium channel blockers. Reprod Toxicol 1997;11:207.

269. Magee LA, Schick B, Donnenfeld AE, et al: The safety of calcium channel blockers in human pregnancy: A prospective, multicenter cohort study. Am J Obstet Gynecol 1996;174:823.

270. Childress CH, Katz VL: Nifedipine and its indications in obstetrics and gynecology. Obstet Gynecol 1994;83:616.

271. Ismail AAA, Medhat I, Tawfic TAS, Kholief A: Evaluation of calcium antagonist (nifedipine) in the treatment of pre-eclampsia. Int J Gynaecol Obstet 1993;40:39.

272. American Academy of Pediatrics Committee on Drugs: The transfer of drugs and other chemicals into human milk. Pediatrics 1994;93:137.

273. Carcas AJ, Abad-Santos F, de Rosendo JM, Frias J: Nimodipine transfer into human breast milk and cerebrospinal fluid. Ann Pharmacother 1996;30:148.

274. Briggs GC, Freeman RK, Yaffe SJ: Amiloride. In Mitchell CW (ed): Drugs in Pregnancy and Lactation: A Guide to Fetal and Neonatal Risk, 5th ed. Baltimore, Williams & Wilkins, 1998, pp 35-36.

275. Messina M, Biffignandi P, Ghigo E, et al: Possible contraindication of spironolactone during pregnancy. J Endocrinol Invest 1990;2:222.

276. Lapinsky SE, Kruczynski K, Slutsky AA: Critical care in the pregnant patient. Am J Respir Crit Care Med 1995;152:427.

277. Clark RB, Brunner JA: Dopamine for the treatment of spinal hypotension during cesarean section. Anesthesiology 1980;53:514.

278. Santos AC, Pedersen H: Current controversies in obstetric anesthesia. Anesth Analg 1994;78:753.

279. Ramsay B, DeBelder A, Campbell S, et al: A nitric oxide donor improves uterine artery diastolic blood flow in normal early pregnancy and in women with high risk for pre-eclampsia. Eur J Clin Invest 1994;24:76.

280. Lees C, Campbell S, Jauniax E, et al: Arrest of preterm labour and prolongation of gestation with glyceryl trinitrate, a nitric oxide donor. Lancet 1994;343:1325.

281. Grunewald C, Kublickas M, Carlstrom K, et al: Effects of nitroglycerin on the uterine artery and umbilical circulation in severe preeclampsia. Obstet Gynecol 1995;86:600.

282. Cotton DB, Longmire S, Jones MM, et al: Cardiovascular alterations in severe pregnancy-induced hypertension: Effects of intravenous nitroglycerin coupled with blood volume expansion. Am J Obstet Gynecol 1986;154:1053.

283. Manson JM, Freyssinges C, Ducrocq MB, Stephenson WP: Postmarketing surveillance of lovastatin and simvastatin exposure during pregnancy. Reprod Toxicol 2001;10:439.

284. Perry KG, Morrison JC, Rust OA, et al: Incidence of adverse cardiopulmonary effects with low-dose continuous terbutaline infusion. Am J Obstet Gynecol 1995;173:1273.

285. Sciscione AC, Ivester T, Largoza M, et al: Acute pulmonary edema in pregnancy. Obstet Gynecol 2003;101:511.

286. Braun U, Weyland A, Bartmus D, et al: Anesthesiology aspects of pregnancy and delivery in a patient following a modified Fontan procedure. Anaesthesist 1996;45:545.

287. Bamber JH, Dresner M: Aortocaval compression in pregnancy: The effect of changing the degree and direction of lateral tilt on maternal cardiac output. Anesth Analg 2003;97:256.

288. Belfort MA, Rokey R, Saade GR, Moise KJ: Rapid echocardiographic assessment of left and right heart hemodynamics in critically ill obstetric patients. Am J Obstet Gynecol 1994;171:884.

7

THYROID DISEASE DURING PREGNANCY

Lauren H. Golden and Gerard N. Burrow

Diseases of the thyroid are, in general, much more prevalent in women than in men, and it is not surprising that thyroid disorders are relatively common among pregnant women. The hormonal changes and increasing metabolic demands of pregnancy effect complex compensatory alterations in maternal thyroid function. Despite these changes, normal pregnancy is considered a euthyroid state. Studies of thyroid function in pregnant women with underlying autoimmune thyroid disease or marginal iodine intake suggest that increased demand may result in thyroid "strain" during pregnancy. Whether there is any significant effect on normal thyroid function is not clear. Reports that hypothyroid women require an increased dosage of L-thyroxine during pregnancy to maintain the euthyroid state raise the question of whether normal women have difficulty in maintaining thyroid function during pregnancy.

The spectrum of thyroid disorders that may affect pregnant women spans the functional gamut from hypothyroidism to hyperthyroidism. Euthyroid pregnant women may exhibit a number of nonspecific signs that mimic those of thyroid dysfunction, which makes clinical diagnosis difficult. For example, pregnant women experience progressive fatigue and de facto weight gain, which may mask underlying thyroid hypofunction. In addition, euthyroid pregnant women may manifest mild tachycardia, an increase in cardiac output, and a widened pulse pressure, signs of a hyperdynamic state that are also common to hyperthyroidism.

An understanding of the normal physiologic processes of the thyroid gland during pregnancy facilitates the understanding of pathologic processes in pregnancy.

MATERNAL THYROID PHYSIOLOGY

During pregnancy, maternal thyroid function is modulated by three independent but interrelated factors (Table 7–1)[1,2]: (1) an increase in human chorionic gonadotropin (hCG) concentrations that stimulate the thyroid gland[3];

(2) significant increases in urinary iodide excretion, resulting in a fall in plasma iodine concentrations; and (3) an increase in thyroxine-binding globulin (TBG) during the first trimester, resulting in increased binding of thyroxine (T_4). In the aggregate, these factors may be responsible for the increased thyroid demand, or thyroid "strain," observed during pregnancy.

Human Chorionic Gonadotropin

The complex hormonal and metabolic changes that follow conception help ensure the continuation of pregnancy. There is a constant hormonal interplay among fetus, mother, and placenta with regard to steroid production in fetal adrenals and gonads, as well as polypeptide hormones produced by the fetal pituitary gland and the placenta. Concentrations of hCG increase rapidly after implantation, ensuring sufficient progesterone concentrations to maintain the pregnancy until placental production is adequate.

hCG is a peptide hormone responsible for the production of adequate concentrations of progesterone early in gestation, until progesterone production by the developing placenta is sufficient to fulfill that function. Thus, hCG concentrations increase dramatically during the first trimester of pregnancy and plateau gradually thereafter. The hCG peptide exhibits structural similarity to thyroid-stimulating hormone (TSH), composed of an α chain and a β chain. Whereas the molecules of the β chains of the two substances differ, the α chain of hCG is identical to that of TSH. This partial structural homology anticipates at least a partial overlap in function, and it has been established that hCG does possess intrinsic, weak thyroid-stimulating activity. In addition, homology exists between the TSH and luteinizing hormone/hCG receptors.

TSH levels fall predictably during the first trimester, paralleling, in a reciprocal manner, the concomitant rise in hCG (Fig. 7–1). The overall effect of hCG on the degree of thyroid stimulation and TSH suppression reflects an

TABLE 7–1   Factors Affecting Maternal Thyroid Function

↑ β–human chorionic gonadotropin
↑ Urinary iodide excretion
↑ Thyroxine-binding globulin

integration of both the amplitude and the duration of the hCG peak. Despite hCG-mediated stimulation of the thyroid gland, free (unbound) serum hormone concentrations generally remain within, or slightly above, the normal range during the first trimester. The stimulatory effects of hCG on normal pregnancy are not significant and are normally confined to the first half of pregnancy. In certain pathologic conditions, however, including hyperemesis gravidarum and trophoblastic tumors, hCG concentrations may increase into the range sufficient to induce biochemical hyperthyroidism.

Iodine Excretion during Pregnancy

The increase in glomerular filtration rate associated with pregnancy results in a sustained rise in the renal clearance of iodine, beginning early in pregnancy. This is a major factor in the decreased plasma inorganic iodine concentration that occurs during pregnancy.[4] The thyroid gland compensates by enlarging and by increasing the plasma clearance of iodine to produce sufficient thyroid hormone to maintain the euthyroid state. Whether subsequent development of a goiter ensues depends on the plasma

concentration of inorganic iodide, because thyroid volume varies as a function of iodine intake.[1,5]

Numerous studies have evaluated changes in maternal thyroid size and function during pregnancy, in settings of varying iodine sufficiency. In geographic regions of relative iodine deficiency,[6] studies have documented an increased prevalence of pregnancy-associated goiter. For example, Glinoer and associates observed an 18% increase in thyroid volume during pregnancy in iodine-deficient Belgium.[7] A follow-up randomized intervention study was performed, in which pregnant women were treated with placebo, with 100 μg of potassium iodide, or with 100 μg of iodide in addition to 100 μg of L-thyroxine daily.[8] A 30% increase in thyroid volume was seen in the placebo recipients, in comparison with a 15% increase in thyroid volume in the patients taking iodide. The patients receiving both L-thyroxine and potassium iodide therapy manifested the smallest change in thyroid volume, an increase of only 8%.

In a large study of 606 pregnant women in an area of marginal iodine intake (50 to 75 μg/day), ultrasonographically determined thyroid volume increased by an average increment of 20%.[7] A cross-sectional study in Scotland, an area of relative iodine deficiency, diagnosed goiter in 70% of pregnant women, in contrast to 38% of nonpregnant women.[9] Goiters were also found in 39% of nulliparous women and 35% of nonpregnant parous women, which suggests that previous pregnancies did not affect the incidence of goiter. The investigators repeated the study in Iceland under the same experimental conditions. In this iodine-replete setting, they noted no increase in goiter during pregnancy,[10] inasmuch as goiter was found in 19% of nonpregnant and 23% of pregnant Icelandic women.

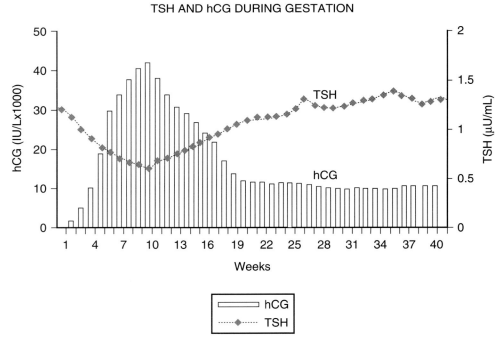

Figure 7–1. Thyroid-stimulating hormone (TSH) and human chorionic gonadotropin (hCG) during gestation. Note the reciprocal relationship between TSH and hCG. (Adapted from Glinoer D: The regulation of thyroid function in pregnancy: Pathways of endocrine adaptation from physiology to pathology. Endocr Rev 1997;18:404.)

A prospective study in the iodine-replete Netherlands also failed to demonstrate a significant change in thyroid volume or size during pregnancy.[11]

These studies provide ample evidence that thyroid volume increases during pregnancy in regions of moderate or marginal iodine intake, whereas no significant changes in thyroid size or volume occur in iodine-replete conditions. Intervention studies suggest that thyroid enlargement during pregnancy is a physiologic, compensatory adaptation to the increased demands for iodine associated with pregnancy.

Iodine-deficiency goiter is unlikely to occur at a plasma iodine concentration above 0.08 µg/dL.[12] In many regions of Europe, the plasma inorganic iodine concentration ranges from 0.10 to 0.15 µg/dL and during pregnancy may fall below 0.08 µg/dL.[13] In residents of North America and Iceland, in contrast, the plasma inorganic iodine concentration is approximately 0.30 µg/dL and remains above 0.08 µg/dL, even during pregnancy.

An iodine balance study in the United States revealed no difference between pregnant and nonpregnant women.[14] Despite the fact that pregnant women in North America manifest increased renal clearance of iodine, ample dietary intake prevents excess iodine loss. Iodized salt should be sufficient to supply the intake of 200 µg of iodine needed during pregnancy, and the iodine in most prenatal vitamin supplements ensures an adequate intake.[15] In areas of marginal iodine intake (i.e., 50 µg/day), supplementary iodine (160 µg/day) given to pregnant women reduced neonatal goiter from 33% to 7%.[16] An excessive iodine intake because of unusual dietary practices (e.g., 2000 µg/day) may cause difficulties for both mother and child and is discussed later.

Thyroxine-Binding Globulin

As noted previously, an increase in TBG, resulting in increased binding of T_4, is a third modulating factor that influences thyroid function during pregnancy. It is discussed in further detail later.

DETERMINATION OF THYROID FUNCTION IN PREGNANCY

The physiologic hormonal changes and alterations in metabolic demand that occur in the pregnant woman complicate the determination of thyroid function. The same changes make the clinical diagnosis of thyroid disease difficult and increase the reliance on laboratory determinations.

Basal Metabolic Rate

Before the development of accurate biochemical determinations of thyroid function, basal metabolic rate was monitored as a reflection of overall thyroid function. Early studies indicated that the basal metabolic rate was elevated in pregnant women, increasing 15% to 20% by the eighth month of pregnancy. Under scrupulous basal conditions,

it was demonstrated that the uterus and its contents could account for 70% to 80% of the rise in oxygen consumption above those of nonpregnant values. Although clinical laboratory tests are now the standard method of appraisal of thyroid function, a true basal metabolic rate is still a good indicator of integrated thyroid function.

Thyroxine-Binding Globulin

Thyroid hormone transport in serum is accomplished by three thyroid hormone transport proteins: TBG, albumin, and transthyretin (T_4-binding prealbumin). TBG is the least abundant of the three transport proteins, although it binds T_4 with the highest affinity.[17] In nonpregnant patients, approximately two thirds of serum T_4 is bound by TBG. In steady-state conditions, the bound hormone fraction is in equilibrium with the unbound (free) fraction.

During pregnancy, TBG concentrations rise to about twice normal values, a direct result of the increased estrogen levels. Estrogens stimulate hepatic synthesis of TBG and cause a fall in transthyretin-binding capacity, increasing the fraction of serum T_4 bound to TBG.[18,19] Thus, the proportion of circulating T_4 bound to TBG may be in excess of 75% throughout pregnancy. Estrogens also prolong the circulatory half-life of TBG by stimulating increased TBG sialylation. The integrated result of these effects is an increase in serum TBG concentrations, and pregnancy is considered a state of TBG excess.

TBG concentration can be measured directly by radioimmunoassay[20] and has a normal range of 12 to 30 µg/L, which increases to 30 to 50 µg/L during pregnancy.[21] TBG has a normal binding capacity that ranges from 19 to 30 µg/dL of T_4 and increases to 40 to 60 µg/dL of T_4 during pregnancy.[22] TBG has a greater affinity for T_4 and actually binds more T_4 in vivo than does transthyretin, although the latter has a greater overall binding capacity for T_4. Of note, TBG binds T_4 more tightly than 3,5,3'-triiodothyronine (T_3), and this difference in affinity is the basis for the resin T_3 uptake test.

In a study of patients with partial or total TBG deficiency,[19] no significant changes in TBG concentration were noted during pregnancy. In keeping with this finding, there were also no significant changes in thyroid function in these patients; that is, the increase in serum T_4 that occurs during normal pregnancy is a direct compensation for a concomitant rise in TBG. Conversely, adequate amounts of thyroid hormone must be produced in order to maintain normal thyroid function in the presence of increased binding.

In one large study of 606 women, serum T_3 and T_4 concentrations during pregnancy did not increase as much as would be predicted from the increase in serum TBG.[7] This relative hypothyroxinemia was accompanied by a serum TSH concentration that was increased, although well within the normal range. The question arises as to whether changes in other binding proteins must be considered when TBG saturation is studied.[23]

In addition to changes in TBG concentration, mutations in the transthyretin and the albumin genes may alter T_4/T_3 binding.[24] The most frequent disorder, familial dysalbuminemic hyperthyroxinemia, is the result of a mutation in the albumin gene, in which affinity for T_4 but not T_3 is increased. The total serum T_4 concentration is elevated, whereas the serum T_3 and TSH concentrations are normal. The resin method does not accurately determine serum free T_4 concentration in these patients.

Total Serum Thyroxine and Triiodothyronine

Radioimmunoassays measure the total T_4 and T_3 content in the serum, and these measurements are elevated in pregnancy because of increased thyroid hormone binding to TBG. It is estimated that serum T_4 concentrations increase by 1% to 3% per day over the trimester to compensate for the aforementioned increase in TBG.[7] Serum T_4 and T_3 concentrations rise significantly in early pregnancy, and T_4 concentrations rise sharply between 6 and 12 weeks of pregnancy, stabilizing by midpregnancy. In areas of iodine sufficiency, T_4 and TBG concentrations rise in tandem. The rise in serum T_3 is more gradual, although it also stabilizes at approximately 20 weeks of pregnancy.[17] Once midpregnancy plateaus have been reached, serum T_4 and T_3 concentrations remain elevated throughout pregnancy, returning to normal shortly after delivery.[25-27]

Free Thyroid Hormone

The unbound (free) fraction of thyroid hormone is metabolically active.[28] Only a small fraction of the total thyroid hormone is unbound: less than 0.05% of the circulating T_4 and less than 0.5% of the circulating T_3. Despite an increase in total T_4 and T_3 during pregnancy, free thyroid hormone concentrations generally remain within the normal range for nonpregnant women.[29-31] However, in areas of marginal iodine intake, mean serum free T_4 and T_3 concentrations may decrease, which is suggestive of relative hypothyroxinemia.[7]

Equilibrium dialysis is considered the "gold standard" reference method of measuring free thyroid hormone concentrations. Because of the expense and the laborious nature of the assay, many commercially available measurements of free thyroid hormone rely on indirect calculations, which may not be reliable in pregnancy. The most common measure of unbound thyroid hormone is the free T_4 index, an arithmetic product of the total serum T_4 determination and a measure of thyroid hormone binding.[32] Of note, many of the binding methods that are used underestimate the large increases in TBG concentration that may occur during pregnancy, resulting in falsely high free T_4 index values in some euthyroid pregnant women.[33] Direct measurement of free thyroid hormones with radioimmunoassays is now available, but there is significant variability among the different tests, which may also be influenced by the presence of elevated concentrations of TBG. If a discrepancy arises, evaluation of the free T_4 values in the context of the total T_4 and ultrasensitive TSH measurement may help clarify the situation.

When accurate measurements of serum free T_4 and free T_3 concentrations are used, most thyrotoxic women have elevated values, women with mild hypothyroidism have low-normal free T_4 values, and women with moderate to severe hypothyroidism have low serum free T_4 values. Serum free T_3 concentrations may remain within the normal range in the patients with severe hypothyroidism as a result of increased T_4-to-T_3 conversion in this setting. Diagnostic accuracy declines with the use of less accurate methods of detection, such as the T_4 index.

Thyroxine Production and Metabolism

Free thyroid hormones exert their effect by binding to nuclear receptors and initiating new protein synthesis. In the steady state, T_4 degradation is a reflective measure of thyroid hormone production. Degradation can be measured with radioisotope-labeled T_4, although the use of radioisotopes is contraindicated in pregnancy. In the presence of an estimated volume of distribution of 10 L and a normal serum T_4 of 8 µg/dL, the entire thyroidal pool of T_4 is approximately 800 µg. T_4 has a half-life of 6 to 8 days in the serum of a euthyroid nonpregnant adult, which results in a fractional turnover of approximately 10% per day. Therefore, approximately 10% of the extrathyroidal pool of T_4, or approximately 80 µg, turns over per day. Thus, in a steady state, 80 µg of T_4 is produced daily to maintain euthyroid status.

Peripheral metabolism of thyroid hormones in human tissues is accomplished by three deiodinase enzymes: types I, II, and III (Fig. 7–2). Both type II and type III deiodinase are expressed in the placenta, whereas type I is not.

Outer ring deiodination of T_4 by type I deiodinase is responsible for the production of the majority of circulating T_3, whereas inner ring deiodination produces reverse T_3 (rT_3). Levels of both T_3 and rT_3 may be elevated in pregnancy in proportion to the increase in serum T_4. There is no direct evidence for up-regulation of type I deiodinase activity in pregnancy.[34-36]

Type II deiodinase acts on the outer ring to produce T_3, and its preferential substrates are T_4 and rT_3. There is

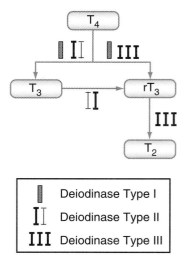

Figure 7–2. Thyroxine (T_4) concentrations during gestation. (Adapted from Burrow GN, Fisher DA, Larsen PR: Maternal and fetal thyroid function. N Engl J Med 1994;331:1072. Copyright 1994 Massachusetts Medical Society. All rights reserved.)

evidence of type II deiodinase expression by the placenta, and it plays an important role in maintenance of local T_3 production. In the setting of relative maternal hypothyroxinemia,[37] the activity of type II deiodinase increases, ensuring adequate availability of T_3 for the developing fetus.

Type III deiodinase converts T_4 to rT_3 and T_3 to diiodothyronine (T_2). It, too, is highly expressed at many maternal-fetal interfaces, including the placenta, fetal epithelium, and fetal endothelium.[38] Type III deiodinase is integral to modulation of fetal thyroid status and may be responsible for the low concentrations of T_3 and high concentrations of rT_3 typically seen in fetal thyroid hormone metabolism.

When TBG capacity is increased by estrogen administration, the fractional rate of T_4 turnover decreases, although the absolute rate of thyroid hormone disposal is unchanged because of increases in total serum T_4 concentration.[39] In one study, net T_4 turnover and, presumably, thyroid hormone requirements were unchanged in normal human pregnancy.[40] Net T_4 turnover was 90 µg/day in the nonpregnant woman and 97 µg/day in the pregnant woman. The two values were identical when expressed as the daily turnover per square meter of body surface. These findings are for one period in pregnancy, but because of necessary restrictions on the use of radioisotopes in pregnant woman, further data will not be available. Increased T_4 turnover has been reported during pregnancy in monkeys.

Triiodothyronine Sulfate

Studies indicate that sulfation of iodothyronines plays a significant role in thyroid hormone metabolism. Despite the fact that T_3 sulfate circulates bound to TBG, values are in the low-normal range in pregnant women. T_3 is not an active hormone, as it binds poorly to nuclear receptors. However, if an active T_3 or T_4 sulfatase were present, T_3 or T_4 sulfate could serve as an active hormone.

The reason why the serum T_3 sulfate concentration is not increased in pregnancy is unclear. Factors such as decreased production, increased clearance, or increased fetal transfer may play a role singly or in combination. The elevated serum T_3 sulfate concentration in the neonate may reflect increased production or decreased metabolism by fetal tissue. In any case, the values represent another example of the changes in thyroid hormone metabolism that occur in pregnancy.

Determination of Serum Thyroid-Stimulating Hormone

The current availability of specific, ultrasensitive, third-generation immunoradiometric assays of serum TSH has brought clarity to the study of TSH values during pregnancy.[32,33] These assays can accurately detect TSH values as low as 0.002 mU/L, and their widespread institution into clinical laboratory usage enables the distinction of normal pregnant women from pregnant women with thyrotoxicosis, because the latter manifest truly suppressed TSH concentrations. For example, during the first trimester, rising concentrations of hCG effect a mild, reciprocal depression in serum TSH concentrations as a result of the intrinsic thyroid-stimulating activity of

hCG (see Fig. 7–1). The TSH values in these patients are typically *not* fully suppressed, and TSH values recover and remain well within the normal range during the remainder of a normal pregnancy.[29,41]

Thus, although more expensive than T_4 determinations, the sensitive TSH determination is the best measure of thyroid function in pregnancy.[42]

Radioactive Iodine Uptake

Administration of radioactive iodine to a pregnant woman is contraindicated because of the potentially harmful effects of radiation on the fetus. Whether there is a threshold dose for radiation effects is not clear, and all radiation to the fetus should be regarded as harmful.[43]

However, early studies in pregnant women, performed in the 1950s, revealed that three of five women had an elevated radioactive iodine thyroid uptake at 12 weeks of pregnancy.[44] A second study showed similar results, with increased iodine isotope ^{131}I uptakes documented at 12, 24, and 36 weeks of pregnancy, as well as 1 week post partum. The radioactive iodine uptake returned to normal by 6 weeks post partum. The reasons for this elevation in radioactive iodine thyroid uptake are clear: Thyroid radioiodine uptake depends on both thyroid-stimulating activity and the size of the iodine pool. Thyroid-stimulating activity is enhanced during pregnancy, particularly during the first trimester. In addition, plasma inorganic iodine concentrations decline during pregnancy as a result of an increase in glomerular filtration rate. In response to a decrease in size of the iodine pool, there is an increase in thyroid clearance of iodine. Therefore, radioactive iodine thyroid uptake is elevated in pregnancy as a result of both enhanced thyroid-stimulating activity and increased thyroid clearance of iodine.

Urinary excretion of radioactive iodine is also useful as an indirect reflection of thyroid uptake. Indeed, in 22 women in the third trimester, the mean urinary excretion of radio-iodine was in the range between normal and thyrotoxic values.[44] However, this method does not distinguish maternal and fetal thyroid uptake.

Hypothalamic-Pituitary-Thyroid Axis

TSH secretion by the pituitary stimulates thyroid hormone secretion. TSH secretion itself is suppressed by increasing concentrations of circulating thyroid hormone. Thyroid function is therefore an example of the classic negative feedback mechanism. The level of thyroid hormone—particularly pituitary T_3—at which TSH secretion is inhibited is determined by thyrotropin-releasing hormone (TRH), a tripeptide, L-pyroglutamyl-L-histidyl-L-proline amide. This hypothalamic releasing hormone determines the set point at which circulating thyroid hormone suppresses TSH secretion by the pituitary gland.

There are conflicting reports about the responsiveness of the hypothalamic-pituitary-thyroid axis during pregnancy. Early studies of thyroid-pituitary suppressibility during pregnancy were performed with a T_3 suppression test. Pregnant women in the second and third trimesters underwent T_3 suppression with 75 to 125 µg T_3 daily for 7 days.

Thyroid uptake of ^{131}I was suppressed to the same extent in pregnant women as in nonpregnant women after exposure to T_3.[45] The increase in ^{131}I uptake with administration of TSH was also similar in pregnant and nonpregnant women. Serum protein-bound iodine values, reflective of thyroid hormone suppression, fell more than 1 µg/dL at all time periods studied, but more T_3 was needed to lower the serum protein-bound iodine concentration in the latter months of pregnancy. In addition, some patients failed to suppress T_3, regardless of the dose. Thus, overall, ^{131}I uptake appears to be normally responsive to thyroid hormone suppression during pregnancy, but the serum protein-bound iodine concentration is not. This apparent lack of responsiveness may result in part from the increase in TBG during pregnancy.

Burrow and colleagues administered TRH to patients in different stages of pregnancy who were to undergo therapeutic abortion.[46] Women in the 16th to 20th weeks of pregnancy had an increased TSH response to TRH in comparison with patients in the 6th to 12th weeks of pregnancy. This increase may have been an estrogen-mediated effect, because nonpregnant women taking oral contraceptive steroids showed a comparable increase in TSH response to TRH. Other investigators, however, have not found an increased TSH response to TRH in pregnant women.[47-49] The discrepancies in these findings may arise from differences in iodine sufficiency among the subjects studied; that is, the failure to find an increase in the TSH response to TRH may be attributable to iodine deficiency,[50] although the mechanism is not clear.

TRH has been shown to cross the placenta and stimulate the fetal pituitary gland in animal studies.[51] TRH activity was found in the human placenta, and lower levels of TRH-degrading activity were found in both cord and maternal sera[52] than in sera from euthyroid nonpregnant adults. All these data suggest that TRH may play a role in the modulation of thyroid function during pregnancy. However, fetal pituitary TSH secretion appears to be controlled independently of both the maternal and the fetal hypothalamus.

FETAL THYROID FUNCTION

The fetal thyroid gland and hypothalamic-pituitary-thyroid axis develop and mature throughout gestation (Table 7–2). Fetal TSH and T_4 are first detectable at 10 weeks' gestation. Before the fetal thyroid gland is able to produce sufficient amounts of endogenous hormone, the maternal thyroid gland provides all thyroid hormone necessary for fetal development. In the setting of maternal hypothyroxinemia, this early dependence on maternal thyroid hormone production exposes the fetus to potential risks.

Ontogenesis of Fetal Thyroid Function

The fetal thyroid gland forms during weeks 7 to 9 of gestation, originating as an epithelial proliferation in the floor of the pharynx at the site of the foramen caecum linguae.[53] The gland descends into the neck, attached to the thyroglossal duct, and reaches its final position by week 9. At this point, the thyroid is a bilobed structure with the lobes connected by the isthmus, but structural maturity of the gland is not achieved until week 17.

Control of the fetal thyroid system develops through maturation of the hypothalamic-pituitary-thyroid axis.[54-56] Maturation of hypothalamic TRH production and pituitary portal function occurs between weeks 18 and 40 of gestation. Extrahypothalamic tissues, such as the placenta, fetal pancreas, and fetal gastrointestinal tissues support TRH production before hypothalamic maturation.[57] Serum TSH is detectable in fetal serum as early as week 10, although levels remain relatively low until about week 18. Fetal serum TSH concentrations increase in parallel with increasing concentrations of TRH. Between weeks 18 and 28, TSH levels increase up to 15 µU/mL and then fall to approximately 10 µU/mL near term.[58] At birth, the exposure of the neonate to the cold extrauterine environment stimulates an acute surge of TSH release that results in increased secretion of thyroid hormones.

Fetal thyroid follicles and T_4 synthesis are first demonstrable approximately 10 weeks after conception. Immaturity of the negative feedback system is implied by increased TSH secretion despite higher serum free T_4 concentrations. The biosynthetic process is also immature at this point. As the thyroid gland matures, the secretory response to stimulation with TSH matures as well. In a study of normal fetuses between 12 and 37 weeks' gestation,[59,60] with blood obtained via cordocentesis (ultrasonographically guided blood sampling from the umbilical cord), fetal serum TSH, TBG, and total free T_4 and T_3 were found to increase significantly with the length of gestation. However, the predicted rise and fall of serum TSH between 18 and 28 weeks was not seen.

Fetal pituitary control of thyroid function may commence as early as 12 weeks' gestation but does not mature until midgestation. As the hypothalamic-pituitary-thyroidal axis develops, elevated levels of TSH may be found in the presence of elevated serum free T_4, reflecting early immaturity of the negative feedback system. After midgestation, elevations in fetal TSH result in appropriate, coincident increases in fetal serum T_4 concentrations. T_4 levels increase from 2 to 3 µg/dL at 10 weeks to 10 µg/dL at 30 weeks (Fig. 7–3). Progressive, incremental increases in serum free T_4 parallel the increases in total serum T_4 concentrations. Second trimester increases in fetal serum TSH, TBG, T_4, and T_3 concentrations are thought to reflect maturation of the pituitary gland, liver, and thyroid gland, respectively. As gestation progresses, the increase in thyroid hormone probably reflects the functional thyroid maturation and increasing serum TBG.

TABLE 7–2	Maturation of Fetal Thyroid Function
Weeks 7-9	Thyroid gland begins forming
Week 10	TSH and T_4 detectable
	Thyroid follicles detectable
Week 17	Structural maturity of thyroid gland
Week 20	Types II and III deiodinases present
Weeks 18-40	Maturation of TRH production, fetal pituitary function, and fetal thyroid response to TSH stimulation

T_4, thyroxine; TRH, thyrotropin-releasing hormone; TSH, thyroid-stimulating hormone.

T₄ CONCENTRATIONS DURING GESTATION

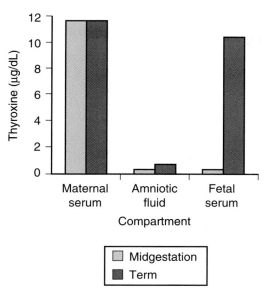

Figure 7–3. Peripheral metabolism of thyroid hormone.

The discovery that anencephalic fetuses have the ability to synthesize iodotyrosines was initially cited as evidence that TSH is not necessary for thyroid hormone production. However, careful studies suggest that pituitary tissue is usually present in these fetuses despite absence of the hypothalamus. In fact, it was demonstrated that anencephalic fetuses have a hyperresponse of TSH to TRH.[61]

The ontogeny of the three deiodinases (see Fig. 7–2) that catalyze the progressive deiodination of T_4 varies in the fetus. Type I deiodinase does not appear until late in gestation, whereas type II and type III deiodinases are present at midgestation.[62] As noted earlier, regulation of fetal exposure to maternal thyroid hormones may be effected by type II and type III deiodinase activity present in placental tissue. This may help with local conversion of T_4 to T_3, T_4 to rT_3, and T_3 to T_2, in addition to providing a source of iodine for the fetus. rT_3 is the predominant fetal metabolite of T_4, produced by inner ring deiodination of T_4 by type III deiodinase. The rT_3 concentration in fetal serum is three times the maternal serum concentration.[63]

Activity levels of the three deiodinases are modulated by the hormonal milieu. In the hypothyroid fetus, activity of the type I and type III deiodinases is decreased, whereas activity of the type II deiodinase, in placenta, brain, and other tissues, is enhanced. These changes favor shunting of T_4 to brain tissues, where deiodination to T_3 is increased, the local concentration of T_3 is increased, and T_3 degradation is decreased. Because of these adaptive responses, even limited transfer of maternal thyroid hormone to the fetus may be sufficient to protect brain maturation.[62]

Maternal Contribution

The maternal thyroid gland provides all thyroid hormone necessary for fetal development until the fetal thyroid gland is able to produce sufficient amounts of endogenous hormone. Investigations into the effects of maternal thyroid status on pregnancy outcome suggest that there *are* perinatal consequences of maternal hypothyroxinemia during pregnancy, including effects on fetal neuropsychologic development. Past studies have demonstrated that maternal thyroid hormone transfer to the fetus occurs but is limited. Measurements of cord-serum total T_4 concentrations in the athyreotic fetus reveal T_4 levels that are approximately 30% of those found in a normal fetus. This finding supports transfer of maternal thyroid hormone to the fetus throughout pregnancy.[64]

Placental Transfer of Thyroid Hormone

The ability of an agent to affect fetal thyroid function is dependent on its ability to cross the placental barrier. Likewise, any effect of maternal thyroid hormone on the fetus must depend on placental transfer.

How effectively T_3 and T_4 cross the placenta is controversial. Early studies, in which radioisotopes were used in pregnant women at term or before pregnancy termination between 11 and 26 weeks, suggested that limited transfer of thyroid hormones occurred across the placenta. However, only serum-precipitable radioactivity was measured. Studies have also been performed in which women at term were infused with large doses of T_4. These studies have limitations, however, inasmuch as placental transfer of thyroid hormone may change with duration of pregnancy and aging of the placenta.

The amniotic cavity containing the developing embryo is surrounded by the extraembryonic coelomic fluid, which is in turn surrounded by the placenta.[65] T_4 concentration in the coelomic fluid at 6 to 12 weeks is low but varies directly with the maternal serum T_4 concentration. In a study of fetuses up to midgestation, concentrations of total T_4 in fetal compartments (coelomic fluid, amniotic fluid and fetal blood) were documented as low as 1% of maternal concentrations, although fetal compartment free T_4 concentrations consistently reached values up to one third of those in maternal blood.[66]

During the second and third trimesters, there are marked maternal-to-fetal gradients of free T_4 and T_3. T_3 appears to cross more easily than T_4; however, fetal serum T_3 concentrations are normally low. The available evidence suggests that thyroid hormone transfer across the placenta reaches the fetus, but not in adequate amounts. A study of antenatal diagnosis and treatment of fetal goitrous hypothyroidism successfully employed intraamniotic injections of T_4 at a dosage of 10 µg/kg/day every 7 days. Investigators documented improvement in the fetal goiter with intraamniotic T_4 therapy.[67]

In a study of 25 neonates born with a complete organification defect and whose mothers also had a complete organification defect, the amount of maternal transfer of physiologic amounts of administered T_4 was examined.[64] The serum T_4 concentration at birth in the affected neonates was 20% to 50% (35 to 70 nmol/L versus 80 to 170 nmol/L) that of normal neonates. The serum T_4 concentration in these infants reflected placental transfer of maternal thyroid hormone. This transfer may be inadequate for inducing euthyroidism in the fetus. Whether it can ensure T_3 concentrations in the fetal brain adequate to promote psychoneurologic development remains to be determined.

Animal studies suggest that it may be possible to modify the structure of the thyroid hormone molecule to increase placental transfer. Placental transfer depends on molecular weight, protein binding, and lipid solubility.[68] We found that dimethyl-isopropyl thyronine (DIMIT), a nonhalogenated thyroid hormone analog, is 20 times as effective as T_4 in preventing fetal rat goiter without inducing maternal thyrotoxicosis.[69] DIMIT is smaller, more lipid soluble, and less tightly protein bound than T_4.

Amniotic Fluid

The accessibility of the amniotic fluid compartment via amniocentesis in pregnant women has led to an interest in TSH and thyroid hormone concentrations in amniotic fluid. Whereas TSH has been difficult to detect in amniotic fluid and results have been unreliable,[62] thyroid hormone concentrations, and their iodothyronine metabolites, have been measured (see Fig. 7–3). Amniotic fluid iodothyronine concentrations reflect both maternal and fetal metabolism.[70] Maternal iodothyronines in amniotic fluid can enter the fetal circulation. In late gestation, this appears to be accomplished by fetal swallowing of amniotic fluid.

The pattern of iodothyronines in amniotic fluid reflects a predominance of type III deiodinase activity in fetal and placental tissue, although significant type II deiodinase activity may be demonstrated as well. As described earlier, type III deiodinase catalyzes the inner ring monodeiodination of T_4 to rT_3 and of T_3 to T_2. Type II deiodinase catalyzes outer ring deiodination, converting T_4 to T_3 and rT_3 to T_2.

rT_3, T_4, and their sulfated conjugates account for more than 95% of thyroid hormones in amniotic fluid. The majority of the T_3 in amniotic fluid is generated from outer ring monodeiodination of T_4 by type II deiodinase. Reverse T_3 concentrations are markedly increased in the amniotic fluid, reaching peak levels at 17 to 20 weeks, again reflecting an increase in 5′-iodothyronine monodeiodinase activity in the fetal compartment. rT_3 has minimal biologic activity. Throughout the course of gestation, amniotic T_3 concentrations decrease progressively, whereas T_4 concentrations increase. At term, T_4 concentrations in amniotic fluid are approximately 0.6 µg/dL lower than those in maternal or fetal serum.[62]

The question has been raised as to whether the amount of thyroid hormone transferred is physiologically significant, particularly early in pregnancy.[71,72] As mentioned earlier, one study measured TSH and thyroid hormone levels in maternal blood (maternal compartment), as well as in coelomic fluid, amniotic fluid, and fetal blood (fetal compartments), in order to evaluate fetal tissue exposure to maternal thyroid hormones up to midgestation.[66] It was revealed that the concentrations of total T_4 in the fetal compartments were as low as 1% of maternal concentrations. Interestingly, however, free T_4 concentrations in the fetal and maternal compartments were more similar: Fetal fluid free T_4 concentrations reached values up to one third of maternal concentrations. This suggests that fetal tissues are exposed to *biologically relevant* concentrations of free T_4 during the first trimester. Fetal free T_4 concentrations are determined by maternal T_4 and free T_4 concentrations, as well as by available concentrations of thyroid hormone–binding proteins. Thus, maternal hypothyroxinemia

would directly affect the thyroid status of the developing fetus, resulting in relative hypothyroxinemia and potentially resulting in adverse developmental effects.

Despite insights into the importance of thyroid hormone for normal fetal development, the specific role of thyroid hormone in development remains unclear.[73] Fetal tissues appear to be exposed to biologically relevant concentrations of free T_4 during early gestation, the result of transfer of maternal thyroid hormone to the fetus. T_3 receptors have been documented in the brain at early stages of fetal development. Adequate maternal serum T_4 concentrations are thus important for the provision of adequate substrate to the fetus. Conversion of T_4 to T_3 in the fetal brain is accomplished by the activity of the 5′D-II isoform of iodothyronine deiodinase.[74] In rat studies, 17.5% of T_4 in fetal tissues of near-term rats came from the mother, which is evidence of the continued importance of maternal serum T_4 transfer throughout gestation.[75] Whether the rat model is directly applicable to pregnant humans is not clear.

Detection of Fetal Thyroid Dysfunction

In a fetus at risk for thyroid dysfunction, surveillance with ultrasonography may be performed, directed at detecting the presence of fetal goiter. This is of clinical relevance, because fetal goiter may result in local airway compromise during delivery. Measurement of maternal serum levels of thyroid-stimulating immunoglobulins, TSH-receptor blocking antibodies, or TSH-binding inhibitory immunoglobulins (TBII) may also be useful in predicting development of fetal thyroid disorders. For example, one study suggests that the fetus is at risk for hypothyroidism if TBII results show inhibition of TSH binding of 50-fold or greater.[76] Likewise, if the TBII value is greater than 30%, or if the thyroid-stimulating immunoglobulin concentration is in excess of 300%, the fetus is at increased risk for hyperthyroidism.[77]

Iodothyronine concentrations in amniotic fluid surrounding fetuses with congenital hypothyroidism predominantly reflect maternal thyroid function. Percutaneous umbilical cord sampling (cordocentesis) is currently the most reliable means to determine *fetal* thyroid status and may be used to evaluate fetuses at risk for thyroid dysfunction.[78,79] For example, amniotic fluid rT_3 concentrations were measured in a fetus whose mother had inadvertently received a therapeutic dose of ^{131}I at 10 to 11 weeks' gestation. This dose would be expected to abolish fetal thyroid function. The amniotic fluid rT_3 concentration was normal at first measurement, and the fetus was treated with an intraamniotic injection of T_4. Investigators documented a rise in amniotic fluid rT_3 concentrations after the T_4 injection, which was suggestive of preservation of function of placental deiodinases. The neonate was euthyroid at birth.[80] Another study employed intraamniotic injections of T_4 in the treatment of fetal goitrous hypothyroidism.[67] Fetal plasma T_3 sulfate concentrations have been found to be normal in fetal hypothyroidism, and T_3 sulfate may help attenuate the effect of hypothyroidism during intrauterine life, perhaps functioning as a local source of T_3 in tissues containing T_3 sulfatase.[62,81]

Neonatal Thyroid Function

As noted previously, at birth, the fetus emerges in the cold extrauterine world, which stimulates an acute release of TSH from the pituitary gland that peaks 30 minutes post partum. TSH levels decrease rapidly during the first 24 hours after birth and more gradually over the next 2 days (Fig. 7–4).[82] The TSH surge elicits increased secretion of thyroid hormones, and, as a result, total and free T_4 concentrations are increased at birth. rT_3 concentrations are also elevated at birth. In contrast, serum T_3 concentrations are low at birth and increase dramatically thereafter. Part of the neonatal increase in T_3 appears to be TSH independent and may be attributed to the rapidly increasing capacity of neonatal tissues to monodeiodinate T_4 to T_3. This capacity is reflected in the progressively changing serum T_3/T_4 and rT_3/T_4 ratios between 30 weeks' gestation and the first postnatal month.[83]

Preterm infants exhibit a decreased TSH response at parturition, which reflects persistent immaturity of the hypothalamic-pituitary-thyroid axis. Although serum T_4 concentration increases during the first few weeks of life, it remains lower than that found in full-term infants. All neonates exhibit elevated radioactive iodine thyroid uptake as early as 10 hours post partum. This increased uptake reaches a peak by the second day and drops to adult normal limits by the fifth day post partum. Iodide kinetic studies suggest that the plasma inorganic iodine and iodine pool are increased, as is the absolute amount of iodide taken up by the thyroid gland.[84] The factors responsible for this stimulation of iodide transport are unknown.

MATERNAL THYROTOXICOSIS

Cause

Thyrotoxicosis occurs in approximately 2 of every 1000 pregnancies.[85,86] Small studies suggest that hyperthyroidism during pregnancy appears to be associated with a significant increase in the frequency of delivery of infants with low birth weight and a slight increase in the neonatal mortality rate.[77] The differential diagnosis of hyperthyroidism in pregnant women includes Graves' disease, hyperemesis gravidarum, transient gestational thyrotoxicosis, and molar pregnancy. Of these, Graves' disease is the most common form of hyperthyroidism occurring in conjunction with pregnancy. In view of the differential diagnosis, the presence of infiltrative ophthalmopathy, pretibial myxedema, goiter, or a family history of autoimmune thyroid disease should be carefully investigated, because these would favor the diagnosis of Graves' disease.

As noted previously, there is considerable overlap between the nonspecific signs and symptoms associated with the hypermetabolic state of pregnancy and those of thyrotoxicosis. An increase in cardiac output, mild tachycardia, widened pulse pressure, systolic flow murmur, and complaints of heat intolerance may be associated with both thyrotoxicosis and normal pregnancy. However, weight

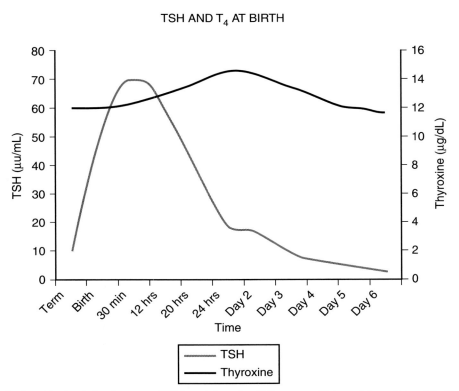

Figure 7–4. Changes in thyroid-stimulating hormone (TSH) and thyroxine (T_4) at term. (Adapted from Fisher DA, Klein AH: Thyroid development and disorders of thyroid function in the newborn. N Engl J Med 1981;304:702.)

loss and sinus tachycardia above 100 beats per minute that is unresponsive to the Valsalva maneuver are not commonly seen in normal pregnancy and are suggestive of underlying thyrotoxicosis (Table 7–3).

Graves' Disease

Graves' disease is a complex autoimmune disorder, consisting of thyrotoxicosis, ophthalmopathy, and dermopathy. It is mediated by thyroid-stimulating immunoglobulins. It has been observed that patients with a known history of Graves' disease tend to undergo remission during pregnancy and exacerbation in the postpartum period.[87] Studies on the immunologic processes of pregnancy provide possible explanations for these observations. Pregnancy has been described as a successful allograft of foreign tissue,[88] and maternal blocking antibodies have been postulated as the primary mechanism for protecting the fetal allograft.[89] Systemic immunomodulatory changes are reflected in the decreased CD4+/CD8+ ratio seen in pregnancy.[90] Both humoral and cell-mediated immunity have been reported to be depressed during normal pregnancy. Thus, several factors are likely to be operative, and a cumulative effect results in survival of the fetal allograft.

Thyroid antibodies have been observed to decrease during pregnancy in patients with Graves' disease, which is concordant with the overall down-regulation of the maternal immune system. The amelioration of Graves' disease during pregnancy with exacerbation after delivery is thought to result from these immunologic changes. The fetal immune system also contributes to suppression of the maternal immune system. An increase in fetal suppressor T cell function is necessary to prevent immunologic rejection by the mother. Soluble factors produced by activated fetal suppressor cells presumably cross the placenta and decrease the maternal autoimmune process. A byproduct of this general down-regulation may be a transient decrease in the intensity of the maternal Graves' disease during pregnancy. Delivery, with loss of the fetal suppressor T cells, is accompanied by restoration of normal maternal immune vigilance and may thus account for the clinically recognized postpartum exacerbation of Graves' disease.[91]

Hyperemesis Gravidarum

Hyperemesis gravidarum is marked by profound vomiting during early pregnancy, which may result in electrolyte imbalance and dehydration. Biochemical evaluation of affected patients reveals hyperthyroxinemia; elevated serum T_4 concentrations and decreased serum TSH concentrations are found in as many as half of pregnant women with hyperemesis gravidarum.[13,92-95] Measurement of serum TSH with ultrasensitive, third-generation assays aids in the differentiation of hyperemesis-associated hyperthyroxinemia from other possible causes, inasmuch as the TSH is not fully suppressed in this condition. There is confusion about the extent to which hyperemesis gravidarum is associated with thyrotoxicosis, because patients rarely manifest overt symptoms, despite their hyperthyroxinemia.[96] The hyperthyroxinemia is usually transient, resolving by 18 weeks of pregnancy without antithyroid therapy.[97]

Patients with hyperemesis tend to have higher serum concentrations of hCG than do pregnant patients without hyperemesis, and this may suggest a mechanism to explain the hyperthyroxinemia observed in this condition. As noted earlier, hCG possesses intrinsic, weak thyroid-stimulating activity, and its presence, at higher concentrations, may account for the hyperthyroxinemia found on biochemical evaluation. The best evidence supports this

TABLE 7–3   Differential Diagnosis of Gestational Maternal Thyrotoxicosis

Causes	Symptoms	Signs	Laboratory Findings	Course
Graves' disease	Heat intolerance Weight loss Palpitations Sweats	Sinus tachycardia > 100 ↑ Cardiac output ↑ Pulse pressure Systolic murmur Ophthalmopathy Dermopathy	↑↑ T_4, free T_4 ↓↓ TSH (suppressed) (+) Antithyroid antibodies	May remit during pregnancy Postpartum flare

Hyperemesis gravidarum	Nausea/vomiting (profound)
	Weight loss
		Often clinically euthyroid in appearance
		Dehydration
			↔/↑ T_4, free T_4
			  "high-normal"
			  or minimally elevated
			No frank elevation in T_4
			  unless hCG > 50,000 IU/L
			↓ TSH minimally low, but
			  not fully suppressed
			↑ β-hCG
			Ketonuria, electrolyte imbalance,
			  hepatic and renal abnormalities
				Resolves by 18 weeks without therapy

Molar pregnancy	Nausea/vomiting First trimester bleeding	Toxemia Absent fetal development	↑ T_4, free T_4 ↓ TSH (suppressed) ↑↑↑ β-hCG	Evacuation of molar pregnancy Hyperthyroidism resolves with normalization of β-hCG

hCG, human chorionic gonadotropin; T_4, thyroxine; TSH, thyroid-stimulating hormone.
↑, mildly increased; ↑↑, moderately increased; ↑↑↑, severely increased; ↓, mildly decreased; (+), positive.

hypothesis that hCG is the cause of the thyroid stimulation in hyperemesis gravidarum and is closely linked to the cause of the hyperemesis itself.[94] It has been shown that the degree of thyroid stimulation varies with the hCG concentration and correlates with the symptoms of hyperemesis. Increased estradiol levels, found in women with hyperemesis gravidarum, may provide a plausible connection between the elevated hCG concentrations and the clinical manifestations of nausea and vomiting. The hyperemesis and hyperthyroxinemia should resolve by 18 to 20 weeks of pregnancy. If it persists beyond 20 weeks, antithyroid therapy should be considered.

In addition, there is debate about the occurrence of hyperthyroxinemia during the common "morning sickness" of pregnancy.[98,99] No goiter is present, and these patients, too, rarely manifest classic symptoms of thyrotoxicosis. Serum TSH values may decrease slightly during the first trimester in response to increased hCG activity, but they are not fully suppressed.[7,94] This transient hyperthyroxinemia is probably another manifestation of the interplay between TSH and hCG during the first trimester. Therefore, a sensitive second- or third-generation TSH determination is the best single indication of thyroid function in the pregnant woman.[100,101]

Diagnosis of Hyperthyroidism in Pregnancy

The clinical diagnosis of thyrotoxicosis in the pregnant woman may be difficult. The euthyroid woman may have a number of hyperdynamic systems and signs, including an increase in cardiac output with systolic flow murmur and tachycardia, skin warmth, and heat intolerance. Diagnostic difficulties are further compounded because the usual diagnostic laboratory tests of thyrotoxicosis may yield results that easily give rise to suspicion but are confirmed only with difficulty. Signs of hyperthyroidism, such as weight loss, may be obscured by the weight gain of pregnancy. The presence of the eye changes of Graves' disease or pretibial myxedema may be suggestive but do not necessarily indicate thyrotoxicosis. A resting pulse above 100 is suggestive, and if the pulse fails to slow during a Valsalva maneuver, thyrotoxicosis is more likely. The presence of onycholysis, or separation of the distal nail from the nailbed, may also be useful in making the clinical diagnosis of thyrotoxicosis.

Despite complications in the interpretation of thyroid function tests because of the elevated TBG concentration during pregnancy, the diagnosis of thyrotoxicosis rests on the laboratory values, particularly on the estimation of serum TSH concentration by a sensitive assay. Unfortunately, because of the elevated TBG during pregnancy, the free T_4 index is not an accurate measure of the actual free T_4 concentration.[102] The newer nonequilibrium dialysis methods for the estimation of free T_4 may be helpful, although some of them are also affected by changes in TBG.

Pregnant women tolerate mild to moderate degrees of hyperthyroidism relatively well. If the diagnosis is in doubt, the thyroid function tests can be repeated in 3 or 4 weeks before a final decision is made. Determination of thyroid-stimulating immunoglobulin may be helpful in alerting the physician to the possibility of fetal thyrotoxicosis or neonatal Graves' disease. It has not been particularly helpful in making the diagnosis of thyrotoxicosis in the pregnant woman.[103,104]

Morbidity/Mortality

Despite the difficulties inherent in confirming the diagnosis of hyperthyroidism in pregnant women, prompt diagnosis is important, because there is potential morbidity associated with untreated maternal thyrotoxicosis (Table 7–4). Studies suggest that uncontrolled hyperthyroidism during pregnancy may be associated with numerous adverse outcomes, including an increase in neonatal mortality rate, delivery of infants with low birth weight, risk of premature labor, and frequency of preeclampsia.[77,105] In a retrospective study of 60 thyrotoxic pregnant women, maternal congestive heart failure, preterm delivery, and perinatal infant mortality were increased among women who remained thyrotoxic.[106] Because pregnancy is a hyperdynamic state, the superimposition of thyrotoxicosis upon the already increased cardiac output and relative tachycardia of pregnancy may explain some of these findings.[107] However, socioeconomic conditions may have played a role in the severity of the complications in this study. In general, women in whom thyrotoxicosis was diagnosed during pregnancy had a higher incidence of morbidity and perinatal infant mortality than did thyrotoxic women treated before conception.

An increased incidence of toxemia has been reported in thyrotoxic pregnancies, but, again, the studies were not well controlled.[108] There is evidence, however, that lack of control of hyperthyroidism significantly increases the risks of severe preeclampsia and of low birth weight in infants.[109] There is also the suggestion that there is an increased incidence of congenital malformations in the offspring of mothers with untreated Graves' disease.[110,111] Down's syndrome has been reported to occur more frequently in the offspring of thyrotoxic mothers, but the studies were not well controlled.[112] Furthermore, one study concluded that the presence of thyroid antibodies in the serum of a pregnant woman has no prognostic value for the birth of a child with Down's syndrome.[113] In general, the small numbers of women included in these studies preclude definitive statements.

There is a lack of convincing evidence that fertility is impaired in mild to moderate hyperthyroidism, although menstrual irregularity is frequent.[114] The balance of available evidence suggests that mild to moderate thyrotoxicosis is not

---

TABLE 7–4 Morbidity and Mortality of Gestational Thyrotoxicosis

Fetal
  ↑ Neonatal mortality
  ↑ Low birth weight
Maternal
  ↑ Risk of premature labor
  ↑ Frequency of preeclampsia
  ↑ Congestive heart failure

inimical to the continuation of pregnancy. Hyperthyroidism during pregnancy may complicate the management of diabetes mellitus with erratic glycemic control and an increased insulin requirement.[115] In view of all of the potential morbid conditions and mortality associated with untreated thyrotoxicosis in pregnancy, treatment of hyperthyroidism during pregnancy is clearly indicated. There is no evidence that pregnancy makes the thyrotoxicosis more difficult to control. In fact, hyperthyroidism tends to be more easily controlled during pregnancy, whereas relapses tend to occur post partum.[30,116] This may be related to the immunologic suppression associated with pregnancy.

Management of Hyperthyroidism in Pregnancy

Therapy of the pregnant, thyrotoxic woman is limited to antithyroid drugs or surgery, in view of the absolute contraindication to the use of radioactive iodine.[30] Antithyroid drugs include the thionamides propylthiouracil (PTU) and methimazole (MMI) (Table 7–5). Their use during pregnancy and lactation has been problematic, because questions have arisen regarding the potential risks to the fetus of thionamide therapy. There have been no prospective clinical trials to address this issue, which remains embroiled in controversy.

Thionamide Therapy

There are arguments for and against both drug therapy and surgery. In the final analysis, the individual decision and course of treatment depends on the physician's treatment bias and recent experience. Even if the decision is made to operate, thyrotoxicosis must first be controlled by antithyroid drug therapy before surgery.

The mainstay of antithyroid drug therapy involves thionamides, which inhibit thyroid hormone synthesis by blocking iodination of the tyrosine molecule. Because these drugs block the synthesis, but not the release, of thyroid hormone, the clinical response to thionamides is not immediate. In fact, a clinical response to thionamides does not occur until colloid stores are depleted. Therefore, the time required to achieve control of the thyrotoxicosis is variable and depends on the amount of colloid stored in the thyroid gland. Commonly, the patient notices some initial clinical improvement after the first week of therapy and approaches euthyroidism by 4 to 6 weeks of therapy. Both PTU and MMI have a short duration of action that is generally not thought to be altered by either pregnancy or thyrotoxicosis.[117] Initial drug requirements may be high; some women require thionamide dosing every 8 hours or even more frequently for adequate control of the thyrotoxicosis. Ultimately, most patients can be maintained on a single daily dose.

In general, PTU and MMI have been used interchangeably without evidence that one or the other has clear therapeutic advantages. However, PTU does have the advantage of partially blocking the peripheral conversion of T_4 to T_3, in addition to inhibiting thyroid hormone synthesis. In theory, this might allow the patient to be rendered euthyroid more quickly. Furthermore, case reports have suggested that treatment with MMI may be associated with aplasia cutis, a scalp defect, in the offspring.[118-122] For these reasons, PTU is preferred as first-line therapy of thyrotoxicosis in pregnancy. However, there is no formal contraindication to the use of MMI.

Dosage

Once the diagnosis of hyperthyroidism has been made, the patient should be given PTU, 100 to 150 mg orally, every 8 hours. Serial serum T_4, free T_4, and TSH determinations

TABLE 7–5   Acute Management of Thyrotoxicosis

Drug	Dosage	Side Effects/Complications	Monitoring
Thionamides			
Propylthiouracil	100-150 mg PO q8h (preferred)	Maternal: Rash Agranulocytosis (0.5%) Hepatitis	TFTs every 4 wk and adjust antithyroid medication
Methimazole (Tapazole)	10-15 mg PO q8h	Fetal: hypothyroidism	Same as for propylthiouracil
Adrenergic Blockers			
Propanolol (Inderal)	20-40 mg PO q6h	Fetal: Intrauterine growth restriction Respiratory distress Bradycardia Hypoglycemia Hypothermia	Heart rate or pulse
Atenolol (Tenormin)	50-100 mg PO every day	Same as for propanolol	Heart rate or pulse
Surgery			
Thyroidectomy		Maternal: Miscarriage Hypoparathyroidism Laryngeal nerve paralysis	Serum calcium TFTs

PO, per os (orally); TFT, thyroid function tests.

should be obtained on a monthly basis, because they may be helpful in monitoring the course of the disease, and dosage adjustments can be made, if indicated. There appears to be a strong correlation between fetal and maternal free T_4 concentrations, and maintenance of the maternal free T_4 concentration at or slightly above the upper range of the normal limit appears to be optimal for fetal thyroid function.[123] After control of thyrotoxicosis has been achieved—as determined by an improvement in symptoms and signs, by a fall in serum T_4, and by an increase in the serum TSH—the dosage of PTU should be decreased to 50 mg four times a day. If the patients remains clinically euthyroid, the PTU dosage could be decreased to 150 mg/day and then, after 3 weeks, to 50 mg twice a day. Pregnant women with thyrotoxicosis should be maintained on as low a dosage of PTU as possible, preferably less than 100 mg/day. Of note, the serum TSH concentration may remain suppressed for several weeks or months after the serum free T_4 has been brought within the optimal range. This is not an indication to further increase the dosage of PTU; it simply represents a lag in the correction of hyperthyroidism-induced pituitary suppression. In contrast, however, serum T_4 concentrations may increase before clinical signs of thyrotoxicosis recur; therefore, vigilance remains paramount.

If thyrotoxicosis recurs, the PTU dosage should again be increased to 300 mg/day in divided doses. As mentioned earlier, a recurrence is particularly likely post partum, and the PTU dosage could be preemptively increased to 300 mg/day at that time. If control of thyrotoxicosis in the pregnant woman is not achieved on this treatment schedule, the PTU dosage should be increased to 600 mg/day and given more frequently (e.g., every 4 to 6 hours). Rarely is it necessary to prescribe more than 600 mg of PTU daily.[106] The need for large amounts of PTU to treat thyrotoxicosis in late pregnancy may relate to low serum concentrations of PTU. Despite the fact that the duration of action of PTU is not generally thought to be altered by pregnancy,[117,124] serum PTU concentrations in one study were consistently lower in the late third trimester than postpartum values.[125] In addition, if compliance is a problem, the slow intrathyroidal turnover of MMI would allow the drug to be used on a once- or twice-daily dose regimen.

Complications of Thionamide Therapy

The most common complications associated with thionamide therapy tend to occur within the first 4 weeks of therapy, affecting approximately 2% of patients. They include a mild, occasionally purpuric rash, pruritus, drug fever, and nausea. There is incomplete cross-reactivity between PTU and MMI. If a drug reaction occurs with PTU, an attempt may be made to continue therapy with MMI.

Agranulocytosis is an idiosyncratic reaction that occurs during treatment with thionamides. It is rare, affecting approximately 0.5% of the treated population. As a result of bone marrow suppression, patients typically present with severe sore throat, oral ulcers, and high fevers. Although agranulocytosis typically manifests within the first 8 to 12 weeks of treatment, it is important to recognize that this idiosyncratic reaction may occur at any time during treatment with a thionamide. The development of agranulocytosis mandates immediate discontinuation of thionamide drug therapy. In most patients, bone marrow

function recovers upon withdrawal of the offending agent, but fatal outcomes have been reported, although they occur in fewer than 1 per 10,000 treated patients. A leukocyte count should be obtained before initiation of thionamide therapy, because approximately 10% of patients with Graves' disease may have leukopenia upon presentation. However, weekly monitoring of the patient's leukocyte count during therapy is probably not helpful, because the white blood cell count may fall precipitously over several days, in between evaluations.

Hepatitis and vasculitis have also been reported as side effects of thionamide therapy. When abnormalities on liver function tests (LFTs) occur, the pattern is that of a transaminitis, rather than of a cholestatic insult. Liver biopsies confirm hepatocellular injury, rather than cholestatic hepatic injury.[126] Severe hepatic dysfunction is rare. Gurlek and colleagues studied the liver function test results of 43 hyperthyroid patients before and after 6 weeks of treatment with PTU at a dosage of 100 mg three times a day.[127] Approximately 60% of patients had at least one LFT abnormality at baseline, before the initiation of treatment. In order of decreasing frequency, the most common baseline elevations were seen in alkaline phosphatase, alanine aminotransferase (ALT), aspartate aminotransferase, and γ-glutamyl-transpeptidase. After 6 weeks of treatment with PTU, 16% of patients had persistent LFT abnormalities, possibly related to therapy, defined as a continued increase in ALT values from baseline or ALT elevations above the upper limit of normal. No patients had any symptoms referable to the LFT abnormalities, and the transaminitis resolved in 60% of affected patients despite continued therapy with PTU. There was no correlation between pretreatment thyroid function test results and the development of a transaminitis. Likewise, the presence or absence of LFT abnormalities at baseline was not a predictor for the subsequent development of LFT abnormalities. Liaw and associates found similar results in 54 hyperthyroid patients treated with PTU, although the PTU dosage was decreased in patients with LFT abnormalities for the duration of the study.[128] In this study, there was a correlation between higher baseline TFTs and degree of subsequent ALT elevation. In addition, Huang and colleagues found that 75% of their 95 hyperthyroid patients had at least one baseline LFT abnormality.[129] Of these, 61% experienced normalization despite continued treatment with PTU.

Effect on the Fetus

Although neonatal hepatitis has been described, the major concern with the use of PTU during pregnancy is the induction of fetal hypothyroidism.[46,130-132] Both PTU and MMI cross the placenta and inhibit fetal thyroid production.[133] Earlier in vitro data suggested that MMI crossed the placenta more easily than PTU,[134] although with the more recent reporting of in vivo data, this belief has been challenged.[135] Reviews of the subject have concluded that there is probably no significant difference in either the efficiency or rate of placental transfer of PTU and MMI.[136] Because of this concern, however, some suggest that thyrotoxic pregnant women should be treated with iodides rather than thionamides.[137]

Many women have given birth to normal children even after receiving large amounts of antithyroid drugs during pregnancy. There does not appear to be an independent relationship between the dose of thionamide used and neonatal thyroid function,[138] which suggests that maternal thyroid stimulating immunoglobulins may play a role in modulating fetal thyroid function. In the Quebec Neonatal Thyroid Screening Program, of 400,000 children screened, 4 had transient hypothyroidism caused by PTU. It was estimated that only 1% to 5% of children exposed to PTU have transient hypothyroidism, although the exact number of mothers receiving antithyroid drugs was unknown. Under ordinary circumstances, sufficient maternal thyroid hormone may cross the placenta to prevent fetal goiter.[139] As mentioned earlier, pregnant women tolerate mild degrees of hyperthyroidism without great difficulty, and the goal of antithyroid therapy during pregnancy is to maintain the free T_4 at or slightly above the upper limit of the normal range to preserve this safe-guarding effect. In general, an attempt should be made to treat the pregnant thyrotoxic woman with the lowest possible dosage of antithyroid medication.[140] This dictum, combined with the evidence that neonatal hypothyroidism is associated with cognitive developmental deficits, suggests that it is better to err by giving too low a dosage of antithyroid medication than to give too large a dosage. Finally, if early diagnosis and treatment of neonatal hypothyroidism prevent the sequelae of in utero hypothyroidism, these affected children can be successfully treated after birth. Fetal blood sampling is possible but involves fetal risk.[141]

Possible Long-Term Effects

In view of the risk of fetal hypothyroidism, is there any evidence that children who are exposed to thionamides in utero fail to develop full intellectual capacity? To study this problem, Burrow and coworkers compared 18 children exposed to PTU in utero with 17 nonexposed siblings.[142] The ages of the children ranged from 2 to 12 years, and there were no important differences in their physical or mental characteristics. Thyroid function tests were normal in both groups, and there was no evidence of abnormal physical development or delayed bone growth. Subsequent psychologic testing revealed no marked differences between the groups, either in overall intellectual development or in patterning of various mental skills.

The small size of the sample precludes definite conclusions, but, in a subsequent study, intelligence tests administered to 29 children who had been exposed to PTU in utero and 32 nonexposed siblings also showed no important differences between the groups.[143] Two other studies have reported similar results.[144,145] It therefore appears that, with careful attention to maintenance of maternal euthyroid status, thionamides can be given to pregnant women without interfering with subsequent intellectual development in the offspring.

Thionamides and Lactation

Thionamides are transferred into the breast milk of women receiving these drugs. This is clinically relevant, because Graves' disease often worsens during the postpartum period, and antithyroid drugs may need to be reinitiated, or the dosage increased, at that time. In addition, some women first present with Graves' disease during the postpartum period. Initial studies suggested that the amount of PTU transferred to the breast-feeding infant is lower than the amount of MMI and would not be expected to have any significant effect on neonatal thyroid function.[146,147] Eleven thyrotoxic women were treated with carbimazole, which is similar to MMI, or with PTU.[148] The amount of thionamide did not exceed 15 mg of carbimazole or 150 mg of PTU. The authors concluded that breast-feeding under these conditions does not pose a risk to the neonate. It has been postulated that pharmacokinetic differences between PTU and MMI might explain their different efficiencies of transfer into breast milk. Whereas PTU is extensively bound to serum proteins (namely, albumin), MMI exhibits minimal protein binding.[149] Differences in ionization and acidity may also play a role.

Similar results have been reported in 35 infants of lactating mothers with thyrotoxicosis who were receiving 5 to 20 mg of MMI daily. Azizi and associates reported on serum MMI levels, thyroid function tests, and intellectual development of 88 infants who were breast-fed by mothers being treated with MMI at a dose of 10 to 20 mg/day.[150] Values of T_4, T_3, and TSH were not significantly different between children in the treatment group and controls. In addition, serum MMI levels were drawn in six of the infants of thyrotoxic, lactating mothers receiving MMI. Although the number of infants studied was small, serum MMI levels in all infants were well below the therapeutic range. Fourteen of these children subsequently underwent extensive psychologic and performance testing between 48 and 74 months of age. No significant differences were found with regard to performance intelligence quotient (IQ) scores in comparison with controls.[151] As with all drugs, there is the theoretic risk of fetal drug reaction with thionamides, but none has been reported so far.[152] Overall, breast-feeding appears to be safe in mothers receiving 450 mg/day of PTU or less or receiving 20 mg/day of MMI or less. In summary, if a mother receiving PTU or MMI has a strong desire to breast-feed, there should be a full explanation of the potential risks and close monitoring of neonatal thyroid function.

Iodine is also excreted into the breast milk. Thus, radioiodine given to the mother is transferred to the infant. Radioactive ^{131}I may remain in the milk for a prolonged period and should be avoided if breast-feeding is desired.[153]

Adrenergic Blockers

Because of the potential risks associated with treatment with PTU, there has been interest in alternative therapy that would have fewer side effects. β-blocking agents do not alter the nonadrenergic actions of thyroid hormone, but they do have ability to blunt many of the adrenergically mediated physiologic sequelae of thyrotoxicosis. For this reason, they have traditionally been used as adjunctive agents in the treatment of thyrotoxicosis, and there has been interest in the use of β-blocking agents, particularly propranolol, in the management of thyrotoxicosis during pregnancy.[154] Concerns have been raised, however, because the use of β-blocking agents during pregnancy has been associated with adverse outcomes, including small placenta; intrauterine growth restriction; neonatal respiratory distress; impaired responses to anoxic stress; and postnatal bradycardia, hypothermia, and hypoglycemia.[155-158] Spontaneous abortion has also been reported more frequently in pregnant women with thyrotoxicosis who were treated with propranolol and carbimazole in comparison with carbimazole alone.[159]

On the basis of these studies, which were often retrospective, β blockers have not been recommended for long-term treatment of thyrotoxicosis during pregnancy. One review addressed the use of β blockers to treat hypertension in pregnancy, and the results may be extrapolated to some degree to address the use of these agents in the management of thyrotoxicosis during pregnancy.[160] The overview consisted of randomized trials in which (1) patients with preexisting mild hypertension received continuous treatment with oral β blockers throughout pregnancy, (2) treatment with oral β blockers was initiated during late pregnancy because of the development of mild-moderate late-onset hypertension (i.e., patients manifested chronic hypertension late in pregnancy or experienced the onset of pregnancy-induced hypertension), or (3) patients received intravenous β blockers as treatment of severe, pregnancy-induced hypertension. Of the two trials specifically addressing the question of intrauterine growth restriction, Butters and associates showed a dramatic increase in the number of infants small for gestational age delivered by patients treated with atenolol for chronic hypertension.[161] Conversely, Sibai and colleagues found no evidence of an adverse effect of labetalol on fetal growth.[162] No effect of duration of therapy was seen on infants small for gestational age. Overall, β blockers were associated with a borderline increase in the number of infants small for gestational age delivered by patients receiving chronic β blocker therapy for mild hypertension. There was also a borderline increased incidence of infants small for gestational age in patients who received oral β-blocking agents late in pregnancy. No excess perinatal mortality was observed in patients with severe, late-onset hypertension who required short-term treatment with intravenous β-blocking agents. Overall, it was unclear that the benefits of β blocker therapy outweighed the risks with regard to treatment of hypertension. The available data suggest that pregnant women may be treated with β-blocking agents if indicated, although the potential for adverse effects on the fetus must be acknowledged.[163] Whether selective β blockers have any advantage in long-term therapy remains to be determined.[164,165]

For rapid control of thyrotoxicosis, propranolol, 20 to 40 mg every 6 hours, or atenolol, 50 to 100 mg/day, are usually adequate to control the maternal cardiac heart rate at 80 to 90 beats per minute. Esmolol, an ultra–short-acting cardioselective β_1-adrenergic blocker, was effective in a thyrotoxic pregnant woman who was unresponsive to propranolol.[166] Whether agents that inhibit the conversion of T_4 to T_3, such as ipodate, have any role in the rapid control of thyrotoxicosis in the pregnant woman is not clear.[167] However, escape from these agents does occur.

Surgery

If an elective subtotal thyroidectomy is to be performed, surgery is often delayed until after the first trimester.

The rationale for this delay is to minimize the risk of spontaneous abortion, inasmuch as the rate of spontaneous abortion is highest during the first trimester and surgery may represent an additional risk. However, if urgent thyroid surgery is indicated, it probably need not be avoided. The arguments against performing a subtotal thyroidectomy in the pregnant woman are based on concerns for potential surgical complications. As with any surgical procedure, there is a minimal but definite surgical risk, and it is probably higher than the risk of fatal complications encountered with medical therapy.[42,168] In addition, the surgical complications of hypoparathyroidism and recurrent laryngeal nerve paralysis are disabling and difficult to treat. These do occur, albeit uncommonly, and with increasing frequency as fewer thyroidectomies are performed. Because of the efficacy of standard medical therapy, non-surgical management is increasingly common. However, studies have indicated that subtotal thyroidectomy after appropriate preparation results in no surgical complications.[169] If surgery is indicated, the patient should be observed carefully for signs of postoperative hypothyroidism. A reasonable approach is to commence immediate replacement therapy with 0.05 mg of T_4 in order to avoid development of hypothyroxinemia.

Because surgical complications do occur, and because the majority of patients who receive PTU have uncomplicated pregnancies, medical therapy seems to be the preferred treatment of hyperthyroidism during pregnancy. Subtotal thyroidectomy should probably be reserved for patients with antithyroid drug hypersensitivity, poor compliance, and the rare instance in which the drugs are ineffective.

Thyroid Storm

The major immediate risk of thyrotoxicosis in the pregnant woman is the development of thyroid storm.[170] This life-threatening complication is uncommon, manifesting as an amplification of the typical signs and symptoms of hyperthyroidism. Patients typically present with a fever as high as 106° F, marked tachycardia, prostration, and severe dehydration. Thyroid storm is more likely to occur when there is some precipitating factor such as labor, cesarean section, or infection.[171] There is a 25% mortality rate, despite aggressive and appropriate medical management. Thyroid storm is more commonly seen in patients in whom the hyperthyroidism has not been recognized and is thus untreated. Of importance is that it may also occur in patients receiving treatment with thionamides in subtherapeutic doses.

Management of thyroid storm should focus on alleviation of identifiable precipitating factors, as well as aggressive pharmacologic therapy. Treatment regimens should include (1) propranolol, 40 mg by mouth every 6 hours to control the β-adrenergic activity (if necessary, the drug can be given intravenously in doses of 1 to 2 mg); (2) sodium iodide, 1 g intravenously, to block the secretion of thyroid hormone; (3) PTU, 1200 mg orally in divided doses, to block the formation of thyroid hormone and the deiodination of T_4 to T_3; (4) dexamethasone, 8 mg/day, to block further the deiodination of T_4 to T_3; (5) sufficient replacement of severe fluid losses; and (6) hypothermia for malignant hyperpyrexia.[172,173] As noted earlier, there is a delay in the onset of clinical efficacy with the thionamides. Therefore, adjunctive, supportive measures are important early in the course of thyroid storm. Plasma exchange remains an option and has been carried out successfully in three pregnant women with severe thyrotoxicosis.[172] If hyperthyroidism is considered in the differential diagnosis of a symptomatic pregnant woman, and if adequate therapy initiated expeditiously, this frightening complication of thyrotoxicosis can be avoided.

Administration of Radioactive Iodine during Pregnancy

As mentioned previously, radioactive iodine is absolutely contraindicated during pregnancy. However, on occasion, patients not known to be pregnant are given a dose of radioactive iodine. Although all women of childbearing age should have a pregnancy test before receiving therapeutic doses of radiation, this is not always done.

Effects of Maternal Irradiation

Hyperthyroidism is the only common nonmalignant disease for which patients receive significant doses of ionizing radiation. During a radioisotope thyroid uptake test, both mother and fetus are exposed to small amounts of radiation. The amount of radiation that the mother receives during an uptake scan is relatively insignificant, in terms of radiation exposure to the thyroid or ovaries. Treatment doses, however, are up to 1000-fold greater than the doses used in uptake studies. There does not appear to be an increased incidence of secondary leukemia or thyroid malignancy in thyrotoxic patients receiving radioactive iodine.[174] However, subsequent repercussions of the gonadal dose are less clear.[175,176]

Persistent chromosomal abnormalities have been found in the white blood cells of patients who had received 5 mCi of ^{131}I for the treatment of thyrotoxicosis. Similar changes probably also occur in gonadal chromosomes, but definitive evidence is lacking. The radiation dose to the maternal and fetal thyroid glands, as well as gonads, has been estimated.[177,178] A thyrotoxic woman receiving a therapeutic dose of 10 mCi of ^{131}I would receive a total body dose of approximately 14.5 rad and a dose to the gonads of approximately 1.3 rad. Whether this radiation dose is sufficient to cause genetic defects is not clear.

Effects of Fetal Irradiation

As noted earlier, the fetal thyroid gland begins to concentrate iodine at approximately the 10th to 12th week of gestation and at that time has an increased avidity for iodine, up to 20 to 50 times that of the maternal thyroid gland. As a result of this increased avidity, any dose of radioiodine is more concentrated per gram of thyroid tissue in the fetus than in the mother. The average absorbed dose in the whole fetus has been estimated to be highest at 1 month of gestation, declining steadily thereafter throughout the remainder of gestation. Therefore, the highest total fetal dose would be expected to occur from the administration of ^{131}I to the mother who is 4 weeks' pregnant. The dose to the fetal thyroid gland is predicted to be highest during the sixth month of gestation.[178] Depending on biologic half-time and maternal thyroid uptake, estimation of the absorbed dose of ^{131}I is approximately 3 rad from 10 mCi of ^{131}I administered to the mother. Inadvertent administration of 14.5 μCi of ^{131}I to a thyrotoxic mother at the end of the first trimester was estimated to have delivered a dose of 20,000 rad to her thyroid gland and 250,000 rad to the fetal thyroid gland, with resulting fetal hypothyroidism. Additional case reports of congenital hypothyroidism have been reported in offspring of mothers who received therapeutic doses of radioiodine.[179-181]

Not only is the fetal thyroid gland more avid for iodine, but fetal tissues in general are also more radiosensitive. In general, the risk of congenital defects has been considered to be negligible at 5 rad.[182] However, studies have demonstrated a causal relationship between prenatal irradiation and the subsequent development of malignant disease. Ultimate risk appears to be related to both the dose and the timing of exposure.[183,184] A study of children who were in utero in or near Hiroshima and Nagasaki at the time of the atomic bombing revealed that radiation exposure in utero resulted in a higher prevalence of microcephaly and mental retardation and an increased rate of fetal and infant mortality. Microcephaly was most common among children irradiated at between 7 and 15 weeks' gestation. Evaluation of growth and development in these children demonstrated that those exposed to ionizing radiation in utero lagged behind nonexposed peers during adolescence in several important areas of development. These findings suggested that radiation exposure may result in subtle defects that are difficult to detect. Significantly, most of the long-term effects occurred with whole-body irradiation above 50 rad. Whether there is a threshold effect for radiation damage or whether the damage is linear is important, because the whole-body radiation dose to the fetus from a therapeutic dose of ^{131}I for thyrotoxicosis is well below 50 rad. At least some of the effects may be linear, and all radiation should be regarded as harmful.

Management after Inadvertent Radioactive Iodine Administration

Before the administration of radioactive iodine to a woman capable of childbearing, it is recommended that nonpregnant status be confirmed. If a woman is found to be pregnant after a radioactive iodine uptake study, nothing further need be done. In a pregnant woman who has inadvertently received a *therapeutic dose* of ^{131}I for treatment of hyperthyroidism, the question of termination of the pregnancy arises. Although administration of radiation is absolutely contraindicated in the pregnant woman, the amount received during a diagnostic thyroid study is not sufficient to cause concern with regard to effects on the fetal thyroid gland. This is particularly true early in pregnancy, when the fetal thyroid is not trapping iodine (i.e., before 10 to 12 weeks). The relatively low fetal whole-body irradiation is probably not sufficient to justify pregnancy termination. If the administration of ^{131}I occurs at a time when the fetal thyroid gland is trapping iodine, there is a definite risk of subsequent fetal hypothyroidism. However, the neonatal thyroid screening program is predicated on the supposition that prompt postnatal thyroid hormone therapy prevents the sequelae of in utero hypothyroidism.

As noted previously, if a woman with thyrotoxicosis not known to be pregnant is given a therapeutic dose of ^{131}I, further intervention is not mandated. However, if pregnancy is discovered within 1 week of administration, and intervention is desired, she may be treated with PTU, 300 mg/day for 7 days, to block the recycling of the ^{131}I in the fetal gland. Administration of cold iodides would dilute the uptake pool, but this would also delay the release of radioactivity, resulting in prolonged exposure. Intervention more than 10 days after treatment is not helpful, because more than 90% of a dose of ^{131}I has been delivered within this time frame. The mother's underlying thyrotoxicosis remains to be treated, and this will further complicate fetal thyroid function. Regardless of the initiation of possible preventive measures, the infant should be carefully monitored for hypothyroidism at birth and immediate treatment begun if indicated. In utero hypothyroidism can be diagnosed by periumbilical blood sampling and T_4 treatment delivered by the amniotic fluid, but the procedure has some risk and is still experimental.

Long-Term Management of Thyrotoxicosis

The long-term management of a young thyrotoxic patient who is planning subsequent pregnancies represents a challenging therapeutic issue. A medical remission in this age group is possible, although sustained remission is unlikely, and therapy during the subsequent pregnancies will probably be indicated. Active consideration should be given to radioactive iodine therapy, despite concerns about administering radioactive iodine to a woman capable of childbearing. It is critical that the decision involve the patient. A sufficient number of young women have been treated with appropriate follow-up to indicate that this is a relatively safe therapy. Although there are no definitive data, women desiring future pregnancies are frequently told to wait 4 to 6 months after ^{131}I treatment before becoming pregnant. Long-term antithyroid drug therapy in such a situation may be undesirable. Despite the attendant risks, subtotal thyroidectomy must also be actively considered in this situation.

POSTPARTUM THYROIDITIS

Systemic immunomodulatory changes occur during pregnancy in order to ensure the survival of the developing fetus. Both humoral and cell-mediated immunity have been reported to be depressed during normal pregnancy, with recovery of immune function in the postpartum period. It follows that the immunologic changes that occur during pregnancy may affect the course of autoimmune thyroid diseases after pregnancy, including Graves' disease, Hashimoto's thyroiditis, and postpartum thyroiditis. Estimates suggest that postpartum thyroiditis develops in approximately 1 per 20 women.[185]

Postpartum thyroiditis classically occurs 3 to 6 months after delivery and evolves as a triphasic manifestation of transient hyperthyroidism, followed by hypothyroidism and spontaneous recovery in 90% of cases (Fig. 7–5).[186,187] Laboratory evaluation classically reveals the presence of microsomal antibodies, and thyroid hormone concentrations are elevated during the thyrotoxic phase. Concurrent radioactive iodine uptake is low, in contrast to that seen in Graves' disease. On physical examination, a small goiter is documented in half the cases. The signs and symptoms of postpartum thyroiditis are often subtle and difficult to detect, particularly because many of them, such as fatigue, fluctuations in weight, and irritability, are common in the postpartum period.

Cause

The exacerbation of immune-mediated disease post partum is common to a variety of autoimmune disease states.

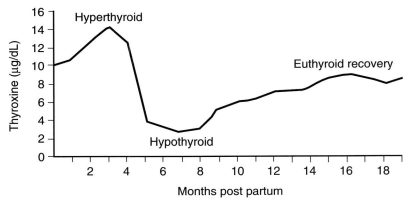

POSTPARTUM THYROIDITIS

Figure 7–5. Postpartum thyroiditis. Note the triphasic presentation: (1) thyrotoxic phase 2 to 4 months post partum; (2) hypothyroid phase 4 to 8 months post partum; and (3) euthyroid recovery phase. Euthyroid recovery occurs in 90% of patients. Women with positive thyroid autoantibodies are at increased risk of developing postpartum thyroiditis. (Reference range for thyroxine: 5.0 to 10.6 mg/dL.)

The down-regulation of immune vigilance in normal pregnancy is characterized by a significant fall in the CD4$^+$/CD8$^+$ ratio in late pregnancy and into the postpartum period. In a carefully performed study, the development of postpartum thyroiditis was associated with a triad of immune markers: (1) a reduction in the normal immune suppression of pregnancy, (2) enhanced postpartum T cell activation, and (3) elevated thyroid autoantibodies. Women with positive thyroid autoantibodies during the first trimester had a 30% chance of subsequently developing postpartum thyroiditis.[90] Serum immunoglobulin G antibody titers, including microsomal antibodies, typically decrease during pregnancy, with a nadir in the third trimester and a rebound in the postpartum period.[188]

Diagnosis

The signs and symptoms of postpartum thyroiditis are often minimal. Monthly postpartum assessment of 152 women with positive antithyroid peroxidase antibodies elicited nonspecific symptoms of hypothyroidism and hyperthyroidism from all affected women.[189] In one study, only excessive fatigue and palpitations distinguished women with postpartum thyroiditis from euthyroid but harried new mothers.[190] In addition, it is important to recognize that women are seen for postpartum evaluation 6 weeks after parturition, which is earlier than the expected manifestation of postpartum thyroiditis, classically occurring at 3 to 6 months. Therefore, suspicion of postpartum thyroiditis should be raised in women with a family history of thyroid disease who present with fatigue, palpitations, emotional lability, or goiter during the first 12 months after delivery. Often, however, these patients do not present for medical evaluation.

The laboratory diagnosis of thyrotoxicosis in postpartum thyroiditis consists of hyperthyroxinemia with suppression of TSH on thyroid function tests. In contrast to Graves' disease, the radioiodine uptake in postpartum thyroiditis is low. As noted previously, however, special consideration must be given to breast-feeding mothers, in whom administration of radioiodine should be avoided.

The subsequent hypothyroid phase is diagnosed in the same way as primary hypothyroidism, with an increased serum TSH and decreased serum T$_4$ levels. Approximately 90% of affected patients experience spontaneous recovery of thyroid function. The remaining 10% require long-term thyroid hormone supplementation. There is also evidence that children of pregnant women who had thyroid peroxidase antibodies but normal thyroid function are at risk for impaired emotional, cognitive, and motor development.[191]

Course

As noted earlier, postpartum thyroiditis typically has a triphasic manifestation. The thyrotoxic phase generally occurs 6 to 12 weeks post partum, running a course of 4 to 8 weeks before resolving spontaneously.[192] The thyrotoxic symptoms and signs are usually milder than in Graves' disease and may be overlooked or attributed to the stress and demands common to the postpartum period. A painless goiter develops in approximately half the cases. Severe hypertension is a rare, associated manifestation.[193]

Primary hypothyroidism typically manifests 3 to 6 months post partum. There may not be a clear history of a preceding thyrotoxic episode. Classical symptoms of hypothyroidism, including lethargy, cold intolerance, and difficulty with memory and concentration, are present and are also mild in nature. Spontaneous recovery occurs in 90% of patients, usually by the first year post partum. However, the risk of recurrence in subsequent pregnancies may be as high as 25%. In addition, these patients, particularly those with high titers of microsomal antibody, are at increased risk of developing permanent hypothyroidism; therefore, long-term follow-up is mandated.[87,194]

Screening

The frequency of postpartum thyroiditis and the difficulty in diagnosis raise the question of screening. Thyroid autoantibodies are predictors of the development of subsequent hypothyroidism both during pregnancy and in the postpartum period. The risks to the fetus of maternal hypothyroidism during gestation and the prevalence of postpartum thyroiditis raise the question of whether all pregnant women should be screened for thyroid autoantibodies. Whether the screening can be justified on a cost-benefit basis is not clear, and further study is required.[2,195] Patients with a personal or family history of autoimmune thyroid disease should certainly undergo evaluation for microsomal antibodies and should be counseled. In addition, women with a history of other autoimmune diseases should be evaluated for thyroid autoantibodies. For example, women with insulin-dependent diabetes mellitus have been shown to be at high risk for postpartum thyroiditis, with an incidence of 25% in one study, a threefold increase in comparison with a similar study in patients without insulin-dependent diabetes mellitus.[196]

Depression

Postpartum depression occurs in 10% to 20% of women in the year after delivery.[197,198] Although thyroid dysfunction is not associated with postpartum psychosis, there are several studies that indicate that postpartum depression is more common in women with thyroid dysfunction.[2,198,199] Because the hyperthyroidism and hypothyroidism of postpartum thyroiditis may be subclinical in their manifestation, it is critical to consider a diagnosis of thyroid dysfunction in women with postpartum depression.

Management of Postpartum Thyroiditis

Because the signs and symptoms of postpartum thyroiditis are frequently mild and transient, specific therapy is usually not indicated.[192] Treatment of thyrotoxicosis with thionamides is deferred, unless the thyrotoxicosis is unduly prolonged. Symptomatic relief of associated tachycardia may be achieved with short-term treatment with β$_1$-adrenergic blocking agents.

Likewise, administration of T$_4$ during the hypothyroid phase is recommended only if the symptoms and signs are severe or prolonged. Typically, the hypothyroid phase is more protracted than the hyperthyroid phase. If treatment is initiated for relief of severe hypothyroid symptoms, it is reasonable to institute a 3-month course of T_4 replacement, followed by withdrawal, in order to assess recovery of endogenous thyroid function. If the hypothyroidism persists, T_4 replacement may be resumed. Administration of T_4 does not alter the course of postpartum thyroiditis other than to treat the hypothyroidism.[200]

NEONATAL THYROTOXICOSIS

Neonatal thyrotoxicosis typically manifests as transient hyperthyroidism in the newborn. It is critical that neonatal thyrotoxicosis be recognized promptly, because it is associated with a 16% mortality rate.[201] Infants of mothers with a history of Graves' disease are at increased risk of developing neonatal thyrotoxicosis. Approximately 1% of pregnant women with a history of Graves' disease give birth to affected infants.[202] For surviving infants, premature craniosynostosis is one serious long-term sequela of neonatal thyrotoxicosis and may result in inadequate cerebral development.[203]

Cause

Placental transfer of thyroid-stimulating immunoglobulins from a mother with Graves' disease to the fetus is the most common cause of neonatal thyrotoxicosis. It is important to note that the mothers may not appear clinically thyrotoxic during pregnancy, although the majority do display some clinical or laboratory manifestations of Graves' disease. Neonatal thyrotoxicosis in this setting is typically transient, inasmuch as the presence of maternal antibodies in the fetus wanes over a period of 2 to 3 months.

Studies have documented a correlation between high maternal-fetal (cord) concentrations of antibodies and subsequent immunoglobulin-mediated induction of neonatal thyrotoxicosis. A decline in antibody titers is typically accompanied by resolution of the neonatal thyrotoxicosis.[103,202] This lends credence to the pathogenic role of thyroid-stimulating immunoglobulins in this condition. The incidence of neonatal thyrotoxicosis is equal among infant boys and girls, which supports the concept of a placentally transferred etiologic agent.

The potential presence of both stimulatory and inhibitory immunoglobulins, each with different binding affinities, makes it difficult to predict the development and course of neonatal thyrotoxicosis.[204,205] Assessment for the presence of thyroid-binding inhibitory immunoglobulins (TSH radioreceptor assay) and a sensitive cyclic adenosine monophosphate accumulation assay (thyroid-stimulating antibody) may provide some insight.[206-208] Antibody titers may decline at different rates. If both inhibitory and stimulatory immunoglobulins are present, their relative abundance and activity determine subsequent development of neonatal thyrotoxicosis. Cases have been reported in which neonatal thyrotoxicosis did not develop until levels of inhibitory immunoglobulins declined, thus unmasking the presence of thyroid-stimulating immunoglobulins.[209]

The duration of neonatal thyrotoxicosis is determined by (1) the initial neonatal serum concentration of the thyroid-stimulating immunoglobulin, (2) the rate of degradation of the thyroid-stimulating immunoglobulin, and (3) the presence or absence of inhibitory antibodies. The estimated half-life of the antibody in the serum of the thyrotoxic neonate is between 4 and 10 days, based on studies with a 7S immunoglobulin, long-acting thyroid stimulator protector.[210,211]

In some children, neonatal thyrotoxicosis persists after 1 year of age.[201,212] Some of these patients may inherit Graves' disease as an autosomal dominant trait. This condition is more common in girls than in boys. In general, in most patients with neonatal thyrotoxicosis, the condition is transient.

Congenital hyperthyroidism, which is distinct from neonatal hyperthyroidism associated with Graves' disease, has been reported but is rare. Case reports demonstrate hyperthyroidism resulting from a mutation in the thyrotropin receptor gene.[213]

Diagnosis and Management

Neonatal thyrotoxicosis should be suspected when a hyperirritable infant has goiter, exophthalmos, and tachycardia (Table 7–6). The presence of an elevated serum T_4 concentration further supports the diagnosis. Infants with neonatal thyrotoxicosis may also present with low birth weight, hepatosplenomegaly, jaundice, cardiac failure, and thrombocytopenia.[214] The presence of low birth weight does not necessarily reflect prematurity in these infants; it is secondary to the thyrotoxicosis. Indeed, on the basis of bone age, these children appear to have accelerated maturity.[215]

A thorough maternal history often reveals a history of maternal Graves' disease, although, as noted earlier, the mother may not have active thyrotoxicosis and may be euthyroid or hypothyroid.

Further complicating the diagnosis of neonatal thyrotoxicosis is the potential exposure of neonates to anti-thyroid drugs in utero. These children may appear euthyroid at birth, because antithyroid drugs effectively block clinical manifestations of thyrotoxicosis in neonates, as well as in their mothers. This may delay both the manifestation of symptoms and the diagnosis in some children.[216]

Screening programs for neonatal hypothyroidism, in which the T_4 radioimmunoassay is used, should also be effective at detecting hyperthyroxinemia in neonates.[217] Positive assays for thyroid-stimulating immunoglobulins strengthen the diagnosis. A high titer is diagnostic in the infant and virtually predictive in the mother.[212]

TABLE 7–6   Clinical Presentation of Neonatal Thyrotoxicosis

Hyperirritability
Tachycardia
Goiter
Exophthalmos
Low birth weight
Cardiac failure
Jaundice

The neonatal narcotic withdrawal syndrome shares features with neonatal thyrotoxicosis, inasmuch as affected neonates may present with tremulousness and irritability. The serum T_4 may also be elevated in this setting.[218] Toxicology screening may be useful in distinguishing the two but is not diagnostic, because both conditions may coexist in the same patient.

Therapy

Because neonatal thyrotoxicosis is transient and self-limiting in most cases, no specific antithyroid therapy is required for mild disease. For more severely affected infants, treatment with Lugol's solution (one drop [8 mg iodine] three times a day), and propranolol (2 mg/kg/day) may be effective.[219,220] Antithyroid drugs are reserved for children whose condition cannot be controlled with iodides or propranolol. If required, PTU (10 mg every 8 hours) can be added to the regimen. If the thyrotoxicosis persists, the iodide may actually exacerbate the condition.

The majority of affected children recover without incident. The serum titer of thyroid-stimulating immunoglobulin determines the duration of treatment in infants who require pharmacologic intervention. Most of the infants who require treatment do so for 3 to 6 weeks. Patients with neonatal thyrotoxicosis who have died have usually been premature and have had severe hyperthyroidism accompanied by congestive heart failure.

FETAL THYROTOXICOSIS

Fetal thyrotoxicosis is caused by the placental transfer of thyroid-stimulating immunoglobulins.[174] Maternal thyroid-stimulating antibodies may be present because they may persist even when the maternal thyroid gland has been ablated or when the mother is in remission.[221,222] Thus, the possibility of fetal thyrotoxicosis should be considered in all pregnant women with a history of Graves' disease, regardless of the current thyroid status. This population includes mothers with a history of Graves' disease who are not currently receiving antithyroid medication.

The diagnosis of fetal thyrotoxicosis is suggested by persistent fetal tachycardia faster than 160 beats per minute with beat-to-beat variations and elevated concentrations of maternal thyroid-stimulating immunoglobulins. Periumbilical blood sampling may also be helpful in assessing fetal thyroid function and should be considered (Fig. 7–6).[141] Ultrasonography may detect the presence of a goiter in a thyrotoxic fetus.[223,224]

Management

Fetal thyrotoxicosis is associated with increased fetal morbidity and mortality. Therefore, prompt identification is crucial, and consideration should be given to thioamide treatment directed specifically toward the fetus. Dosages of 5 to 10 mg/day of MMI are typically employed,[174] although the recognition of a specific phenotype of MMI-induced malformations supports the use of PTU, rather than MMI, during early gestation.[225] Overtreatment with antithyroid

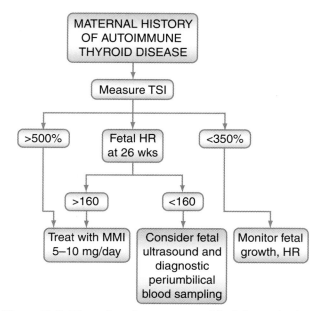

Figure 7–6. Diagnosis and management of fetal thyrotoxicosis. HR, fetal heart rate; MMI, methimazole; TSI, thyroid-stimulating immunoglobulin. (Adapted from Wallace G, Couch R, Ginsberg J: Fetal thyrotoxicosis: A case report and recommendations for prediction, diagnosis, and treatment. Thyroid 1995;5:125.)

agents may induce the development of fetal hypothyroidism, which is associated with future psychoneurologic and developmental delay. It is important to note that fetal hypothyroidism may develop after only 1 week of therapy, despite the presence of a persistent fetal tachycardia.[226] Close monitoring is mandatory. After delivery, the neonate should continue to be treated for thyrotoxicosis, which should be self-limited.

MATERNAL HYPOTHYROIDISM

Estimates of the incidence of maternal hypothyroidism in iodine-sufficient areas are in the range of 0.1% to 0.3%.[227,228] The most common cause is related to thyroid autoimmunity (Table 7–7), although iatrogenic causes must not be overlooked. The requirement for thyroid hormone replacement therapy is increased during pregnancy, which is suggestive of an increased demand on the thyroid gland.[229-232]

Diagnosis of Hypothyroidism

Hypothyroidism is most commonly iatrogenic, the result of either thyroid surgery or prior administration of radioactive iodine therapy. Idiopathic hypothyroidism is most often attributable to underlying Hashimoto's disease, and its onset may be more insidious. Hashimoto's disease is more common in patients with diabetes mellitus; in one study of 100 diabetic women, 20% of patients with type I diabetes also had Hashimoto's disease.[233]

The symptoms referable to underlying hypothyroidism are common to all of the underlying causes, and there is significant overlap with complaints common to euthyroid pregnant women, which makes the clinical diagnosis difficult.

TABLE 7–7   Maternal Hypothyroidism

Causes	Symptoms	Signs	Laboratory Findings	Course	Outcome
Autoimmune thyroid disease	Cold intolerance	Periorbital edema	$\uparrow$ TSH	Worsens during pregnancy as demands on thyroid increase	Maternal: Increased risk of fetal loss
Iodine deficiency	Constipation	Myxedema	$\downarrow$ T$_4$		
	Fatigue	Hoarse voice	$\downarrow$ Free T$_4$		Fetal:
Prior RAI treatment	Dry skin/hair	Macroglossia	Antithyroid antibodies		Psychoneurologic defects
Thyroidectomy	Paresthesias	Delayed DTR	(TPO, TG)		Cretinism
		HTN			

DTR, deep tendon reflex; HTN, hypertension; RAI, radioactive iodine; T$_4$, thyroxine; TG, thyroglobulin; TPO, thyroid peroxidase; TSH, thyroid-stimulating hormone.

Patients complain of constipation; cold intolerance; cool, dry skin; coarse hair; irritability; and inability to concentrate. The presence of paresthesias may be helpful in the diagnosis, because it is an early symptom in approximately 75% of patients with hypothyroidism. The presence of delayed deep tendon reflexes is also suggestive of hypothyroidism. In addition, signs of gross myxedema, including a low body temperature, large tongue, hoarse voice, and periorbital edema are not found in normal pregnancy, and their presence should prompt an immediate evaluation for hypothyroidism. Patients may complain of excessive fatigue. Maternal hypertension is common.[234] Postpartum amenorrhea and galactorrhea associated with hyperprolactinemia may be indicative of hypothyroidism.[235,236]

The most sensitive indicator of primary hypothyroidism is an elevated TSH in association with a low serum T$_4$ concentration. Because of the elevated TBG of pregnancy, the serum T$_4$ determination may not be as low as would be expected and may appear inappropriate in the setting of an elevated TSH. Thyroid autoantibody positivity provides supporting evidence for the presence of hypothyroidism, particularly in the absence of a history of thyroidectomy or radioactive iodine therapy. Elevated serum cholesterol concentrations are common in hypothyroidism but are not helpful in the diagnosis, inasmuch as serum cholesterol concentrations increase during pregnancy, up to 60% above prepregnancy values. Screening for hypothyroidism, with a serum TSH, should be performed during the first 2 months of pregnancy in selected patients with a personal or family history of hypothyroidism or other autoimmune disorders. Screening the entire population is not cost effective and currently is not recommended, although it is the subject of much debate.

Pregnancy in Hypothyroid Women

Myxedematous patients have been reported to carry their pregnancies to term successfully.[237-240] Before the second trimester, thyroid hormone requirements necessary for normal fetal growth are provided by the maternal thyroid gland, with associated transplacental passage of thyroid hormone. In severely hypothyroid mothers, this hormone is lacking. There is no evidence for an increased risk of birth defects and a history of maternal hypothyroidism,[241] although an interesting association has been made between the presence of high titers of thyroid autoantibodies in women and Down's syndrome in their children.[112] A hypothetical explanation for this is that maternal thyroid autoimmunity may predispose to aneuploidy in the mother's gametes and may play a major role in the birth of children with Down's syndrome in younger mothers. In addition, as mentioned previously, there is increasing evidence that maternal thyroid hormone plays a role in the development of the fetal brain.[242,243] Inadequate thyroid hormone replacement during pregnancy may result in psychoneurologic and developmental deficits in the progeny.[244,245]

Outcome

Animal data suggest that mild or moderate hypothyroidism has minimal effect on fertility, although hypothyroid animals do have difficulty maintaining pregnancy. A study of 244 pregnant hypothyroid women found the rate of stillbirth was double that in control subjects.[85] Another study evaluated the outcome of a group of children whose mothers had proven or suspected thyroid disorders during pregnancy. This smaller study revealed that outcomes were poor in six of seven pregnancies in women with clinically suspected hypothyroidism and low butanol-extractable iodine.

The work of Man and coworkers suggested that the progeny of inadequately treated "hypothyroxinemic" women suffer psychoneurologic deficits. Developmental deficits are demonstrable as early as 8 months of age.[244] A 7-year follow-up study revealed that these children had persistent deficits and manifested in lower psychologic test scores, although confounding factors, such as socioeconomic status, may have played a role in the poor outcome. More recently, a 7- to 9-year follow-up study of 62 euthyroid children of hypothyroid mothers confirmed these findings. Children of hypothyroid mothers who remained untreated during pregnancy achieved lower IQ scores than did controls. In addition, a larger percentage (15%) of children of untreated mothers had IQ scores of 85 or less, in comparison with 5% of controls.[245] Animal studies demonstrate that early maternal hypothyroxinemia alters fetal brain histogenesis and the cytoarchitecture of the fetal cortex[246,247]; this provides a potential mechanistic explanation for these findings. Together these findings suggest that thyroid hormone influences the developing fetal brain, affecting neuronal differentiation and multiplication, among other events.

Management of Hypothyroidism during Pregnancy

Full replacement doses of T_4 should be given immediately upon the diagnosis of hypothyroidism in the pregnant woman, regardless of the degree of thyroid function. This treatment minimizes further fetal exposure to the hypothyroid milieu. Therapy can be titrated rapidly[240] in young pregnant women with no other comorbid conditions. One reasonable schedule is to start with 0.100 mg of T_4 daily for 3 to 5 weeks, with subsequent dosage adjustments depending on thyroid function test results. T_4 need be given only once a day because of the long half-life. With adequate treatment, the serum TSH concentration should decrease to values less than 6 μU/mL, usually within 4 weeks, and the serum T_4 concentration should increase to normal values for pregnancy. The optimal range for TSH during pregnancy is less than 3.0 μU/mL. Note that normal serum T_4 concentrations in pregnancy may be at the upper limit of the normal range for nonpregnant women. This results from an increase in T_4 binding in the setting of pregnancy-induced increases in serum TBG concentrations. The free T_4 concentrations should be brought into the upper range of normal. If the values do not return to normal, the dosage of T_4 should be increased by 0.05-mg increments. The serum TSH concentration may take longer to return to normal values.

Pregnant Women Receiving Continuous Thyroid Hormone Replacement Therapy

In the majority of pregnant women receiving thyroid hormone during pregnancy, hypothyroidism has been diagnosed before conception. In many cases, the initial diagnosis of hypothyroidism may be obscure. The number of women in whom hypothyroidism is diagnosed during pregnancy is small. To ensure that the pregnant woman is receiving adequate thyroid hormone, full replacement doses must be given. As mentioned previously, the dosage of thyroid hormone commonly has to be increased by up to 50% during pregnancy.[231] The recommended replacement dose of T_4 is approximately 0.10 mg/day, according to the amount of T_4 necessary to suppress the elevated serum TSH concentration.[248] Women receiving thyroid hormone therapy require close follow-up during pregnancy to maintain optimal thyroid hormone concentrations.[229-232]

In women with no history of hypothyroidism in whom the diagnosis is made during pregnancy, thyroid hormone therapy may be discontinued during the postpartum period and thyroid function reassessed 5 to 6 weeks later. Recovery may be delayed, because normal thyroid function may remain suppressed for a number of weeks after prolonged thyroid hormone therapy. Some women remain hypothyroid and ultimately require chronic replacement therapy.

Thyroid Function and Fetal Loss

It has been observed that hypothyroid women experience increased rates of fetal loss. As a result of this observation, serum thyroid hormone determinations were evaluated in women who aborted spontaneously, and the levels were found to be low.[136] Normal values were found in the majority of patients who had elective abortions, although a minority of these women did have low thyroid hormone levels as well. Follow-up studies in patients with low thyroid hormone levels who had undergone elective abortions determined that they were euthyroid and presumably had not been hypothyroid during pregnancy. The data suggested that lower estrogen levels after termination were associated with concomitant decreases in TBG and serum thyroid hormone concentration. Therefore, the low serum thyroid values were believed to be secondary to the abortion, rather than the cause. Because the low serum T_4 merely reflects the decreased estrogen production and TBG, there is no reason to suppose that thyroid hormone would be helpful in these situations.[249]

The balance of evidence suggests that the great majority of women with early spontaneous abortions have normal thyroid function. However, an association has been made between the presence of thyroid autoantibodies (antithyroid peroxidase and antithyroglobulin antibodies) and an increased risk of spontaneous abortion. In a study of 552 antibody-positive women in the first trimester of pregnancy, the rate of spontaneous abortion was 17%, in comparison with 8.4% in antibody-negative women.[250] The miscarriage rate was found to be unrelated to the titer of autoantibody or the level of serum TSH. It is important to note that secondary causes of abortion were not excluded in this study and may have had a confounding effect on the results. Nonetheless, this initial observation prompted further investigation into the potential association between thyroid autoantibodies and pregnancy loss.[251] A review of the available evidence[252] cited successive corroborative studies in Belgium[253] and Japan,[254] involving hundreds of women, in which rates of spontaneous abortion were found to be increased twofold to fourfold in autoantibody-positive women in comparison with controls. Subsequent studies in smaller study populations found an increased incidence of thyroid antibodies only in patients with repeated spontaneous abortions.[255-257] The cause of pregnancy loss in women who are thyroid antibody–positive remains unknown. It has been hypothesized that the presence of thyroid autoantibodies reflects a generalized activation of the immune system and that the antibodies are not the causative agents of spontaneous abortion. It is also possible that subtle, subclinical deficiencies in thyroid hormone levels occur in these women, predisposing them to pregnancy loss. The question of intervention has been raised. Small studies[258-261] have addressed the issue of immunomodulation with intravenous immune globulin. Because of suboptimal study designs and size constraints, its impact is unclear, and the results are inconclusive.

NEONATAL HYPOTHYROIDISM

Generalized neuropsychologic developmental delay has been reported in children who experience thyroid hormone deficiency during early fetal and neonatal periods.[244,245,262] Studies suggest that *maternal* hypothyroxinemia alone, even in the setting of a normal TSH, is a risk factor for poor neuropsychologic developmental outcomes in the progeny.[263] Optimal development of brain structures early in gestation is dependent on the presence of adequate concentrations of serum T_4, which is converted to T_3 locally by the fetus. Whether subclinical hypothyroidism, defined as serum T_4 concentrations within normal limits in association with a minimally elevated TSH, can affect fetal brain development is the question.

The diagnosis of *primary* hypothyroidism in infants appears to be associated with a higher incidence of congenital anomalies.[264] A population-based study of more than 1300 infants found that the prevalence of major anomalies was 8.4% among infants with congenital hypothyroidism, in comparison with 1% to 2% of the general population.[265] Cardiac anomalies were the most common associated congenital anomalies, although anomalies of the nervous system and eyes were noted as well. The mechanisms underlying these associations remain to be elucidated.

If left untreated, neonatal and early childhood hypothyroidism results in profound mental and developmental retardation. It is important to note that both the severity of thyroid hormone deficiency and the time of onset during development determine the degree and potential reversibility of the ensuing brain damage. As would be expected, the earlier hypothyroidism occurs during fetal development, the more severely affected the neonate is. Onset of hypothyroidism after the age of 2 years appears to exert few if any irreversible effects on mental development.

Intrauterine hypothyroidism is detected from the presence of elevated TSH concentrations and low serum T_4 concentrations.[266] Clinically, neonates with hypothyroidism, even those with thyroid agenesis, are usually normal with regard to appearance, size, weight, behavior, and immediate postnatal development. Of note, however, is that bone maturation is delayed at birth in approximately 60% of affected infants. Because of the absence of pathognomonic features at birth, the condition is diagnosed in fewer than 5% of affected patients in the neonatal period on the basis of clinical presentation alone.

Prompt identification and treatment of newborns with congenital hypothyroidism is vital to ensure their appropriate neuropsychologic development. Identification through screening programs, with immediate institution of replacement therapy, leads to a normal IQ at 5 to 7 years of age.[71,107,153,267] Aggressive early treatment with thyroid hormone may be beneficial (e.g., 8 to 10 µg of T_4/kg body weight).

Cause

The causes of congenital fetal and neonatal thyroid dysfunction are varied, ranging from thyroid dysgenesis to thyroid hormone resistance. The various causes of congenital hypothyroidism are outlined in Table 7–8. The most common cause of congenital fetal/neonatal thyroid dysfunction is primary hypothyroidism, estimated to occur in approximately 1 per 4000 births.[268] Thyroid dysgenesis may result from thyroid aplasia, hypoplasia, or ectopy. Of children with thyroid dysgenesis, approximately 40% have ectopic thyroid tissue, 40% have thyroid aplasia, and 20% have thyroid hypoplasia.[269] Rare disorders of thyroid function include dyshormonogenesis, hereditary TSH deficiency, TSH receptor mutations, and thyroid hormone resistance. The presence of thyroid growth–blocking antibodies has been reported in mothers who give birth to hypothyroid infants.[70,205,270-272] However, seasonal variation

Cause	Incidence
Congenital Hypothyroidism	**1:4,000**
Primary Hypothyroidism	**1:4,400**
Thyroid dysgenesis	
Thyroid aplasia (40%)	
Thyroid hypoplasia (20%)	
Thyroid ectopy (40%)	
Drug-induced	1:10,000
Dyshormonogenesis	1:30,000
Secondary Hypothyroidism	**1:75,000**
Other	**1:60,000**
TSH receptor mutations	
Thyroid hormone resistance	

TABLE 7–8   Congenital Hypothyroidism

TSH, thyroid-stimulating hormone.

in the incidence of congenital hypothyroidism implies that environmental factors may play a role. It is important to consider potential fetal exposure to antithyroid drugs or other agents when neonatal hypothyroidism is evaluated.

A reduction in maternal serum T_4 as a result of maternal iodine deficiency during early pregnancy compromises the development of the fetal nervous system and can lead to profound neurologic impairment (neurologic cretinism).[267,273] Iodine deficiency in later pregnancy or infancy that results in fetal or neonatal hypothyroidism exerts effects on somatic development (myxedematous cretinism). Neonatal thyroid screening programs have been instituted to ensure prompt detection and treatment of neonatal thyroid dysfunction.

Thyroid Dysgenesis

The cause of thyroid dysgenesis is unknown. Various mechanisms have been implicated, including single-gene mutations and familial autoimmune factors. The term *athyreotic cretinism* has been used, although some thyroid tissue is usually present.[274] It has been postulated that thyrocytotoxic factors may be transferred across the placenta, resulting in destruction of the fetal thyroid gland. However, it seems more likely that these antibodies represent a reaction to thyroid injury rather than a primary event.[275] Transplacental transfer of a thyrosuppressive factor has been observed in one family.[4]

In addition, families have been identified with a mutation in the Pit-1 gene, a pituitary transcription factor that activates expression of TSH and growth hormone genes. Hypopituitarism results, in association with in utero TSH deficiency.[276]

Inborn Errors of Thyroid Function

Defects in thyroid hormone synthesis occur in approximately 1 child per 30,000. Usually these defects in thyroid hormone biosynthesis are inherited as autosomal recessive traits. Biochemical defects that correspond to each step in hormone biosynthesis, including defects in organification, iodide transport, and thyroglobulin and deiodinase synthesis, have been identified. Affected children may not have significant thyroid enlargement at birth, because maternal-fetal transfer of thyroid hormone supplies the fetus with sufficient concentrations of thyroid hormone to suppress goiter formation. Progressive, defective thyroid hormone synthesis, if left untreated, ultimately results in goitrous cretinism.[277] A family history of goitrous cretinism should alert the physician to this possibility in the neonate.

Drug-Induced Hypothyroidism

Numerous compounds that possess antithyroid activity, including thioamides, amiodarone, lithium, and potassium iodide, have been identified. Maternal exposure to these compounds results in fetal exposure and may adversely affect fetal thyroid function. The effects are usually transient. Neonatal thyroid screening program data suggest that transient hypothyroidism may occur in 1 per 10,000 births.

Children who have been exposed to PTU in utero may be born with a small goiter and transient hypothyroidism.[130,152,278] Screening data indicate that, of 100 infants exposed to PTU in utero, one may develop transient hypothyroidism. The hypothyroidism resolves post partum, as exposure of the neonate to the antithyroid medication is eliminated.

Maternal iodide ingestion during pregnancy is an important cause of neonatal hypothyroidism and goiter. It is important to note that fetal goiter may develop with maternal ingestion of as little as 12 mg of iodide daily.[279] Studies of neonatal response to therapy with iodides document sensitivity to relatively low doses of iodide therapy. Indeed, one case report of oral iodide therapy for neonatal hyperthyroidism secondary to maternal Graves' disease demonstrated rapid normalization of neonatal thyroid indices with doses of 8 mg of potassium iodide three times a day (total, 24 mg/day).[280] Thus, administration of iodides to euthyroid fetuses/neonates might induce hypothyroidism. Radiopaque dyes used for radiologic procedures, including amniography, contain large amounts of iodides and may result in transient neonatal hypothyroidism.[13]

The antiarrhythmic drug amiodarone contains 75 mg of iodine in each 200-mg capsule. There have been case reports of women who have received the amiodarone throughout pregnancy. The majority of the resulting offspring have been euthyroid without goiter, but there have been exceptions.[281-286] The hypothyroidism is usually transient, but mental retardation has occurred. Maternal iodide ingestion may result in significant enlargement of the fetal thyroid, and the goiters may be large and obstructive.[125] Large goiters may be detected in utero through ultrasonography. The presence of a large goiter makes maintenance of an adequate airway difficult. Extremely large goiters may necessitate surgery. Treatment with intraamniotic injection of thyroid hormone may also be of benefit in reducing the size of the goiter and restoring euthyroid status.[67]

Diagnosis

To ensure adequate treatment of neonatal hypothyroidism and abrogation of the deleterious effects of the hypothyroid state, it is crucial that the diagnosis of hypothyroidism be made during the first weeks after birth.

Unfortunately, clinical features of hypothyroidism are uncommon at this point, and the diagnosis is rarely suspected on the basis of clinical presentation alone. Clinical features of neonatal hypothyroidism are variable and include prolonged gestation with macrosomia, feeding and respiratory difficulties, protracted icterus, abdominal distention with vomiting, and constipation. In addition, delayed bone age, hypothermia, cyanosis, umbilical hernia, dry skin, and a large posterior fontanel have been observed.[287-289]

Laboratory evaluation revealing a low serum T_4 concentration (<6 μg/dL), in association with an elevated TSH level (>80 μU/dL), is diagnostic of hypothyroidism. Neonatal screening may detect borderline T_4 or borderline TSH in infants. Radiographs for bone age estimation may be helpful, inasmuch as hypothyroidism is associated with low osteoblastic activity. This is reflected in bone radiographs as delayed bone/skeletal maturation. Specifically, a lack of ossification of the distal femoral epiphysis on the proximal tibial epiphysis is suggestive of a history of in utero thyroid hormone deficiency.[290]

Epiphyseal dysgenesis, commonly affecting the proximal femoral epiphysis, has also been described. Of note, any center of endochondral ossification may be affected.[291] The ossification center originates as multiple small centers scattered throughout the epiphysis. These centers eventually coalesce to form a single center with an irregular shape and a stippled appearance.

Full assessment of neonates with borderline thyroid function should include a thyroid scan. Infants who have residual thyroid tissue, no signs or symptoms of hypothyroidism, normal serum T_3 concentration, and normal bone age have an excellent prognosis for normal development. In contrast, infants lacking visible thyroid tissue, with low serum T_4 and T_3 concentrations and with detectable signs of bone age retardation, have a more guarded prognosis for entirely normal development, even with early treatment.

It is important to distinguish cretinism from other syndromes with which it may share common features. Both cretinism and Down's syndrome are characterized by short stature and mental retardation. However, the child with Down's syndrome is more active and has specific stigmata. Cretinism may also be confused with the Beckwith-Wiedemann syndrome, which includes umbilical hernia and macroglossia.[292]

Management of Congenital Hypothyroidism

The efficacy of thyroid hormone replacement therapy depends on the promptness of its institution. Numerous studies have documented minimization of mental retardation and neuropsychologic delay with early neonatal treatment.[266,293] Instituting therapy in utero appears beneficial, if the diagnosis of fetal hypothyroidism has been made.

In Utero Therapy

Because of the mounting evidence that in utero hypothyroidism is associated with irreversible central nervous system damage and developmental delay,[245] there has been interest in intrauterine treatment of fetal hypothyroidism. Although the intrauterine diagnosis of hypothyroidism is difficult,[63,294] evaluation of cord blood via cordocentesis can help clarify the clinical situation. In addition, fetal ultrasonography is useful in identifying the presence of fetal goiter.

It has been estimated that third trimester fetal T_4 requirements are in the range of 6 µg/kg/day.[295] Therapeutic interventions have been designed to take advantage of the fact that the fetus effectively absorbs T_4 from amniotic fluid. Numerous case reports document intraamniotic injection of T_4 for treatment of fetal hypothyroidism.[78,296,297] One early study utilized such therapy in a pregnant woman who had inadvertently received 150 mCi of ^{131}I during weeks 10 to 11 of pregnancy.[80] Because of the potential risks of fetal hypothyroidism, an amniocentesis was performed weekly from week 33 until delivery, with an injection of 500 µg of T_4 each week. The concentration of T_4 in the cord serum was in the hypothyroid range, and the TSH concentration was low. At birth, however, the infant was not hypothyroid.

In one study of antenatal diagnosis and treatment of fetal goitrous hypothyroidism, intraamniotic injections of T_4 were successfully employed at a dose of 10 µg/kg/day every 7 days. Investigators documented improvement in the fetal goiter with this therapy.[67] Current recommendations cite intraamniotic administration of 250 to 500 µg of L-thyroxine at 7- to 10-day intervals for the management of fetal hypothyroidism.

THYROID NODULE AND THYROID CARCINOMA

Relative iodine deficiency during pregnancy may result in the development of a nontoxic diffuse goiter, as discussed earlier. Of more concern, in both pregnant and nonpregnant women, is the discovery of a solitary thyroid nodule.[298]

Management of the Thyroid Nodule

Evaluation of the solitary thyroid nodule during pregnancy relies on the use of ultrasonography and fine-needle aspiration, because the radioisotope thyroid scan is contraindicated. Ultrasonographic evaluation provides information about the size of the nodule and characterizes the nodule as solid or cystic. Ultrasonography is also useful in identifying the presence of diffuse thyroid disease and in revealing the presence of previously undetected, nonpalpable nodules. Fine-needle aspiration biopsy is indicated in women before 20 weeks of pregnancy for nodules that are (1) rapidly enlarging, (2) associated with palpable cervical lymph nodes, (3) solid and larger than 2 cm, or (4) cystic and larger than 4 cm. Aspiration should be performed after 20 weeks if a nodule increases in size on suppression therapy (Fig. 7–7).[299,300] If the biopsy specimen is adequate and does not reveal suspect cells, then thyroid hormone suppression

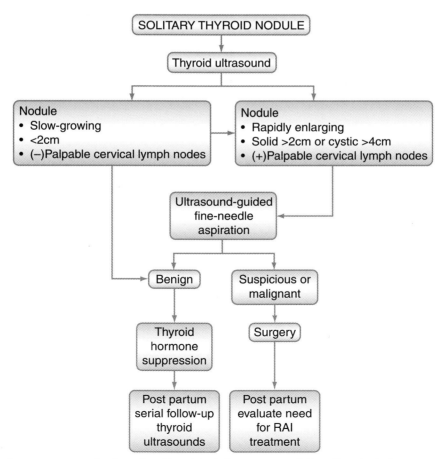

Figure 7–7. Algorithm for management of solitary thyroid nodule during pregnancy. RAI, radioactive iodine.

should be instituted for the duration of the pregnancy. A dosage of 0.10 mg of T_4 per day is used. If the biopsy findings are suggestive of malignancy, surgery is indicated even though the patient is pregnant. The nodule must be reevaluated post partum.

A small study assessed 26 pregnant women who had undergone surgery for solitary nodules that had arisen during, or were affected by, pregnancy.[301] At surgery, nine nodules were found to be true adenomas; the majority represented nontoxic nodular goiter. Parity seemed to have no influence on the development of thyroid nodules, although in areas of marginal iodine intake, thyroid nodularity does increase with parity.[302]

Thyroid Carcinoma and Pregnancy

The diagnosis of thyroid carcinoma during pregnancy is not an absolute indication for termination of the pregnancy. Studies of pregnant women with histories of past and current thyroid carcinoma suggest that pregnancy does not have a direct effect on the natural history of thyroid carcinoma. In one study, 70 women with thyroid carcinoma who became pregnant were compared with 109 women with thyroid carcinoma who did not.[303] The overall recurrence rate did not differ between the two groups; this finding prompted the conclusion that pregnancy occurring after the diagnosis of thyroid carcinoma had no effect on the course of the disease.

It has also been observed that the presence of thyroid carcinoma does not appear to have any significant effect on the pregnancy itself.[155,304] In a study of 60 pregnant women who had concurrent thyroid carcinoma, 22 women with a history of thyroid carcinoma had been pregnant multiple times with this condition. The other 38 women had been treated and were free of disease for 2 to 15 years before becoming pregnant.[305] In this study, the presence of extensive metastases in one patient, and the need for radioactive iodine therapy in another, resulted in the performance of two therapeutic abortions.

Treatment options for thyroid carcinoma during pregnancy are more limited than in the nongravid state. Radioactive iodine is contraindicated, but thyroid surgery remains an option, when necessary.[306] There is no evidence to suggest that a past exposure to radioactive iodine precludes future pregnancy or affects the outcome of subsequent pregnancies and offspring.[307]

References

1. Glinoer D, Lemone M: Goiter and pregnancy: A new insight into an old problem. Thyroid 1992;2:65.
2. Hall R, Richards C, Lazarus J: The thyroid and pregnancy. Br J Obstet Gynaecol 1993;100:512.
3. Hershman J, Lee H, Sugawara M, et al: Human chorionic gonadotropin stimulates iodide uptake, adenylate cyclase, and deoxyribonucleic acid synthesis in cultured rat thyroid cells. J Clin Endocrinol Metab 1988;67:74.
4. Aboul-Khair SA, Crooks J, Turnbull AC, Hytten FE: The physiological changes in thyroid function during pregnancy. Clin Sci 1964;27:195.
5. Smyth PPA, Hetherton MT, Smith DF, et al: Maternal iodine states and thyroid volume during pregnancy: Correlation with neonatal iodine intake. J Clin Endocrinol Metab 1997;82:2840.
6. Berghout A, Wiersinga W: Thyroid size and thyroid function during pregnancy: An analysis. Eur J Endocrinol 1998;138:536.
7. Glinoer D, De Nayer P, Bourdoux P, et al: Regulation of maternal thyroid during pregnancy. J Clin Endocrinol Metab 1990;71:276.
8. Glinoer D, De Nayer P, DeLange F, et al: A randomized trial for the treatment of mild iodine deficiency during pregnancy: Maternal and neonatal effects. J Clin Endocrinol Metab 1995;80:258.
9. Crooks J, Aboul-Khair SA, Turnbull AC, Hytten FE: The incidence of goiter during pregnancy. Lancet 1964;2:334.
10. Crooks J, Tulloch MI, Turnbull AC, et al: Comparative incidence of goiter in pregnancy in Iceland and Scotland. Lancet 1967;2:625.
11. Berghout A, Endert E, Ross A, et al: Thyroid function and thyroid size in normal pregnant women living in an iodine replete area. Clin Endocrinol 1994;41:375.
12. Alexander WD, Koutras DA, Crooks J, et al: Quantitative studies of iodine metabolism in thyroid disease. Q J Med 1972;31:281.
13. Becroft DMO, Smeeton WMI, Stewart JH: Fetal thyroid hyperplasia, rhesus isoimmunization, and amniography. Arch Dis Child 1980;55:213.
14. Dworkin HJ, Jacquez JA, Beierwaltes WH: Relationship of iodine ingestion to iodine excretion in pregnancy. J Clin Endocrinol Metab 1966;26:1329.
15. Delange F, Bourdoux P, Chanoine JP, Ermans AM: Physiopathology of iodine nutrition during pregnancy, lactation, and early postnatal life. In Berger H (ed): Vitamins and Minerals in Pregnancy and Lactation. Nestle Nutrition Workshop Series, vol 16. New York, Raven Press, 1988, p 205.
16. Wespi-Eggenberger HJ: Untersuchungen uber das Vorkommen und die Verhuntung des Neugeborenkropfes im Eizugsgebiet. Schweiz Med Wochenschr 1948;78:130.
17. Glinoer D: The regulation of thyroid function in pregnancy: Pathways of endocrine adaptation from physiology to pathology. Endocr Rev 1997;18:404.
18. Glinoer D, Gershengorn MC, Dubois A, Robbins J: Stimulation of thyroxine-binding globulin synthesis by isolated rhesus monkey hepatocytes after in vitro estradiol administration. Endocrinology 1977;100:807.
19. Premachandra BN, Gossain WV, Perlstein IB: Effect of pregnancy on thyroxine binding globulin (TBG) in partial TBG deficiency. Am J Med Sci 1977;274:189.
20. Spencer C: Thyroid Function Tests: Assay of thyroid hormones and related substances. Revised Aug. 1, 1999, www.thyroidmanager.org/Functiontests/assaytext.htm
21. Burr WA, Ramsden DB, Evans SE, et al: Concentration of thyroxine-binding globulin: Value of direct assay. BMJ 1977;1:485.
22. Oppenheimer JH, Squef R, Surks MI, Hauer H: Binding of thyroxine by serum proteins evaluated by equilibrium dialysis and electrophoretic techniques: Alteration in nonthyroidal illness. J Clin Invest 1963;42:1769.
23. Gow SM, Kellet HA, Seth J, et al: Limitations of new thyroid function tests in pregnancy. Clin Chim Acta 1985;152:325.
24. Sachmechi IA, Schussler GC: Familial hyperthyroxinase in pregnancy. Eur J Endocrinol 1995;153:729.
25. Harada A, Hershman J, Reed A, et al: Comparison of thyroid stimulators and thyroid hormone concentrations in the sera of pregnant women. J Clin Endocrinol Metab 1979;48:793.
26. Osathanondh R, Tulchinsky D, Chopra IJ: Total and free thyroxine and triiodothyronine in normal and complicated pregnancy. J Clin Endocrinol Metab 1976;42:98.
27. Yamamoto R, Amino N, Tanizawa O, et al: Longitudinal study of serum thyroid hormones, chorionic gonadotropin and thyrotropin during and after normal pregnancy. Clin Endocrinol 1979;10:459.
28. Robbins J: Thyroid hormone transport proteins and the physiology of hormone binding. In: Gray CH, James VHT (eds): Hormones in Blood. London: Academic Press, 1996, pp 96-110.
29. Pacchiarotti A, Martino E, Bartalena L, et al: Serum thyrotropin by ultrasensitive immunoradiometric assay and serum free thyroid hormones in pregnancy. J Endocrinol Invest 1986;9:185.
30. Burrow G: Thyroid function and hyperfunction during gestation. Endocrinol Rev 1993;14:194.
31. Ball R, Freedman DB, Holmes JC, et al: Low-normal concentrations of free thyroxin in serum in late pregnancy: Physiological fact, not technical artefact. Clin Chem 1989;35:1891.
32. Hay I, Klee G: Thyroid dysfunction. Endocrinol Metab Clin North Am 1988;17:473.

33. Kaplan M: Assessment of thyroid function during pregnancy. Thyroid 1992;2:57.

34. Larsen PR, Silva JE, Kaplan MM: Relationships between circulating and intracellular thyroid hormones: Physiological and clinical implications. Endocr Rev 1981;2:87.

35. Meinhold H, Dudenhausen JW, Wenzel KW, Saling E: Amniotic fluid concentrations of 3,3′5′-tri-iodothyronine (reverse T_3), 3,3′-di-iodothyronine, 3,5,3′-tri-iodothyronine (T_3) and thyroxine (T_4) in normal and complicated pregnancy. Clin Endocrinol 1979;10:355.

36. Cooper E, Aickin CM, Burke CW: Serum concentration of 3,3′5′-dei-iodothyronine (reverse T_3) in normal pregnancy. Clin Chim Acta 1980;106:347.

37. Hidal JT, Kaplan MM: Characteristics of thyroxine 5′-deiodination in cultured human placental cells: Regulation by iodothyronines. J Clin Invest 1985;76:947.

38. Huang SA, Dorfman DM, Genest DR, et al: Type 3 Deiodinase is highly expressed in the human uteroplacental unit and in fetal epithelium. J Clin Endocrinol Metab 2003;88:1384.

39. Dowling JT, Freinkel N, Ingbar SH: The effect of estrogens upon the peripheral metabolism of thyroxine. J Clin Invest 1960;39:1119.

40. Dowling JT, Appleton WG, Nicoloff JT: Thyroxine turnover during human pregnancy. J Clin Endocrinol Metab 1967;27:1749.

41. Weeke J, Dybkjaer L, Granlie K, et al: A longitudinal study of serum TSH, and total and free iodothyronines during normal pregnancy. Acta Endocrinol (Copenh) 1982;101:531.

42. Brodsky JB, Cohen EN, Brown BW Jr, et al: Surgery during pregnancy and fetal outcome. Am J Obstet Gynecol 1980;138:1165.

43. Sternberg J: Irradiation and radiocontamination during pregnancy. Am J Obstet Gynecol 1970;108:490.

44. Noble MJD, Rowlands S: Utilization of radioiodine during pregnancy. J Obstet Gynaecol Br Emp 1953;60:892.

45. Pochin EE: The iodine uptake of the human thyroid throughout the menstrual cycle and in pregnancy. Clin Sci 1952;11:441.

46. Burrow GN, Polackwich R, Donabedian R: The hypothalamic-pituitary-thyroid axis in normal pregnancy. In Fisher DA, Burrow GN (eds): Perinatal Thyroid Physiology and Disease. New York, Raven Press, 1975, p 1.

47. Guillaume J, Schussler GC, Goldman J: Components of the total serum thyroid hormone concentrations during pregnancy: High free thyroxine and blunted thyrotropin (TSH) response to TSH-releasing hormone in the first trimester. J Clin Endocrinol Metab 1985;60:678.

48. Vandalem JL, Pirens G, Hennen G, Gaspard J: Thyroliberin and gonadoliberin tests during pregnancy and the puerperium. Acta Endocrinol (Copenh) 1977;86:695.

49. Yikorkala O, Kivinen S, Reinila MI: Serial prolactin and thyrotropin responses to thyrotropin-releasing hormone throughout normal human pregnancy. J Clin Endocrinol Metab 1979;48:288.

50. Koutras DA, Phamakoitis AD, Koliopoulos N, et al: The plasma inorganic iodine and the pituitary thyroid axis in pregnancy. J Endocrinol Invest 1978;1:227.

51. Kojima A, Hershman JM: Effects of thyrotropin-releasing hormone (TRH) in maternal, fetal and newborn rats. Endocrinology 1974;94:1133.

52. Shambaugh G III, Kubek M, Wilber JF: Thyrotropin-releasing hormone activity in the human placenta. J Clin Endocrinol Metab 1979;48:483.

53. Girling JC: Thyroid disease and pregnancy. Br J Hosp Med 1996;56:316.

54. Chapman EM, Corner GW Jr, Robinson D, Evans RD: The collection of radioactive iodine by the human fetal thyroid. J Clin Endocrinol Metab 1948;8:717.

55. Evans TC, Kretschmar RM, Hodges RE, Song CW: Radioiodine uptake studies of the human fetal thyroid. J Nucl Med 1967;8:157.

56. Hershman JM, Hershman FK: Development of the thyroid control system. In Stanbury JB, Kroc RL (eds): Human Development and the Thyroid Gland: Relation to Endemic Cretinism. Proceedings. Symposium on Endemic Cretinism, Kroc Foundation. New York, Plenum Press, 1972, p 417.

57. Fisher DA: Endocrinology of fetal development. In Wilson JD, Foster DW (eds): Textbook of Endocrinology, 8th ed. Philadelphia, WB Saunders, 1992, pp 1049-1077.

58. Fisher D, Klein A: Medical progress: Thyroid development and disorders of thyroid function in the newborn. N Engl J Med 1981;304:702.

59. Ballabio M, Nicolini U, Jowett T, et al: Maturation of thyroid function in normal human foetuses. Clin Endocrinol (Oxf) 1989;31:565.

60. Thorpe-Beeston J, Nicolaides K, Felton C, et al: Maturation of the secretion of thyroid hormone and thyroid-stimulating hormone in the fetus. N Engl J Med 1991;324:531.

61. Hennen C, Pierce JG, Freychet P: Human chorionic thyrotropin: Further characterization and study of its secretion during pregnancy. J Clin Endocrinol Metab 1969;29:581.

62. Burrow GN, Fisher DA, Larsen PR: Maternal and fetal thyroid function. N Engl J Med 1994;331:1074.

63. Landau H, Sack J, Frucht H, et al: Amniotic fluid 3,3′,5′-triiodothyronine in the detection of congenital hypothyroidism. J Clin Endocrinol Metab 1980;50:799.

64. Vulsma T, Gons M, De Vijlder J: Maternal-fetal transfer of thyroxine in congenital hypothyroidism due to a total organification defect or thyroid agenesis. N Engl J Med 1989;321:13.

65. Contempre B, Jauniaux E, Calvo R, et al: Detection of thyroid hormones in human embryonic cavities during the first trimester of pregnancy. J Clin Endocrinol Metab 1993;77:1719.

66. Calvo RM, Jauniaux E, Gulbis B, et al: Fetal tissues are exposed to biologically relevant free thyroxine concentrations during early phases of development. J Clin Endocrinol Metab 2002;87:1768.

67. Abuhamad AZ, Fisher DA, Warsot SL, et al: Antenatal diagnosis and treatment of fetal goitrous hypothyroidism: Case report and review of the literature. Ultrasound Obstet Gynecol 1995;6:368.

68. Asling J, Way EL: Placental transfer of drugs. In La Du BN, Mandel HG, Way EL (eds): Fundamentals of Drug Metabolism and Drug Disposition. Baltimore, Williams & Wilkins, 1971, p 88.

69. Comite F, Burrow GN, Jorgensen EC: Thyroid hormone analogs and fetal goiter. J Clin Endocrinol Metab 1978;102:1670.

70. Brown RS, Bellisaro AL, Botero D, et al: Incidence of transient congenital hypothyroidism due to maternal thyrotropin receptor-blocking antibodies in over one million babies. J Clin Endocrinol Metab 1996;81:1147.

71. Ekins R: Roles of serum thyroxine-binding proteins and maternal thyroid hormones in fetal development. Lancet 1985;1:1129.

72. Obregon M, Mallol J, Pastor R, et al: L-Thyroxine and 3,5,3′-triiodo-L-thyronine in rat embryos before onset of fetal thyroid function. Endocrinology 1984;114:305.

73. Porterfield SP, Hendrich CE: Tissue iodothyronine levels in fetuses of control and hypothyroid rats of 13 and 16 days' gestation. Endocrinology 1992;131:200.

74. Calvo R, Obregon MJ, Ruiz de Ona C, et al: Congenital hypothyroidism as studied in rats. J Clin Invest 1990;86:889.

75. Morreale de Escobar G, Calvo R, Obregon M, et al: Contribution of maternal thyroxine to fetal thyroxine pools in normal rats near term. Endocrinology 1990;126:2765.

76. Matsuura N, Konishi J, Harada S, et al: The prediction of thyroid function in infants born to mothers with chronic thyroiditis. Endocrinol Jpn 1989;36:865.

77. Mitsuda N, Tamaki H, Amino N, et al: Risk factors for developmental disorders in infants born to women with Graves' disease. Obstet Gynecol 1992;80:359.

78. Davidson K, Richards D, Schatz D, Fisher D: Successful in utero treatment of fetal goiter and hypothyroidism. N Engl J Med 1991;324:543.

79. Wenstrom K, Weiner C, Williamson R: Prenatal diagnosis of fetal hypothyroidism using funipuncture. Obstet Gynecol 1990;76:513.

80. Lightner ES, Fismer DA, Giles H, Woolfenden J: Intra-amniotic injection of thyroxine (T_4) to a human fetus. Am J Obstet Gynecol 1977;127:487.

81. Santini F, Cortelazzi D, Baggiani AM, et al: A study of the serum 3,5,3′-triiodothyroxine sulfate concentration in normal and hypothyroid fetuses at various gestational stages. J Clin Endocrinol Metab 1993;72:1583.

82. Fisher D, Foley B: Early treatment of congenital hypothyroidism. Pediatrics 1989;83:785.

83. Fisher DA: Thyroid function in the premature infant. Am J Dis Child 1977;131:842.

84. Ponchon G, Beckers C, DeVisscher M: Iodide kinetic studies in newborns and infants. J Clin Endocrinol Metab 1966;26:1392.

85. Niswander KR, Gordon M, Berendes HW: The Women and Their Pregnancies. Philadelphia, WB Saunders, 1972.

86. Glinoer D: Thyroid hyperfunction during pregnancy. Thyroid 1998;8(9):859.

87. Burrow G: Thyroid function and hyperfunction during gestation. Endocrinol Rev 1993;14:194.

88. Nelson J, Hughes K, Smith A, et al: Maternal-fetal disparity in induced amelioration of rheumatoid arthritis. N Engl J Med 1993;329:466.

89. Salvi M, How J: Pregnancy and autoimmune thyroid disease. Endocrinol Metab Clin North Am 1987;16:431.

90. Stagnaro-Green A, Roman S, Cobin R, et al: A prospective study of lymphocyte-initiated immunosuppression in normal pregnancy: Evidence of a T-cell etiology for postpartum thyroid dysfunction. J Clin Endocrinol Metab 1992;74:645.

91. Sridama V, Pacini F, Yang S, et al: Decreased levels of helper T cells: A possible cause of immunodeficiency in pregnancy. N Engl J Med 1982;307:352.

92. Bouillon R, Naesens M, Van Assche F, et al: Thyroid function in patients with hyperemesis gravidarum. Am J Obstet Gynecol 1982;143:922.

93. Chin R, Lao T: Thyroxine concentrations and outcome of hyperemetic pregnancies. Br J Obstet Gynaecol 1988;95:507.

94. Goodwin T, Montoro M, Mestman J, et al: The role of chorionic gonadotropin in transient hyperthyroidism of hyperemesis gravidarum. J Clin Endocrinol Metab 1992;75:1333.

95. Goodwin T, Hershman JM: Hyperthyroidism due to inappropriate production of human chronic gonadotropism. Clin Obstet Gynecol 1997;40:32.

96. Thomson J, Wilson R, Gray C, et al: Hyperemesis gravidarum and thyrotoxicosis: A diagnostic problem. Scot Med J 1989;34:472.

97. Goodwin T, Montoro M, Mestman J: Transient hyperthyroidism and hyperemesis gravidarum: Clinical aspects. Am J Obstet Gynecol 1992;167:648.

98. Evans A, Li T, Selby C, Jeffcoate W: Morning sickness and thyroid function. Br J Obstet Gynaecol 1986;93:520.

99. Mori M, Amino N, Tamaki H, et al: Morning sickness and thyroid function in normal pregnancy. Obstet Gynecol 1988;72:355.

100. Bassett F, Eastman C, Ma G, et al: Diagnostic value of thyrotropin concentrations in serum as measured by a sensitive immunoradiometric assay. Clin Chem 1986;32:461.

101. de los Santos E, Mazzaferri E: Sensitive thyroid-stimulating hormone assays: Clinical applications and limitations. Compr Ther 1988;14:26.

102. Souma JA, Niejadlik DC, Cottrell S, Rankle S: Comparison of thyroid function in each trimester of pregnancy with the use of triiodothyronine uptake, thyroxine iodine, free thyroxine and free thyroxine index. Am J Obstet Gynecol 1973;116:905.

103. McKenzie J, Zakarija M: Clinical review 3: The clinical use of thyrotropin receptor antibody measurements. J Clin Endocrinol Metab 1989;69:1093.

104. Smith S, Bold A: Interpretation of in vitro thyroid function tests during pregnancy. Br J Obstet Gynaecol 1983;90:532.

105. Drury MI: Hyperthyroidism and pregnancy. J R Soc Med 1986;79:317.

106. Davis L, Lucas M, Hankins G, et al: Thyrotoxicosis complicating pregnancy. Am J Obstet Gynecol 1989;160:63.

107. Easterling T, Schmucker B, Carlson K, et al: Maternal hemodynamics in pregnancies complicated by hyperthyroidism. Obstet Gynecol 1991;78:348.

108. McLaughlin CW Jr, McGoogan LS: Hyperthyroidism complicating pregnancy. Am J Obstet Gynecol 1943;45:591.

109. Millar LK, Wingda, Leung AS, et al: Low birth weight and preeclampsia in pregnancies complicated by hyperthyroidism. Obstet Gynecol 1994;84:946.

110. Momotani N, Ito K, Hamada N, et al: Maternal hyperthyroidism and congenital malformation in the offspring. Clin Endocrinol 1984;20:695.

111. Roti E, Minelli R, Saloi M: Management of hyperthyroidism in the pregnant woman. J Clin Endocrinol Metab 1996;81:1679.

112. Dinami S, Carpenter S: Down's syndrome and thyroid disorder. J Ment Def Res 1990;34:187.

113. Gustafsson J, Anneten G, Ericsson U, et al: Thyroid antibodies are not a risk factor for pregnancies with Down's syndrome. Prenat Diagn 1995;15:451.

114. Thomas R, Reid R: Thyroid disease and reproductive dysfunction: A review. Obstet Gynecol 1987;70:789.

115. Bruner J, Landon M, Grabbe S: Diabetes mellitus and Graves' disease complicated by maternal allergies to antithyroid drugs. Obstet Gynecol 1988;72:443.

116. Mestman JH: Hyperthyroidism in pregnancy. Clin Obstet Gynecol 1997;40:45.

117. Sitar D, Abu-Bakare A, Gardiner R: Propylthiouracil disposition in pregnant and postpartum women. Pharmacology 1982;25:57.

118. Bachrach L, Burrow G: Aplasia cutis congenita and methimazole. Can Med Assoc J 1984;130:1264.

119. Kalb R, Grossman M: The association of aplasia cutis congenita with therapy of maternal thyroid disease. Pediatr Dermatol 1986;3:327.

120. Mandel SJ, Brent GA, Larsen PR: Review of antithyroid drug use during pregnancy and report of a case of aplasia cutis. Thyroid 1994;4:129.

121. Stephan MF, Smith DW, Ponzi JW, Alden ER: Origin of scalp vertex aplasia cutis. J Pediatr 1982;101:850.

122. Van Dijke C, Heydendael R, de Keline M: Methimazole, carbimazole, and congenital skin defects. Ann Intern Med 1987;106:60.

123. Gardner DF, Cruikshank DP, Hays PM, Cooper DS: Pharmacology of propylthiouracil (PTU) in pregnant hyperthyroid women: Correlation of maternal PTU concentrations with cord serum thyroid function tests. J Clin Endocrinol Metab 1986;62:217.

124. Sato K, Mimura H, Kato S, et al: Serum propylthiouracil concentration in patients with Graves' disease with various clinical courses. Acta Endocrinol (Copenh) 1983;104:189.

125. Galina MP, Arnet ML, Einhorn A: Iodides during pregnancy. N Engl J Med 1962;267:1124.

126. Vitug AC, Goldman JM: Hepatotoxicity from antithyroid drugs. Horm Res 1985;21:229.

127. Gurlek A, Cobankara V, Bayraktar M: Liver tests in hyperthyroidism: Effect of antithyroid therapy. J Clin Gastroenterol 1997;24:180.

128. Liaw YF, Huang MJ, Fan KD, et al: Hepatic injury during propylthiouracil therapy in patients with hyperthyroidism. Ann Intern Med 1993;118:424.

129. Huang MJ, Li KL, Wei JS, et al: Sequential liver and bone biochemical changes in hyperthyroidism: Prospective controlled follow-up study. Am J Gastroenterol 1994;89:1071.

130. Hadi H, Strickland D: In utero treatment of fetal goitrous hypothyroidism caused by maternal Graves' disease. Am J Perinatol 1995;12:455.

131. Hayashida C, Duarte A, Sato A, Hamashiro-Kanashiro E: Neonatal hepatitis and lymphocyte sensitization by placental transfer of propylthiouracil. J Endocrinol Invest 1990;13:937.

132. Momotani N, Noh J, Oyanagi H el al: Antithyroid drug therapy for Graves' disease during pregnancy. N Engl J Med 1986;315:24.

133. Soliman S, McGrath F, Brennan B, Glazebrook K: Color Doppler imaging of the thyroid gland in a fetus with congenital goiter: A case report. Am J Perinatol 1994;11:21.

134. Marchant B, Brownlie BEW, McKay HD, et al: The placental transfer of propylthiouracil, methimazole and carbimazole. J Clin Endocrinol Metab 1977;45:1187.

135. Mortimer RH, Cannell GR, Addison RS, et al: Methimazole and propylthiouracil equally cross the perfused human term placental lobule. J Clin Endocrinol Metab 1997;82:3099.

136. Mandel SJ, Cooper DS: The use of antithyroid drugs in pregnancy and lactation. J Clin Endocrinol Metab 2001;86:2354.

137. Momotani N, Hisaoka T, Noh J, et al: Effects of iodine on thyroid status of fetus versus mother in treatment of Graves' disease complicated by pregnancy. J Clin Endocrinol Metab 1992;75:738.

138. Momotani N, Noh JY, Ishikawa N, Ito K: Effects of propylthiouracil and methimazole on fetal thyroid status in mothers with Graves' hyperthyroidism. J Clin Endocrinol Metab 1997;82:3633.

139. Burrow G: Thyroid status in normal pregnancy: An editorial. J Clin Endocrinol Metab 1990;71:274.

140. Lamberg BA, Idonen E, Teramo K, et al: Treatment of hyperthyroidism with antithyroid agents and changes in thyrotropin and thyroxine in the newborn. Acta Endocrinol 1981;97:186.

141. Porreco R, Bloch C: Fetal blood sampling in the management of intrauterine thyrotoxicosis. Obstet Gynecol 1990;76:509.

142. Burrow GN, Bartsocas C, Klatskin EH, Grunt JA: Children exposed in utero to propylthiouracil. Arch Dis Child 1968;116:161.

143. Burrow GN, Klatskin EH, Genel M: Intellectual development in children whose mothers received propylthiouracil during pregnancy. Yale J Biol Med 1978;51:151.

144. McCarroll AM, Hutchinson M, McAuley R, Montgomery DAD: Long-term assessment of children exposed in utero to carbimazole. Arch Dis Child 1976;51:531.

145. Messer P, Hauffa B, Olbricht T, et al: Antithyroid drug treatment of Graves' disease in pregnancy: Long-term effects of somatic growth, intellectual development and thyroid function of the offspring. Acta Endocrinol (Copenh) 1990;123:311.

146. Cooper DS, Bode HH, Nath B, et al: Methimazole pharmacology in man: Studies using a newly developed radioimmunoassay for methimazole. J Clin Endocrinol Metab 1984;58:473.

147. Kampmann JP, Hansen JM, Johansen K, Helweg J: Propylthiouracil in human milk. Lancet 1980;1:736.

148. Lamberg BA, Ikonen I, Osterlund K, et al: Anti-thyroid treatment of maternal hypothyroidism during lactation. Clin Endocrinol 1984;21:81.

149. Zaton A, Martinez A, DeGandaris JM: The binding of thiourethylene compounds to human serum albumin. Biochem Pharmacol 1988;37:3127.

150. Azizi F: Effect of methimazole treatment of maternal thyrotoxicosis on thyroid function in breast-feeding infants. J Pediatr 1996;128:855.

151. Azizi F, Khoshniat M, Bahrainian M, Hedayati M: Thyroid function and intellectual development of infants nursed by mothers taking methimazole. J Clin Endocrinol Metab 2000;85:3233.

152. Momotani N, Yamashita R, Yoshimoto M, et al: Recovery from foetal hypothyroidism: Evidence for the safety of breast-feeding while taking propylthiouracil. Clin Endocrinol 1989;31:591.

153. Dydek G, Blue P: Human breast milk excretion of iodine-131 following diagnostic and therapeutic administration to a lactating patient with Graves' disease. J Nucl Med 1988;29:407.

154. Bullock J, Harris RE, Young R: Treatment of thyrotoxicosis during pregnancy with propranolol. Am J Obstet Gynecol 1975;121:242.

155. Gladstone GR, Hordof A, Gersony WM: Propranolol administration during pregnancy: Effects on the fetus. J Pediatr 1975;86:962.

156. Habib A, McCarthy JS: Effects on the neonate of propranolol administered during pregnancy. J Pediatr 1977;91:808.

157. Pruyn SC, Phelan JP, Buchanan GC: Long-term propranolol therapy in pregnancy: Maternal and fetal outcome. Am J Obstet Gynecol 1979;135:485.

158. Briggs GG, Freeman RK, Yaffe SH (eds): Drugs in Pregnancy and Lactation, 4th ed. Baltimore, Williams & Wilkins, 1994.

159. Sherif IH, Oyan WT, Bosairi S, Carrascal SM: Treatment of hyperthyroidism in pregnancy. Acta Obstet Gynecol Scand 1991;70:461.

160. Magee LA, Elran EI, Bull SB, et al: Risks and benefits of β-receptor blockers for pregnancy hypertension: Overview of the randomized trials. Eur J Obstet Gynecol Reprod Biol 2000;88:15.

161. Butters L, Kennedy S, Rubin PC: Atenolol in essential hypertension during pregnancy. BMJ 1990;301:587.

162. Sibai BM, Mabie WC, Shamsa F, et al: A comparison of no medication versus methyldopa or labetalol in chronic hypertension during pregnancy. Am J Obstet Gynecol 1990;162:960.

163. Rubin PC: Beta-blockers in pregnancy. N Engl J Med 1983;18:73.

164. Rubin PC, Butters L, Clark DM, et al: Placebo-controlled trial of atenolol in treatment of pregnancy-associated hypertension. Lancet 1983;1:431.

165. Sandstrom B: Antihypertensive treatment with the adrenergic beta-receptor blocker metoprolol during pregnancy Gynecol Invest 1978;9:195.

166. Isely W, Dahl S, Gibbs H: Use of esmolol in managing a thyrotoxic patient needing emergency surgery. Am J Med 1990;89:122.

167. Wu SY, Shyh TP, Chopra U, et al: Comparison of sodium ipodate (Oragrafin) and propylthiouracil in early treatment of hyperthyroidism. J Clin Endocrinol Metab 1982;54:630.

168. Weingold AB: Surgical diseases in pregnancy. Clin Obstet Gynecol 1983;26:793.

169. Emslander RF, Weeks RE, Malkasian GD Jr: Hyperthyroidism and pregnancy. Med Clin North Am 1974;58:835.

170. Prihoda J, Davis L: Metabolic emergencies in obstetrics. Obstet Gynecol Clin North Am 1991;18:301.

171. Guenter KE, Friedland GA: Thyroid storm and placenta previa in a primigravida. Obstet Gynecol 1965;26:403.

172. Derksen RHWV, van der Wiel A, Poortman J, et al: Plasma exchange in the treatment of severe thyrotoxicosis in pregnancy. Eur J Obstet Gynecol Reprod Biol 1984;18:139.

173. Ingbar SH: Management of emergencies. IX. Thyrotoxic storm. N Engl J Med 1966;274:1252.

174. Robinson PL, O'Mullane NM, Alderman B: Prenatal treatment of fetal thyrotoxicosis. BMJ 1979;1:383.

175. Farrar J, Toft A: Iodine-131 treatment of hyperthyroidism: Current issues. Clin Endocrinol 1991;35:207.

176. Safa AM, Schumacher OP, Rodriguez-Antunez A: Long-term follow-up results in children and adolescents treated with radioactive iodine (131I) for hypothyroidism. N Engl J Med 1975;292:167.

177. Robertson JS, Gorman CA: Gonadal radiation dose and its genetic significance in radioiodine therapy of hypothyroidism. J Nucl Med 1976;17:826.

178. Stabin M, Watson E, Marcus C, Salk R: Radiation dosimetry for the adult female and fetus from iodine-131 administration in hyperthyroidism. J Nucl Med 1991;32:808.

179. Fisher WD, Voorhess ML, Gardner LI: Congenital hypothyroidism in infant following maternal I-131 therapy. J Pediatr 1963;62:132.

180. Klein AH, Hobel CJ, Sack J, Fisher DA: Effect of intraamniotic fluid thyroxine injection on fetal serum and amniotic fluid iodothyronine concentrations. J Clin Endocrinol Metab 1978;47:1034.

181. Stoffer SS, Hamburger JI: Inadvertent ^{131}I therapy for hypothyroidism in the first trimester of pregnancy. J Nucl Med 1976;17:146.

182. National Council on Radiation Protection and Measurements [NCRP]: Medical Radiation Exposure of Pregnant and Potentially Pregnant Women. NCRP Report 54. Bethesda, MD, NCRP, 1977.

183. MacMahon B: Prenatal x-ray exposure and childhood cancer. J Natl Cancer Inst 1962;28:1173.

184. Stewart A, Webb J, Hewitt D: A survey of childhood malignancies. BMJ 1958;1:1495.

185. Gerstein H: How common is postpartum thyroiditis? Arch Intern Med 1990;150:1397.

186. Browne-Martin K, Emerson CH: Postpartum thyroid dysfunction. Clin Obstet Gynecol 1997;40:90.

187. Walfish P, Chan J: Postpartum hyperthyroidism. J Endocrinol Metab 1985;14:417.

188. Learoyd D, Fung H, McGregor A: Postpartum thyroid dysfunction. Thyroid 1992;2:73.

189. Lazaros JH, Hall B, Othman S, et al: The clinical spectrum of postpartum thyroid disease. Q J Med 1996;89:429.

190. Amino N, Mori H, Iwatani Y, et al: High prevalence of transient postpartum thyrotoxicosis and hypothyroidism. N Engl J Med 1982;306:849.

191. Pop UJ, deVries E, van Baar AL, et al: Maternal thyroid peroxidase antibodies during pregnancy: A marker for impaired child development. J Clin Endocrinol Metab 1995;80:3561.

192. Roti E, Emerson C: Clinical review 29: Postpartum thyroiditis. J Clin Endocrinol Metab 1992;74:3.

193. White W, Andreoli J: Severe accelerated postpartum hypertension associated with hyperthyroxinemia. Br J Obstet Gynaecol 1986;93:1297.

194. Othman S, Phillips D, Parkes A, et al: A long-term follow-up of postpartum thyroiditis. Clin Endocrinol (Oxf) 1990;32:559.

195. Glinoer D, Riahi M, Grun J, Kinthaert J: Risk of subclinical hypothyroidism in pregnant women with asymptomatic autoimmune thyroid disorders. J Clin Endocrinol Metab 1994;79:197.

196. Alvarez-Marfany M, Roman SH, Drexler AN, et al: Long-term prospective study of postpartum thyroid dysfunction in women with insulin dependent diabetes mellitus. J Clin Endocrinol Metab 1994;79:1.

197. Pop LT, DeRooy H, Vader H, et al: Postpartum thyroid dysfunction and depression in an unselected population. N Engl J Med 1991;324:1815.

198. Stewart D, Addison A, Robinson G, et al: Thyroid function in psychosis following childbirth. Am J Psychiat 1988;145:1579.

199. Harris B, Othman S, Davies JA, et al: Association between postpartum thyroid dysfunction and thyroid antibodies and depression. BMJ 1992;305:152.

200. Kimpe O, Jansson R, Karlsson F: Effects of L-thyroxine and iodide on the development of autoimmune postpartum thyroiditis. J Clin Endocrinol Metab 1990;70:1014.

201. Hollingsworth DR, Mabry CC: Congenital Graves' disease: Four familial cases with long-term follow-up and perspective. Am J Dis Child 1976;130:148.

202. Munro DS, Dirmikis SM, Humphries H, et al: The role of thyroid stimulating immunoglobulins of Graves' disease in neonatal thyrotoxicosis. Br J Obstet Gynaecol 1978;85:837.

203. Menking M, Wiebel J, Schmid WU, et al: Premature craniosynostosis associated with hypothyroidism in 4 children with reference to 5 further cases in the literature. Monatsschr Kinderheilkd 1972;120:106.

204. Yagi H, Takeuchi M, Nagashima K, et al: Neonatal transient thyrotoxicosis resulting from maternal TSH-binding inhibitor immunoglobulins. Clin Lab Observ 1983;103:591.

205. Yoshida S, Takamatsu J, Kuma K, Ohsawa N: Thyroid-stimulating antibodies and thyroid stimulation-blocking antibodies during the pregnancy and postpartum period: A case report. Thyroid 1992;2:27.

206. Clavel S, Madec A-M, Bornet H, et al: Anti TSH-receptor antibodies in pregnant patients with autoimmune thyroid disorder. Br J Obstet Gynaecol 1990;97:1003.

207. Tamaki H, Amino N, Aozasa M, et al: Universal predictive criteria for neonatal overt thyrotoxicosis requiring treatment. Am J Perinatol 1988;5:152.

208. Tamaki H, Amino N, Iwatani Y, et al: Evaluation of TSH receptor antibody by "natural in vivo human assay" in neonates born to mothers with Graves' disease. Clin Endocrinol 1989;30:493.

209. Zakarija M, McKenzie JM, Nunro DS: Immunoglobulin G inhibitor of thyroid stimulating antibody is a cause of delay in the onset of neonatal Graves' disease. J Clin Invest 1983;72:1352.

210. Maisey MN, Stimmler L: The role of long acting thyroid stimulator in neonatal thyrotoxicosis. Clin Endocrinol 1972;1:81.

211. Munro DS, Cooke ID, Kirmikis SM, et al: Neonatal thyrotoxicosis. Q J Med 1976;45:689.

212. Hollingsworth DR, Mabry CC, Eckerd JM: Hereditary aspects of Graves' disease in infancy and childhood. J Pediatr 1972;81:446.

213. Kopp P, Van Sande J, Parma J, et al: Brief report: Congenital hyperthyroidism caused by a mutation in the thyrotropin-receptor gene. N Engl J Med 1995;332:150.

214. Elsas LJ, Whitemore R, Burrow GN: Maternal and neonatal Graves' disease. JAMA 1967;200:250.

215. Farrehi C: Accelerated maturity in fetal thyrotoxicosis. Clin Pediatr 1968;7:134.

216. Wilkin TJ, Kenyon E, Isles TE: The behaviour of thyroid hormones in an infant with untreated neonatal thyrotoxicosis. Clin Endocrinol 1977;7:227.

217. Walter P, Dussault JH, Hart IR, et al: Thyrotoxicosis detected in a mass-screening program for neonatal hypothyroidism: Demonstration of placental transfer for an immunoglobulin with marked lipolytic activity. J Pediatr 1977;91:400.

218. Jhaveri RC, Glass L, Evans HE, et al: Effects of methadone on thyroid function in mother, fetus, and newborn. Pediatrics 1980;65:557.

219. Hayek A, Brooks M: Neonatal hyperthyroidism following intrauterine hypothyroidism. J Pediatr 1975;87:446.

220. Smith CS, Howard NJ: Propranolol in treatment of neonatal thyrotoxicosis. J Pediatr 1973;83:1046.

221. Cove DH, Johnston P: Fetal hyperthyroidism: Experience of treatment in four siblings. Lancet 1985;1:430.

222. Maxwell KD, Kearney KK, Johnson JWC, et al: Fetal tachycardia associated with intrauterine fetal thyrotoxicosis. Obstet Gynecol 1980;55:18S.

223. Belfar H, Foley T, Hill L, Kislak S: Sonographic findings in maternal hyperthyroidism: Fetal hyperthyroidism/fetal goiter. J Ultrasound Med 1991;10:281.

224. Pekonen F, Teramo K, Makinen T, et al: Prenatal diagnosis and treatment of fetal thyrotoxicosis. Am J Obstet Gynecol 1984;64:893.

225. Di Gianantonio ED, Schaefer C, Mastroiacovo PP et al: Adverse effects of prenatal methimazole exposure. Teratology 2001;64:262.

226. Wallace C, Couch R, Ginsberg J: Fetal thyrotoxicosis: A case report and recommendations for prediction, diagnosis and treatment. Thyroid 1995;5:125.

227. Klein R, Haddow J, Faix J, et al: Prevalence of thyroid deficiency in pregnant women. Clin Endocrinol 1991;35:41.

228. Moosa M, Mazzaferri EL: Outcome of differentiated thyroid cancer diagnosed in pregnant women. J Clin Endocrinol Metab 1997;82:2862.

229. Kaplan M: Monitoring thyroxine treatment during pregnancy. Thyroid 1992;2:147.

230. Larsen P: Monitoring thyroxine treatment during pregnancy. Thyroid 1992;2:153.

231. Mandel S, Larsen P, Seely E, Brent G: Increased need for thyroxine during pregnancy in women with primary hypothyroidism. N Engl J Med 1990;323:91.

232. Tamaki H, Amino N, Takeoka K, et al: Thyroxine requirement during pregnancy for replacement therapy of hypothyroidism. Obstet Gynecol 1990;76:230.

233. Soler NG, Nicholson H: Diabetes and thyroid disease during pregnancy. Obstet Gynecol 1979;54:318.

234. Leung A, Millar L, Koonings P, et al: Perinatal outcome in hypothyroid pregnancies. Obstet Gynecol 1993;81:349.

235. Kinch RA, Plunkett ER, Devlin MC: Postpartum amenorrhea-galactorrhea of hypothyroidism. Am J Obstet Gynecol 1969;105:766.

236. Thorner MO: Prolactin. Clin Endocrinol Metab 1977;6:201.

237. Hodges RE, Hamilton HE, Keettel WC: Pregnancy of myxedema. Arch Intern Med 1952;90:863.

238. Kennedy AL, Montgomery DAD: Hypothyroidism in pregnancy. Br J Obstet Gynecol 1978;85:225.

239. Lachelin GC: Myxedema and pregnancy: A case report. J Obstet Gynaecol Br Commonw 1970;77:77.

240. Monturo MN Collea JA, Frasier SN, Mestman JH: Successful outcome of pregnancy in women with hypothyroidism. Ann Intern Med 1981;94:31.

241. Khoury M, Becerra J, d'Almada P: Maternal thyroid disease and risk of birth defects in offspring: A population-based case-control study. Paediatr Perinatol Epidemiol 1989;3:402.

242. Boyages S, Halpern J-P: Endemic cretinism: Toward a unifying hypothesis. Thyroid 1993;3:59.

243. Larsen P: Maternal thyroxine and congenital hypothyroidism. N Engl J Med 1989;321:44.

244. Man EB, Brown JF, Serunian SA: Maternal hypothyroxinemia: Psychoneurological deficits of progeny. Ann Clin Lab Sci 1991;21:227.

245. Haddow JE, Palomaki GE, Allan WC, et al: Maternal thyroid deficiency during pregnancy and subsequent neuropsychological development of the child. N Engl J Med 1999;341:549.

246. Lavado-Autric R, Auso E, Garcia-Velasco JV, et al: Early maternal hypothyroxinemia alters histogenesis and cerebral cortex cytoarchitecture of the progeny. J Clin Invest 2003;111:1073.

247. Zoeller RT: Transplacental thyroxine and fetal brain development. J Clin Invest 2003;111:954.

248. Stock JM, Surks MI, Oppenheimer JH: Replacement dosage of L-thyroxine in hypothyroidism. N Engl J Med 1974;290:529.

249. Nicoloff JT, Nicoloff R, Dowling JT: Evaluation of vaginal smear, serum gonadotropin, protein-bound iodine and thyroxine-binding as measures of placental adequacy. J Clin Invest 1998;41:1962.

250. Stagnaro-Green A, Roman S, Cobin R, et al: Detection of at-risk pregnancy by means of highly sensitive assays for thyroid autoantibodies. JAMA 1990;264:1422.

251. Poppe K, Glinoer D: Thyroid autoimmunity and hypothyroidism before and during pregnancy. Hum Reprod Update 2003;9:149.

252. Stagnaro-Green A, Abramson J: Thyroid antibodies and fetal loss: An evolving story. Thyroid 2001;11:57.

253. Glinoer D, Solo M, Bourdoux P, et al: Pregnancy in patients with mild thyroid abnormalities: Maternal and neonatal repercussions. J Clin Endocrinol Metab 1991;73:421.

254. Iijima T, Tada H, Hidaka Y, et al: Effects of autoantibodies of the course of pregnancy and fetal growth. Obstet Gynecol 1997;90:364.

255. Roberts J, Jenkins C, Wilson R, et al: Recurrent miscarriage is associated with increased numbers of CD5/20 positive lymphocytes and an increased incidence of thyroid antibodies. Eur J Endocrinol 1996;134:84.

256. Bussen S, Steck T: Thyroid autoantibodies in euthyroid nonpregnant women with recurrent spontaneous abortions. Hum Reprod 1995;10:2938.

257. Bussen S, Steck T: Thyroid antibodies and their relation to antithrombin antibodies, anticardiolipin antibodies and lupus anticoagulant in women with recurrent spontaneous abortions (antithyroid, anticardiolipin and antithrombin autoantibodies and lupus anticoagulant in habitual aborters). Eur J Obstet Gynecol Reprod Biol 1997;74:139.

258. Stricker RB, Steinleitner A, Bookoff CN: Successful treatment of immunologic abortion with low dose intravenous immunoglobulin. Fertil Steril 2000;73:536.

259. Kiprov DD, Nactigall RD, Weaver RC, et al: The use of intravenous immunoglobulin in recurrent pregnancy loss associated with combined alloimmune and autoimmune abnormalities. Am J Reprod Immunol 1996;36:228.

260. Sher G, Maassarani G, Zouves C, et al: The use of combined heparin/aspirin and immunoglobulin G therapy in the treatment

of in vitro fertilization patients with thyroid antibodies. Am J Reprod Immunol 1998;39:223.

261. Vaquero E, Lazzarin CD, Valensise H, et al: Mild thyroid abnormalities and recurrent spontaneous abortion: Diagnostic and therapeutical approach. Am J Reprod Immunol 2000;43:204.

262. Hetzel BS, Hay ID: Thyroid function, iodine nutrition and fetal brain development. Clin Endocrinol 1979;11:445.

263. Morreale de Escobar G, Obregon MJ, Escobar del Rey E: Is neuropsychological development related to maternal hypothyroidism or to maternal hypothyroxinemia? J Clin Endocrinol Metab 2000;85:3975.

264. Congenital concomitants of infantile hypothyroidism. New England Congenital Hypothyroidism Collaborative. J Pediatr 1988;112:244.

265. Olivieri A, Stazi MA, Mastroiacovo P, et al: A population-based study on the frequency of additional congenital malformations in infants with congenital hypothyroidism: Data from the Italian Registry for Congenital Hypothyroidism (1991-1998). J Clin Endocrinol Metab 2002;87:557.

266. Dussault JH, Letarte J, et al: Psychological development of hypothyroid infants at age 12 and 18 months: Experience after neonatal screening. In Burrow GN, Dussault JH (eds): Neonatal Thyroid Screening. New York, Raven Press, 1980, pp 62.

267. Eastman C, Phillips D: Endemic goiter and iodine deficiency disorders: Aetiology, epidemiology and treatment. Baillieres Clin Endocrinol Metab 1988;2:719.

268. Fisher DA: Fetal thyroid function: Diagnosis and management of fetal thyroid disorders. Clin Obstet Gynecol 1997;40:16.

269. La Franchi SH, Harma CE, Krainz PL, et al: Screening for congenital hypothyroidism with specimen collection at two time periods: Results of the northwest regional screening program. Pediatrics 1995;76:734.

270. Fort P, Lifshitz F, Pugliese M, Klein I: Neonatal thyroid disease: Differential expression in three successive offspring. J Clin Endocrinol Metab 1988;66:645.

271. Tamaki H, Amino N, Aozasa M, et al: Effective method for prediction of transient hypothyroidism in neonates born to mothers with chronic thyroiditis. Am J Perinatol 1989;6:396.

272. Tamaki H, Amino N, Takeoka K, et al: Prediction of later development of thyrotoxicosis or central hypothyroidism from the cord serum thyroid-stimulating hormone level in neonates born to mothers with Graves' disease. J Pediatr 1989;115:318.

273. Pharoah P, Connolly K, Ekins R, Harding A: Maternal thyroid hormone levels in pregnancy and the subsequent cognitive and motor performance of the children. Clin Endocrinol (Oxf) 1984;21:265.

274. Little G, Meador CK, Cunningham R, Pittman JA: "Cryptothyroidism," the major cause of sporadic "athyreotic" cretinism. J Clin Endocrinol Metab 1965;25:1529.

275. Chandler JW, Blizzard RM, Hung W, Kyle J: Thyroid antibodies passing to fetus. N Engl J Med 1962;267:376.

276. de Zegher F, Pernasetti F, Vanhole G, et al: The prenatal role of thyroid hormone evidenced by fetomaternal Pit-1 deficiency. J Clin Endocrinol Metab 1995;80:3127.

277. Bongiovanni AM, Eberlein WR, Thomas PZ, Anderson WB: Sporadic goiter of the newborn. J Clin Endocrinol Metab 1956;16:146.

278. Van Loon AJ, Derksen JTM, Bosa F, Rouwe CW: In utero diagnosis and treatment of fetal goitrous hypothyroidism caused by maternal use of propylthiouracil. Prenat Diagn 1995;15:599.

279. Black JA: Neonatal goiter and mental deficiency: The role of iodides taken during pregnancy. Arch Dis Child 1963;38:526.

280. Maragliano G, Zuppa AA, Florio MG, et al: Efficacy of oral iodide therapy on neonatal hyperthyroidism caused by maternal Graves' disease. Fetal Diagn Ther 2000;15:122.

281. Carswell F, Kerr MM, Hutchison JH: Congenital goitre and hypothyroidism produced by maternal ingestion of iodides. Lancet 1970;1:1241.

282. DeWolf D, De Schepper J, Verhaaren H, et al: Congenital hypothyroid goiter and amiodarone. Acta Paediatr Scand 1988;77:616.

283. Magee L, Dowmar E, Sermer M, et al: Pregnancy outcome after gestational exposure to amiodarone in Canada. Am J Obstet Gynecol 1995;172:1307.

284. Matsumura L, Born D, Kunii I, et al: Outcome of thyroid function in newborns from mothers treated with amiodarone. Thyroid 1992;2:279.

285. Plomp T, Vulsma T, de Vijlder J: Use of amiodarone during pregnancy. Eur J Obstet Gynecol Reprod Biol 1992;43:201.

286. Rey E, Bachrach L, Burrow G: Effects of amiodarone during pregnancy. Can Med Assoc J 1987;136:959.

287. Klein AH, Foley TP Jr, Larsen PR, et al: Neonatal thyroid function in congenital hypothyroidism. J Pediatr 1976;89:545.

288. Letarte J, Guyda H, Dussault JH: Clinical biochemical, and radiological features of neonatal hypothyroid infants. In Burrow GN, Dussault JH (eds): Neonatal Thyroid Screening. New York, Raven Press, 1980, pp 225-236.

289. Smith DW, Kelin AM, Henderson JR, Nyrianthopoulos NC: Congenital hypothyroidism: Signs and symptoms in the newborn period. J Pediatr 1975;87:958.

290. Lusted LB, Pickering DE: The hypothyroid infant and child: The role of roentgen evaluation in therapy. Radiology 1956;66:708.

291. Wilkins L: Epiphysial dysgenesis associated with hypothyroidism. Arch Dis Child 1941;61:13.

292. Fillippi G, McKusick VA: The Beckwith-Wiedemann syndrome. Medicine 1970;49:279.

293. Klein AH, Meltzer S, Kenny FM: Improved prognosis in congenital hypothyroidism treated before age three months. J Pediatr 1972;81:912.

294. Klein AH, Murphy BEP, Artal R, et al: Amniotic fluid thyroid hormone concentration during human gestation. Am J Obstet Gynecol 1980;136:626.

295. Van Wassenaer AG, Kok JH, Ender TE, et al: Thyroxine administration to infants of less than 30 weeks gestational age does not increase plasma triiodothyronine concentrations. Acta Endocrinol (Copenh) 1993;129:139.

296. Nicolini U, Vemegoni E, Acia B, et al: Prenatal treatment of fetal hypothyroidism: Is there more than one option? Prenat Diagn 1996;16:443.

297. Perelman A, Johnson R, Clemons R, et al: Intrauterine diagnosis and treatment of fetal goitrous hypothyroidism. J Clin Endocrinol Metab 1990;71:618.

298. Rosen IB, Korman M, Walfish PG: Thyroid nodular disease in pregnancy: Current diagnosis and management. Clin Obstet Gynecol 1997;40:81.

299. Mazzaferri EL: Evolution and management of common thyroid disorders in women. Am J Obstet Gynecol 1997;176:507.

300. Marley EF, Oertel YC: Fine-needle aspiration of thyroid lesions in 57 pregnant and post partum women. Diagn Cytopathol 1997;16:122.

301. Cunningham MP, Slaughter DP: Surgical treatment of disease of the thyroid gland in pregnancy. Surg Gynecol Obstet 1970;131:486.

302. Struve C, Haupt S, Ohlen S: Influence of frequency of previous pregnancies on the prevalence of thyroid nodules in women without clinical evidence of thyroid disease. Thyroid 1993;3:7.

303. Hill CS Jr, Clark FI, Wolf M: The effect of subsequent pregnancy on patients with thyroid carcinoma. Surg Gynecol Obstet 1966;122:1219.

304. Preston-Martin S, Bernstein L, Pike M, et al: Thyroid cancer among young women related to prior thyroid disease and pregnancy history. Br J Cancer 1987;55:191.

305. Rosvoll RV, Winship T: Thyroid carcinoma and pregnancy. Surg Gynecol Obstet 1965;121:1039.

306. Choew AN, McDougall R: Thyroid cancer in pregnant women: Diagnostic and therapeutic management. Thyroid 1994;4:433.

307. Schlumberger M, Devathalve F, Ceccarellie C, et al: Exposure to radioactive iodine-131 therapy does not preclude pregnancy in thyroid cancer patients. J Nucl Med 1996;37:606.

8

PITUITARY AND ADRENAL DISORDERS OF PREGNANCY

Peter R. Garner* and Gerard N. Burrow

PITUITARY DISORDERS OF PREGNANCY

Physiologic and Anatomic Changes of the Pituitary during Pregnancy

In pregnancy, the normal pituitary gland enlarges from 660 mg in the nonpregnant state to 760 mg by term. This occurs mainly because of an increase in the number and size of the lactotrophic cells. This increase in pituitary size does not result in visual field changes if a woman has a normal pituitary gland before the pregnancy. Therefore, visual changes that occur for the first time in pregnancy should be fully investigated. Serial magnetic resonance imaging (MRI) of the pituitary gland has been done by various investigators. Gonzales and colleagues[1] showed an increase in pituitary volume of about 136% overall and an increase in the vertical and anteroposterior diameter of 2.6 mm on average. They also found that the MRI signal intensity was increased in relation to that in the nonpregnant state. Therefore, physicians and radiologists should be aware of these normal changes, particularly the increased signal density, because this may lead to misrepresentation. Dinc and colleagues found on MRI that the pituitary gland enlarges in three dimensions throughout pregnancy. The maximum height of the gland does not exceed 10 mm during pregnancy but actually may exceed 10 mm during the 3 days immediately post partum.[2] In conclusion, therefore, the pituitary gland enlarges throughout pregnancy but should probably not exceed 10 mm in height during most of this period. A size of up to 12 mm may be acceptable immediately post partum.

Changes in Pituitary Physiology in Normal Pregnancy

Because of the normal physiologic changes in pituitary hormone concentrations in pregnancy, it is very difficult to diagnose pituitary hypersecretion or hyposecretion during pregnancy itself; therefore, confirmation must wait until the postpartum period. The results of dynamic pituitary function testing (e.g., triple-bolus testing) in pregnancy are difficult to interpret because no pregnancy standard exists (Table 8–1). Lactotrophic cell secretion of prolactin increases (Fig. 8–1) during the first trimester. This is because both estrogen and progesterone simulate the lactotrophic cells. In the second and third trimesters, the decidua is a source of much increased prolactin production. Decidual prolactin secretion is not suppressible

TABLE 8–1   Changes in Pituitary Function during Pregnancy

Hormone	Basal Serum Level Changes	Dynamic Testing
LH	Suppressed	Flat response to GnRH
FSH	Suppressed	Flat response to GnRH
Prolactin	Elevated	—
GH	Suppressed	Blunted response to hypoglycemia
TSH	Unchanged	Increased response to TRH
ACTH	Small rise	Blunted response to metyrapone
BMSH	Elevated	—
Vasopressin	Unchanged	Normal response to water deprivation
Oxytocin	Vary considerably	Variable increase during labor

From Garner PR: Pituitary disorders in pregnancy. Curr Obstet Med 1991;1:48. ACTH, adrenocorticotropic hormone; BMSH, β-melanocyte–stimulating hormone; FSH, follicle-stimulating hormone; GH, growth hormone; GnRH, gonadotropin-releasing hormone; TRH, thyrotropin-releasing hormone; TSH, thyroid-stimulating hormone.

*Shortly after completing this chapter, Peter R. Garner, MD, FRCP(C), succumbed to cancer. He leaves the legacy of a distinguished and productive career in Obstetric Medicine.

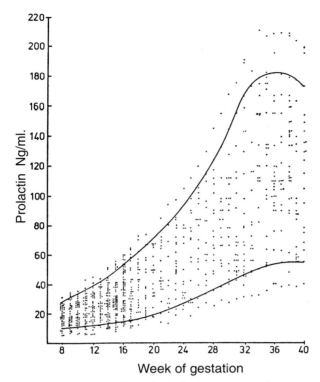

Figure 8–1. Plasma prolactin levels during pregnancy. (From Biswas S, Rodeck CH: Plasma prolactin levels during pregnancy. Br J Obstet Gynaecol 1976;83:684.)

Maternal adrenocorticotropic hormone (ACTH) levels increase progressively throughout pregnancy and increase further during labor. The progressive increase in ACTH is a response to elevated corticotropin-releasing hormone (CRH) concentrations in pregnancy, which increase several hundred-fold by term. The elevated CRH levels in pregnancy are of placental origin.[6] Of diagnostic importance is that placental ACTH is not suppressible by corticosteroids such as dexamethasone. This leads to difficulties in the interpretation of dexamethasone suppression test results during pregnancy. There is also a blunted response to metyrapone, but this test is not recommended during pregnancy. There is also good evidence that opioids regulate the production of ACTH secretion during pregnancy and parturition.[7]

Luteinizing hormone (LH) and follicle-stimulating hormone (FSH) levels are suppressed during pregnancy. The FSH levels remain low post partum, possibly because of prolactin suppression. LH levels are in the luteal phase range. Gonadotropin-releasing hormone (GnRH) stimulation shows a flattened response. Postpartum FSH levels return to normal more predictably than do LH levels; they begin to rise by 14 days after delivery and return to normal by 21 days post partum.[8] In the third trimester, low levels of amniotic fluid FSH are found in fetuses of both sexes. LH levels rise in amniotic fluid in the second trimester in both sexes but become undetectable by term. The source of amniotic fluid LH and FSH is thought to be fetal, inasmuch as maternal levels remain low throughout pregnancy.

by dopamine agonists. Prolactin responses to thyrotropin-releasing hormone (TRH) infusion are similar in all three trimesters, but they are probably greater than the non-pregnant response.

Maternal serum growth hormone levels during early pregnancy are similar to those in the nonpregnant state. They increase in late pregnancy as a result of increasing levels of human placental growth hormone. However, maternal pituitary growth hormone levels decrease. Thus, during pregnancy, placental growth hormone levels increase progressively, but the regulation of placental growth hormone secretion remains unknown. Insulin-like growth factor 1 is produced in response to growth hormone, and its level is elevated in pregnancy. Growth hormone release and response to hypoglycemia are suppressed during pregnancy and up to 1 week post partum, but testing for this during pregnancy is not advised, because of the potential fetal danger of hypoglycemia. Growth hormone–releasing hormone (GHRH) stimulation testing in pregnancy is safe and the response is unaltered.[3]

Levels of thyroid-stimulating hormone (TSH) decrease during the first trimester with a reciprocal relationship to β–human chorionic gonadotrophin (β-hCG).[4] TSH levels then rise by the third trimester but usually remain in the upper normal range.[5] In fact, the higher the β-hCG levels are in the first trimester, the lower the TSH level is, and this may lead to an erroneous diagnosis of hyperthyroidism in the first trimester, particularly in conditions associated with high first trimester β-hCG levels, such as hyperemesis gravidarum.

Normal Changes in Posterior Pituitary Function during Pregnancy

Vasopressin release by the hypothalamus is controlled by alterations in plasma osmolality, blood volume, and several other stress factors, both in pregnancy and in nonpregnant states. During pregnancy, plasma osmolality decreases from 285 to 275 mOsm/kg.[9] This has been called "resetting of the osmostat." Also during pregnancy, both the plasma levels of vasopressin and the release of vasopressin after dehydration or water loading remain unchanged. Because plasma osmolality decreases during pregnancy, this suggests that there is a true resetting of the threshold of vasopressin secretion during pregnancy in association with the downward adjustment of the thirst threshold. The mechanism by which osmoregulatory changes occur during pregnancy is not known, but there have been several hypothetical suggestions. Hyperventilation in pregnancy leads to hypocapnia, which leads to bicarbonate wasting. This is accompanied by sodium loss and a decrease in plasma osmolality. Acute administration of estradiol has also been reported to decrease plasma osmolality. Changes in the renin-angiotensin-aldosterone system may change osmoregulation in pregnancy, but further investigation is required.[10]

Oxytocin is a nine–amino acid peptide secreted mainly by the supraoptic nucleus of the hypothalamus. Oxytocin levels increase in pregnancy from 10 pg/mL in the first trimester to 30 pg/mL in the third trimester. Around term, there is a dramatic increase to approximately 75 pg/mL which may be due to an estrogen stimulatory effect.

Plasma oxytocin levels rise dramatically during labor and peak during the second stage. There is an increase in oxytocin receptors in the myometrium, with the resultant increase in uterine sensitivity to oxytocin. In spite of this, endogenous oxytocin seems to play only a facilitatory role in human labor, inasmuch as labor is not altered by hypophysectomy. Pulsatile release of oxytocin in patients with diabetes insipidus also is not correlated with uterine contractions.

The supraoptic and paraventricular nuclei of the hypothalamus also synthesize neurophysins, which are carrier proteins for both oxytocin and vasopressins. Neurophysins bind oxytocin and are stimulated by estrogen. Plasma neurophysin levels rise during pregnancy but do not increase during breast-feeding.[11]

Dynamic Pituitary Function Testing in Pregnancy (Triple-Bolus Test)

A normal triple-bolus test consists of GnRH and TRH stimulation with added hypoglycemia induced by insulin for release of ACTH and growth hormone. To avoid hypoglycemia, CRH and GHRH may be used in place of insulin. TRH, GnRh, and CRH seem to be safe in pregnancy in addition to GHRH, but no standardized response range has been obtained in pregnant patients. Hypoglycemia can be dangerous to the fetus and should not be used in a case of suspected hypopituitarism (e.g., Sheehan's syndrome). This test should therefore be delayed until the postpartum period, preferably until at least 6 weeks after delivery.

Imaging of the Pituitary Gland during Pregnancy

It is safe to undergo MRI during pregnancy; thin-section (2.5- to 3.0-mm) MRI is superior to computed tomographic (CT) scanning. To date, there is no evidence of embryo sensitivity to magnetic or radiowave frequency at the intensities encountered during MRI. The National Radiological Protection Board, however, suggests avoiding MRI during the first trimester if possible. High-resolution CT scan of the pituitary produces a radiation dose to the pelvis of less than 10 mGy. The acceptable upper limit of radiation to the pelvis is 25 mGy, but if CT is done during pregnancy, abdominal shielding measures are required.[12]

Diabetes Insipidus in Pregnancy

Diabetes insipidus in pregnancy is caused by an abnormality of vasopressin secretion or action or by a change in vasopressin degradation. Presenting features are polydipsia, polyuria, and dehydration. Three types of diabetes insipidus can be encountered during pregnancy: central, nephrogenic, and the transient vasopressin-resistant type (Table 8–2).

Central Diabetes Insipidus

Central diabetes insipidus is caused by decreased production of vasopressin by the paraventricular nuclei of

TABLE 8–2   Causes of Diabetes Insipidus in Pregnancy

Type of Diabetes Insipidus	Cause
Central	Pregnancy worsening of prior diabetes insipidus
	Central nervous system tumor (e.g., prolactinoma)
	Granuloma (e.g., sarcoid)
	Histiocytosis X
	Aneurysm
	Lymphocytic hypophysitis
	Sheehan's syndrome
Nephrogenic	X-linked abnormality of vasopressin V_2 receptor
Transient vasopressin-resistant	Increased vasopressinase activity resulting from decreased vasopressinase degradation caused by hepatic disease (e.g., acute fatty liver, HELLP syndrome, hepatitis B)

HELLP, hemolysis, elevated liver enzyme levels, and low platelet counts.

the hypothalamus. It complicates 1 per 15,000 deliveries. The most common scenario is that of a woman with preexisting central diabetes insipidus who becomes pregnant. Central diabetes insipidus often worsens with pregnancy because of increased clearance of endogenous vasopressin by vasopressinase. Vasopressinase (cystine aminopeptidase) is produced by the placenta, and its concentration dramatically increases in pregnancy in proportion to placental weight. It is metabolized by the liver; therefore, its activity increases in liver disease. Subclinical central diabetes insipidus may be unmasked for the first time during pregnancy, because of increased clearance of vasopressin. During pregnancy, 60% of established cases of central diabetes insipidus worsened, but 25% improved and 15% remained the same.[10] Central diabetes insipidus may manifest for the first time during pregnancy; this has been reported in the setting of the Sheehan's syndrome and as a result of enlargement of a prolactinoma and lymphocytic hypophysitis. It has also been reported as a complication of a ventriculoperitoneal shunt during pregnancy.

Diagnosis of central diabetes insipidus occurring for the first time during pregnancy requires a modification of the standard water deprivation test. Nonpregnant patients are normally required to lose up to 5% of their total body weight before dehydration adequately stimulates vasopressin release. Such dehydration can be dangerous in pregnancy and should not be instituted. The use of 1-deamino(8-D-arginine) vasopressin (DDAVP) as a test of urinary concentrating ability is preferred. Maximum urine osmolality over the next 11 hours is assessed, and any value greater than 700 mOsm/kg is considered normal.[13]

Treatment of central diabetes insipidus in pregnancy is best achieved by using DDAVP, 2 to 20 µg intranasally twice daily. This treatment can be given parenterally after cesarean section, but intravenous dosing is 5- to 20-fold more potent than the intranasal spray. DDAVP is used because it is not degraded by vasopressinase. The amount of DDAVP in breast milk is small, and breast-feeding is not contraindicated. Treatment of central maternal diabetes insipidus with DDAVP throughout pregnancy does not pose a risk to the infant.[14]

Labor proceeds normally in women with central diabetes insipidus, and surges of oxytocin can be detected during labor and the puerperium. This suggests that women with central diabetes insipidus, although they are vasopressin deficient, still secrete oxytocin normally. Lactation is not impaired.

Nephrogenic Diabetes Insipidus

The second type of diabetes insipidus seen in pregnancy is the nephrogenic type. Nephrogenic diabetes insipidus is a rare X-linked disorder caused by a mutation in the vasopressin V_2 receptor gene. At least six mutations in this gene have been identified, and direct mutation analysis can now be used for carrier detection and early prenatal diagnosis.[15] The discovery of aquaporin-1 has answered the long-standing biophysical question of how water specifically crosses biologic membranes: Aquaporin-1 and aquaporin-2 act as water channels. In the kidney, at least seven aquaporins are expressed at distal sites. They are extremely abundant in the proximal tubule and the descending thin limb and are essential for urinary concentration. Aquaporin-2 is found mainly in the connecting tubule and collecting duct and is a predominant vasopressin-regulating water channel. Lack of functional aquaporin-2 is seen in primary forms of diabetes insipidus, and reduced expression of the aquaporin-2 and targeting is seen in diseases associated with urinary concentrating defects.[16] Nonpregnant women with nephrogenic diabetes insipidus are usually treated with a thiazide diuretic or chlorpropamide. Chlorpropamide stimulates vasopressin release and enhances its action on the renal tubule. If used during pregnancy, it may cause fetal hypoglycemia and neonatal diabetes insipidus, and therefore it should not be taken by pregnant women. Thiazide diuretics are the treatment of choice in nephrogenic diabetes insipidus in pregnancy.[17]

Transient Vasopressin-Resistant Diabetes Insipidus in Pregnancy

Transient vasopressin-resistant diabetes insipidus in pregnancy is caused by increased vasopressinase activity, which is caused by either increased placental production of the enzyme or the decreased hepatic vasopressinase metabolism from liver damage. The latter is the most common type and occurs in the third trimester in the setting of transient disturbances of liver function, such as acute fatty liver of pregnancy, preeclampsia (particularly the syndrome of hemolysis, elevation of liver enzyme levels, and low platelet counts [HELLP]), and hepatitis.[18] Treatment of transient vasopressin-resistant diabetes insipidus in pregnancy requires DDAVP, because DDAVP is not degraded by vasopressinase. Close attention to electrolyte and fluid balance is important in the postpartum period. The symptoms of transient vasopressin-resistant diabetes insipidus resolve in a few days to a few weeks after delivery or when hepatic function returns to normal.

The Empty Sella Syndrome in Pregnancy

The empty sella syndrome is a radiographic diagnosis made when there is incompetence of the diaphragma sellae, which allows cerebrospinal fluid to enter the sella and flatten the pituitary gland. The incompetence of the diaphragma sellae may be congenital or it may follow tumor erosion, increased intracranial pressure surgery, or even irradiation. Pituitary function is usually normal, and fertility is not impaired. The empty sella syndrome has been described with varying degrees of hypopituitarism, and hyperprolactinemia has been reported. Pregnancy in a woman with the empty sella syndrome is usually uneventful, although a case of pregnancy-associated osteoporosis in conjunction with the empty sella syndrome has been described.[19]

Pituitary Tumors in Pregnancy

Several distinct types of tumors can occur in the pituitary gland, but pituitary adenomas derived from the adenohypophyseal cells are the most common in pregnancy and represent 15% of all intracranial tumors. Pituitary adenomas are often classified on the basis of either immuno-electromicroscopic features or size (e.g., microadenomas are less than 10 mm in diameter and macroadenomas are larger than 10 mm in diameter). Classification on the basis of size has a practical application with regard to the management of prolactinomas in pregnancy.

The incidence of prolactinoma is approximately 1 case per 1000 women. Estrogen produced by the placenta can stimulate lactotroph DNA synthesis and mitotic activity. Because estrogen stimulates lactotroph function, the effects of both pregnancy and estrogen therapy, including oral contraceptive use, have been intensively studied by several groups. The Pituitary Adenoma Study Group suggested that no increase in risk for prolactinoma formation occurs as a result of oral contraceptive use.[20] The benign course of pituitary microadenoma that secretes prolactin in pregnancy has been emphasized by large series, including that of Molitch (Table 8–3).[21]

Prolactin-Secreting Pituitary Microadenomas

All the large series of cases in particular found that pregnant women in whom ovulation was induced by bromocriptine usually had an uneventful course, although about 1% had symptomatic complications such as headache or visual field defects. Serial MRI studies of women with microadenoma in pregnancy have shown that most

TABLE 8–3   Effect of Pregnancy on Prolactin-Secreting Microadenomas and Macroadenomas

| Type of Prolactinoma | Number | Tumor Enlargement | |
		Symptomatic (%)	Asymptomatic (%)
Microadenoma, untreated	246	1.6	4.5
Macroadenoma, treated	46	4.4	0
Macroadenoma, untreated	45	15.5	8.9

From Molitch ME: Pregnancy and the hyperprolactinemic woman. N Engl J Med 1985;312:1366. Reprinted by permission from the New England Journal of Medicine.

microadenomas enlarged slightly during pregnancy but did not become symptomatic. Molitch, in a survey of 16 prolactinomas in pregnancy, illustrated well the difference between prolactin-secreting microadenoma and the macroadenoma responses to pregnancy (see Table 8–3).[21] These large series of cases have also provided a rational approach to management.

Women who have hyperprolactinemia caused by microadenoma can conceive after the use of dopamine agonists such as bromocriptine, pergolide, or the longer acting cabergoline, as well as quinagolide. Some women have adverse effects from all of these or are resistant to dopamine agonist therapy; for this group, other options include GnRH pulsatile therapy or human menopausal gonadotropin induction of ovulation or transsphenoidal surgery. Bromocriptine is the treatment of choice because it produces a high ovulation rate (80% to 90%) and carries a low risk for adenoma enlargement. Transsphenoidal surgery carries a high morbidity rate and induced ovulation in only 60% of treated women; the rate of recurrence of hyperprolactinemia was 25% to 50% over 4 or 5 years of follow-up.[22]

If ovulation induction is achieved with a dopamine agonist, then microadenomas have a low risk (less than 1%) of complications related to pituitary expansion during pregnancy. In view of this low risk, the use of the dopamine agonist can be discontinued upon confirmation of pregnancy. Because of the low risk for microadenoma enlargement, routine periodic visual field testing is not cost effective. In addition, because prolactin production in pregnancy is both pituitary and decidual, prolactin levels are variable, and monitoring of microadenoma activity by serial estimation of prolactin has little value. Visual field testing or MRI should be reserved for the rare woman with a microadenoma who develops symptoms of tumor enlargement, such as headaches or visual field changes.

Unexpected spontaneous remission of hyperprolactinemia has been noted after delivery in 40% to 65% of women with microadenoma, particularly if their prepregnancy levels of prolactin were lower than 60 µg/L. It is therefore ironic that for many women with a microadenoma, pregnancy may be more of a treatment than a hazard. Breast-feeding should be encouraged because postpartum tumor regression has been seen on radiologic evaluation in lactating women.[23]

Because dopamine agonists are often used both to induce ovulation in hyperprolactinemic women and prophylactically during pregnancy to prevent macroadenoma enlargement, there has been a great interest in the safety of bromocriptine in pregnancy. Bromocriptine freely crosses the placenta, and a report on fetal and neonatal outcome were published by Krupp and Turkalj from the Bromocriptine Registry.[24] The rates of spontaneous abortion (11.2%), multiple pregnancies (1.8%), congenital malformations (major, 1%; minor, 2.5%) were similar to the corresponding rates seen in unexposed pregnancies. Long-term follow-up studies have confirmed these initial findings, and postnatal development of children up to 5 years of age is normal. Fewer data are available on the safety of cabergoline, quinagolide, and pergolide; initial studies have shown no adverse effects of these agents on fetal or neonatal outcome, but there are no long-term follow-up studies.

Prolactin-Secreting Macroadenoma in Pregnancy

Management of prolactin-secreting macroadenoma differs from the management of microadenoma during pregnancy because symptomatic tumor enlargement is greater (16%) in women with macroadenoma (see Table 8–3). The risk is still low in women who were treated with either irradiation or surgery before conceiving (4%). In untreated women with macroadenoma larger than 1 cm, visual field defects often occur during pregnancy (Fig. 8–2).

The Bromocriptine Study Group suggested that bromocriptine or another dopamine agonist be the initial choice for the management of women with macroadenoma who wish to conceive. Surgery or irradiation should be reserved for cases in which bromocriptine fails to reduce

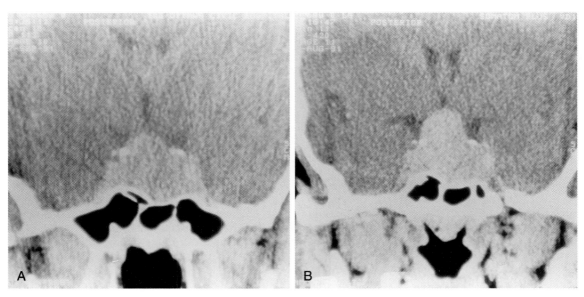

Figure 8–2. Prolactin-secreting pituitary macroadenoma during pregnancy. **A,** Computed tomographic scan before pregnancy. **B,** Computed tomographic scan at 34 weeks, showing onset of bitemporal hemianopsia.

tumor size or causes excessive adverse effects, or for cases with sudden visual deterioration. Response to dopamine agonist therapy should be documented by repeated imaging before conception. Although it may be safe to discontinue bromocriptine for the first trimester, the risk of tumor enlargement and the safety record of bromocriptine make it more desirable to continue the therapy throughout the pregnancy, or at least to restart it in the second or third trimester. De Wit and Coelingh Bennink showed that bromocriptine prophylaxis during pregnancy in women with prolactin-secreting macroadenoma prevents symptomatic enlargement.[25] If bromocriptine prophylactic therapy is not used during pregnancy, women with macroadenoma require careful monitoring, including monthly Goldmann perimetric visual-field assessment and MRI confirmation in cases of suspected macroadenoma enlargement (see Fig. 8-2). Clinically, macroadenoma enlargement in pregnancy manifests with headache, visual-field defects, diabetes insipidus, or, in rare cases, pituitary apoplexy. The last sign can occur at any time during pregnancy but it is more likely to occur during the third trimester. If enlargement of the macroadenoma is proven, bromocriptine should be the initial treatment of choice. Other therapeutic possibilities include dexamethasone treatment, transsphenoidal pituitary surgery, or delivery if deterioration occurs late in the third trimester.

Labor and delivery are usually uneventful, although it has been suggested that women with evidence of macroadenoma expansion should deliver electively by forceps because intracerebral pressure may be markedly increased by maternal pushing. Breast-feeding does not cause macroadenomas to enlarge and should therefore be encouraged.

Acromegaly in Pregnancy

Acromegaly complicating a pregnancy is rare, the prevalence being 5 cases per 100,000 persons. Pregnancy in patients with acromegaly are uncommon because 85% of these women have disturbances of ovulation, associated primarily with hyperprolactinemia and impaired gonadotropin secretion. Excess growth hormone may also result in maternal diabetes, hypertension, and left ventricular hypertrophy, which may deter the woman from attempting a pregnancy. Acromegaly is usually caused by a growth hormone–secreting pituitary adenoma. In rare cases, it may be caused by a GHRH-secreting tumor of the pancreas. Enlargement of growth hormone–secreting pituitary adenomas has been reported in pregnancy but is unusual; it manifests with visual field impairment, which often resolves spontaneously after delivery.[26]

Before pregnancy is considered, active acromegaly should be treated by surgical removal of the adenoma, followed by adjunct radiation or medical therapy if complete surgical ablation is not possible. Bromocriptine therapy normalizes growth hormone levels in only 50% of acromegalic women, and it has little effect on tumor size. Long-acting somatostatin analogs are the medical treatment of choice in acromegaly, and successful pregnancies after treatment with the analog octreotide have been reported. Data on the use of octreotide during pregnancy are limited, but most publications show no side effects of mother or fetus.[27] Conventional radioimmunoassays for growth hormone cannot distinguish between normal pituitary growth hormone and the placental growth hormone variant. Therefore, these assays may yield misleading results, especially in the latter half of the pregnancy, when basal levels of the variant are considerably higher than normal nonpregnant growth hormone levels. There are two physiologic differences between placental growth hormone secretion and pituitary growth hormone secretion in acromegaly: (1) Pituitary growth hormone in acromegaly is highly pulsatile, whereas secretion of the pregnancy growth hormone variant is nonpulsatile, and (2) placental growth hormone also does not respond to TRH stimulation.[21]

Maternal growth hormone does not cross the placenta, and elevated maternal growth hormone levels have little effect on fetal growth and development. Macrosomia has been reported in infants of mothers with active acromegaly, but this is because acromegaly is associated with elevated maternal glucose levels. Overt diabetes mellitus has been noted in 10% to 20% of patients with acromegaly.

Adrenocorticotropic Hormone–Secreting Pituitary Tumors

Cushing's disease caused by a pituitary ACTH-secreting pituitary adenoma is discussed in the section "Adrenal Disorders."

Thyrotropin-Secreting Pituitary Adenomas

A successful pregnancy in an infertile woman with a TSH-secreting pituitary macroadenoma has been reported. Before the pregnancy, the woman was treated with octreotide, which resulted in a euthyroid state and reduced the size of the macroadenoma. Octreotide therapy was discontinued during pregnancy, but symptomatic adenoma enlargement occurred in the second trimester and octreotide therapy was restarted. It thus seems that octreotide is effective in controlling TSH-secreting macroadenoma during pregnancy, and in spite of transplacental passage of octreotide, no abnormalities in neonatal thyroid variables were found.[28]

Gonadotropin-Secreting Pituitary Adenomas in Pregnancy

Pregnancy has been reported in a woman with a combined FSH- and prolactin-secreting pituitary macroadenoma after cabergoline treatment.[29]

Clinically Nonfunctioning Pituitary Tumors in Pregnancy

Although clinically "nonfunctioning" tumors appear to be functionless, most do produce glycoprotein subunits. Often these tumors are quite large, and they can produce mass effects. There have been reports of visual field defects in women with clinically nonfunctioning tumors larger than 1.2 cm in height. Thus, in pregnancy, these patients need to be monitored in a manner similar to that of patients presenting with prolactin-secreting macroadenoma.[30]

Craniopharyngioma can manifest in pregnancy. A 39-year-old woman experienced symptoms from a craniopharyngioma diagnosed during a pregnancy that had resulted from in vitro fertilization. An MRI scan from 4 years previously had disclosed nothing abnormal. The patient underwent a right frontotemporal craniotomy with total resection of the suprasellar tumor, and the pregnancy was otherwise unremarkable. This case suggests that there might be a possible link in the adult patient between the growth of the supposedly congenital tumor and hormone stimulation of pregnancy.[31]

Pituitary Surgery during Pregnancy

Transsphenoidal surgery has become the treatment of choice of all microadenomas and also of macroadenomas that are not responsive to medical treatment or that are producing signs or symptoms of enlargement. At least 10 instances of transsphenoidal surgery during pregnancy have been reported (in five women with Cushing's disease, one woman with Nelson's syndrome, one woman with acromegaly, and three women with enlarging prolactinomas). There was no increase in fetal or maternal morbidity or mortality in any of these cases.[22]

Nelson's Syndrome in Pregnancy

In 1958, Nelson and colleagues reported the occurrence of an ACTH-secreting pituitary adenoma with associated hyperpigmentation and visual field disturbances after bilateral adrenalectomy for Cushing's disease.[31a] The occurrence of Nelson's syndrome is rarely reported in pregnancy. The pregnancy can be complicated by symptomatic enlargement of the tumor. Transsphenoidal surgery has been performed in pregnancy in this situation with a successful outcome for both mother and fetus.[32]

Lymphocytic Hypophysitis

Lymphocytic hypophysitis is a rare but intriguing autoimmune condition of the pituitary gland that usually manifests in the peripartum period. Most autoimmune diseases improve during pregnancy; thus, an autoimmune disorder of the pituitary that manifests, in most instances, in association with pregnancy, during pregnancy, or after delivery is highly unusual. Clinically in the peripartum period, the manifestation is that of a mass lesion that is indistinguishable from a pituitary adenoma. The pituitary gland is infiltrated by lymphocytes and plasma cells with associated destruction of the normal tissue. Affected women therefore present with symptoms of various degrees of hypopituitarism, headaches, or visual field defects and occasionally hyperprolactinemia and diabetes insipidus.[33] In terms of the hypopituitarism, ACTH-, TSH-, and prolactin-producing cells seem to be most affected. Indeed, severe lymphocytic adenohypophysitis with selective disappearance of prolactin cells has been reported.[34] The pathophysiologic process seems to be that of circulating antihypophyseal antibodies.[35] One of the antibodies has been identified as the 49-kDa autoantigen that has also been identified as an α-enolase. α-Enolase autoantibodies

are not specific to pituitary autoimmune disease and have been reported in other autoimmune diseases. This disorder can progress to chronic panhypopituitarism, but in some cases, it is reversible; subsequent spontaneous pregnancies have been reported. Pregnancy-related relapse of the disease does not seem to occur in subsequent pregnancies. The differential diagnosis includes an enlarging pituitary adenoma and the Sheehan's syndrome. Absolute differentiation from pituitary adenoma requires a pituitary biopsy. In most cases, CT scanning shows uniform contrast enhancement. Because of the preferential destruction of some cells, early striking diffuse homogenous contrast enhancement on MRI has been noted; therefore, MRI seems to be more helpful than CT scanning in differentiating between this disorder and an enlarging pituitary adenoma. On occasion, the pituitary stalk is involved, and MRI shows thickening of the pituitary stalk. This condition is known as "stalkitis" and has been associated with recurrent optic neuritis.[36]

Treatment of lymphocytic hypophysitis, once it has been diagnosed, requires correction of the hypopituitarism. A short course of high-dosage corticosteroids can produce a dramatic resolution of visual field defects in some women, but this response is not always obtained.[37] Postpartum response to corticosteroids can be dramatic, and medical management may be more suitable than previously thought.[38] In women who do not respond to corticosteroids, surgical decompression by partial hypophysectomy may be required. Unless the patient has visual field defects, uncontrollable headaches, or radiologic evidence of progressive enlargement of the sellar mass, rapid surgical intervention is not warranted, because some women may undergo spontaneous regression of the mass and have regained pituitary function post partum.

Hypopituitarism in Pregnancy

Women with chronic hypopituitarism, regardless of the cause (Table 8–4), have a normal pregnancy and spontaneous labor after induction of ovulation if they receive adequate replacement with corticosteroids, thyroxine, and vasopressin alone.[39] Women whose hypopituitarism is diagnosed before they conceive generally have a good pregnancy outcome. Undiagnosed or poorly treated hypopituitarism carries an increased risk of spontaneous abortion, stillbirth, and maternal morbidity from hypotension and hypoglycemia.[40] Hypopituitarism may manifest for the first time during a pregnancy, particularly during the third trimester, and the most likely causes of hypopituitarism in pregnancy are shown in Table 8–4. Making a clinical diagnosis of hypopituitarism occurring for the first time

TABLE 8–4   Hypopituitarism Associated with Pregnancy

Diabetic peripartum necrosis
Enlarging prolactin-secreting macroadenoma
Lymphocytic hypophysitis and "stalkitis"
Histiocytosis X
Sheehan's syndrome

in pregnancy is difficult because the symptoms in most include vomiting and fatigue and are common in normal pregnancy. Presenting clinical features are often severe such as central frontal headaches, visual field changes, or diabetes insipidus. Dynamic testing of pituitary function during pregnancy is very difficult to interpret, as there are no standard ranges but the hypothalamic-pituitary-adrenal and pituitary-thyroidal axes can be tested by a combined CRH/TRH challenge test. The physiologic changes that occur in ACTH and TSH levels during normal pregnancy should be considered when the test results are interpreted. MRI is most useful in distinguishing a pituitary adenoma from lymphocytic hypophysitis.

The treatment of hypopituitarism during pregnancy consists of hormone replacement therapy. Secondary hypoadrenalism requires maintenance doses of a corticosteroid such as cortisone acetate 25 mg AM and 12.5 mg PM. Parenteral corticosteroids are required to cover the stress of labor and cesarian section, emesis, intercurrent disease and infection that may occur during pregnancy. An added mineralocorticoid is not usually required because the renin-angiotensin-aldosterone system is intact. Normal thyroid function is maintained by thyroxine replacement. There is some controversy as to whether the dosage of thyroxine requires an increase in pregnancy, but because of the increased thyroxine turnover that occurs during pregnancy some investigators have found the main increase of thyroxine needs to be about 0.05 mg per day.[41] The management of diabetes insipidus requires DDAVP.

Sheehan's Syndrome

Severe hemorrhage, shock, or hypotension at delivery may lead to postpartum pituitary necrosis or the Sheehan's syndrome (Table 8–4).[42] The syndrome is, fortunately, less common now as a result of improved obstetric practice and a reduction in postpartum hemorrhage. Sheehan himself estimated the incidence at less than 1 per 10,000 deliveries.[43]

The pathogenesis of Sheehan's syndrome is still not completely clear. Sheehan believed that the primary vascular disturbance is spasm of the arterial supply to the anterior lobe of the pituitary gland. This results in pituitary gland ischemia and edema, which further compromises the circulation, leading to cellular necrosis and thrombosis in the portal sinuses and capillaries.

Usually, only anterior pituitary function is affected, because the posterior pituitary gland and hypothalamus are supplied by the inferior hypophyseal arteries and the circle of Willis, which makes them less vulnerable to ischemic necrosis. However, some women with Sheehan's syndrome have an impairment of antidiuretic hormone secretion that may lead to partial or overt diabetes insipidus.[44]

After destruction of 95% to 99% of the anterior pituitary gland, the disease is characterized by postpartum failure of lactation, secondary amenorrhea, loss of axillary and pubic hair, genital and breast atrophy, and increasing signs of secondary hypothyroidism and adrenocortical insufficiency. Because mineralocorticoid secretion is not impaired, there are usually no electrolyte disturbances. However, hyponatremia has been reported in conjunction with

Sheehan's syndrome and appears to be secondary to inappropriate antidiuretic hormone secretion.[45]

Less extensive pituitary destruction (50% to 95%) is associated with an atypical form of the disease with loss of one or more trophic hormones. The pattern of loss of trophic hormones is unpredictable, but in some instances, gonadotropin secretion may be preserved and pregnancy is possible.[46] Postpartum diagnosis of Sheehan's syndrome requires dynamic provocative testing of both anterior and posterior lobes of the pituitary. The anterior pituitary gland function is best assessed with pituitary hormone response to standard stimulatory tests in conjunction with pituitary imaging with axial CT scanning or MRI. Posterior pituitary function in Sheehan's syndrome can be studied with plasma vasopressin response to osmotic stimuli either during 5% hypotonic saline infusion or after a water deprivation test. Spontaneous recovery from hypopituitarism caused by postpartum hemorrhage has also been reported.

ADRENAL DISORDERS IN PREGNANCY

The Adrenal Cortex

During pregnancy, increased steroid hormone production is essential for meeting both the maternal need for increased levels of estrogens and cortisol and the fetal need for reproductive and somatic growth development. In addition, alterations in the renin-angiotensin-aldosterone cascade are necessary to allow for a 50% increase in maternal blood volume without resulting in hypertension. These changes occur through a complex interaction among maternal and fetal endocrine systems in the placenta.

Changes in Adrenal Anatomy and Physiology during Pregnancy

The normal adult adrenal gland weighs approximately 5 g, and during pregnancy it increases only slightly in size. Histologically, the zona fasciculata (glucocorticoids) widens during pregnancy, which is suggestive of increased secretion. The zona glomerulosa (mineralocorticoids) and the zona reticularis (androgens) remain unchanged in width.

Control of the Adrenal Cortex during Pregnancy

CRH is secreted from the hypothalamus as well as from the lungs, liver, gastrointestinal tract, adrenal glands, and placenta.[47] CRH releases pro-opiomelanocortin and its breakdown products, including ACTH from the anterior pituitary gland. Release of CRH from the hypothalamus is stimulated by stress, volume contraction, and other factors and is inhibited by glucocorticoids and ACTH.

During pregnancy, maternal CRH levels increase dramatically, predominantly as a result of placental production.[48] Placental CRH enters both the maternal and fetal circulation. Placental CRH production is stimulated by circulating glucocorticoids, which is in contrast to the negative feedback of the hypothalamic production of CRH.

Placental CRH entering the fetal circulation may stimulate the fetal hypothalamic-pituitary-adrenal axis, and this in turn may play a role in fetal organ maturation and also parturition.[49]

During pregnancy, ACTH levels increase approximately twofold after the first trimester (Table 8–5). This increase is, in part, placental in origin and may be a local paracrine effect of placental CRH production. Placental ACTH is not suppressible by glucocorticoids. The normal circadian rhythm of high morning and low evening levels of ACTH and cortisol continues throughout pregnancy.[6] The stress of labor causes ACTH levels to increase rapidly and then decrease within 2 days post partum.

Cortisol circulates both free and bound (primarily to cortisol-binding globulin). Both total cortisol (as measured by serum cortisol) and free cortisol (as measured by 24-hour urinary free cortisol) increase in pregnancy. Serum cortisol levels increase twofold to threefold during pregnancy. The increase in serum cortisol in pregnancy results mainly from the increase in corticosteroid-binding globulin levels. However, increased free and total cortisol levels in pregnancy may also be related to resetting of the sensitivity of the hypothalamic-pituitary-adrenal axis and not merely to raised corticosteroid-binding globulin, progesterone, or CRH levels.[50]

Exogenous corticosteroids are variably affected by placental enzymatic activity, and thus have different rates of placental transfer (Table 8–6) when these medications are prescribed, because maternal and fetal availabilities differ. Because glucocorticoids such as dexamethasone increase placental CRH and placental ACTH activity, the dexamethasone suppression test is unreliable in pregnancy.[51]

The Renin-Angiotension-Aldosterone System in Pregnancy

The renin-angiotensin-aldosterone system is a cascade of events that regulates blood pressure, circulating blood volume, and sodium-potassium homeostasis. Renin production from the juxtaglomerular apparatus in the kidney is controlled by a renal arteriolar blood pressure, sodium concentration in the distal tubule, and β-adrenergic receptors.

Aldosterone is the major circulating mineralocorticoid and controls reabsorption of sodium and excretion of potassium and bicarbonate in the distal renal tubule. Its secretion is controlled primarily by angiotensin II, but hyperkalemia, ACTH, and vasopressin are also stimulants.[52]

During pregnancy, the woman must increase plasma volume and, thus, also sodium reabsorption without increasing blood pressure. Despite the increase in extracellular fluid volume, plasma renin activity levels increase fourfold between 8 and 20 weeks of pregnancy, after which they plateau (Table 8–7).

Angiotension II levels are increased threefold as a result of increased renin and angiotensinogen. However, resistance to the pressure effect of angiotensin II develops by 7 weeks of pregnancy and reaches a maximum at 28 weeks; after 30 weeks, there is some return of sensitivity. This does not reach values seen in the nonpregnant state.[53]

Aldosterone levels in pregnancy increase fourfold by 8 weeks and continue to increase, reaching a 10-fold increase by term. This is in response to increased renin and angiotensin II levels.[54]

Disorders of the Adrenal Cortex

Cushing's Syndrome

Cushing's syndrome is caused by excess glucocorticoid production of any cause. It may be caused by excess ACTH

TABLE 8–6 Maternal and Fetal Distribution of Synthetic Steroids

Steroid	Maternal : Fetal Concentration Ratio
Prednisone	10 : 1
Hydrocortisone	6 : 1
Betamethasone	3 : 1
Dexamethasone	2 : 1

Adapted from Garner PR: Disorders of the adrenal cortex. In Lee R (ed): Current Obstetric Medicine, vol 2. St. Louis, Mosby, 1993, pp 183-220.

TABLE 8–5 Normal Plasma Free Cortisol, Urinary Free Cortisol, and Plasma ACTH Concentrations in Pregnancy

	Nonpregnant	Third Trimester
Total cortisol		
09.00 hr	11.34 ± 3.5 mg/mL (324 ± 100 nmol/L)	36.0 ± 7 mg/mL (1029 ± 200 nmol/L)
24.00 hr	3.6 ± 2.6 mg/mL (103 ± 76 nmol/L)	23.5 ± 4.34 mg/mL (470 ± 124 nmol/L)
Plasma free cortisol		
09.00 hr	0.63 ± 0.3 mg/mL (18 ± 9 nmol/L)	1.33 ± 0.4 mg/mL (38 ± 12 nmol/L)
24.00 hr	0.2 ± 0.14 mg/mL (6 ± 4 nmol/L)	0.59 ± 0.17 mg/mL (17 ± 5 nmol/L)
Urinary free cortisol	4.7-95 mg/day (13-256 nmol/day)	82.4-244.8 mg/day (229-680 nmol/day)
Plasma ACTH	15-70 pg/mL (3.3-15.4 pmol/L)	20-120 pg/mL (4.4-26.4 pmol/L)

ACTH, adrenocorticotropic hormone.

TABLE 8–7 Renin-Aldosterone System in Normal Pregnancy

	Nonpregnant State	First Trimester	Second Trimester	Third Trimester
Plasmin renin activity (mg/mL/hr)	1.4 ± 0.3	4.1 ± 0.4	4.1 ± 0.7	4.2 ± 0.6
Plasma aldosterone (mg/dL)	6.2 ± 2.2	22 ± 2	30 ± 5	60 ± 12
Urinary aldosterone (mg/day)	10 ± 8	34 ± 8	80 ± 14	105 ± 20

Data from Wilson M, Morganti AA, Zervoudakis I, et al: Blood pressure, the renin-aldosterone system and sex steroids throughout normal pregnancy. Am J Med 1980;68:97, and Hsueh WA, Leutscher JA, Carlson EJ, et al: Changes in active and inactive renin throughout pregnancy. J Clin Endocrinol Metab 1982;54:1010.

stimulation of the adrenal cortex (ACTH-dependent Cushing's syndrome). If the ACTH is from a pituitary adenoma, the disorder is known as Cushing's disease. ACTH may also come from ectopic sources. Cushing's syndrome may be independent of ACTH, as seen in adrenal adenoma or carcinoma and glucocorticoid therapy. Cushing's syndrome in pregnancy is rare, because women with ACTH-dependent cases have a 75% to 95% incidence of menstrual irregularities and anovulation.[55] The causes of Cushing's syndrome in pregnancy are very different from those in the nonpregnant state, and adrenal causes of Cushing's syndrome are overrepresented in relation to ACTH-dependent causes (Table 8–8).

Clinical diagnosis of Cushing's syndrome in pregnancy may be difficult because several features of hypercortisolemia such as moon facies, abdominal striae, and glucose intolerance are common during pregnancy. Clues to diagnosis of Cushing's syndrome in pregnancy are that the striae tend to be wider, greater than 1 cm, and darker than normal and tend to occur in sites other than the abdominal wall. The presence of proximal myopathy, hypertension, neuropsychiatric disturbances, hirsutism, acne and spontaneous bruising are all informative clues.

Diagnosis

The diagnosis of Cushing's syndrome is often difficult to make in the nonpregnant state, and its diagnosis is even more challenging during pregnancy because of the altered hypothalamic-pituitary-adrenal axis and placental production of CRH and ACTH. As in the nonpregnant state, investigation should occur in three stages: (1) screening test for hypercortisolemia; (2) biochemical diagnosis; and (3) determination of the cause.

The best screening test in pregnancy is a 24-hour urine collection for free cortisol. Because the urinary free cortisol range differs in pregnancy, the higher reference range found in Table 8–6 should be utilized. The diurnal variation of plasma cortisol may also be used because it is unaffected by pregnancy. The 1.0-mg overnight dexamethasone suppression test does not yield accurate results in patients during pregnancy because placental ACTH is not suppressed by glucocorticoids.

If the urinary free cortisol tests suggest hypercortisolemia, a 2-day low-dose dexamethasone test can be used (0.5 mg every 6 hours). Dexamethasone is safer to use in pregnancy because the maternal:fetal concentrations

are 2:1.[56] During pregnancy, urinary free cortisol concentrations should be suppressed to less than 55 nmol for 24 hours.

After hypercortisolemia is confirmed, its cause must be established. ACTH is measured to differentiate ACTH-dependent from ACTH-independent causes. Because of placental production, levels of ACTH are increased in pregnancy. If Cushing's syndrome is ACTH dependent, then MRI of the pituitary gland should follow. If Cushing's syndrome is ACTH independent, MRI of the adrenal glands is indicated. MRI is preferred for both pituitary and adrenal lesions because of its specificity and lack of ionizing radiation. Bilateral inferior petrosal sinus corticotropin sampling with CRH stimulation may also be helpful in the differential diagnosis of Cushing's syndrome. An increase of more than 50% in ACTH or more than 20% in cortisol after 1 μg of ovine CRH per kilogram of body weight suggests a pituitary source. Comparison of plasma ACTH levels in the venous drainage of the pituitary gland with peripheral values allows localization and lateralization within the pituitary gland. A modified approach through brachial rather than femoral veins to reduce the radiation exposure is preferred. However, case reports have demonstrated that the procedure of bilateral simultaneous inferior petrosal corticotropin sampling can safely be performed in pregnancy.[57]

Treatment

Untreated Cushing's syndrome during pregnancy has a poor fetal and maternal outcome. The outcome is greatly improved when hypercortisolemia is treated. Transsphenoidal surgery is preferred for ACTH-dependent pituitary adenoma. For adrenal lesions, unilateral adrenalectomy during pregnancy decreases neonatal complications. This should be undertaken unless a diagnosis is made late in pregnancy.[58] Cortisol replacement is required after both adrenal and pituitary surgery and should be continued until the hypothalamic-pituitary axis has had time to recover. High-dosage corticosteroid therapy should be utilized at times of stress such as delivery.

If surgical therapy is contraindicated, then medical therapy may be considered. Both metyrapone and ketoconazole have been used in pregnancy but in only a few cases. Therefore, the fetal risks of both these agents are not fully known.[59]

The optimal treatment for adrenal carcinoma in pregnancy has not been established. If the carcinoma is diagnosed during the first trimester, therapeutic termination of pregnancy should be considered, with definitive therapy after surgery and chemotherapy. If the carcinoma is identified during the second trimester, adrenalectomy may be performed, followed by postoperative ketoconazole or metyrapone therapy. In the third trimester, ketoconazole or metyrapone can be used until delivery is feasible and then followed by definitive surgery and chemotherapy post partum. Unfortunately, in spite of the use of surgery and chemotherapy, the maternal prognosis remains grim, although fetal prognosis is good.

Primary Hyperaldosteronism in Pregnancy

Primary hyperaldosteronism is the excess production of aldosterone from the adrenal cortex that causes

---

TABLE 8–8   Causes of Cushing's Syndrome in Nonpregnant and Pregnant Women

Cause	Nonpregnant Women (%)	Pregnant Women (%)
ACTH-dependent ectopic tumor	16	2
Pituitary adenoma	59	33
ACTH-independent adrenal adenoma	16	50
ACTH-independent adrenal carcinoma	9	10
Unknown	—	5

Adapted from Buescher MA, McClamrock HD, Adashi EY: Cushing syndrome in pregnancy. Obstet Gynecol 1992;79:130.

hypertension, hypokalemia, and bicarbonate retention (metabolic alkalosis). It is a very rare cause of secondary hypertension in pregnancy. Between 60% and 70% of cases during pregnancy are caused by a unilateral benign adrenal adenoma.[60]

Clinical Presentation and Diagnosis

Hypertension in association with hypokalemia is a classic presentation but 40% of women have normal potassium levels. Very low potassium levels may cause their symptoms of a headache, muscular weakness and cramps, and fatigue. Serum sodium levels are high normal and metabolic alkalosis is present. Normally in pregnancy, there is a respiratory alkalosis with a compensatory decrease in bicarbonate of 4 mEq/L. Thus, in pregnancy, bicarbonate levels must be compared to the reference range of 18 to 22 mEq/L. If hypokalemia is present, urinary potassium levels greater than 30 mmol/24 hours are necessary to confirm renal potassium wasting. Before further biochemical testing is done, the hypokalemia should be corrected and the use of any medications that suppress renin, such as β blockers, calcium-channel blockers, and spironolactone, must be discontinued. Methyldopa (Aldomet) may be used to control the hypertension during investigations.[61]

The normal increase in aldosterone into the hyperaldosteronism range during pregnancy makes baseline plasma aldosterone levels difficult to interpret (see Table 8–7). Plasma renin levels should be decreased in primary hyperaldosteronism and are increased during pregnancy. In pregnant patients with primary hyperaldosteronism, renin levels are suppressed and are therefore helpful in diagnosis.

Ordinarily, to confirm autonomous mineralocorticoid secretion, salt-loading studies are done. In pregnancy, however, there is a risk of volume overload and worsening hypokalemia, and there is also a lack of established diagnostic criteria, all of which limit the usefulness of this test in pregnancy. The response to the upright position is maintained in pregnancy, but, again, normal values for renin stimulation have not yet been established in pregnancy.

Imaging should be done after biochemical confirmation, and MRI is the preferred imaging tool.

Treatment

In pregnancy, the use of medical therapy to reduce the risk of inhibiting production or inhibiting the action of aldosterone is difficult because of the risk of adverse fetal effects. In the nonpregnant situation, spironolactone has been used, but in pregnancy there is a concern about the risk of feminization of the male fetus, inasmuch as the drug is a mild antiandrogen. The angiotensin-converting enzyme inhibitors are helpful in nonpregnant women, but they are contraindicated in pregnancy because they carry risks of fetal malformations and neonatal renal failure. Calcium channel blockers have a reducing effect on aldosterone synthesis and release, are safe to use in pregnancy, and are more effective than methyldopa and β blockers.[62]

Surgical removal of an unidentified adrenal adenoma is the treatment of choice. Adrenalectomy performed at 15 and 17 weeks of pregnancy normalized maternal blood pressure, and healthy full-term infants were delivered.

Therefore, if hypertension or if hypokalemia cannot be controlled medically, surgery during the second trimester is definitely warranted.[63]

Androgen-Producing Adrenal Adenomas in Pregnancy

Virilizing adrenal adenomas are rare during the reproductive years. Some androgen-producing adrenal adenomas have been gonadotropin-responsive, but most are associated with amenorrhea and infertility.[64] Androgen-producing adrenal adenomas are very rare in pregnancy. Virilization of infant girls was reported in each case; this suggested that a high maternal-fetal placental transfer of testosterone occurred during the first trimester (7 to 12 weeks), which is when labial fusion and clitoromegaly can develop. Between the second and third trimesters, maternal-fetal transfer of testosterone is minimal as a result of placental aromatization.[65] Maternal signs of androgen-producing adrenal adenomas usually includes increasing hirsutism, alopecia, and vocal change. However, a definitive diagnosis in all the reported cases was undertaken only after the delivery of a virilized female fetus. Surgical therapy at the time of diagnosis is the treatment of choice.

Addison's Disease

Adrenocortical insufficiency (ACIS) is a result of inadequate production of adrenocorticosteroid hormones and may be acute or chronic and primary or secondary. Primary ACIS (Addison's disease) is caused by deficient steroid production as a result of an adrenal lesion, whereas secondary ACIS is a result of understimulation of the adrenal cortex by ACTH. The clinical presentation of ACIS may be insidious, with a prolonged period of partial hormone deficiency that becomes chronic ACIS. This may end in an abrupt crisis of acute ACIS when hormone production falls below a critical point or when the affected individual is stressed by intercurrent illness. Hormone deficiency usually is combined as a result of disease that affects all the three adrenal zones, with decreased production of aldosterone, glucocorticoids, and androgens. On occasion, ACIS may be a result of isolated steroid deficiency, but only decreased production of aldosterone and cortisol have important clinical sequelae. Autoimmune adrenalitis causes 85% of primary ACIS. All three zones of the adrenal cortex exhibit diffuse mononuclear cell infiltration histologically, and adrenal autoantibodies are found in the serum of two thirds of these patients.[66] In addition, more than half of all affected patients show cell immunity against the adrenal cortex. ACTH receptor-blocking antibodies have also been isolated.[67]

The diagnosis of Addison's disease manifesting for the first time in pregnancy may be difficult because some clinical features, such as vomiting, weakness, syncope, and hyperpigmentation, may also accompany normal pregnancies. As mentioned, undiagnosed chronic ACIS may develop into an acute crisis after stress such as hyperemesis gravidarum, infection, or a delivery. Before corticosteroid therapy, the rate of maternal mortality was 77%.[68] With full corticosteroid replacement therapy, maternal morbidity and mortality are substantially lower.

The clinical diagnosis should be contemplated in a pregnancy complicated by excessive vomiting during the first two trimesters or by weakness, hypotension, and hyperpigmentation during early pregnancy or the postpartum period. Hyperpigmentation can be differentiated from the chloasma of pregnancy when the pigmentation is found in the mucous membranes of the mouth, rectum, or vagina; over nonexposed areas; or over extensor surfaces of the body.

Diagnosis of Addison's Disease in Pregnancy

Laboratory diagnosis can be made more difficult by the normal physiologic changes that accompany a pregnancy. Common findings include hyponatremia, hyperkalemia, eosinophilia, hypoglycemia, hypercalcemia, and an elevated blood urea nitrogen level. Plasma cortisol levels may be in the normal nonpregnant range because of the rise in the corticosteroid-binding globulin concentrations in pregnancy. Low baseline plasma or urinary corticosteroid estimation are not adequate for the diagnosis of chronic ACIS. Diagnosis is best made by finding high plasma ACTH levels and low plasma cortisol levels for the stage of pregnancy (Table 8-9). In chronic ACIS, plasma cortisol levels do not respond to cosyntropin (Synacthen), 0.25 mg, given intramuscularly. Basal plasma cortisol levels normally double within 30 minutes of cosyntropin administration.[69]

TABLE 8-9   Diagnosis and Management of Acute Adrenal Insufficiency in Pregnancy

Clinical Signs
Weakness
Hyperpigmentation
Anorexia
Nausea
Vomiting
Hypotension
Abdominal pain

Laboratory Data
Hypoglycemia
Hyponatremia
Hyperkalemia
Azotemia

Diagnosis
Baseline plasma cortisol
ACTH
Electrolytes
BUN
Creatinine
Dexamethasone, 4-6 mg IV
Tetracosactrin, 0.25 mg IM or IV
Plasma cortisol 30 minutes after tetracosactrin

Treatment
Fluid replacement: 5% dextrose/1 L normal saline, over 1-2 hr; then, according to response, 2-5 L over 24 hr
Cortisol replacement: hydrocortisone, 100-200 mg IM or IV; then 100 mg q8h for 24 hr
Taper steroid dosage over 2-3 days, then maintenance

Identification of Precipitating Cause
Coagulation studies
Blood and urine cultures
Antiadrenal antibodies
Adrenal MRI

ACTH, adrenocorticotropic hormone; BUN, blood urea nitrogen; IM, intramuscularly; IV, intravenously; MRI, magnetic resonance imaging.

The traditional methods of evaluating the hypothalamic-pituitary-adrenal axis by a metyrapone test or an insulin-induced hypoglycemia stress test should be avoided in pregnancy. A CRH stimulation test has been found to be of value in diagnosis of primary ACIS in nonpregnant research subjects. Reports suggest a hyperresponsiveness of ACTH to CRH in primary ACIS but a diminished response in pituitary disease. There are no reports of this test being used in pregnancy to date.

Demonstration of adrenal antibodies in the plasma confirms an autoimmune cause, but the concentration of these antibodies may fall during pregnancy. MRI of the adrenal glands may reveal calcification suggestive of a tuberculous or fungal infection as the cause.

Management of Addison's Disease in Pregnancy

As in the nonpregnant state, replacement of glucocorticoids during pregnancy is carried out with cortisol (30 mg/day), cortisone (37.5 mg/day), prednisone (7.5 mg/day), or dexamethasone (0.75 mg/day). The latter two glucocorticoids have very little mineralocorticoid activity. Women with mineralocorticoid deficiency should also receive fludrocortisone, 0.075 to 0.10 mg/day, in addition to the glucocorticoids. Fludrocortisone is usually not necessary in secondary adrenal insufficiency, because mineralocorticoid secretion is not primarily under pituitary control. In primary adrenal insufficiency, the fludrocortisone dosage should be decreased during pregnancy if hypertension or hypokalemia occurs. Careful monitoring of electrolyte levels is required if hyperemesis gravidarum or preeclampsia complicates pregnancy. Glucocorticoid therapy in human pregnancy is not associated with an increase in congenital malformations, although cleft palate has been reported in rabbits. There has been a theoretical concern that the maternal steroid therapy could suppress the fetal hypothalamic-pituitary-adrenal axis, but this has not been upheld on neonatal ACTH stimulation testing.[70] The maternal and fetal distributions of the synthetic steroids are found in Table 8-6.

Long-term follow-up in children exposed to glucocorticoid therapy during gestation has been undertaken. Results of neurologic assessment at 3 and 6 years of age are normal, and psychometric testing reveals no deficit. Somatic growth is also similar to that of control children of similar ages. Maternal glucocorticoid administration should be changed from oral to the parenteral route at times of stress during pregnancy, such as during severe hyperemesis gravidarum, infection, or delivery. A suitable regimen is hydrocortisone sodium succinate, 200 to 300 mg/day intramuscularly or intravenously.

Effect of Chronic Adrenocortical Insufficiency on the Fetal/Neonatal Outcome

In women with undiagnosed chronic ACIS, fetal growth patterns have been found to be suboptimal, but this is not a uniform finding. Maternal antibodies to the adrenal cortex do cross the placenta but not in sufficient concentrations to cause fetal or neonatal adrenal insufficiency. Neonatal hypoglycemia has been reported in rare cases but seldom necessitates intervention, and glucocorticoid therapy in the newborn is not indicated.[71]

Acute Adrenocortical Insufficiency in Pregnancy

Acute ACIS, or addisonian crisis, can occur in pregnancy in women with chronic ACIS who are undergoing stress or in those in whom the disease is undiagnosed. It also may result from any obstetric complication that results in disseminated intravascular coagulation, such as eclampsia, amniotic fluid embolus, or postpartum hemorrhage. The resultant bilateral massive adrenal hemorrhage is an acute emergency manifesting with nausea, vomiting, abdominal pain, and shock, and it is frequently fatal. Death can be prevented by early recognition and treatment. A similar manifestation has been noted in the third trimester of pregnancy or in the postpartum period in association with acute pyelonephritis, gram-negative bacillemia, and fulminant meningococcal infection (Waterhouse-Friderichsen syndrome). The largest series of acute ACIS in pregnancy has been reported by MacGillivray.[72]

Emergency treatment of acute ACIS in pregnancy should include cortisol hemisuccinate, 200 mg intravenously as a bolus, followed by 100 mg in each liter of normal saline solution. The first liter should be given over 30 minutes, and hydration might take 5 to 6 liters. Hypoglycemia should be avoided by a 15-g glucose infusion. Because these patients receive up to 600 mg of cortisol by this method, no additional mineralocorticoid is required.

Congenital Adrenal Hyperplasia in Pregnancy

The congenital adrenal hyperplasias (CAHs) are a group of inherited enzymatic defects of adrenal steroid biosynthesis (Fig. 8–3). Deficiencies of each enzyme required in the steroid biosynthesis pathway are known, and these deficiencies are all inherited as autosomal recessive disorders. During pregnancy, maternal and fetal problems are confined to women who have 21-hydroxylase deficiency (21-OHD), 11-hydroxylase deficiency (11β-OHD), and 3β-hydroxysteroid dehydrogenase deficiency (3β-HSD)

because the other adrenal enzyme deficiencies are not compatible with fertility. The interposition of the placenta on the hypothalamic-pituitary-adrenal axis and other endocrine changes during pregnancy considerably influence the clinical evaluation of the congenital adrenal hyperplasias. Successful management of CAH in pregnancy requires a firm knowledge of normal adrenal, anatomic, and endocrine changes that occur during pregnancy. Women with severe forms of CAH have decreased fertility rates because of oligoovulation, and successful conception often requires a combination of good therapeutic compliance, careful endocrine monitoring, and, often, ovulation induction. Accurate prenatal diagnosis of these three enzyme deficiencies is now possible, which allows prenatal treatment in an attempt to minimize clinical problems in the neonate. Prevention of masculinization of affected female fetuses (i.e., corticosteroid suppression) has been attempted in all three enzyme deficiency states with variable degrees of success. CAH is a relatively common disease occurring 1 per 5000 to 1 per 15,000 births in most populations.[73] 21-OHD has a particularly high frequency among Hispanic persons. Carrier rates of 21-OHD vary between 1.2% and 6% of the population. The gene responsible for the 21-OHD was isolated in 1984; since then, knowledge of the mutations that cause different forms of CAH has grown rapidly. Of clinical importance is that the clinical expression of endocrine disease is not always correlated with the mutations of the primary structural gene. Clinicians therefore cannot accurately predict the cause of the disease or base their decisions on genotype alone.[73]

Pathophysiology of Congenital Adrenal Hyperplasia

CAH is an abnormality of steroid biosynthesis. Most steroidogenetic enzymes belong to the cytochrome P450 group of oxidases.[74] Most cytochrome P450 enzymes can act on multiple substrates and can also catalyze many oxidation steps. This accounts in part for the broad clinical spectrum of steroid hormone deficiency seen in association

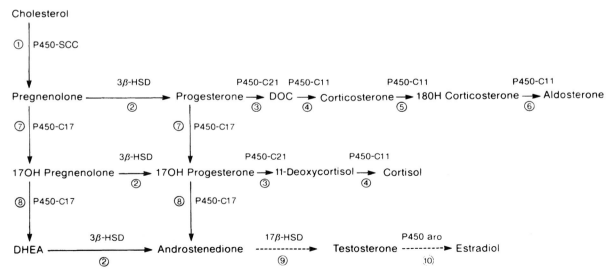

Figure 8–3. Adrenal steroid biosynthesis. HSD, hydroxysteroid dehydrogenase; DOC, deoxycorticosterone; DHEA, dehydroepiandrosterone (8-9).

with a single cytochrome P450 enzyme defect. The P450-C21 enzyme is found in the cellular endoplasmic reticulum. The P450-C11 enzyme is located in the mitochondria. The 3β-HSD enzyme is a non–cytochrome P450 enzyme and is also found in endoplasmic reticulum. The P450-C21 genes (P450-C21A and P450-C21B) are located on the short arm of the chromosome 6 in the middle of the region of the major histocompatibility complex. The P450-C21A gene is nonfunctional and is known as a pseudogene. The P450-C21A pseudogene can exert an effect on the active P450-C21B gene by exchanging DNA, which is known as gene conversion. Because the P450-C21 genes are linked to the HLA locus, this association was used clinically to assess whether the fetus was a CAH carrier or would be affected. However, HLA typing has now been superseded by molecular genetic techniques. Because of the large number of different defects in the P450-C21B gene, this means that most subjects affected with this type of CAH are "compound heterozygotes" and have different genetic lesions found in association with each of the two P450-C21 genes. Thus, the very clinical manifestation of this form of CAH is also determined partly by the different genetic lesions of the P450-C21B gene. Gene conversions are the most common lesions found, but 10% of women with severe forms of CAH have macroconversions that change the P450-C21B gene sequence into one that resembles the P450-C21A sequence. The majority of women with severe disease (75%) have microconversions. Random gene deletions, insertions, and point mutations are rare in 21-OHD deficiency.[75]

Deficiency of 11β-OHD is responsible for 15% of CAH cases in Muslim and Ashkenazi Jewish women but is uncommon in women of European descent. The genes of the P450-C11 enzyme are located on the long arm of chromosome 8 and are therefore not HLA linked. The gene encoding 3β-HSD has been cloned and is located on chromosome 1. The 3β-HSD enzyme is not a cytochrome P450 enzyme and is also not HLA linked.

21-Hydroxylase Deficiency: Pregnancy Considerations

Historically, different forms of 21-OHD CAH have been identified clinically. Although this was practically convenient, terms such as "salt-wasting," "simple virilizing," "nonclassic," "late-onset," and "cryptic" all refer to different presentations of the same disease. Women with all manifestations of the disease should receive prepregnancy counseling, which must include reference to fertility concerns, possible pregnancy complications, prenatal diagnosis, and prenatal treatment.

Fertility in Congenital Adrenal Hyperplasia

Menarche in girls with CAH may be delayed up to 2 years in comparison with that in normal girls. Women with severe forms of CAH have decreased fertility rates (32%) because of several factors[76]:

1. Oligoovulation rates are high (30%) in 21-OHD CAH, which may reflect either noncompliance with therapy or perhaps abnormal brain androgen imprinting both in utero and before puberty. There is a possibility that women with 21-OHD CAH have oligoovulation on the basis of a masculinized center nervous system, but this is a controversial area.

2. Inadequate vaginal introitus can contribute to the low fertility rate (35%). The presence of the salt-losing 21-OHD CAH is often associated with marked masculinization and the necessity of major plastic surgery. In spite of the surgery, the vaginal introitus was inadequate for intercourse in 35% of markedly masculinized women.[34]

3. Women with 21-OHD CAH also exhibit less sexual activity than normal women and tend to have a more negative body image.

4. Women with severe 21-OHD CAH have a low marriage rate (32%).

5. 21-OHD is associated with other medical conditions that may reduce fertility, such as Turner's syndrome. This association may be a reason for diminished endometrial receptivity.[35]

6. In women with milder forms of 21-OHD CAH, fertility may actually reach normal rates, particularly in the "late-onset" group. Even in this group, the increased rates of oligoovulation may resemble polycystic ovarian disease.[77] Successful conception in this group requires good compliance with therapy, careful endocrine monitoring, and, often, induction of ovulation.

7. Spontaneous first trimester abortion rates are high (30%) in comparison with those in the normal population (12% to 15%). The mechanism behind the increased rate of spontaneous abortion is not known, but the possibilities include inadequate corpus luteum activity and endometrial implantation difficulties caused by the presence of elevated androgen levels.[36]

Pregnancy Outcome in 21-Hydroxylase Deficiency Congenital Adrenal Hyperplasia

Women with 21-OHD CAH should be prescribed glucocorticoids, usually hydrocortisone, prednisone, or dexamethasone, and (if the condition is salt losing) a mineralocorticoid. In the nonpregnant state, 17α-hydroxyprogesterone levels are measured to assess the effectiveness of this treatment in lowering ACTH levels and thus stimulation to the adrenal cortex. However, 17α-hydroxyprogesterone levels normally increase throughout pregnancy. Free testosterone levels do not change and may be used as a marker for adequate suppression. Blood pressure, edema, and electrolytes should be monitored for adequacy of mineralocorticoid replacement. Most women do not require any change in either mineralocorticoid or glucocorticoid therapy, except at times of stress (e.g., hyperemesis, labor, delivery), when parenteral stress dosages are required.

Prevention of Virilization in an Affected Fetus

In most situations, the fetus is at risk for virilization, as discovered when the condition is diagnosed in a sibling in infancy or in childhood. This diagnosis confirms that both parents are carriers of the enzymatic defect, of which they were probably unaware previously. Each subsequent pregnancy therefore carries a 1-in-4 risk for an affected child and a 1-in-8 risk for an affected girl.

Prenatal Treatment to Avoid Virilization

The first course of treatment is to prevent virilization in female fetuses; thus, 1 in 8 fetuses may benefit for in utero intervention. The fetal adrenal gland synthesizes and secretes testosterone from 6 to 12 weeks of gestation, which is the time of masculinization of female genitalia. If the excess androgen can be decreased by reducing ACTH stimulation to the fetal adrenal glands, the need for genital corrective surgery and the potential masculinization of the female brain may be avoided. Because of the early development of the external genitalia, treatment must be initiated before anyone knows whether the child is affected and what sex the child is; thus, eight fetuses must be treated to prevent virilization in one. New and colleagues developed an algorithm for prenatal diagnosis and treatment of 21-OHD (Fig. 8–4) to suppress fetal ACTH; glucocorticoids are given to the mother.[77a] Dexamethasone is the agent of choice because it has the greatest transplacental passage. Dosages of 0.5 mg three times daily or 20 μg per kilogram of prepregnancy body weight per day in two or three doses are recommended. To obtain the best results, treatment must be started with confirmation of pregnancy and continued throughout the pregnancy. Fetal response to dexamethasone is very variable, and although masculinization may be reduced, it is often not eliminated. Two thirds of treated affected girls and women nonetheless need some reconstructive surgery for the external genitalia.

There are several theoretical and actual disadvantages to the use of fetal adrenal corticosteroid suppressive therapy.[78]

Glucocorticoid therapy in human pregnancy is not associated with an increase in congenital malformations. Suppression of the fetal hypothalamic-pituitary-adrenal axis is a theoretical concern, but neonatal ACTH stimulation test results have generally been normal. Dexamethasone has been assigned a risk factor C by the U.S. Food and Drug Administration.

Another disadvantage of fetal adrenal suppression by first trimester corticosteroid use is the blanket coverage of all potentially affected fetuses that is required until fetal sex is known and whether the fetus is affected. No long-term effects of psychomotor development or intrauterine death has been seen. However, there have been reports of low birth weight and a reduction in central nervous system DNA content in animal studies. The full consequence may not yet be apparent, in view of the small numbers in young infants exposed to date. This treatment should therefore be considered experimental, and parents must be informed that the risk/benefit ratio has not been clearly established and that the controversy over the effectiveness of treatment continues.

Sonographic Prenatal Diagnosis of Congenital Adrenal Hyperplasia

Ultrasonography of the fetal perineum can demonstrate ambiguous genitalia in affected female fetuses. Ultrasound examination of the adrenal glands of three newborns with

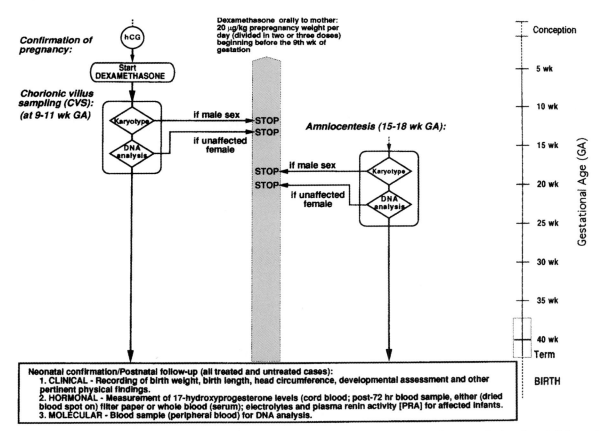

Figure 8–4. Procedure for management of pregnancies at risk for congenital adrenal hyperplasia due to 21-hydroxylase deficiency. hCG, human chorionic gonadotropin. (From Mercado AB, Wilson RC, Cheng KC, et al: Prenatal treatment and diagnosis of congenital adrenal hyperplasia owing to steroid 21-hydroxylase deficiency. J Clin Endocrinol Metab 1995;80:2014. © The Endocrine Society.)

CAH demonstrated a cerebriform pattern. In fetuses of mothers in whom CAH is treated with glucocorticoids, the adrenal glands are much smaller.[79]

11β-Hydroxylase Deficiency Congenital Adrenal Hyperplasia

11β-OHD CAH is the second most common cause of CAH and results in a hypertensive form of the disease. 11β-OHD is inherited as an autosomal recessive condition. The enzyme is a mitochondrial P450 enzyme and is coded by the CYP11B1 gene, which is situated on chromosome 8q22 in tandem with the gene for aldosterone synthase. Deficiency of 11β-hydroxylase results in the inability to convert 11-deoxycortisol, and this deficiency accounts for 5% to 8% of cases of CAH. 11β-OHD causes a decrease in cortisol production, and virilization develops in affected women. Salt-losing forms are not found because the substrate for 11β-hydroxylase is 11-deoxycortisol, which has mineralocorticoid activity. 11β-OHD CAH can be caused by one of several mutations in the CYP11B1 gene.[80] The diagnosis of 11β-hydroxylase deficiency is based on the findings of elevated plasma deoxycorticosterone levels and an exaggerated response of plasma deoxycorticosterone to ACTH stimulation.

This form of CAH is uncommon in North America, but the incidence of the defect is higher in certain populations from Morocco, Tunisia, Turkey, Iran, and Israel. There is marked clinical variability in manifestation, varying from modest masculinization with clitoromegaly to extreme forms with fused labial scrotal folds. Menstrual disturbances are common. The degrees of hirsutism and acne are variable. Many women with 11β-OHD CAH who are treated with adequate dosages of glucocorticoids appear to have normal fertility, and uneventful pregnancies have been reported. Severe forms of 11β-OHD show a poor response to glucocorticoid suppressive therapy and have been treated by laparoscopic bilateral adrenalectomy with marked clinical and biochemical improvement. Therefore, more aggressive management with early bilateral adrenalectomy may be appropriate in selected difficult cases before pregnancy.[81] In spite of the association of 11β-OHD with hypertension, pregnancies reported do not appear to have been complicated by an increased incidence of any other type of hypertensive disease.

Prenatal Diagnosis of Affected Female Fetuses in 11β-Hydroxylase Deficiency Congenital Adrenal Hyperplasia

Masculinization of the external genitalia may affect female fetuses during the first trimester, but the extent of the genital ambiguity is extremely variable. Prenatal diagnosis and treatment have met with some success. Initially, endocrine diagnosis involved utilization of amniotic fluid levels of 11-deoxycortisol and tetrahydro-11-deoxycortisol, which are elevated in pregnancies with affected fetuses.[82] Better distinction between affected and unaffected fetuses was obtained when sequential maternal urine and amniotic fluid levels were obtained in parallel. More accurate diagnosis can now be achieved by the application of the new molecular genetic techniques. Dexamethasone suppressive therapy has been used in an attempt to prevent genital masculinization of affected female fetuses but has not always been successful.[83]

3β-Hydroxysteroid Dehydrogenase Deficiency and Pregnancy

Classical 3β-HSD deficiency is a rare form of congenital CAH that impairs steroidogenesis in both the adrenal glands and gonads, resulting from mutations in the HSD 3B2 gene, causing varying degrees of salt loss in both sexes and in complete masculinization of the external genitalia in genetically male persons. The condition causes decreases in steroid synthesis in three pathways: (1) reducing the conversion of pregnenolone to progesterone, (2) reducing the conversion of 17α-pregnenolone to 17α-hydroxyprogesterone, and (3) reducing the conversion of dehydroepiandrosterone to androstenedione. The genes encoding 3β-HSD are located on chromosome 1. The type 1 gene that is expressed in peripheral tissues does not appear to mutate, unlike the type 2 gene that is expressed almost exclusively in the adrenal glands and gonads. Mutations identified include nonsense, frame shift, and missense mutations.[84] The type 1β-HSD gene is also expressed in the placenta, as well as peripheral tissues.

The 3β-HSD deficiencies are characterized by varying degrees of salt wasting and normal female sexual differentiation or mild virilization. Clinically, there is a very broad spectrum of the disease, varying from acute severe neonatal presentation to a mild form manifesting up to puberty with features suggestive of polycystic ovarian disease.[85] Women with mild 3β-HSD deficiency often are infertile because of oligoovulation, but menstrual regularity occurs after dexamethasone suppression. The 3β-HSD deficiency is uncommon in North America but has been found in up to 12% of Israeli women presenting with hyperandrogenism. Successful pregnancies have been reported after both dexamethasone therapy and in vitro fertilization.[86] Affected female fetuses may have variable degrees of labial fusion and clitoromegaly, but masculinization is usually mild because dehydroepiandrosterone is a weak androgen.

References

1. Gonzales JG, Elizondo G, Saldivar D, et al: Pituitary gland growth during normal pregnancy: An in vivo study using magnetic resonance imaging. Am J Med 1988;85:217.
2. Dinc H, Esen F, Demisci A, et al: Pituitary dimensions and volume measurements in pregnancy and post-partum MRI assessment. Acta Radiol 1998;39:64.
3. Von Werder K, Muller OA, Harth R, et al: Growth hormone releasing factor stimulation tests in normal controls. J Enderinol Invest 1984;7:185.
4. Glinoer D, de Nayer P, Bourdoux P, et al: Regulation of maternal thyroid during pregnancy. J Clin Endocrinol Metab 1990;71:276.
5. Kotarba DD, Garner PR, Perkins SL: Changes in serum free thyroxine and free tri-iodothyronine and TSH reference intervals in normal pregnant women. J Obstet Gynecol 1995;15:5.
6. Rees LH, Burke CW, Chard T, et al: Possible placental origin of ACTH in normal pregnancy. Nature 1975;254:620.
7. Douglas AJ, Russell JA: Endogenous opioid regulation of oxytocin and ACTH secretion during pregnancy and parturition. Progr Brain Res 2001;133:67.
8. Garner PR: Pituitary disorder in pregnancy. Curr Obstet Med 1991;1:143.
9. Davison JA, Valloton MB, Lindenheimer MD: Plasma osmolality and urinary concentrations and dilution during and after pregnancy. Br J Obstet Gynaecol 1998;88:472.
10. Hime MC, Williams DJ: Osmoregulatory adaptation in pregnancy and its disorders. J Endocrinol 1992;132:7.
11. Dawood MY, Ylikorkala O, Tivedi D, et al: Oxytocin in maternal circulation and amniotic fluid during pregnancy. J Clin Endocrinol Metab 1979;49:429.

12. National Radiological Protection Board: Advice on acceptable limits of exposure to nuclear magnetic resonance clinical imaging. Radiography 1984;50:220.

13. Huchon DJR, VanZijl JAWM, Campbell-Brown MB, et al: Desmopressin as a test of urinary concentrating ability in pregnancy. J Obstet Gynecol 1982;2:206.

14. Kallen BA, Carlsson SS, Bergen BK: Diabetes insipidus and the use of DDAVP during pregnancy. Eur J Endocrinol 1995;132:144.

15. Cheong HI, Park HW, Ha IS, et al: Six novel mutations in the vasopressin V_2 receptor gene causing diabetes insipidus. Nephron 1997;75:431.

16. Kwon TH, Hager H, Nejsom LN, et al: Physiology and pathophysiology of renal aquaporins. Semin Nephrol 2001;21:231.

17. Uhrig JD, Hurley RM: Chlorpropamide in pregnancy and transient neonatal diabetes insipidus. Can Med Assoc J 1983;128:368.

18. Usta IM, Barton J, Amon EA, et al: Acute fatty liver in pregnancy: An experience in the diagnosis and management of fourteen cases. Am J Obstet Gynecol 1994;171:1342.

19. Kinsella P, O'Brien T, Brosnan E, O'Sullivan DJ: A case of pregnancy associated with osteoporosis and the empty sella syndrome. Ir Med J 1991;84:25.

20. Pituitary Adenoma Study Group: Pituitary adenomas and oral contraceptives. A multicentre case-control study. Fertil Steril 1983;39:753.

21. Molitch M: Evaluation and management of pituitary tumors during pregnancy. Endocr Pract 1996;2:287.

22. Zervas NT: Surgical results for pituitary adenoma: Results of an international survey. In Black PM, Zevas NT, Ridgway EC, Martiz JB (eds): Secretory Tumors of the Pituitary Gland. New York, Raven Press, 1984, pp 377-385.

23. Bergh T, Nillius SJ: Prolactinomas: follow up medical treatment. In Molliatt GM (ed): A Clinical Problem: Microadenoma. Oxford, U.K., Excerpta Medica, 1982, pp 115-131.

24. Krupp T, Turkalj I: Surveillance of bromocriptine in pregnancy and offspring. In Jacobs HS (ed): Prolatinomas in Pregnancy. Lancaster, U.K., MTP Press, 1984, pp 45-50.

25. De Wit W, Coelingh Bennink HJT, Gerards LJ: Prophylactic bromocriptine treatment during pregnancy in women with macroprolactinomas: Report of 13 pregnancies. Br J Obstet Gynaecol 1984;91:1059.

26. Herman-Bonert V, Seliverstov M, Melmed S: Pregnancy in acromegaly: Successful therapeutic outcome. J Endocrinol Metab 1998;83:727.

27. Fassnacht M, Cappeller B, Art W, et al: Octreotide LAR treatment throughout pregnancy in an acromegalic woman. Clin Endocrinol 2001;55:411.

28. Caron P, Gesbeau C, Pradayrol L, et al: Successful pregnancy in an infertile woman with a TSH-secreting macroadenoma treated with octreotide. J Clin Endocrinol Metab 1996;81:1164.

29. Paoletti AM, Depan GF, Meis V, et al: Effectiveness of cabergoline in reducing FSH and prolactin hypersecretion from a pituitary macroadenoma in an infertile woman. Fertil Steril 1994;62:882.

30. Kupersmith MJ, Rosenberg C, Kleinberg D: Visual loss in pregnant women with pituitary adenomas. Ann Intern Med 1994;121:473.

31. Magge SN, Brunt M, Scott RM: Craniopharyngioma presenting during pregnancy 4 years after a normal pituitary MRI. Neurosurgery 2001;49:1014.

31a. Nelson DH, Meakin JW, Dealy JB Jr, et al: ACTH-producing tumor of the pituitary gland. N Engl J Med 1958;259:161.

32. Surrey ES, Chang RJ: Nelson's syndrome in pregnancy. Fertil Steril 1985;44:548.

33. Nakamura Y, Okada H, Wada Y, et al: Lymphocytic hypophysitis: Its expanding features. J Endocrinol Invest 2001;24:267.

34. Horvath E, Vidal S, Syro LV, et al: Severe lymphocytic hypophysitis with selective disappearance of prolactin cells: A histologic ultrastructural and immunoelectron microscopic study. Acta Neuropathologica 2001;101:631.

35. Nishiki M, Murakomi Y, Ozawa Y, Kato Y: Serum antibodies to human pituitary membrane antigens in patients with autoimmune lymphocytic hypophysitis. Clin Endocrinol 2001;54:327.

36. Tamiya A, Saeki N, Mizota A: Lymphocytic infundibulo-neurohypophysitis associated with recurrent optic neuritis. Br J Neurosurg 2001;15:180.

37. Reusch JE, Kleinschmidt-De Master BU, Lillehei KO, et al: Preoperative diagnosis of lymphocytic hypophysitis unresponsive to short course dexamethasone. Neurosurgery 1992;30:268.

38. Tubridy N, Molloy J, Saunders D, et al: Postpartum hypophysitis. J Neuropath 2001;21:106.

39. Kaplan NM: Successful pregnancy following hypophysectomy during the twelfth week of gestation. J Endocrinol Metab 1962;21:1139.

40. Israel SL, Cornstrain AS: Unrecognized pituitary necrosis: A sudden cause of death. JAMA 1952;148:189.

41. Mandel SJ, Larsen PR, Seely EW, Brent GA: Increased need for thyroxin during pregnancy in women with primary hypothyroidism. N Engl J Med 1990;323:91.

42. Sheehan HL: Postpartum necrosis of the anterior pituitary. J Pathol Bactiol 1937;45:189.

43. Sheehan HL: The recognition of chronic hypopituitarism resulting from post-partum pituitary necrosis. Am J Obstet Gynecol 1971;111:852.

44. Jialal I, Desai RK, Rajput MC: An assessment of posterior pituitary function in patients with Sheehan syndrome. Clin Endocrinol 1987;27:91.

45. Lust K, McIntyre HD, Morton A: Sheehan syndrome—acute presentation with hyponatremia and headache. Aus N Z J Obstet Gynaecol 2001;41:348.

46. Moreira AC, Maciel LMZ, Foss MC, et al: Gonadotropin secretory capacity in a patient with Sheehan syndrome with successful pregnancies. Fertil Steril 1984;42:303.

47. Taylor AL, Fishman LM: Corticotropin-releasing hormone. N Engl J Med 1988;319:213.

48. Sasaki A, Shinkawa O, Yoshinaaga K: Placental corticotropin-releasing hormone may be a stimulator of maternal pituitary adrenocorticotropin hormone secretion in humans. J Clin Invest 1989;84:1997.

49. McLean M, Smith R: Corticotropin-releasing hormone and human parturition. Reproduction 2001;121:493.

50. Scott EM, McGasrigle HHG, Lachelin GCL: The increase in plasma and saliva cortisol levels in pregnancy is not due to the increased corticosteroid-binding globulin levels. J Clin Endocrinol Metab 1990;71:639.

51. Anderson KJ, Walters WAW: Cushing's syndrome in pregnancy. Aust N Z J Obstet Gynaecol 1974;43:861.

52. Kaplan NM: Endocrine hypertension. In Wilson JD, Foster DW (eds): Williams Textbook of Endocrinology, 8th ed. Philadelphia, WB Saunders, 1992, pp 707-731.

53. Wilson M, Morganti AA, Zervoudakis I, et al: Blood pressure, the renin-aldosterone system and sex steroids throughout normal pregnancy. Am J Med 1980;68:97.

54. Demey-Ponsart E, Foidart JM, Sulon J, et al: Serum CBG, free and total cortisol and circadian patterns of adrenal function in normal pregnancy. J Steroid Biochem 1982;16:165.

55. Buescher MA, McClanrock HD, Adashi EY: Cushing syndrome in pregnancy. Obstet Gynecol 1992;79:130.

56. Collaborative Group of Antenatal Steroid Therapy: Effects of antenatal dexamethasone administration in the infant: Long term follow-up. J Paediatr 1984;104:259.

57. Pinette MG, Pan YQ, Oppenheim D, et al: Bilateral inferior petrosal sinus corticotropin sampling with CRH stimulation in a pregnant patient with Cushing's syndrome. Am J Obstet Gynecol 1994;171:563.

58. Pricolo VE, Monchik JM, Prinz RA, et al: Management of Cushing's syndrome secondary to an adrenal adenoma in pregnancy. Surgery 1990;108:1072.

59. Harra V, Dokoupilova M, Marek J, Plavka R: Recurrent ACTH-independent Cushing's syndrome in multiple pregnancies and its treatment with metyrapone. Clin Endocrinol (Oxf) 2001;54:277.

60. Solomon GC, Thiet M, Moore F, Seely EW: Primary hyperaldosteronism in pregnancy. Obstet Gynecol 1996;41:255.

61. Hammond TG, Buchanan JG, Scoggins BA, et al: Primary hyperaldosteronism in pregnancy. Aust N Z J Med 1982;12:537.

62. Laurel MT, Kabadi UM: Primary hyperaldosteronism. Endocr Pract 1997;3:47.

63. Baron F, Sprauve ME, Hiddlestone JF, Fisher AJ: Diagnosis and surgical treatment of primary hyperaldosteronism in pregnancy. Obstet Gynecol 1995;86:644.

64. Smith HC, Posen S, Clifton-Bligh P, Casey J: A testosterone-secreting adrenal cortical adenoma. Aust N Z J Med 1978;8:171.

65. Simmer HH, Frankland MV, Greipel M: Plasma testosterone in maternal peripheral blood and in cord venous blood after administration of testosterone enanthate to the mother. Steroids 1972;19:229.

66. Volpe R: Autoimmunity in the endocrine system. Monogr Endocrinol 1981;20:149.

67. Kendall-Taylor P, Lambert A, Mitchell R, et al: Antibody that blocks stimulation of cortisol secretion by ACTH in Addison's disease. BMJ 1988;296:1489.

68. Khundra S: Pregnancy and Addison's disease. Obstet Gynecol 1972;39:431.

69. Clayton RN: Diagnosis of adrenal insufficiency [Editorial]. BMJ 1989;298:271.

70. Arad I, Landau H: Adrenocortical reserve of neonatal born of long term steroid treated mothers. Eur J Pediatr 1984;298:279.

71. Osler M: Addison's disease and pregnancy. Acta Endocrinol (Copenh) 1962;41:67.

72. MacGillivray I: Acute suprarenal insufficiency in pregnancy. BMJ 1951;2:212.

73. Kalaitzoglou G, New MI: Congenital adrenal hyperplasia. Molecular insights learned from patients. Receptor 1993;3:211.

74. Gonzales FJ: The molecular biology of cytochrome P450's. Pharmacol Rev 1989;40:243.

75. Garner PR: Congenital adrenal hyperplasia in pregnancy. Semin Perinatol 1998;22:446.

76. Mulaikal RM, Migeon CJ, Rock JA: Fertility rates in female patients with congenital adrenal hyperplasia due to 21-hydroxylase deficiency. N Engl J Med 1987;316:178.

77. Hague WM, Adams J, Rodda C, et al: The prevalence of polycystic ovaries in patients with congenital adrenal hyperplasia and their close relatives. Clin Endocrinol (Oxf) 1990;36:53.

77a. Mercado AB, Wilson RC, Cheng KC, et al: Prenatal treatment and diagnosis of congenital adrenal hyperplasia owing to steroid 21-hydroxylase deficiency. J Clin Endocrinol Metab 1995;80:2014.

78. Fainstat T: Cortisone-induced congenital cleft palate in rabbits. Endocrinol 1954;55:502.

79. Avni EF, Rypens F, Smet MH, Galletty E: Sonographic demonstration of congenital adrenal hyperplasia in the neonate: The cerebriform pattern. Pediatr Radiol 1993;23:88.

80. Geley S, Kapelari K, Johrer K, et al: CYP11B1 mutations causing congenital adrenal hyperplasia due to 11 beta-hydroxylase deficiency. J Clin Endocrinol Metab 1996;81:2896.

81. Nasir J, Royston C, Walton C, White MC: 11 beta-hydroxylase deficiency: Management of a difficult case by laparoscopic bilateral adrenalectomy. Clin Endocrinol 1996;45:225.

82. Schumert Z, Rosenmann A, Landau H, Rosler: 11-Deoxycortisol in amniotic fluid. Prenatal diagnosis of congenital adrenal hyperplasia due to 11 beta-hydroxylase deficiency. Clin Endocrinol 1980;12:257.

83. Bouchard M, Forest MG, David M, et al: Familial congenital adrenal hyperplasia caused by 11 beta-hydroxylase deficiency: Failure of prevention of sexual ambiguity and prenatal diagnosis. Pediatric 1989;44:637.

84. Ricketts SJ, Moisan AM, Tardy V, et al: A new insight into the molecular basis of 3 beta-hydroxysteroid dehydrogenase deficiency. Endocr Res 2000;26:761.

85. Lobo RA, Goebelsman V: Evidence for reduced 3 beta-HSD activity in some hirsute women thought to have polycystic ovarian disease. J Clin Endocrinol Metab 1981;55:394.

86. Rojansky N, Shushan A, Rosler A, et al: Long term infertility in late-onset 3 beta-HSD deficiency: Successful pregnancy following dexamethasone and in vitro fertilization. J In Vitro Fert Embryo Transf 1991;8:298.

9

Calcium Homeostasis and Disorders of Calcium Metabolism during Pregnancy and Lactation

Urszula S. Masiukiewicz and Karl L. Insogna

In adult life, adaptation to acute and subacute alterations in calcium homeostasis is largely accomplished through the actions of parathyroid hormone (PTH) and 1,25-dihydroxyvitamin D. During pregnancy and lactation, other, "nonclassical" hormones, such as parathyroid hormone–related protein (PTHrP) appear to contribute to the alterations in calcium and skeletal homeostasis that occur in this setting. Maternal calcium homeostasis is geared to provide sufficient calcium flux across the placenta during pregnancy and into breast milk during lactation to ensure normal fetal and neonatal skeletal mineralization. These requirements are substantial and cannot be met solely by augmented intestinal calcium absorption; therefore, pregnancy and lactation are typically accompanied by increased rates of bone resorption and declines in bone density. As a consequence of these changes, the clinical course of diseases associated with hypercalcemia or hypocalcemia is altered during pregnancy. Recognizing this is critical to successful management of these diseases and to ensuring good maternal and fetal outcomes.

The physiologic alterations that occur in mineral and skeletal metabolism during pregnancy and lactation are reviewed below. This is followed by a discussion of common clinical disorders of mineral homeostasis that can occur during this period and their appropriate management. Although there is an extensive literature on experimental animal models of pregnancy and lactation, the focus of this review is solely human physiology and pathophysiology.

MATERNAL CALCIUM HOMEOSTASIS DURING PREGNANCY AND LACTATION

Pregnancy

Changes in Serum Minerals

As a consequence of hemodilution, the total serum calcium concentration falls during a normal pregnancy. This fall largely reflects the fall in serum albumin and the albumin-bound fraction of the total calcium.[1] Ionized calcium levels, when measured directly, are not different from values in nonpregnant women.[2-11] Serum concentrations of phosphate are normal throughout pregnancy.[5,8,12,13]

Changes in Calcitropic Hormones

The normal fetus accumulates approximately 21 g of calcium (range, 13 to 33 g)[14] during gestation; 80% of this accrues to the rapidly mineralizing skeleton in the third trimester.[14,15] A key adaptive change in response to this dramatic strain on maternal calcium metabolism is an increase in production of 1,25-dihydroxyvitamin D [1,25(OH)$_2$-vitamin D, or calcitriol]. 1,25-Dihydroxyvitamin D is the active form of vitamin D, and its main site of action is the proximal intestine, in which it increases calcium absorption. Pregnancy is associated with an approximately twofold increase in circulating levels of 1,25-dihydroxyvitamin D.[3,11,12,16-21] This increase occurs early in the first trimester and is sustained throughout pregnancy.

The source and regulatory events that mediate this increase in 1,25-dihydroxyvitamin D production has been the topic of much debate. The principal site of increased production appears to be the maternal kidney, with contributions from maternal decidua, placenta, and fetal kidneys.[22] PTH, which is the primary regulator of 1,25-dihydroxyvitamin D synthesis in the nonpregnant state, plays little role in mediating this increase; several prospective studies have shown that the level of immunoreactive PTH is in a low-normal range early in pregnancy when 1,25(OH)$_2$-vitamin D levels are high, and PTH levels reach the midnormal range only by the end of pregnancy.[5-7,11,12,23] Furthermore, women without functioning parathyroid glands still evidence a rise in circulating 1,25(OH)$_2$-vitamin D during pregnancy.

Increased 1,25-(OH)$_2$-vitamin D production during pregnancy leads to a marked increase in intestinal calcium absorption and, as a consequence, hypercalciuria. The increase in intestinal calcium absorption has been demonstrated as early as week 12 of gestation, well before fetal skeletal mineralization is maximal.[12,24,25] This suggests that the increase in 1,25-dihydroxyvitamin D is an independent phenomenon and may allow the maternal skeleton to store calcium in advance of peak fetal demands later in pregnancy. Urinary calcium excretion rates in the hypercalciuric range (i.e., >4 mg/kg body weight) are not uncommon.[3,5,11,12,26,27]

A role for calcitonin and PTHrP in mediating mineral metabolism in pregnancy has also been suggested. Serum calcitonin levels during pregnancy are generally higher than values in nonpregnant women; at least 20% of values exceed the normal range.[22] It has been speculated that elevated calcitonin levels protect the maternal skeleton from excessive bone resorption, but the experimental data that address this issue are scant, and it deserves further study.

Several studies have documented elevated levels of PTHrP as early as the first trimester of pregnancy.[23,28] PTHrP was discovered in the early 1980s when it was found to be overexpressed by tumors that cause hypercalcemia; thus, it was called *humoral hypercalcemia of malignancy.*[29-31] It is a product of a gene distinct from that for PTH. It is processed into multiple forms, including an amino- (N-) terminal fragment with structural similarity to the N-terminus of PTH, and structurally unique middle and carboxyl- (C-) terminal fragments. Unlike PTH, PTHrP does not normally circulate in detectable concentrations. It is widely expressed and appears to be an important paracrine signal in several tissues. Absence of PTHrP leads to a failure of normal skeletal development caused by accelerated mineralizing of cartilage. PTHrP can relax smooth muscle, and stretch induces its expression in the bladder, vascular smooth muscle, and uterus. Potential sources of PTHrP production during pregnancy include the placenta, decidua, amnion, fetal parathyroid glands, and umbilical cord.[32-35] PTHrP is also produced by breast tissue.[36,37] Elevations in N-terminal fragments of PTHrP may contribute to the increase in 1,25-dihydroxyvitamin D and to the suppression of PTH noted during pregnancy. It has also been suggested that N-terminal forms of PTHrP may play a role in regulating the onset of labor, inasmuch as PTHrP levels decline in myometrium at the onset of labor.[32] A midmolecular form of PTHrP stimulates placental calcium transport[38] and may

be important in ensuring that adequate calcium gets to the developing fetus. The C-terminal portion of PTHrP, termed *osteostatin,* is able to inhibit osteoclastic bone resorption in some in vitro assays and in rats in vivo. Therefore, this fragment of PTHrP could have a role in protecting the maternal skeleton from excessive bone loss during pregnancy.[22]

Lactation

Although accurate estimates of the calcium loss during lactation are difficult to quantify precisely because of inherent variations in the calcium content of breast milk, as well as because of other factors,[39,40] the daily loss of calcium in breast milk has been estimated to range from 280 to 400 mg.[40] Losses up to 1000 mg calcium per day have been reported.[41] In contrast to the pregnant state, lactation is not associated with intestinal calcium hyperabsorption, and the skeleton appears to be the primary source from which lactating women meet these requirements. The underlying mechanisms responsible for this demineralization are not fully understood, but a prominent role for PTHrP in mediating this process has been proposed. Total and ionized calcium[42-46] and serum phosphate[5,13,44,47-50] are high-normal or slightly elevated in lactating mothers in comparison with nonlactating women. The majority of studies have found that PTH levels are low in lactating women in comparison with nonlactating women, and levels rise to normal or just above normal after weaning.[12,44-49,51-54] The postweaning increase in PTH levels may be sustained for up to 3 months,[12,44] but whether this increase contributes to rebuilding of bone after weaning remains unknown. Levels of 1,25-dihydroxyvitamin D, elevated in pregnancy, fall into the normal range within days of delivery and remain normal during lactation.[11,12,18,21,43,48,54-56] As a consequence of this, the intestinal calcium hyperabsorption and hypercalciuria seen during pregnancy resolve within days after delivery. In addition, the renal excretion of calcium has been reported to be low during lactation.[3,5,12,13,23,26,48,57] After weaning, there is an increase in intestinal absorption of calcium,[50] whereas low urinary calcium excretion persists.[48] These changes probably contribute to rebuilding the maternal skeleton after weaning.

PTHrP is expressed in lactating mammary tissue and plays a key role in mammary gland development.[58] In its absence, the mammary gland does not develop. PTHrP is secreted into milk in large quantities.[59-61] In fact, the concentration of PTHrP in milk is 1000-fold higher than that measured in hypercalcemic cancer patients.[59] The role of PTHrP in milk remains unclear. It is possible that, as in the placenta, it augments transport of calcium into breast milk, although this has not been established. In support of this notion, PTHrP concentrations in the milk have been found to correlate positively with a total milk calcium content.[62] PTHrP, like PTH, stimulates bone resorption through the PTH receptor expressed in bone,[63] and emerging evidence suggests that breast milk–derived PTHrP may reach the maternal circulation and may be an important mediator of maternal skeletal resorption during lactation. In accordance with this, PTHrP levels have been found to correlate positively with serum ionized calcium levels[46,47,64] as well as with the degree of bone loss during lactation.[65] Hypercalcemia associated with low PTH levels has been reported in lactating women, and it has resolved after weaning[66] or reduction mammoplasty,[67] which suggests breast milk–derived PTHrP may be responsible. Calcitonin is also secreted into breast milk at concentrations significantly higher than in the maternal serum,[68] but its functions if any are not known.

In summary, maternal calcium homeostasis is geared to provide sufficient calcium flux across the placenta during pregnancy and into breast milk during lactation to ensure normal fetal and neonatal skeletal mineralization. These requirements are substantial and are met by alterations in calcitropic hormone profile and effects of "nonclassical" hormones, such as PTHrP, on calcium homeostasis, as summarized in Table 9-1.

FETAL-PLACENTAL PHYSIOLOGY

Among the many functions of the fetal-placental unit is to provide sufficient calcium for the fetal skeleton to mineralize and to maintain the fetal extracellular calcium concentration in the appropriate range. Serum calcium levels are higher in the fetus than in the mother. Human cord blood calcium levels exceed maternal values by 1 and 0.5 mEq/L for total and ionized calcium, respectively.[69] Therefore, placental calcium transport occurs against a concentration gradient, especially at the end of gestation, when the difference between maternal and fetal blood calcium is greatest. As noted, there is evidence that the active placental transport mechanism for calcium is regulated by a midmolecule portion of PTHrP.[22,70] Fetal hypercalcemia is also maintained by the effects of PTrP: in this instance, the N-terminal fragment of PTHrP stimulates fetal renal tubular calcium reabsorption, thereby helping to maintain a high serum level of calcium. Unlike calcium, PTH, 1,25-dihydroxyvitamin D, and calcitonin apparently do not cross the placenta in appreciable amounts. Circulating 25-hydroxyvitamin D freely crosses the placenta, where placental 1α-hydroxylases convert it to the active 1,25-dihydroxyvitamin D.

The fetal-placental unit functions relatively independently of the maternal calcium needs. For example, the fetal skeleton mineralizes normally, and the fetal calcium concentration is unaffected even in the presence of moderate hypocalcemia and vitamin D deficiency in the mother.[71-73] The circulating concentration of intact PTH in the fetus has been reported to be one fourth that of maternal values,[74] presumably because of the relative hypercalcemia of the fetus. At birth, the neonate has relatively elevated serum levels of total and ionized calcium, calcitonin, and PTHrP and suppressed levels of PTH. Serum calcium levels fall by about 1 mEq/L and reach a nadir at 1 or 2 days of age. In normal infants, secretion of PTH is stimulated at this point, and recovery of normal serum calcium levels generally occurs by 1 week of age.

BONE PHYSIOLOGY AND DISEASE STATES IN PREGNANCY AND LACTATION

Pregnancy

Effect of Pregnancy on Markers of Bone Turnover and Bone Density

Studies examining the effects of pregnancy on bone turnover markers in humans are limited, but the existing evidence suggests that bone turnover is low in the first half of pregnancy and increases towards the end of pregnancy, which coincides with the increased demands of the mineralizing fetal skeleton. Markers of bone resorption (pyridinoline and deoxypyridinoline crosslinks and hydroxyproline) are low in the first trimester and increase steadily throughout pregnancy, peaking at about twice the normal levels in the third trimester.[12,23,51,75] Markers of bone formation, such as osteocalcin and procollagen I carboxypeptides, are low or undetectable in early pregnancy but rise to normal levels by the end of pregnancy.[6,12,51,75-77] Alkaline phosphatase, which is routinely used to evaluate bone turnover in a nonpregnant patient, is not a helpful marker during the pregnancy because of the contribution of placental alkaline phosphatase to maternal levels.

Despite several studies and case reports describing changes in bone mineral density (BMD) during pregnancy, there exists controversy regarding the time course and extent of BMD changes during and after gestation. Because of concerns about radiation exposure to the fetus, few studies have examined BMD during the pregnancy by precise techniques such as dual-energy x-ray absorptiometry (DEXA). Older prospective studies with either single- or dual-photon absorptiometry did not find a significant change in BMD during the pregnancy.[13,26,78,79] One study found a significant decrease in BMD of the femoral neck and radial shaft, but no change in lumbar bone density, by comparing single- and dual-photon absorptiometry measurements before conception with those 6 weeks post partum.[80] More recent studies with DEXA measurements before and after pregnancy reported conflicting results; two studies showed declines in lumbar bone density ranging

TABLE 9-1	Summary of Calcitropic Hormone Profile during Pregnancy and Lactation						
	Serum Calcium Total	Serum Calcium Ionized	Serum Phosphate	Urine Calcium	1,25-Dihydroxy-vitamin D	Parathyroid Hormone	Parathyroid Hormone–Related Protein
Pregnancy	↓	Normal	Normal	↑	↑	Low normal	↑
Lactation	Normal	Normal	High normal	↓	Normal	Low normal	↑

from 3.5% to 4.5%,[81,82] whereas a third study reported no change in bone density during pregnancy.[83] These results may be divergent because, in the first two studies, bone density was measured 4 to 6 weeks post partum and lactation-induced bone loss may have confounded the results (see later discussion under "Lactation"). A few investigators have used ultrasonography to measure bone density and have reported a decrease in BMD according to this technique during pregnancy.[75,84,85] Whether parity has any long-term effect on the maternal skeleton is unclear, although the majority of studies have found no effect of parity on bone density or fracture risk,[22] and several other studies have found increased parity to have a beneficial effect on bone mass. Few studies have linked parity to decreased bone density.[86-88] In summary, it has not been clearly established whether the increased bone turnover seen in late pregnancy has any long-term effects on the maternal skeleton. The discrepancies in data are attributable to a number of factors, including small sample sizes in study populations, differences in gestational weight gain, body composition, pattern of physical activity, and whether the mothers breast-fed. On balance, the existing evidence suggests either no effect or a very small negative effect of pregnancy on bone density over the long term.

Osteoporosis and Pregnancy

Osteoporosis with accompanying fragility fracture is extremely rare in pregnancy. When it does occur, it is usually assumed that the woman's bone density was very low before conception and that the additional physiologic and physical stress of pregnancy (i.e., back strain) unmasks rather than causes the osteoporosis. There are rare cases of women presenting in the third trimester with transient osteoporosis of the knee or hip.[89-93] The pathophysiologic mechanism in these unusual cases is unknown, but the normal calcitropic hormone profile in these patients and the fact that this condition is usually localized suggest that mechanisms other than generalized bone loss are the underlying causes. Local factors, such as reflex sympathetic dystrophy, ischemia, trauma, viral infections, marrow hypertrophy, immobilization, and fetal pressure on the obturator nerve, have been proposed. Affected patients typically present with hip pain and/or insufficiency fractures of the hip.[89,91,94,95] Osteopenia is seen on plain films,[90,96] and DEXA measurements of the symptomatic femoral head and neck document reduced bone mass.[94] Magnetic resonance imaging of the affected femoral head has demonstrated joint effusions and increased water content of the femoral head and marrow cavity.[97] The condition is typically self-limiting and necessitates no treatment except for analgesia. The decreased BMD and magnetic resonance imaging findings usually resolve within 2 to 6 months post partum.[89,94,95,97]

Lactation

Effect of Lactation on Bone Turnover and Bone Density

In the aggregate, studies examining the rate of bone turnover indicate that both bone resorption and formation

are increased during lactation. Markers of bone resorption are elevated twofold to threefold during lactation and are higher than values observed during pregnancy.[12,13,46,48,51,52,75,98] Similarly, markers of bone formation have been reported to be high during lactation and to increase over the levels observed during pregnancy, with the exception of alkaline phosphatase, which typically falls immediately after delivery of the placenta.[13,46,48,51,52,75,98] Several longitudinal studies of bone density during lactation have documented 3% to 8.0% declines in trabecular bone mass (i.e., at sites such as the lumbar spine) after 2 to 6 months; smaller losses have been recorded at cortical sites when lactating women are compared with women who are feeding their infants formula.[13,26,46,48,51,52,54,80,98-107] It is not clear whether the lactation-induced bone loss results from the relative estrogen deficiency that occurs during lactation or from the combined effects of estrogen deficiency and PTHrP-induced skeletal resorption. Several studies have suggested that estrogen withdrawal and the intensity and duration of lactation are factors that predict the degree of bone loss during lactation.[53,94,106,108,109] Early resumption of menses or use of supplemental estrogen can reduce skeletal losses during lactation.[106,108] Conversely, bone density may continue to decrease during extended lactation, even after resumption of menses,[94,109] which suggests that estrogen deficiency alone cannot fully account for lactation-induced bone loss. In selected studies, PTHrP levels were found to correlate with loss of BMD at the lumbar spine and femoral neck in lactating women, even after serum estradiol and PTH levels were controlled.[65] PTHrP has also been reported to be elevated in patients with hyperprolactinemia[47,110]; in these patients, PTHrP correlated negatively with bone density of the lumbar spine, which lends further support to the notion that PTHrP is a mediator of lactation-induced bone resorption. The majority of studies have reported that the bone loss associated with lactation is completely reversed during weaning.[48,51,54,109] Recovery of skeletal mass occurs quickly, because women who breast-fed for at least 6 months and had a second pregnancy within 18 months of their prior delivery did not have lower bone density after the second pregnancy.[107,111] Further extended lactation was not associated with lower BMD in a cross-sectional study of 30 multiparous women who had breast-fed, in comparison with a control population.[112] There is no convincing evidence in the literature that increasing dietary calcium intake prevents lactation-induced bone loss.[113,114] In addition, the majority of epidemiologic studies of premenopausal and postmenopausal women have found that a history of lactation has no adverse or salutatory effect on peak bone mass or hip fracture risk.

Osteoporosis of Lactation

Osteoporosis with accompanying fragility fractures has occasionally been described to occur during lactation. As is the case for osteoporosis during pregnancy, it is difficult to distinguish patients with preexisting low bone mass from those with significant pregnancy- and lactation-induced bone loss. Typically, women with lactation-associated osteoporosis present several months post partum with vertebral crush fractures, bone pain, loss of height, and, in rare instances, hypercalcemia.[66,115] Histologic evaluation of bone shows either normal cellular activity or evidence of increased resorption.[115] Serum PTH levels have been reported to be normal or reduced, and 1,25-dihydroxyvitamin D levels are normal.[66,115] It has been postulated that PTHrP released from the lactating breast into the maternal circulation contributes to the excessive bone resorption, osteoporosis, and fractures in these cases.[66,116]

HYPERCALCEMIA DURING PREGNANCY

Primary Hyperparathyroidism

Hypercalcemia during pregnancy poses a risk to both the mother and fetus and can present a complex management issue. Hypercalcemia from any cause can occur during pregnancy (Table 9–2); however, because women of child-bearing years are young and healthy, primary hyper-parathyroidism is the most common cause. The incidence of hyperparathyroidism during pregnancy is not known, but it is uncommon; less than 200 cases have been reported in the literature.[117] This may reflect underreporting or a failure to recognize all cases. Furthermore, it is possible that pregnancy-related changes in calcium and PTH physiology (as outlined previously) with a physiologic fall in total serum calcium level, as well as the pregnancy-related hypercalciuria, obscure the diagnosis of mild primary hyperparathyroidism in some women. As noted, calcium easily crosses the placenta, and hypercalcemia in a pregnant woman with hyperparathyroidism may be further masked by the ability to "dispose" of calcium in the mineralizing fetus. Up to 80% of pregnant women with hyperparathyroidism are asymptomatic,[118-121] and the condition is detected on routine prenatal biochemical tests or post partum when the newborn develops symptomatic hypocalcemia. Although most patients with hyperparathyroidism are asymptomatic, this disease can be associated with a significantly increased risk of maternal and fetal complications. Earlier studies (conducted largely before automated blood sampling of calcium) reported maternal complication rates as high as 67% in patients with hyperparathyroidism.[122] Because the hypercalciuria of pregnancy can be exacerbated by hyperparathyroidism, nephrolithiasis is the most common symptomatic manifestation of hyperparathyroidism during pregnancy, with an estimated incidence of 24% to 36%.[118,123] Pancreatitis, which poses a significant risk, occurs in 7% to 13% of pregnant women with hyperparathyroidism.[118,122,124-127] Hyperemesis gravidarum also occurs with a significantly increased frequency in pregnant patients with primary hyperparathyroidism.

In the past, fetal complications have occurred with a frequency as high as 53%,[128-130] and the incidence of neonatal death has been reported to be as high as 27% to 31%.[128,129,131] Fortunately, neonatal death is rare now. Nonfatal complications of hyperparathyroidism in pregnancy have included intrauterine growth restriction, low birth weight, and preterm delivery.[118,128,129,131-133]

Although less serious, neonatal hypocalcemia and unrecognized hypocalcemic tetany are common in off-spring of women with hyperparathyroidism and may be seen in up to 50% of such infants.[130,134-137] Even mild asymptomatic hypercalcemia in the mother has been reported to cause neonatal parathyroid suppression and tetany.[134-136] This can largely be avoided if calcium supplementation is started promptly after birth. Neonatal hypocalcemia is usually transient, but it can persist for several months, and cases of permanent neonatal hypoparathyroidism have been reported.[131,138,139]

Because of the potential for serious complications, women with a diagnosis of hyperparathyroidism who wish to conceive should be treated surgically before pregnancy. When the hyperparathyroidism is discovered during the pregnancy, management is influenced by the degree of hypercalcemia, gestational age, and presence of complications. Surgical correction of primary hyperparathyroidism during the second trimester, to prevent fetal and neonatal complications, was recommended in early studies.[140-143] However, many of the women in those early cases were symptomatic and had nephrocalcinosis or renal insufficiency. Available evidence, although limited, suggests that the typical mildly hypercalcemic asymptomatic pregnant woman with primary hyperparathyroidism can be safely managed conservatively[144-147] if neonatal hypocalcemia is sought and treated. A proposed algorithm for managing pregnant women with primary hyperparathyroidism is presented in Figure 9–1. In general, it is reasonable to manage patients with mild asymptomatic primary hyperparathyroidism conservatively, simply by discontinuing the use of calcium supplements and encouraging good hydration. Medications often used to treat nonpregnant hypercalcemic patients, such as loop diuretics (e.g., furosemide) and bisphosphonates, readily cross the placenta and should be avoided during pregnancy.[121,127] As noted for conservatively managed patients, the neonate must be monitored closely for the development of hypocalcemia. In patients in whom conservative management fails or who present with complications during

---

TABLE 9–2   Differential Diagnosis of Hypercalcemia

Primary hyperparathyroidism
Malignant disease
Familial hypocalciuric hypercalcemia
Granulomatous diseases
  Sarcoidosis
  Tuberculosis
  Histoplasmosis
  Coccidioidomycosis
Endocrine disorders
  Thyrotoxicosis
  Pheochromocytoma
  Adrenal crisis
Drug induced
  Vitamin D
  Thiazide diuretics
  Lithium
  Vitamin A
  Aluminum intoxication (in chronic renal failure)
  Aminophylline
Miscellaneous
  Milk-alkali syndrome
  Renal failure (tertiary hyperparathyroidism)
  Total parenteral nutrition
  Hypophosphatasia

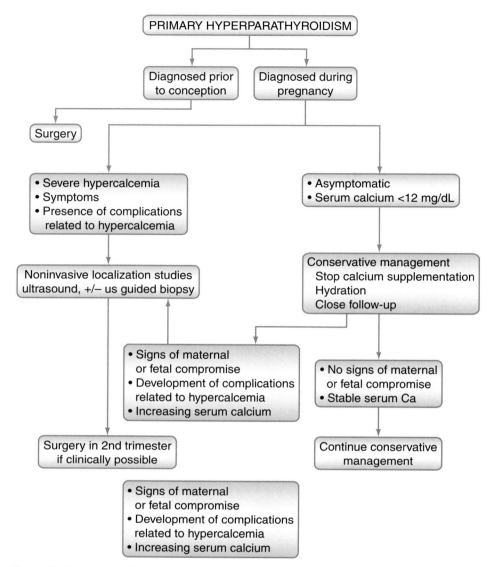

Figure 9-1. Proposed algorithm for managing pregnant women with primary hyperparathyroidism.

pregnancy, surgical therapy is indicated. To limit the extent and duration of surgery, noninvasive preoperative localization studies can be helpful. Radionuclide localizing studies (sestamibi scan) are contraindicated during pregnancy, but ultrasonography, when performed by an experienced clinician, can be helpful in localizing a parathyroid adenoma.[148,149] In selected cases, ultrasonographically guided biopsy of a suspect lesion with measurement of PTH in the aspirate can confirm the diagnosis. Such fine-needle aspirates carry minimal risk and, if successful, provide the opportunity to limit surgery to a minimally invasive parathyroidectomy. Intraoperative measurement of serum PTH, available in most major centers in which parathyroid surgery is performed, should be done to ensure the success of the procedure.[150] If necessary, a pregnant patient should undergo parathyroid adenomectomy during the second trimester, when the rate of surgical complications and risk of preterm labor are generally considered low.[151]

Familial Hypocalciuric Hypercalcemia

Familial hypocalciuric hypercalcemia (FHH), is an autosomal dominant disorder resulting from heterozygous inactivation of the calcium-sensing receptor gene. This receptor is expressed in the parathyroid gland and kidney, and loss of its function leads to a failure of the parathyroid gland to appropriately sense serum calcium and to suppress secretion of the hormone when serum calcium rises. Therefore, patients with FHH evidence mild elevations in serum calcium with concomitant elevations in serum PTH. Urine calcium is paradoxically low because the kidney cannot sense the level of calcium in the blood and inappropriately reclaims excessive amounts of filtered calcium. It is important not to confuse FHH with primary hyperparathyroidism because parathyroidectomy is not indicated in patients with FHH. Although FHH usually poses no risk to the mother, infants of mothers with the disease can have suppressed parathyroid glands and are at risk for neonatal hypocalcemia and seizures or tetany. Neonatal hypocalcemia can have a delayed presentation in this setting and may necessitate prolonged treatment while parathyroid function recovers.[139]

HYPOCALCEMIA DURING PREGNANCY

The many causes of hypocalcemia are summarized in Table 9–3. The specific causes and management of these diseases have been reviewed in detail elsewhere.[152,153] However, because pregnancy and lactation can alter the clinical course and management of some of these diseases, a selected few are discussed as follows.

Hypoparathyroidism

Hypoparathyroidism results from inadequate secretion of PTH. Absent or diminished action of PTH in the kidney and in bone leads to hypocalcemia and hyperphosphatemia. Multiple causes of hypoparathyroidism have been described[153]; autoimmune causes and inadvertent removal of the parathyroid glands during thyroid surgery are relatively more common. Patients with mild hypoparathyroidism may be asymptomatic or may experience only subtle manifestations of the disease. In more severe forms of the disorder, symptoms and signs related to decreased serum ionized calcium concentrations may occur. Increased neuromuscular excitability with a positive Chvostek or Trousseau sign can be observed. Muscle weakness and paresthesias can progress to the development of seizures, tetany, or laryngospasm. Papilledema, elevated cerebrospinal fluid pressure, and neurologic signs that mimic a cerebral tumor may be found. A spectrum of mental status changes, from irritability to psychosis, can also occur. Abnormalities in cardiac conduction, particularly prolongation of the QT interval and T wave changes, may be present.

TABLE 9–3 Causes of Hypocalcemia

Hypoparathyroidism/abnormal parathyroid hormone secretion
  Autoimmune
  Neck surgery
  Activating mutations in calcium-sensing receptor
  Developmental abnormalities (DiGeorge's sequence)
  Severe magnesium deficiency
  Hypermagnesemia
Pseudohypoparathyroidism/parathyroid hormone resistance
  Pseudohypoparathyroidism (types 1a, 1b, 2)
  Severe magnesium deficiency
Disorders of vitamin D metabolism
Medication-induced
  Bisphosphonates, calcitonin, phosphate, anticancer agents, pentamidine, foscarnet
Increased osteoblastic activity
  Hungry bone syndrome (after parathyroidectomy)
  Osteoblastic tumor metastases
Miscellaneous
  Hyperphosphatemia
  Massive blood transfusion
  Pancreatitis
  Sepsis

Radiographs of the skull may demonstrate intracranial calcifications. Uncorrected hypocalcemia in pregnancy can lead to maternal, fetal, and neonatal complications.[154] As a consequence of decreased availability of maternal calcium, the fetus of a hypocalcemic woman develops compensatory secondary hyperparathyroidism (with measurable elevations of serum PTH). Generalized skeletal demineralization can result.[155] Although the secondary hyperparathyroidism is usually transient and resolves in the neonatal period, the infant may not achieve normal bone mineralization until age 6 months.[154] These complications can be avoided if the maternal serum calcium level is maintained in a low-normal range during pregnancy. Because of PTH-independent production of 1,25(OH)$_2$-vitamin D during pregnancy, hypoparathyroid women have fewer hypocalcemic symptoms and reduced requirements for supplemental 1,25(OH)$_2$-vitamin D to maintain a serum calcium in the desired range.[156-164] Despite a few reports to the contrary,[165-167] there is general agreement that in *late* pregnancy, the dose of 1,25(OH)$_2$-vitamin D must be reduced or discontinued altogether to avoid the appearance of hypercalcemia.[22,156,157,160,165,166,168]

Severe hypomagnesemia, in the setting of diabetes mellitus, alcoholism, aminoglycoside use, or malabsorptive syndrome, may cause an acquired hypoparathyroidism. Hypomagnesemia is thought to impair release of PTH from the parathyroid gland, although impaired PTH bioactivity or end-organ resistance may contribute to the hypocalcemia in some hypomagnesemic patients. Calcium and vitamin D supplementation may not be effective in treating hypocalcemia associated with hypomagnesemia, and correction of the hypomagnesemia is the preferred approach. Magnesium supplementation is safe and effective in pregnancy.

Women with hypocalcemia (regardless of cause) are at increased risk of tetany during labor, presumably because of the frequent occurrence of hyperventilation leads to an acute fall in ionized calcium. Intravenous calcium should be available at the bedside of women with documented hypocalcemia or who are at risk for developing hypocalcemia.

Pseudohypoparathyroidism

Pseudohypoparathyroidism is a heterogeneous group of genetic syndromes characterized by hypocalcemia caused by PTH resistance.[153] Pseudohypoparathyroidism has been described in pregnancy, and Breslau and Zerwekh,[169] in their report of pregnant patients with pseudohypoparathyroidism, noted a normalization of serum calcium levels as pregnancy progressed. These patients remained normocalcemic without the use of supplemental calcium or vitamin D. During pregnancy, the circulating level of 1,25-dihydroxyvitamin D increased twofold to threefold, whereas PTH levels fell to nearly half the prepregnancy values. Again, this is largely a result of the PTH-independent rise in circulating levels of 1,25(OH)$_2$-vitamin D. Therefore, the requirement for vitamin D and calcium supplementation should be reevaluated frequently in pregnant patients with pseudohypoparathyroidism to avoid hypercalcemia.

In both patients with hypoparathyroidism and those with pseudohypoparathyroidism, the requirement for supplemental 1,25(OH)$_2$-vitamin D and calcium after delivery increases rapidly as placental 1,25(OH)$_2$-vitamin D production ceases.

Magnesium Sulfate Therapy

Parenteral magnesium sulfate, used in the treatment of women with eclampsia, preeclampsia, or preterm labor, can cause alterations in calcium homeostasis. In women treated for as little as 24 hours, hypocalcemia, hyperphosphatemia, and hypercalciuria, can occur. The mechanism by which magnesium sulfate causes hypocalcemia is unclear, although a plausible explanation is that magnesium ions compete with calcium for common reabsorptive sites in Henle's loop. A loading dose of 4 to 6 g intravenously, followed by infusion of 1 to 2 g/hour, has been shown to cause serum ionized calcium concentrations to fall. A compensatory secondary hyperparathyroidism develops with a rise in circulating levels of PTH and 1,25-dihydroxyvitamin D, which tends to limit the degree of hypocalcemia.[170] Umbilical venous levels of 1,25-dihydroxyvitamin D and PTH are also found to be elevated during maternal treatment with magnesium sulfate. The elevated levels of 1,25-dihydroxyvitamin D may be caused by placental transport of maternal 1,25(OH)$_2$-vitamin D; however, the PTH is of fetal origin. These hormonal changes, in addition to other placental protective mechanisms, shield the fetus somewhat from the hypermagnesemia and hypocalcemia experienced by the mother. However, at birth these infants can be mildly hypermagnesemic and hypocalcemic. Usually neither condition is clinically significant, and both typically resolve during the first 2 days after birth.

Although the effects of short-term magnesium sulfate therapy on calcium homeostasis appear benign and reversible, the use of long-term, higher dose magnesium sulfate for tocolysis has raised safety concerns. A prospective study of women treated with magnesium sulfate for a mean of 26 days revealed alterations in calcium homeostasis that parallel those described previously with short-term magnesium therapy.[171] The frequency of significant side effects in neonates born to mothers receiving long-term magnesium sulfate therapy are largely unknown. There are, however, a few case reports of neonatal hypocalcemia, osteopenia, and rickets,[172,173] although it appears that these are rare complications.

References

1. Pitkin RM, Gebhardt MP: Serum calcium concentrations in human pregnancy. Am J Obstet Gynecol 1977;127:775-778.
2. Davis OK, Hawkins DS, Rubin LP, et al: Serum parathyroid hormone (PTH) in pregnant women determined by an immunoradiometric assay for intact PTH. J Clin Endocrinol Metab 1988;67:850-852.
3. Gertner JM, Coustan DR, Kliger AS, et al: Pregnancy as state of physiologic absorptive hypercalciuria. Am J Med 1986;81:451-456.
4. Cruikshank DP, Pitkin RM, Reynolds WA, et al: Calcium-regulating hormones and ions in amniotic fluid. Am J Obstet Gynecol 1980;136:621-625.
5. Dahlman T, Sjoberg HE, Bucht E: Calcium homeostasis in normal pregnancy and puerperium. A longitudinal study. Acta Obstet Gynecol Scand 1994;73:393-398.
6. Seki K, Makimura N, Mitsui C, et al: Calcium-regulating hormones and osteocalcin levels during pregnancy: A longitudinal study. Am J Obstet Gynecol 1991;164:1248-1252.
7. Rasmussen N, Frolich A, Hornnes PJ, Hegedus L: Serum ionized calcium and intact parathyroid hormone levels during pregnancy and postpartum. Br J Obstet Gynaecol 1990;97:857-859.
8. Saggese G, Baroncelli GI, Bertelloni S, Cipolloni C: Intact parathyroid hormone levels during pregnancy, in healthy term neonates and in hypocalcemic preterm infants. Acta Paediatr Scand 1991;80:36-41.
9. Pitkin RM, Reynolds WA, Williams GA, Hargis GK: Calcium metabolism in normal pregnancy: A longitudinal study. Am J Obstet Gynecol 1979;133:781-790.
10. Frolich A, Rudnicki M, Fischer-Rasmussen W, Olofsson K: Serum concentrations of intact parathyroid hormone during late human pregnancy: A longitudinal study. Eur J Obstet Gynecol Reprod Biol 1991;42:85-87.
11. Seely EW, Brown EM, DeMaggio DM, et al: A prospective study of calciotropic hormones in pregnancy and post partum: Reciprocal changes in serum intact parathyroid hormone and 1,25-dihydroxyvitamin D. Am J Obstet Gynecol 1997;176:214-217.
12. Cross NA, Hillman LS, Allen SH, et al: Calcium homeostasis and bone metabolism during pregnancy, lactation, and postweaning: A longitudinal study. Am J Clin Nutr 1995;61:514-523.
13. Kent GN, Price RI, Gutteridge DH, et al: Effect of pregnancy and lactation on maternal bone mass and calcium metabolism. Osteoporos Int 1993;3(Suppl 1):44-47.
14. Givens MH, Macy IC: The chemical composition of the human fetus. J Biol Chem 1933;102:7-17.
15. Trotter M, Hixon BB: Sequential changes in weight, density, and percentage ash weight of human skeletons from an early fetal period through old age. Anat Rec 1974;179:1-18.
16. Whitehead M, Lane G, Young O, et al: Interrelations of calcium-regulating hormones during normal pregnancy. BMJ 1981;283:10-12.
17. Wieland P, Fischer JA, Trechsel U, et al: Perinatal parathyroid hormone, vitamin D metabolites, and calcitonin in man. Am J Physiol 1980;239:E385-E390.
18. Lund B, Selnes A: Plasma 1,25-dihydroxyvitamin D levels in pregnancy and lactation. Acta Endocrinol (Copenh) 1979;92:330-335.
19. Fleischman AR, Rosen JF, Cole J, et al: Maternal and fetal serum 1,25-dihydroxyvitamin D levels at term. J Pediatr 1980;97:640-642.
20. Bikle DD, Gee E, Halloran B, Haddad JG: Free 1,25-dihydroxyvitamin D levels in serum from normal subjects, pregnant subjects, and subjects with liver disease. J Clin Invest 1984;74:1966-1971.
21. Wilson SG, Retallack RW, Kent JC, et al: Serum free 1,25-dihydroxyvitamin D and the free 1,25-dihydroxyvitamin D index during a longitudinal study of human pregnancy and lactation. Clin Endocrinol (Oxf) 1990;32:613-622.
22. Kovacs C, Kronenberg H: Maternal-fetal calcium and bone metabolism during pregnancy, puerperium and lactation. Endocr Rev 1997;18:832-872.
23. Gallacher SJ, Fraser WD, Owens OJ, et al: Changes in calciotrophic hormones and biochemical markers of bone turnover in normal human pregnancy. Eur J Endocrinol 1994;131:369-374.
24. Heaney RP, Skillman TG: Calcium metabolism in normal human pregnancy. J Clin Endocrinol Metab 1971;33:661-670.
25. Kent GN, Price RI, Gutteridge DH, et al: The efficiency of intestinal calcium absorption is increased in late pregnancy but not in established lactation. Calcif Tissue Int 1991;48:293-295.
26. Klein CJ, Moser-Veillon PB, Douglass LW, et al: A longitudinal study of urinary calcium, magnesium, and zinc excretion in lactating and nonlactating postpartum women. Am J Clin Nutr 1995;61:779-786.
27. Pedersen EB, Johannesen P, Kristensen S, et al: Calcium, parathyroid hormone and calcitonin in normal pregnancy and preeclampsia. Gynecol Obstet Invest 1984;18:156-164.
28. Bertelloni S, Baroncelli GI, Pelletti A, et al: Parathyroid hormone–related protein in healthy pregnant women. Calcif Tissue Int 1994;54:195-197.
29. Martin TJ: Properties of parathyroid hormone–related protein and its role in malignant hypercalemia. Q J Med 1990;76:771-786.
30. Wysolmerski JJ, Broadus AE: Hypercalcemia of malignancy: The central role of parathyroid hormone–related protein. Annu Rev Med 1994;45:189-200.

31. Strewler GJ: The physiology of parathyroid hormone–related protein. N Engl J Med 2000;342:177-185.

32. Ferguson JE II, Gorman JV, Bruns DE, et al: Abundant expression of parathyroid hormone–related protein in human amnion and its association with labor. Proc Natl Acad Sci U S A 1992;89: 8384-8388.

33. Senior PV, Heath DA, Beck F: Expression of parathyroid hormone–related protein mRNA in the rat before birth: Demonstration by hybridization histochemistry. J Mol Endocrinol 1991;6:281-290.

34. Ferguson JE, Seaner R, Bruns DE, et al: Expression of parathyroid hormone–related protein and its receptor in human umbilical cord: Evidence for a paracrine system involving umbilical vessels. Am J Obstet Gynecol 1994;170:1018-1024.

35. MacIsaac RJ, Caple IW, Danks JA, et al: Ontogeny of parathyroid hormone–related protein in the ovine parathyroid gland. Endocrinology 1991;129:757-764.

36. Budayr AA, Halloran BP, King JC, et al: High levels of a parathyroid hormone-like protein in milk. Proc Natl Acad Sci U S A 1989; 86:7183-7185.

37. Van Heerden JA, Gharib H, Jackson IT: Pseudohyperparathyroidism secondary to gigantic mammary hypertrophy. Arch Surg 1988; 123:80-82.

38. Kronenberg HM, Lanske B, Kovacs CS, et al: Functional analysis of the PTH/PTHrP network of ligands and receptors. Recent Prog Horm Res 1998;53:283-303.

39. Laskey MA, Prentice A, Shaw J, et al: Breast-milk calcium concentrations during prolonged lactation in British and rural Gambian mothers. Acta Paediatr Scand 1990;79:507-512.

40. Neville MC, Keller RP, Seacat J, et al: Studies on human lactation. Within-feed and between-breast variation in selected components of human milk. Am J Clin Nutr 1984;40:635-646.

41. Hunscher HA: Metabolism of women during the reproductive cycle. II. Calcium and phosphorus utilization in two successive lactation periods. J Biol Chem 1930;86:37-57.

42. Mull JW, Bill AH: Variations in serum calcium and phosphorus during pregnancy. Am J Obstet Gynecol 1934;27:510-517.

43. Hillman L, Sateesha S, Haussler M, et al: Control of mineral homeostasis during lactation: Interrelationships of 25-hydroxyvitamin D, 24,25-dihydroxyvitamin D, 1,25-dihydroxyvitamin D, parathyroid hormone, calcitonin, prolactin, and estradiol. Am J Obstet Gynecol 1981;139:471-476.

44. Specker BL, Tsang RC, Ho ML: Changes in calcium homeostasis over the first year postpartum: Effect of lactation and weaning. Obstet Gynecol 1991;78:56-62.

45. Grill V, Hillary J, Ho PM, et al: Parathyroid hormone–related protein: A possible endocrine function in lactation. Clin Endocrinol (Oxf) 1992;37:405-410.

46. Dobnig H, Kainer F, Stepan V, et al: Elevated parathyroid hormone–related peptide levels after human gestation: Relationship to changes in bone and mineral metabolism. J Clin Endocrinol Metab 1995;80:3699-3707.

47. Kovacs CS, Chik CL: Hyperprolactinemia caused by lactation and pituitary adenomas is associated with altered serum calcium, phosphate, parathyroid hormone (PTH), and PTH-related peptide levels. J Clin Endocrinol Metab 1995;80:3036-3042.

48. Kent GN, Price RI, Gutteridge DH, et al: Human lactation: Forearm trabecular bone loss, increased bone turnover, and renal conservation of calcium and inorganic phosphate with recovery of bone mass following weaning. J Bone Miner Res 1990;5: 361-369.

49. Lippuner K, Zehnder HJ, Casez JP, et al: PTH-related protein is released into the mother's bloodstream during lactation: Evidence for beneficial effects on maternal calcium-phosphate metabolism. J Bone Miner Res 1996;11:1394-1399.

50. Kalkwarf HJ, Specker BL, Heubi JE, et al: Intestinal calcium absorption of women during lactation and after weaning. Am J Clin Nutr 1996;63:526-531.

51. Cross NA, Hillman LS, Allen SH, Krause GF: Changes in bone mineral density and markers of bone remodeling during lactation and postweaning in women consuming high amounts of calcium. J Bone Miner Res 1995;10:1312-1320.

52. Affinito P, Tommaselli GA, di Carlo C, et al: Changes in bone mineral density and calcium metabolism in breastfeeding women: A one year follow-up study. J Clin Endocrinol Metab 1996;81: 2314-2318.

53. Zinaman MJ, Hickey M, Tomai TP, et al: Calcium metabolism in postpartum lactation: The effect of estrogen status. Fertil Steril 1990;54:465-469.

54. Krebs NF, Reidinger CJ, Robertson AD, Brenner M: Bone mineral density changes during lactation: Maternal, dietary, and biochemical correlates. Am J Clin Nutr 1997;65:1738-1746.

55. Reddy GS, Norman AW, Willis DM, et al: Regulation of vitamin D metabolism in normal human pregnancy. J Clin Endocrinol Metab 1983;56:363-370.

56. Greer FR, Tsang RC, Searcy JE, et al: Mineral homeostasis during lactation—relationship to serum 1,25-dihydroxyvitamin D, 25-hydroxyvitamin D, parathyroid hormone, and calcitonin. Am J Clin Nutr 1982;36:431-437.

57. Kent GN, Price RI, Gutteridge DH, et al: Acute effects of an oral calcium load in pregnancy and lactation: Findings on renal calcium conservation and biochemical indices of bone turnover. Miner Electrolyte Metab 1991;17:1-7.

58. Dunbar ME, Wysolmerski JJ: Parathyroid hormone–related protein: A developmental regulatory molecule necessary for mammary gland development. J Mammary Gland Biol Neoplasia 1999;4:21-34.

59. Ratcliffe WA, Green E, Emly J, et al: Identification and partial characterization of parathyroid hormone–related protein in human and bovine milk. J Endocrinol 1990;127:167-176.

60. Yamamoto M, Fisher JE, Thiede MA, et al: Concentrations of parathyroid hormone–related protein in rat milk change with duration of lactation and interval from previous suckling, but not with milk calcium. Endocrinology 1992;130:741-747.

61. Thiede MA: The mRNA encoding a parathyroid hormone-like peptide is produced in mammary tissue in response to elevations in serum prolactin. Mol Endocrinol, 1989;3:1443-1447.

62. Uemura H, Yasui T, Yoneda N, et al: Measurement of N- and C-terminal-region fragments of parathyroid hormone–related peptide in milk from lactating women and investigation of the relationship of their concentrations to calcium in milk. J Endocrinol 1997;153:445-451.

63. Gardella TJ, Juppner H: Molecular properties of the PTH/PTHrP receptor. Trends Endocrinol Metab 2001;12:210-217.

64. DeSantiago S, Alonso L, Larrea F, et al: Negative calcium balance during lactation in rural Mexican women. Am J Clin Nutr 2002;76:845-851.

65. Sowers MF, Hollis BW, Shapiro B, et al: Elevated parathyroid hormone–related peptide associated with lactation and bone density loss. JAMA 1996;276:549-554.

66. Reid IR, Wattie DJ, Evans MC, Budayr AA: Post-pregnancy osteoporosis associated with hypercalcaemia. Clin Endocrinol (Oxf) 1992;37:298-303.

67. Khosla S, van Heerden JA, Gharib H, et al: Parathyroid hormone–related protein and hypercalcemia secondary to massive mammary hyperplasia [Letter]. N Engl J Med 1990;322:1157.

68. Bucht E, Telenius-Berg M, Lundell G, Sjoberg HE: Immunoextracted calcitonin in milk and plasma from totally thyroidectomized women. Evidence of monomeric calcitonin in plasma during pregnancy and lactation. Acta Endocrinol (Copenh) 1986;113:529-535.

69. Saxe A, Dean S, Gibson G, et al: Parathyroid hormone and parathyroid hormone–related peptide in venous umbilical cord blood of healthy neonates. J Perinat Med 1997;25:288-291.

70. MacIsaac RJ, Heath JA, Rodda CP, et al: Role of the fetal parathyroid glands and parathyroid hormone–related protein in the regulation of placental transport of calcium, magnesium and inorganic phosphate. Reprod Fertil Dev 1991;3:447-457.

71. Campbell DE, Fleischman AR: Rickets of prematurity: Controversies in causation and prevention. Clin Perinatol 1988;15:879-890.

72. Pereira GR, Zucker AH: Nutritional deficiencies in the neonate. Clin Perinatol 1986;13:175-189.

73. Specker BL: Do North American women need supplemental vitamin D during pregnancy or lactation? Am J Clin Nutr 1994;59(Suppl):484S-490S.

74. Seki K, Makimura N, Mitsui C, et al: Calcium-regulating hormones and osteocalcin levels during pregnancy: A longitudinal study. Am J Obstet Gynecol 1991;164:1248-1252.

75. Yamaga A, Taga M, Minaguchi H, Sato K: Changes in bone mass as determined by ultrasound and biochemical markers of bone

turnover during pregnancy and puerperium: A longitudinal study. J Clin Endocrinol Metab 1996;81:752-756.

76. Rodin A, Duncan A, Quartero HW, et al: Serum concentrations of alkaline phosphatase isoenzymes and osteocalcin in normal pregnancy. J Clin Endocrinol Metab 1989;68:1123-1127.

77. Karlsson R, Eden S, Eriksson L, von Schoultz B: Osteocalcin 24-hour profiles during normal pregnancy. Gynecol Obstet Invest 1992;34:197-201.

78. Sowers M, Crutchfield M, Jannausch M, et al: A prospective evaluation of bone mineral change in pregnancy. Obstet Gynecol 1991;77:841-845.

79. Drinkwater BL, Chesnut CH III: Bone density changes during pregnancy and lactation in active women: A longitudinal study. Bone Miner 1991;14:153-160.

80. Paparella P, Giorgino R, Maglione A, et al: Maternal ultrasound bone density in normal pregnancy. Clin Exp Obstet Gynecol 1995;22:268-278.

81. Naylor KE, Iqbal P, Fledelius C, et al: The effect of pregnancy on bone mineral density and bone turnover. J Bone Miner Res 2000;15:129-137.

82. Black AJ, Topping J, Durham B, et al: A detailed assessment of alterations in bone turnover, calcium homeostasis and bone density in normal pregnancy. J Bone Miner Res 2000;15:557-563.

83. Ritchie LD, Fung EB, Halloran BP, et al: A longitudinal study of calcium homeostasis during human pregnancy and lactation and after resumption of menses. Am J Clin Nutr 1998;67:693-701.

84. Paparella P, Giorgino R, Maglione A, et al: Maternal ultrasound bone density in normal pregnancy. Clin Exp Obstet Gynecol 1995;22:268-278.

85. Gambacciani M, Spinetti A, Gallo R, et al: Ultrasonographic bone characteristics during normal pregnancy: Longitudinal and cross-sectional evaluation. Am J Obstet Gynecol. 1995;173:890-893.

86. Lissner L, Bengtsson C, Hansson T: Bone mineral content in relation to lactation history in pre- and postmenopausal women. Calcif Tissue Int 1991;48:319-325.

87. Biberoglu KO, Yildiz A, Kandemir O: Bone mineral density in Turkish postmenopausal women. Int J Gynaecol Obstet 1993; 41:153-157.

88. Parra-Cabrera S, Hernandez-Avila M, Tamayo-y-Orozco J, et al: Exercise and reproductive factors as predictors of bone density among osteoporotic women in Mexico City. Calcif Tissue Int 1996;59:89-94.

89. Goldman GA, Friedman S, Hod M, Ovadia J: Idiopathic transient osteoporosis of the hip in pregnancy. Int J Gynaecol Obstet 1994;46:317-320.

90. Longstreth PL, Malinak LR, Hill CS Jr: Transient osteoporosis of the hip in pregnancy. Obstet Gynecol 1973;41:563-569.

91. Brodell JD, Burns JE Jr, Heiple KG: Transient osteoporosis of the hip of pregnancy. Two cases complicated by pathological fracture. J Bone Joint Surg Am 1989;71:1252-1257.

92. Guerra JJ, Steinberg ME: Distinguishing transient osteoporosis from avascular necrosis of the hip. J Bone Joint Surg Am 1995;77:616-624.

93. Stamp L, McLean L, Stewart N, et al: Bilateral transient osteoporosis of the knee in pregnancy. Ann Rheum Dis 2001;60:721-722.

94. Funk JL, Shoback DM, Genant HK: Transient osteoporosis of the hip in pregnancy: Natural history of changes in bone mineral density. Clin Endocrinol (Oxf) 1995;43:373-382.

95. Lose G, Lindholm P: Transient painful osteoporosis of the hip in pregnancy. Int J Gynaecol Obstet 1986;24:13-16.

96. Curtiss PH Jr, Kincaid WE: Transitory demineralization of the hip in pregnancy: A report of three cases. J Bone Joint Surg Am 1959;41:1327-1333.

97. Takatori Y, Kokubo T, Ninomiya S, et al: Transient osteoporosis of the hip. Magnetic resonance imaging. Clin Orthop 1991;271:190-194.

98. Sowers M, Eyre D, Hollis BW, et al: Biochemical markers of bone turnover in lactating and nonlactating postpartum women. J Clin Endocrinol Metab 1995;80:2210-2216.

99. Lamke B, Brundin J, Moberg P: Changes of bone mineral content during pregnancy and lactation. Acta Obstet Gynecol Scand 1977;56:217-219.

100. Atkinson PJ, West RR: Loss of skeletal calcium in lactating women. J Obstet Gynaecol Br Commonw 1970;77:555-560.

101. Sorenson JA, Cameron JR: A reliable in vivo measurement of bone mineral content. J Bone Joint Surg Am 1967;49:481-497.

102. Hayslip CC, Klein TA, Wray HL, Duncan WE: The effects of lactation on bone mineral content in healthy postpartum women. Obstet Gynecol 1989;73:588-592.

103. Chan GM, Slater P, Ronald N, et al: Bone mineral status of lactating mothers of different ages. Am J Obstet Gynecol 1982;144:438-441.

104. Chan GM, Ronald N, Slater P, et al: Decreased bone mineral status in lactating adolescent mothers. J Pediatr 1982;101:767-770.

105. Chan GM, Roberts CC, Folland D, Jackson R: Growth and bone mineralization of normal breast-fed infants and the effects of lactation on maternal bone mineral status. Am J Clin Nutr 1982;36:438-443.

106. Caird LE, Reid-Thomas V, Hannan WJ, et al: Oral progestogen-only contraception may protect against loss of bone mass in breast-feeding women. Clin Endocrinol (Oxf) 1994;41:739-745.

107. Laskey MA, Prentice A: Effect of pregnancy on recovery of lactational bone loss [Letter]. Lancet 1997;349:1518-1519.

108. Kalkwarf HJ, Specker BL: Bone mineral loss during lactation and recovery after weaning. Obstet Gynecol 1995;86:26-32.

109. Sowers M, Corton G, Shapiro B, et al: Changes in bone density with lactation. JAMA 1993;269:3130-3135.

110. Stiegler C, Leb G, Kleinert R, et al: Plasma levels of parathyroid hormone–related peptide are elevated in hyperprolactinemia and correlated to bone density status. J Bone Miner Res 1995;10:751-759.

111. Sowers M, Randolph J, Shapiro B, Jannausch M: A prospective study of bone density and pregnancy after an extended period of lactation with bone loss. Obstet Gynecol 1995;85:285-289.

112. Henderson P 3rd, Sowers M, Kutzko K, Jannausch M: Bone mineral density in grand multiparous women with extended lactation. Am. J Obstet. Gynecol. 2000;182:1371-1377.

113. Kalkwarf H, Specker B, Bianch D, et al: The effect of calcium supplementation on bone density during lactation and after weaning. N Engl J Med 1997;337:523-528.

114. Prientice A: Calcium supplementation during breast-feeding. N Engl J Med 1997;337:558-559.

115. Yamamoto N, Takahashi HE, Tanizawa T, et al: Bone mineral density and bone histomorphometric assessments of postpregnancy osteoporosis: A report of five patients. Calcif Tissue Int 1994;54:20-25.

116. Ratcliffe WA: Role of parathyroid hormone–related protein in lactation. Clin Endocrinol (Oxf) 1992;37:402-404.

117. Schnatz P, Curry S: Primary hyperparathyroidism in pregnancy: Evidence-based management. Obst Gynecol Surv 2002;57:365-376.

118. Carella MJ, Gossain VV: Hyperparathyroidism and pregnancy. Case report and review. J Gen Intern Med 1992;7:448-453.

119. Silverberg SJ, Shane E, Jacobs TP, et al: Primary hyperparathyroidism: 10-year course with or without parathyroid surgery. N Engl J Med 1999;341:1249-1255.

120. Heath H, Hodgson SF, Kennedy MA: Primary hyperparathyroidism—incidence, morbidity, and potential economic impact in a community. N Engl J Med 1980;302:189-193.

121. Mundy GR, Cove DH, Fisken R: Primary hyperparathyroidism: Changes in the pattern of clinical presentation. Lancet 1980;1:1317-1320.

122. Kort KC, Schiller HJ, Numann PJ: Hyperparathyroidism and pregnancy. Am J Surg 1999;177:66-68.

123. Kristoffersson A, Dahlgren S, Lithner F, Jarhult J: Primary hyperparathyroidism in pregnancy. Surgery 1985;97:326-330.

124. Croom RD, Thomas CG: Primary hyperparathyroidism during pregnancy. Surgery 1984;96:1109-1118.

125. Purnell DC, Smith LH, Scholz DA, et al: Primary hyperparathyroidism: A prospective clinical study. Am J Med 1971;50:670-678.

126. Mestman JH: Parathyroid disorders of pregnancy. Semin Perinatol 1998;22:485-496.

127. Clark D, Seeds JW, Cefalo RC: Hyperparathyroid crisis and pregnancy. Am J Obstet Gynecol 1981;140:840-842.

128. Kelly TR: Primary hyperparathyroidism during pregnancy. Surgery 1991;110:1028-1034.

129. Delmonico FL, Neer RM, Cosimi AB, et al: Hyperparathyroidism during pregnancy. Am J Surg 1976;131:328-337.

130. Wagner G, Transhol L, Melchior JC: Hyperparathyroidism and pregnancy. Acta Endocrinol 1964;47:549-564.

131. Ludwig GD: Hyperparathyroidism in relation to pregnancy. N Engl J Med 1962;267:637-642.

132. Pedersen NT, Permin H: Hyperparathyroidism and pregnancy. Report of a case and review of the literature. Acta Obstet Gynecol Scand 1975;54:281-283.

133. Graham EM, Freedman LJ, Forouzan I: Intrauterine growth retardation in a woman with primary hyperparathyroidism. A case report. J Reprod Med 1998;43:451-454.

134. Thomas BR, Bennett JD: Symptomatic hypocalcemia and hypoparathyroidism in two infants of mothers with hyperparathyroidism and familial benign hypercalcemia. J Perinatol 1995;15:23-26.

135. Marx SJ, Attie MF, Levine MA, et al: The hypocalciuric or benign variant of familial hypercalcemia: Clinical and biochemical features in fifteen kindreds. Medicine 1981;60:397-412.

136. Powell BR, Buist NR: Late presenting, prolonged hypocalcemia in an infant of a woman with hypocalciuric hypercalcemia. Clin Pediatr 1990;29:241-243.

137. Beattie GC, Ravi NR, Lewis M, et al: Rare presentation of maternal primary hyperparathyroidism. BMJ 2000;321:223-224.

138. Bruce J, Strong JA: Maternal hyperparathyroidism and parathyroid deficiency in the child. Q J Med 1955;96:307-319.

139. Mitchell TG: Chronic hypoparathyroidism associated with multicystic kidney. Arch Dis Child 1954;29:349-353.

140. Shangold MM, Dor N, Welt SI, et al: Hyperparathyroidism and pregnancy: A review. Obstet Gynecol Surv 1982;37:217-228.

141. Kaplan EL, Burrington JD, Klementschitsch P, et al: Primary hyperparathyroidism, pregnancy, and neonatal hypocalcemia. Surgery 1984;96:717-722.

142. Johnstone RE, Kreindler T: Hyperparathyroidism during pregnancy. Obstet Gynecol 1972;40:580-585.

143. Wilson DT, Martin T, Christensen R, et al: Hyperparathyroidism in pregnancy: Case report and review of the literature. Can Med Assoc J 1983;129:986-989.

144. Lueg MC, Dawkins WE: Primary hyperparathyroidism and pregnancy. South Med J 1983;76:1389-1392.

145. Lowe DK, Orwoll ES, McClung MR, et al: Hyperparathyroidism and pregnancy. Am J Surg 1983;145:611-614.

146. Tollin S: Course and outcome of pregnancy in a patient with mild, asymptomatic, primary hyperparathyroidism diagnosed before conception. Am J Med Sci 2000;320:144-147.

147. Haenel L, Mayfield R: Primary hyperparathyroidism in a twin pregnancy and review of fetal/maternal calcium homeostasis. Am J Med Sci 2000;319:191-194.

148. Reading CC, Charboneau JW, James EM, et al: High-resolution parathyroid sonography. AJR Am J Roentgenol 1982;139:539-546.

149. Sauer M, Steere A, Parsons MT: Hyperparathyroidism in pregnancy with sonographic documentation of a parathyroid adenoma. A case report. J Reprod Med 1985;30:615-617.

150. Udelsman R: Surgery in primary hyperparathyroidism: The patient without previous neck surgery. J Bone Min Res 2002;17(Suppl 2):N126-N132.

151. Visser BC, Glasgow RE, Mulvihill KK, Mulvihill SJ: Safety and timing of nonobstetric abdominal surgery in pregnancy. Dig Surg 2001;18:409-417.

152. Favus M (ed): Primer on the Metabolic Bone Diseases and Disorders of Mineral Metabolism, 4th ed. Philadelphia, Lippincott-Raven, 1999, pp 223-241.

153. Downs, RW: Hypoparathyroidism in the differential diagnosis of hypocalcemia. In Belizikan J, Levine M, Marcus R (eds): The Parathyroids, 2nd ed. New York, Academic Press, 2001, pp 755-835.

154. Kohlmeier L, Marcus R: Calcium disorders of pregnancy. Endocrinol Metab Clin North Am 1995;24:15-39.

155. Loughead JL, Mughal Z, Mimouni F, et al: Spectrum and natural history of congenital hyperparathyroidism secondary to maternal hypocalcemia. Am J Perinatol 1990;7:350-355.

156. Rude RK, Haussler MR, Singer FR: Postpartum resolution of hypocalcemia in a lactating hypoparathyroid patient. Endocrinol Jpn 1984;31:227-233.

157. Cundy T, Haining SA, Guilland-Cumming DF, et al: Remission of hypoparathyroidism during lactation: Evidence for a physiological role for prolactin in the regulation of vitamin D metabolism. Clin Endocrinol (Oxf) 1987;26:667-674.

158. Bronsky D, Kiamko RT, Moncada R, Rosenthal IM: Intra-uterine hyperparathyroidism secondary to maternal hypoparathyroidism. Pediatrics 1968;42:606-613.

159. Grant DK: Papilloedema and fits in hypoparathyroidism. Q J Med 1953;22:243-259.

160. Wright AD, Joplin GF, Dixon HG: Post-partum hypercalcaemia in treated hypoparathyroidism. BMJ 1969;1:23-25.

161. Blickstein I, Kessler I, Lancet M: Idiopathic hypoparathyroidism with gestational diabetes. Am J Obstet Gynecol 1985;153:649-650.

162. Redell G: Parathyroprival tetany and pregnancy. Acta Obstet Gynecol Scand 1946;26:1-10.

163. Blohm RW, Wurl OA, Gillespie JO, Escamilla RF: Refractoriness to antitetanic therapy in a case of surgical hypoparathyroidism. J Clin Endocrinol Metab 1953;13:519-533.

164. Graham WP III, Gordon CS, Loken HF, et al: Effect of pregnancy and of the menstrual cycle on hypoparathyroidism. J Clin Endocrinol Metab 1964;24:512-516.

165. Markestad T, Ulstein M, Bassoe HH, et al: Vitamin D metabolism in normal and hypoparathyroid pregnancy and lactation. Case report. Br J Obstet Gynaecol 1983;90:971-976.

166. Caplan RH, Beguin EA: Hypercalcemia in a calcitriol-treated hypoparathyroid woman during lactation. Obstet Gynecol 1990;76:485-489.

167. Salle BL, Berthezene F, Glorieux FH, et al: Hypoparathyroidism during pregnancy: Treatment with calcitriol. J Clin Endocrinol Metab 1981;52:810-813.

168. Caplan RH, Wickus GG: Reduced calcitriol requirements for treating hypoparathyroidism during lactation. A case report. J Reprod Med 1993;38:914-919.

169. Breslau NA, Zerwekh JE: Relationship of estrogen and pregnancy to calcium homeostasis in pseudohypoparathyroidism. J Clin Endocrinol Metab 1986;62:45-51.

170. Cruickshank DP, Pitkin RM, Reynolds WA, et al: Effects of magnesium sulfate treatment on perinatal calcium metabolism. Am J Obstet Gynecol 1979;134:243-249.

171. Cruickshank DP, Chan GM, Doerrfeld D: Alterations in vitamin D metabolism with magnesium sulfate treatment of pre-eclampsia. Am J Obstet Gynecol 1993;168:1170-1177.

172. Cumming WA, Thomas VJ: Hypermagnesemia: A cause of abnormal metaphases in the neonate. AJR Am J Roentgenol 1989;152:1071-1072.

173. Lamm CI, Norton KI, Murphy RJ, et al: Congenital rickets associated with magnesium sulfate infusion for tocolysis. J Pediatr 1988;113:1078-1082.

CLINICAL GENETICS

Margretta R. Seashore

10

The impact of genetic disorders on health and disease has been increasingly recognized since the 1950s. The overall frequency of inherited conditions, including those with single-gene, chromosomal, and nonclassical genetic causes, has been estimated to be just over 5%.[1] Two percent of infants have a major congenital malformation, many of which have a genetic component to their cause.[2] Genetic or gene-influenced conditions also contribute a substantial amount to infant and childhood morbidity and mortality. Hall and colleagues showed that 5% to 10% of hospital admissions in children are accounted for by these conditions,[3] and Roberts and associates estimated that almost 40% of childhood deaths are caused by conditions with a genetic component.[4] It is estimated that genetic disorders affect about 12% of hospitalized adults.[5,6] The knowledge about inherited conditions has expanded significantly as scientific understanding of many genetic conditions has increased. The completion of the draft sequence of the human genome in the current phase of the Human Genome Project has expanded the understanding of the structure and function of human genes, and the National Human Genome Research Institute is moving forward into the genomic era.[7] This expansion of knowledge in human genetics and genomics is providing new understanding of the role of genes in human disease. It signals the arrival of genomic medicine.[8] New molecular genetic tools have expanded diagnostic capabilities and will improve the ability to define risks to individuals and families on the basis of genotype. This increase in knowledge has begun to give the physician caring for women in the childbearing years the ability to provide anticipatory guidance and a timely assessment of risks when a woman is contemplating pregnancy, as well as advice and management when a woman is already pregnant. The physician requires enhanced understanding of these molecular genetic tools to provide up-to-date information to the pregnant woman. Genetic disorders that can affect pregnancy generate risks to the fetus on the basis of maternal or paternal factors and risks to maternal health resulting from the maternal genetic disease. Interventions that are available to the physician caring for the woman of childbearing age can address risk to the fetus as well as to the health of the mother.

When risk to the fetus or the mother is identified, the family can make reproductive decisions ahead of time.

GENETIC MECHANISMS THAT AFFECT PREGNANCY MANAGEMENT

Several genetic mechanisms are relevant to the care of the pregnant woman. In monogenic disorders, the clinical signs and symptoms are caused by a mutation in a single gene that significantly affects function. These conditions are individually rare and, in the aggregate, affect somewhat fewer than 1% of the population. Nevertheless, they cause significant morbidity and mortality. A considerable amount has been learned about these genes and the mechanisms by which they cause disease. Many common disorders aggregate in families but do not follow classical mendelian genetic patterns. The role that genes play in these conditions is that of conferring susceptibility to the disorder, and other factors that include different genes and environmental factors must also play a role. Although these mechanisms are still poorly understood,[9-11] much research is currently being devoted to their identification. Of the 30,000 to 35,000 genes currently estimated to make up the human genome,[7] many must play this kind of role. In addition, some genes follow a developmental timetable; time of expression during fetal life may play an important role in fetal growth and development.

The expansion of genetic knowledge has increased scientific understanding of many genetic conditions. Traditionally, the physician was limited to the use of pedigree analysis and estimation of risk with statistical methods for most mendelian conditions. Diagnosis was often based on phenotype, because it could be defined by physical examination, imaging tools such as radiography and ultrasonography, linkage to protein markers, and the measurement of analytes in body fluids such as blood and urine. In the 1990s, the understanding of the molecular genetic pathologic mechanisms of a large number of genetic conditions was advanced. The draft sequence of the human genome has been completed, and the understanding of the genetics and genomics of both rare and common disorders is expanding rapidly. Physicians will be able to use this information to make specific genetic diagnoses of the single-gene disorders and to identify genetic factors that influence the development of common disorders. Specific molecular testing now complements earlier methods for identifying genetic risk. New cytogenetic techniques have augmented earlier methods for detecting chromosome abnormalities.

Genetic factors that affect pregnancy outcome and management of the pregnant woman may be viewed as mechanisms that cause disease and as tools for identifying risk. In addition, the risks identified may be to the health of the fetus or the health of the mother. Risks to maternal health that arise from maternal genetic disease can involve any organ system. In addition, many genetic conditions affect more than one organ system, and the management plan must account for this. The mechanisms considered in this chapter include chromosomal (cytogenetic) and molecular mechanisms. Patterns of inheritance that are considered include mendelian single-gene patterns and familial aggregation in which the genetic mechanisms are not yet understood. The chapter addresses the ways in which increased genetic risk is recognized. Finally, it addresses the use of genetic tests in assessing the genetic effect on pregnancy and pregnancy outcome.

Cytogenetic Disorders

In every cell, the genetic material resides in chromosomes that contain DNA and nucleoproteins such as histones. Each human cell contains 23 pairs of chromosomes: 22 pairs of autosomes and 1 pair of sex chromosomes.[12,13] Abnormality in the structure or number of chromosomes is a major cause of fetal demise and contributes substantially to perinatal morbidity and mortality. In addition, chromosomal abnormalities are an important cause of mental retardation and of congenital malformations. Chromosomal abnormalities are thoroughly reviewed in several texts.[12-14]

Lymphocytes are the usual source of cells for preparing a karyotype. Cells are stimulated to divide so that mitosis can be stopped in metaphase. Microscopic slides are then prepared from the cells, and stains are applied. Chromosomes thus prepared demonstrate alternating dark and light bands, each of which contains a number of genes. By convention, the chromosomes are numbered according to size and position of the centromere[15] (Fig. 10–1).

New techniques for identifying chromosomes involve fluorescent in situ hybridization (FISH), in which fluorochromes and specific molecular probes are used.[16-19] These methods allow the identification of deletions,

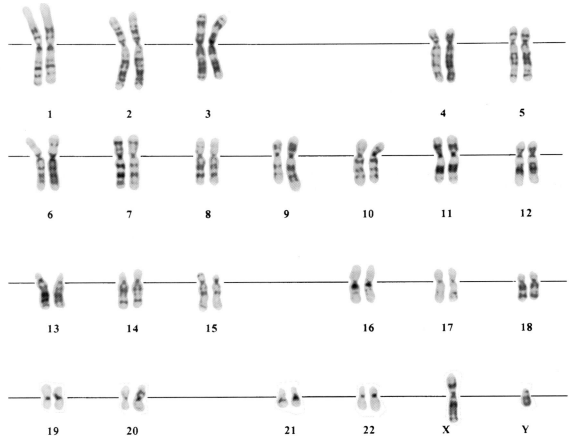

Figure 10–1. Normal karyotype, 46,XX. The distinctive bands of each chromosome can easily be seen. (Courtesy of Teresa Yang-Feng, PhD, Yale University.)

insertions, and rearrangements that cannot be appreciated with banding alone. Diagnostic testing for contiguous gene syndromes, microdeletions, and mosaicism involves the use of metaphase preparations and FISH methods in interphase preparations, such as cells obtained by chorionic villus sampling (CVS). Such FISH studies may provide a preliminary diagnosis of chromosome abnormalities. The full karyotype is normally used for confirmation. Multicolor spectral imaging enables visualization of the entire chromosome complement.[20,21]

Chromosomal abnormalities can be divided into abnormalities in number and abnormalities in structure. Abnormalities in number represent deviations from the normal number of 46, a situation known as aneuploidy. Trisomy, an extra chromosome from one of the pairs, occurs with autosomes and with sex chromosomes (Fig. 10–2). The most common trisomies are listed in Table 10–1. Monosomy, the loss of one chromosome from a pair, occurs with sex chromosomes; monosomy of X is the most common example. Autosomal monosomy is not seen in liveborn individuals; it is a cause of fetal demise. Other chromosomal abnormalities found in spontaneously aborted fetuses are listed in Table 10–2. Integral multiples of the haploid set of 23 chromosomes can also be seen. The most commonly recognized are three sets

(triploidy, or 69 chromosomes in each cell) and four sets (tetraploidy, or 92 chromosomes in each cell). These abnormalities are seen in spontaneously aborted fetuses and stillborn infants, and they are incompatible with life.

Structural rearrangements of chromosomal material can be balanced or unbalanced. In the balanced situation, the correct amount of genetic material is present, but it is rearranged. Structural chromosomal abnormalities have phenotypic consequences if there is deletion or duplication of genetic material or disruption of genes. In general, deletions have a worse effect on the phenotype than do duplications. Deleted euchromatic material contains a number of genes; thus, it is not surprising that such deletions result in a complex phenotype. The mechanisms by which these rearrangements occur are not well understood.

Translocations result from breakage and reassembly between two nonhomologous chromosomes. If no material is either gained or lost, these translocations are referred to as *balanced.* If the breaks occur at the centromere, the rearrangement is called *robertsonian;* if the breaks are on either the long or short arm, the translocation is called *reciprocal.* Figure 10–3 demonstrates a male karyotype with a translocation involving chromosomes 14 and 21. This translocation results in trisomy of chromosome 21 when the translocation is unbalanced. The possible chromosome

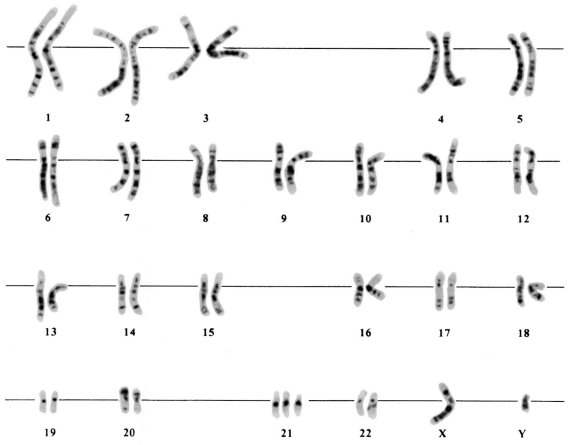

Figure 10–2. Karyotype demonstrating trisomy for chromosome 21, 47,XY +21. This is the karyotype found in the most common autosomal trisomy, Down's syndrome. (Courtesy of Teresa Yang-Feng, PhD, Yale University.)

TABLE 10–1 The Most Common Chromosome Abnormalities in Liveborn Infants

Types of Chromosomal Abnormalities	Frequency (per 1000 Liveborn Infants)
Autosomal trisomies (13, 18, and 21)	1.5
Sex chromosomes	
Male: (all types)	2.6 (of boys)
Female:	
XXX	1.04 (of girls)
45,X and mosaics	0.5 (of girls)
Structural rearrangements	
Balanced	1.9
Unbalanced	0.6
Total abnormalities	6.2
Abnormalities with phenotypic effects	4.0

Data from Hassold TJ, Jacobs PA: Trisomy in man. Annu Rev Genet 1984;18:69.

constitutions with this translocation are shown in Figure 10-4. Inversions occur when one chromosome undergoes two breaks and reassembly takes place with one piece inverted. Usually this has no phenotypic consequences, but it may have serious reproductive consequences when the inverted chromosome attempts to line up with its homologue at meiosis. The consequences of deletions have been recognized more clearly since the development of techniques that resolve the chromosome into discrete bands, because the correlation between phenotype and specific deleted bands can be made. A number of specific deletion and duplication syndromes are now recognized. Some of these are undoubtedly the result of the deletion of several important genes and have come to be called *contiguous gene syndromes*.[22,23] Insertions result from nonhomologous recombination between chromosomes. These are rare and cause no phenotypic effect but may have reproductive consequences because of their behavior at meiosis. Very small deletions and duplications undetected on light microscopy but identifiable through molecular techniques can be recognized by using specific probes for regions where deletions are known to occur and to result in clinical syndromes. Unbalanced rearrangements that occur at the telomeric ends of chromosomes are increasingly being recognized as a cause of mental retardation

TABLE 10–2 The Most Common Chromosomal Abnormalities in Spontaneously Aborted Fetuses

Chromosomal Abnormality	Karyotype
Monosomy X	45,X
Monosomy 21	45,XY, −21
Trisomy	47, + autosome
Double trisomy	48, + two autosomes
Mosaic trisomy	46/47, + autosome or 48, + two autosomes
Triploidy	69,XXX, XXX, or XYY
Tetraploidy	92,XXXX, XXXY, or XXYY
Structural abnormalities	Translocations, unbalanced

Data from Hassold TJ, Jacobs PA: Trisomy in man. Annu Rev Genet 1984;18:69.

and congenital malformations.[24,25] In some families, this event has occurred for the first time in the affected child. In other families, a balanced rearrangement is carried by a parent; this may lead to an unbalanced rearrangement in a child. When such a child is identified, a subtelomeric FISH study on both parents can identify whether such a rearrangement exists in a parent. FISH testing for subtelomeric rearrangements has been effective in prenatal diagnosis in families at risk for such disorders. FISH studies of both cultured and interphase cells obtained with CVS have achieved prenatal diagnosis of affected fetuses.[26,27]

The syndromes listed in Table 10-3 are associated with deletions or duplications, some of which are not detected at the light microscopic level.[23,28]

Trisomies account for more than 25% of spontaneous abortions and about 4% of stillbirths.[29] Trisomies occur in the fetus de novo as a result of nondisjunction of a pair of homologous chromosomes during meiosis in a parental gamete. The result is that the gamete, which should contain only one copy of each chromosome of the pair, instead contains two chromosomes of that pair. These can be the two homologous chromosomes of the pair or two copies of one of the homologues, depending on the stage of meiosis at which the error occurs. The mechanism of nondisjunction is not understood. There is some evidence for reduced meiotic recombination,[30] and techniques involving molecular cytogenetics are being developed to study the stage at which nondisjunction occurs.[31] The only well-recognized risk factor is maternal age.[32] The incidence of trisomies in live births and spontaneously aborted fetuses increases as maternal age advances, with an exponential rise beginning around the age of 35 years.[29] The frequency of trisomy has been estimated to exceed 30% in recognized pregnancies at maternal age 42.[29] Hook and Regal estimated the incidence of all trisomies at live birth at the same age to be approximately 2.5%.[33] This is in contrast to much lower frequencies at younger ages. Paternal age has also been examined as a factor in the cause of nondisjunction trisomy 21 (Down's syndrome),[34] a challenge because of the correlation of paternal age with maternal age. Nevertheless, the data show no significant effect of paternal age on nondisjunction.[33] Cross and Hook found an odds ratio of 1.5 (observed to expected paternal age) at paternal age 55, and this did not reach statistical significance.[34]

Uniparental disomy (UPD) is also now recognized as a cause of genetic disease.[35-38] In this situation, both of the chromosomes in a pair come from one parent with no contribution from the other parent. The total number of chromosomes is normal. The child may inherit two copies of the same homologue (isodisomy) or both chromosomes of a homologous pair (heterodisomy), depending on the stage of meiosis at which the error occurs. The mechanism probably involves a phenomenon called *trisomy rescue*.[39] The original zygote is trisomic, and the cell then loses one of the extra chromosomes without regard to the parental origin of that chromosome.[40-42] Isodisomy for chromosome 7 caused cystic fibrosis (CF) in a child whose mother was heterozygous for the CF mutation.[43] Another example of UPD accounting for a rare recessive disorder is a child with the fatty acid oxidation disorder trifunctional protein deficiency who inherited both chromosomes

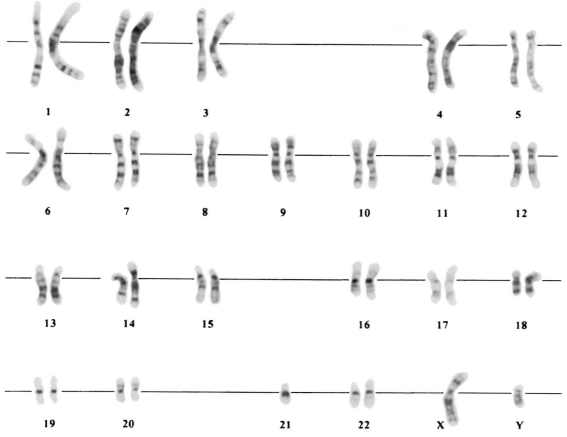

Figure 10–3. Karyotype demonstrating translocation of chromosomes 14 and 21, 45,XY, t(14q21q). The individual with this genotype has a balanced karyotype with the normal amount of material from chromosomes 14 and 21 and thus has a normal phenotype.

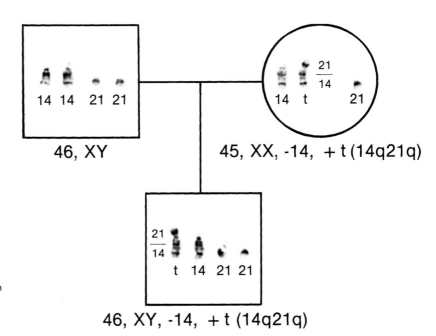

Figure 10–4. Reproductive consequences for an individual with the balanced translocation shown in Figure 10-3. (From Thompson MW, McInnis RR, Willard HF: Thompson and Thompson Genetics in Medicine. Philadelphia, WB Saunders, 1991, p 223.)

TABLE 10–3   Contiguous Gene Syndromes

Syndrome	Region	Critical Chromosomal Location
Greig's cephalopolysyndactyly	GCPS	del 7p13
Holoprosencephaly	HOLO	del 7q34
Trichorhinophalangeal/Langer-Giedion syndrome	TRP	del 8q24.1
Wilms' tumor, aniridia, genital abnormalities, retardation	WAGR	del 11p13
Beckwith-Wiedemann syndrome	BWS	dup 11p15
Retinoblastoma	RB	del 13q14.11
Prader-Willi/Angelman's syndrome	PWS/AS	del 15q12
HbH/α-thalassemia–mental retardation	ATMR	del 16p13.3
Rubinstein-Taybi syndrome	RTS	del 16p13.3
Miller-Dieker syndrome	MDS	del 17p13
Smith-Magenis syndrome	SMS	del 17p11.2
Charcot-Marie-Tooth disease type 1A	CMT1A	dup 17p11.2p12
Arteriohepatic dysplasia (Alagille's syndrome)	AHD	del 20p11.23p12.2
DiGeorge's/velocardiofacial syndrome	DGS	del 22q11
Cat-eye syndrome	CES	dup 22q11
Duchenne's muscular dystrophy/contiguous genes	DMD	del Xp21
Kallmann's syndrome/contiguous genes	KAL	del Xp22.3
Choroideremia, deafness, clefting, retardation	CDCR	del Xq21

Data from Greenberg F: Contiguous gene syndromes. Growth Genet Horm 1993;9:5; Schmickel R: Contiguous gene syndromes: A component of recognizable syndromes. J Pediatr 1986;109:231; and Eman BS: Molecular cytogenetics: Towards dissection of the contiguous gene syndromes. Am J Hum Genet 1988;43:575.

from one parent.[44] Although these events are important and their identification changes the estimates of genetic recurrence risks in affected families, they appear not to be a common mechanism for causing mental retardation and malformations. Heterodisomy has been recognized as a cause of Prader-Willi syndrome[45-47] and some growth retardation syndromes such as Russell-Silver syndrome. The genes involved in these conditions represent examples of parental imprinting, a poorly understood process by which the expression of a gene depends on the sex of the parent from whom it was inherited.[37] A number of genes involved in fetal growth exhibit imprinting.[48] Studies suggest that the role of UPD as a cause of early spontaneous abortion is not large.[40]

The overall effect of chromosomal abnormalities on pregnancy outcome derives from the frequency of trisomies caused by nondisjunction, the consequences of balanced rearrangements in a parent, and the occurrence of de novo structural rearrangements in the fetus. Trisomies involving autosomes and sex chromosomes are not rare. Hassold and Jacobs[29] reported an overall incidence of trisomy of 0.3% (1 per 333) of live births. The effect of chromosomal abnormalities on pregnancy outcome is summarized in Table 10–4.

Because maternal age is a well-known factor in the cause of nondisjunction, it is of interest to know the parental origin of the extra chromosome. Morphologic polymorphisms have been used to determine the parent of origin and, when informative, have shown that the extra chromosome is of maternal origin in more than 75% of cases.[25,49,50] More recently, the use of molecular techniques[51,52] has confirmed this conclusion and demonstrated that the extra chromosome is of maternal origin in about 95% of cases, independently of maternal age. The factors that lead to this phenomenon are poorly understood.[53-56]

The risk of recurrence of trisomy 21 in a subsequent pregnancy for a woman who has had a child with trisomy 21 is about 1%.[57,58] Several studies have addressed the rate

of trisomy 21 in second- and third-degree relatives of individuals with trisomy 21.[59,60] The results of these studies generally agree that the risk is below 1%, but it is unclear whether the age-related risk is increased over that in the general population. Speculation about the possibility of familial nondisjunction continues, and mechanisms such as mitochondrial DNA mutations have been proposed, but no convincing data exist.[61,62]

Balanced translocations in a parent have reproductive consequences because chromosomal segregation cannot take place normally during meiosis. The consequences of this in the fetus depend on whether the segregation in the parental gamete results in a balanced or unbalanced state in the fetus. The magnitude of the risk depends on the sex of the parent who carries the translocation; the risks are higher if the affected parent is the mother. If the fetal chromosomes contain a balanced amount of genetic material, the child will be like the parent with regard to the affected chromosome. This will have reproductive consequences for the child later in life, but no phenotypic effects. The most common example is illustrated by the parent with a robertsonian translocation involving chromosomes 14 and 21. The parent has 45 chromosomes, of which one is a translocation chromosome in which

TABLE 10–4   Effect of Cytogenetic Abnormalities on Pregnancy Outcome

Outcome	Trisomy 13 (%)	Trisomy 18 (%)	Trisomy 21 (%)
Spontaneous abortions	1.1	1.1	2.3
Stillbirths	0.3	1.1	1.3
Livebirths	0.005	0.01	0.13
All recognized pregnancies	0.18	0.18	0.45
Percentage that are liveborn	2.8	5.4	23.8

Data from Hassold TJ, Jacobs PA: Trisomy in man. Annu Rev Genet 1984;18:69.

14 and 21 are attached at the centromere (see Fig. 10–3). The small amount of centromeric material that is missing from one of those two chromosomes does not contribute to the phenotype. Gametes from such a parent can have the constitutions and consequences listed in Figure 10–4. The monosomies and trisomy 14 are not viable; these may result in early miscarriages even before the woman recognizes that she is pregnant. Trisomy 21 occurs in fewer than 5% of liveborn infants if the father is the translocation carrier and in about 10% of liveborn infants if the mother is the translocation carrier.[12] The reason for this difference is not known. Unbalanced translocations account for about 3% to 6% of all individuals with trisomy 21.[63] Other translocations occur, but they are considerably less frequent than 14;21 translocation (Table 10–5). If the situation is unbalanced in the fetus, the phenotype depends on the specific additional genetic material. Careful banding and molecular studies may be needed to define the expected phenotype. Other, more complex chromosomal rearrangements also occur and similarly have reproductive consequences. The risk of having chromosomally unbalanced offspring can vary from as much as 50% with some insertions to 0%, depending on the nature of the rearrangement.[64] Experience with subtelomeric rearrangements has shown an increased risk of an unbalanced offspring when a parent carries a balanced subtelomeric rearrangement.[26]

Abnormal chromosomal constitution in a parent is a cause of pregnancy loss and should be investigated when a couple has had more than two miscarriages. One study noted that in 10% of couples who have had recurrent miscarriages, one of the members of the couple had a chromosomal abnormality.[65] Tharapel and colleagues reviewed the literature and, combining data from 79 studies and their own study, they found that the frequency of chromosomal abnormalities in couples with two or more pregnancy losses was 2.9%, five to six times the frequency in the general population.[66] They defined pregnancy loss as spontaneous abortion, stillbirth, and early neonatal death. The types of chromosomal abnormalities found include translocations (both reciprocal and robertsonian), inversions, mosaicism, and extra sex chromosomes (both 47,XXX and 47,XXY karyotypes). It is clear that when any couple has a history of reproductive failure, including repeated miscarriage, stillbirth, or early infant death, the chromosomes of both members of the couple should be carefully evaluated. Identification of an abnormality has implications for the reproductive future of that couple, and it may also lead to the identification of extended family members at similar risk. Prenatal diagnosis with any method that provides

a fetal karyotype can be offered for a fetus at risk in a subsequent pregnancy.

Molecular Genetics

It has been said that the physician of the future must know the molecular anatomy, physiology, and biochemistry of the human genome if real understanding of inherited disorders is to be possible.[67,68] New understanding has been added to the traditional concepts of gene structure and function. DNA directs the synthesis of RNA, which in turn directs the synthesis of protein.[12,13] Genes, originally believed to be linear arrays of DNA, are now known to have a more complex structure. The coding regions of DNA (called *exons*) are interrupted by noncoding regions (called *introns*), which are transcribed to RNA but removed during RNA processing by a complex splicing mechanism. This mechanism then puts the RNA together as a continuous string of exons that are translated into protein.[69,70]

A number of ways of studying gene structure and function have been developed, and many of these are now being used for clinical diagnosis.[71,72] Several classes of mutations influence both gene expression and phenotype, and specific molecular abnormalities have been increasingly defined in a number of disorders.[73,74] Classes of mutations are listed in Table 10–6. Specific mutations result in specific abnormalities, and methods for identifying them have improved diagnostic precision. Mechanisms such as mosaicism in phenotypically normal parents of affected individuals, gonadal mosaicism, and gene expansion are being identified. Gene expansion changes gene structure and leads to abnormal or absent protein because of a number of repeated trinucleotide elements within the gene or in the untranslated region of the gene.[75,76] Mutations can affect protein function in a variety of ways, some of which may depend on the kind of protein involved. Examples of specific disorders and their molecular pathologic processes are listed in Table 10–7.

A number of new techniques provide molecular diagnosis of many genetic conditions.[71,77] Techniques that separate DNA into identifiable fragments,[78] cloning technology,[79] direct DNA sequencing,[80] and DNA amplification techniques[81] have revolutionized genetic diagnosis. As positional cloning has located and specified more disease genes, greater understanding of pathophysiologic processes, improved diagnosis, and possibilities for treatment have resulted. With increasing diagnostic specificity, heterogeneity at the genetic level is being recognized in a greater number of disorders. When direct DNA analysis does not give adequate information, new methods of protein analysis may yield answers. Duchenne's muscular dystrophy has been diagnosed by immunocytochemical analysis of the dystrophin made in muscle cells.[82] Such innovative methods that take advantage of molecular tools continue to be developed. Microarray technology, although not yet in wide use, is helpful in cancer diagnosis.[83] Examples of disorders for which molecular testing is available are listed in Table 10–8.

The increase in molecular understanding of genetic disorders has also led to new therapeutic ideas. Several investigators have suggested that understanding of the

TABLE 10–5   Translocations: Consequences of 14;21 Translocation in a Parent

Ovum/Sperm Cell Chromosomes	Phenotype of Offspring
Normal 21, normal 14	Normal
Normal 21, 14;21	Trisomy 21
Normal 14, 14;21	Trisomy 14 (nonviable)
14;21	Balanced 14;21 carrier
21, no 14	Monosomy 14 (nonviable)

TABLE 10–6　Classes of Mutations

Single base changes
　　Substitution (missense)
　　Nonsense
　　Premature stop codons
Messenger RNA processing mutations
　　Splice site mutations
　　Cryptic splice site activation
Deletions, insertions
　　Frameshift
　　Codon insertions, deletions
　　Gene deletions, duplications
　　Repeat element insertions, deletions
Fusion genes

CF mutation may lead to both pharmacologic interventions and to gene therapy for that disorder.[84,85] Major effort is being made to develop methods of gene transfer that could be clinically useful and result in normal functioning of the defective pathway in a genetic disorder.[86] Strategies involving retroviral vectors and direct or conjugated DNA injection are being investigated. For a number of disorders, animal models are being studied and clinical trials are being developed.[87,88] Experience with gene therapy approaches in congenital immune disorders have raised significant concerns, however, because of the development of leukemia in several recipients.[89]

INHERITED DISORDERS THAT AFFECT A PARENT

Inherited disorders that affect a parent confer risk on the unborn child, the magnitude of which depends on the mechanism of inheritance of the condition. Both mendelian inheritance and nonmendelian inheritance operate to cause the child to be at risk for developing the parent's condition.

The principle underlying mendelian inheritance is that a mutation at a single genetic locus results in the synthesis of an abnormal protein, the effects of which are expressed as an abnormality in a structural protein, an enzyme, a transport mechanism, or a regulatory mechanism.[12,13] If the gene involved is located on one of the 22 autosomes, the condition is called *autosomal*, and if it is located on the X chromosome, it is called *X-linked* or *sex-linked*. Known genes on the Y chromosome that lead to a clinical phenotype

TABLE 10–7　Examples of Specific Molecular Pathology

Disorder	Molecular Pathology
Duchenne's muscular dystrophy	Deletions, duplications
Cystic fibrosis	Codon deletion, point mutations
Phenylketonuria	Point mutations, splice site mutations
Huntington's disease	Trinucleotide repeat
Myotonic dystrophy	Trinucleotide repeat
Hemophilia A	Deletions, point mutations

TABLE 10–8　Examples of Disorders for which Molecular Testing Is Available*

Disorder	Testing
Duchenne's musclular dystrophy	Deletion analysis, linkage studies, dystrophin analysis in transformed cells
Phenylketonuria (PKU)	Specific mutation analysis, linkage analysis
Myotonic dystrophy	Trinucleotide repeat analysis
Fragile X syndrome	Trinucleotide repeat analysis
Neurofibromatosis	Linkage analysis, specific mutation analysis
Contiguous gene syndromes	Fluorescent in situ hybridization
Adult polycystic kidney disease	Linkage analysis
Thalassemias	Allele-specific oligonucleotide analysis
α_1-Antitrypsin deficiency	Allele-specific oligonucleotide analysis
Hemophilia A	Specific mutation analysis, linkage analysis

*A comprehensive list can be found in Phillips and Vnencak-Jones.[351] The list increases daily; several hundred disorders can be diagnosed with molecular tools.

are limited to the sex-determining genes on the short arm, but much research is being done to refine the Y map.[90] In the case of autosomal genes, if the deficit caused by this abnormal protein is clinically significant when only one of the two alleles is abnormal, the condition is called *dominant*. When both alleles must be abnormal for clinical expression, the condition is termed *recessive*. In the case of genes on the X chromosome, the mechanism is somewhat different. Boys and men with XY chromosome constitution have only a single X, and a mutant gene on that X chromosome is expressed. Girls and women, however, have two X chromosomes, and thus the definition of dominant and recessive holds. Single-gene disorders have an inheritance pattern that follows from these principles. Little is known as yet about the modifying effects of other genes on the expression of mutant genes that cause mendelian disorders.

The catalog published by McKusick includes more than 3000 traits inherited as single-gene traits.[91,92] This catalog now has more than 14,000 entries of phenotypes and gene loci related to human phenotypes. An increasing number of conditions have been shown to be inherited in a mendelian way. The chromosomal mapping strategy and location of more than 700 genetic disorders has been reviewed according to what McKusick called the "morbid anatomy of the human genome."[74,93] From a clinical point of view, autosomal dominant conditions can present problems for the physician caring for the pregnant woman. Often, a family history reveals a vertically inherited pattern of many members of the family affected with the same condition; this makes the diagnosis and assessment of risk fairly straightforward. More commonly, the patient represents the first affected member of a family, and the challenge is to establish the correct pattern of inheritance in order to establish risk. The first step is making the specific diagnosis in the individual. The phenomenon of genetic heterogeneity must be kept in mind during this process. As the molecular mechanisms of genetic disorders are established, it is increasingly recognized that in an autosomal dominant pattern, many conditions have similar phenotypes but different genetic mechanisms. Sometimes the specific genetic diagnosis may need to rely on molecular testing for certainty. Once the diagnosis is established, the literature must then be reviewed to establish the pattern of inheritance. In the case of autosomal dominant inheritance without a family history, the affected individual has a new mutation of the gene that can then be passed on to the offspring at the same 50% risk as if there were a family history. The other issue is the variability that some dominantly inherited conditions display both within and between families. This must be recognized and taken into account in discussions of the phenotype that the child at risk might develop. Figures 10-5 to 10-8 illustrate the mendelian patterns of inheritance.

The conditions that are inherited in an autosomal recessive manner do not show vertical inheritance; rather, they appear in multiple affected members in the same sibship. Whether there are also affected cousins depends on the frequency of the gene involved. The challenge is that of determining the correct diagnosis and whether recessive inheritance or consanguinity is involved. As in autosomal dominant inheritance, multiple affected members of the family may suggest the inheritance pattern, but specificity of the diagnosis is important, because genetic heterogeneity also operates here. In a family in which one child already suffers from an autosomal recessive condition, the 25% risk that another child will be affected must be represented as a new risk to that pregnancy. There is much less phenotypic variability within sibships in autosomal recessive conditions.

When the condition is X-linked, the family history demonstrates matrilineal inheritance, in which all affected individuals are related through their mothers. In the case of genes expressed in a single copy, the pattern is X-linked dominant and both sexes are affected, but affected men have only affected daughters, not affected sons. Because of X inactivation and random lyonization,[94] there is more phenotypic variability among affected girls and women. If the condition is X-linked recessive, affected boys and men express the condition, but girls and women usually do not. The risk to the unborn child depends on which parent has a personal or family history of an X-linked condition. If only the father has a positive family history, the risk depends on whether he too is affected. If so, he can pass his X chromosome, which bears the mutation, on to a daughter, who will be either affected or a carrier, depending on whether the condition is expressed in a dominant or recessive way. He cannot have an affected son, because he passes his Y and not his X chromosome on to a son. If the mother has a family history of an X-linked condition, it must be determined whether she is a heterozygote for this mutation. For many conditions, molecular testing is available. For others, reliance must be made on empirical risk calculations. If she already has an affected son, she is a heterozygote if she has such a family history. If she does not have a family history, the birth of an affected child may be the result of a new mutation or she may be heterozygous. Again, molecular testing may be helpful. Otherwise, clinical testing or empirical risk data must be used.

Mental retardation is more common in boys and men, and genes have been sought on the X chromosome to explain this observation. The first recognition of a specific causal gene on the X chromosome was marked by the observation cytogenetically of an abnormal-appearing X chromosome that was called a fragile site,[95] or "fragile X." In the past, cytogenetic techniques were used to diagnose this condition. The gene, FMR1, has been identified, and direct DNA analysis is used to diagnose this condition both postnatally and prenatally.[76,96,97] The number of repeats determines the severity of the phenotype. In normal individuals, the number of repeats ranges from about 5 to 44. Affected boys and men generally have more than 200 repeats, known as a full mutation.[98] An intermediate range of about 45 to 58 repeats is not usually associated with expansion or with a clinical phenotype. A repeat number of about 58 to 200 is called a premutation. Women who carry a premutation on one of their X chromosomes are at risk for expansion of the repeat number to more than 200; if a woman transmits that expanded

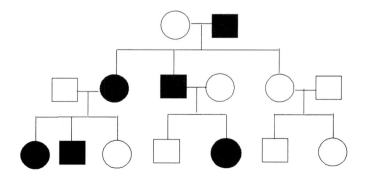

Figure 10–5. Prototype pedigree of autosomal dominant inheritance. Note that there is male-to-male transmission of the trait and that both sexes are affected. Unaffected persons do not have affected children.

Affected   Normal

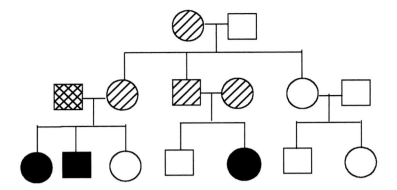

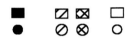

Affected   Heterozygous Normal

Figure 10–6. Prototype pedigree of autosomal recessive inheritance. Note that both male and female family members are affected. Cousins in the same generation can be affected. Affected persons do not have affected children unless the affected person's partner is heterozygous for the mutation, a situation that occurs if there is consanguinity or if the gene is very common.

X chromosome to her son, he will have fragile X mental retardation. The larger the number of repeats she has, the higher will be the risk that her offspring will have the full mutation. Maternal age and parental origin of the FMR1 gene may also be factors.[99,100]

Careful molecular diagnosis and genetic counseling are crucial for helping such a woman assess the risks to her offspring. The most significant risk is the 50% risk of transmitting her X chromosome with the expanded allele to a son. If she transmits the normal X chromosome, her son will not be affected. However, girls and women with an expanded FMR1 gene have an increased frequency of mental retardation; for this reason, if an affected woman's daughter inherits the X chromosome with an expanded allele, she is at risk for being affected. In addition, premature ovarian failure has been reported in women with a premutation.[101,102] Other fragile sites on the X chromosome have

now been identified, including fragile X (E), for which molecular testing is becoming available. A family history of boys and men with mental retardation or girls and women with mild mental retardation should prompt investigation of fragile X syndrome.[103]

Nonmendelian inheritance is a term used to refer to situations in which genes are involved but the pattern is not that of mendelian or single-gene inheritance. Several genetic mechanisms can explain this kind of family history. UPD for a chromosome that bears a mutation expressed as an autosomal recessive is one.[104] The recurrence risk in such a family would not be 25%, as predicted by autosomal recessive inheritance; in the case of UPD, risk for recurrence would be quite low. This has been reported in CF.[43]

In other situations, there may be genes that confer susceptibility to disease, but these genes alone are not enough to cause the disease. Major work is being done to

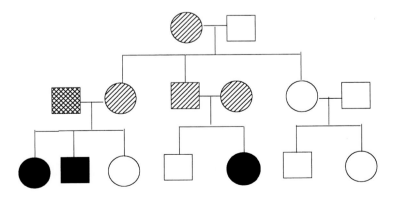

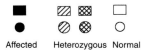

Affected   Heterozygous Normal

Figure 10–7. Prototype pedigree of X-linked recessive inheritance. The pattern is matrilineal. Affected men can have affected grandsons, but not affected sons.

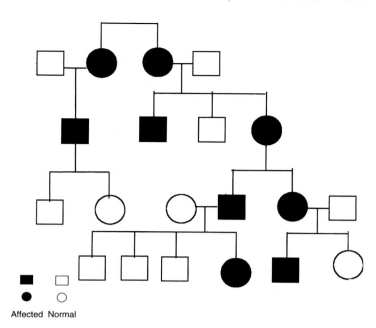

Figure 10–8. Prototype pedigree of X-linked dominant inheritance. The pattern is matrilineal. Affected men can have affected daughters and grandsons, but not affected sons. Women are also affected and can have affected sons and daughters.

Affected Normal

search for these kinds of susceptibility genes for hypertension, diabetes, obesity, and cancer. Current examples largely still include rare alleles that account for a small percentage of these disorders. Disorders in which such genes play a role include type II diabetes[105] and heart disease.[106] Similarly, such genes are being sought in relation to congenital malformations. Examples include Hirschsprung's disease,[107] in which mutations in the *RET* protooncogene and in SOX 10 have been identified,[108] and neural tube defects,[109,110] in which folic acid metabolism is being implicated. Such susceptibility genes probably have to act in concert with environmental factors, most of which are still largely unknown.

The phenomenon of maternal inheritance is recognized when the mutation responsible resides in the mitochondrial genome. The small mitochondrial genome encodes 13 polypeptides, all of which are subunits of enzymes involved in oxidative phosphorylation. This genome is entirely maternally inherited; mutations in mitochondrial DNA are passed from an affected mother to all her children regardless of sex.[111] In segregation during mitosis, mitochondria behave as populations; therefore, if cells contain both normal and mutated mitochondrial genomes, progeny cells may be normal or may contain mutated mitochondrial genomes. The segregation process is random. This segregation accounts for the clinical variability seen in these conditions. The most prominent mitochondrial disorders that are maternally inherited include the following disorders: Leber's hereditary optic neuropathy, a disorder characterized by loss of central vision and cardiac arrhythmias, has been associated with at least one specific mutation in mitochondrial DNA.[112] Both the syndrome of mitochondrial encephalomyopathy, lactic acidosis, and stroke-like symptoms (MELAS) and myoclonus epilepsy with ragged red fibers (MERRF) have been associated with maternally inherited mitochondrial mutations.[113-115] Diagnosis is accomplished by microscopy and molecular studies of muscle tissue from affected individuals. The inheritance pattern is demonstrated in Figure 10–9. Prenatal diagnosis may pose a challenge,[116] because a small sample of heteroplasmic fetal cells may not be representative of the rest of the body.

Risks to the Fetus Because of Maternal Genetic Conditions

Phenylketonuria

Phenylketonuria (PKU) is a recessively inherited inborn error of phenylalanine metabolism that, until the early 1960s, caused irreparable brain damage in the affected individual, resulting in severe mental retardation. It results from a deficiency in phenylalanine hydroxylase. The gene has been mapped to chromosome 12q24.1 and has been cloned.[68,117,118] If identified in the first weeks after birth and treated with a phenylalanine-restricted diet, children who have PKU can undergo normal intellectual development.[119,120] Since the development of neonatal screening for PKU, a generation of women who were diagnosed in the neonatal period and treated with the restricted diet have grown up. These women have not suffered the ravages of untreated PKU. Over the years, it has been observed that infants born to women with PKU suffer the teratogenic effects of high concentrations of phenylalanine circulating in the blood of the affected woman who does not follow the restricted diet during pregnancy.[120,121] Congenital heart defects, severe microcephaly, and mental retardation with a cerebral palsy–like picture are the most commonly seen effects.[119] In Lenke and Levy's study, 95% of mothers whose blood phenylalanine

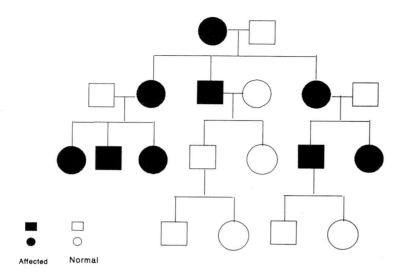

Affected   Normal

Figure 10–9. Prototype pedigree of mitochondrial inheritance. Note that male and female family members can be affected. All offspring of affected mothers are affected. Affected men cannot have affected offspring.

concentrations exceeded 20 mg/dL had one or more infants with mental retardation, 72% had infants with microcephaly, and 17% had infants with congenital heart disease. The Maternal PKU Collaborative Study[122] reported on a total of 468 pregnancies in 227 women with hyperphenylalaninemias. The data indicate that the blood phenylalanine levels through the first 8 weeks of pregnancy play an important role in the development of congenital malformations; levels during weeks 8 to 12 of pregnancy are a determinant of brain, fetal, and body growth. An influence on nervous system development continues through the rest of pregnancy. It is clear that the best outcome occurs when phenylalanine restriction results in good control before pregnancy begins.[120,122] It is crucial, however, that the diet be followed during the early weeks, which are extremely important in embryonic development.[123,124] In practical terms, this means before the onset of pregnancy. Major efforts are being made throughout the United States by the Maternal PKU Collaborative to identify women in whom PKU was diagnosed in neonatal screening programs to be sure that they are aware of the importance of the diet during pregnancy. In a report from the Centers for Disease Control and Prevention,[125] only 33% of pregnant women with PKU had confidence that their obstetrician was knowledgeable about PKU management during pregnancy; this prompted a call for improved education of obstetricians in this area. A National Institute of Child Health and Human Development (NICHD) Consensus Development Conference on Phenylketonuria[126] emphasized the importance of anticipatory management and dietary control for pregnant women with PKU. The physician who cares for a woman undertaking pregnancy should assess for this condition when obtaining the medical history and should test for it by measuring serum phenylalanine concentration if the woman has a history of two or more infants with microcephaly of unknown cause.[125,127]

Other Inborn Errors of Metabolism

Other inborn errors of metabolism have been studied for the kind of teratogenesis that occurs in PKU. Histidinemia,[128] Hartnup's disease,[128] propionic acidemia,[129] and lysinuric protein intolerance[130] have been specifically exonerated.

Folate Availability

Folate has been implicated in the origin of neural tube defects. Although it has not been shown that women who deliver infants with neural tube defects (spina bifida or anencephaly) are deficient in folate, evidence that folate supplementation can reduce the incidence of neural tube defects in offspring of women who have previously had such an affected child has accumulated.[131,132] Current recommendations for folate intake for pregnant women to prevent neural tube defects address women who have never had a child with a neural tube defect and those who have previously given birth to a child with a neural tube defect.[133] All women should supplement their diet with 0.4 mg/day of folate during their reproductive years. Women who have had a previous child with a neural tube defect should receive counseling regarding the risk for a recurrence and the appropriate amount of folate to take. Current recommendations include 4 mg/day of folate before the start of pregnancy.[134-136] Currently, food supplementation with folate provides more folic acid to prospective mothers.[137]

Skeletal Dysplasias

Infants of women who are affected with any of the skeletal dysplasias incur two kinds of risks: (1) the genetic risk during gestation of being affected with the condition and (2) the possible difficulty during delivery, which may necessitate operative delivery. The genetic risk to the fetus is best addressed by ascertaining the specific genetic diagnosis and mode of inheritance. The decision to undertake operative delivery depends on the anatomic changes that the skeletal dysplasia has produced. Of major concern are the skeletal dysplasias that cause pelvic contraction: most particularly, achondroplasia (Table 10-9).

TABLE 10–9   Skeletal Dysplasias with Obstetric Implications

Condition	Mode of Inheritance
Achondroplasia	Autosomal dominant
Osteogenesis imperfecta	Autosomal dominant and recessive
Pseudoachondroplasia	Autosomal dominant
Cartilage-hair hypoplasia	Autosomal recessive
Spondyloepiphyseal dysplasia	Autosomal dominant and recessive
Epiphyseal dysplasia	Autosomal dominant

Data from Allanson JE, Hall JG: Obstetric and gynecologic problems in women with chondrodystrophies. Obstet Gynecol 1986;67:74.

Maternal Epilepsy

Maternal epilepsy is associated with risks to maternal health and fetal well-being.[138-140] Anticonvulsant treatment of mothers raises special concerns.[141-143] Maternal health may be threatened because of a change in the metabolism of anticonvulsants during pregnancy and resultant increase in seizure frequency. An increased risk of toxemia, vaginal bleeding, hyperemesis gravidarum, and abruptio placentae have been reported.[144] Fetal malformations, low birth weight, prematurity, and neonatal drug withdrawal complicate fetal and neonatal life. A serious concern is the risk to the fetus posed by the teratogenic effects of some of the anticonvulsants. Hanson and associates[145,146] first reported a constellation of dysmorphic features in children born to mothers taking diphenylhydantoin during pregnancy; thus, fetal hydantoin syndrome was an additional cause of congenital malformations and mental retardation. Further studies on other anticonvulsants have shown that anticonvulsant exposure during fetal life increases the frequency of congenital malformations, microcephaly, mental retardation, growth restriction, and fetal death. Not all infants exposed to anticonvulsants are affected: Time of exposure, maternal dosage, maternal pharmacokinetics, and the specific drug are all factors.[144,147,148] The most common malformations identified are congenital heart disease, cleft lip and palate, and neural tube defects. Neural tube defects are particularly associated with exposure to valproic acid or carbamazepine. The frequency of minor malformations ranges from 6% to 20%, about a twofold increase in relative risk over that in the general population. Major malformations occur in 4% to 6% of the offspring of women with epilepsy, in comparison with about 1% to 2% in the general population.[144,147,148]

The woman with epilepsy needs to be informed of these associations, and her treatment must be tailored to her individual situation. Prevention of seizures contributes to maternal health and well-being. Because seizures increase the risk of miscarriage, their prevention also contributes to fetal well-being.[147,148] In addition, because the risk of adverse fetal outcome is relatively low when pregnancy is carefully managed, pregnant women should not automatically change or discontinue therapy because of concern about fetal risk.[144] Prenatal diagnostic tests, such as ultrasonography, that assess fetal anatomy should be offered to evaluate the fetus for evidence of malformations.

There is some evidence that folate supplementation may not be as protective against neural tube defects in pregnant women with epilepsy who are taking anticonvulsants,[147,148] particularly valproic acid and carbamazepine.

Vitamin A Toxicity

Two circumstances expose the pregnant woman to the teratogenic effects of vitamin A and other retinols. Intake of vitamin supplements has become popular, and such supplements are widely available; some calcium supplements also contain vitamin A. In addition, the synthetic retinol, isotretinoin, is used in the treatment of severe acne. Isotretinoin has been recognized as a teratogen since the early 1990s; estimates are that fetal exposure to this agent confers a 25-fold increase in risk for congenital malformations involving the head, face, heart, and central nervous system.[149,150] Other data[151] suggest that mothers who consume more than 10,000 IU per day of vitamin A as dietary supplements during pregnancy have an approximately threefold increased risk of having a child with craniofacial, central nervous system, thymic, and cardiac defects.

Wilson's Disease

Wilson's disease is a disorder of copper metabolism that is inherited in an autosomal dominant manner. The gene has been mapped to chromosome 13q14-21.[152] The mainstay of treatment has consisted of a copper-restricted diet and administration of agents that chelate copper, chiefly penicillamine and now trientine.[153] Current therapy for Wilson's disease includes the use of zinc acetate, which competes for copper transport.[154] The effect of Wilson's disease on pregnancy raised concern because of two case reports of infants born with connective tissue abnormalities to mothers receiving penicillamine during pregnancy.[155,156] The evidence is not clear that this outcome had anything to do with penicillamine. It has been reported that good pregnancy outcome can be achieved with careful management in patients with Wilson's disease treated with each of these preparations.[153,157-159] The risk of fetal abnormality in pregnancies complicated by Wilson's disease is probably very low, and treatment should continue because of the recognized dangers of treatment withdrawal.[153,160]

Myotonic Dystrophy

Myotonic dystrophy is an autosomal dominant condition with an estimated incidence of 1 per 8000.[161] Although age at onset of neurologic symptoms has usually been in the second decade, a congenital severe neonatal form has been recognized, and most often such a child is born to an affected mother.[161,162] The disorder results from a C-T-G trinucleotide repeat in the 3' untranslated region of the myotonic dystrophy protein kinase gene located on chromosome 19q13.3.[163-168] The number of repeats is increased in affected individuals in comparison with normal persons, and the size of the repeat may be correlated with clinical age at onset.[169,170] Expansion from generation to generation occurs and may account for the more severe phenotype of congenital hypotonia seen in the infant of an affected mother. Both clinical diagnosis and prenatal diagnosis can be made with molecular techniques; direct mutation analysis is preferred when possible.[76,116,168,171]

Risks to the Fetus Because of Paternal Genetic Conditions Disorders

The genetic risk to a fetus of being affected because of inherited parental genetic conditions, heterozygote status, or chromosomal translocations has already been discussed. There are few other risks to the fetus that result from paternal genetic disorders. Paternal PKU has been studied, and no effects on the fetus have been identified.[172]

Risks to Maternal Health Based on Maternal Genetic Disease

There are a number of genetic conditions in which the mother can experience worsening of disease during pregnancy or catastrophic events during delivery. It is important to be aware of these conditions so that the woman can be aware of the risks associated with pregnancy if she is not already pregnant or so that she can be managed expectantly if pregnancy is already under way. The following sections describe examples of specific genetic disorders with known risks associated with pregnancy. Other chapters in this textbook consider a variety of serious medical conditions that affect pregnancy. Textbooks of general medical management during pregnancy should be reviewed, or experts in management of the specific disorder should be consulted, for more detailed recommendations on specific management issues.

Hematologic Disorders

Alterations in physiology associated with pregnancy can complicate both the inherited hematologic disorders and the management of these disorders. Sickle cell anemia is an example of such a disorder. In addition, the use of pain medications to control painful crises can place the neonate at risk for withdrawal symptoms.[173] Children of mothers who are heterozygous for the either α- or β-thalassemia gene may be at risk for having severe forms of thalassemia if the fathers are also heterozygous for a deleterious mutation.

Connective Tissue and Skeletal Disorders

Marfan's Syndrome This disorder affects connective tissue, with manifestations in the ocular, skeletal, and vascular systems. The cardinal features are tall stature, scoliosis, joint hypermobility, arachnodactyly, dislocation of ocular lenses, mitral valve regurgitation, and dilatation of the aortic root.[174] The syndrome is inherited in an autosomal dominant manner and is associated with mutations in the gene for fibrillin (FBN1), which is located on chromosome 15q21.1.[175-177] Fibrillin is an important component of connective tissue. Point mutations as well

as deletions have been reported in FBN1 in patients with Marfan's syndrome. The diagnosis is based on clinical criteria and, in families in which a specific mutation has been identified, on molecular analysis of FBN1. Studies are beginning to make correlations between fibrillin abnormalities and the prognosis in Marfan's syndrome and the related fibrillinopathies that may prove useful for prognosis and treatment planning.[178] Women with Marfan's syndrome are at risk for catastrophic aortic rupture during pregnancy and delivery, as well as during the puerperium, if they have preexisting aortic root dilatation, aortic valve regurgitation, or other severe cardiovascular compromise. They can be managed well throughout pregnancy if these problems have not occurred.[179] Data suggest that aggressive medical and surgical management can mitigate risks of early death from cardiovascular complications. Treatment with β-adrenergic blockade and use of surgical techniques including mitral valve repair and composite aortic graft[180] are among the interventions that have been reported. The pregnant patient with Marfan's syndrome requires careful management by a team experienced with this condition.

Ehlers-Danlos Syndrome This name is applied to a number of disorders that involve the connective tissue of the skin and vascular system. At least 10 types have been identified, some of which are more severe than others and some of which have implications for the affected pregnant patient. Diagnosis is based on clinical grounds, except in families in which a molecular lesion can be identified in one of the collagen genes or in lysyl hydroxylase. The greatest risk to the pregnant woman is that of vascular rupture and uterine rupture (Ehlers-Danlos syndrome type IV).

Pseudoxanthoma Elasticum This genetically heterogeneous condition has been associated with gastrointestinal bleeding during pregnancy[181] and with abnormal placentation.[182]

Skeletal Dysplasias These conditions may complicate pregnancy. Allanson and Hall showed that pregnancy occurs in women with a variety of chondrodystrophies and that mean age at conception is no different from that in the general population.[183] In this group of disorders, an increased rate of poor pregnancy outcome, including spontaneous abortion, neonatal death, and prematurity, has been reported, but that was not substantiated in Allanson and Hall's study.[183] Pelvic abnormalities may necessitate operative delivery in the affected mother, and this is the preferred method of delivery in patients with achondroplasia. Respiratory distress based on thoracic contraction may make early delivery necessary. Care should be taken to evaluate the mother's spine before attempting any kind of spinal anesthesia, because of the danger of complications, especially spinal cord damage.

Pulmonary Disorders

Cystic Fibrosis This recessively inherited condition is associated with chronic, usually severe pulmonary disease and pancreatic insufficiency. It occurs in about 1 per 2500 white persons.[67] The gene has been mapped to chromosome 7q31.2. It codes for a protein, CFTR, which is a cell membrane protein essential for ion transport. Women with CF can survive to childbearing age and become pregnant. Clinton and associates' review suggested that pregnancy outcome is related to severity of maternal disease before the onset of pregnancy.[184] Increased fetal wastage, premature labor, and worsening of the mother's pulmonary status can all occur. Hypoxemia, cor pulmonale, and a decreased vital capacity all are predictive of difficulty with maternal tolerance of the increased cardiac load typical of pregnancy.[185,186] Other reports suggest that at least 75% of women with CF wishing to become pregnant can do so successfully.[187,188] Although prematurity is reported, outcome in the infant is generally good.[189] Good outcomes have been reported around the world. Pregnancy, however, is a stress on maternal lung function. Management during pregnancy requires attention to nutritional, infectious, and pulmonary functional needs and collaboration with CF specialists. Women who have CF transmit one CF mutation to their offspring; they should be offered testing for paternal CF carrier status. Prenatal screening for carrier status for CF is discussed in the section on genetic testing in this chapter.

Neurologic Disorders

Myotonic Dystrophy The implications of myotonic dystrophy for fetal well-being have been discussed earlier. The condition can worsen in the mother during pregnancy.[190] The myotonic process affects the myometrium, resulting in premature labor and postpartum complications.

Neurofibromatosis This autosomal dominant condition is associated with café au lait spots, neurofibromas, Lisch nodules, and, in some persons, optic neuroma and skeletal manifestations.[191,192] It occurs in about 1 per 3000 individuals; about 30% to 50% of cases represent new mutations in the neurofibromatosis type 1 (NF1) gene.[193,194] There is much clinical variability both within and between families. Diagnosis is made on the basis of the presence of two or more of the following: café au lait spots, neurofibromas, axillary or groin freckling, Lisch nodules, distinctive bone lesions, and the existence of an affected first-degree relative.[195] The central and the peripheral nervous systems can be involved. The NF1 gene has been mapped and cloned.[196,197] It is a very large gene and codes for a protein that is homologous to guanosine triphosphatase activating protein.[198] Mutations in the NF1 gene located on chromosome 17q11.2 have been identified and associated with the disease. Since the cloning of the NF1 gene, the clinical diagnosis has been augmented by DNA analysis in families in which a specific mutation has been identified and molecular diagnosis can be performed. DNA probes can be used for prenatal or postnatal diagnosis[199] when the family is informative with linkage markers or specific mutations or deletions.[200-202] The implications of this diagnosis for the health of the pregnant patient have been reviewed by several authors.[203-206] The early literature referred to increase in the size and number of neurofibromas during pregnancy,[207]

and these changes are still observed. If these are superficial, this growth may be of only cosmetic significance, but if they are located in areas where compression is a significant problem, such as the spinal canal, symptoms can progress rapidly. Rapid growth of intraspinal tumors has been reported in pregnancy with progression to paraplegia.[208] Hypertension has been a frequent problem in pregnant patients with NF1. Frequency has varied in several studies from half to nearly all patients.[209-212] Eclampsia has been noted,[212] as have thrombocytopenia[213] and occasional cases of malignant tumors such as neurofibrosarcoma and malignant schwannoma.[214-216] Molecular testing has been applied to preimplantation diagnosis.[217-220]

Disorders of Intermediary Metabolism

Ornithine Transcarbamylase Deficiency There have been several reports of women with ornithine transcarbamylase deficiency suffering acute ammonia intoxication that results in coma after delivery.[221] Ornithine transcarbamylase deficiency is an X-linked disorder of ammonia disposal that causes severe hyperammonemia and death if untreated in the affected boy or man.[222] Ornithine transcarbamylase is a mitochondrial enzyme crucial to the disposal of ammonia; the gene has been mapped to Xp21.1. More than 60 mutations in the gene have been identified, and molecular diagnosis is possible for some families.[223] Girls and women who, because of unfavorable lyonization, have a partial deficiency of this enzyme are intolerant of protein and can develop hyperammonemia under conditions of stress.[224] Because this condition is X-linked, its existence in a heterozygous woman could go undiagnosed as until the birth of an affected son or the occurrence of acute ammonia intolerance in the mother during the postpartum period. A family history of early infant death, especially of boys, should prompt investigation of this possibility. Other disorders of ammonia disposal could perhaps behave in the same manner, and careful monitoring is advisable.

Lysinuric Protein Intolerance This disorder has been reported[130] to be associated with anemia and thrombocytopenia in pregnancy and in at least one case of a stormy perinatal course for mother and child.

Homocystinuria It is possible that patients with homocystinuria caused by cystathionine synthase deficiency might be at risk for thromboembolic phenomena during operative delivery, much as they are during any surgery,[225] and thrombophlebitis has been reported during pregnancy. Women with pyridoxine-responsive cystathionine synthase-deficient homocystinuria have been reported to withstand pregnancy successfully.[226] With pyridoxine-unresponsive women and men, fewer conceptions occur.[227] No untoward effects on offspring have been noted.[226,227]

Porphyria Porphyria has been reported to worsen during pregnancy.[228-230] Causal factors that operate during pregnancy include poor caloric intake because of hyperemesis and increased estrogen and progesterone. It is important that the drugs known to precipitate attacks not be used and that caloric restriction be avoided.[231] Some drugs to be avoided include metoclopramide, ergot preparations, barbiturates, and sulfonamides. Aggarwal and associates emphasized the need for careful management in achieving good outcome of pregnancy.[230]

COMPLEX COMMON DISORDERS

Understanding of the genetics of common complex disorders such as heart disease and diabetes lags behind that of the rare single-gene disorders. The management of diabetes in pregnancy is addressed in Chapter 2, but the pregnant woman with diabetes may be concerned about the risk that her child will also develop diabetes. This risk is estimated to be about 2% for children of women with type 1 (insulin-dependent) diabetes mellitus; if the father has type 1 diabetes, the risk to the offspring is slightly higher, about 6%. Studies of susceptibility genes continue, but genetic testing is not yet practical. The frequency of type 2 (non–insulin-dependent) diabetes mellitus in the first-degree relatives of individuals who have type 2 diabetes has been estimated to be about 10% to 15%.[232]

COMMON PREGNANCY-RELATED CONDITIONS WITH A GENETIC COMPONENT

Hypertension in Pregnancy

Geller and colleagues described a genetic mechanism that accounts for pregnancy-induced hypertension in at least one family.[233] In this family, a mutation in the mineralo-corticoid receptor resulted in activation of this receptor in the presence of increased progesterone, exacerbating hypertension during pregnancy. It is unclear how common this mechanism may be, but it is an important model. Similarly, in glucocorticoid-remediable aldosteronism, a hereditary form of primary hyperaldosteronism that manifests with hypokalemia and hypertension, there is aggravation of existing hypertension without frank eclampsia or apparent increase in the frequency of preeclampsia during pregnancy.[234]

Preeclampsia/Eclampsia

The ongoing search for possible genetic mechanisms in preeclampsia and eclampsia has not yet led to conclusive results. Family studies have suggested that genetic factors are involved,[235] and attention has centered on maternal susceptibility and on maternal-fetal interactions. Immunogenetic mechanisms in particular have been sought but not yet found. Increased frequency of the thrombophilic disorders, including hyperhomocystinemia, factor V Leiden, and activated protein C resistance have been linked, as have procoagulant factors, but, again, the associations are not definitive. Numerous family studies and genetic considerations have been explored,[235,236] and familial aggregation has been confirmed. A positive family history that includes female first-degree relatives increases the risk in the primigravida by about fourfold in some studies.[237] Although many candidate loci have been proposed, none has been proved. Ultimately, this condition is likely to be heterogeneous, and a genetic contribution from both the mother and the fetus will probably be found.

Acute Fatty Liver of Pregnancy and HELLP Syndrome

Acute fatty liver of pregnancy and HELLP (hemolysis, elevated liver enzymes, and low platelets) syndrome[44] can be devastating illnesses in the mother. Some mothers with either of these conditions are carrying infants with deficient activity of mitochondrial trifunctional protein (TFP) (long-chain 3-hydroxyacyl–coenzyme A dehydrogenase [LCHAD] deficiency), an inherited disorder of fatty acid degradation.[238] This fetal-maternal combination has also been described in women with placental floor infarction. This condition appears to require the combination of a heterozygous mother and a homozygous affected infant. LCHAD deficiency can be successfully treated in the infant, but the mortality rate for these infants is high when it is unrecognized, and early treatment is therefore important. Although the carrier frequency in pregnant women with HELLP syndrome is probably low,[239] evaluation of the infant for LCHAD/TFP deficiency should be considered. In addition, the mother may be at risk during future pregnancies because LCHAD/TFP deficiency is inherited in an autosomal recessive manner.

INTERVENTIONS IN PREGNANCY COMPLICATED BY A GENETIC DISORDER

Before establishment of pregnancy, it is helpful to establish the risk to the fetus and the mother so that choices about reproductive management are available to the family. It is important to discuss the risks to both the mother and the baby. Referral to a genetic specialist may be of value, particularly if the diagnosis is in question or if complex genetic processes or testing is involved. The physician should discuss alternative methods of reproduction that may mitigate the risk to the health of mother or child. The family may wish to consider adoption if there is risk to the mother or the fetus. Assisted reproduction may be helpful if the risk is to the fetus. Strategies include artificial insemination by donor, in vitro fertilization with donor egg or sperm, or in vitro fertilization with the husband's sperm and then diagnostic testing of the blastocyst.[240] Intracytoplasmic sperm injection is also being used to address male disorders in which sperm production is abnormal.[241]

Tests that Address Risk to the Fetus

The interventions that address the risk to the fetus depend on the nature of the concern about that fetus. When the risk is for a condition with major anatomic or functional correlates, the use of only one modality for fetal diagnosis may suffice. Often, more than one modality is needed. The assessment of fetal anatomy, chromosome status, and biochemical and molecular status may all be needed to evaluate the fetus for the presence of a specific genetic abnormality.[242] Anatomy and functional correlates of anatomic structures such as the heart and kidneys can be assessed with ultrasonography. Specific diagnosis may often be accomplished by applying biochemical, molecular, and cytogenetic techniques to fetal cells.

Ultrasound examination can provide anatomic and functional information through noninvasive methods. Current ultrasound techniques entail the use of real-time scanners and provide information about fetal growth and movement. Specialized examinations can provide detailed information about cardiac structure and activity and about the anatomic structure of the head, chest, skeleton, and abdominal organs.[243] It is important that the sonologist be experienced in the diagnosis of congenital malformations if false-positive and false-negative results are to be avoided in ultrasound diagnosis of genetic conditions. In addition, it is crucial that the sonologist be familiar with the associations of congenital malformations within genetic syndromes; in particular, knowledge of the association between congenital cardiac malformations and other anatomic malformations should lead to further evaluation when one of these is identified. When the fetus is at known risk for a genetic syndrome, the examination can be planned to look for all associated malformations. The fetal skeleton can be assessed by ultrasonography, making it possible to diagnose a large number of skeletal dysplasias. Congenital heart disease is amenable to fetal diagnosis. The use of real-time transducers allows a functional assessment of valvular movement, and a four-chamber view provides more anatomic definition.[244,245] In addition, the great vessels can also be imaged. Other structures within the chest can be identified, and abnormalities such as diaphragmatic hernia can be diagnosed. The body wall can be well imaged, and defects such as omphalocele and intraabdominal masses such as polycystic kidneys can be seen. Hydrocephalus and microcephaly can be detected, as can absence of the corpus callosum and holoprosencephaly. Defects in development of the fetal spine, such as spina bifida and anencephaly, can also be seen. Ultrasonographic equipment continues to become more sophisticated, and increasingly finer anatomic detail is recognized. Second trimester ultrasound examination as a screening tool to identify pregnancies at high risk for chromosomal abnormalities may allow women to select more invasive testing such as amniocentesis to confirm or rule out a chromosomal disorder if such abnormalities are found.

Fetal biometry may be helpful in identifying the fetus at risk for trisomy 21. Ultrasound features that suggest the presence of trisomy 21 include short humerus and femur lengths,[246] increased nuchal fold thickness, echogenic bowel, echogenic intracardiac focus, and renal pyelectasis.[247-249]

The presence of *cystic hygroma* increases the risk that the fetus is affected with Turner's syndrome.[250,251] Other ultrasound abnormalities seen in Turner's syndrome include short femur length, subcutaneous edema, and narrow aortic arch.[251]

The presence of *fetal choroid plexus cysts* alerts the obstetrician to the increased risk of trisomy 18, and some studies have suggested that this risk may be as high as about 1 per 200.[252,253] However, isolated choroid plexus cysts may be seen in as many as 1% of pregnancies during the second trimester. For this reason, the risk of trisomy 18 must be refined to help the woman decide about the option for further invasive testing, such as amniocentesis. Ultrasound algorithms have been suggested, in which maternal age is taken into account and measurements of femur length, presence of other gross anomalies, and presence of a two-vessel umbilical cord are included.[254]

The risk for a chromosome abnormality can be refined with multiple serum markers. Protocols have been developed to use ultrasound markers and results of maternal serum markers to calculate a combined risk that can guide the decision to use more invasive testing such as amniocentesis, in view of its attendant risks.[255,256] These calculations can decrease the number of amniocenteses performed, but they must be carefully designed so that the detection of chromosomally abnormal fetuses is not substantially reduced.[249,252,257,258] Ultrasonography is being used to individualize risk estimates for trisomy 18, in combination with results of maternal serum screening.[254,259] Testing strategies that can be used earlier in pregnancy are under development.[260]

Longitudinal follow-up of children exposed to diagnostic ultrasonography in utero has shown no evidence of harm from this exposure. In a study performed by Stark and colleagues,[261] detailed neurologic and physical examination was performed on children who were monitored up to 12 years of age; no differences between these children and a control group were noted either at birth or at 12 years of age. Further reports continue to show the lack of association with significant effects on neurologic outcome, growth, development or cancer.[262] However, there are reports of an increase in left-handedness in boys exposed to fetal ultrasonography, which indicates the need for further research.[262,263] Examples of conditions that can be diagnosed in the fetus with ultrasonography are listed in Table 10–10.

Maternal blood is a source of both *proteins and cells* that reflect fetal status. The most prominent protein of fetal origin is α-fetoprotein (AFP). First recognized as a component of fetal serum, AFP was later measured in maternal serum through radioimmunoassay. Several large clinical studies have documented the association of greater-than-normal amounts of AFP in maternal serum when the fetus has a neural tube defect, open body wall defects, and skin abnormalities or when fetal well-being is compromised.[264-268] The U.K. study[268] and others demonstrated overlap between maternal serum concentrations and the presence of fetal defects, but the differences were sufficient to allow this measurement to become a useful screening test. When followed by careful ultrasound examination, AFP screening can detect 80% to 85% of open neural tube defects.[267] Because elevated maternal serum AFP can be associated with maternal diabetes, twin pregnancy, impending fetal demise, or no abnormality at all, and because the concentration is correlated with

TABLE 10–10 Fetal Diagnosis by Ultrasonography	
Congenital heart disease	Renal anomalies
Arrhythmias	Polycystic disease
Valvular anomalies	Renal agenesis obstructive
Hypoplastic left heart syndrome	uropathy
Neural tube defects	Skeletal dysplasias
Spina bifida	Ellis–van Creveld syndrome
Anencephaly	Thanatophoric syndrome
Gastrointestinal anomalies	Jeune's syndrome
Diaphragmatic hernia	Achondroplasia
Duodenal atresia	Osteogenesis imperfecta
Body wall defects	Camptomelic dysplasia
Omphalocele	Jarcho-Levin syndrome
Gastroschisis	Diastrophic dysplasia
	Robinow's syndrome
	Tetraphocomelia
	Craniosynostosis syndromes

gestational age and maternal weight, careful evaluation of the test result is crucial to its usefulness.

The observation that decreased concentrations of AFP in maternal serum were associated with an increased frequency of Down's syndrome[269] has led to efforts to refine maternal serum screening for fetal chromosomal abnormalities.[254,270-272] The addition of maternal age and history of a previous child with Down's syndrome were considered by Cuckle and Wald[273] to improve the risk estimates, but further refinement with three or four biochemical markers is now becoming widely used. Measurement of AFP, human chorionic gonadotropin, and unconjugated estrogen allows detection of an estimated 60% to 70% of fetuses with Down's syndrome or trisomy 18, regardless of maternal age.[274,275] Research is being directed at separation of fetal cells from the maternal circulation, but the problems relating to fetal cell enrichment have not yet been solved to make this a clinical reality.[276,277]

The three serum biochemical markers now in wide use are AFP, human chorionic gonadotropin, and unconjugated estriol. Statistical studies indicate that as many as 60% to 70% of fetuses with Down's syndrome can be detected through the combination of measuring these three analytes. This triple analyte screening does have a significant false-positive rate, which necessitates amniocentesis, with its entailed risks, to exclude cytogenetic abnormalities in the fetus. Adjusting the cutoff rate that is considered to be normal reduces the false-positive rate at the expense of also decreasing the number of abnormal fetuses identified. The decision to use these screening methods as an alternative to amniocentesis in the mother at higher risk should be made only after thorough genetic counseling with discussion of the predictive value of both kinds of testing.[278] Serum analyte screening is less reliable in predicting chromosome abnormalities in twin pregnancies, and the changes in each analyte are not consistent; therefore, this testing is unreliable in twin and higher order multiple pregnancies.[279] Studies continue in the efforts to develop more serum markers that would increase the precision of maternal serum screening.[280] Maternal serum screening with four serum markers by the addition of inhibin to the panel (quadruple testing, or "quad screen") is now entering clinical practice.[281]

Evidence is accumulating that the quadruple testing may have greater efficacy in detecting Down's syndrome.[282-284]

Amniocentesis in midtrimester has been performed for prenatal diagnosis for more than three decades. As the earliest of the techniques used to diagnose disease in the fetus, its safety and effectiveness have been carefully studied since the early 1970s. The procedure depends on obtaining amniotic fluid from the uterine cavity, most commonly through a transabdominal approach. Many studies have documented the safety and accuracy of midtrimester amniocentesis.[285-288] The percentage of fetal losses was not different from that in pregnant women who did not undergo amniocentesis. No significant differences were seen between newborns born after amniocentesis and those without amniocentesis. The pregnancy loss rate varied from 1.5%[82] to 4.7%.[288] Other collaborative studies have found similar data,[289] and the usual risk for fetal loss quoted for amniocentesis is 0.5%. Diagnostic errors were rare in all of the studies; Golbus and associates reported a karyotyping error rate of 0.07%.[285] The technique was further improved when Romero and colleagues showed that real-time ultrasonographic guidance could reduce the number of needle insertions necessary to obtain an adequate sample.[287] There is evidence that experience of the operator is also a factor.[289] The major drawback to midtrimester amniocentesis is the timing.

CVS can be used between weeks 10 and 13 of gestation to obtain fetal cells that can be studied directly or cultured to provide information about the fetus.[290-293] The advantage of CVS is the ability to obtain fetal cells in the first trimester, when the pregnancy is not far advanced. Information gained can be used for decisions about pregnancy termination at a time when there are fewer obstetric and social complications.[291] Because some studies can be done directly without the need for culturing cells, the time between the test and the result is minimal, thus reducing parental anxiety. The technique is performed under ultrasound guidance. In the transcervical approach, a flexible catheter is introduced into the chorion frondosum, and, under negative pressure, villi are aspirated.[294] Samples can also be obtained through the maternal abdomen using a 19-gauge spinal needle. The villi can then be dissected under a microscope, and cells can be examined directly or submitted for culture. Most data suggest that the fetal loss rate is lowest if the procedure is performed between the 9th and 11th weeks of pregnancy.[294,295] The collaborative study sponsored by NICHD[296] demonstrated the safety of CVS from the standpoint of maternal complications and fetal loss rate. Maternal complications are few. The fetal loss rate was estimated to be 3.8%, only 0.6% higher than the miscarriage rate for amniocentesis, and very close to the rate of spontaneous abortion at that gestational age of about 4%.[294] Brambati noted a range in fetal loss rates in various collaborative studies of 6.2% to 13.6%, some variation being related to gestational age and some to experience of the operator.[297]

Other reviews suggest that the risk of CVS for procedure-induced pregnancy loss is little different from that for amniocentesis.[298] Long-term follow-up studies have shown no difference in health status of children exposed to CVS in comparison with those who underwent amniocentesis, other than the increased frequency of limb deficiency abnormalities after early CVS. After scattered case reports appeared, Burton and coworkers first called attention to the association of limb anomalies in infants born after CVS had been performed early in the pregnancy.[299] They observed four infants with limb-reduction defects involving both hands and feet; the mothers had undergone CVS between 9.5 and 11 weeks of pregnancy. No technical factors could be identified to explain the observation, and no specific syndrome could be identified to explain the findings. After a study in Germany, Schloo and colleagues concluded that the incidence in large series might be no greater than population incidence and recommended further study.[300] In a study of 4300 pregnancies in which CVS was performed between 9 and 12 weeks' gestation, Jahoda and associates observed three cases of transverse limb defects—in two, CVS had been performed before 11 weeks—and concluded that further study was needed to clarify the safety of CVS, especially in early pregnancy.[301] In a workshop held at the NICHD, in which clinicians of worldwide expertise gathered to address this question,[302] the data from several large studies,[303] including the United States and Canadian collaborative studies, was reviewed.[296,304-306] This workshop showed that oromandibular limb hypoplasia was more common in CVS-exposed infants, perhaps correlated with performance of the procedure before 9 weeks' gestation. Holmes included early CVS among the causes of congenital limb defects.[307]

Current data suggest no increase in limb defects in comparison with the population risk if CVS is performed after 10 weeks' gestation.[298] The ethical issues involved in the use of CVS before 8 weeks' gestation[308] center on the increased risks of such early CVS and ethical and religious views surrounding pregnancy termination.

Observations of the outcome of pregnancies in which chromosomal mosaicism was noted in samples obtained at CVS have led to new uncertainties regarding the interpretation of the results of prenatal karyotyping.[46,309-313] Normally, the expectation is that both fetal and placental tissues should reflect the status of the fetus. However, at CVS, mosaicism is noted in 1% to 2% of pregnancies. When mosaicism is noted, two issues are paramount. The first is the need to distinguish between mosaicism confined to the placenta and mosaicism affecting the fetus; this risk has been ranged from 10% to 40% of the fetuses with confined placental mosaicism.[298,314] The second issue is assessing the risk that the embryo was initially trisomic and that rescue of this trisomic embryo has resulted in uniparental disomy of a pair of chromosomes in the fetus. Further studies that are indicated include fetal ultrasound examination,[315] to assess growth and anatomic structures, and amniocentesis, to confirm the fetal karyotype. Normal karyotype suggests that the fetus is not aneuploid, but true fetal mosaicism can never be completely ruled out. Molecular studies that identify maternal and paternal origin of the chromosome that was trisomic in the CVS study can confirm or rule out uniparental disomy. Certain chromosomes are of particular concern for uniparental disomy because of the presence of imprinted genes on them. These chromosomes include 7, 11, 14, and 15.[316] Fetal growth failure and malformations have been reported with confined placental mosaicism of chromosome 16.[317,318] If mosaicism is identified on CVS, amniocentesis should

be offered to the woman to confirm the status of the fetus.[298]

Percutaneous fetal blood sampling, also called *cordocentesis,* has been used to provide access to fetal blood when fetal cells obtained by other means are unrevealing or fetal serum is critical to the diagnostic study.[319,320] The technique involves the introduction of a needle into the umbilical cord near its insertion into the placenta and the withdrawal of fetal blood.[320] Volumes obtained vary from 1 to 4 mL. Real-time ultrasound guidance is used. The risks of the procedure are being assessed; rates of fetal loss range from 0% to 1.6%.[320,321] The advantage of this technique is that both cells and serum can be obtained, which widens the range of studies that can be performed. The technique is limited at present to a few specialized centers.

Fetal cells (whether obtained by CVS, amniotic fluid cell culture, or cordocentesis) can provide information through the use of cytogenetic, biochemical, or molecular tools. These cells can be used for karyotype analysis, enzyme measurement, or DNA analysis.[322] Analytes measured in amniotic fluid or fetal serum can include metabolites reflective of inborn errors of metabolism, proteins that leak from compromised body wall surfaces, kidneys affected by nephrosis, proteins known to be associated with pathologic conditions, and evidence of infections. Various prenatal diagnostic techniques are listed in Table 10-11.

A number of options for actions based on diagnostic information exist, and these should be discussed before any testing is undertaken. Although it is no longer considered important that parents decide on a course of action before prenatal testing, it is valuable to have considered the many possibilities before the crisis of decision making. Termination of pregnancy may be the option favored by a family confronted with the diagnosis in a fetus of a disorder that is incompatible with life or normal development. Undertaking this option should be accompanied by sensitivity to the feelings of the parents. Confirmatory studies

TABLE 10-11 Fetal Diagnostic Modalities

Method	Increased Risk of Fetal Loss*	Identified Pathologic Process
Maternal serum triple screening	0%	Open body wall defects; chromosomal abnormalities; impending fetal demise
Fetal ultrasonography	0%	Skeletal abnormalities; CNS, renal, body wall abnormalities; other anatomic features
Amniocentesis	0.5%	Biochemical abnormalities; enzymatic abnormalities; specific mutations; linkage markers for genetic disease; chromosomal abnormalities
Chorionic villus sampling	0.6%	Enzymatic abnormalities; specific mutations; linkage markers for genetic disease; chromosomal abnormalities

*Versus control group.
CNS, central nervous system.

should be considered on the abortus after the termination of pregnancy. The option of postabortion counseling should be presented. Delivery at a center that can address the fetal condition needs to be considered if a serious condition has been identified and the pregnancy is continued. Such a strategy has two important advantages: (1) the availability of skills and interventions to address the fetal problem, and (2) the lack of need for separation of the mother from the infant. This approach has been valuable in managing congenital heart disease and other congenital malformations such as omphalocele, diaphragmatic hernia, and neural tube defects.

As more treatment modalities become available, it may be possible to provide therapy in utero for genetically determined disorders. Treatment of a rare inborn error of metabolism has been reported[323] after prenatal diagnosis of vitamin B_{12}-responsive methylmalonic acidemia by providing the mother with large amounts of vitamin B_{12}. Packman and colleagues[324] successfully treated a fetus in whom biotin-responsive multiple carboxylase deficiency was prenatally diagnosed, by administering biotin to the mother. Prenatal diagnosis of congenital adrenal hyperplasia, followed by treatment of the mother with dexamethasone can reduce or even prevent virilization of the female fetus.[247,325] Fetal surgery has been performed in an effort to correct anatomic abnormalities in the fetus before they produce permanent damage. Efforts at catheter drainage for hydrocephalus, hydronephrosis, and hydrothorax have been reported,[326,327] but the outcome has been mixed. Lung expansion was seen in six of eight infants treated for hydrothorax.[327] For the uropathies, the chance of survival was good for posterior urethral valves but poor for other categories of uropathy. The outcome in the patients with hydrocephalus was less encouraging.[326] Open fetal surgery has been performed in both primate models and humans.[328] Wilson reported that the conditions for which fetal surgery is currently being considered include myelomeningocele, sacrococcygeal teratoma, cystic adenomatoid malformation of the lung with fetal hydrops, twin-to-twin transfusion syndrome, and other monochorionic twin abnormalities (severe discordant birth defects or twin reversed arterial perfusion sequences).[329] Maternal safety has been well demonstrated in the small number of cases reported, and no adverse effects on future reproductive capacity have been seen. Limiting factors have been the difficulty in preventing premature labor and the less-than-ideal outcome in the infants thus far treated.

Tests that Address Risk to the Mother

Confirmation of a genetic diagnosis in the mother is the first step needed to assess the risk and determine a diagnostic and therapeutic plan. Consultation with a genetic specialist may be of value in completing this part of the evaluation. After that, assessment of baseline status can be done with the involvement of appropriate specialists. The importance of counseling and follow-up cannot be overemphasized. In some cases, a new diagnosis may result from the assessment. The patient may require more information and longitudinal care, or specific

disease-related intervention during the pregnancy may be crucial. If the risk to the pregnant mother's life or health is determined to be high, she may elect termination of pregnancy.

IDENTIFICATION, GENETIC TESTING, AND COUNSELING OF PATIENT AND FAMILY AT RISK

Careful assessment of maternal health, as discussed earlier, is a keystone of the identification of the family at risk for a genetic condition in the fetus. Questions about paternal health history and age may turn up information that is also important to this assessment. A thorough family history, obtaining information about the families of both parents, should be documented with particular attention to early infant deaths, neurologic disorders, mental retardation, congenital malformations, skeletal disorders, and renal disorders.

Ethnic Background

All ethnic groups have genes that are more common in them than in other segments of the population. The reasons for this include geographic or religious isolation, founder effect, and genetic drift. If a mutation appears in a group that is socially or geographically isolated, it tends to be perpetuated in that group and is eventually common in that group than in others. It is important for the physician caring for the pregnant mother to recognize that she may be at a higher risk for a given condition on the basis of her ethnic background or that of the baby's father. The ability to determine heterozygote status for recessive conditions by means of screening tests is improving, and this kind of testing can be offered to provide knowledge to the family and to mitigate risk.[330] A list of disorders with increased prevalence in particular ethnic groups is provided in Table 10–12.

TABLE 10–12 **Heterozygote Screening in Ethnic Groups**

Ethnic Group	Disorder at Risk	Prenatal Diagnostic Test
European and U.S. populations	Cystic fibrosis	DNA analysis
White persons	Phenylketonuria	DNA analysis
Ashkenazi Jews	Tay-Sachs disease	Enzyme measurement, DNA analysis
	Canavan's disease	DNA analysis
	Gaucher's disease (adult)	DNA analysis
West African populations	Sickle cell anemia	DNA analysis
Mediterranean peoples	Thalassemia	DNA analysis
	Sickle cell anemia	DNA analysis
Asian peoples	α-Thalassemia	DNA analysis
	Sickle cell anemia	DNA analysis
French-Canadians	Tay-Sachs disease	Enzyme measurement, DNA analysis

Consanguinity

The offspring of consanguineous parents are at risk for recessively inherited conditions by virtue of inheriting two copies of a mutant gene from the shared ancestor of the parents. An affected child thus inherits two copies of a gene identical by descent. The more remote in generation the shared ancestor is, the lower the risk is. Siblings, who share two parents, have the highest risk of sharing the same recessive gene inherited from a parent, a chance of 50%. Distant cousins, on the other hand, whose shared relative may be many generations removed, have a much smaller risk of sharing a gene inherited from the common relative. These risks are recognized by U.S. law, in that most (but not all) states prohibit marriage between relatives closer than first cousins. Consanguineous marriage is, however, practiced among many populations around the world.[331] Empirical data exist to assess the risk of abnormal offspring to consanguineous parents when there is no genetic condition segregating in the family. These data demonstrate that the risks are high in siblings and other first-degree relatives. The empirical data suggest that when the relationship is further removed than first cousins, the risks are not greatly different from the risks in the general population. The empirical risk that first cousins will have a child with an abnormality is estimated to be 4.5% to 5%,[332] in comparison to the general population incidence of congenital malformations of 2% to 3%.[2] Decreased birth weight, stillbirth, early infant death, and congenital malformations are all increased among the offspring of cousins.[332-334] The offspring of siblings or father-daughter matings have a high risk of mental retardation, congenital malformations, and early death.[335]

Genetic Counseling and Testing

Risks in a Fetus Based on Parental or Family History

Information obtained from the family history may alert the physician to a number of kinds of risk in the fetus. A single-gene condition that follows mendelian principles may become obvious from the pedigree. On the other hand, the family history may reveal an individual who has a condition known to be inherited in a mendelian manner. In either case, careful assessment of the pedigree may establish the risk to the fetus. Alternatively, further testing of at-risk individuals may be needed.

Nonmendelian inheritance, discussed earlier, can also account for a family history of disorders that would be of concern to the couple planning a family or the woman already pregnant. In the case of the multifactorial situations, conditions in which genes and environment are operating, empirical risk figures must guide genetic assessment counseling. Because the risk in relatives for these conditions is low, there may be only one or two such affected persons in a family. Review of what is known about inheritance in the specific condition is helpful in assessing risk in the unborn child. In general, risks are low if the affected relative is more remote than second degree.

Maternal inheritance of a mitochondrial mutation should be considered when the clinical picture of myopathy or other neurologic symptoms, diabetes and deafness, or certain eye disorders is seen or when a family history is suggestive of maternal inheritance.

Balanced chromosomal translocations should also be considered when there is familial aggregation that does not fit a mendelian or maternally inherited pattern. The medical history of the affected individual may provide information as to whether a karyotype was obtained. If there is no information, the phenotype of the individual should be assessed to determine whether it is consistent with a chromosomal abnormality. Examples include multiple congenital malformations, mental retardation, or the combination of these. Further testing can be performed on the affected individual or on the parent of the unborn child at risk if the situation cannot be clarified.

Maternal health can affect the health of the unborn child. Mendelian conditions, nonmendelian conditions, chromosomal translocations, and maternal age have already been discussed. All these represent genetic risks. In addition, the maternal disease state may represent a risk to the fetus because of either direct effects of the disease on the baby or effects of the treatment.

Two opportunities for imparting information about genetic risks present themselves: before pregnancy has occurred and after pregnancy has been established. The challenges are somewhat different for each time, but the principles are the same. The importance of communication cannot be overemphasized.

The physician should take time to hear and understand the concerns and questions of the patient and family. A careful and thorough family history needs to be obtained, along with supporting data regarding any possible genetic diagnosis in other family members.[192] Thorough explanation of the genetic mechanisms involved and the factors that explain the risks should be made (Tables 10-13 to 10-16). Diagrams and other educational material may be helpful. Care should be taken to use terms that the patient and family can understand and to explain scientific terms that are unfamiliar. The physician needs to be sensitive to the concerns that the family may have about confidentiality and to the need to avoid stigmatization. Risks and probability statements should be clear. There should be ample opportunity for the patient and family to ask questions and to clarify areas of confusion. Empathic concern for the fear and anxiety that genetic risks raise is a crucial part of the communication process. It is also crucial that the patient and family use the information provided to arrive at their own choice of action.[336]

Prenatal Carrier Screening, Specialized Genetic Testing, and Neonatal Screening

As discussed in the section on ethnic background, carrier screening for heterozygosity for deleterious genes is an important way of identifying families at risk for an inherited disorder. Carrier screening for disorders that are highly prevalent within a particular ethnic group is routinely offered to women who are pregnant or contemplating pregnancy. Carrier screening for additional conditions is

TABLE 10-13   Congenital Malformations, Not Mendelian or Chromosomal

Malformation	Frequency Per 1000 Live Births	Recurrence Risk (%)
Spina bifida	2.5	3–5
Anencephaly	2	3–5
Congenital heart disease	6	3–10*
Pyloric stenosis	3	2–12†
Cleft lip/palate	1	3–5

Data from Carter CO: Genetics of common single malformations. Br Med Bull 1976;32:21.
*Depending on specific lesion.
†Depends on the sex of the index patient and of the siblings.

recommended in many centers. The American College of Obstetricians and Gynecologists and the American College of Medical Genetics (ACMG) published clinical guidelines for carrier screening for CF.[337-339] CF is a recessively inherited disorder that affects gastrointestinal and pulmonary function. When both members of a couple carry a CF mutation, the risk of having a child affected with CF is 25% with each pregnancy. The guidelines recommend offering CF screening to individuals with a history of CF, reproductive partners of persons with CF, and couples with one or both partners of European or Ashkenazi Jewish ancestry. The standard screening test should include a pan-ethnic panel of at least 25 mutations; this will identify 80% of white persons of European descent, 90% of white persons of northern European descent, and 97% of Ashkenazi Jews who are heterozygous.[338,340] The predictive value for persons who are members of other ethnic groups varies; the CF mutation is rare in Native Americans and in persons of Asian ethnicity. Although the frequency of CF in African Americans is lower than in white persons in general and Ashkenazi Jews, they may want to consider testing after being informed of the predictive value of testing for them. Molecular testing for CF heterozygosity is highly complex, and it is important that the physician select a laboratory that participates in the relevant quality assurance and proficiency testing programs provided by the College of American Pathologists and the ACMG. On occasion, test results can be equivocal because particular variants may be complicated to interpret. In such cases, referral to a genetic specialist may be needed if the laboratory report does not clarify the situation. Before choosing

TABLE 10-14   Factors in the Medical History to Consider in Assessing Genetic Risks

Consanguinity
Ethnic background
Maternal age
Medical history of known genetic condition
Family history of
    Early infant deaths
    Congenital malformations
    Mental retardation
    Multiply affected individuals, same disorder
    Known genetic condition

TABLE 10-15   Incidence, Prevalence, and Morbidity of Genetic Disorders

Estimated Incidence at Birth of Diseases with a Major Heritable Component

Disorder	Percentage of All Births
Chromosomal abnormalities at birth	0.5–1
Most common single-gene disorders	1–2
Major congenital anomalies (3% of births) with a genetic component	1.2
Nonspecific mental retardation (3% of births) with a genetic component	1.8
Total	4.5–6

Estimated Prevalence of Morbidity and Mortality Caused by Genetic Diseases

Perinatal Morbidity and Mortality	Percentage of All Cases
Chromosomal disorders	
Spontaneous abortions	50
Stillbirths/neonatal deaths	5
Surviving live births	0.5
Genetic disorders	
Genetic variation potentially handicapping: liveborn	10

Late Morbidity	Percentage of All Cases
Pediatric hospital admissions attributable to	
Single-gene diseases	
Chromosomal diseases	12
Multifactorial diseases	
Pediatric hospital admissions attributable to multifactorial congenital malformations	18
Adult hospital admissions with a significant genetic component	12
Severe mental retardation with a significant genetic component	60
15% single-gene defect	
45% other genetic component	

to be tested, patients should be fully informed about CF and factors to consider in screening, including the fact that CF genotype is not perfectly predictive of the clinical course in an affected individual. The American College of Obstetricians and Gynecologists provides educational material for patients that is helpful to the practitioner. Preconception testing allows the couple to discuss the options before undertaking a pregnancy. Prenatal testing is available through molecular testing on material obtained at CVS or amniocentesis.

Because the fragile X syndrome is the second most common cause of mental retardation after Down's syndrome, screening for fragile X carrier status is being offered to all women in some prenatal diagnostic centers. A recent Cochrane review reported that no clinical trials have been performed to show how effective this is in identifying families who would not be identified on the basis of family history.[341] However, patients with fragile X syndrome may have few clinical symptoms, and the condition may go undiagnosed. Pembrey and associates estimated that clinical case-finding followed by carrier testing may identify only half of premutation carriers.[342] Testing is accurate with molecular methods that detect the C-G-G repeat number.

TABLE 10–16 Categories of Biochemical Disorders for Which Prenatal Diagnosis Is Feasible, and Examples of Specific Disorders*

Amino Acid Metabolic Disorders
Argininosuccinic aciduria
Maple syrup urine disease
Methylmalonic acidemia
Propionyl-CoA carboxylase deficiency
Cystinosis
Homocystinuria

Carbohydrate Metabolic Disorders
Galactosemia
Glycogen storage diseases, types II–IV
Glucose-6-phosphate dehydrogenase deficiency
Mucolipidoses, types I–IV

Lipid Metabolic Disorders
Lipidosis Group
Gaucher's disease
Fabry's disease (XL)
Tay-Sachs disease
Sandhoff's disease
G_{M1} gangliosidosis
Krabbe's disease
Metachromatic leukodystrophy
Niemann-Pick disease
Farber's disease

Other Lipid Disorders
Familial hypercholesterolemia (AD)
Cholesterol ester storage disease
Refsum's syndrome
Wolman's disease

Mucopolysaccharide Metabolic Disorders
Hurler's syndrome
Hunter's syndrome (XL)
Sanfilippo's syndrome
Scheie's syndrome
Morquio's syndrome
β-Glucuronidase deficiency

Miscellaneous Disorders
Cystic fibrosis
Orotic aciduria
Lesch-Nyhan syndrome (XL)
Testicular feminization (XL)
Xeroderma pigmentosum
Hypophosphatasia (AR or AD)
Adenosine deaminase deficiency
Congenital adrenal hyperplasia
Porphyrias (AR and AD)
Sickle cell anemia
Thalassemia

*Mode of inheritance: autosomal recessive (AR) except when noted AD (autosomal dominant) or XL (X-linked).
CoA, coenzyme A.

As in other genetic testing, patients need to have accurate information before deciding whether to undergo this testing. The ACMG published guidelines on fragile X testing that discussed prenatal diagnostic testing[343]; material from both CVS and amniocentesis can be used, but the unique properties of CVS cells need to be recognized.

Neonatal screening represents another kind of genetic screening that is of interest to the pregnant woman. Although she will not be confronted with this until her newborn arrives, the obstetrician-gynecologist is in a unique position to prepare her for this testing, which takes place in the first days after her baby's birth.[344] Newborn screening for a battery of conditions is mandated in all 50 of the United States, in the uniformed services, in Puerto Rico, and throughout the developed world.[345,346] An increasing number of states has expanded the disorders tested for to include about 30 conditions, a large proportion of which are genetic. In some states, screening for CF[347] and congenital hearing loss are provided.[348] In all states in the United States, these programs are mandated by public health law and carried out in collaboration with Departments of Public Health. Some states require informed consent from the mother, but most do not. Information provided in a late prenatal visit can help a mother prepare for these tests and the possibility of a positive test result that will warrant further testing.

With the increasing recognition of molecular heterogeneity, the use of molecular diagnostic tools has become more complex.[349,350] The physician caring for the pregnant woman who has a genetic disorder or whose fetus is at risk for one may have an increased need for consultation with genetic specialists in diagnosis and management.[192] Clinicians should expect such specialists to provide up-to-date information on the availability of molecular diagnosis, the role of genetic heterogeneity, the modalities for prenatal testing, the availability of presymptomatic or heterozygote testing, and the prognosis for the fetus. Consultation with such specialists can be made available to the patient and family when the information and testing required are complex. Access to Internet resources can be of valuable help to the physician. Genetics resources on the Internet include the following:

Genetests: *http://genetests.org/*
National Human Genome Research Institute: *http://www.genome.gov/*
ACMG: *http://www.acmg.net/*
National Newborn Screening and Genetics Resource Center: *http://genes-r-us.uthscsa.edu/*
Cystic Fibrosis Mutation Database: *http://www.genet.sickkids.on.ca/cftr/*

SUMMARY

The physician caring for the woman who is pregnant or contemplating pregnancy has a unique opportunity to affect the health of both mother and child as well as to provide information of potential value to the mother's family. To take advantage of this opportunity to address genetic risks, the physician needs to be informed in all the major areas of diagnosis and management. Genetic conditions affect all organ systems without regard for age or class. Knowledge of new molecular diagnostic tools and of classical genetic mechanisms is necessary to provide the patient with information and available options. Communication skills and compassionate support are crucial in helping the patient understand and use the means that can be provided to ensure her health and the health of her unborn child.

References

1. Baird PA, Anderson TW, Newcombe HB, Lowry RB: Genetic disorders in children and young adults: A population study. Am J Hum Genet 1988;42:677.

2. Marden PM, Smith DW, McDonald MJ: Congenital anomalies in the newborn infant, including minor variations. J Pediatr 1964;64:357.

3. Hall JG, Powers EK, McIlvaine RT, Ean VH: The frequency and financial burden of genetic disease in a pediatric hospital. Am J Med Genet 1978;1:417.

4. Roberts DF, Chavez J, Court SDM: The genetic component in child mortality. Arch Dis Child 1970;45:33.

5. Day N, Holmes LB: The incidence of genetic disease in a university hospital population. Am J Hum Genet 1973;25:237.

6. Emery AEH, Rimoin D (eds): Principles and Practice of Medical Genetics, 2nd ed. Edinburgh, Churchill Livingstone, 1990.

7. Guttmacher AE, Collins FS: Genomic medicine—a primer. N Engl J Med 2002;347:1512.

8. Gerling IC, Solomon SS, Bryer-Ash M: Genomes, transcriptomes, and proteomes: Molecular medicine and its impact on medical practice. Arch Intern Med 2003;163:190.

9. Holtzman, NA, Marteau TM: Will genetics revolutionize medicine? N Engl J Med 2000;343:141.

10. Scriver CR: Mutation analysis in metabolic (and other genetic) disease: How soon, how useful. Eur J Pediatr 2000;159(Suppl 3):S243.

11. Scriver CR: Why mutation analysis does not always predict clinical consequences: Explanations in the era of genomics. J Pediatr 2002; 140:502.

12. Gelehrter TD, Collins FS: Principles of Medical Genetics. Baltimore, Williams & Wilkins, 1990.

13. Thompson MW, McInnis RR, Willard HF: Thompson and Thompson Genetics in Medicine, 6th ed. Philadelphia, WB Saunders, 2000.

14. deGrouchy J, Turleau C: Clinical Atlas of Human Chromosomes. New York, John Wiley, 1984.

15. International System for Human Cytogenetic Nomenclature: An international system for human cytogenetic nomenclature—high resolution banding. In Birth Defects: Original Article Series, vol 21, no. 1. New York, March of Dimes Birth Defects Foundation, 1985.

16. Lichter P, Boyle A, Cremer T, Ward D: Analysis of genes and chromosomes by nonisotopic in situ hybridization. Genet Anal Tech Appl 1991;8:24.

17. Mark H, Meyers-Seifer C, Seifer D, et al: Assessment of sex chromosome composition using fluorescent in situ hybridization as an adjunct to GTC-banding. Ann Clin Lab Sci 1995;25:402.

18. Trask B: Fluorescence in situ hybridization. Trends Genet 1991;7:149.

19. Anderlid BM, Schoumans J, Anneren G, et al: Subtelomeric rearrangements detected in patients with idiopathic mental retardation. Am J Med Genet 2002;107:275.

20. Schrock E, du Manoir S, Veldman T, et al: Multicolor spectral karyotyping of human chromosomes. N Engl J Med 1996;273:494.

21. Heng HH, Ye CJ, Yang F, et al: Analysis of marker or complex chromosomal rearrangements present in pre- and post-natal karyotypes utilizing a combination of G-banding, spectral karyotyping and fluorescence in situ hybridization. Clin Genet 2003;63:358.

22. Greenberg F: Contiguous gene syndromes. Growth Genet Horm 1993;9:5.

23. Schmickel R: Contiguous gene syndromes: A component of recognizable syndromes. J Pediatr 1986;109:231.

24. Fan YS, Zhang Y, Speevak M, et al: Detection of submicroscopic aberrations in patients with unexplained mental retardation by fluorescence in situ hybridization using multiple subtelomeric probes. Genet Med 2001;3:416.

25. Helias-Rodzewicz Z, Bocian E, Stankiewicz P, et al: Subtelomeric rearrangements detected by FISH in three of 33 families with idiopathic mental retardation and minor physical anomalies. J Med Genet 2002;39:e53.

26. Kilby MD, Brackley KJ, Walters JJ, et al: First-trimester prenatal diagnosis of a familial subtelomeric translocation. Ultrasound Obstet Gynecol 2001;17:531.

27. Pettenati MJ, Von Kap-Herr C, Jackle B, et al: Rapid interphase analysis for prenatal diagnosis of translocation carriers using subtelomeric probes. Prenat Diagn 2002;22:193.

28. Emanuel BS: Molecular cytogenetics: Towards dissection of the continuous gene syndromes. Am J Hum Genet 1988;43:575.

29. Hassold TJ, Jacobs PA: Trisomy in man. Annu Rev Genet 1984;18:69.

30. Warren AC, Chakravarti A, Wong C, et al: Evidence for reduced recombination on the non-disjoined chromosomes 21 in Down syndrome. Science 1987;237:652.

31. Stewart GD, Hassold TJ, Berg A, et al: Trisomy 21 (Down syndrome): Studying nondisjunction and meiotic recombination by using cytogenetic and molecular polymorphisms that span chromosome 21. Am J Hum Genet 1988;42:227.

32. Petersen MB, Mikkelsen M: Nondisjunction in trisomy 21: Origin and mechanisms. Cytogenet Cell Genet 2000;91:199.

33. Hook EB, Regal RR: A search for a paternal-age effect upon cases of 47, +21 in which the extra chromosome is of paternal origin. Am J Hum Genet 1984;36:413.

34. Cross PK, Hook EB: An analysis of paternal age and 47, +21 in 35,000 new prenatal cytogenetic diagnosis data from the New York State Chromosome Registry: No significant effect. Hum Genet 1987;77:307.

35. Moore GE, Ali Z, Khan RU, et al: The incidence of uniparental disomy associated with intrauterine growth retardation in a cohort of thirty-five severely affected babies. Am J Obstet Gynecol 1997;176:294.

36. Robinson WP, Langlois S, Schuffenhauer S, et al: Cytogenetic and age-dependent risk factors associated with uniparental disomy 15. Prenat Diagn 1996;16:837.

37. Schinzel A: Genomic imprinting: Consequences of uniparental disomy for human disease. Am J Med Genet 1993;46:683.

38. Webb AL, Sturgiss S, Warwicker P, et al: Maternal uniparental disomy for chromosome 2 in association with confined placental mosaicism for trisomy 2 and severe intrauterine growth retardation. Prenat Diagn 1996;16:958.

39. Sirchia SM, Garagiola I, Colucci G, et al: Trisomic zygote rescue revealed by DNA polymorphism analysis in confined placental mosaicism. Prenat Diagn 1998;18:201.

40. Fritz B, Aslan M, Kalscheuer V, et al: Low incidence of UPD in spontaneous abortions beyond the 5th gestational week. Eur J Hum Genet 2001;9:910.

41. Sanlaville D, Aubry MC, Dumez Y, et al: Maternal uniparental heterodisomy of chromosome 14: Chromosomal mechanism and clinical follow up. J Med Genet 2000;37:525.

42. Yong PJ, Marion SA, Barrett IJ, et al: Evidence for imprinting on chromosome 16: the effect of uniparental disomy on the outcome of mosaic trisomy 16 pregnancies. Am J Med Genet 2002;112:123.

43. Spence JE, Perciaccante RG, Greig GM, et al: Uniparental disomy as a mechanism for human genetic disease. Am J Hum Genet 1988;42:217.

44. Strauss AW, Bennett MJ, Rinaldo P, et al: Inherited long-chain 3-hydroxyacyl–CoA dehydrogenase deficiency and a fetal-maternal interaction cause maternal liver disease and other pregnancy complications. Semin Perinatol 1999;23:100.

45. Nicholls R, Knoll J, Butler M, et al: Genetic imprinting suggested by maternal heterodisomy in nondeletion Prader-Willi syndrome. Nature 1989;342:281.

46. Robinson WP, Christian SL, Kuchinka BD, et al: Somatic segregation errors predominantly contribute to the gain or loss of a paternal chromosome leading to uniparental disomy for chromosome 15. Clin Genet 2000;57:349.

47. Christian SL, Smith AC, Macha M, et al: Prenatal diagnosis of uniparental disomy 15 following trisomy 15 mosaicism. Prenat Diagn 1996;16:323.

48. Miozzo M, Simoni G: The role of imprinted genes in fetal growth. Biol Neonate 2002;81:217.

49. Mikkelsen M, Poulsen H, Grinsted J, Lange A: Nondisjunction in trisomy 21: Study of chromosomal heteromorphisms in 110 families. Ann Hum Genet 1980;44:17.

50. Thomas NS, Ennis S, Sharp AJ, et al: Maternal sex chromosome non-disjunction: Evidence for X chromosome–specific risk factors. Hum Mol Genet 2001;10:243.

51. Antonarakis SE: Parental origin of the extra chromosome in trisomy 21 as indicated by analysis of DNA polymorphisms. Down Syndrome Collaborative Group. N Engl J Med 1991;324:872.

52. Ballesta F, Queralt R, Gomez D, et al: Parental origin and meiotic stage of non-disjunction in 139 cases of trisomy 21. Ann Genet 1999;42:11.

53. Franco GC, Lucio PS, Parra FC, Pena SD: A probability model for the meiosis I non-disjunction fraction in numerical chromosomal anomalies. Stat Med 2003;22:2015.
54. Lamb NE, Freeman SB, Savage-Austin A, et al: Susceptible chiasmate configurations of chromosome 21 predispose to non-disjunction in both maternal meiosis I and meiosis II. Nat Genet 1996;14:400.
55. Sherman SL, Petersen MB, Freeman SB, et al: Non-disjunction of chromosome 21 in maternal meiosis I: Evidence for a maternal age-dependent mechanism involving reduced recombination. Hum Mol Genet 1994;3:1529.
56. Touil N, Elhajouji A, Thierens H, et al: Analysis of chromosome loss and chromosome segregation in cytokinesis-blocked human lymphocytes: non-disjunction is the prevalent mistake in chromosome segregation produced by low dose exposure to ionizing radiation. Mutagenesis 2000;15:1.
57. Daniel A, Hook EB, Wulf G: Risks of unbalanced progeny at amniocentesis to carriers of chromosome rearrangements: Data from United States and Canadian laboratories. Am J Med Genet 1989;31:14.
58. Stene J, Stene E, Mikkelsen M: Risk for chromosome abnormality at amniocentesis following a child with a noninherited chromosome aberration. Prenat Diagn 1984;4:81.
59. Eunpu DL, McDonald DM, Zackai EH: Trisomy 21: Rate in second-degree relatives. Am J Med Genet 1986;25:361.
60. Tamaren J, Spuhler K, Sujanksy E: Risk of Down syndrome among second- and third-degree relatives of a proband with trisomy 21. Am J Med Genet 1983;15:393.
61. Arbuzova S, Cuckle H, Mueller R, Sehmi I: Familial Down syndrome: Evidence supporting cytoplasmic inheritance. Clin Genet 2001;60:456.
62. Schon EA, Kim SH, Ferreira JC, et al: Chromosomal non-disjunction in human oocytes: Is there a mitochondrial connection? Hum Reprod 2000;15(Suppl 2):160.
63. Albright SG, Hook EB: Estimates of the likelihood that a Down syndrome child of unknown genotype is a consequence of an inherited translocation. Am J Med Genet 1980;17:272.
64. Daniel A, Stewart L, Saville T, et al: Prenatal diagnosis in 3000 women for chromosome, X-linked, and metabolic disorders. Am J Med Genet 1982;11:61.
65. Sachs ES, Jahoda MGJ, Van Hemel JO, et al: Chromosome studies of 500 couples with two or more abortions. Obstet Gynecol 1985;65:375.
66. Tharapel A, Tharapel S, Bannerman R: Recurrent pregnancy losses and parental chromosome abnormalities: A review. Br J Obstet Gynaecol 1985;92:899.
67. Boat T, Welsh M, Beaudet A: Cystic fibrosis. In Scriver C, Beaudet A, Sly W, Valle D (eds): The Metabolic Basis of Inherited Disease, 6th ed. New York, McGraw-Hill, 1989, pp 2649-2680.
68. Scriver C: Presidential address: Physiological genetics—who needs it? Am J Hum Genet 1987;40:199.
69. Singer M, Berg P: Genes and Genomes. Mill Valley, CA, University Science Books, 1991.
70. Beaudet A: Genetics, biochemistry, and molecular bases of variant human phenotypes. In Beaudet AL, Scriver CR, Sly WS, et al (eds): The Metabolic Basis of Inherited Disease, 8th ed. New York, McGraw-Hill, 2001, pp 3-128.
71. Caskey CT: Molecular medicine: A spin-off from the helix. JAMA 1993;269:1986.
72. Burke W: Genetic testing. N Engl J Med 2002;347:1867.
73. McKusick VM: Mendelian Inheritance in Man: Catalogs of Autosomal Dominant, Autosomal Recessive, and X-Linked Phenotypes, 10th ed. Baltimore, Johns Hopkins University Press, 1992.
74. McKusick VM: The morbid anatomy of the human genome: Chromosomal location of mutations causing disease. J Med Genet 1993;30:1.
75. Mandel JL: Questions of expansion. Nat Genet 1993;4:8.
76. Wenstrom KD: Fragile X and other trinucleotide repeat diseases. Obstet Gynecol Clin North Am 2002;29:367.
77. Landegren U, Kaiser R, Caskey CT, Hood L: DNA diagnostics—molecular techniques and automation. Science 1988;242:229.
78. Southern EM: Detection of specific sequences among DNA fragments separated by gel electrophoresis. J Molec Biol 1975;98:503.
79. Maniatis T, Hardison RC, Lacy E, et al: The isolation of structural genes from libraries of eucaryotic DNA. Cell 1975;15:687.
80. Ansorge W, Sproat B, Stegeman J, et al: Automated DNA sequencing: Ultrasensitive detection of fluorescent bands during electrophoresis. Nucleic Acids Res 1987;15:4593.
81. Mullis K, Faloona F, Scharf S, et al: Specific enzymatic amplification of DNA in vitro: The polymerase chain reaction. Cold Spring Harb Symp Quant Biol 1986;51:263.
82. Uchino M, Araki S, Miike T, et al: Localization and characterization of dystrophin in muscle biopsy specimens from Duchenne muscular dystrophy and various neuromuscular disorders. Muscle Nerve 1989;12:1009.
83. Tefferi A, Bolander ME, Ansell SM, et al: Primer on medical genomics. Part III: Microarray experiments and data analysis. Mayo Clin Proc 2002;77:927.
84. Collins FC: Cystic fibrosis: Molecular biology and therapeutic implications. Science 1992;256:774.
85. Tizzano EF, Buchwald M: Cystic fibrosis: Beyond the gene to therapy. J Pediatr 1992;120:337.
86. Mulligan RC: The basic science of gene therapy. Science 1993;260:926.
87. Ledley FD: Clinical considerations in the design of protocols for somatic genetic therapy. Hum Gene Ther 1991;2:77.
88. Ledley FD: Designing clinical trials of somatic gene therapy. Ann N Y Acad Sci 1994;716:283.
89. Check E: Harmful potential of viral vectors fuels doubts over gene therapy. Nature 2003;423:573.
90. Rozen S, Skaletsky H, Marszalek JD, et al: Abundant gene conversion between arms of palindromes in human and ape Y chromosomes. Nature 2003;423:873.
91. National Center for Biotechnology Information: Online Mendelian Inheritance in Man, *http://www3.ncbi.nlm.nih.gov:80/Omim/searchomim.html*. Bethesda, Md, National Library of Medicine, 2000.
92. McKusick VA: Mendelian Inheritance in Man. A Catalog of Human Genes and Genetic Disorders, 12th ed. Baltimore: Johns Hopkins University Press, 1998.
93. McKusick VA: The anatomy of the human genome: A neo-Vesalian basis for medicine in the 21st century. JAMA 2001;286:2289.
94. Lyon M: Gene action in the X-chromosome of the mouse (*Mus musculus*). Naturwissenschaften 1961;190:372.
95. Lubs HA: A marker X chromosome. Am J Hum Genet 1969;21:231.
96. Oostra BA, Willemsen R: Diagnostic tests for fragile X syndrome. Expert Rev Mol Diagn 2001;1:226.
97. Willemsen R, Oostra BA: FMRP detection assay for the diagnosis of the fragile X syndrome. Am J Med Genet 2000;97:183.
98. Backes M, Genc B, Schreck J, et al: Cognitive and behavioral profile of fragile X boys: correlations to molecular data. Am J Med Genet 2000;95:150.
99. Sherman S, Meadows K, Ashley A: Examination of factors that influence the expansion of the fragile X mutation in a sample of conceptuses from known carrier females. Am J Med Genet 1996;64:256.
100. Geva E, Yaron Y, Shomrat R, et al: The risk of fragile X premutation expansion is lower in carriers detected by general prenatal screening than in carriers from known fragile X families. Genet Test 2000;4:289.
101. Marozzi A, Vegetti W, Manfredini E, et al: Association between idiopathic premature ovarian failure and fragile X premutation. Hum Reprod 2000;15:197.
102. Bussani C, Papi L, Sestini R, et al: Premature ovarian failure and fragile X premutation: A study on 45 women. Eur J Obstet Gynecol Reprod Biol 2004;112:189.
103. GeneTests: Medical Genetics Information Resource (database online: *http://genetests.org/*). Copyright, University of Washington and Children's Health System, Seattle, 2003.
104. Hall JG: The clinical behavior of hereditary syndromes, with a precis of medical genetics. In Beighton P (ed): McKusick's Heritable Disorders of Connective Tissue, 5th ed. St. Louis, CV Mosby, 1993, pp 1-32.
105. Rich SS, Concannon P: Challenges and strategies for investigating the genetic complexity of common human diseases. Diabetes 2002;51(Suppl 3):S288.
106. Nabel EG: Cardiovascular disease. N Engl J Med 2003;349:60.
107. Eng C: The RET proto-oncogene in multiple endocrine neoplasia type 2 and Hirschsprung's disease. N Engl J Med 1996;335:943.

108. Amiel J, Lyonnet S: Hirschsprung disease, associated syndromes, and genetics: A review. J Med Genet 2001;38:729.

109. Gordon N: Folate metabolism and neural tube defects. Brain Dev 1995;17:307.

110. Steegers-Theunissen RP: Folate metabolism and neural tube defects: A review. Eur J Obstet Gynecol Reprod Biol 1995;61:39.

111. Kroon AM, Van den Bogert C: Biogenesis of mitochondria and genetics of mitochondrial defects. J Inherited Metab Dis 1987;10(Suppl 1):54.

112. Singh G, Lott MT, Wallace DC: A mitochondrial DNA mutation as a cause of Leber's hereditary optic neuropathy. N Engl J Med 1989;320:1300.

113. Inui K, Fukushima H, Tsukamoto H, et al: Mitochondrial encephalomyopathies with mutation of the mitochondrial tRNALeu(URR) gene. J Pediatr 1992;120:62.

114. Rosing HS, Hopkins LC, Wallace DC, et al: Maternally inherited mitochondrial myopathy and myoclonic epilepsy. Ann Neurol 1985;17:228.

115. Shoffner JM, Lott MT, Lezza AMS, et al: Myoclonic epilepsy and ragged-red fiber disease (MERFF) is associated with a mitochondrial DNA tRNALys mutation. Cell 1990;61:931.

116. Amiel J, Gigarel N, Benacki A, et al: Prenatal diagnosis of respiratory chain deficiency by direct mutation screening. Prenat Diagn 2001;21:602.

117. Kwok SC, Ledley FD, DiLella AG, et al: Nucleotide sequence of a full-length complementary DNA clone and amino acid sequence of human phenylalanine hydroxylase. Biochemistry 1985;24:556.

118. Waters PJ, Parniak MA, Akerman BR, Scriver CR: Characterization of phenylketonuria missense substitutions, distant from the phenylalanine hydroxylase active site, illustrates a paradigm for mechanism and potential modulation of phenotype. Mol Genet Metab 2000;69:101.

119. Lenke RR, Levy HL: Maternal phenylketonuria and hyperphenylalaninemia. An international survey of the outcome of untreated and treated pregnancies. N Engl J Med 1980;303:1202.

120. Smith I, Glossop J, Beasley M: Effects of dietary treatment and maternal phenylalanine concentrations around the time of conception. J Inherited Metab Dis 1990;13:651.

121. Mabry CC, Dennistron JC, Nelson TL, Son CD: Maternal phenylketonuria: A cause of mental retardation in children with the metabolic defect. N Engl J Med 1963;269:1404.

122. Rouse B, Azen C, Kock R, et al: Maternal Phenylketonuria Collaborative Study (MPKUCS) offspring: Facial anomalies, malformations, and early neurological sequelae. Am J Med Genet 1997;69:89.

123. American Academy of Pediatrics Committee on Genetics: Maternal phenylketonuria. Pediatrics 1991;88:1284.

124. Platt LD, Koch R, Azen C, et al: Maternal Phenylketonuria Collaborative Study, obstetric aspects and outcome: The first 6 years. Am J Obstet Gynecol 1992;166:1150.

125. From the Centers for Disease Control and Prevention. Barriers to dietary control among pregnant women with phenylketonuria—United States, 1998-2000. JAMA 2002;287:1258.

126. U.S. Department of Health and Human Services, Public Health Service, National Institutes of Health: Report of the NIH Consensus Development Conference on Phenylketonuria (PKU): Screening and Management. Washington, D.C., U.S. Government Printing Office, 2001.

127. Hanley WB: Prenatal testing for maternal phenylketonuria (MPKU). Int Pediatr 1994;9(Suppl):33.

128. Levy H: Hartnup disorder. In Beaudet AL, Scriver CR, Sly WS, et al (eds): The Metabolic Basis of Inherited Disease, 8th ed. New York, McGraw-Hill, 2001, pp 4957-4970.

129. Van Calcar SC, Harding CO, Davidson SR, et al: Case reports of successful pregnancy in women with maple syrup urine disease and propionic acidemia. Am J Med Genet 1992;44:641.

130. Simell O: Lysinuric protein intolerance and other cationic aminodacidurias. In Scriver C, Beaudet A, Sly W, Valle D (eds): The Metabolic Basis of Inherited Disease, 6th ed. New York, McGraw-Hill, 1989, pp 2497-2513.

131. Recommendations for the use of folic acid to reduce the number of cases of spina bifida and other neural tube defects. MMWR Recomm Rep 1992;41:1.

132. Prevention of neural tube defects: Results of the Medical Research Council Vitamin Study. MRC Vitamin Study Research Group. Lancet 1991;338:131.

133. Butterworth CE Jr, Bendich A: Folic acid and the prevention of birth defects. Annu Rev Nutr 1996;16:73.

134. Czeizel AE: Nutritional supplementation and prevention of congenital abnormalities. Curr Opin Obstet Gynecol 1995;7:88.

135. Oakley GP Jr, Adams MJ, Dickinson CM: More folic acid for everyone, now. J Nutr 1996;126:751S.

136. Rayburn WF, Stanley JR, Garrett ME: Periconceptional folate intake and neural tube defects. J Am Coll Nutr 1996;15:121.

137. Olney RS, Mulinare J: Trends in neural tube defect prevalence, folic acid fortification, and vitamin supplement use. Semin Perinatol 2002;26:277.

138. Bruno MK, Harden CL: Epilepsy in pregnant women. Curr Treat Options Neurol 2002;4:31.

139. Morrell MJ: Guidelines for the care of women with epilepsy. Neurology 1998;51(5, Suppl 4):S21.

140. Morrow JI, Craig JJ: Anti-epileptic drugs in pregnancy: Current safety and other issues. Expert Opin Pharmacother 2003;4:445.

141. Pack AM, Morrell MJ: Treatment of women with epilepsy. Semin Neurol 2002;22:289.

142. Zahn CA, Morrell MJ, Collins SD, et al: Management issues for women with epilepsy: a review of the literature. Neurology 1998;51:949.

143. Zahn C: Neurologic care of pregnant women with epilepsy. Epilepsia 1998;39(Suppl 8):S26.

144. Pennell PB: Pregnancy in the woman with epilepsy: maternal and fetal outcomes. Semin Neurol 2002;22:299.

145. Hanson JW, Myrianthopoulos NC, Harvey MAS, Smith DW: Risks to the offspring of women treated with hydantoin anticonvulsants, with emphasis on the fetal hydantoin syndrome. J Pediatr 1976;89:662.

146. Hanson JW, Smith DW: The fetal hydantoin syndrome. J Pediatr 1975;87:285.

147. Yerby MS: Special considerations for women with epilepsy. Pharmacotherapy 2000;20:159S.

148. Yerby MS: The use of anticonvulsants during pregnancy. Semin Perinatol 2001;25:153.

149. Lammer E, Chen D, Hoar R: Retinoic acid embryopathy. N Engl J Med 1985;313:837.

150. Rosa F: Teratogenicity of isotretinoin. Lancet 1983;2:513.

151. Rothman KJ, Moore LL, Singer MR, et al: Teratogenicity of high vitamin A intake. N Engl J Med 1995;333:1369.

152. Cox DW: Disorders of copper transport. Br Med Bull 1999;55:544.

153. Sternlieb I: Wilson's disease and pregnancy. Hepatology 2000;31:531.

154. Anderson LA, Hakojarvi SL, Boudreaux SK: Zinc acetate treatment in Wilson's disease. Ann Pharmacother 1998;32:78.

155. Linares A, Zarranz JJ, Rodrequez-Alarcon J, Diaz-Perez JL: Reversible cutis laxa due to maternal D-penicillamine treatment. Lancet 1979;2:43.

156. Mjolnerod OK, Rasmussen K, Dommerud SA, Gjeruldsen ST: Congenital connective-tissue defect probably due to D-penicillamine treatment in pregnancy. Lancet 1971;1:673.

157. Tarnacka B, Rodo M, Cichy S, Czlonkowska A: Procreation ability in Wilson's disease. Acta Neurol Scand 2000;101:395.

158. Brewer GJ, Johnson VD, Dick RD, et al: Treatment of Wilson's disease with zinc. XVII: Treatment during pregnancy. Hepatology 2000;31:364.

159. Furman B, Bashiri A, Wiznitzer A, et al: Wilson's disease in pregnancy: Five successful consecutive pregnancies of the same woman. Eur J Obstet Gynecol Reprod Biol 2001;96:232.

160. Scheinberg IH, Sternlieb I: Pregnancy in penicillamine-treated patients with Wilson's disease. N Engl J Med 1975;293:1300.

161. Harper PS: Myotonic Dystrophy. London, WB Saunders, 1989.

162. Ptacek LJ, Johnson KJ, Griggs RC: Genetics and physiology of the myotonic muscle disorders. N Engl J Med 1993;328:482.

163. Brook JD, McCurrach ME, Harley HG, et al: Molecular basis of myotonic dystrophy: Expansion of a trinucleotide (CTG) repeat at the 3' end of a transcript encoding a protein kinase family member. Cell 1992;68:799.

164. Buxton J, Sherbourne P, Davies J: Detection of an unstable fragment of DNA specific to individuals with myotonic dystrophy. Nature 1992;355:547.

165. Fu YH, Pizzuti A, Fenwick RG Jr, et al: An unstable triplet repeat in a gene related to myotonic muscular dystrophy. Science 1992;255:1253.

166. Harley HG, Brook JD, Rundle SA, et al: Expansion of an unstable DNA region and phenotypic variation in myotonic dystrophy. Nature 1992;355:545.

167. Fokstuen S, Myring J, Meredith L, et al: Eight years' experience of direct molecular testing for myotonic dystrophy in Wales. J Med Genet 2001;38:E42.
168. New nomenclature and DNA testing guidelines for myotonic dystrophy type 1 (DM1). The International Myotonic Dystrophy Consortium (IDMC). Neurology 2000;54:1218.
169. Hunter A, Tsilfidis C, Mettler G, et al: The correlation of age on onset with CTG trinucleotide repeat amplification in myotonic dystrophy. J Med Genet 1992;29:774.
170. Redman JB, Fenwick RG, Fu YH, et al: Relationship between parental trinucleotide GCT repeat length and severity of myotonic dystrophy in offspring. JAMA 1993;269:1960.
171. Zuhlke C, Atici J, Martorell L, et al: Rapid detection of expansions by PCR and non-radioactive hybridization: Application for prenatal diagnosis of myotonic dystrophy. Prenat Diagn 2000;20:66.
172. Fisch RO, Matalon R, Weisberg S, Michals K: Children of fathers with phenylketonuria: An international survey. J Pediatr 1991;118:739.
173. Browne I, Byrne H, Briggs L: Sickle cell disease in pregnancy. Eur J Anaesthesiol 2003;20:75.
174. Beighton P (ed): McKusick's Heritable Disorders of Connective Tissue, 5th ed. St. Louis, CV Mosby, 1993.
175. Dietz HC, Cutting GR, Pyeritz RE, et al: Marfan syndrome caused by a recurrent de novo missense mutation in the fibrillin gene. Nature 1991;352:337.
176. Dietz HC, Pyeritz RE, Hall BD, et al: The Marfan syndrome locus: Confirmation of assignment to chromosome 15 and identification of tightly linked markers at 15q15-q21.3. Genomics 1991;9:355.
177. Kainulainen K, Pulkkinen L, Savolainen A, et al: Location on chromosome 15 of the gene defect causing the Marfan syndrome. N Engl J Med 1990;323:935.
178. Aoyama T, Francke U, Gasner C, Furthmayr H: Fibrillin abnormalities and prognosis in Marfan syndrome and related disorders. Am J Med Genet 1995;58:169.
179. Pyeritz RE, Francke U: Conference report: The second international symposium on the Marfan syndrome. Am J Med Genet 1993;47:127.
180. Shores J, Berger K, Murphy E, Pyeritz R: Progression of aortic dilatation and the benefit of long-term β-adrenergic blockage in Marfan's syndrome. N Engl J Med 1994;330:1335.
181. Goodman RM: Pseudoxanthoma elasticum and related disorders. In Emery AEH, Rimoin D (eds): Principles and Practice of Medical Genetics, 2nd ed. Edinburgh, Churchill Livingstone, 1990, pp 1083-1096.
182. Elejalde BR, Mercedes de Elejalde M, Samter T, et al: Manifestations of pseudoxanthoma elasticum during pregnancy. Am J Med Genet 1984;18:755.
183. Allanson JE, Hall JG: Obstetric and gynecologic problems in women with chondrodystrophies. Obstet Gynecol 1986;67:74.
184. Clinton MJ, Niederman MS, Matthay RA: Maternal pulmonary disorders complicating pregnancy. In Reece EA, Hobbins JC, Mahoney MJ, Petrie RH (eds): Medicine of the Fetus and Mother. Philadelphia, JB Lippincott, 1992, pp 955-981.
185. Gillet D, de Braekeleer M, Bellis G, et al: Cystic fibrosis and pregnancy. Report from French data (1980-1999). BJOG 2002;109:912.
186. Gilljam M, Antoniou M, Shin J, et al: Pregnancy in cystic fibrosis. Fetal and maternal outcome. Chest 2000;118:85.
187. Odegaard I, Stray-Pedersen B, Hallberg K, et al: Maternal and fetal morbidity in pregnancies of Norwegian and Swedish women with cystic fibrosis. Acta Obstet Gynecol Scand 2002;81:698.
188. Odegaard I, Stray-Pedersen B, Hallberg K, et al: Prevalence and outcome of pregnancies in Norwegian and Swedish women with cystic fibrosis. Acta Obstet Gynecol Scand 2002;81:693.
189. Edenborough FP, Mackenzie WE, Stableforth DE: The outcome of 72 pregnancies in 55 women with cystic fibrosis in the United Kingdom 1977-1996. BJOG 2000;107:254.
190. Jaffe R, Mock M, Abramowicz J: Myotonic dystrophy and pregnancy: A review. Obstet Gynecol Surv 1986;31:272.
191. Rubenstein AE, Korf BR: Neurofibromatosis: A Handbook for Patients, Families, and Healthcare Professionals. New York, Thieme, 1990.
192. Seashore MR: Genetic counseling. In Wyngarden JB, Smith LH, Bennett JC (eds): Cecil Textbook of Medicine. Philadelphia, WB Saunders, 1988, pp 143-146.
193. Riccardi VM: Von Recklinghausen neurofibromatosis. N Engl J Med 1981;305:1617.
194. Riccardi VM: Neurofibromatosis: Phenotype, Natural History and Pathogenesis, 2nd ed. Baltimore, Johns Hopkins University Press, 1992.
195. American Academy of Pediatrics Committee on Genetics. Health supervision for children with neurofibromatosis. Pediatrics 1995;96:368-372.
196. Collins FC, Ponder BAJ, Seizinger BR, Epstein CJ: The von Recklinghausen neurofibromatosis region on chromosome 17-genetic and physical maps come into focus [Editorial]. Am J Hum Genet 1989;44:1.
197. Fountain JW, Wallace MR, Brereton AM, et al: Physical mapping of the von Recklinghausen neurofibromatosis region on chromosome 17. Am J Hum Genet 1989;44:58.
198. Collins FC: Of needles and haystacks: Finding human disease genes by positional cloning. Clin Res 1991;39:615.
199. Origone P, Bonioli E, Panucci E, et al: The Genoa experience of prenatal diagnosis in NF1. Prenat Diagn 2000;20:719.
200. Rodenheiser DI, Ainsworth PJ, Coulter-Mackie MB, et al: A genetic study of neurofibromatosis type 1 (NF1) in south-western Ontario. II: A PCR based approach to molecular and prenatal diagnosis using linkage. J Med Genet 1993;30:363.
201. Ward K, O'Connel P, Carey JC, et al: Diagnosis of neurofibromatosis 1 by using tightly linked, flanking DNA markers. Am J Hum Genet 1990;46:943.
202. Ars E, Kruyer H, Gaona A, et al: Prenatal diagnosis of sporadic neurofibromatosis type 1 (NF1) by RNA and DNA analysis of a splicing mutation. Prenat Diagn 1999;19:739.
203. Criado E, Izquierdo L, Lujan S, et al: Abdominal aortic coarctation, renovascular, hypertension, and neurofibromatosis. Ann Vasc Surg 2002;16:363.
204. Isikoglu M, Has R, Korkmaz D, Bebek N: Plexiform neurofibroma during and after pregnancy. Arch Gynecol Obstet 2002;267:41.
205. Segal D, Holcberg G, Sapir O, et al: Neurofibromatosis in pregnancy. Maternal and perinatal outcome. Eur J Obstet Gynecol Reprod Biol 1999;84:59.
206. Smith BL, Munschauer CE, Diamond N, Rivera F: Ruptured internal carotid aneurysm resulting from neurofibromatosis: Treatment with intraluminal stent graft. J Vasc Surg 2000;32:824.
207. Kusher JI: Pregnancy as a complication of neurofibromatosis (von Recklinghausen's disease). Am J Obstet Gynecol 1931;21:116.
208. Ansari AH, Nagamani M: Pregnancy and neurofibromatosis (von Recklinghausen's disease). Obstet Gynecol 1976;47:25.
209. Blickstein I, Lancet M, Shoham Z: The obstetric perspective of neurofibromatosis. Am J Obstet Gynecol 1988;158:385.
210. Edwards JNT, Fooks M, Davey DA: Neurofibromatosis and severe hypertension in pregnancy. Br J Obstet Gynaecol 1983;90:528.
211. Sharma JB, Gulati N, Malik S: Maternal and perinatal complications in neurofibromatosis during pregnancy. Int J Gynaecol Obstet 1991;34:221.
212. Sherman SJ, Schwartz DB: Eclampsia complicating a pregnancy with neurofibromatosis. J Reprod Med 1992;37:469.
213. Wiznitzer A, Katz M, Mazor M, et al: Neurofibromatosis in pregnancy. Isr J Med Sci 1986;22:579.
214. Baker VV, Hatch KD, Shingleton HM: Neurofibrosarcoma complicating pregnancy. Gynecol Oncol 1989;34:237.
215. Puls LE, Chandler PA: Malignant schwannoma in pregnancy. Acta Obstet Gynecol Scand 1991;70:243.
216. Posma E, Aalbers R, Kurniawan YS, et al: Neurofibromatosis type I and pregnancy: A fatal attraction? Development of malignant schwannoma during pregnancy in a patient with neurofibromatosis type I. BJOG 2003;110:530.
217. Verlinsky Y, Rechitsky S, Verlinsky O, et al: Preimplantation diagnosis for neurofibromatosis. Reprod Biomed Online 2002;4:218.
218. Verlinsky Y, Kuliev A: Preimplantation diagnosis for diseases with genetic predisposition and nondisease testing. Expert Rev Mol Diagn 2002;2:509.
219. Harper JC, Wells D, Piyamongkol W, et al: Preimplantation genetic diagnosis for single gene disorders: Experience with five single gene disorders. Prenat Diagn 2002;22:525.
220. Goossens V, Sermon K, Lissens W, et al: Clinical application of preimplantation genetic diagnosis for cystic fibrosis. Prenat Diagn 2000;20:571.

221. Arn PW, Hauser ER, Thomas GH, et al: Hyperammonemia in women with a mutation at the ornithine carbamoyltransferase locus: A cause of postpartum coma. N Engl J Med 1990;322:1652.

222. Brusilow SW, Horwich AL: Urea cycle enzymes. In Scriver C, Beaudet A, Sly W, Valle D (eds): The Metabolic Basis of Inherited Disease, 6th ed. New York, McGraw-Hill, 1989, pp 629-663.

223. Tuchman M, Plante R: Mutations and polymorphisms in the human ornithine transcarbamylase gene: Mutation update addendum. Hum Mutat 1995;5:293.

224. Horwich AL, Fenton WA: Precarious balance of nitrogen metabolism in women with a urea-cycle defect. N Engl J Med 1990;322:1668.

225. Parris WCV, Quimby CW: Anesthetic considerations for the patient with homocystinuria. Anaesth Analg 1982;61:708.

226. Brenton DP, Cusworth DC, Biddle SA, et al: Pregnancy and homocystinuria. Ann Clin Biochem 1977;14:161.

227. Mudd SH, Skovby F, Levy HL, et al: The natural history of homocystinuria due to cystathionine β-synthase deficiency. Am J Hum Genet 1985;37:1.

228. Brodie MJ, Moore MR, Thompson GG, Goldberg A: Pregnancy and the porphyrias. Br J Obstet Gynaecol 1977;84:726.

229. Desnick RJ, Roberts AG, Anderson KE: The inherited porphyrias. In Emery AEH, Rimoin D (eds): Principles and Practice of Medical Genetics, 2nd ed. Edinburgh, Churchill Livingstone, 1990, pp 1747-1770.

230. Aggarwal, N, Bagga R, Sawhney H, et al: Pregnancy with acute intermittent porphyria: A case report and review of literature: Acute intermittent porphyria with seizure and paralysis in the puerperium. J Obstet Gynaecol Res 2002;28:160.

231. Milo R, Neuman M, Klein C, et al: Acute intermittent porphyria in pregnancy. Obstet Gynecol 1989;73:450.

232. Scheuner MT, Wang SJ, Raffel LJ, et al: Family history: A comprehensive genetic risk assessment method for the chronic conditions of adulthood. Am J Med Genet 1997;71:315.

233. Geller DS, Farhi A, Pinkerton N, et al: Activating mineralocorticoid receptor mutation in hypertension exacerbated by pregnancy. Science 2000;289:119.

234. Wyckoff JA, Seely EW, Hurwitz S, et al: Glucocorticoid-remediable aldosteronism and pregnancy. Hypertension 2000;35:668.

235. Lachmeijer AM, Dekker GA, Pals G, et al: Searching for preeclampsia genes: The current position. Eur J Obstet Gynecol Reprod Biol 2002;105:94.

236. Pridjian G, Puschett JB: Preeclampsia. Part 2: Experimental and genetic considerations. Obstet Gynecol Surv 2002;57:619.

237. Cincotta RB, Brennecke SP: Family history of pre-eclampsia as a predictor for pre-eclampsia in primigravidas. Int J Gynaecol Obstet 1998;60:23.

238. Ibdah JA, Yang Z, Bennett MJ: Liver disease in pregnancy and fetal fatty acid oxidation defects. Mol Genet Metab 2000;71:182.

239. den Boer ME, Ijlst L, Wijburg FA, et al: Heterozygosity for the common LCHAD mutation (1528G>C) is not a major cause of HELLP syndrome and the prevalence of the mutation in the Dutch population is low. Pediatr Res 2000;48:151.

240. Handyside AH, Lesko JG, Tarin JJ, et al: Birth of a normal girl after in vitro fertilization and preimplantation diagnostic testing for cystic fibrosis. N Engl J Med 1992;327:905.

241. Silber SJ: Intracytoplasmic sperm injection today: A personal review. Hum Reprod 1998;13(Suppl 1):208.

242. Chervenak FA, Issacson G, Mahoney MJ: Advances in the diagnosis of fetal defects. N Engl J Med 1986;315:305.

243. Buskens E, Grobbee DE, Frohn-Mulder IM, et al: Efficacy of routine fetal ultrasound screening for congenital heart disease in normal pregnancy. Circulation 1996;94:67.

244. Blaas HG, Eik-Nes SH, Berg S: Three-dimensional fetal ultrasound. Baillieres Best Pract Res Clin Obstet Gynaecol 2000;14:611.

245. Todros T: Prenatal diagnosis and management of fetal cardiovascular malformations. Curr Opin Obstet Gynecol 2000;12:105.

246. Tannirandorn Y, Manotaya S, Uerpairojkit B, et al: Value of humerus length shortening for prenatal detection of Down syndrome in a Thai population. J Obstet Gynaecol Res 2002;28:89.

247. Benn PA, Kaminsky LM, Ying J, et al: Combined second-trimester biochemical and ultrasound screening for Down syndrome. Obstet Gynecol 2002;100:1168.

248. Souter VL, Nyberg DA, El-Bastawissi A, et al: Correlation of ultrasound findings and biochemical markers in the second trimester of pregnancy in fetuses with trisomy 21. Prenat Diagn 2002;22:175.

249. Bahado-Singh R, Shahabi S, Karaca M, et al: The comprehensive midtrimester test: High-sensitivity Down syndrome test. Am J Obstet Gynecol 2002;186:803.

250. Taipale P, Hiilesmaa V, Salonen R, Ylostalo P: Increased nuchal translucency as a marker for fetal chromosomal defects. N Engl J Med 1997;337:1654.

251. Bronshtein M, Zimmer EZ, Blazer S: A characteristic cluster of fetal sonographic markers that are predictive of fetal Turner syndrome in early pregnancy. Am J Obstet Gynecol 2003;188:1016.

252. Walkinshaw SA: Fetal choroid plexus cysts: Are we there yet? Prenat Diagn 2000;20:657.

253. Bird LM, Dixson B, Masser-Frye D, et al: Choroid plexus cysts in the mid-trimester fetus—practical application suggests superiority of an individualized risk method of counseling for trisomy 18. Prenat Diagn 2002;22:792. [Published erratum appears in Prenat Diagn 2003;23:268.]

254. Bahado-Singh RO, Choi SJ, Oz U, et al: Early second-trimester individualized estimation of trisomy 18 risk by ultrasound. Obstet Gynecol 2003;101:463.

255. Rosen DJ, Kedar I, Amiel A, et al: A negative second trimester triple test and absence of specific ultrasonographic markers may decrease the need for genetic amniocentesis in advanced maternal age by 60%. Prenat Diagn 2002;22:59.

256. Vintzileos AM, Guzman ER, Smulian JC, et al: Second-trimester genetic sonography in patients with advanced maternal age and normal triple screen. Obstet Gynecol 2002;99:993.

257. Benn PA: Advances in prenatal screening for Down syndrome: II first trimester testing, integrated testing, and future directions. Clin Chim Acta 2002;324:1.

258. Benn PA: Advances in prenatal screening for Down syndrome: I. general principles and second trimester testing. Clin Chim Acta 2002;323:1.

259. Palomaki GE, Neveux LM, Knight GJ, Haddow JE: Maternal serum-integrated screening for trisomy 18 using both first- and second-trimester markers. Prenat Diagn 2003;23:243.

260. Spencer K: Accuracy of Down syndrome risks produced in a first-trimester screening programme incorporating fetal nuchal translucency thickness and maternal serum biochemistry. Prenat Diagn 2002;22:244.

261. Stark CR, Orleans M, Haverkamp AD, Murphy J: Short- and long-term risks after exposure to diagnostic ultrasound in utero. Obstet Gynecol 1984;63:194.

262. Salvesen KA: EFSUMB: Safety tutorial: Epidemiology of diagnostic ultrasound exposure during pregnancy-European committee for medical ultrasound safety (ECMUS). Eur J Ultrasound 2002;15:165.

263. Marinac-Dabic D, Krulewitch CJ, Moore RM Jr: The safety of prenatal ultrasound exposure in human studies. Epidemiology 2002;13(3 Suppl):S19.

264. Ferguson-Smith MA, May HM, Vince JD, et al: Avoidance of anencephalic and spina bifida births by maternal serum-α-fetoprotein screening. Lancet 1978;1:1330.

265. Haddow JE, Kloza EM, Smith DE, Knight GJ: Data from an α-fetoprotein pilot screening program in Maine. Obstet Gynecol 1983;62:556.

266. Macri JN, Haddow JE, Weiss RR: Screening for neural tube defects in the United States. Am J Obstet Gynecol 1979;133:119.

267. Milunsky A, Alpert E: Results and benefits of a maternal serum α-fetoprotein screening program. JAMA 1984;252:1438.

268. Wald NJ, Cuckle H: Maternal serum-α-fetoprotein measurement in antenatal screening for anencephaly and spina bifida in early pregnancy: Report of U.K. collaborative study on α-fetoprotein in relation to neural-tube defects. Lancet 1977;1:1323.

269. Palomaki GE, Haddow J: Maternal serum α-fetoprotein, age and Down syndrome risk. Am J Obstet Gynecol 1987;156:460.

270. Muller F, Forestier F, Dingeon B: Second trimester trisomy 21 maternal serum marker screening. Results of a countrywide study of 854,902 patients. Prenat Diagn 2002;22:925.

271. Muller F, Sault C, Lemay C, et al: Second trimester two-step trisomy 18 screening using maternal serum markers. Prenat Diagn 2002;22:605.

272. Summers AM, Huang T, Wyatt PR: Pregnancy outcomes of women with positive serum screening results for Down syndrome and trisomy 18. Prenat Diagn 2002;22:269.

273. Cuckle HS, Wald NJ: Screening for Down's syndrome. In Lilford RJ (ed): Prenatal Diagnosis and Prognosis. London, Butterworth-Heinemann, 1990, pp 67-92.

274. Milunsky A: The use of biochemical markers in maternal serum screening for chromosome defects. In Milunsky A (ed): Genetic Disorders and the Fetus. Baltimore, Johns Hopkins University Press, 1992, pp 565-592.

275. Christiansen M, Hogdall EV, Larsen SO, Hogdall C: The variation of risk estimates through pregnancy in second trimester maternal serum screening for Down syndrome. Prenat Diagn 2002;22:385.

276. Pertl B, Bianchi DW: First trimester prenatal diagnosis: Fetal cells in the maternal circulation. Semin Perinatol 1999;23:393.

277. Bischoff FZ, Hahn S, Johnson KL, et al: Intact fetal cells in maternal plasma: Are they really there? Lancet 2003;361:139.

278. Mennuti M: A 35-year-old pregnant woman considering maternal serum screening and amniocentesis. JAMA 1996;275:1440.

279. O'Brien J, Dvorin E, Yaron Y, et al: Differential increases in AFP, hCG, and uE3 in twin pregnancies: Impact on attempts to quantify Down syndrome screening calculations. Am J Med Genet 1997;73:109.

280. Wald N, Smith G, Densem J, Petterson K: Serum screening for Down syndrome between 8 and 14 weeks of pregnancy. Br J Obstet Gynaecol 1996;103:407.

281. Wald NJ, Huttly WJ, Hackshaw AK: Antenatal screening for Down's syndrome with the quadruple test. Lancet 2003;361:835.

282. Benn PA, Ying J, Beazoglou T, Egan JF: Estimates for the sensitivity and false-positive rates for second trimester serum screening for Down syndrome and trisomy 18 with adjustment for cross-identification and double-positive results. Prenat Diagn 2001;21:46.

283. Benn PA, Fang M, Egan JF, et al: Incorporation of inhibin-A in second-trimester screening for Down syndrome. Obstet Gynecol 2003;101:451.

284. Azuma M, Yamamoto R, Wakui Y, et al: A novel method for the detection of Down syndrome with the use of four serum markers. Am J Obstet Gynecol 2002;187:197.

285. Golbus MS, Loughman WD, Epstein CJ, et al: Prenatal genetic diagnosis in 3000 amniocenteses. N Engl J Med 1979;300:157.

286. Midtrimester amniocentesis for prenatal diagnosis: Safety and accuracy. JAMA 1976;236:1471.

287. Romero R, Jeanty P, Reece EA, et al: Sonographically monitored amniocentesis to decrease intraoperative complications. Obstet Gynecol 1985;65:426.

288. Simpson NE, Dallaire L, Miller JR, et al: Prenatal diagnosis of genetic disease in Canada: Report of a collaborative study. Can Med Assoc J 1976;115:739.

289. Elias S, Simpson JL: Amniocentesis. In Milunsky A (ed): Genetic Disorders and the Fetus. Baltimore, Johns Hopkins University Press, 1992, pp 33-57.

290. Brambati B, Simoni G: Diagnosis of fetal trisomy 21 in first trimester. Lancet 1983;1:586.

291. Brambati B, Simoni G, Danesino C, et al: First trimester fetal diagnosis of genetic disorders: Clinical evaluation of 250 cases. J Med Genet 1985;22:92.

292. Kazy Z, Rozovsky IS, Bakharev VA: Chorion biopsy in early pregnancy: A method of early prenatal diagnosis for inherited disorders. Prenat Diagn 1982;2:39.

293. Simoni G, Brambati B, Danesino C, et al: Efficient direct chromosome analyses and enzyme determinations from chorionic villi samples in the first trimester of pregnancy. Hum Genet 1983;63:349.

294. Golbus MS, Appelman Z: Chorionic villus sampling. In Eden RD, Boehm FH (eds): Assessment and Care of the Fetus: Physiological, Clinical, and Medicolegal Principles. E. Norwalk, Conn, Appleton & Lange, 1990, pp 259-265.

295. Hogge WA, Schonberg SA, Golbus MS: Chorionic villus sampling: Experience of the first 1000 cases. Am J Obstet Gynecol 1986;154:1249.

296. Multicentre randomised clinical trial of chorionic villus sampling and amniocentesis. First report. Canadian Collaborative CVS-Amniocentesis Clinical Trial Group. Lancet 1989;1:1.

297. Brambati B: Genetic diagnosis through chorionic villus sampling. In Milunsky A (ed): Genetic Disorders and the Fetus. Baltimore, Johns Hopkins University Press, 1992, pp 123-153.

298. Eisenberg B, Wapner RJ: Clinical procedures in prenatal diagnosis. Best Pract Res Clin Obstet Gynaecol 2002;16:611.

299. Burton BK, Schulz CJ, Burd LI: Limb anomalies associated with chorionic villus sampling. Obstet Gynecol 1992;79:726.

300. Schloo R, Miny P, Holzgreve W, et al: Distal limb deficiency following chorionic villus sampling? Am J Med Genet 1992;42:404.

301. Jahoda MGJ, Brandenburg H, Cohen-Overbeek T, et al: Terminal transverse limb defects and early chorionic villus sampling: Evaluation of 4,300 cases with completed follow-up. Am J Med Genet 1993;46:483.

302. de la Cruz F: Report of NICHHD workshop on chorionic villus sampling and limb and other defects, October 20, 1992. Am J Obstet Gynecol 1993;169:1.

303. Froster UG, Jackson L: Limb defects and chorionic villus sampling: Results from an international registry, 1992-94. Lancet 1996;347:489.

304. Jackson LG, Zachary JM, Fowler SE: A randomized comparison of transcervical and transabdominal chorionic-villus sampling. N Engl J Med 1992;327:594.

305. Mahoney MJ: Limb abnormalities and chorionic villus sampling. Lancet 1991;337:1422.

306. Rhoads GG, Jackson LG, Schlessman SE, et al: The safety and efficacy of chorionic villus sampling for early prenatal diagnosis of cytogenetic abnormalities. N Engl J Med 1989;320:609.

307. Holmes LB: Teratogen-induced limb defects. Am J Med Genet 2002;112:297.

308. Wapner RJ, Evans MI, Davis G, et al: Procedural risks versus theology: Chorionic villus sampling for Orthodox Jews at less than 8 weeks' gestation. Am J Obstet Gynecol 2002;186:1133.

309. Hahnemann JM, Vejerslev LO: European collaborative research on mosaicism in CVS (EUCROMIC)—fetal and extrafetal cell lineages in 192 gestations with CVS mosaicism involving single autosomal trisomy. Am J Med Genet 1997;70:179.

310. Johnson A, Wapner RJ: Mosaicism: Implications for postnatal outcome. Curr Opin Obstet Gynecol 1997;9:126.

311. Kalousek DK, Langlois S, Robinson WP, et al: Trisomy 7 CVS mosaicism: Pregnancy outcome, placental and DNA analysis in 14 cases. Am J Med Genet 1996;65:348.

312. Robinson WP, Barrett IJ, Bernard L, et al: Meiotic origin of trisomy in confined placental mosaicism is correlated with presence of fetal uniparental disomy, high levels of trisomy in trophoblast, and increased risk of fetal intrauterine growth restriction. Am J Hum Genet 1997;60:917.

313. Wolstenholme J: Confined placental mosaicism for trisomies 2, 3, 7, 8, 9, 16, and 22: Their incidence, likely origins, and mechanisms for cell lineage compartmentalization. Prenat Diagn 1996;16:511.

314. Phillips OP, Tharapel AT, Lerner JL, et al: Risk of fetal mosaicism when placental mosaicism is diagnosed by chorionic villus sampling. Am J Obstet Gynecol 1996;174:850.

315. Shipp TD, Benacerraf BR: Second trimester ultrasound screening for chromosomal abnormalities. Prenat Diagn 2002;22:296.

316. Hsu LY, Yu MT, Neu RL, et al: Rare trisomy mosaicism diagnosed in amniocytes, involving an autosome other than chromosomes 13, 18, 20, and 21: Karyotype/phenotype correlations. Prenat Diagn 1997;17:201.

317. Kalousek DK, Vekemans M: Confined placental mosaicism. J Med Genet 1996;33:529.

318. Sanchez JM, Lopez de Diaz S, Panal MJ, et al: Severe fetal malformations associated with trisomy 16 confined to the placenta. Prenat Diagn 1997;17:777.

319. Hobbins JC, Grannum PA, Romero R, et al: Percutaneous umbilical blood sampling. Am J Obstet Gynecol 1985;152:1.

320. Nicolaides KH, Thorpe-Beeston JG, Noble P: Cordocentesis. In Eden RD, Boehm FH (eds): Assessment and Care of the Fetus: Physiological, Clinical, and Medicolegal Principles. E. Norwalk, Conn, Appleton & Lange, 1990, pp 291-306.

321. Ludomirski A, Weiner S: Percutaneous fetal umbilical blood sampling. Clin Obstet Gynecol 1988;31:19.

322. Bryndorf T, Christensen B, Vad M, et al: Prenatal detection of chromosome aneuploidies in uncultured chorionic villus samples by FISH. Am J Hum Genet 1996;59:918.

323. Ampola MG, Mahoney MJ, Nakamura E, Tanaka K: Prenatal therapy of a patient with vitamin-B_{12}-responsive methylmalonic acidemia. N Engl J Med 1975;293:313.

324. Packman S, Cowan MJ, Golbus MS, et al: Prenatal treatment of biotin-responsive multiple carboxylase deficiency. Lancet 1982;1:1435.

325. Carlson AD, Obeid JS, Kanellopoulou N, et al: Congenital adrenal hyperplasia: Update on prenatal diagnosis and treatment. J Steroid Biochem Mol Biol 1999;69:19.

326. Manning FA, Harrison MR, Rodeck C, et al: Catheter shunts for fetal hydronephrosis and hydrocephalus. N Engl J Med 1986; 315:336.

327. Rodeck CH, Fisk NM, Fraser DI, Nicolini U: Long-term in utero drainage of fetal hydrothorax. N Engl J Med 1988;319:1135.

328. Longaker MT, Golbus MS, Filly RA, et al: Maternal outcome after open fetal surgery. JAMA 1991;265:737.

329. Wilson RD: Prenatal evaluation for fetal surgery. Curr Opin Obstet Gynecol 2002;14:187.

330. Motulsky A: Screening for genetic diseases. N Engl J Med 1997; 336:1314.

331. Jaber L, Merlob P, Gabriel R, Shohat M: Effects of consanguineous marriage on reproductive outcome in an Arab community in Israel. J Med Genet 1997;34:1000.

332. Stoltenberg C, Magnus P, Skrondal A, Lie RT: Consanguinity and recurrence risk of birth defects: a population-based study. Am J Med Genet 1999;82:423.

333. Magnus P, Berg K, Bjerkedal T: Association of parental consanguinity with decreased birth weight and increased rate of early death and congenital malformations. Clin Genet 1985;28:335.

334. Stoltenberg C, Magnus P, Skrondal A, Lie RT: Consanguinity and recurrence risk of stillbirth and infant death. Am J Public Health 1999;89:517.

335. Adams MS, Neel JV: Children of incest. Pediatrics 1967;40:55.

336. Rucquoi J: Genetic counselling and prenatal genetic evaluation. Med Clin North Am 1983;36:3359.

337. American College of Obstetricians and Gynecologists, American College of Medical Genetics, and National Institutes of Health: Preconception and Prenatal Carrier Screening for Cystic Fibrosis: Clinical and Laboratory Guidelines. Washington, D.C., American College of Obstetricians and Gynecologists, 2001, p. 31.

338. Grody WW, Cutting GR, Klinger KW, et al: Laboratory standards and guidelines for population-based cystic fibrosis carrier screening. Genet Med 2001;3:149.

339. Richards CS, Bradley LA, Amos J, et al: Standards and guidelines for CFTR mutation testing. Genet Med 2002;4:379.

340. Doherty RA, Bradley LA, Haddow JE: Prenatal screening for cystic fibrosis: An updated perspective. Am J Obstet Gynecol 1997;176:268.

341. Kornman L, Chambers H, Nisbet D, Liebelt J: Pre-conception and antenatal screening for the fragile site on the X-chromosome. Cochrane Database Syst Rev 2002(1):CD001806.

342. Pembrey ME, Barnicoat AJ, Carmichael B, et al: An assessment of screening strategies for fragile X syndrome in the UK. Health Technol Assess 2001;5:1.

343. Maddalena A, Richards CS, McGinniss MJ, et al: Technical standards and guidelines for fragile X: The first of a series of disease-specific supplements to the Standards and Guidelines for Clinical Genetics Laboratories of the American College of Medical Genetics. Quality Assurance Subcommittee of the Laboratory Practice Committee. Genet Med 2001;3:200.

344. Larsson A, Therrell BL: Newborn screening: The role of the obstetrician. Clin Obstet Gynecol 2002;45:697.

345. Therrell BL Jr: U.S. newborn screening policy dilemmas for the twenty-first century. Mol Genet Metab 2001;74:64.

346. Levy HL, Albers SK: Genetic screening of newborns. Annu Rev Genomics Hum Genet 2000;1:139.

347. Wheeler PG, Smith R, Dorkin H, et al: Genetic counseling after implementation of statewide cystic fibrosis newborn screening: Two years' experience in one medical center. Genet Med 2001;3:411.

348. Garganta C, Seashore MR: Universal screening for congenital hearing loss. Pediatr Ann 2000;29:302.

349. Bryant-Greenwood P: Molecular diagnostics in obstetrics and gynecology. Clin Obstet Gynecol 2002;45:605.

350. Collins FS: Medical and societal consequences of the Human Genome Project. N Engl J Med 1999;341:28.

351. Phillips JA III, Vnencak-Jones CL: Molecular genetic techniques for prenatal diagnosis. In Milunsky A (ed): Genetic Disorders and the Fetus. Baltimore, Johns Hopkins University Press, 1992, pp 257-301.

11

ETHICAL ISSUES IN OBSTETRICS

Mark R. Mercurio

The study of ethics involves the determination of whether a proposed action is morally acceptable, or which among various proposed actions is morally preferable. The branch of ethics known as *normative ethics* involves the search for fundamental principles or theories on which to base these judgments. The branch known as *applied ethics,* of which medical ethics is one example, refers to the application of those principles to specific difficult cases.[1]

In medical ethical dilemmas, many people share in the responsibility to identify a morally acceptable solution, but the President's Commission for the Study of Ethical Problems in Medicine has stated that "the primary responsibility for ensuring that morally justified decisions are made lies with the physician."[2] In accordance with that view, training in ethics is now a required part of all postgraduate medical education in the United States. The American College of Obstetricians and Gynecologists (ACOG) also recommends that physicians have general background knowledge in the discipline of ethics.[3]

Essential to ethical discourse is an individual's ability to articulate the principles or theories upon which his or her judgment is based, and the ability to apply them in a rational and consistent manner. There are some widely accepted basic principles of medical ethics that should be understood by all physicians, and a brief overview of those principles is presented. The review of fundamental principles is followed by a discussion of some specific problems of particular interest to the practicing obstetrician, including how the principles might be applied to those problems.

LEGAL VERSUS ETHICAL ANALYSIS

The principles described in this chapter are ethical ones and not necessarily legal ones. Although there may be laws in place that are based on some or all of these principles, an understanding and application of the principles does not necessarily provide the correct answer to the question "Is it legal?" Although references to court rulings and legal issues are made in the following discussion, these are intended to provide an historical and societal perspective; a true legal analysis is beyond the scope of this chapter. The reader with legal questions is encouraged to seek the guidance of an attorney familiar with the laws in the relevant state that pertain to the practice of medicine. The focus of this chapter is to establish an approach to answering a fundamental question that is surely no less important than the legal one: "Is it morally acceptable?"

THE INFLUENCE OF RELIGION

Agreement on basic principles is no easy matter in a pluralistic society with no universally accepted set of beliefs.[4,5] How, for example, should religious beliefs be incorporated into our fundamental principles? For many individuals, including many physicians, moral behavior is based largely or entirely on adherence to specific religious precepts. For some people, faith itself stands as the justification for their principles and beliefs, and reason or logic is not necessarily required. The philosophical discourse typically employed in ethics to defend or reject a position may then become difficult or impossible between individuals who hold disparate religious beliefs. Many medical ethicists seek to justify their positions on rational rather than religious grounds, which seems the most appropriate approach for this textbook. Therefore, the ethical principles and arguments presented in this chapter are not based on any specific religious belief or tradition. Nevertheless, the reader should have the self-awareness to understand that religious beliefs may have a significant effect on his or her own ethical viewpoint, and the insight to realize that this is often true of patients and colleagues as well.

FUNDAMENTAL PRINCIPLES

Although there are many possible approaches to ethical questions in medicine, an approach based on the application of four fundamental principles is widely (although not universally) accepted. These principles have been described in detail by Beauchamp and Childress in their text *Principles of Biomedical Ethics.*[6] The four principles are respect for patient autonomy, nonmaleficence, beneficence, and justice.

Respect for Autonomy

The word *autonomy* is of Greek origin, meaning "self-rule."[7] In the medical context, it refers to the patient's right to determine what is done to his or her body.

The importance of patient autonomy was noted by the United States Supreme Court in 1914, when reviewing the case of a surgical procedure that was medically indicated and was performed but to which the patient had not agreed. Judge Benjamin Cardoza noted, "Every human being of adult years and sound mind has the right to determine what shall be done with his body."[8] In 1947, the Nuremberg Code addressed the issue of autonomy in clinical research, stating unequivocally that "the voluntary consent of the human subject is absolutely essential."[9] In recent decades, the central role of patient autonomy has been widely accepted, and it has become for many ethicists the dominating principle.

At first look, it seems quite reasonable that the patient should have the final say on what is done to his or her body. There are, nevertheless, circumstances in which deference to a patient's wishes is not appropriate. One generally accepted example is the very young child, who may strenuously object to immunizations or life-saving surgery. A justification for overriding the child's wishes is that he or she is unable to adequately understand the nature of the situation or the consequences of his or her decision. This justification may rightly be extended to some adults with an inadequate ability to understand, such as some with mental retardation or certain mental illnesses. Children or adults lacking the capacity for understanding, communication, and reasoning in light of their own conception of the good are deemed incompetent to make medical decisions. Although small children are generally believed incompetent to make major medical decisions, there is a *legal and societal presumption of competence for all adults;* that is, adults are presumed competent to make their own health care decisions until proven otherwise. A decision inconsistent with the values or advice of the physician is not adequate evidence of incompetence.[10]

If a patient is truly not able to decide for himself or herself, a qualified *surrogate decision maker* should be identified. The surrogate decision maker should be able to understand the situation and the therapeutic options and should make decisions for the patient by using the *substituted judgment standard.* This standard calls for the decision to be based on what the patient would have wanted if he or she were competent. If the surrogate lacks adequate knowledge of the patient to use substituted judgment, then the decision should be based on optimizing the balance of benefits and burdens to the patient, referred to as the *patient's best interest standard.*[11] The role of surrogate decision maker is usually filled by a close family member or, less often, someone designated by the court. It is generally inadvisable for the physician to assume the role of surrogate decision maker when making major decisions for a patient in a nonemergency situation.

The need for patient understanding, the prohibition of coercion, and the objective provision of relevant information form the basis of the concept of *informed consent.*[4,12] A patient unable to understand his or her current situation or the possible consequences of his or her decision cannot make a truly autonomous decision and therefore cannot give informed consent. In addition, a patient who gives consent under coercion cannot be said to have made a truly autonomous decision. One example of this would be a prisoner who agrees to a treatment or participation in a clinical study, out of fear of reprisals should he or she refuse.

Beneficence

The principle of beneficence directs the physician to act for the benefit of the patient. This is consistent with the basic virtues of *self-effacement* and *self-sacrifice,* as described by McCullough and Chervenak, which rightly call upon the physician to place his own interests secondary to those of the patient.[13] A conflict of principles may arise when the interests of the patient, as perceived by the physician, conflict with the patient's autonomous decision. The physician can choose a path consistent with respect for autonomy and thereby seemingly violate the principle of beneficence. Conversely, the physician can do what he or she believes is best for the patient, despite the patient's wishes, thereby being in accord with the principle of beneficence but violating the patient's autonomy.

Dissonance between these two central principles often arises and illustrates why a working knowledge of some fundamental principles does not ensure avoidance of all ethical dilemmas. However, familiarity with the principles does provide a framework within which to consider and discuss a problem. Although there is no simple answer to such conflicts, a course acceptable to all involved can nearly always be found, through communication, compassion, and patience. The physician should also bear in mind that even a well-informed patient often makes decisions that are based on misperceptions, fears, or experiences that may or may not be relevant. This, too, highlights the importance of communication.

Ultimately, if the physician believes it is unethical to provide the treatment the patient has chosen, there are other avenues that can be pursued. These might include consultation with a colleague, a formal second opinion, withdrawal from the case, and/or consultation with the Hospital Ethics Committee. In general, the presumption in such conflicts is in favor of respect for autonomy, particularly when a competent, informed patient refuses a recommended treatment. There may be valid exceptions to this presumption, such as when a patient demands a treatment the physician believes is futile or is not medically indicated.[14]

Nonmaleficence

The principle of nonmaleficence calls for the clinician to avoid harming the patient. This is one of the central dogmas in medicine, as stated in the Physician's Credo, "*Primum non nocere*" ("First do no harm"). Whereas beneficence implies the positive obligation to provide benefit (or remove harm), nonmaleficence seems less demanding, calling upon the physician only to avoid doing harm. Beauchamp and Childress provide examples of harming another, including killing, causing pain or offense, or depriving one of the goods of life.[15] They recognize, however, that in some circumstances the dictates of nonmaleficence may be overruled by another relevant principle, such as beneficence. For example, it is sometimes acceptable to cause pain if that pain is part of a treatment that is in the patient's overall best interest and the patient has agreed to it.

Justice

Justice may be viewed as requiring that each person be treated fairly or receive what they are entitled to receive.[16] Justice for the worker may include fair pay; for the accused criminal, a fair trial. What each patient is necessarily entitled to has been explored at length by ethicists and physicians and remains unclear. For example, whether justice requires that all patients receive free medical care at some level or what that level might be, is a subject of much debate and is not explored here. At the very least, however, justice requires that equals be treated equally.[4] Justice therefore seems to dictate a measure of consistency in medical practice; that is, patients with similar clinical status should be treated similarly, without regard to ethnic, social, or financial characteristics. In support of this concept of justice, the ACOG Code of Professional Ethics prohibits "discrimination on the basis of race, color, national origin, or any other basis that would constitute illegal discrimination."[17]

A particularly important aspect of justice in the medical setting is distributive justice, which refers to the fair distribution of scarce or limited resources. The search for a just means of prioritizing candidates for the receipt of organ transplants represents one example. Other, perhaps less obvious, examples may include the allotting of beds in the intensive care unit on a busy night or the distribution of research funds.

VERACITY

Veracity, or devotion to the truth, is described as a "moral rule" rather than a fundamental principle[18] and is essential to the field of medical ethics. Respect for another individual generally (although not always) includes a duty to be honest, and the physician-patient relationship is typically built in large part on the patient's trust in the physician's honesty. As with each of the principles previously discussed, there may be situations in which the requirements of veracity are outweighed by other ethical concerns. Nevertheless, there is generally a clear obligation to be truthful with patients. As stated by the ACOG Committee on Ethics, "Because human interaction and self-determination depend upon use of accurate information, there is a strong presumption that deception either by imparting or withholding information is unethical."[19]

This obligation extends beyond the simple prohibition of lying. Deception may also take the form of omitting information. Although it is often impractical for the physician to share every bit of information that may be relevant to a given patient, this should not be used as an excuse to avoid disclosing information that is both relevant and significant. Another violation of the rule of veracity occurs when a physician fails to disclose a conflict of interest. Examples might include a financial incentive to prescribe (or withhold) a certain treatment, or a relationship the physician has with a colleague or institution to which the patient is being referred.

Deception may also take the form of implication. For example, the physician may not provide misinformation directly to the patient; however, it is possible for the physician to give a false impression by actions or words. If the physician has reason to believe that the patient is proceeding under a false assumption, there is an obligation to address that assumption and clarify the situation.

Lastly, the physician should avoid self-deception, such as an unrealistic view of his or her own clinical capabilities or a failure to appreciate the impact of outside influences, such as gifts from vendors.

VIRTUES

McCullough and Chervenak define virtues in the context of medical ethics as traits of character that blunt self-interest and direct a physician's concern to the interests of others. It is the essential "other-regarding" nature of these traits that makes them a central component of morality in medicine. These authors describe four basic virtues that promote a sound ethical basis for the physician's relationship with the patient: self-effacement, self-sacrifice, compassion, and integrity. *Self-effacement* is the tendency of the physician to focus on the needs and interests of the patient rather than his or her own. *Self-sacrifice* may refer to a sacrifice of financial well-being, time, energy, or, in some cases, even personal safety in order to serve the interests of the patient. Realism and practicality suggest that there are necessarily limits to even the most dedicated physician's self-sacrifice, but the importance of this virtue remains. *Compassion* toward another person in that person's time of distress motivates an individual to act on that person's behalf. *Integrity* may be seen as adherence to certain moral and professional standards.[20] A fifth virtue worthy of consideration is *courage*. Pellegrino has advocated for the "courage to pursue the good in the face of today's commercialization, depersonalization, and industrialization of professional life."[21]

PHYSICIAN-PATIENT RELATIONSHIP

The sanctity of the physician-patient relationship is at the core of medical ethics, and as a special relationship, it carries special duties. These duties can be derived from the principles and virtues just described. For example, the duty of the physician to place the interests of the patient ahead of his or her own interests correlates with the virtues of self-effacement and self-sacrifice. It is in light of this special relationship that the unique nature of medical ethics in the field of obstetrics is observed. In caring for a pregnant woman, it is commonly argued, the obstetrician cares for two patients. If the fetus is truly a patient, then it seems to follow that the same duties that apply to the physician's relationship with the mother apply to the physician's relationship with the fetus as well.

The point at which a fetus becomes a patient, thereby acquiring the right to be treated according to the precepts governing the physician-patient relationship, is controversial. McCullough and Chervenak suggest that a human being becomes a patient when presented to the physician for the purpose of providing clinical care and interventions, which are expected to promote the interests of the patient.[22] Thus, when a pregnant woman presents to the obstetrician for the care of herself and her fetus, the fetus becomes (along with the woman) the obstetrician's patient. The woman, therefore, essentially confers the status of patient on her fetus. These authors differentiate between the viable and previable fetus, stating that the pregnant woman is free to withhold or withdraw the moral status of patient from her previable fetus but not necessarily from the viable fetus.[23] This moral distinction between the viable and previable fetus, however, is not universally held.

MORAL STANDING OF THE FETUS

Moral standing may be thought of as a measure of how much an individual's interests should count.[24] The rights attributed to an individual may be said to derive from that individual's moral standing. Throughout most of human history, societies have accorded what can be considered different moral standing to different individuals on the basis of ethnicity, social stratum, gender, age, and many other criteria. Much of modern political and ethical thought, however, is based on the concept that every person should have equal or "full" moral standing. The moral standing (and therefore the rights) of the fetus, however, remains unclear and is a central question in medical ethics.

Should a fetus be accorded the same rights as an infant? At the time of this writing, the Supreme Court seems to have determined that early in gestation the fetus should not be accorded full human moral standing (or at least full legal standing), as evidenced by rulings permitting abortion. Later in gestation, particularly at the age of viability, a greater standing is generally accorded the fetus, as evidenced by laws limiting or forbidding termination of pregnancy at that time. However, even late in gestation, the fetus may not be seen as having full moral standing, equivalent to that of a child or adult.

Two commonly held views are that the fetus has full standing or no standing. A third viewpoint, based on the work of Sumner and others, is that there is a gradual increase in moral standing through gestation. This suggests that the fetus has less standing than an adult but nevertheless has some moral standing and therefore some rights.[24] The rights of the viable fetus would therefore exceed those of the previable fetus, which would be consistent with the views of McCullough and Chervenak as discussed previously, and with current laws allowing termination of pregnancy early but not late in gestation. Similarly, the rights of the newborn may then exceed the rights of the viable fetus.

Most readers have an opinion regarding the moral standing and rights of the fetus but should recognize that, at the time of this writing, society's inability to come to agreement on this issue remains a source of conflict. Each obstetrician should have an understanding of the moral question, his or her own views on the matter, and the views of other professionals with whom he or she works closely. Some colleagues (physicians and/or nurses) may refuse to participate in procedures that do not, in their perception, adequately respect the rights of the fetus, and this is best discovered in a nonurgent setting. An obstetrician with firmly held convictions in this area should also have an understanding of the views of the pregnant patient, and potential conflicts are, again, better discussed in advance, in a nonurgent setting.

MATERNAL-FETAL CONFLICT

The term *maternal-fetal conflict* has been used to describe situations in which a pregnant woman's actions are thought to be inconsistent with the interests of her fetus. Examples of this may include the use of illegal drugs, excessive nicotine or alcohol intake, and noncompliance with prescribed treatment regimens. Among the most dramatic examples is the refusal of cesarean section when, in the opinion of the obstetrician, the well-being or even the survival of the fetus may be jeopardized. Opinions on this issue have evolved considerably, and specific recommendations have been made by professional organizations and the courts. Before recommendations are presented, the relevant principles and the most recent history of the question are briefly reviewed.

Principles Relevant to Maternal-Fetal Conflict

Two basic principles that appear to conflict in this situation are respect for the woman's autonomy and the beneficence-based obligation to act in the best interest of the fetus. The pregnant woman and the physician may each have a beneficence-based obligation to the fetus, but this chapter focuses on the physician's obligations. Surely the physician has an obligation to respect the autonomy of the pregnant patient, but is there a point at which that obligation is essentially trumped by the needs of the fetus? This question might be approached in light of the rights, or moral standing, of the fetus. However, as noted previously, on this question there are a spectrum of strongly held beliefs, endless debate in the philosophical, theologic, and popular writings, and no clear consensus.

Three possible approaches to this conflict may be considered, and their relative merit probably depends largely on the reader's opinion regarding fetal rights. One approach grants absolute autonomy to the competent pregnant woman, without considering the interests of the fetus. A second view is that they have equal moral standing, and in this case the vital interests of the fetus in some situations may outweigh the woman's autonomy. According to this view, a procedure that poses a relatively low risk to the woman but may offer great benefit to the fetus (e.g., cesarean section in certain settings) would be appropriate, even over the woman's objection. A third approach is based on the view that the fetus has some (but less than full) moral standing. In that case, the woman's autonomy would generally trump fetal interests, but in certain extreme situations, fetal interests may override the mother's.

Even for people who recognize some moral standing for the fetus, however, overruling a pregnant woman's autonomy remains problematic from an ethical standpoint, on the basis of consideration of a third relevant principle: justice. Justice requires that equals be treated equally, and unless society is willing to state that a woman, upon becoming pregnant, abdicates her claim to equality within society, she must be accorded the same rights as her equals, who are men and nonpregnant women. This understanding of justice suggests that a pregnant woman should never be forced to undergo a procedure without her consent, even to benefit another person (in this case, her fetus) unless a similar demand could be made of a nonpregnant adult. As Burrows has pointed out, it is most unlikely that a court would order a father to donate bone marrow without his consent.[25] Indeed, a Pennsylvania court in 1978 refused to order an adult to donate bone marrow to a family member who would presumably die without it.[26] In fact, no adult in the United States has ever been forced to donate tissue or organs to another person, regardless of the severity of the need or the safety of the procedure.[27] An appeal to justice, therefore, would suggest that society should not compel a pregnant woman to undergo a procedure (even one of relatively low risk) to save the life of another, unless it would similarly compel nonpregnant adults to undergo the same procedure, which has not been the case.

One potential response to this justice-based argument is that pregnancy is a unique circumstance, both physiologically and morally. It could be argued that analogies to other situations, such as bone marrow donation, are therefore not entirely valid. The validity of the justice-based argument seems to be predicated on the reader's acceptance of the moral equality of pregnant and nonpregnant adult patients.

Historical Background and Landmark Cases

The performance of invasive treatments on competent pregnant patients without consent has been practiced in the United States, long after court rulings presumably put an end to it for competent nonpregnant adults. In 1987, Kolder published the results of a survey of program directors in Maternal-Fetal Medicine regarding coerced interventions.[28] Nearly half the physicians surveyed believed that a pregnant woman could be detained to ensure compliance and that she could be required to undergo a procedure to save the life of her fetus. Many respondents reported having obtained a court order to perform a cesarean section against a competent patient's wishes. In 2003, Adams and colleagues published a subsequent survey of Maternal-Fetal Medicine fellowship directors, which showed a significant change.[26] In this more recent survey, only 4% agreed that women should be compelled to undergo surgery for the sake of the fetus. However, eight respondents reported cases in which pregnant patients were compelled to undergo procedures, usually cesarean section, against their wishes, all with a court order.[26,28]

Perhaps the best-known case of maternal-fetal conflict and refusal of treatment is that of Angela Carder, a 28-year-old pregnant woman who was dying of cancer. She was undergoing chemotherapy in an effort to survive until her fetus could be delivered at 28 weeks' gestation. At 25 weeks, as her condition deteriorated, lawyers for George Washington University Hospital sought a court order to perform a cesarean section in an effort to maximize the chances of survival for the baby. The patient, her husband, and her physician were all opposed to the procedure, but the court ordered surgical delivery over their objections. The baby died within hours of birth, and Angela Carder died 2 days later. In 1990, after the deaths of Angela Carder and her baby, the District of Columbia Court of Appeals overturned the original court order. With the benefit of written legal briefs, formal oral arguments from both sides, and time to reflect on the question in the absence of a perceived emergency, the court stated that the informed decision of a competent pregnant patient should "control in virtually all cases."[26,29]

Similar rulings in Illinois have emphasized that a woman's right to autonomy cannot be subordinated to the interests of her fetus, even for less invasive procedures such as blood transfusion. An Illinois Appeals Court has stated that "a woman's right to refuse invasive medical treatment … is not diminished during pregnancy…. The potential impact on the fetus is not legally relevant."[26] In the view of the Illinois judges, the right to bodily integrity emphasized by Judge Cardoza more than a half-century before clearly included pregnant women. Similarly, in the United Kingdom, the Court of Appeal in 1997 pronounced that a competent woman had the right to refuse an intervention even if the consequence of that refusal may be death or disability for her fetus or herself.[25]

Patient Incompetence

A potential loophole in the legal support of the pregnant woman's autonomy is the question of incompetence. Even in keeping with the court rulings and ethical arguments in favor of respect for autonomy, a physician could legitimately seek to override a pregnant woman's objections to invasive treatment, if the physician could show that the woman was incompetent to make decisions. However, many ethicists, clinicians, and jurists have cautioned against the abuse of this argument. Specifically, a patient is not shown to be incompetent simply because she disagrees with the recommendation of her physician or because she makes a decision that is based on a value system different from that of her physician or of most individuals in her society. The patient who refuses intervention (e.g., transfusion) on religious grounds, for example, should not be deemed incompetent solely on that basis.

Any physician seeking to override a patient's wishes on the basis of presumed incompetence should obtain confirmation of that assessment by a qualified colleague, preferably a psychiatrist or psychologist, and the involvement of the courts may be needed in contested cases. If the patient is truly incompetent to make the decision, then a surrogate decision maker should be identified to speak (and decide) for her. As with nonpregnant patients deemed incompetent, the surrogate should usually be the spouse or another close relative. The physician should generally not serve as the surrogate decision maker.

Potential Pitfalls

A retrospective look at court-ordered obstetric interventions yields two important observations that should influence any physician considering a court order to override a patient's refusal. First, as many as one third of those interventions in the United States may have been, in retrospect, based on poor medical judgment.[25,28,30] In every medical specialty, there is ample experience in which physicians were convinced that one outcome would occur, only to subsequently observe a different outcome. Obstetrics is no exception. An understanding that any good physician will, over time, make mistakes in judgment and prognosis should provide each physician with an appropriate measure of humility, particularly when he or she considers overriding a patient's fundamental right to autonomy.

An additional concern is that there appears to be an increased tendency to seek court orders to override the refusal of pregnant woman of ethnic minorities and/or low socioeconomic status.[27,28,30] Justice requires that equals be treated equally; that is, in order to justify treating two groups differently, a *morally relevant* difference between them must be identified. Because no such difference has been identified, there is no moral justification for what appears to be a difference in respect for the right to autonomy on the basis of ethnic background or social standing.

Professional Organizations

In the position statement entitled "Patient Choice and the Maternal-Fetal Relationship,"[31] ACOG describes recommendations for scenarios in which maternal and fetal interests may be divergent: (1) when the pregnant woman refuses a procedure or therapy intended to benefit the fetus and (2) when the pregnant woman engages in behavior thought by the physician to be potentially harmful to the fetus. In either case, according to these guidelines, once the physician has made a thorough effort to persuade the patient to accept the recommendation and she refuses, the physician has three options. The first option is to accept the woman's refusal. The second is to help the patient find a different physician willing to accept her refusal and assume responsibility for her medical care. This, of course, is less practical in an emergency and is best handled as a preventive approach by identifying areas of conflict before a crisis. The third option is to seek a court order to override the patient's refusal of the recommended treatment.

A court order, per the ACOG guidelines, should be sought only on very rare occasions and only when *all* the following four scenarios are present: (1) There is high probability of serious harm to the fetus if the woman's refusal is accepted, (2) there is high probability that the treatment will substantially reduce harm to the fetus, (3) no other comparatively effective but less intrusive way to reduce the harm to the fetus is available, and (4) the recommended treatment poses little or no risk to the pregnant woman. Furthermore, even if a court order is obtained and the patient continues to refuse, ACOG has stated that the use of force against a competent resistant patient is still not justified.

The International Federation of Gynecology and Obstetrics, in their ethical guidelines regarding interventions for fetal well-being, are even stronger in their emphasis on patient autonomy: "... No woman should be forced to undergo an unwished-for medical or surgical procedure to preserve the life or health of her fetus since this would be a violation of her autonomy and fundamental human rights. Resort to the courts ... is inappropriate and usually counterproductive."[32]

Specific maternal-fetal conflict guidelines were developed by the University of Virginia Health Sciences Center and can serve as a model for other hospitals.[33] Several elements of the following recommendations are drawn from the University of Virginia maternal-fetal conflict guidelines:

1. Conflict may arise when the pregnant woman refuses a recommended medical or surgical intervention that the physician believes is in her best interest and/or that of her fetus.
2. The physician may have a beneficence-based obligation to the fetus, and the pregnant woman may herself have a beneficence-based obligation to act in the best interest of her fetus. However, neither her denial of that obligation nor the physician's obligations provide sufficient ethical grounds for the physician to overrule the woman's right to autonomy in refusing a recommended therapy. In other words, her right to autonomy is ultimately the deciding factor in virtually all cases.
3. The physician should present the relevant data in a clear and objective manner. If the physician perceives a moral compulsion to then advocate for a given therapeutic course, it is appropriate to do so. If a conflict is not resolved by careful deliberation, a second medical opinion is advised. If conflict persists, consultation with the Hospital Ethics Committee (as time allows) is recommended. Both the physician and the patient should be afforded the opportunity to meet with the committee in an effort to reach an agreement. The Ethics Committee and/or the physician may also seek administrative and legal counsel from hospital authorities.
4. In nonemergency situations, the patient should be offered the option of transferring care to another physician and/or hospital.
5. Ultimately, if the competent patient continues to refuse the recommended intervention despite the efforts just listed, her refusal should be respected.
6. Court intervention in the case of a competent patient is very rarely, if ever, appropriate. Some authorities have argued, and the ACOG guidelines also suggest,

that in rare, extreme cases, in which the physician feels an overwhelming ethical obligation to provide the proposed intervention (e.g., the therapy would be lifesaving for mother or fetus, with a relatively low risk to the mother), a court order may be sought. It is not clear, however, that this can be justified on ethical grounds. The court order may be used as a means to persuade the pregnant woman, but even with a court order, physical force (including forced anesthesia) should never be used on a competent patient. If the patient continues to refuse the recommended therapy, even in the event of a court order, the refusal should ultimately be respected.

7. In emergencies, there may be no time to pursue the avenues just discussed, and in those cases the competent patient's refusal should not be overridden.

8. If a physician believes that the patient is not competent to decide the question at hand, the physician should obtain confirmation of that assessment by a qualified colleague, preferably a psychiatrist or psychologist, before seeking to overrule the refusal. If a patient is incompetent, a surrogate decision maker (a person other than the physician) should be identified.

PRENATAL DIAGNOSIS AND WITHHOLDING OBSTETRIC AND NEONATAL INTERVENTIONS

In nearly every delivery, the obstetrician and the neonatologist proceed with the assumption that every effort should be made to preserve the life of the newborn. A valid exception to this approach may exist when there is a prenatal diagnosis that carries a very poor prognosis and the physicians and the expectant parents agree that resuscitation of the newborn should not be performed. That decision should generally be based on an assessment of the child's best interests.[34] A very poor prognosis may similarly be used to decide against obstetric interventions, such as operative delivery or electronic fetal monitoring. The American Academy of Pediatrics *Textbook of Neonatal Resuscitation* specifically cites anencephaly, trisomy 13, and trisomy 18 as examples in which it is appropriate not to perform resuscitation. This textbook does not exclude the possibility of other diagnoses that warrant this approach as well.[35]

A decision to withhold resuscitation requires confidence in the prenatal diagnosis (typically confirmed by serial ultrasonograms and/or chromosomal analysis) and a willingness to change the plan in the delivery room if physical examination of the newborn raises significant doubt about the diagnosis. The obstetrician must be forthright about any degree of diagnostic uncertainty with the parents, the neonatologist, and himself or herself when making plans for the management of labor and of the newborn immediately after birth. The expectant parents should be fully informed about the diagnosis, including the possibility of error, and about the short- and long-term consequences of the diagnosis and of various management options.

In many circumstances, it is helpful for the expectant parents to discuss the prenatal diagnosis with a neonatologist and/or other appropriate pediatric subspecialist. Although it is appropriate for the physicians to make a recommendation, all relevant information should first be presented to the expectant parents in an objective manner. If there are any concerns about legality, consultation with a hospital attorney is recommended. Consultation with a hospital ethics committee may be helpful and reassuring to the parents and/or the physician, and should be available, but should not necessarily be required if parents and clinicians are in agreement about the most appropriate management. Nonphysician members of the clinical team who are expected to take part in the management—notably, obstetric or neonatal nurses—should also be included in planning.

When a decision is reached not to provide resuscitation, all efforts should be made to minimize pain and discomfort in the newborn. Parents should be offered the option of holding their child, and staff familiar with bereavement support should be involved. In addition, support from clergy should be available if the parents desire it.

When there is uncertainty regarding the diagnosis or the most appropriate course, aggressive obstetric management is recommended, and neonatal resuscitation should generally be carried out. Examination of the infant immediately after birth may, in some circumstances, yield findings that indicate that withholding resuscitation is appropriate. It is generally accepted that withholding and withdrawing a treatment are ethically equivalent, and any treatment that could potentially improve the outcome should not be withheld in the delivery room out of fear that, once initiated, it cannot later be withdrawn.[34] The neonatology team, in conjunction with the parents, may make the determination to continue or withdraw support after more information becomes available.

DELIVERY AT THE EDGE OF VIABILITY

Preterm delivery may be necessitated by maternal illness or injury or by fetal illness, or it may occur as a result of premature labor, amnionitis, or incompetent cervix. Anticipated delivery at the edge of viability, currently 22 to 24 completed weeks' gestation, may pose a difficult dilemma. It could be viewed as another situation in which prognosis may be poor and the advisability of certain obstetric interventions and/or neonatal resuscitation is not clear. Should cesarean section or newborn resuscitation be recommended at 22 weeks? At 23 weeks? Should a woman expected to deliver at 22 weeks be moved to a facility with neonatal intensive care capability? The obstetrician's approach should be based on accurate data and on full and honest communication with the expectant parents, typically in conjunction with a neonatologist. The data considered should be current and relevant to the institution where delivery will take place.

Predicted Survival

Lorenz's review of the medical literature revealed mean survival rates of 10% at 22 completed weeks' gestation

($n = 151$), 28% at 23 weeks ($n = 490$), 51% at 24 weeks ($n = 1295$), and 71% at 25 weeks ($n = 1608$).[36] Similar results were published by the National Institutes of Child Health and Human Development (NICHD) Neonatal Research Network for infants born at its 14 participating academic medical centers, although a somewhat higher rate of survival (21%) was noted at 22 weeks. There were no survivors among those born at less than 22 weeks' gestation in the NICHD study.[37] Lorenz noted a wide range of reported survival rates at the lowest gestational ages: for example, ranging from 0% to 21% at 22 weeks. Different levels of skill with these most fragile patients may account for some of the variability in survival rates observed. Perhaps an even larger influence on the data, particularly at 22 weeks, is the varying degree of clinical aggressiveness for these newborns practiced at different institutions. Variability in survival rate among different institutions for the lowest gestational ages underscores the importance of knowing and communicating the recent data from the relevant institution when expectant parents are counseled.[36] An obligation of veracity would also suggest that if predicted survival is significantly better at another available facility, the expectant parents deserve that information as well.

The steep slope of the survival curve at 22 to 25 weeks' gestation makes it particularly difficult to predict newborn survival for a pending delivery. The published data are usually based on best obstetric estimates of gestational age for the subjects studied, and a margin of error as small as 1 week may have had a significant impact on results. Moreover, the exact gestational age of the specific infant about to be delivered is also often unknown.

Resnick and Moore noted that the classical obstetric methods of estimating gestational age, such as last menstrual period and first trimester uterine size, are accurate only to within 2 weeks. They also stated that a single sonographic study at 16 to 22 weeks "affords acceptable dating accuracy (±10 days)."[38] Although it may be acceptable in most situations, an error of ±10 days represents a major difference in predicted outcome at the edge of viability. Physicians often give a false sense of accuracy when describing the gestational age, for example, as "$22\frac{4}{7}$ weeks." If that estimate were based on ultrasonograms at 16 weeks, a more appropriate description would be "21 to 24 weeks." This margin of error reveals a predicted rate of survival ranging from 0% to 50%! Sometimes more accurate dating is available, such as after in vitro fertilization or ultrasonography in the earliest weeks of gestation. Planning and counseling can then be made with this greater accuracy in mind. Because of the inherent difficulties in determining the exact gestational age of most newborns, many prefer to use survival data based on birth weight. Of course, the exact weight is not available before birth, and estimation of fetal weight from ultrasonograms has its own inherent error.

Self-Fulfilling Prophecy

One potential pitfall in the use of survival statistics is the creation of a self-fulfilling prophecy. In an institution in which newborns younger than 23 weeks' gestation are not resuscitated or given intensive care measures, the survival rate for this gestational age at that institution will remain at 0%. The staff could then honestly report that "there has never been a survivor under 23 weeks at our institution" and withhold resuscitation on that basis, thus maintaining a survival rate of 0% and perpetuating the rationale. This is flawed logic, as illustrated by the fact that 0% survival could be perpetuated among infants born at 25 weeks' gestation and thus justify withholding support in such infants by using the same approach.

This faulty reasoning might be employed by individual physicians, but it could also be used by institutions or on a much wider scale. Thus, when the chances of success of therapy is considered, it is important to distinguish what has not been successful at one institution from what has not been successful anywhere and to distinguish each of these from what has not been successful because it has not been tried. This is not to suggest that every physician or institution is obligated to attempt resuscitation regardless of the infant's gestational age. The decision not to attempt resuscitation in infants younger than 23 weeks, for example, may be appropriate but cannot be justified solely by this flawed rationale.

Long-Term Morbidity

Many authorities argue that decisions about providing obstetric interventions or newborn resuscitation at borderline gestational ages should also take long-term morbidity into account. Significant problems found on follow-up have included cerebral palsy, low scores on the Bayley Mental and Psychomotor Developmental Indices, visual impairment, and hearing impairment. Wood and associates studied 314 infants born at 22 to 25 completed weeks' gestation in the United Kingdom and Ireland in 1995, including a neurologic and developmental evaluation at 30 months.[39] Of the infants born at 22 completed weeks, there were only two survivors; one had severe disability, and the other had no disability. Of those born at 23 to 25 weeks, "severe disability" was noted at 30 months in 23%. Just fewer than half had no detectable disability. In Lorenz's review of the literature on follow-up of infants born at 22 to 26 completed weeks, 24% had "at least one major disability."[36] The NICHD Neonatal Research Network presented their follow-up data by birth weight rather than gestational age, based on evaluation at 18 to 22 months of corrected age. Approximately 60% of all newborns with birth weight less than 800 g had at least one "major deficit" at follow-up.[40]

Variation in reported morbidity may arise from differences in assessment of gestational age, in clinical proficiency, in age and assessment tools used at follow-up, and in clinical aggressiveness. For example, the NICHD study showed an increase in neurodevelopmental morbidity associated with grade 3 or 4 intraventricular hemorrhage; thus, a center that is likely to withdraw support from patients with severe hemorrhage may have a lower incidence of neurologic morbidity among survivors. The NICHD investigators also observed an association between later neurodevelopmental morbidity and other neonatal findings, including chronic lung disease, necrotizing enterocolitis, periventricular leukomalacia, male gender, and steroid therapy for chronic lung disease. Lorenz argued that these associations are not strong enough to provide guidance for withdrawal of support.[36] Nevertheless, some clinicians may consider these findings, particularly severe intraventricular hemorrhage and widespread periventricular leukomalacia, when discussing possible withdrawal of intensive care measures.

Decisions under Uncertainty

Ultimately, when physicians and expectant parents consider whether to provide interventions such as cesarean section or newborn resuscitation at the edge of viability, the decision is often made in the setting of uncertainty that exists on many levels. There may be uncertainty regarding the exact gestational age of the fetus. Even if the exact gestational age is known, despite ample statistical data, it would generally not be clear how an individual newborn would fare.

An additional layer of uncertainty exists surrounding the infant's best interest. It has been recommended that decisions regarding withholding or withdrawing support be based on the best interest of the patient.[34] Is it in the child's best interest to actively resuscitate at 23 weeks? Does the benefit of potential survival outweigh the burden of invasive procedures, prolonged intensive care, and a probable poor outcome? The answer may be far from clear, and an assessment of best interest ultimately becomes more of a value judgment than a medical one. Finally, although most physicians and medical ethicists recognize the patient's best interest standard, there exists some disagreement about that standard itself. It has been argued that the benefits and burdens to family members should also be considered in the decision-making process.[41,42]

Recommendations

ACOG has acknowledged that it may be appropriate to withhold support from certain newborns with extremely low birth weight, placing particular emphasis on parents' preferences.[43] The American Academy of Pediatrics has similarly emphasized the central role of parents, as well as the physician's responsibility to be certain that the parents are well informed and competent to decide. The physician should generally defer to the wishes of the parents, unless their preferences clearly conflict with the best interests of the child or they are requesting a therapy that the physician believes cannot benefit the patient.[34,44,45] An example of the latter would be a request to resuscitate a newborn that was clearly previable. The American Academy of Pediatrics *Textbook of Neonatal Resuscitation* suggests that withholding resuscitation is appropriate for newborns with a confirmed gestational age of less than 23 weeks or a birth weight of less than 400 g.[35] This recommendation, however, does not prohibit attempted resuscitation in infants younger than 23 weeks, nor does it preclude withholding resuscitation from slightly larger or more mature newborns (e.g., those weighing less than 600 g or aged younger than 24 weeks) if informed parents so request.

A large survey of neonatologists in the United States indicated support for parental decisions for infants at borderline gestational ages. Most neonatologists believed that parents have a right to demand that aggressive resuscitation be provided to a newborn weighing less than 600 g with a fair prognosis. A majority also believed that parents have a right to demand that aggressive resuscitation be withheld in the same situation.[46] Ultimately, 22 to 24 completed weeks of gestation may be perceived as an area of ethical uncertainty, wherein the predicted survival, long-term morbidity, and balance of benefits and burdens to the patient are unclear. The physicians should provide medical information and data in an objective and thorough manner. It is also appropriate to provide an opinion and recommendations regarding obstetric intervention and newborn resuscitation, but within this area of uncertainty, the wishes of competent, well-informed parents should prevail.[47]

It is strongly recommended that delivery of a newborn of borderline viable gestational age take place in a setting in which neonatology support is immediately available and that planning for obstetric interventions and newborn resuscitation be made in concert with the neonatologist. It is reasonable to advise parents that the agreed-upon plan might be altered in the delivery room once the child is born, on the basis of size, apparent maturity, and response to resuscitation, if the newborn appears to be much different than anticipated. However, there are no data to suggest that neonatologists can accurately determine gestational age in this range, or that presentation or initial response to resuscitation is predictive of long-term outcome.[48]

In the event that time does not permit the parents to provide an informed opinion regarding resuscitation, aggressive care should be provided until it is clear that the child cannot survive or until the parents have been adequately informed and have requested that intensive care measures be withdrawn.

CONFLICT RESOLUTION AND THREE PRACTICAL GUIDELINES

Much of the ethics literature, including this chapter, may be helpful to the obstetrician who finds himself or herself in conflict with the requests or demands of the pregnant patient. An analysis of the situation and the search for the best course of action may be guided by an understanding of the principles of medical ethics described previously. Alternatively, some ethicists have rejected this "principlism" in favor of other theories. There are many theories, principles, or approaches that the ethicist may endorse, but ultimately it is the physician who is left with the responsibility of finding an acceptable solution to the specific conflict at hand. Toward that end, three practical guidelines are provided.

The first guideline is to avoid acting alone. A physician in conflict with a patient or other caregivers over the morally acceptable course of action should, at the very least, seek the opinion of a respected colleague. Moreover, consultation with the hospital ethics committee should be strongly considered when the obstetrician is faced with ongoing conflict. That committee, which ideally includes physicians, nurses, clergy, and others, may provide valuable objective insight. They may also help construct a compromise proposal that is acceptable to all parties involved. In some situations, other resources, such as a hospital attorney or the courts, may be an appropriate source of help. The essence of the guideline is that, except perhaps in rare emergencies in which no help is available, a physician should not take unilateral action in the presence of conflict but rather should seek the counsel of other appropriate individuals.

The second practical guideline is for the physician to be open to the possibility that he or she is wrong. When the obstetrician seeks the advice of a colleague or the ethics committee, he or she should not do so just to have "covered that base," although in retrospect the physician's justification of his or her actions might well be aided by having done so. Rather, he or she should do so while mindful of the possibility that the other viewpoint, on further reflection, is in fact valid and that it may be morally acceptable to yield.

The third practical guideline is to remember that many conflicts, or what are perceived as "ethical dilemmas," require no special intervention from outside the physician-patient relationship but, rather, can be resolved through the use of compassion and communication. Often a consideration of the emotional state of the patient and/or family may make it most appropriate for the physician to yield. Moreover, many (perhaps most) conflicts brought to the attention of hospital ethics committees can be resolved simply by facilitating better communication among the parties involved. That communication remains one of the physician's central responsibilities.

References

1. Kagan S: Normative Ethics. Boulder, Co, Westview Press, 1998, pp 1-3.
2. President's Commission for the Study of Ethical Problems in Medicine and Biomedical and Behavioral Research: Deciding to Forego Life-Sustaining Treatment: A Report on the Ethical, Medical, and Legal Issues in Treatment Decisions. Washington, D.C., U.S. Government Printing Office, 1983.
3. American College of Obstetricians and Gynecologists: Technical Bulletin: Ethical Decision-Making in Obstetrics and Gynecology. Washington, D.C., American College of Obstetricians and Gynecologists, November 1989.
4. Finnerty J, Pinkerton J, Moreno J, Ferguson J: Ethical theory and principles: Do they have any relevance to problems arising in everyday practice? Am J Obstet Gynecol 2000;183:301.
5. McCullough L, Chervenak F: Ethics in Obstetrics and Gynecology. New York, Oxford University Press, 1994, p 6.
6. Beauchamp T, Childress J: Principles of Biomedical Ethics, 5th edition. Oxford, United Kingdom, Oxford University Press, 2001, pp 57-282.
7. Beauchamp T, Childress J: Principles of Biomedical Ethics, 5th edition. Oxford, United Kingdom, Oxford University Press, 2001, p 57.
8. McCullough L, Chervenak F: Ethics in Obstetrics and Gynecology. New York, Oxford University Press, 1994, p 50.
9. Shuster E: The Nuremberg code: Hippocrates and human rights. Lancet 1998;351:974.
10. Buchanan A, Brock D: Deciding for Others. Cambridge, United Kingdom, Cambridge University Press, 1990, p 21.
11. Buchanan A, Brock D: Deciding for Others. Cambridge, United Kingdom, Cambridge University Press, 1990, p 112.
12. Beauchamp T, Childress J: Principles of Biomedical Ethics, 5th edition. Oxford, United Kingdom, Oxford University Press, 2001, p 59.
13. McCullough L, Chervenak F: Ethics in Obstetrics and Gynecology. New York, Oxford University Press, 1994, p 11.
14. American Medical Association Council on Ethical and Judicial Affairs: Medical futility in end-of-life care. JAMA 1999;281:937.
15. Beauchamp T, Childress J: Principles of Biomedical Ethics, 5th edition. Oxford, United Kingdom, Oxford University Press, 2001, p 117.
16. Beauchamp T, Childress J: Principles of Biomedical Ethics, 5th edition. Oxford, United Kingdom, Oxford University Press, 2001, p 226.
17. American College of Obstetricians and Gynecologists: Code of professional ethics. In Compendium of Selected Publications. Washington, D.C., American College of Obstetricians and Gynecologists, 2002, p 97.
18. Beauchamp T, Childress J: Principles of Biomedical Ethics, 5th edition. Oxford, United Kingdom, Oxford University Press, 2001, p 39.
19. American College of Obstetricians and Gynecologists Committee on Ethics Committee Opinion: Deception. Washington, D.C., American College of Obstetricians and Gynecologists, 1990.
20. McCullough L, Chervenak F: Ethics in Obstetrics and Gynecology. New York, Oxford University Press, 1994, pp 11-16.
21. Pellegrino E: The internal morality of clinical medicine: A paradigm for the ethics of the helping and healing professions. J Med Philos 2001;26:559.
22. McCullough L, Chervenak F: Ethics in Obstetrics and Gynecology. New York, Oxford University Press, 1994, p 59.
23. McCullough L, Chervenak F: Ethics in Obstetrics and Gynecology. New York, Oxford University Press, 1994, p 105.
24. Sumner L: Abortion and Moral Theory. Princeton, NJ, Princeton University Press, 1981.
25. Burrows J: The parturient woman: Can there be room for more than one person with full and equal rights inside a single human skin? J Adv Nursing 2001;33:689.
26. Adams S, Mahowald M, Gallagher J: Refusal of treatment during pregnancy. Clin Perinatol 2003;30:127.
27. Mahowald M: Maternal-fetal conflict: Positions and principles. Clin Obstet Gynecol 1992;35:729.
28. Kolder V: Court-ordered obstetrical interventions. N Engl J Med 1987;316:1192.
29. Catlin A: When pregnant women and their physicians disagree on the need for cesarean section: No simple solution. Adv Prac Nurs Q 1998;4:23.
30. Harris L: Rethinking maternal-fetal conflict: Gender and equality in perinatal ethics. Obstet Gynecol 2000;96:786.
31. American College of Obstetricians and Gynecologists Committee on Ethics Committee Opinion: Patient Choice and the Maternal-Fetal Relationship. Washington, D.C., American College of Obstetricians and Gynecologists, 1999.
32. International Federation of Gynecology and Obstetrics Committee for the Ethical Aspects of Human Reproduction and Women's Health: Ethical guidelines on human reproduction and women's health. J Reprod Med 1999;44:482.
33. Pinkerton J, Finnerty J: Resolving the clinical and ethical dilemma involved in fetal-maternal conflicts. Am J Obstet Gynecol 1996;175:289.
34. American Academy of Pediatrics Committee on Bioethics: Guidelines on forgoing life-sustaining medical treatment. Pediatrics 1994;93:532.
35. American Academy of Pediatrics and American Heart Association: Textbook of Neonatal Resuscitation, 4th ed. Elk Grove Village, IL, American Academy of Pediatrics, 2000.
36. Lorenz J: The outcome of prematurity. Semin Perinatol 2001;25:348.
37. Lemons J, Bauer CR, Oh W, et al: Very low birth weight outcomes of the National Institute of Child Health and Human Development Neonatal Research Network, January 1995 through December 1996. NICHD Neonatal Research Network. Pediatrics 2001;107:E1.
38. Resnick R, Moore T: Obstetric management of the high risk patient. In Burrow G, Duffy T (eds): Medical Complications during Pregnancy, 5th ed. Philadelphia, WB Saunders, 1999, p 5.
39. Wood N, Marlow N, Costeloe K, et al: Neurologic and developmental disability after extremely preterm birth. New Engl J Med 2000;343:378.
40. Vohr B, Wright LL, Dusick AM, et al: Neurodevelopmental and functional outcomes of extremely low birth weight infants in the National Institute of Child Health and Human Development Neonatal Research Network, 1993-1994. Pediatrics 2000;105:1216.
41. Duff R, Campbell A: Moral and ethical dilemmas in the special-care nursery. New Engl J Med 1973;289:890.
42. Hardwig J: Is There a Duty to Die? New York, Routledge, 2000.

43. American College of Obstetricians and Gynecologists Practice Bulletin: Perinatal Care at the Threshold of Viability. Washington, D.C., American College of Obstetricians and Gynecologists, September 2002.

44. American Academy of Pediatrics Committee on Fetus and Newborn: The initiation or withdrawal of treatment for high-risk newborns. Pediatrics 1995;96:362.

45. American Academy of Pediatrics Committee on Fetus and Newborn: Perinatal care at the threshold of viability. Pediatrics 2002;110:1024.

46. Ballard D, Li Y, Evans J, et al: Fear of litigation may increase resuscitation of infants born near the limits of viability. J Pediatr 2002;140:713.

47. Campbell D, Fleischman A: Limits of viability: Dilemmas, decisions, and decision makers. Am J Perinatol 2001;18:117.

48. Leuthner S: Decisions regarding resuscitation of the extremely premature infant and models of best interest. J Perinatol 2001;21:193.

12

EMERGENCY MANAGEMENT OF THE OBSTETRIC PATIENT

Debra Houry and Jean T. Abbott

Emergency care of the pregnant patient involves recognition of the needs of two organisms: mother and fetus. In general, optimizing maternal physiology results in optimal outcome for the fetus. This is true for medical cardiopulmonary resuscitation (CPR), resuscitation from traumatic injury, and acute surgical or toxicologic emergencies. Physiologic changes in pregnancy, however, change some aspects of emergency assessment of the mother and some of the resuscitation needs of both mother and fetus. This chapter reviews general and specific aspects of maternal resuscitation in the context of pregnancy.

PHYSIOLOGIC CHANGES THAT ALTER RESUSCITATION IN PREGNANCY

Pregnancy is a hypermetabolic state characterized by a hyperdynamic, low-resistance cardiovascular profile and respiratory alkalosis. In spite of an expanded plasma volume and anemia, hypercoagulability is present. The uterus grows to use one fourth to one third of the maternal cardiac output, and its physical mass distorts abdominal anatomy, decreases residual volume, and compresses venous return. The important changes that affect resuscitation are listed in Table 12–1. In the critically ill pregnant woman, airway and ventilatory control should be maintained aggressively and cardiovascular volume must be supported because disproportionate fetal sequelae of metabolic derangements and decreased maternal reserve can occur.

MEDICAL CARDIOPULMONARY COLLAPSE IN PREGNANCY

Cardiopulmonary arrest occurs infrequently in pregnancy. Maternal cardiac arrest is most often related to events that occur at time of delivery (i.e., eclampsia, amniotic fluid embolus, iatrogenic drug toxicity) or as a result of physiologic changes (i.e., cardiomyopathy).[1] In patients in whom resuscitation is possible, the outcome is clearly time dependent. The clinician caring for the obstetric woman with cardiac arrest must therefore have a preplanned approach that ensures the following:

1. Basic life support algorithms and a management plan based on primary rhythm disturbance (advanced cardiopulmonary life support [ACLS]).
2. Consideration of the potential reversible etiologies for the cardiac arrest.
3. Rescue of the fetus if maternal resuscitation fails but fetal survival is possible.

Principles of Basic and Advanced Life Support

Basic life support and ACLS are based primarily on recommendations and cardiac rhythm algorithms published

---

TABLE 12–1 Physiologic Changes That Affect Resuscitation in Pregnancy

Uteroplacental vasoconstriction in response to hypercarbia and hypoxia

Increased minute ventilation and decreased lung residual volume

Normal P_{CO_2} of 30 to 32 mm Hg with physiologic "hyperventilation"

Expanded plasma volume and physiologic anemia

Hypercoagulability: increased levels of multiple coagulation factors and fibrinogen

Lack of autoregulation of uterine blood flow in response to changing maternal blood pressures

Obstruction of venous return in the supine position after 20 weeks' pregnancy

Uterine vasoconstriction in response to α-adrenergic stimulation and maternal hypovolemia

Impaired fetal carbon dioxide excretion with maternal hypercarbia

Generalized smooth muscle relaxation and increased abdominal pressure with risk of aspiration

---

Data derived from Buchsbaum[14]; Lee et al[56]; Neufeld et al[57]; Nolan et al[58]; Patterson[59]; Pearlman et al[32]; and Satin et al.[5]
P_{CO_2}, partial pressure of carbon dioxide.

and updated periodically by the American Heart Association. The current recommendations are based on consensus statements published by the AHA in 2000[2] and a review of modifications, particularly in pregnancy.[1] The cornerstones of resuscitation consist of the following factors: early institution of CPR, rapid identification and electrical conversion of ventricular fibrillation (VF), early intubation and establishment of effective ventilation, and use of epinephrine to restore coronary perfusion pressure (Fig. 12–1). In pregnancy, reversible causes of cardiac arrest should be sought early because these may be more common than in the general population[1] and the majority of successes (particularly if initial defibrillation efforts are not successful) come from this group of patients with *secondary* cardiac arrest. Only the special considerations of resuscitation in pregnancy are reviewed here.

Early Cardiopulmonary Resuscitation

Institution of rescuer ventilation and closed cardiac massage results in improved survival rates in out-of-hospital cardiac arrests when initiated within 4 minutes. Optimal CPR techniques generate a maximum of only 30% of normal cardiac output and therefore should be immediately followed by further methods of restoring effective cardiac output. In the operating room, open cardiac massage can generate a more satisfactory cardiac output and may therefore be preferable.[2,3]

Uterine compression of the inferior vena cava in the second half of pregnancy can decrease cardiac output by 20% to 30% in the supine position, in which women are placed during standard resuscitation and CPR. This may be even more critical in the low-flow states that accompany critical illness, and impaired venous return to the heart may either precipitate cardiac arrest or prevent restoration of effective circulation in established cardiac arrest.[4] CPR in the second half of pregnancy should therefore be modified to displace the uterus off the inferior vena cava by one of the following methods: manual displacement of the uterus to the left of the midline by the rescuer, tilting of the patient to the left by at least 15 degrees on a secure backboard, wedging of the patient's trunk and pelvis, or use of the Cardiff tilt table. Performance of CPR at an angle of at least 15 degrees diminishes the effectiveness of CPR and increases rescuer effort but has been shown to minimize supine hypotensive changes.[5]

Early Defibrillation

The most successful outcome from adult cardiac arrest in the general population occurs with identification of VF and rapid defibrillation.[6] VF is probably a less common initial rhythm in the pregnant patient, because secondary causes of arrest may be more common than sudden primary cardiac events. However, defibrillation of VF is the highest priority of advanced life support when VF is identified, taking precedence in the monitored in-hospital patient

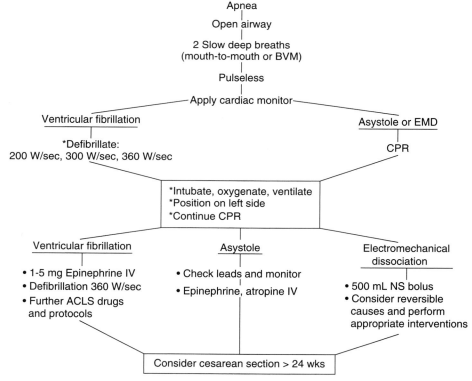

*For doses and specific details, see text reference AHA, 2000.[2]

Figure 12–1. Cardiopulmonary arrest in pregnancy. ACLS, advanced cardiopulmonary life support; BVM, bronchovascular markings; CPR, cardiopulmonary resuscitation; EMD, esophageal motility disorder; IV, intravenous; NS, normal saline; W, watts.

over even airway management and initiation of CPR.[6] Physiologic changes during pregnancy may affect transthoracic impedance, but no studies have found a significant difference in the "dose" required for effective defibrillation.[7]

The safety of direct current electric shock to the fetus has been demonstrated in several series of case reports. In cases in which maternal defibrillation at 200 to 300 W/second has been accompanied by fetal monitoring, neither disruption of the fetal rhythm nor stimulation of uterine contractions has been reported.[8] Fetal monitoring is desirable during countershock, although it often is not possible in an arrest situation. It is currently believed that the fetus is protected because the direct energy received is small and that fetal hearts have a high fibrillatory threshold.[9]

Early Establishment of Airway and Ventilation

In all patients in cardiac arrest, inadequate ventilation is the major cause of acidosis, particularly in the first 10 minutes of resuscitation. Therefore, early normalization of respiratory function is a priority. Because the risk of aspiration is increased as a result of gastroesophageal sphincter relaxation and decreased lower gastrointestinal motility, intubation should be performed early in the affected pregnant patient. Maternal hypoxia and hypercarbia are disproportionately reflected in decreased fetal blood flow, fetal acidosis, and hypoxia.

Medications to Restore Circulation and Coronary Perfusion Pressure

Epinephrine has remained a useful vasoactive drug in cardiac resuscitation, probably because of its α-sympathetic effect of increasing arterial pressure and creating a perfusion gradient across the coronary vascular bed. In addition, vasopressin was added to ACLS protocols as a treatment for ventricular fibrillation.[2] Vasopressin is a class B drug that directly stimulates smooth muscle receptors, resulting in vasoconstriction. Establishment of at least a 30–mm Hg gradient for coronary perfusion pressure is currently the best predictor of successful resuscitation from cardiac arrest.[6] Although theoretical concerns might make the clinician hesitate to administer drugs that will cause uterine vasoconstriction, this should not be a consideration in the pregnant patient in cardiac arrest. The best hope for fetal survival is restoration of spontaneous maternal circulation.[6]

Discovery and Treatment of Reversible Causes of Cardiac Arrest

In pregnancy, several secondary causes of cardiac arrest need to be rapidly identified and addressed. The most common of these are listed in Table 12-2. Clues to the presence of a reversible cause include the clinical setting and the presence of a pulseless organized electric rhythm (pulseless electrical activity).[6] In cardiac arrest, time constraints mandate that interventions, such as intravenous (IV) fluids or chest decompression, be performed rapidly if these causes are suspected, without the luxury of time-consuming diagnostic studies.

Perimortem Cesarean Section

Basic management during the first minutes of cardiac arrest is outlined in Figure 12-1. If VF is not present or cannot be converted to an organized rhythm, CPR should be started with the uterus at a 15-degree tilt to the left, if the pregnancy is at least 24 weeks along. Intubation, oxygenation, and ventilatory support are performed, and a fluid bolus may be indicated if hypovolemia is suspected. If this fails to restore maternal circulation, emergency cesarean section is suggested in the woman with a fetus of more than 24 weeks' gestation, to maximize survival of both the mother and the fetus.[1,10] Fetal survival is optimal when delivery is performed within 5 to 10 minutes of the cardiac arrest, although cases with normal fetal outcome have been reported after prolonged resuscitations.[4,11]

TABLE 12-2   Potentially Reversible Causes of Cardiopulmonary Arrest in Pregnancy

Cause	Setting	Intervention
Pulmonary embolus	Late pregnancy	Oxygen, CPR
	Peripartum	Consideration of thrombolytics
	Hypoxia, cyanosis, respiratory distress	
Amniotic fluid embolus	Labor	Inotropic support
	Uterine evacuation or procedure	Coagulation factor replacement
Hypovolemia	External blood loss	Fluid bolus: 500-1000 mL NS or RL
	Suspected abruptio placentae	Coagulation factor support
	GI bleeding; ruptured liver, spleen, or other bleeding source	
Anaphylaxis	Anesthetic or IV pharmacologic agents	Fluid bolus: 500-1000 mL NS or RL
	Radiographic dye procedures	IV epinephrine
Tension pneumothorax	Intubation, positive-pressure ventilation	Chest decompression
Pericardial tamponade	Chronic renal failure, TB	Fluid bolus, 500 mL NS or RL Needle aspiration of pericardium
Sepsis	Infection: pyelonephritis; pelvic, septic emboli	Oxygen, CPR, bicarbonate
Primary respiratory failure	Magnesium toxicity; pulmonary infection or emboli or congestive heart failure	Positive-pressure ventilatory support
	Seizure, eclampsia, intracranial bleeding	Suctioning, hyperventilation

CPR, cardiopulmonary resuscitation; GI, gastrointestinal; IV, intravenous; NS, normal saline; RL, Ringer's lactated solution; TB, tuberculosis.

Other Rhythms and Drugs in Cardiac Arrest in Pregnancy

Asystole

Asystole is an ominous rhythm from which resuscitation is uncommon. It is often the end result of prolonged cardiac ischemia. Mechanical difficulties, such as disconnected leads, should always be considered. The monitor gain should be turned up, and leads should be changed by 90 degrees to detect the rare fine VF that appears to be asystolic. Initial management includes CPR, airway control, and use of epinephrine and atropine to restore cardiac activity.

Cardiac Resuscitation Drugs

The majority of standard ACLS pharmaceutical agents, including atropine and lidocaine, are safe in pregnancy.[12] Amiodarone has been linked with fetal/neonatal hypothyroidism and thus should be used only in life-threatening situations.[13] All medications should be used according to standard ACLS protocols. Dosages may need to be increased because maternal blood volume in late pregnancy is increased. Per-kilogram dosages usually allow adequate drug levels, at least as these are currently known. In the intubated patient, epinephrine, diazepam, and lidocaine may be given (usually in double dosages) through the endotracheal tube if IV access has not been established.[2]

Sodium Bicarbonate

Sodium bicarbonate usage in cardiac resuscitation has been increasingly discouraged for several reasons, including the following: (1) The major cause of acidosis in the first 15 minutes of a cardiac arrest is respiratory; (2) the ability to resuscitate is poorly correlated with bicarbonate administration, even in the presence of a low serum pH; and (3) serum alkalinization is associated with a paradoxic brain acidosis as carbon dioxide rapidly crosses the blood-brain barrier but the bicarbonate ion diffuses poorly.[2] In pregnancy the fetal circulation, likewise affected by a blood-membrane barrier, experiences a similar paradoxic increase in acidosis with sodium bicarbonate administration. Thus, ventilation should be the mainstay of management for metabolic and respiratory acidosis in the pregnant patient in cardiac arrest, and bicarbonate therapy should only be used in specific situations. Current indications for sodium bicarbonate use are cardiac arrest caused by hyperkalemia (from renal failure or iatrogenic), cyclic antidepressant overdose, and preexistent metabolic acidosis, as from sepsis or drug ingestion (methanol, ethanol, salicylates).[2,5]

Treatment of Nonarrest Cardiac Rhythm Disturbances

Supraventricular Tachycardias

Paroxysmal tachycardias of supraventricular origin (PSVTs) are not uncommon in young women, and their frequency may increase with the stress of pregnancy. Management of the patient with PSVT depends on the cardiovascular stability of the mother. Rapid conversion is often a greater priority in pregnancy, because the fetus is particularly sensitive to decreases in maternal cardiac output. Placental blood flow may decrease 20% in the presence of normal maternal blood pressure, as the uterine vasculature has no ability to autoregulate and maintain perfusion pressure in the presence of decreases in cardiac output.[14] In the treatment of PSVTs, care should always be taken to exclude sinus tachycardia, which is a secondary rhythm necessitating management of the following underlying conditions: sepsis, hypovolemia, hypoxia, pain, pulmonary embolus, or congestive failure. Sinus tachycardia rarely exceeds a rate of 180 bpm, and is characterized by gradual rate changes over time. For the patient with primary PSVT, the following treatments should be considered:

1. *Cardioversion* has been reported to be safe for the fetus and effective in pregnancy.[9,15] Usual "doses" for PSVTs start at 50 W/second, with the defibrillator in the "synchronized" mode. If no conversion occurs, rates can be increased in increments of 50 to 100 W/second to the maximum of the unit. If transient conversion occurs, higher electricity levels should not be used, but medications may be necessary to maintain the converted rhythm. Cardioversion is the first line of treatment in the unstable woman with impaired cardiac output secondary to PSVT.[2,15]

2. *Adenosine* is the treatment of choice for the stable patient with a narrow-complex tachycardia. A direct vagal-receptor stimulator with an onset of action of 10 to 20 seconds and a duration of effect of 30 to 60 seconds, adenosine is ideal, even in the patient with some measure of hypotension: 6 mg should be rapidly given intravenously. If that dose is not effective, 12 mg are given. Patients frequently experience a transient wave of flushing or warmth; only reassurance is necessary for it. Adenosine does not affect the fetal heart rate and is well tolerated in pregnancy.[12]

3. In general, *verapamil* has become a second-line drug because of its longer duration of action and hypotensive calcium channel blocker effects. Although no adverse outcomes have been reported in pregnancy, fetal bradycardia has been reported.[16]

Wide-Complex Tachycardias

Wide-complex tachycardias, which are much rarer in young patients, can be caused either by ventricular tachycardia or by supraventricular tachycardia with aberrant rate-related conduction. Often the two cannot be differentiated. Treatment is, again, dependent on maternal cardiovascular status: In the pulseless patient, the treatment is defibrillation as with VF. In the unstable patient, synchronized cardioversion is used, as described previously. In the stable patient, a trial of lidocaine (1 mg/kg), amiodarone (150 mg in an IV bolus over 10 minutes), or IV procainamide is recommended. If these fail, sedation and synchronized cardioversion can be used in the awake patient.[2,12]

Bradycardias

Bradycardia is defined as a pulse less than 60 bpm. Although sometimes normal in healthy nonpregnant adults, slow rates are particularly poorly tolerated in pregnancy, in which resting pulse rates are more commonly in the range of 90 to 100 bpm. Sinus bradycardias and even asystole may occur while patients undergo instrumentation, when overstimulation of vagal pathways through pain or visceral organ manipulation occurs. Bradycardia rates less than 60 bpm in pregnancy should be treated if associated with hypotension (systolic blood pressure <80 mm Hg or less than the patient's known normal level), fetal distress, or other signs of hypoperfusion. Treatment in patients with a pulse is IV atropine in 0.5-mg increments every 5 minutes, to a total of 3 mg. In pulseless bradyarrhythmias, 1 mg intravenously is used. Pacing, with a transcutaneous pacer, may be necessary, particularly in the peripartum patient with significant myocardial or conduction system disease.

ASSESSMENT AND MANAGEMENT OF THE PREGNANT TRAUMA PATIENT

Physiology and Response to Hypovolemia

Injury is currently the leading cause of death in women of reproductive age and is a leading cause of maternal mortality in several urban series. Homicide accounts for the majority of fatalities; motor vehicle accidents, suicides, and intentional assault injury account for the rest.[17,18]

The same physiologic changes in pregnancy that are seen in medical cardiopulmonary arrest confound assessment in the pregnant trauma victim. The capacities of the maternal respiratory and circulatory systems to respond to injury are impaired (see Table 12–1). Also of importance in trauma is that abdominal anatomy is distorted. The diaphragm is higher, and the location of the bowel shifts as the uterus displaces structures into the upper abdomen. The uterus itself becomes the leading target for anterior abdominal forces beyond the first trimester. In addition, peritoneal bleeding is less likely to cause the nonpregnant response of guarding, tenderness, and rigidity, because the abdominal muscles are stretched and the anterior peritoneum and abdominal wall are distanced from organs such as the liver and spleen.[19]

Hypovolemia is a common consequence of blunt or penetrating injury. The fetus is not protected from maternal blood loss, because autoregulation of uterine perfusion does not occur. Confounding the problem is the vasoconstrictive effect of maternal hypoxia, acidosis, and sympathetic stimulation (α-adrenergic) often seen in hypovolemic shock.[14,20] Maternal vital signs can remain normal until up to 30% of blood volume is lost; the fetus, however, may have markedly impaired perfusion. Resuscitation of the pregnant trauma victim in the second half of pregnancy is also impaired by the effects of prolonged supine positioning on venous return. Supine hypotension is a clear danger in the gravid patient who requires immobilization for potential spinal injury, and such danger may be accentuated in the setting of decreased blood volume.

Fetal and Maternal Injury in Blunt Trauma

Both the mother and the fetus are susceptible to lethal injury in assaults, falls, and motor vehicle accidents.

Mortality in pregnant women, as in nonpregnant blunt trauma, is most commonly caused by uncontrolled hemorrhage or head injury, and this risk is probably not altered in pregnancy.

The most common cause of *fetal* death is maternal death or sustained hypotension.[19,21] Other causes of fetal death include direct uterine trauma, hypoxia, pelvic fracture, and severe head injury. One study found that a maternal injury severity score of 25 or higher was correlated with at least 50% fetal mortality.[22] However, correlation of fetal outcome with the severity of maternal injuries is not entirely predictable, and the fetus may survive after severe maternal insult, or it may die after relatively minor maternal injury.[23]

In the trauma victim without fatal injuries, the most common mechanism of fetal death is abruptio placentae.[22] Forces on the gravid uterus can result from assault, falls, impact with the steering wheel, or ejection from a vehicle. The likelihood of uterine trauma increases as the size and prominence of the uterus increase. It is thought that frontal impact and rapid distortion of the uterine shape causes shear forces between the elastic uterus and the nonelastic placenta, resulting in separation. Whereas abruptio placentae is seen in only a small percentage of minor injuries in pregnant women, the incidence is as high as 50% in major injuries.[24] Fetal death most often occurs rapidly, particularly if a large percentage of the placenta is involved.[19] Delayed fetal distress and death can also occur from placental abruption, even with injuries that are minor.[22] In such cases, vaginal bleeding, amniotic fluid leakage, and abdominal contractions are less common than abnormal fetal heart tracings as early warning signs of abruption.[25]

Uterine rupture is rare and occurs in 1% or fewer cases of severe trauma. It almost always results in fetal death. Rupture is usually associated with severe frontal abdominal trauma; it is more common with pelvis fractures and with increased gestational age. Direct injury to the fetus may also occur during trauma. Although more common with penetrating injury, blunt injury has also been associated with fractures and head injury in the fetus. Such injuries are more common as the fetus approaches term and the head becomes engaged within the pelvis. Associated maternal pelvis fractures are commonly present.[18]

Approach to the Blunt Trauma Patient

Maternal Resuscitation

Aggressive maternal resuscitation provides the best assurance of fetal well-being, both because the best fetal environment is a physiologic maternal one and because the fetus is frequently affected disproportionately by maternal injury. The principles of blunt trauma resuscitation have been well outlined in more specific references.[19,26] Primary assessment and resuscitation of the mother consist of ensuring a patent *airway* (while keeping the cervical spine immobilized), assessment and control of *breathing* if needed to ensure adequate oxygenation and acid-base balance, followed by control of bleeding and restoration of adequate *circulation*. These principles apply in pregnancy to an equal if not greater extent because the fetus may be the first to become impaired if there is inadequate oxygenation or hypovolemia. After 20 weeks of pregnancy, the patient should be tilted onto her left side, either with a 15-degree wedge under the right side of the backboard or by supporting the right hip and pelvis, to protect against the effects of supine hypotension.[26]

Monitoring the Fetus

In the patient pregnant more than 24 to 26 weeks, evaluation of the fetus should be added to the primary assessment of the injured patient, because emergency surgical intervention (a "D" for *delivery* to add to the initial "ABCs" of resuscitation) may be necessary to save the fetus. Although auscultation of the fetus can sometimes be managed, both cardiotocographic monitoring and bedside sonography are usually necessary to accurately diagnose fetal death or distress, particularly in the setting of a multiply injured patient with hypovolemia undergoing major resuscitation.[27,28] The fetal heart rate is moderately accurate as an indicator of fetal health. However, decreases in baseline variability are more sensitive markers and necessitate continuous monitoring.[21,23] Two indications for emergency cesarean section have been described. The first is a distressed but live fetus if abruptio placentae or uterine rupture is suspected. The second is a moribund mother who does not respond to initial primary interventions of trauma resuscitation. As in a medical cardiac arrest, delivery may allow not only fetal rescue but also restoration of maternal venous return. Perimortem cesarean section in the trauma resuscitation room has been suggested in such circumstances, although only rare case reports of successful fetal and maternal resuscitation in trauma exist.[29]

Secondary Assessment and Management of the Pregnant Woman

After initial stabilization of the mother, a complete assessment for injuries is sought, because multiple and often occult injuries are common in blunt trauma. Hypovolemia and head injury are the most common causes of death. Radiographs of the cervical spine are standard to rule out cervical spine fracture. Chest and pelvis radiographs are indicated in the significantly injured patient and should never be withheld because of fetal risk if they are indicated. When the beam edge is more than 10 cm from the fetus, radiation exposure is negligible.[30] Lead shielding can also be used to protect the fetus from unnecessary exposure. Thoracic and lumbar films should be taken if the physical examination or symptoms dictate, because half of all spinal injuries in blunt trauma occur below the cervical vertebrae.

In the hypovolemic trauma patient, the location of internal bleeding must be sought aggressively at the same time as crystalloid and blood are being used to replace losses. The common sites of occult blood loss include the chest cavity, peritoneum, retroperitoneum, pelvis, and femur fractures. In pregnancy, uterine bleeding from abruptio placentae may also be occult but significant. Plain radiographic diagnosis of long bone fractures, pelvic fractures, and intrathoracic injuries can be made rapidly. Emergency laparotomy may be the diagnostic procedure

of choice in the critically injured patient with blunt abdominal trauma and hypovolemic shock, but more commonly peritoneal lavage, computed tomography (CT), or ultrasonography are first used to detect intra-abdominal sources of bleeding. Successful peritoneal lavage has been reported even in the third trimester with an open, supraumbilical approach. Sensitivity ranges from 80% to 90%, equivalent to that in the nonpregnant woman.[31] Because of the oversensitivity and lack of specificity of a positive lavage for injuries necessitating laparotomy, CT of the abdomen is usually preferred in the stable patient.[32] An added advantage of CT is the ability to determine the extent of solid organ injuries and to assess the retroperitoneum, the other potential source of occult blood loss. Fetal radiation dosage with abdominal CT and a modern scanner is on the order of 5 to 10 rad.[29] Ultrasonography has also been reported as a newer method of assessment of intraperitoneal bleeding in trauma, and it is particularly suitable for pregnancy, because fetal assessment can be done concomitantly with no radiation exposure to the fetus. Ultrasonography has been reported to have a sensitivity of 83% and a specificity of 98% for detecting intraperitoneal fluid in pregnant patients who have suffered blunt abdominal trauma.[33]

Initial laboratory tests in major trauma include complete blood cell count, blood typing and crossing, baseline hepatic and renal function studies, toxicology studies as indicated, and a Kleihauer-Betke smear to detect large-volume fetomaternal transfusion.[26] Coagulation studies, including fibrinogen and fibrin split product levels, should be performed if abruptio placentae is suspected, because this may trigger disseminated intravascular coagulation. Baseline fibrinogen levels in the third trimester are normally 400 to 500 mg/dL. Levels less than 300 mg/dL are abnormal, and levels less than 150 mg/dL are associated with significant coagulopathy.[14,19]

Cardiotocographic monitoring should be an integral part of the early and ongoing evaluation of the fetus older than 20 weeks' gestation after maternal trauma. Early auscultation for abnormal fetal heart rate is useful as a screening procedure; abnormal rates may be present with maternal shock, abruptio placentae, uterine rupture, or direct fetal injury. Cardiotocographic monitoring allows early recognition of fetal distress and response to volume therapy and can also detect uterine irritability or contractions. Monitoring should be continued for at least 4 to 6 hours if significant abdominal forces have occurred. Abnormal fetal heart rates and loss of beat-to-beat variability are believed to be the most sensitive clues to occult abruptio placentae.[25,27,34]

Bedside sonography can be useful to detect fetal heart activity that often cannot be readily heard with simple auscultation in a busy resuscitation room, as well as uterine rupture, gestational age, and amniotic fluid volume.[28] Sensitivity for recognizing placental abruption is only fair, but when a separation is seen, sonography is useful for monitoring subchorionic clots to see whether they are stable or expanding.[21]

Several other complications of blunt trauma should be anticipated. *Uterine contractions* are probably the most common consequence of trauma in pregnancy and developed in 5% of women with nonadmissible injuries in one series.[35] These usually stop spontaneously but may be an early indicator of abruptio placentae. The role of tocolytic agents is uncertain.[19,21]

Fetomaternal transfusion is also a risk after blunt abdominal trauma. Although it occurs spontaneously in normal pregnancies, fetomaternal transfusion occurs more frequently after trauma, particularly to the abdomen. In one prospective series, 30% of women with significant abdominal trauma had evidence of fetal cells in the maternal circulation, with a 6% control rate.[36] In another series of patients with dischargeable injuries, a 9% incidence of fetomaternal hemorrhage occurred.[34] The Kleihauer-Betke test has been used to detect fetal hemorrhage into the maternal circulation, but its sensitivity is much less than the volume of fetal cells necessary to sensitize an Rh-negative mother with an Rh-positive fetus.[34] As few as 0.01 mL of fetal red blood cells can trigger a maternal immune response; therefore, it has been recommended that $Rh_O(D)$ immune globulin (RhoGAM), 300 μg, be given to all Rh-negative mothers without antibodies, and whose fetuses have no known Rh-negative father, who sustain abdominal trauma. The Kleihauer-Betke assay can be used to detect the rare instances of massive fetomaternal transfusion that may result in fetal anemia. The dose of $Rh_O(D)$ immune globulin may need to be increased if large-volume transfusion is detected in an Rh-negative mother (300 μg/30 mL of fetal whole blood).[32,34]

One of the most difficult questions in maternal trauma management is how to predict and anticipate the risk to the fetus in mothers who are uninjured or who have minor injuries. Several series have emphasized that fetal death, usually from placental abruption, can occur with minor injury to the mother.[25,34] Although isolated case reports have indicated that fetal death can occur several days after blunt trauma, prospective studies have determined that signs of fetal distress are usually immediate. For the fetus that initially appears healthy, frequent uterine activity (more than eight contractions per hour) in the first 4 to 6 hours is a sensitive if nonspecific predictor of later fetal complications and mandates a longer period of monitoring.[24,32,34] In the mother who is admitted for other indications or in whom cardiotocographic abnormalities are seen, monitoring should be continued until contractions are resolved and abruptio placentae has been ruled out.[21,27,34] Pregnant patients involved in motorcycle or pedestrian collisions or patients with absent fetal heart tones or a fetal heart rate of less than 120 bpm or more than 160 bpm have an increased risk of fetal demise.[27]

Prevention of maternal and fetal injury is always important for primary care providers such as obstetricians. Women should be encouraged to wear three-point restraint systems. A significant percentage of women never use seat belts in pregnancy, many because they are uncomfortable or afraid of causing injury.[37] As with nonpregnant trauma victims, seat belts prevent ejection from a motor vehicle. Their use is associated with a fivefold decrease in mortality for both the mother and fetus. Seat belts should always be worn snugly, with the lap portion against the anterior iliac crests and with the shoulder strap above the uterine fundus.[38] Reports of air bag deployment in pregnancy have not shown risk to the fetus.[39] In the general population, driver fatalities are decreased overall in vehicles with air bags by about 28% in frontal crashes over fatality rates in vehicles with manual belts only.[40] Frontal impact of the gravid uterus against the steering wheel is a significant risk to the unbelted pregnant driver; thus, air bags have the potential to decrease the risk of abruption and fetal injury.

Other Traumatic Injuries in Pregnancy

Penetrating Trauma

Protocols for managing penetrating abdominal trauma in the *general* population have evolved since the mid-1990s. Exploration by radiography or examination is mandated by maternal instability, gunshot wound with penetration of the peritoneal cavity, evisceration, or signs of peritoneal irritation. In the stable patient, stab wounds are explored locally, as are gunshot wounds that do not appear to penetrate the peritoneum, and peritoneal lavage is performed on all wounds whose extent cannot be ascertained or that penetrate the peritoneum.

In pregnancy, the uterus is more often involved in penetrating trauma, and the viscera are relatively protected, particularly in late pregnancy. Fetal mortality rates approach 50% in some penetrating trauma series, whereas the incidence of maternal visceral injury is only 20% in gunshot wounds when penetrating trauma occurs below the uterine fundus.[41] Because of the low incidence of visceral injury necessitating repair, observation alone has been recommended in anterior penetrating abdominal trauma below the uterine fundus, if the fetus does not appear compromised or is dead (because spontaneous delivery can be anticipated).[41] Even when fetal injury is suspected, survival is more likely in the premature fetus, unless fetal distress is seen. Exploratory laparotomy is still recommended if the mother is unstable, if injury is above the fundus, or if there is evidence of maternal visceral injury. Even when laparotomy is indicated, hysterotomy may not need to be part of the surgical procedure.[20,35,41]

Burns

In general, the pregnant patient who sustains burns is managed as any other burn patient. Fetal prognosis in general parallels maternal prognosis; about an 80% rate of mortality is reported in major burns of 30% maternal body surface area or greater.[42] Loss of a significant percentage of dermal integrity is associated with massive fluid losses, and the major causes of early mortality are hypoxia from inhalation injury or hypovolemia from inability to keep up with fluid losses.[43] Premature labor may be a problem in pregnancy complicated by burns. Early delivery of the fetus in third trimester patients with severe burns is recommended, and an emergency cesarean section is indicated for maternal distress.[43] Magnesium sulfate has been suggested as a tocolytic because β-sympathomimetics may be countertherapeutic in the context of volume resuscitation.[42]

Electrical Injury

Although direct current countershock has been reported to be safe in pregnancy (as with cardioversion), fetal risk has been reported with exposure to alternative current electrical shocks, such as household current, that may appear minor.[44] Fetal death has been reported without maternal injury, and in surviving fetuses, decreased movement, oligohydramnios, or growth restriction may be evident over time. All patients who experience electrical exposures should be evaluated for fetal health, and fetal activity should be monitored periodically thereafter, although the risk to the fetus is probably low.[44,45]

POISONINGS AND OVERDOSES IN PREGNANCY

Epidemiology

The pattern of drug ingestion in pregnancy parallels that in the general adult population: Intentional overdoses usually involve a single substance, the majority of overdoses in adults are intentional, and medically dangerous overdoses are rare. In a series of 111 pregnant women with intentional overdoses reported by the Michigan Poison Control Center, 55% had mild or no symptoms, 45% had major symptoms, and no fatalities were reported. Most overdoses were associated with depression and situational stresses. The most common substances involved in overdose were nonnarcotic analgesics (26%), nutritional supplements (12%), antianxiety agents (11%), sedative/hypnotic drugs (10%), controlled analgesics (8%), antibiotics (7%), and antihistamines/decongestants (6%).[46] As with other adult overdoses, these substances are usually readily available (if not over the counter) and are commonly used during pregnancy.

Pregnancy Effects on Toxicity

Several changes in maternal physiology would be expected to alter the toxicity of various poisonings in pregnancy. Increased ventilatory needs are more susceptible to narcotic- and sedative-induced depression. Increased blood volume and maternal fat stores lead to a larger volume of drug distribution. The glomerular filtration rate is increased, resulting in more rapid handling of renally excreted drugs. Experience is limited with poisonings in pregnancy; thus, the exact balance of protection and increased risk of overdose in pregnancy is often not clear.

General Approach to the Poisoned Patient

The pregnant patient with an acute drug ingestion should be handled in the same manner as a nonpregnant patient. A history of the ingestion should be elicited to give an idea of the type of toxicity that may be encountered. Accuracy of the history is compromised by both accidental and deliberate errors by the patient. In most cases, a toxicology screen on blood or urine, directed at the most likely substances (e.g., hallucinogens, drugs of abuse, sedative/hypnotics) is useful for confirming which substances are present. The time of ingestion is likewise important, as is the reason for the overdose. Although medical management takes precedence, the psychologic

background must always be addressed when the patient is recovered from medical effects. Seemingly benign ingestions must be taken seriously from a psychiatric standpoint because this pattern of "communication" for help commonly repeats itself and may be fatal, even if that was not the patient's intention. Among pregnant women, more than 50% of suicidal ingestions occur in the first trimester.[46] Learning to deal constructively with the stresses of continued pregnancy and eventual parenting or seeking counsel to decide whether pregnancy termination is best are important aspects of the complete care of the patient.

Consultation with a regional poison control center should be a routine part of management of poisoned patients.[47] Poison control centers provide information about signs and symptoms to expect, delayed toxicity, specific antidotes, and general management. The obstetrician should be aware of the following common principles of toxicologic management.

Initial Stabilization

Opening and protection of the airway, assessment of breathing and support as needed, and circulatory support are the first interventions needed, as with any unknown and potentially critically ill patient. The breathing patient should be assessed with pulse oximetry, and oxygen should be applied liberally to keep the maternal oxygen saturation more than 90%. Arterial blood gas analyses should be obtained if the adequacy of ventilation is in question. The pregnant patient is at higher risk of aspiration because of slower gut motility and higher intragastric pressures[19] and normally has a respiratory alkalosis with a partial pressure of carbon dioxide of 30 to 35 mm Hg. Thus, intubation should be performed in a poisoned pregnant patient to support fetal oxygenation, increased metabolism, and carbon dioxide excretion. Vasodilation is a common cause of hypotension in drug overdose; therefore, the first step in circulatory support should be fluid administration to expand the circulating volume. Vasopressors should be avoided unless fluid resuscitation is insufficient. In pregnancy, the α-adrenergic effects of pressors have the potential risk of increasing uterine contractility and decreasing uterine blood flow.

Three standard antidotes are commonly given to the patient with altered consciousness who may have taken an overdose.[47] IV dextrose, 50 mL of a 50% solution in water, is given to treat potential hypoglycemia. The pregnant diabetic may be more susceptible to accidental hypoglycemia than she is when not pregnant; thus, this guideline is particularly appropriate in pregnancy. IV naloxone, 2 mg, is given for a suspected narcotic overdose. In addition, thiamine, 50 to 100 mg intramuscularly or intravenously, is given to alcoholic or nutritionally deficient patients with suspected thiamine deficiency to prevent adverse effects from glucose administration, which can precipitate Wernicke-Korsakoff syndrome in such patients.[47]

General Measures to Prevent Absorption

Traditionally, gastric emptying with either syrup of ipecac or gastric lavage has been a standard method of preventing absorption of ingested substances. However, no benefit and some hazards of both of these interventions have been shown. The most effective gastrointestinal decontaminant is activated charcoal. Administration of at least one dose of activated charcoal (50 to 100 g in a slurry, or 10 times the mass of the ingested substance) is currently recommended.[47] Charcoal is an inert substance with a large surface area that absorbs a wide range of toxic substances, including most pharmacologic compounds that are commonly ingested, preventing absorption from the gastrointestinal tract into the systemic circulation. Substances for which charcoal is not effective include ethanol, lithium, and strong acids or bases.[47] Cathartics may be used with the charcoal to speed transit through the gastrointestinal tract, thus also limiting drug absorption.

Specific Diagnosis and Treatment

Diagnosis of specific poisonings by use of toxicology screening tests on blood or urine is not necessary in the patient who is not sick. Serum drug levels are useful in only a small number of poisonings in which symptoms are subtle or initially absent, in which toxicity may be severe, or for which specific antidotes exist. Selectively, blood levels are indicated to detect acetaminophen, salicylates, antiepileptic medications, lithium, alcohols, iron, theophylline, or digoxin. An electrocardiogram to screen for cyclic antidepressant overdose (serum levels are not useful in general) is commonly performed.[47]

The care of most poisoned patients is supportive. In the unknown ingestion, it is frequently useful to group symptoms to guide supportive and specific therapy. In pregnancy, the most common syndromes are those associated with sedatives (narcotics), anticholinergic symptoms associated with cyclic antidepressants or antihistamines (over-the-counter sleep medications), and those associated with sympathomimetic medications.[47]

Specific Poisonings in the Pregnant Patient

In all patients with toxic ingestions or exposures, treatment should be guided by the complete and up-to-date databases available through a regional poison control center. The following discussions highlight the current specifics of treatment for common or potentially dangerous poisonings in the pregnant patient but should never be substituted for detailed management according to such protocols.

Acetaminophen

Acetaminophen is one of the safest and most commonly used over-the-counter drugs currently available. It is part of many multidrug combinations and in therapeutic doses has a wide toxic-therapeutic ratio. Deliberate overdose, however, can be fatal.[47,48] In general, ingestion of about 7.5 g of drug is potentially toxic, although nomograms based on blood levels taken at 4 hours after ingestion (or later) should be used to guide specific treatment. Acetaminophen poisoning is important for three reasons: (1) the overdose may be fatal, (2) early symptoms may be subtle or absent, and (3) an excellent antidote is available

if the diagnosis is recognized early. For these reasons and because patients are often confused about which over-the-counter pain medication they have ingested, routine serum screening for acetaminophen is usually part of the initial workup of the poisoned patient.[47]

In pregnancy, toxicity of acetaminophen to the fetus may be enhanced over that of the mother. Toxicity occurs in the maternal liver when the serum load of acetaminophen overwhelms the normal metabolic pathways and a toxic metabolite, usually detoxified by glutathione, builds up in the blood. Injury to hepatocytes occurs, which may result in fatal liver injury. The specific antidote, *N*-acetyl-L-cysteine (NAC), administered in a loading dose of 140 mg/kg orally, via nasogastric tube, or intravenously and continued at 70 mg/kg every 4 hours for 48 to 72 hours, causes regeneration of glutathione, which metabolizes the toxic intermediary compound and protects the liver, particularly when administered within 10 hours of an acute ingestion.[48]

Acetaminophen freely crosses the placenta into the fetal circulation and is metabolized by the fetal liver. In a series of 60 pregnant patients with acetaminophen poisoning, increased incidence of spontaneous abortion or fetal death was noted in patients with delayed NAC administration.[49] As with nonpregnant patients, it is recommended that NAC be administered as soon as possible after ingestion, preferably within 10 hours.

Salicylates

Although salicylate poisonings are less common than in previous years, significant toxicity still occurs, either as deliberate or accidental overdose. The narrow toxic-therapeutic ratio of salicylates makes unintentional poisoning common, usually in the setting of repeated therapeutic doses in a patient with dehydration from vomiting or poor oral intake (common in pregnancy). Major symptoms of salicylate intoxication include tachypnea, tinnitus or decreased hearing, gastrointestinal upset, vomiting and dehydration, and alterations in consciousness. Although acute single-ingestion toxicity can be estimated from serum salicylate levels, clinical variability is great. With chronic toxicity from multiple ingestions, toxicity may be present at a salicylate level only slightly above therapeutic.

Treatment consists of alkaline diuresis, repletion of potassium and phosphate depletion, and dialysis for severe toxicity. Salicylates cross into the fetal circulation and cannot be metabolized by the fetus efficiently. Fetal toxicity may therefore be greater, and fetal deaths due to salicylism have been reported.[50]

Antidepressants

Antidepressant drugs are currently the second leading cause of adult overdose fatalities.[47] Intentional overdose causes both (1) neurotoxicity in the form of agitation, delirium, seizures, and coma and (2) cardiac toxicity in the form of serious conduction disturbances, arrhythmias, and even cardiac arrest. Peripheral anticholinergic signs such as dry mucous membranes, mydriasis, fever, flushing, and tachycardia are also commonly seen. Serious symptoms can develop rapidly and with little warning; thus, antide-pressant overdose is particularly dangerous. Alterations in mental status, sinus tachycardia greater than 120 bpm, or QRS widening greater than 100 milliseconds on the electrocardiogram suggest significant potential for complications.[51]

Little experience in managing pregnant patients with cyclic antidepressant overdoses has been reported. Such patients should be watched and monitored for at least 6 hours, and poison control center consultation should be prompt. In addition to general treatment measures, emergency treatment of arrhythmias and seizures consists of intubation, hyperventilation, benzodiazepines, and serum alkalinization with sodium bicarbonate to a pH of 7.55.[51]

Iron

Iron is the second most commonly ingested overdose in pregnancy, probably because of the accessibility to iron in maternal vitamins.[52] Iron overdose may be fatal, and treatment is complex, based on serum iron levels and evidence of free iron in the serum. Initial treatment consists of IV fluids and gastrointestinal decontamination. Deferoxamine is commonly used as a chelating agent to bind free iron and is used in moderate to severe overdoses. Deferoxamine does not cross the placenta and is safe for use in pregnancy. No fetal injury directly attributable to iron has been reported.[52]

Carbon Monoxide

Carbon monoxide exposure is the most common cause of fatal poisoning nationwide. Although not common in pregnancy, cases of fetal death and fetal injury in the presence of maternal survival make therapeutic decisions critical. The fetus may be more susceptible to the effects of hypoxia from carbon monoxide poisoning than is the mother because fetal hemoglobin has a greater affinity for carbon monoxide than does adult hemoglobin. In addition, because the fetus operates on the steep part of a left-shifted oxygen-hemoglobin dissociation curve, small decreases in oxygenation may cause significant fetal hypoxia. Carbon monoxide uptake and excretion by the fetus, however, are slower than in the mother, and therefore effects are more sustained.[53]

In the nonpregnant patient, the use of hyperbaric oxygen is an effective method of rapidly unloading carbon monoxide from hemoglobin and restoring its ability to carry oxygen to the tissues. The half-life of carboxyhemoglobin can be reduced from 240 minutes at room air to 90 minutes breathing 100% oxygen and to 20 minutes with treatment at three atmospheres, resulting in significant attenuation of the hypoxic insult.[54] In pregnancy, many hours of extended treatment with 100% oxygen are required to achieve washout from the fetus. Hyperbaric oxygen treatment in pregnancy has been prospectively described in one small, nonrandomized series of 44 women, in which two miscarriages and 34 normal deliveries were reported.[55] Other pathophysiologic benefits of hyperbaric oxygen have been proposed but are not yet well accepted.

In pregnancy, theoretical concerns with hyperoxia include retinal injury to the fetus, premature closure of the ductus arteriosus, cardiovascular alterations in uterine flow, and fetal anomalies. Elkharrat and colleagues used hyperbaric oxygen irrespective of the maternal carbon monoxide level and clinical features because of the enhanced fetal concerns, although current recommendations are to use hyperbaric oxygen in carbon monoxide poisoning treatment in pregnancy with significant carbon monoxide levels (>20%), signs of fetal distress, or maternal central nervous system symptoms.[53,55]

References

1. Part 8: Advanced challenges in resuscitation. Section 3: Special challenges in ECC. 3F: Cardiac arrest associated with pregnancy. European Resuscitation Council. Resuscitation 2000;46:293.
2. American Heart Association: 2000 Handbook of Emergency Cardiovascular Care for Health Care Providers, 4th ed. Dallas, American Heart Association, 2000.
3. Rosenthal RE, Turbiak TW: Open-chest cardiopulmonary resuscitation. Am J Emerg Med 1986;4:248.
4. DePace NL, Betesh JS, Kotler MN: "Postmortem" cesarean section with recovery of both mother and offspring. JAMA 1982;248:971.
5. Satin AJ, Hankins GDV: Cardiopulmonary resuscitation in pregnancy. In Clark SL, Cotton DB, Hankins GDV, Phelan JP (eds): Critical Care Obstetrics, 2nd ed. Oxford, UK, Blackwell Scientific, 1991.
6. Cairns CB, Bender PR: Management of cardiac arrest and resuscitation. In Markovchick VJ, Pons PT (eds): Emergency Medicine Secrets. Philadelphia, Hanley & Belfus, 1999.
7. Nanson J, Elcock D, Williams M, Deakin CD: Do physiological changes in pregnancy change defibrillation energy requirements? Br J Anaesth 2001;87:237.
8. Sanchez-Diaz CJ, Gonzalez-Carmona VM, Ruesga-Zamore E, et al: Electric cardioversion in the emergency service. Arch Inst Cardiol Mex 1987;57:387.
9. Rosemond RL: Cardioversion during pregnancy. JAMA 1993;269:3167.
10. Rees GA, Willis BA: Resuscitation in late pregnancy. Anesthesia 1988;43:347.
11. Oates S, Williams GL, Rees GA: Cardiopulmonary resuscitation in late pregnancy. BMJ 1988;297:404.
12. Joglar JA, Page RL: Treatment of cardiac arrhythmias during pregnancy. Drug Safety 1999;20:85.
13. Batalena L, Bogazzi F, Braverman LE, et al: Effects of amiodarone administration during pregnancy on neonatal thyroid function and subsequent neurodevelopment. J Endocrinol Invest 2001;24:116.
14. Buchsbaum HJ: Trauma in Pregnancy. Philadelphia, WB Saunders, 1979.
15. Brown O, Davidson N, Palmer J: Cardioversion in the third trimester of pregnancy. Aust N Z J Obstet Gynaecol 2001;41:241.
16. Byerly WG, Hartmann A, Foster DE, et al: Verapamil in the treatment of maternal paroxysmal supraventricular tachycardia. Ann Emerg Med 1991;20:552.
17. Corsi PR, Rasslan S, Bechelli de Oliveira L, et al: Trauma in pregnant women: Analysis of maternal and fetal mortality. Injury 1999;30:239.
18. Harper M, Parsons L: Maternal deaths due to homicide and other injuries in North Carolina: 1992-1994. Obstet Gynecol 1997;90:920.
19. Lavery JP, Staten-McCormick F: Management of moderate to severe trauma in pregnancy. Obstet Gynecol Clin North Am 1995;22:69.
20. Dudley DJ, Cruikshank DP: Trauma and acute surgical emergencies in pregnancy. Semin Perinatol 1990;14:42.
21. Pearlman MD, Tintinalli JE, Lorenz RP: A prospective controlled study of outcome after trauma during pregnancy. Am J Obstet Gynecol 1990;162:1502.
22. Rogers FB, Rozycki GS, Osler TM, et al: A multi-institutional study of factors associated with fetal death in injured pregnant patients. Arch Surg 1999;134:1274.
23. Kissinger DP, Rozycki GS, Morris JA Jr, et al: Trauma in pregnancy. Predicting pregnancy outcome. Arch Surg 1991;126:1079.
24. Dahmus MA, Sibai BM: Blunt abdominal trauma: Are there any predictive factors for abruptio placentae or maternal-fetal distress? Am J Obstet Gynecol 1993;169:1054.
25. Kettel LM, Branch DW, Scott JR: Occult placental abruption after maternal trauma. Obstet Gynecol 1988;71:449.
26. Committee on Trauma: Advanced Trauma Life Support for Doctors Program. Chicago, American College of Surgeons, 1997.

27. Curet MJ, Schermer CR, Demarest GB, et al: Predictors of outcome in trauma during pregnancy: Identification of patients who can be monitored for less than 6 hours. J Trauma 2000;49:18.

28. Drost TF, Rosemurgy AS, Sherman HF, et al: Major trauma in pregnant women: Maternal/fetal outcome. J Trauma 1990;30:574.

29. Lopez-Zeno JA, Carlo WA, O'Grady JP, et al: Infant survival following delayed postmortem cesarean delivery. Obstet Gynecol 1990;76:991.

30. Mossman KL, Hill LT: Radiation risks in pregnancy. Obstet Gynecol 1982;60:237.

31. Esposito TJ, Gens DR, Smith LG, et al: Evaluation of blunt abdominal trauma occurring during pregnancy. J Trauma 1989;29:1628.

32. Pearlman MD, Tintinalli JE, Lorenz RP: Blunt trauma in pregnancy. N Engl J Med 1990;323:1609.

33. Goodwin H, Homes JF, Wisner DH: Abdominal ultrasound examination in pregnant blunt trauma patients. J Trauma 2001;50:689.

34. Goodwin TM, Breen MT: Pregnancy outcome and fetomaternal hemorrhage after noncatastrophic trauma. Am J Obstet Gynecol 1990;162:665.

35. Goff BA, Muntz HG: Gunshot wounds to the gravida uterus. J Reprod Med 1990;35:436.

36. Rose PG, Strohm PL, Zuspan FP: Fetomaternal hemorrhage following trauma. Am J Obstet Gynecol 1985;153:844.

37. Pearlman MD, Phillips ME: Safety belt use during pregnancy. Obstet Gynecol 1996;88:1026.

38. Schoenfeld A, Ziv E, Stein L, et al: Seat belts in pregnancy and the obstetrician. Obstet Gynecol Surv 1987;42:275.

39. Sims CJ, Boardman CH, Fuller SJ: Airbag deployment following a motor vehicle accident in pregnancy. Obstet Gynecol 1996;88:726.

40. Zador PL, Ciccone MA: Automobile driver fatalities in frontal impacts: Air bags compared with manual belts. Am J Public Health 1993;83:661.

41. Awwad JT, Azar GB, Seoud MA, et al: High-velocity penetrating wounds of the gravid uterus: review of 16 years of civil war. Obstet Gynecol 1994;83:259.

42. Rayburn W, Smith B, Feller I, et al: Major burns during pregnancy: Effects on fetal well-being. Obstet Gynecol 1984;64:611.

43. Guo SS, Greenspoon JS, Kahn AM: Management of burn injuries during pregnancy. Burns 2001;27:394.

44. Lieberman JR, Mazor M, Molcho J, et al: Electrical accidents during pregnancy. Obstet Gynecol 1986;67:861.

45. Fish RM: Electric injury: Cardiac monitoring indications, the pregnant patient, and lightning. J Emerg Med 2000;18:181.

46. Rayburn W, Aronow R, DeLancey B, et al: Drug overdose in pregnancy: An overview from a metropolitan poison control center. Obstet Gynecol 1984;64:611.

47. Kulig K: Initial management of ingestions of toxic substances. N Engl J Med 1992;326:1677.

48. Zed PJ, Krenzelok EP: Treatment of acetaminophen overdose. Am J Health Syst Pharm 1999;56:1081.

49. Riggs BS, Bronstein AC, Kulig KW, et al: Acute acetaminophen overdose during pregnancy. Obstet Gynecol 1989;74:247.

50. Balakas TN: Common poisons. In Gleicher N (ed): Principles and Practice of Medical Therapy in Pregnancy, 2nd ed. E. Norwalk, Conn, Appleton & Lange, 1992.

51. Walter FG, Bilden EF: Antidepressants. In Marx J, Hockberger R (eds): Rosen's Emergency Medicine: Concepts and Clinical Practice, 5th ed. St. Louis, Mosby-Year Book, 2002.

52. Tran T, Wax JR, Philput C, et al: Intentional iron overdose in pregnancy—management and outcome. J Emerg Med 2000;18:225.

53. Van Hoesen KB, Camporesi EM, Moon RE, et al: Should hyperbaric oxygen be used to treat the pregnant patient for acute carbon monoxide poisoning? JAMA 1989;261:1039.

54. Aubard Y, Magne I: Carbon monoxide poisoning in pregnancy. Br J Obstet Gynecol 2000;107:833.

55. Elkharrat D, Raphael JC, Korach JM, et al: Acute carbon monoxide intoxication and hyperbaric oxygen in pregnancy. Intensive Care Med 1991;17:289.

56. Lee RV, Rodgers BD, White LM, et al: Cardiopulmonary resuscitation of pregnant women. Am J Med 1986;81:311.

57. Neufeld JD, Moore EE, Marx JA, et al: Trauma in pregnancy. Emerg Med Clin North Am 1987;5:623.

58. Nolan TE, Hankins GD: Acute pulmonary dysfunction and distress. Obstet Gynecol Clin North Am 1995;22:39.

59. Patterson RM: Trauma in pregnancy. Clin Obstet Gynecol 1984;27:32.

RENAL DISEASE IN PREGNANCY

13

John P. Hayslett

PHYSIOLOGIC CHANGES IN PREGNANCY

Renal disease in pregnancy, resulting from either primary renal disease or systemic disorders, may threaten fetal development as well as the health of the mother. Because assessment of renal function must account for the significant and unique functional and morphologic changes that occur in the kidney during normal pregnancy, it is important to understand the dynamic changes that occur in the peripheral vasculature during pregnancy. In human pregnancy, there is a marked expansion of extracellular fluid volume, associated with a cumulative retention of 500 to 700 Eq of sodium and a 1.5-fold increase in plasma volume.[1] Concurrently, a pronounced peripheral vascular dilatation begins early in pregnancy and persists until term, resulting in a 40% decrease in total peripheral arterial resistance.[2] Blood pressure declines modestly in the second trimester and returns to baseline values near term. Additional hemodynamic changes include a 50% increase in cardiac output and similar rises in blood flow to the visceral organs, such as the kidney and uterus.[2,3] It is assumed that these changes occur to provide an optimal environment for the growth and development of the fetus, but the mechanisms that cause these changes are not fully understood.

The renin-angiotensin-aldosterone system has attracted attention for its possible role in the control of sodium balance in pregnancy. A striking increase in adrenal secretion of aldosterone is observed by the eighth week of pregnancy and continues to rise throughout pregnancy until plasma aldosterone levels reach 80 to 100 ng/dL by the third trimester,[4] fourfold to sixfold above the upper level observed in euvolemic nonpregnant adults. Although renin activity also increases, the time of change does not correlate with that of aldosterone. Special interest is also directed toward progesterone, produced by the placenta, because the progressive rise during pregnancy parallels that of aldosterone and a level of about 200 ng/dL is reached by term,[4] and because progesterone is an antagonist for aldosterone. The administration of progesterone, in physiologic amounts, to adults with normal adrenal function induces natriuresis, but not in subjects with adrenal insufficiency[5]; this suggests that progesterone blocks the action of aldosterone to retain sodium.

Some investigators postulate that high plasma levels of aldosterone during pregnancy reflect a compensatory response to salt-losing factors, such as the 50% increase in filtered sodium and the inhibitory action of progesterone. An alternative proposal, however, is that aldosterone secretion is adjusted to support the expanded vasculature as a result of the direct action of a vasodilating factor.[6] Studies in the rat model of pregnancy suggest that that factor may be relaxin, a peptide hormone belonging to the insulin family, which stimulates vascular dilatation by inducing the production of nitric oxide in vascular endothelial cells.[7,8] Relaxin is normally produced in the corpus luteum and in larger amounts by the placenta and decidua during pregnancy.

Notwithstanding evidence that progesterone can antagonize the action of aldosterone, numerous studies indicate that aldosterone is independently poised to maintain sodium balance and extracellular fluid volume at a level appropriate for the stage of pregnancy. When sodium balance is perturbed by decreases or increases in dietary sodium, there are immediate and appropriate changes in plasma aldosterone levels.[9] At high sodium loads, the aldosterone level falls to values observed in euvolemic nonpregnant adults. The administration of mineralocorticoid hormones to pregnant women stimulate sodium retention and an increase in body weight[10]; this shows that the mineralocorticoid receptor is capable of responding to the ligand by becoming activated and that the signaling mechanism to stimulate the epithelial sodium channel is intact. All these responses occur in the presence of high, stable plasma levels of progesterone. Together, these data support the notion that aldosterone is critical in maintaining sodium balance in pregnancy.

As noted previously, the peripheral vascular dilatation results in a marked increase in renal blood flow.

Renal plasma flow increases by about 80% between conception and the third trimester and subsequently falls to a level about 60% higher than the nonpregnant norm.[3] The glomerular filtration rate (GFR), as shown in Figure 13-1, achieves an incremental increase of 30% to 50% by the ninth week of pregnancy; this level is then sustained until term, after which the rate falls to nongravid levels.[11] In a study performed on 10 healthy women, with inulin as marker, the GFR rose from the nonpregnant level of 105 ± 24 mL/minute (mean ± standard deviation) to 168 ± 22 mL/minute. The mechanism responsible for this remarkable alteration in renal function probably relates to the generalized dilatation that characterizes pregnancy, because micropuncture studies performed in the rat model of pregnancy showed that GFR correlates solely with the increase in glomerular plasma flow and not with a rise in intraglomerular capillary pressure.[12] These findings were subsequently corroborated in human pregnancy, in which gestational hyperfiltration was caused primarily by renal plasma flow, with only a minor contribution from a reduction in capillary oncotic pressure.[13]

In addition to changes in sodium metabolism, pregnancy alters the mechanism for water metabolism. In health, the volume of body water is regulated within narrow limits by the kidney through the action of a vasopressin that maintains serum osmolality at about 280 mOsm/kg H_2O in the nongravid state; a rise above that level induces a release of the hormone, whereas a fall inhibits release. In contrast, the plasma osmolality in pregnancy falls to about 270 mOsm/kg H_2O.[14] Studies in pregnant women show that the fall in plasma osmolality is caused by a reduction in the set point of the osmostat that regulates vasopressin release.[15] The physiologic response to changes in osmolality above or below the new level is comparable with that in the nonpregnant state. In addition, changes

in the thirst threshold, which is set approximately 10 mOsm/kg H_2O above the osmostat level in the nongravid individual, parallels that of the osmostat in pregnancy and falls from about 290 to 280 mOsm/kg H_2O. Furthermore, studies have shown that the metabolic clearance of vasopressin is accelerated during pregnancy severalfold and reaches a peak at weeks 22 to 24, apparently because of the progressive increase in the production of the enzyme vasopressinase, produced by the placenta.[16] Serum levels of vasopressin, however remain normal. Together, these data suggest that the production of vasopressinase rapidly degrades circulating vasopressin, which is compensated by an increased production and release of vasopressin from the posterior pituitary gland to maintain normal plasma vasopressin levels. Some rare individuals fail to fully compensate for the rapid degradation of vasopressin or excess production of vasopressinase and develop the syndrome of diabetes insipidus.[17,18] The ability to concentrate urine can be restored by the administration of 1-deamino-8-D-arginine-vasopressin (DDAVP), the synthetic V_2 vasopressin agonist, which is resistant to the action of vasopressinase. Despite these physiologic changes in water metabolism, however, the ability to concentrate urine and, alternatively, to excrete a water load during gestation is unchanged in comparison to the nongravid state.[15]

Pregnancy also alters renal tubular function. The fractional absorption of glucose,[19] amino acids,[20] and β microglobulin is decreased, which results in higher rates of urinary excretion; this is consistent with the notion that renal absorption of nonelectrolyte solutes is reduced in the proximal tubule in pregnancy. This phenomenon may have clinical relevance in some patients who exhibit glucosuria during pregnancy in the absence of hyperglycemia. In addition, total urinary protein excretion also rises in normal pregnancy, from a nonpregnant level of

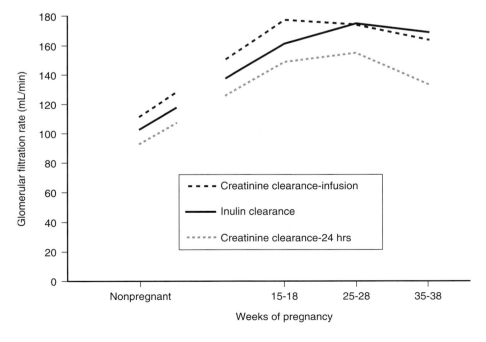

Figure 13-1. Mean glomerular filtration rate measured by three methods in 10 healthy women at 15 to 18, 25 to 28, and 35 to 38 weeks of pregnancy, and again at 8 to 12 weeks post partum. (Adapted from Davison JM, Hytten FE: Glomerular filtration during and after pregnancy. J Obstet Gynaecol Br Commonw 1974;81:588-595.)

97 ± 52 mg per 24 hours to 180 ± 50 mg per 24 hours in the third trimester.[21] Another study confirmed that protein excretion can reach a level of approximately 250 mg/day but also showed that albumin excretion does not exceed 30 mg/day, the upper limit of the normal range in nonpregnant women.[22]

These insights into the physiologic alterations that occur in normal pregnancy indicate that a different scale of values should be considered in determining normal renal function. For example, screening techniques for estimating the level of GFR usually rely on measurements of serum levels of urea nitrogen and creatinine. Because of the expansion of extracellular fluid and the increased GFR, levels of these substances are substantially lower during pregnancy than in nonpregnant women. In comparison with nonpregnancy values of 13 ± 3 mg/dL (mean $\pm$ standard deviation) of serum urea nitrogen and 0.67 ± 0.2 mg/dL of plasma creatinine, levels fall to 8.7 ± 1.5 mg/dL and 0.46 ± 0.1 mg/dL, respectively. Concentrations that exceed 13 mg/dL for urea nitrogen or 0.8 mg/dL for creatinine suggest the possibility of renal insufficiency. In patients with known or suspected renal insufficiency, formal estimates of GFR are required. In early pregnancy, the GFR can be estimated from creatinine clearance, performed on a 24-hour urine collection. In the latter half of pregnancy, however, a 24-hour urine collection may yield underestimates of the true GFR because of edema formation in the lower extremities, shown in Figure 13–1. If that is a concern, a short-term creatinine clearance should be measured with the subject lying on her side, after hydration with water to increase urine flow rate to about 5 mL per minute.

EFFECT OF RENAL DISEASE ON PREGNANCY

When renal disease occurs during pregnancy, three questions are inevitably raised:

1. Does pregnancy adversely affect the course of the underlying renal disease?
2. Is the outcome of pregnancy adversely affected?
3. What are the maternal complications?

Regardless of the type of renal injury, the functional consequences may take one or two nonexclusive forms: namely, the nephrotic syndrome and renal insufficiency. Each of these clinical expressions of renal disease is considered separately, although in many cases they occur concurrently, and I attempt to provide insights for the questions that have been posed.

Nephrotic Syndrome

The nephrotic syndrome is defined as proteinuria in which protein levels exceed 3 g per 24 hours and a serum albumin level lower than 3 g/dL. Patients with this syndrome inevitably have a reduced capacity for excreting sodium and retain salt and water as edema fluid if sodium intake exceeds the lowered maximum excretory capacity for sodium excretion. The nephrotic syndrome therefore represents symptomatic proteinuria, in contrast to lesser rates of protein excretion that are not associated with clinical symptoms. In many patients with glomerular disease, however, asymptomatic proteinuria progresses to the nephrotic syndrome in the latter part of pregnancy. In addition, and apparently as a consequence of hypoalbuminuria, these patients usually also exhibit elevated cholesterol and triglyceride levels as a result of increased lipid production. The GFR may be normal or reduced, depending on the severity of renal injury. The nephrotic syndrome always results from an injury reaction that affects the glomerulus in both primary and systemic diseases.

The nephrotic syndrome in pregnancy may be caused by preexisting renal disease, renal disease that develops de novo during pregnancy, or preeclampsia. The distinction between intrinsic renal disease and preeclampsia has important clinical implications because of differences in patient management. In patients with established renal disease before pregnancy or in whom proteinuria is documented before the 20th week of pregnancy, the diagnosis of intrinsic renal disease is easily made because preeclampsia rarely occurs before the 20th week. The onset of proteinuria in the latter part of pregnancy or when there is no information on protein excretion in early pregnancy, however, is of diagnostic uncertainty because of the similarities in clinical features of primary renal disease and preeclampsia: namely, the clinical features of hypertension and proteinuria. In this case, it may be possible to confirm the diagnosis of preeclampsia because of hemolysis, thrombocytopenia, and/or liver function abnormalities. With regard to management of patients with nephrotic syndrome caused by intrinsic renal disease, in the absence of renal insufficiency or significant hypertension, it is usually possible to achieve full-term delivery. In contrast, delivery in preeclamptic patents is usually indicated as soon as fetal maturity is achieved.

In patients with nephrotic syndrome caused by primary renal disease, several analyses of relatively large numbers of patients have concluded that, in the absence of moderate or severe renal insufficiency, pregnancy does not seem to affect the natural course of the underlying renal disease or fetal survival rate.[23,24] In regard to maternal morbidity, the accumulation of edema can cause massive edema, especially near term, and may aggravate or cause hypertension; vaginal delivery has been reported to be complicated by vulvar edema. One report showed that women with preeclampsia-induced nephrotic syndrome may develop dilutional hyponatremia.[25] This impairment in water excretion was ascribed to the nonosmotic mechanism for release of vasopressin, activated by a reduction in plasma volume. Therefore, these results suggest that serum sodium levels should be monitored in patients with preeclampsia, especially when complicated by nephrotic syndrome, because the neurologic effects of hyponatremia can resemble the features of impending eclampsia, although clinical management differs markedly. Although the usual guidelines for severe preeclampsia are indicated when premonitory signs of preeclampsia are exhibited, a delay in delivery is indicated, if possible, in women with significant hyponatremia, until serum sodium concentration is raised by restriction of oral fluid intake and the volume of intravenous fluids. If delivery cannot be delayed, the volume of water in parenterally administered fluids must be reduced.

The clinical management of patients with nephrotic syndrome caused by renal disease should aim to mitigate the severity of edema formation. In this regard, it is important to initiate a low sodium intake (1.5 g/day) to reduce the rate of edema formation. The administration of a low-sodium diet was shown to blunt several of the hemodynamic changes associated with pregnancy, but it did not affect fetal development or pregnancy outcome.[2] Frequently, bed rest promotes a higher GFR and renal plasma flow and, subsequently, an increase in the excretion of sodium. In general, the use of diuretic drugs during pregnancy has been discouraged on the grounds that volume contraction may reduce placental blood flow. When diuretics are used to reduce intractable edema that is resistant to conservative measures, this therapy should aim to reduce only excessive edema and, if needed on a chronic basis, should be administered intermittently to avoid volume contraction, electrolyte abnormalities, and drug resistance. In most cases, a spontaneous diuresis occurs post partum as serum albumin levels improve.

It is important to note that the most common cause of de novo nephrotic syndrome in pregnancy is preeclampsia.[26] In contrast to nephrotic syndrome caused by primary renal disease, preeclampsia-induced nephrotic syndrome is associated with a decrease in fetal survival, probably because the nephrotic syndrome is a sign of severe preeclampsia. Management of affected patients follows the usual guidelines for managing preeclampsia. Unless pulmonary edema occurs, diuretic agents are not used in patients with preeclampsia or the probability of preeclampsia, because this condition has been shown to involve reduced circulating plasma volume.[6]

Primary Renal Disease with Normal or Near-Normal Renal Function

Early reports before the introduction of potent oral anti-hypertensive agents and modern techniques for monitoring fetal growth suggested that the course of pregnancy was relatively benign in patients with preserved renal function. The first of several large series involving patients with primary renal disease and normal or near-normal renal function was reported in 1980.[27] The definition of near-normal renal function was arbitrarily defined as a serum creatinine level lower than 1.4 mg/dL. In that study, 121 pregnancies in 89 women were analyzed. Criteria for inclusion were continuation of pregnancy beyond the first trimester and available data for evaluating its impact on the underlying renal disease. In all patients, a histologic diagnosis was established. The serum creatinine level at onset of pregnancy was lower than 1.4 mg/dL, proteinuria was present in one third of the women, and hypertension was observed in 20%. During pregnancy, hypertension increased or occurred de novo in 28%, and renal function decreased in 16%, most often in women with diffuse glomerulonephritis, as shown in Table 13-1. In addition, protein excretion rose in 50% of cases and exceeded 3.0 g per 24 hours in 39 (68%) of 57 pregnancies. These changes

generally resolved after delivery, and during long-term follow-up, the decline in renal function was judged to be similar to that expected during the natural course of the underlying types of renal disease. As shown in Table 13-2, the live birth rate was 93% and the rate of perinatal mortality (stillbirths and neonatal deaths) was 10%, in comparison with a rate of 2% in the general population. The incidence of preterm deliveries (20%) and growth-restricted infants (24%) were substantially higher than the corresponding rates in normal pregnancies (11% and 10%, respectively). These results therefore indicate a moderate incidence of reversible maternal complications and a moderate decrease in fetal survival, and have, in general, been confirmed subsequently by other large series.[28,29] In all of these studies, the data suggested that pregnancy had not altered the natural course of the underlying renal disease.

Because many of these patients were hypertensive, it is difficult to determine whether the high incidences of fetal growth restriction and preterm delivery were related to hypertension per se or to some factor specifically related to renal disease. On the basis of other reports, however, it seems likely that hypertension did play an important role in the causation of adverse neonatal outcomes. In an analysis of 763 women with chronic hypertension enrolled in a multicenter trial of low-dose aspirin for the prevention of preeclampsia, 81 women had proteinuria at baseline.[30] The frequency of preeclampsia in this subset was not affected by the presence of proteinuria at baseline in comparison with the group as a whole, which involved 25% of the total group with chronic hypertension. Women with proteinuria (and therefore with renal disease) at baseline, however, were more likely to deliver babies at less than 35 weeks of gestation than were controls (36% vs. 16%) and to have infants that were growth restricted (23% vs. 10%).

The safety of newer antihypertensive agents in pregnancy is uncertain because of a lack of well-designed studies involving sufficiently large numbers of patients and the absence of long-term evaluation of the effect of these drugs on the physical and cognitive development of offspring. Early studies proposed restricting antihypertensive therapy to patients with severe hypertension, defined

TABLE 13–1   New Maternal Complications during Pregnancy in Primary Renal Disease with Preserved and Moderately Reduced Renal Function

	Creatinine Level	
	<1.4 mg/dL*	>1.4 mg/dL†
Number of pregnancies	121	82
Reduction in glomerular filtration rate (pregnancy and post partum)	16%	43%
Exacerbation or de novo onset of hypertension	28%	48%
Significant proteinuria	29%	41%

*Data from Katz AI, Davison JM, Hayslett JP, et al: Pregnancy in women with kidney disease. Kidney Int 1980;18:192.
†Data from Jones DC, Hayslett JP: Outcome of pregnancy in women with moderate or severe renal insufficiency. N Engl J Med 1996;335:226.

TABLE 13–2 Obstetric Complications in Primary Renal Disease with Preserved and Moderately Reduced Renal Function

	Creatinine Level		General Population in United States[‡]
	<1.4 mg/dL*	>1.4 mg/dL†	
Number of pregnancies	121	82	
Preterm delivery (<37 wk)	20%	59%	11%
Growth restriction (<10th percentile)	24%	37%	10%
Birth weight	2693 ± 878 g	2239 ± 839 g	3400 g
Stillbirths	5%	5%	0.7%
Fetal deaths	2%	7%	0.7%
Neonatal deaths	4.9%	2%	0.7%
Infant survival	89%	91%	98.6%

*Data from Katz AI, Davison JM, Hayslett JP, et al: Pregnancy in women with kidney disease. Kidney Int 1980;18:192.
†Data from Jones DC, Hayslett JP: Outcome of pregnancy in women with moderate or severe renal insufficiency. N Engl J Med 1996;335:226.
‡Data from Cunningham G, Gant NF, Gilstrap L, et al: Williams Obstetrics, 21st ed. New York, McGraw-Hill, 2001, p 746.

as a diastolic pressure higher than 110 mm Hg, under the assumption that lower levels did not threaten the life of the mother or produce long-term vascular complications.[31] In contrast, the consensus report published by the National Institutes of Health[32] indicates that women with chronic hypertension and renal disease are at increased risk for preeclampsia, perinatal morbidity and death, and the possibility of deterioration of renal function. This report suggests the use of antihypertensive agents if the diastolic pressure exceeds 100 mm Hg. More recent studies, however, have clearly shown that hypertension accelerates the decline in renal function in nonpregnant patients with chronic renal insufficiency, and probably in patients with lesser degrees of renal injury, in comparison with patients with normal blood pressure.[33] Together, these results argue for treatment of all patients with renal disease, especially when chronic hypertension is present at onset of pregnancy.

The consensus report just noted proposed continuation of the same antihypertensive agents that were shown to be effective before conception, except for angiotensin-converting enzyme inhibitors or angiotensin-blocking agents that are fetopathic.[31] Methyldopa has been the preferred antihypertensive agent in pregnancy because there is evidence that it is free of adverse effects in the fetus. Unfortunately, it is not as potent as some of the newer drugs and therefore may not control blood pressure adequately in some patents. Despite the lack of evidence based on scientific studies that affirm the effectiveness and safety of newer agents, β-blocking agents, such as labetalol, and calcium channel blockers are widely used and appear to be safe.[32,34] These drugs can be taken both orally and parenterally and therefore offer the opportunity for outpatient management and control of hypertensive crises.

As noted previously, patients with chronic hypertension with or without renal disease are at increased risk for developing preeclampsia. There has, therefore, been a great interest in developing methods to reduce the risk of preeclampsia in such high-risk pregnancies. In small series of patients at increased risk for preeclampsia, low-dose aspirin was reported to reduce proteinuric hypertension, as well as to reduce preterm birth, intrauterine growth restriction, and perinatal death. Subsequently, a large-scale

prospective, randomized study was performed with 2539 women at high risk for preeclampsia, including women with established diabetes, chronic hypertension, and multiple pregnancies and those with a history of preeclampsia in a previous pregnancy. Women were enrolled between weeks 13 and 26 of pregnancy and received either 60 mg of aspirin or placebo daily. Unfortunately, this study did not confirm the benefits of a reduced incidence of preeclampsia or improved perinatal outcomes.[35]

Primary Renal Disease with Moderate or Severe Renal Insufficiency

In contrast to gravid women with preserved renal function, moderate (serum creatinine level, 1.4 mg/dL to 2.5 mg/dL) and severe (serum creatinine level, >2.5 mg/dL) renal insufficiency have been reported, in earlier case reports and small series, to accelerate the underlying disease and to be associated with markedly reduced fetal survival rates to 50% or less. Maternal and obstetric complications in pregnancy with preexisting primary renal disease and a serum creatinine level exceeding 1.4 mg/dL at the onset of pregnancy were reported in a large series of 82 pregnancies (67 women).[36] The types of renal disease in these women were equally divided between chronic glomerulonephritis and tubulointerstitial diseases. Follow-up on nearly all women at 12 months after delivery enabled an assessment of long-term effects of pregnancy on the natural course of renal disease.

In these patients, maternal complications included a doubling of the incidence of hypertension in the third trimester over that in the first antepartum visit (48% vs. 28%) and significant proteinuria (41% vs. 29%), as shown in Table 13–1. In addition, there was a pregnancy-related loss of renal function (occurring during pregnancy or within 6 weeks of delivery) in nearly half of all cases, and in 23% of this subgroup (10% of the total series), there was a rapid progression to end-stage renal failure within 6 months after delivery. The risk of accelerated progression was higher when the serum creatinine level was higher than 2.0 mg/dL at the beginning of pregnancy. Obstetric complications were also higher than in patients with relatively preserved renal function and included pre-term delivery in 59% and fetal growth restriction in 37%. Despite these complications, the overall fetal survival was 91%, as shown in Table 13-2.

These findings corroborate prior smaller studies, involving 19 to 37 pregnancies, that reported fetal survival rates of 76% to 80%.[37-39] In these studies, 16% to 50% of women had a loss of renal function during pregnancy. The better obstetric outcomes in the more recent studies, in comparison with older studies, probably reflect improved medical and perinatal care and the availability of the intensive care nurseries for infants born before term.

The effect of hypertension on pregnancy outcome was also examined in women with moderate or severe hypertension. In the smaller previous series of patients who exhibited chronic hypertension, higher incidences of superimposed preeclampsia, preterm deliveries, growth restriction, and fetal loss were observed, in comparison with normotensive pregnant women. In the larger study of 82 pregnancies, however, hypertension at onset of pregnancy was not correlated with fetal survival, preterm delivery, or growth restriction.[36] When present in the third trimester, however, hypertension was associated with a higher rate of preterm delivery (72% vs. 46%) but not with increased intrauterine growth restriction (36% vs. 38%) or reduced fetal survival rates. The presence of high-grade protein-uria at any time during pregnancy had no effect on the outcome of pregnancy.

Acute Renal Failure

Acute renal failure in pregnancy in industrialized countries is now relatively uncommon, apparently because of liberalization of abortion laws, aggressive treatment of infections, and improved antepartum care. The marked decline in acute renal failure since the early 1960s is attributed largely to reduction of sepsis caused by nonsterile therapeutic abortion procedures and administration of abortifacients. Although the cause of acute renal failure in pregnant women is similar to the causes in the general population, pregnancy-specific factors account for the majority of cases of acute renal failure and include abortion, volume contraction caused by hyperemesis gravidarum, and severe pyelonephritis in early pregnancy.[40] In late pregnancy, hemorrhage, either overt or concealed by an abruptio placentae, is a leading cause, along with preeclampsia; disseminated vascular coagulation resulting from the syndrome of hemolysis, elevated liver enzymes, and low platelets (HELLP) or postpartum renal failure[41]; and acute fatty liver of pregnancy. In rare cases, renal failure has resulted from bilateral ureteral obstruction caused by massive polyhydramnios.[42]

Bilateral renal cortical necrosis, which is not unique to pregnancy, may result from any cause of acute renal failure.[43] Abruptio placentae is the most common precipitating event in most series, followed by uterine hemorrhage and amniotic fluid embolism. This lesion is characterized by irreversible necrosis of the renal cortex, often in a patchy manner, and may cause varying degrees of renal failure. The clinical presentation is characterized by severe oliguria persisting for 1 month or more and the subsequent identification of calcification in the subcapsular zone of the kidneys. The higher incidence of bilateral cortical necrosis in pregnancy than in the general population is thought to be attributable to the procoagulant properties of serum in pregnant women.

Septic abortion resulting from clostridia can be dramatic and life-threatening within a few days after an attempted or completed abortion. An abrupt rise in temperature, brisk leukocytosis, nausea, vomiting, and generalized muscle pain are often a prelude to shock. Access to aggressive therapy with antibiotics and volume resuscitation in an intensive care setting usually can be lifesaving. Acute tubular necrosis is a frequent sequela.

Renal function can be moderately reduced in severe preeclampsia and usually returns to baseline values within a week or so after delivery. Acute renal failure does occur, however, when preeclampsia progresses to the HELLP syndrome.[44] In an analysis of 442 pregnancies with the HELLP syndrome, 33 (7%) had acute renal failure. The pregnancies of all these patients were complicated with one or more of the following: abruptio placentae, fetal death, disseminated intravascular coagulation, hypotensive shock, or sepsis. Ten patients required dialysis therapy for azotemia or hyperkalemia during hospitalization.

Diabetic Nephropathy

In a classic report from the Joslin Clinic in 1977, Hare and White[45] described morbidity and mortality in women with pregestational diabetes and their products of conception from 1898 to 1975. In the preinsulin era, before 1917, the rate of viable fetal salvage was 40%, and the maternal mortality rate was 33%. Subsequently, the fetal survival rate rose to 90% and the maternal survival rate to 100% by 1975 among diabetic women as a whole. Hare and White commented, however, that "it is striking to note the almost universal incidence of fetal distress or serious neonatal morbidity in class F"(diabetic nephropathy). In 1975, the fetal survival rate in patients with diabetic nephropathy was only 72% in 54 cases in their series. By the 1980s, neonatal intensive care units had been established and modern antepartum care methods were introduced, along with better overall medical treatment to manage diabetic women with vascular complications. Two reports, one from the Joslin Clinic[46] and the other from Yale,[47] were published to describe the effects of diabetic nephropathy on maternal blood chemistry and renal vascular function during pregnancy; they were conducted to assess maternal and neonatal outcome and to evaluate maternal and infant status at long-term follow-up in the combined total of 57 women.

Data from the Yale study is presented because it is representative of the Joslin Clinic report and other, smaller studies. The Yale study involved 31 continuing pregnancies managed at the Yale–New Haven Hospital between 1975 and 1984.[47] At the initial visit, 26% of cases were complicated by the nephrotic syndrome, and 33% of patients had protein excretion rates exceeding 500 mg per 24 hours. Renal insufficiency was present in 48%, and 68% had proliferative retinopathy. During pregnancy, renal function worsened in 39% and blood pressure increased in 29%. Most patients had significant increases in proteinuria, and the incidence of nephrotic syndrome rose to 71% by the third trimester. After delivery, changes in renal function, blood pressure, and protein excretion returned to values similar to those observed in the first trimester. The long-term course was viewed as not differing from the expected course of diabetic nephropathy in subjects who had not become pregnant.

The fetal outcomes reported in the Yale and Joslin Clinic reports on patients with diabetic nephropathy are shown in Table 13-3, and are compared with results in a large series of patients with either nonproteinuric diabetes or primary renal disease.[47a] This table shows that perinatal survival in diabetic patients with renal disease averaged about 90%, a value that was similar to that for patients with primary renal disease. In addition, data derived from patients with primary renal disease and diabetic renal disease indicate similar rates of fetal survival, preterm deliveries, and intrauterine growth restriction. It therefore seems likely that these types of fetal complications in the diabetic population with renal disease were caused primarily by renal injury and/or associated hypertension. In contrast, the high incidences of large size for gestational age, neonatal complications, and major congenital anomalies were confined to the groups with diabetes, which suggests that they were caused by metabolic changes induced by diabetes. Because it has been demonstrated that the latter group of complications can be prevented or markedly reduced by normalizing maternal blood glucose levels from conception through term,[48,49] a strategy is available to reduce diabetes-related fetal complications. Moreover, it appears that in diabetic renal disease, fetal and neonatal disorders reflect the additive effects of renal disease per se and those associated with diabetes.

Not surprisingly, subsequent reports demonstrated that in comparison to the Joslin Clinic and Yale series with a relatively high prevalence of vascular complications, patients with milder forms of diabetic nephropathy generally produce infants who exhibit fewer fetal and neonatal complications, and the pregnancy outcomes are better. This correlation is similar to the findings in women with primary renal disease. For example, in a report from Ohio State University of 49 pregnancies in 45 women, the serum creatinine level exceeded 1.0 mg/dL in only four patients (9%) and heavy proteinuria in six patients (13%) at the initial presentation.[50] A mean blood pressure of less than 108 mm Hg was found in all pregnancies. Fifty three percent of patients developed preeclampsia, and by the third trimester, 58% of patients excreted more than 1.0 g of protein per 24 hours and 36% demonstrated a 15% fall in creatinine clearance. With regard to pregnancy outcome, however, 84% of pregnancies lasted at least 34 weeks, the incidence of fetal growth restriction was only 11%, and the rate of perinatal survival was 100%. Long-term follow-up for 2.8 years indicated that proteinuria had markedly improved from time of delivery and that renal function continued to decline at a rate that probably reflected the rate expected if pregnancy had not occurred.

A more global assessment of pregnancy outcome in women with pregestational diabetes was derived from 462 women in a study designed to determine whether aspirin reduced the incidence of preeclampsia.[51] Preeclampsia frequency and preterm delivery before 35 weeks rose significantly with the increasing severity of diabetes, according to the White classification,[45] and was highest in the 58 women with class F/R (retinopathy/renal disease) diabetes. In women with proteinuria (renal function was not reported), the incidence of preeclampsia was 36%, the incidence of preterm delivery was 29%, and the incidence of fetal growth restriction was 14%.

Preconception evaluation and care of diabetic women with nephropathy is discussed elsewhere.[52] Although maternal death is a rare event, it is clear that in women with diabetic vascular complications, fetuses are at risk for high levels of morbidity. Optimal care requires facilities with a neonatal intensive care unit, because of a high incidence of preterm delivery, and a team of specialists to manage both the obstetric complications and medical issues that include chronic hypertension, renal insufficiency, diabetic retinopathy, heart failure, and kidney failure. For some women, the risk of complications is so high that pregnancy is relatively contraindicated. Most patients, however, can be expected to achieve a satisfactory pregnancy outcome if antepartum care is comprehensive and aggressive.

TABLE 13-3 **Comparison of Perinatal Outcome in Diabetic Patients and in Patients with Primary Renal Disease**

	Diabetes	Diabetic Nephropathy	Nondiabetic Renal Disease
Number of pregnancies	232*	57†	121‡
Fetal death	0.4%	7%	6%
Preterm deliveries	4%	26%	20%
Small for gestational age	2%	19%	24%
Large for gestational age	40%	14%	5%
Major congenital anomalies	9%	9%	—
Neonatal complications			
Respiratory distress syndrome	8%	23%	—
Death	3%	2%	5%
Perinatal survival	97%	91%	89%

*Data derived from Kitzmiller JL, Cloherty JP, Younger MD, et al: Diabetic pregnancy and perinatal morbidity. Am J Obstet Gynecol 1978;131:560-580.
†Data derived from Kitzmiller JL, Brown ER, Phillippe M, Stark AR, et al: Diabetic nephropathy and perinatal outcome. Am J Obstet Gynecol 1981;141:741-751; and from Reece EA, Coustan DR, Hayslett JP, et al: Diabetic nephropathy: Pregnancy performance and fetomaternal outcome. Am J Obstet Gynecol 1988;159:56-66.
‡Data derived from Katz AI, Davison JM, Hayslett JP, et al: Pregnancy in women with kidney disease. Kidney Int 1980;18:192-206.

Systemic Lupus Erythematosus and Pregnancy

Systemic lupus erythematosus (SLE) is an autoimmune disorder that has a predominance among women and occurs in women during their reproductive years. Women with the established diagnosis of SLE may seek counseling with regard to their chances for a successful pregnancy outcome, or the disease may be detected after conception has occurred. In some cases, SLE may first occur during pregnancy. There is some evidence that pregnancy may aggravate this autoimmune disorder. In addition to the fact that 90% of all patients with this disease are women, experimental studies have demonstrated that estrogens activate an animal model of SLE.[53] One large study reported an increase in the rate of exacerbations during pregnancy in women with SLE in comparison with the rates before and after pregnancy.[54]

The first large series of pregnancy associated with lupus nephropathy was published in 1980.[55] In an analysis of 65 pregnancies in 47 patients in whom clinical renal disease was present before pregnancy in 80%, the rate and severity of exacerbations were correlated with disease activity in the mother during the 6 months before conception. Among 35 patients with clinical remission for at least 6 months, the relapse rate during pregnancy was 26%, and clinical flares were usually mild and resolved after delivery. In contrast, among 25 women with evidence of disease at the beginning of pregnancy, SLE remained active in 36% and exacerbations occurred in 32%; these flares were more severe, and did not always resolve post partum. The correlation between disease activity in the mother and pregnancy flares is supported by three subsequent studies[56-58] and were summarized[59] as shown in Figure 13-2A.

The overall fetal and neonatal survival rate was 87% in the same four studies published since 1980,[55-58] as shown in Figure 13-2B. These data, however, reveal a fetal survival rate of 88% to 100% in women with inactive disease at the beginning of pregnancy, in comparison with an incidence of 50% to 82% in women with active disease.

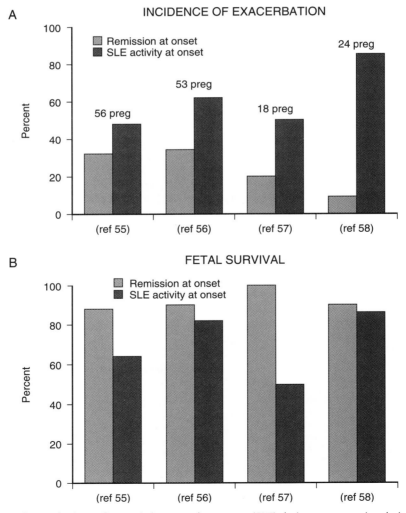

Figure 13–2. A, Correlation of exacerbations of systemic lupus erythematosus (SLE) during pregnancy in relationship to activity of disease at onset of pregnancy. **B,** Incidence of fetal survival in relationship to activity of disease at onset of pregnancy. Data is shown from four individual reports as indicated by the citations in parentheses. (Adapted from Hayslett JP: The effect of systemic lupus erythematosus on pregnancy and pregnancy outcome. Am J Reprod Immunol 1992;28:199-204.)

When SLE begins in pregnancy, maternal disease is usually reported to be severe, and fetal survival rates averaged 50% in the studies mentioned. Patients in these reports were usually treated aggressively with glucocorticoid hormones and immunosuppressive agents. Inspection of these reports failed to reveal an increase in fetal anomalies as a result of treatment. Because fetal morbidity and mortality were correlated with disease activity in the mother, these data suggest that the maternal disease should be aggressively treated.

An important complication of SLE involves transmission of a maternal antibody to the soluble tissue ribonucleoprotein antigen Ro (SS-A) in the fetus.[60] This antibody has been associated with complete heart block in infants born to women with established SLE and to women with this circulating antibody in the absence of clinical features of connective tissue disease. At autopsy, a diffuse and extensive endocardial fibrosis that may involve all four cardiac chambers and replace septal musculature in the area of the atrioventricular node has been described. Tissue-antigen variation in the child may be important because not all children born to anti-Ro (SS-A)–positive women develop heart block.[61] Nevertheless, pregnant women with SLE should be screened for this antibody and, if they are seropositive, fetal echocardiography monitoring should be offered.

DIALYSIS DURING PREGNANCY

Dialysis has been employed during pregnancy when renal failure occurs in women who conceive before the development of severe renal insufficiency and in women receiving chronic dialysis. In the latter case, the diagnosis of pregnancy is usually made in the second trimester because menstrual irregularities are common in women with renal failure and the typical symptoms of pregnancy are usually attributed to other causes. Ultrasonography is useful for diagnosis and assessment of gestational age because human chorionic gonadotropin levels are elevated in severe renal insufficiency as a result of a reduction in metabolic clearance. Information on pregnancy outcome in gravid women supported by dialysis treatment is available only from case reports and small series that may favor pregnancies with better outcomes. The scarcity of data reflects, at least in part, the uncommon use of dialysis in pregnancy. The prevalence of fertility among women on chronic dialysis may, however, be higher than thought, according to a report from Saudi Arabia.[62] In that survey of the incidence of pregnancy in 50% of all women younger than 50 years receiving chronic dialysis during the interval 1985 to 1990, 27 pregnancies were reported in 380 women, an incidence of 7%. Ten pregnancies, including all 8 pregnancies that continued for at least 34 weeks, were successful, representing a survival rate of 37%. This result highlights the importance of counseling women of reproductive age about the necessity for birth control if they wish to avoid pregnancy.

Perinatal death is most commonly related to preterm delivery resulting from premature labor, although abruptio placentae, fetal distress, and maternal bleeding are also frequent causes of early delivery.[63] Both hemodialysis and chronic peritoneal dialysis have been employed with about equal rates of a successful outcome, ranging from 20% to 50%.[64] Peritoneal dialysis may have a theoretical advantage because it avoids dramatic changes in fluid volume, the absence of heparin, and greater ease in continuing an unrestricted diet.

It is common practice to perform hemodialysis more frequently than the usual routine of three times per week. Dialysis is usually performed daily or on an alternating-day basis to maintain the urea nitrogen level below 50 mg/dL and to reduce the likelihood of large changes in fluid volume and electrolytes. The prescription for dialysis, largely based on theoretical considerations, is detailed elsewhere.[64] It proposes using a bicarbonate dialysate, rather than one containing acetate, and the maintenance of normal plasma levels of ionized calcium and 1,25-vitamin D, along with appropriate adjustments in the dialysate calcium level. Only minimal doses of heparin are used to reduce the risk of bleeding. In addition, recommendations include control of hypertension to levels lower than 140/90 mm Hg. Recombinant erythropoietin is used to prevent the hematocrit from falling below 30% to 32%.

In one report, a series of eight consecutive pregnancies were treated with peritoneal dialysis as the primary modality of treatment for end-stage renal failure.[65] The authors showed that it was feasible to implant Tenckhoff catheters intraperitoneally during pregnancy and that sufficient space was available in the peritoneal cavity to accommodate adequate volumes of dialysate.

RENAL TRANSPLANTATION AND PREGNANCY

Because successful renal transplantation restores fertility as well as renal function, it is not surprising that some women have become pregnant after transplantation or desire to do so after their sense of well-being returns. Insights into pregnancy outcome and maternal complications can be derived from careful studies performed at single transplantation centers and also from registries that compile data from many transplantation centers. Sturgiss and Davison reported their study of 34 pregnancies among 18 renal allograft recipients managed at a single medical center between 1967 and 1987, when immunosuppression consisted of azathioprine/prednisone.[66] Of 24 pregnancies in 17 women that continued beyond early pregnancy, 11 had adverse prenatal outcomes: five growth-restricted babies, five stillbirths (fetal survival rate of 79%), and one neonatal death. Preterm delivery was common (46%), and five pregnancies ended at or before 32 weeks.

These patients was compared with 18 women, who underwent transplantation in the same center, who did not become pregnant. They were matched with regard to underlying disease and renal function in order to determine the long-term effect of pregnancy on allograft recipients. The periods of observation averaged 12 years. The incidences of spontaneous abortions in the two groups were similar, and there was no long-term difference in GFR or the prevalence of hypertension between those who conceived and those who did not conceive. When the follow-up was extended to 15 years, the same results were obtained.[67] Although the number of patients in this series was small, this study suggested that pregnancy does not cause a remote adverse affect on renal function or on blood pressure in allograft recipients.

Subsequently, Davison reported a survey obtained from published reports on obstetric outcome and maternal complications in allograft recipients during the interval 1961 to 1987.[68] About 40% of all conceptions did not continue beyond the first trimester because of spontaneous and therapeutic abortions. The overall complication rate in pregnancies beyond the first trimester was 46%. Furthermore, he made the noteworthy observation that a successful obstetric outcome occurred in only 73% of pregnancies associated with complications (usually uncontrolled hypertension, graft rejection, or deterioration in renal function) before 28 weeks, in contrast to a success rate of 92% when complications did not occur before 28 weeks.

On the basis of this experience, Davison stressed the importance of counseling at the time of transplantation because women who were previously infertile may not be aware of the possible change in fertility status if they achieve a well-functioning graft. In addition, he proposed guidelines to reduce maternal complications and enhance a successful obstetric outcome, which included avoiding pregnancy for at least 24 months after surgery and then attempting conception only when the plasma creatinine level is 2.0 mg/dL or less, there is no hypertension, and immunosuppressive therapy is stable at a maintenance dosage.

A National Transplant Registry was established in 1991 to study pregnancy outcomes in transplant recipients in the United States and reflects more current clinical experience. Results from the Registry published in 1995[69] are shown in Table 13–4, according to whether 297 patients were immunosuppressed with or without cyclosporine. In this table, only pregnancies that advanced beyond the early weeks are tabulated, because the rate of spontaneous abortion in an average normal population is about 20% and because a large fraction of pregnancies in allograft recipients are interruption by therapeutic abortion. These data show that the incidence of live births was 97% among the patients not taking cyclosporine and 97% in those taking cyclosporine, because of a 3% incidence of stillbirths in each group. The incidence of low birth weight (<2500 g) was high, at between 37% and 50%, primarily because of preterm delivery. The table also indicates that the incidence of rejection of the graft during pregnancy was between 6% and 11%, and graft loss within 2 years of delivery occurred in 4.5% to 8.9%. Maternal complications, including hypertension, preeclampsia, and infection, were common, as shown in Table 13–4. Multivariate analysis demonstrated that low birth weight was correlated with hypertension, a plasma creatinine concentration exceeding 1.5 mg/dL, and pregnancy within 2 years of operation. These registry data therefore indicate better fetal survival rates than did earlier reports. These data also provide information on the introduction of cyclosporine into graft management and show that the incidence of low birth weight and maternal hypertension is increased, in comparison to the azathioprine era.

The Registry was updated in 2000 and now includes 619 kidney recipients and 947 pregnancies. A comparison of outcomes in recipients treated with two types of cyclosporine (Sandimmune and Neoral) and tacrolimus (FK506, Prograf) showed that the incidences of live births were similar among the three groups and were higher than 95%. As in the earlier report, the incidence of pregnancy complications was high, with 50% preterm deliveries, a 50% cesarean section rate, and 40% neonatal complications.[70]

References

1. Lindheimer MD, Katz AI: The kidney in pregnancy. N Engl J Med 1970;283:1095-1097.
2. Steegers EA, Van Lakwijk HP, Jongsma HW, et al: (Patho)physiological implications of chronic dietary sodium restriction during pregnancy; a longitudinal prospective randomized study. Br J Obstet Gynaecol 1991;98:980-987.
3. Davison JM, Dunlop W: Renal hemodynamics and tubular function normal human pregnancy. Kidney Int 1980;18:152-161.
4. Weinberger MH, Kramer NJ, Petersen LP, et al: Sequential changes in the renin-angiotensin-aldosterone systems and plasma progesterone concentration in normal and abnormal human pregnancy. Perspect Nephrol Hypertens 1976;5:263-269.
5. Landau RL, Bergenstal DM, Lugibihl K, Kascht ME: The metabolic effects of progesterone in man. J Clin Endocrinol Metab 1955;15:1194-1214.
6. Brown MA, Gallery DM: Volume homeostasis in normal pregnancy and preeclampsia: Physiology and clinical implications. In Lindheimer MD, Davison M (eds): Bailliere's Clinical Obstetrics and Gynecology, 2nd ed. London, Bailliere Tindall, 1994, pp 287-310.
7. Conrad KP, Joffe GM, Kruszyna H, et al: Identification of increased nitric oxide biosynthesis during pregnancy in rats. FASEB J 1993;7:566-571.
8. Baylis C: Relaxin may be the "elusive" renal vasodilatory agent of normal pregnancy. Am J Kidney Dis 1999;34:1142-1144.
9. Bay WH, Ferris TF: Factors controlling plasma renin and aldosterone during pregnancy. Hypertension 1979;1:410-415.
10. Ehrlich EN, Lindheimer MD: Effect of administered mineralocorticoids or ACTH in pregnant women. Attenuation of kaliuretic influence of mineralocorticoids during pregnancy. J Clin Invest 1972;51:1301-1309.
11. Davison JM, Hytten FE: Glomerular filtration during and after pregnancy. J Obstet Gynaecol Br Commonw 1974;81:588-595.
12. Baylis C: Glomerular filtration and volume regulation in gravid animals. In Lindheimer MD, Davison M (eds): Bailliere's Clinical Obstetrics and Gynecology, 2nd ed. London, Bailliere Tindall, 1994, pp 235-264.

TABLE 13–4 Obstetric and Maternal Complications in 500 Pregnancies by Transplant Recipients

	No Cyclosporine	Cyclosporine
Number of pregnancies	252	197
Obstetric complications		
Premature (<37 wk)	52%	54%
Low birth weight (<2,500 g)	37%	50%
Live births	97%	97%
Maternal complications		
Hypertension	21%	56%
Preeclampsia	20%	29%
Infection	18%	22%
Rejection	6.5%	11.1%
Graft loss (within 2 yr of delivery)	4.5%	8.9%

Adapted from Radomski JS, Ahlswede BA, Jarrell BE, et al: Outcomes of 500 pregnancies in 335 female kidney, liver, and heart transplant recipients. Transplant Proc 1995;27:1089-1090.

13. Roberts M, Lindheimer MD, Davison JM: Altered glomerular permselectivity to neutral dextrans and heteroporous membrane modeling in human pregnancy. Am J Physiol 1996;270:F338-F343.

14. Lindheimer MD, Barron WM, Davison JM: Osmoregulation of thirst and vasopressin release in pregnancy. Am J Physiol 1989;257:F159-F169.

15. Davison JM, Shiells EA, Philips PR, Lindheimer MD: Serial evaluation of vasopressin release and thirst in human pregnancy. Role of human chorionic gonadotrophin in the osmoregulatory changes of gestation. J Clin Invest 1988;81:798-806.

16. Davison JM, Sheills EA, Barron WM, et al: Changes in the metabolic clearance of vasopressin and in plasma vasopressinase throughout human pregnancy. J Clin Invest 1989;83:1313-1318.

17. Barron WM, Cohen LH, Ulland LA, et al: Transient vasopressin-resistant diabetes insipidus of pregnancy. N Engl J Med 1984;310:442-444.

18. Durr JA, Hoggard JG, Hunt JM, Schrier RW: Diabetes insipidus in pregnancy associated with abnormally high circulating vasopressinase activity. N Engl J Med 1987;316:1070-1074.

19. Davison JM, Hytten FE: The effect of pregnancy on the renal handling of glucose. Br J Obstet Gynaecol 1975;82:374-381.

20. Hytten FE, Cheyne GA: The aminoaciduria of pregnancy. J Obstet Gynaecol Br Commonw 1972;79:424-432.

21. Davison JM: The effect of pregnancy on kidney function in renal allograft recipients. Kidney Int 1985;27:74-79.

22. Higby K, Suiter CR, Phelps JY, et al: Normal values of urinary albumin and total protein excretion during pregnancy. Am J Obstet Gynecol 1994;171:984-989.

23. Strauch BS, Hayslett JP: Kidney disease and pregnancy. BMJ 1974;4:578-582.

24. Studd JW, Blainey JD: Pregnancy and the nephrotic syndrome. BMJ 1969;1:276-280.

25. Magriples U, Laifer S, Hayslett JP: Dilutional hyponatremia in preeclampsia with and without nephrotic syndrome. Am J Obstet Gynecol 2001;184:231-232.

26. Fisher KA, Luger A, Spargo BH, Lindheimer MD: Hypertension in pregnancy: Clinical-pathological correlations and remote prognosis. Medicine (Baltimore) 1981;60:267-276.

27. Katz AI, Davison JM, Hayslett JP, et al: Pregnancy in women with kidney disease. Kidney Int 1980;18:192-206.

28. Jungers P, Forget D, Henry-Amar M, et al: Chronic kidney disease and pregnancy. Adv Nephrol Necker Hosp 1986;15:103-141.

29. Surian M, Imbasciati E, Cosci P, et al: Glomerular disease and pregnancy. A study of 123 pregnancies in patients with primary and secondary glomerular diseases. Nephron 1984;36:101-105.

30. Sibai BM, Lindheimer M, Hauth J, et al: Risk factors for preeclampsia, abruptio placentae, and adverse neonatal outcomes among women with chronic hypertension. National Institute of Child Health and Human Development Network of Maternal-Fetal Medicine Units. N Engl J Med 1998;339:667-671.

31. Naden RP, Redman CW: Antihypertensive drugs in pregnancy. Clin Perinatol 1985;12:521-538.

32. National High Blood Pressure Education Program Working Group report on high blood pressure in pregnancy. Am J Obstet Gynecol 1990;163:1691-1712.

33. Zucchelli P, Gaggi R, Zuccala A: Angiotensin converting enzyme inhibitors and calcium antagonists in the progression of renal insufficiency. Contrib Nephrol 1992;98:116-124.

34. Sibai BM: Treatment of hypertension in pregnant women. N Engl J Med 1996;335:257-265.

35. Caritis S, Sibai B, Hauth J, et al: Low-dose aspirin to prevent preeclampsia in women at high risk. National Institute of Child Health and Human Development Network of Maternal-Fetal Medicine Units. N Engl J Med 1998;338:701-705.

36. Jones DC, Hayslett JP: Outcome of pregnancy in women with moderate or severe renal insufficiency. N Engl J Med 1996;335:226-232. [Published erratum appears in N Engl J Med 1997;336:739.]

37. Imbasciati E, Pardi G, Capetta P, et al: Pregnancy in women with chronic renal failure. Am J Nephrol 1986;6:193-198.

38. Hou S: Pregnancy in women with chronic renal disease. N Engl J Med 1985;312:836-839.

39. Cunningham FG, Cox SM, Harstad TW, et al: Chronic renal disease and pregnancy outcome. Am J Obstet Gynecol 1990;163:453-459.

40. Pertuiset N, Ganeval G, Grunfeld JP: Acute renal failure in pregnancy: An update. Semin Nephrol 1984;4:232-239.

41. Hayslett JP: Current concepts. Postpartum renal failure. N Engl J Med 1985;312:1556-1559.

42. Homans DC, Blake GD, Harrington JT, Cetrulo CL: Acute renal failure caused by ureteral obstruction by a gravid uterus. JAMA 1981;246:1230-1231.

43. Prakash J, Tripathi K, Pandey LK, et al: Renal cortical necrosis in pregnancy-related acute renal failure. J Indian Med Assoc 1994;94:227-229.

44. Sibai BM, Ramadan MK, Usta I, et al: Maternal morbidity and mortality in 442 pregnancies with hemolysis, elevated liver enzymes, and low platelets (HELLP syndrome). Am J Obstet Gynecol 1993;169:1000-1006.

45. Hare JW, White P: Pregnancy in diabetes complicated by vascular disease. Diabetes 1977;26:953-955.

46. Kitzmiller JL, Brown ER, Phillippe M, et al: Diabetic nephropathy and perinatal outcome. Am J Obstet Gynecol 1981;141:741-751.

47. Reece EA, Coustan DR, Hayslett JP, et al: Diabetic nephropathy: pregnancy performance and fetomaternal outcome. Am J Obstet Gynecol 1988;159:56-66.

47a. Kitzmiller JL, Cloherty JP, Younger MD, et al: Diabetic pregnancy and perinatal morbidity. Am J Obstet Gynecol 1978;13:560-580.

48. Jovanovic R, Jovanovic L: Obstetric management when normoglycemia is maintained in diabetic pregnant women with vascular compromise. Am J Obstet Gynecol 1984;149:617-623.

49. Fuhrmann K, Reiher H, Semmler K, et al: Prevention of congenital malformations in infants of insulin-dependent diabetic mothers. Diabetes Care 1983;6:219-223.

50. Gordon M, Landon MB, Samuels P, et al: Perinatal outcome and long-term follow-up associated with modern management of diabetic nephropathy. Obstet Gynecol 1996;87:401-409.

51. Sibai BM, Caritis S, Hauth J, et al: Risks of preeclampsia and adverse neonatal outcomes among women with pregestational diabetes mellitus. National Institute of Child Health and Human Development Network of Maternal-Fetal Medicine Units. Am J Obstet Gynecol 2000;182:364-369.

52. Kitzmiller JL, Combs CA: Diabetic nephropathy and pregnancy. Obstet Gynecol Clin North Am 1996;23:173-203.

53. Melez KA, Reeves JP, Steinberg AD: Regulation of the expression of autoimmunity in NZB × NZW F1 mice by sex hormones. J Immunopharmacol 1978;1:27-42.

54. Zulman JI, Talal N, Hoffman GS, Epstein WV: Problems associated with the management of pregnancies in patients with systemic lupus erythematosus. J Rheumatol 1980;7:37-49.

55. Hayslett JP, Lynn RI: Effect of pregnancy in patients with lupus nephropathy. Kidney Int 1980;18:207-220.

56. Bobrie G, Liote F, Houillier P, et al: Pregnancy in lupus nephritis and related disorders. Am J Kidney Dis 1987;9:339-343.

57. Houser MT, Fish AJ, Tagatz GE, et al: Pregnancy and systemic lupus erythematosus. Am J Obstet Gynecol 1980;138:409-413.

58. Tozman EC, Urowitz MB, Gladman DD: Systemic lupus erythematosus and pregnancy. J Rheumatol 1980;7:624-632.

59. Hayslett JP: The effect of systemic lupus erythematosus on pregnancy and pregnancy outcome. Am J Reprod Immunol 1992;28:199-204.

60. Chameides L, Truex RC, Vetter V, et al: Association of maternal systemic lupus erythematosus with congenital complete heart block. N Engl J Med 1977;297:1204-1207.

61. Brucato A, Frassi M, Franceschini F, et al: Risk of congenital complete heart block in newborns of mothers with anti-Ro/SSA antibodies detected by counterimmunoelectrophoresis: A prospective study of 100 women. Arthritis Rheum 2001;44:1832-1835.

62. Souqiyyeh MZ, Huraib SO, Saleh AG, Aswad S: Pregnancy in chronic hemodialysis patients in the Kingdom of Saudi Arabia. Am J Kidney Dis 1992;19:235-238.

63. Okundaye I, Abrinko P, Hou S: Registry of pregnancy in dialysis patients. Am J Kidney Dis 1998;31:766-773.

64. Hou SH: Pregnancy in women on haemodialysis and peritoneal dialysis. Baillieres Clin Obstet Gynaecol 1994;8:481-500.

65. Redrow M, Cherem L, Elliott J, et al: Dialysis in the management of pregnant patients with renal insufficiency. Medicine (Baltimore) 1988;67:199-208.

66. Sturgiss SN, Davison JM: Effect of pregnancy on the long-term function of renal allografts. Am J Kidney Dis 1992;19:167-172.

67. Sturgiss SN, Davison JM: Effect of pregnancy on the long-term function of renal allografts: An update. Am J Kidney Dis 1995;26: 54-56.

68. Davison JM: Pregnancy in renal allograft recipients: Prognosis and management. Baillieres Clin Obstet Gynaecol 1987;1: 1027-1045.

69. Radomski JS, Ahlswede BA, Jarrell BE, et al: Outcomes of 500 pregnancies in 335 female kidney, liver, and heart transplant recipients. Transplant Proc 1995;27:1089-1090.

70. Armenti VT, Radomski JS, Moritz MJ, et al: Report from the National Transplantation Pregnancy Registry (NTPR): Outcomes of pregnancy after transplantation. Clin Transpl 2000:123-134.

14

GASTROINTESTINAL COMPLICATIONS

Adam F. Steinlauf, Peter K. Chang, and Morris Traube

Gastrointestinal disorders are common during pregnancy. Clinicians treating a pregnant woman must (1) differentiate symptoms that are normal during pregnancy from those that may indicate more serious disorders, (2) understand how the disorder and the pregnancy may affect each other, (3) know how to safely evaluate the pregnant patient, (4) be able to weigh the risks of a disease against the risks of treatment, and (5) be able to safely treat the condition without causing adverse effects on the mother or the fetus. This chapter reviews these issues with regard to some of the major gastrointestinal disorders that can occur during pregnancy.

DIAGNOSTIC TESTING IN PREGNANCY

Radiologic and Related Studies

A clinician can choose among a variety of radiologic techniques to evaluate a pregnant patient with gastrointestinal symptoms. Plain films, computed tomography (CT), barium studies, and radionuclide studies emit ionizing radiation, whereas ultrasonography and magnetic resonance imaging (MRI) do not.

There may be a general belief that any radiation exposure is harmful to the fetus. However, this belief is unwarranted and could potentially lead to either missed diagnoses or unnecessary elective abortions. The main concerns of ionizing radiation exposure are cell death, teratogenic effects, carcinogenesis, and genetic effects[1-3]; however, most radiologic procedures are associated with few, if any, such risks. According to the American College of Radiology, no single diagnostic radiologic procedure results in sufficient radiation to threaten the well-being of the fetus.[2] Fetal risk of anomalies, growth restriction, or abortion is not increased with radiation exposure of less than 5 rad. To put this into perspective, a two-view chest x-ray examination gives an exposure of approximately 0.02 to 0.07 mrad, abdominal radiographs result in exposure of .245 mrad, a barium enema study or a small bowel series results in 2 to 4 rad, and CT of the abdomen or the lumbar spine results in exposure of 2.6 rad and 3.5 rad, respectively.[3] CT pelvimetry, using a low-exposure technique,[4] results in only a 250-mrad exposure.

The risk of carcinogenesis after radiation exposure is also probably small. Exposure to as little as 1 or 2 rad results in a slight increase in childhood malignancies, particularly leukemia.[1,5] The background rate of childhood leukemia is approximately 3.6 per 10,000 children. The rate in those exposed in utero to radiation is approximately 5 per 10,000, representing an increase of about 1 per 10,000 from the background rate.

Nuclear medicine scans with radionuclides are occasionally required during pregnancy. The most common scans—those for the lung, gallbladder, kidney, bone, or for evaluation of intestinal bleeding—all make use of technetium 99m. They deliver doses of less than 0.5 rad to the fetus, much lower than that known to produce detrimental effects. Accordingly, scans involving ^{99m}Tc may be performed with relative safety if medically indicated.[6] However, scans that involve radioactive iodine are contraindicated during pregnancy.

The decision to utilize studies with ionizing radiation should involve a consideration of the gestational age of the fetus. The preimplantation period (days 0 to 9 after conception) is the time during which the fetus is most sensitive to radiation-induced prenatal death. The period of organogenesis (days 15 to 50 after conception) is the time during which the fetus is most sensitive to radiation-induced malformations. Finally, the entire first trimester (days 15 to 90) is the period during which radiation can induce growth and mental retardation, as well as childhood cancer.[7]

In contrast to studies with ionizing radiation, there are no reports of detrimental fetal effects from ultrasound waves, including those produced during duplex Doppler imaging, and ultrasound examinations are not contraindicated during pregnancy. Likewise, there are no documented detrimental fetal effects from MRI, in which magnets are used to alter the energy state of hydrogen protons. Nevertheless, the National Radiological Protection Board has arbitrarily recommended that MRI not be used during the first trimester.[8] Moreover, gadolinium chelates, which can cross the placenta, should be avoided, because their long-term effects are not known.

In summary, attempts should be made to avoid non-emergency radiologic procedures involving ionizing radiation during pregnancy, particularly during the first trimester. However, if a radiologic procedure has already been performed in a patient with undiagnosed pregnancy or is medically required, there is no substantial concern for significant risk.[3] If diagnostic x-ray procedures are indicated, they should be recommended and performed after appropriate discussion with the patient, who may be informed that a single x-ray exposure does not increase the risk of fetal anomalies or pregnancy loss. If diagnostic modalities that do not involve ionizing radiation (i.e., ultrasonography or MRI) are available and appropriate, they should be considered better alternatives, but MRI should be avoided in the first trimester.

Gastrointestinal Endoscopy

A series of reports indicates general safety of endoscopic examinations in pregnancy. In one study of 26 flexible sigmoidoscopic evaluations in 24 pregnant women, there were no complications during the procedures. There were 18 healthy infants, 4 voluntary abortions, 1 involuntary abortion 9 weeks after the procedure in a diabetic hypertensive woman, and an unknown outcome in one patient.[9] In another study of 48 flexible sigmoidoscopic examinations in 46 patients, the outcomes were 38 healthy infants (27 full term), 4 voluntary abortions, 1 unknown outcome, and 3 cases of fetal demise.[10] This study also reported on colonoscopy in eight pregnant women. The outcomes were six normal infants, one voluntary abortion, and one fetal demise 4 months after colonoscopy, which was probably unrelated to the procedure. Thus, diagnostic flexible sigmoidoscopy and colonoscopy appear to be safe in pregnancy and should be undertaken if clinically indicated. However, therapeutic endoscopy was not evaluated in these studies.

Another study evaluated the safety of upper endoscopy in 83 pregnant women.[11] No clinically significant complications occurred during the procedures. The outcomes were 70 healthy infants, 6 voluntary abortions, 3 unknown outcomes, and 4 cases of fetal loss. However, there were eight high-risk pregnancies, and fetal loss was considered unrelated to the procedures. Two of the patients underwent therapeutic endoscopy, and the pregnancies resulted in healthy infants.

The use of endoscopic retrograde cholangiopancreatography (ERCP) should be limited, whenever possible, to *therapeutic* indications, because *diagnostic* information can usually be obtained through noninvasive tests, such as ultrasonography or magnetic resonance cholangiopancreatography. However, when necessary for diagnostic or therapeutic purposes, ERCP appears to be safe for both mother and fetus. One study reported on the safety of 29 ERCP procedures in 23 patients.[12] In this study, 3 patients had diagnostic procedures, and 20 had therapeutic procedures. Fifteen, eight, and six procedures were performed in the first, second, and third trimesters, respectively. There was only one complication, that of post-ERCP pancreatitis. There was one spontaneous abortion 3 months after the ERCP and one neonatal death; however, a causal relationship was not established. With additional intraprocedure safety measures, such as lead shielding of the pelvis, minimizing the fluoroscopy time, and taking hard copy radiographs only when essential, the radiation exposure can be minimized. In a study of 15 patients with a mean length of pregnancy of 25 weeks, the average estimated fetal dose, including exposure from fluoroscopy and spot films, was 310 mrad, a dose substantially below the 5- to 10-rad level that is considered to be of concern for radiation teratogenesis. Labor did not occur within 1 month after any ERCP in these patients. By the end of the study, 11 patients had delivered, with Apgar scores higher than 8, and the continuing pregnancies were uneventful.[13]

The normal practice in the United States is to provide medications for conscious sedation for most endoscopic procedures other than flexible sigmoidoscopy. Table 14–1 lists the Food and Drug Administration (FDA) rating system that is used to describe drug safety during pregnancy[14]; *pregnancy category* is the term used in this chapter to refer to this rating system. Table 14–2 lists medications commonly used for conscious sedation in endoscopy and comments on their safety in pregnancy.[15-18] Finally, the general principles and precautions for performance of endoscopy and the administration of medications during endoscopy have been reviewed[19] and are listed in Tables 14–3 and 14–4.

GASTROINTESTINAL MOTILITY DISORDERS

Nausea, Vomiting, and Hyperemesis Gravidarum

Nausea and vomiting occur frequently during pregnancy, particularly during the first trimester, and affect approximately 70% to 90% of pregnant women.[20-23] Mild to

TABLE 14–1 Food and Drug Administration Categories Used in Pregnancy Rating

Category	Interpretation
A	Controlled studies show no risk
B	No evidence of risk in humans:
	Animal findings show risk but human studies do not
	or
	Animal findings are negative but there are no adequate human studies
C	Risk cannot be ruled out:
	Animal findings are positive or lacking; human studies are lacking
D	Positive evidence of risk:
	Can still be used if benefit outweighs risk
X	Contraindicated during pregnancy

TABLE 14–2   Drugs Used for Conscious Sedation during Endoscopy

Medication	FDA Category	Comments
Meperidine	B	Appears to be safe and nonteratogenic The most commonly used labor narcotic Can cause neonatal respiratory depression when given near the time of labor
Fentanyl	C	Generally safe to use during pregnancy Can cause a brief decrease in fetal heart rate variability Associated with less maternal nausea, vomiting, and prolonged sedation than is meperidine
Diazepam	D	There are case reports of first trimester exposure in utero resulting in facial clefts, cardiac malformations, and other malformations, but no syndrome of defects has been identified Can cause floppy infant syndrome or marked neonatal withdrawal symptoms when exposure is in the third trimester
Midazolam	D	There are no published reports of malformation, but the drug is not as well studied as diazepam during pregnancy
Propofol	B	Considered relatively safe during pregnancy but can cause profound respiratory depression and should therefore be administered by an anesthesiologist

FDA, Food and Drug Administration.

TABLE 14–3   General Endoscopy: Recommendations

Defer endoscopy to after first trimester, when possible
Defer endoscopy to postpartum period, when possible (e.g., postpone surveillance colonoscopy)
Avoid endoscopy for "weak" indications
Terminate poorly tolerated endoscopic procedures
Consider obstetric consultation
Obtain fully informed and written consent after discussion, which should include fetal risk from procedure
Obtain continuous cardiac monitoring and pulse oximetry, as well as intermittent sphygmomanometry
Consider fetal monitoring during endoscopy, if available
Avoid endoscopy during threatened abortion, placental abruption, or other serious obstetric complications
Postpone endoscopy during active labor until post partum
Substitute less invasive procedure if possible: sigmoidoscopy for colonoscopy or possibly MRCP for diagnostic ERCP
Perform procedure expeditiously (e.g., avoid examination of distal duodenum at upper endoscopy or unnecessary endoscopic biopsies)
Avoid polypectomy, hot biopsy, and electrocoagulation, if possible
Restrict performance of endoscopy to highly experienced attending endoscopists
Consider performing ambulatory endoscopy in a hospital endoscopy suite rather than in the physician's office
Avoid fluoroscopy during colonoscopy or EGD, and minimize fluoroscopy during ERCP
Refer patient with complicated biliary disease during pregnancy to a tertiary medical center

EGD, esophagogastroduodenoscopy; ERCP, endoscopic retrograde cholangiopancreatography; MRCP, magnetic resonance cholangiopancreatography.

("morning sickness"), although symptoms can occur any time of the day and have a variable duration.[21,23,24] The prognosis for both mother and infant is excellent; there is no increased risk of fetal death, low birth weight, or congenital malformations.[28]

Hyperemesis gravidarum is a severe, debilitating condition characterized by vomiting severe enough to result in weight loss (>5% of body weight), dehydration, hypokalemia, or acidosis. It occurs in up to 2% of all pregnancies and usually necessitates hospitalization.[29-31] The diagnosis of hyperemesis gravidarum requires the exclusion of other causes of severe vomiting, such as gastroenteritis, cholecystitis, pyelonephritis, primary hyperparathyroidism, and liver dysfunction.[20,32-34] Similar to mild or moderate nausea and vomiting of pregnancy, hyperemesis usually begins early during pregnancy, but it persists after the 14th week. It occurs more often in

TABLE 14–4   Medications for Endoscopy: Recommendations

Use smallest effective dosage of medication
Involve patients in decisions about potentially fetotoxic drugs
When alternative drugs are available, use the drug that is safest for the fetus
Avoid category D drugs
Do not use category X drugs
Avoid optional drugs
Contact pharmacologist or review literature as necessary with regard to drug teratogenicity
Consider involvement of anesthesiologist for administering sedative

moderate nausea and vomiting are physiologically and "statistically" normal in pregnancy. They represent the most common complaints during the first 5 months of pregnancy.[24] Symptoms are more common in younger women, obese women, women from Western cultures, women with fewer than 12 years of formal education,[20] women who experience nausea and vomiting while taking oral contraceptives,[21] and women with a corpus luteum in the right ovary.[25] Increased symptoms have been correlated with heaviness of the placenta, nonsmoking status, history of nausea in previous pregnancies, and history of nausea and vomiting in the pregnant patient's mother.[26] Lower levels of prolactin and, perhaps, higher levels of estradiol contribute to the occurrence of nausea with or without vomiting at any time during the first two trimesters of pregnancy.[27] The nausea and vomiting of later pregnancy are probably the results of mechanical action by the enlarging uterus on the diaphragm or lower esophageal and pyloric sphincters.[24]

Typically, symptoms begin by 4 to 6 weeks of pregnancy, peak in incidence and severity by 8 to 12 weeks, and resolve by the third to fourth month. They usually appear early in the morning and improve later in the day

Western populations, has a higher prevalence in primigravid women, and tends to recur in subsequent pregnancies. One study showed that fetal outcome is not adversely affected by the presence of hyperemesis gravidarum[35]; however, earlier studies demonstrated an increased frequency of low birth weight, antepartum hemorrhage, preterm delivery, and fetal anomalies, including central nervous system malformations, undescended testicles, hip dysplasia, and Down syndrome. Most investigators agree that the vomiting itself is not responsible for the adverse outcomes; rather, they result from the electrolyte disturbances, malnutrition, and maternal weight loss.[29,32,36-39]

The exact cause of hyperemesis gravidarum remains unknown. It is probably related to rising estrogen or human chorionic gonadotropin levels, which are characteristically elevated during the first trimester of pregnancy. Increased progesterone and reduced motilin levels have also been implicated,[23,24,40] as have adrenal dysfunction[41] and thyroid disorders. The hormonal derangement that occurs during pregnancy may result in impaired gastric motility. Indeed, studies comparing gastric emptying in women and men found that premenopausal women and postmenopausal women taking hormone replacement had slower gastric emptying than men; however, postmenopausal women without hormone replacement did not.[42,43] Electrogastrography, which is performed with cutaneous electrodes, has demonstrated gastric dysrhythmias in pregnant women experiencing nausea.[44] Most recently, the presence of antibodies against Helicobacter pylori has been shown to be associated with vomiting during pregnancy.[45] Among patients with hyperemesis gravidarum, the prevalence of H. pylori is twice that among pregnant controls.[46,47] However, a causal relationship has not been established, and it is not known whether eradication of H. pylori improves the vomiting.

The treatment for mild nausea and vomiting is supportive therapy. The ingestion of multiple small-portion meals high in carbohydrates and low in fats has been suggested.[23] As symptoms become more severe, pharmacologic therapy and nutritional support become necessary. Table 14-5 lists medications available for the treatment of nausea and vomiting, along with comments on their safety in pregnancy.[23,48-56]

For more severe cases of nausea and vomiting, as well as hyperemesis gravidarum, antiemetics remain the backbone of treatment, inasmuch as specific therapies or interventions to treat pregnant women with nausea and vomiting are lacking. Doxylamine succinate plus pyridoxine HCL (Bendectin) was one of the first antiemetics approved for use during pregnancy but was subsequently withdrawn from use because of suspected teratogenicity.[57] Metoclopramide (Reglan) has been in use in Europe since the early 1970s. It has no teratogenic effects in animals when given at doses 12 to 250 times the recommended maximal human dose, and anecdotal reports of use in humans have shown no fetal abnormalities.[51,52] Moreover, continuous subcutaneous metoclopramide therapy can be given for at-home treatment of hyperemesis gravidarum. The treatment is safe, effective, associated with mild side effects, and cost effective in comparison with inpatient hospitalization.[53] Other antiemetics, such as antihistamines (e.g., meclizine) and phenothiazine derivatives (e.g., promethazine), may be used if symptoms are severe and intractable.[23] One study in hyperemesis gravidarum found the combination of droperidol and diphenhydramine to be beneficial and cost effective, leading to fewer and shorter hospital admissions. There were no significant differences with regard to maternal or perinatal outcomes in comparison with a group that did not receive treatment.[50] However, droperidol now has a "black box" warning because of associated corrected QT interval prolongation and cardiac arrhythmias.[49] Another study showed that vitamin B_6, 25 mg every 8 hours, was significantly better than placebo in decreasing vomiting in all patients and decreasing nausea in patients with severe symptoms.[48] Because vitamin B_6 has no known teratogenic or adverse side effects, it is a good therapeutic alternative. More recently, case reports have shown some success with ondansetron in treating refractory hyperemesis gravidarum,[54,55] and a double-blind study showed ondansetron not to be worse than promethazine.[56] In very severe cases, total parenteral nutrition may be required.[33] Finally, psychotherapy may be useful in selected cases.[58]

Gastroesophageal Reflux Disease

Gastroesophageal reflux disease (GERD) has been shown to affect 30% to 50% of pregnant women, although it may be up to 80% in some populations.[59,60] One study of 25 patients completing a questionnaire showed that half had symptoms severe enough to change their lifestyles.[61] Of these patients, 53% had heartburn before pregnancy; however, only 30% believed it was severe enough to require H_2 receptor antagonists, and only 20% consulted their physicians for such symptoms.

The symptoms of GERD do not differ from those in nonpregnant patients. Symptoms are typically worse during the third trimester and abate soon after delivery. They typically include retrosternal burning but may also be discomfort in the epigastrium, neck, throat, or back. They usually occur postprandially but also nocturnally and are exacerbated by recumbency or bending over.

TABLE 14–5   Drugs Used for Nausea, Vomiting, and Hyperemesis Gravidarum

Medication	Comments
Vitamin B_6	Considered safe
Metoclopramide	Category B; anecdotal reports show no significant human risk
Meclizine	Category B; epidemiologic studies show no fetal abnormalities
Diphenhydramine	Category B; shown in human study to be safe when combined with droperidol
Promethazine	Category C; animal studies indicate that it is teratogenic, interferes with platelets, and is associated with perinatal wastage, prematurity, premature labor, and fetal anomalies
Droperidol	Category C; slight increase in mortality in rats in high doses; black box warning relating to corrected QT interval abnormalities and cardiac arrhythmias
Ondansetron	Category B; limited data available

Other symptoms are regurgitation, dysphagia, globus sensation, or water brash (reflex esophageal hypersalivation in response to esophageal acid). As in nongravid people, the symptoms are aggravated by dietary factors, such as the ingestion of caffeine, chocolate, fatty foods, peppermint, alcohol, orange and apple juice, large meals or late-night meals, various medications that decrease lower esophageal sphincter (LES) pressure, and smoking. The three main atypical manifestations of GERD are noncardiac chest pain; pulmonary symptoms, such as asthma; and ear, nose, and throat manifestations, such as laryngitis.[62]

The pathophysiologic mechanism of GERD in pregnancy is multifactorial. In the nonpregnant patient, gastroesophageal reflux results from (1) decreases in resting LES pressure, (2) increases in spontaneous relaxation of the LES, (3) increases in volume and acidity of gastric secretions, (4) decreased esophageal clearance of refluxed secretions, and (5) changes in the resistance of the esophageal mucosa to refluxed gastric secretions.[62] In pregnancy, the resting LES pressure is significantly decreased, leading to more frequent regurgitation and reflux episodes. In addition, increased transient LES relaxations are present and are believed to be the effect of hormonal changes. Progesterone has a smooth-muscle relaxant effect on the LES. These changes appear to reverse post partum.[63] Furthermore, the increases in intraabdominal pressure that result from the enlarging uterus may exacerbate reflux as well, particularly when the patient is recumbent.

The diagnosis can usually be established by documenting the patient's medical history carefully. In some of the more vague cases, diagnostic endoscopy can be performed safely, looking for changes in the esophageal mucosa, such as erythema, friability, exudate, erosions, frank ulcerations, and strictures. In the setting of a normal endoscopic result, distal esophageal mucosal biopsies may support a diagnosis of reflux if microscopic inflammatory changes are present. A negative endoscopy and biopsy do not completely exclude reflux, and 24-hour pH monitoring effectively establishes the presence or absence of reflux. However, it is quite unusual to require endoscopic or pH studies to confirm a working diagnosis of esophageal reflux during pregnancy.

Initial treatment of reflux in the pregnant woman should be conservative. Initial recommendations include avoidance of exacerbating medications listed previously, elevation of the head of the bed at night, and the use of non–systemically absorbed medications, such as antacids, as needed.[64] When these measures fail and the patient is bothered sufficiently to affect her quality of life, prescription drugs should be considered. Medications used to treat reflux include H$_2$ receptor antagonists (cimetidine, ranitidine, famotidine, and nizatidine) and the proton pump inhibitors (PPIs) (omeprazole, lansoprazole, rabeprazole, pantoprazole, and esomeprazole) (Table 14–6).[61,65-68]

The H$_2$ receptor antagonists are classified by the FDA as category B. They are considered generally safe for use during pregnancy, including the first trimester. In a prospective study of 178 pregnant women with gestational H$_2$ blocker use during the first trimester, major

TABLE 14–6   Drugs Used for Gastroesophageal Reflux and Peptic Ulcer Disease

Medication	Comments
Antacids	Bicarbonate can cause sodium retention
Sucralfate	Category B; considered safe for use in pregnancy
Cimetidine	Category B
Ranitidine	Category B; no adverse effects in a human study
Famotidine	Category B
Nizatidine	Category B
Omeprazole	Category C; animal studies indicate dose-related lethality in embryos, fetal abortion, pregnancy disruption, postnatal development toxicity; human study indicate safety at 20- to 40-mg doses
Lansoprazole	Category B
Rabeprazole	Category B
Pantoprazole	Category B
Esomeprazole	Category B
Metoclopramide	Category B; anecdotal reports show no significant human risk
Cisapride	Category C; embryotoxic/fetotoxic in animals, no teratogenic effects; available only through a limited access program with the manufacturer
Misoprostol	Category X; causes uterine contraction, bleeding, and miscarriage

malformations, method of delivery, gestational age, prematurity, birth weight, smallness for gestational age, neonatal health problems, and developmental milestones were not different from those in children of an age-matched control group.[68] The dose of the H$_2$ blocker can be oral, once at night or twice daily, but the twice-daily regimen may be better than the single nightly dose.[61]

The PPIs are significantly more effective than H$_2$ blockers for acid suppression. Human studies of PPIs in pregnant women are not as common as studies of H$_2$ blockers, but PPI use is generally safe. PPIs are classified as category B by the FDA, except omeprazole, which is classified category C. Ironically, the majority of studies of PPI safety in pregnancy involve omeprazole. A metaanalysis comprising five cohort studies with almost 600 exposed pregnancies showed that PPI exposure during the first trimester did not pose an important teratogenic risk.[65] A small case series described nine women, including three who continued omeprazole therapy without interruption until delivery, and reported no side effect to the mothers or fetuses.[66]

Other medications used for the treatment of GERD are the prokinetic agents, such as metoclopramide (discussed previously) and cisapride. Cisapride acts by enhancing the cholinergic excitatory process at postganglionic sites at neuromuscular junctions, thereby increasing gastrointestinal motility from the upper gastrointestinal tract down through the colon. It is no longer generally available because of an association with QT interval prolongations and serious cardiac arrhythmias. It is available only through a limited access program developed by the manufacturer and the FDA. Cisapride should not be used by pregnant patients.

Constipation

The prevalence of constipation in the pregnant population varies from 11% to 38%, and symptoms tend to be worse in the first and third trimesters.[69-71] Constipation is probably related to the effects of progesterone on motility of both the small intestine and the colon.[23] Other factors may contribute as well. Motilin, a stimulatory gastrointestinal hormone, is reduced during pregnancy. Progesterone may inhibit motilin release, thus further adversely affecting gastrointestinal motility.[72] Finally, the enlarging uterus may physically affect the small intestinal motility directly, particularly late in pregnancy.

Initial treatment should include patient education, reassurance, increased physical activity, and increased fluid intake. Dietary supplements of fiber in the form of bran or wheat fiber are likely to help.[73] If lifestyle modifications and dietary supplements are inadequate, many agents are available for the treatment of constipation. The bulk-forming preparations containing fiber are the safest, because they are not absorbed. Other relatively safe options include the hyperosmotic agents such as lactulose and sorbitol, saline laxatives (in moderation) such as milk of magnesia, the stimulant bisacodyl, and the docusate sodium stool softeners. The use of polyethylene glycol solution for constipation is increasing, particularly among the pediatric population, primarily because of its efficacy and safety profile.[74] However, there are insufficient data on the use of polyethylene glycol in treating constipation during pregnancy. Tegaserod, a new 5-HT$_4$ receptor partial agonist, has emerged as a new medication indicated for the treatment of constipation-predominant irritable bowel syndrome in women.[75] Animal studies suggest that it would be safe for use during pregnancy; however, human data for evaluating its safety during pregnancy are lacking. It is therefore listed in pregnancy category B. The risks of these and other agents are outlined in Table 14–7.[23,76,77]

Diarrhea

Diarrhea in the pregnant woman can be caused by the same processes as in the nonpregnant patient, such as infection, malabsorption, inflammatory bowel disease (IBD), and drug-related diarrhea. When a pregnant woman presents with new-onset diarrhea, a standard evaluation is indicated.

The workup should begin with a thorough history, because this helps direct any further evaluation and treatment. Careful attention must be paid to comorbid diseases or medications that could cause diarrhea. A history of voluminous diarrhea or of midabdominal cramping suggests a small bowel source, whereas the passage of red blood, tenesmus, or small volumes of stool suggest a colonic source. Stool studies should be obtained; fecal red or white blood cells suggest colonic inflammation, which could be secondary to an infection or idiopathic IBD. Stool cultures should be obtained and, if positive, prompt appropriate treatment. If these measures fail to reveal the cause of the diarrhea, flexible sigmoidoscopy or upper endoscopy can safely be performed for diagnostic purposes.

If the diarrhea appears to be mild and nonspecific but sufficiently bothersome to warrant treatment,

TABLE 14–7   Drugs Used for Constipation

Medication	Comments
Bulk-Forming Agents	
Fiber preparations	Regarded as safe; agents of choice during pregnancy
Osmotic Laxatives	
Sorbitol, lactulose	Regarded as safe
Polyethylene glycol (MiraLax)	Insufficient data on use in pregnancy
Cationic Laxatives	
Milk of magnesia, magnesium citrate, Fleets products	Regarded as safe; can cause electrolyte disturbances and fluid retention
Stimulant Laxatives	
Anthraquinones (cascara, senna)	Excreted in breast milk; may cause diarrhea in neonate. Increased congenital malformations
Phenylmethanes (bisacodyl)	Generally safe
Castor oil	Unsafe; may cause premature uterine contractions
Lubricants	
Mineral oil	Can cause fat-soluble vitamin deficiency
Promotility Agents	
Tegaserod (Zelnorm)	Studies in rats and rabbits demonstrate that it is safe; no human data
Stool Softeners	
Docusate salts (Colace)	Generally safe

Modified from Baron TH, Ramirez B, Richter JE: Gastrointestinal motility disorders during pregnancy. Ann Intern Med 1993;118:336.

non–systemically absorbed medications should be tried first (Table 14–8).[23] Of the systemically absorbed medications listed in Table 14–8, loperamide is probably the least dangerous; however, even this agent, if used, should be given in small and limited doses.

TABLE 14–8   Drugs Used for Diarrhea

Medication	Comment
Nonsystemic	
Kaolin with pectin (Kaopectate)	Safe; not absorbed
Stool-bulking agents	See Table 14–7
Systemic	
Loperamide (Imodium)	Category B; safe in animals at up to 30 × human dose. Limited human data: of pregnancies in nine patients, four were normal, two resulted in infants with congenital malformations, two ended in spontaneous abortions, one resulted in infant with bilateral Erb's palsy
Diphenoxylate/atropine (Lomotil)	Category C; affects fertility; may cause malformations in humans if used in first trimester
Bismuth subsalicylate (Pepto-Bismol)	Unsafe; can be teratogenic and cause bleeding

Data from Baron TH, Ramirez B, Richter JE: Gastrointestinal motility disorders during pregnancy. Ann Intern Med 1993;118:336.

PEPTIC ULCER DISEASE

Pathophysiology

Our understanding of the pathogenesis of peptic ulcer disease (PUD) has changed substantially over time. In the early part of the 20th century, psychosocial stress and dietary factors were thought to be important.[78] In 1910, gastric acid was implicated and remained highest on the list of causes through most of the 20th century. Although acid plays an important role in the pathogenesis of PUD, recurrences of PUD after treatment with H_2 receptor antagonists are frequent.[79] Defective mucosal defenses have been considered to be more likely to be involved in the pathogenesis of most cases of PUD.[80] Specifically, occurrences of most gastric and duodenal ulcers have been attributed to nonsteroidal antiinflammatory drugs (NSAIDs) or to colonization of the stomach by *H. pylori*.

NSAIDs cause gastric mucosal damage, resulting in hemorrhage or perforation.[81] The risk for the need of hospitalization in patients taking NSAIDs has been estimated at 1% to 1.5% per year, and the risk of death from gastrointestinal complications, at 0.13% per year.[82] Risk factors for such complications include increased age, history of PUD, use of more than one NSAID, and concomitant steroid use.[83-86]

NSAIDs cause two types of gastrointestinal lesions.[80] With short-term use, endoscopically visible punctate lesions occur and are replaced by white-based erosions, usually in the antrum, which wax and wane spontaneously. With long-term use, these erosions can become ulcers: again, usually in the antrum but at times anywhere in the gastrointestinal tract. These ulcers result from the inhibition of cyclooxygenase and prostaglandin synthesis.

H. pylori is a unipolar, multiflagellate, spiral-shaped, microaerophilic, gram-negative rod that lives in a portion of the mucous gel where the pH is near neutral. It is the most common chronic bacterial infection in the world and is present in one third of the population.[87] It is most prevalent in underdeveloped countries, where it is common in children and where more than 70% of adults are infected by the age of 25 years. In developed countries, it is uncommon in children but seen in 50% of adults older than 60 years. *H. pylori* causes a superficial type B gastritis.[88,89] Duodenal and gastric ulcers are also closely associated with *H. pylori*. *H. pylori* has been found in 90% to 100% of patients with duodenal ulcers and in 60% to 100% of patients with gastric ulcers.[90] The presence of the bacteria appears to be *essential* for the development of most non–NSAID-induced ulcers; however, its presence alone is not *sufficient* for ulcer formation, because only 1.7% to 20% of patients with *H. pylori* infection acquire ulcers.[91-93] Other factors, such as cytotoxins released by the bacteria, smoking, stress, concurrent NSAID use,[91,94] and underlying genetic predisposition, are important.[95-97] The mechanisms by which *H. pylori* infection leads to PUD are not completely clear. Once *H. pylori* gains access into the mucous layer, it synthesizes phospholipase A_2 and ammonium ions, which destroy the hydrophobic phospholipid surface.[80] Other physiologic alterations associated with PUD, including an increase in gastrin levels,[98] inhibition of antral somatostatin release,[99] and a decrease in the secretion of duodenal bicarbonate release, are produced by *H. pylori*.[100] The net results of these alterations are increased acid secretion, decreased acid neutralization, and gastric metaplasia in the duodenum, resulting in further colonization of *H. pylori*. However, the steps from gastritis and duodenitis to frank ulceration are unclear, but they probably involve host and bacterial virulence factors.

Symptoms of Peptic Ulcer Disease

Duodenal ulcers produce epigastric pain that can be sharp, burning, gnawing, pressure-like, or ill defined. The pain is episodic and recurrent, usually begins 1.5 to 3 hours after eating, frequently awakens the patient from sleep, and is relieved by eating or antacids. Recurrences last days to months and can occur without symptoms. The symptoms of gastric ulcers are less well defined. Epigastric pain is the most common symptom. The pain may not be relieved by food, and, in some patients, the pain may increase after food intake. Antacids relieve the pain less reliably than in duodenal ulcers. Changes in the quality of pain may signal that a complication has occurred. The main complications and their symptoms are penetration, which is usually posterior toward the pancreas (pain radiating to the back); perforation (abrupt increase in abdominal pain); gastric outlet obstruction (pain that increases with food and increased nausea and vomiting); and hemorrhage (hematemesis, Hemoccult-positive stools, melena). Physical examination in uncomplicated cases may reveal mild midepigastric or right upper quadrant tenderness. When complications occur, physical examination may reveal tachycardia or hypotension, cutaneous or mucosal pallor if significant bleeding has occurred, a "surgical abdomen" if perforation or penetration has occurred, or a succussion splash if gastric outlet obstruction has resulted.

The diagnosis of PUD can be made radiologically or endoscopically. In single-contrast barium studies, 70% to 80% of duodenal ulcers found at endoscopy can be seen, whereas 90% can be identified in a double-contrast barium study. With regard to gastric ulcers, barium studies are 80% accurate. Endoscopy is most accurate for the diagnosis of PUD; furthermore, in the case of hemorrhage, the risk of bleeding recurrence can be ascertained and endoscopic therapy can be applied.

The treatment of PUD requires discontinuing offending medications such as NSAIDs, administering antisecretory medications (see Table 14–6), and treating *H. pylori*, if identified, in order to decrease recurrences. If NSAIDs cannot be stopped, concurrent, long-term use of medications aimed at protecting the gastric and duodenal mucosa is necessary. These include misoprostol (a prostaglandin analog), sucralfate, H_2 receptor antagonists, and PPIs. Misoprostol and the PPIs are most effective in protecting against both duodenal and gastric ulcers.

Approach to and Treatment of Peptic Ulcer Disease in Pregnancy

The true incidence of PUD during pregnancy is unknown because indigestion, nausea, heartburn, and vomiting are all common during this time. However, it is believed that the incidence is very low. One study identified only six cases of PUD in 23,000 deliveries.[101] If PUD becomes more clinically apparent during pregnancy, it tends to do so closer to the time of delivery.[102] Pregnancy tends to have a beneficial effect on the course of disease.[103] This beneficial effect may be caused by diminished gastric acid output and increased gastric mucus secondary to progesterone[104] or histaminase release from the placenta.[105] The beneficial effects of pregnancy may also result from the ability of gastric and duodenal mucosa to regenerate, possibly as a result of epidermal growth factor.[103]

When a pregnant woman presents with a prior history of PUD, a detailed history should help determine the certainty of the diagnosis. The patient without typical burning symptoms who has suffered complications without warning should continue with H$_2$ receptor antagonists. The patient with typical symptomatic disease in the past should receive medications only with the onset of recurrent symptoms. In the absence of a history of PUD, symptoms may be confused with GERD, simple nausea and vomiting, or hyperemesis. Treatment should initially be conservative. Recommendations should include dietary measures, such as eating small, frequent meals and avoiding foods known to trigger symptoms, particularly those that promote reflux, such as caffeine, chocolates, fatty foods, and mints. Antireflux measures, as described previously, should also be recommended. When these measures fail to work, antacids are the first line of therapy. They are safe, particularly when used in the second or third trimesters, as well as during breastfeeding. H$_2$ receptor antagonists are considered next in line; they are classified in category B (see Table 14-6). Sucralfate is a sulfated disaccharide with aluminum hydroxide that is minimally absorbed and functions as a topical agent, forming an ulcer-adherent complex that provides an acid barrier. It is also considered safe for use during pregnancy. PPIs are generally safe and classified in category B, except for omeprazole, which is in category C. However, omeprazole has not been found to be associated with major malformations in humans when used during pregnancy.[65] Misoprostol (Cytotec) is a synthetic prostaglandin E$_1$ analog. It exhibits both antisecretory and mucosal protective properties. Because it can cause uterine contraction, bleeding, and miscarriage, misoprostol should be avoided during pregnancy.[67] In fact, it is used to induce labor.[106]

In view of the chronic nature of the infection and the risk of exposing the fetus to multiple medications, it is best to delay treatment of the *H. pylori* infection until the postpartum period. For this reason, the various combinations of antibiotics and their rates of eradication are not discussed here.

INFLAMMATORY BOWEL DISEASE

Pathophysiology

The IBDs are ulcerative colitis (UC) and Crohn's disease (CD). These are two distinct disorders, each with its own varied manifestations. Both are characterized by chronic, relapsing, nonspecific intestinal inflammation. Although of unknown orgin, they have their own constellation of genetic, immunologic, and pathologic characteristics.

There are currently three theories regarding the etiology of IBD: (1) reaction to a persistent intestinal infection, (2) defective intestinal mucosal barrier to bacterial antigens, and (3) dysregulated host immune response to ubiquitous antigens. Whichever theory proves to be true, it can be said that luminal bacteria, either pathogenic or resident, stimulate the immune system, which in turn starts and perpetuates the inflammatory cascade. The chronicity of IBD results from a complex interplay of environmental stimuli, as mentioned (bacterial antigens or other toxins), affecting a patient with genetically predetermined host susceptibility factors and resulting in the person's preprogrammed immune response or mucosal barrier function. When the mucosal barrier is disrupted, the lamina propria immune cells are continually exposed to bacteria and other antigens present in the lumen, thereby perpetuating the immune cascade. Many immunoregulatory abnormalities have been identified, such as increases in helper T cells in relation to suppressor T cells, changes in epithelial antigen presentation, and cytokine alterations that favor continued inflammation. When the T lymphocytes and macrophages are activated, more cytokines are released, attracting and stimulating more cells of inflammation, thereby perpetuating the immune cascade. The end result of all the inflammation is tissue damage.[107]

Many of the therapies available are aimed at correcting the dysregulated immune response in a nonspecific manner. Treatments designed to correct the antigenic drive, such as antibiotics, have also been given a role in the management of IBD. More recently, therapies aimed at proinflammatory cytokines such as tumor necrosis factor α (TNF-α) have attained a role in the management of IBD.

Ulcerative Colitis: General Overview

The main symptom of UC is bloody diarrhea. Other symptoms associated with increasing severity include frequency, pus, crampy abdominal pain, fever, weight loss, dehydration, and anemia. With primary rectal involvement, tenesmus may be a major complaint, and some patients may present with constipation rather than diarrhea.

Findings on physical examination are usually nonspecific. In mild cases, the examination findings may be entirely normal. In more severe cases, the abdomen may be tender along the course of the colon, and fever, tachycardia, and postural hypotension may be present. Extraintestinal manifestations of IBD involve the eyes, skin, and joints (Table 14-9); their presence should increase the clinician's degree of suspicion about the presence of IBD. Laboratory data are also nonspecific and usually reflect the degree and chronicity of inflammation and bleeding. Anemia may be observed, and if chronic bleeding has taken place, iron deficiency may result. Inflammation may lead to leukocytosis and an elevated erythrocyte sedimentation rate. Hypokalemia may result

TABLE 14–9   Extraintestinal Manifestations of Inflammatory Bowel Disease

Rheumatologic
Arthralgias
Nondeforming (peripheral) arthritis
Central arthritis (ankylosing spondylitis)

Dermatologic/Oral
Erythema nodosum
Pyoderma gangrenosum
Aphthous ulcers

Hepatobiliary
Focal hepatitis/fatty infiltration
Pericholangitis
Sclerosing cholangitis
Cholangiocarcinoma
Chronic active hepatitis
Cirrhosis

Ocular
Episcleritis
Recurrent iritis
Uveitis

from fecal loss of potassium and hypoalbuminemia from loss of luminal protein. Liver function test results may be abnormal if the hepatobiliary system is affected (see Table 14–9). Stool testing usually reveals red and white blood cells, reflecting mucosal inflammation; the results of stool cultures are usually negative.

The diagnosis is suspected on the basis of the patient's history, physical examination findings, and laboratory data, as already described. Stool cultures should be obtained to rule out infectious colitis, which can manifest with similar signs and symptoms. Single-contrast barium enema studies may show changes consistent with early disease; however, barium enema study is often nonrevealing at this early stage. In the later stages, barium enema can determine the extent of inflammation and identify associated features such as pseudopolyps, ulcerations, bowel shortening, depression of flexures, loss of haustral markings, and the development of carcinoma. Of course, barium studies should not be done during pregnancy because of radiation exposure.

Direct examination of the colonic mucosa with mucosal biopsies is the best way to make the diagnosis. Sigmoidoscopy in UC shows inflamed mucosa beginning in the rectum and extending proximally in a continuous manner for a variable distance. The findings include erythema, edema, friability, loss of normal vascular pattern, exudate, and shallow ulcerations. As mentioned, the inflammatory changes are continuous; there are no skipped areas. The inflammation may involve only the rectum (proctitis), extend only as far as the sigmoid colon (proctosigmoiditis), or involve the entire colon (pancolitis). In the latter case, a small segment of terminal ileum may be involved in what is known as "backwash ileitis." If this occurs, thickening and narrowing of the terminal ileum rarely develop; this characteristic helps distinguish such disease from CD. During acute inflammation, the goal of the endoscopic evaluation is only to establish a diagnosis, not its anatomic extent. If the patient

experiences discomfort and the disease appears to extend beyond the level of insertion of the scope, the examination should be aborted, and treatment can be initiated. Continuing to advance the sigmoidoscope may result in further patient discomfort and greater risk of perforation related to the acute inflammation. The extent of the disease can be established at a later date, when inflammation is under better control.

Biopsies of the inflamed areas confirm the diagnosis. Microscopically, the inflammation in UC affects the mucosa and submucosa without affecting deeper layers (in contrast to CD). Pathologic findings include neutrophilic infiltration, loss of surface epithelial cells, ulceration, crypt abscesses, loss of crypt epithelium and goblet cells, and bifurcation at crypt bases. Recurrent inflammation results in submucosal fibrosis, shortening of the colon, and regenerative islands of mucosa amidst denuded areas, resulting in pseudopolyps. Dysplasia may be seen in long-standing UC. In very severe cases, when toxic megacolon develops, the bowel wall becomes very thin, and inflammation can extend to the level of serosa.

The main therapies for UC consist of 5-aminosalicylic acid (5-ASA) compounds and corticosteroids, delivered orally or rectally. In more severe cases, other agents may be necessary, such as azathioprine/6-mercaptopurine and cyclosporine. A more detailed discussion of the medications used in IBD follows.

Crohn's Disease: General Overview

CD can affect any part of the gastrointestinal tract, from the mouth to the rectum; most cases involve the small bowel, the colon, or both. The clinical manifestation of CD therefore depends on the area of involvement. The major clinical features of CD are fever, abdominal pain, and diarrhea, often without blood. Diarrhea and rectal pain are the most common colonic manifestations. Anorectal complications, such as fistulas, fissures, and abscesses may develop. Extensive involvement of the colon may lead to colonic dilatation, but this is less common than in UC. Presumably, the transmural involvement of CD results in colonic wall thickening, which makes dilatation less likely. Extraintestinal manifestations of IBD (see Table 14–9) are more common when the colon is involved. With disease of the small bowel, symptoms may consist of fatigue, weight loss, low-grade fever, anorexia, nausea, vomiting, and right lower quadrant pain. The pain may be colicky or crampy, depending on the degree of intestinal narrowing. The diarrhea of small bowel CD may be moderate and without associated blood loss.

The physical examination helps determine the site and severity of disease. Vital signs may be normal in mild cases. The examination may reveal elevated temperature, hypotension, and tachycardia resulting from active inflammation, fistula or abscess formation, dehydration from nausea and vomiting, or diminished oral intake. Extraintestinal manifestations may be evident (see Table 14–9). The abdominal examination may reveal tenderness with or without an associated fullness, reflecting adherent loops of bowel or an inflammatory mass. The perianal examination may reveal skin tags, abscesses, or fistula formation.

Laboratory data may reveal a mild anemia resulting from chronic disease or an iron deficiency, a folate deficiency, or a vitamin B_{12} deficiency resulting from extensive ileal involvement. Leukocytosis with a predominance of immature forms and an elevated erythrocyte sedimentation rate may be found. Abnormal liver function tests reflect hepatobiliary involvement. Extensive diarrhea may lead to electrolyte disturbances, such as hypokalemia and hypomagnesemia. Hypocalcemia may result from vitamin D malabsorption and protein-losing enteropathy. Steatorrhea may be present from bile acid malabsorption. Stool analysis may reveal leukocytes if the colon is involved, but the results of cultures are negative.

Radiologic studies are helpful in delineating extent of disease. A barium enema study shows rectal sparing, skip lesions, small ulcerations, longitudinal fissures, or strictures, the last resulting from irregular bowel wall thickening and fibrosis. A small bowel series may reveal a cobblestone appearance, loss of mucosal detail and rigidity of segments of bowel from submucosal edema or stenosis, and fistulous tracts. CT may identify segments of involved bowel, phlegmons, and abscesses.

Endoscopic examination shows ulcerations (tiny aphthae or longitudinal fissures), a cobblestone appearance, pseudopolyps, or strictures. In view of the noncontinuous nature of the disease, colonoscopy is superior to flexible sigmoidoscopy because it allows evaluation of the entire colon and of the terminal ileum. Biopsies should be undertaken to evaluate for nonspecific findings such as crypt abscesses, inflammatory infiltrates, and ulcerations and for the specific finding of granulomas, which are seen in 30% to 50% of biopsy samples of inflamed areas.

The medications for the treatment of CD are the same as those used for UC. For colonic involvement, an approach similar to UC is appropriate. Antibiotics such as ciprofloxacin and metronidazole have shown benefit.[108] If the small bowel is involved, 5-ASA products in the form of mesalamine, which are released more proximally in the intestinal tract, may be helpful. These include Asacol, a pH-released preparation, and Pentasa, a moisture-released preparation. Corticosteroids can be used to treat acute flares. Other medicines used with success in CD are azathioprine/6-mercaptopurine, infliximab, methotrexate, cyclosporine, tacrolimus, and thalidomide. A more detailed discussion of the drugs used for IBD during pregnancy follows.

Pregnancy and Inflammatory Bowel Disease

It can be difficult to diagnose IBD during pregnancy because many signs and symptoms of IBD are nonspecific and may erroneously be attributed to pregnancy itself. However, a thorough history, physical examination, and appropriate laboratory data should strongly suggest the diagnosis. A limited flexible sigmoidoscopic evaluation can be performed safely.[109] Total colonoscopy is usually not necessary because the findings are not likely to change therapeutic decisions.

Although it is best to achieve and maintain disease remission before conceiving, some patients conceive during the throes of a flare. Many of these patients prefer to struggle through the pregnancy rather than treat the disease medically. Furthermore, some patients prefer to stop maintenance medications before conception.[110] This decision is often based on patients' personal beliefs or on inappropriate advice from ill-advised physicians. Indeed, physicians' reference books, such as the Physician's Desk Reference (PDR), often emphasize risks and side effects without weighing risk/benefit ratios. The FDA pregnancy categories reflect this cautious approach. Although it is important to inform couples contemplating pregnancy about drug risks and warnings, it is equally important to educate and counsel them with regard to the experience and safety of these medications during pregnancy.

Aminosalicylates

This group includes sulfasalazine, in which 5-ASA is the active therapeutic agent linked via a diazo bond to sulfapyridine, and the mesalamine products, which consist of two diazo-linked 5-ASA molecules encapsulated in various vehicles to allow delivery of the drug to different locations in the intestinal tract without the intake of the sulfapyridine moiety, which is responsible for most side effects.[111] These medications are considered first line for the treatment of the IBDs. Table 14–10 summarizes the data on their safety during pregnancy.[112-117]

Antibiotics

The use of antibiotics in IBD is becoming increasingly important not only for the treatment of intercurrent infections but also as first-line therapy for CD.[118] There are limited data regarding the safety of antibiotics for the treatment of CD during pregnancy.

Metronidazole and ciprofloxacin are typically the first antibiotics considered in the treatment of patients with active CD.[119] Both appear to be safe for use during pregnancy (see Table 14–10).[119-127]

Other antibiotics thought to be safe for use in the treatment of CD during pregnancy include penicillins, cephalosporins, and the erythromycins.[128]

Corticosteroids

Corticosteroids are indicated for the treatment of moderate to severely active IBD. During pregnancy, corticosteroids cross the placental barrier, but they are rapidly converted to less active metabolites by placental 11β-dehydrogenase, resulting in lower fetal blood levels. For example, prednisone results in fetal levels that are approximately 10% of maternal levels.[129] For this reason, pituitary adrenal axis suppression is rarely seen. Dexamethasone and betamethasone are less efficiently metabolized by the placenta. Budesonide, a new synthetic glucocorticoid, is released in the small bowel and is indicated for the treatment of CD involving the terminal ileum or ascending colon. It acts topically and has very high first-pass metabolism (80% to 90%), which results in lower plasma levels.

In general, corticosteroids are well tolerated during pregnancy. However, as with all drugs, risks of their use should be carefully weighed against the risks of the disease on the developing fetus, and the drugs

TABLE 14–10   Drugs Used for Inflammatory Bowel Disease

Medication	Pregnancy Category	Comments and Data of Recent Safety during Pregnancy
5–Aminosalicylic Acid		
Sulfasalazine (Azulfidine)	B	All shown to be safe
Mesalamine	B	Kernicterus a potential but rare concern with sulfasalazine
Balsalazide*	B	Sulfasalazine interferes with folate absorption; folate supplements required
		Very high doses of 5–aminosalicylic acid should be used with caution
Antibiotics		
Metronidazole	B	Short courses of metronidazole for *Trichomonas* infection found to be safe
Quinolones	C	Possible arthropathogenicity with ciprofloxacin, but not
Penicillins	B	seen in two major studies
Cephalosporins	B	
Erythromycin	B	
Corticosteroids		
Prednisone	No rating	Generally well tolerated and safe in pregnancy
Prednisolone	No rating	Increased spontaneous abortions, small litter size, and cleft palate in
Hydrocortisone sodium succinate (Solu-Cortef)	No rating	animal studies; none of these outcomes observed in human studies
		Topical agents are safe until third trimester unless miscarriage or preterm
Methylprednisolone sodium succinate (Solu-Medrol)	No rating	delivery is a concern
		Budesonide is teratogenic and embryocidal in rats and rabbits
Budesonide*	C	Safe to women during pregnancy when inhaled
Purine Analogues		
Mercaptopurine	D	Appears safe for use during pregnancy
Azathioprine	D	High doses in animals reveal increased congenital malformations, prematurity, low birth weight, and chromosomal abnormalities
		Only decreased fertility and low birth weight seen in humans
		Paternal use within 3 months before conception associated with spontaneous abortions and congenital abnormalities
Anti–Tumor Necrosis Factor Agents		
Infliximab	B	Infliximab safe in murine models
Thalidomide	X	Postmarketing safety database of 35 pregnancies reveals rates of 74.3% live births, 14.3% miscarriages, 11.4% therapeutic terminations; these data are consistent with those in healthy women
		Thalidomide associated with fetal abnormalities and a high mortality rate of 40%
Immunosuppressive Agents		
Cyclosporine	C	Cyclosporine is safe for use during pregnancy
Tacrolimus	C	Transplantation and rheumatology literature show association with low birth weight and prematurity but high survival rates
		One abstract showed successful pregnancies in 4 of 5 mothers with IBD
		Tacrolimus appears safe; it results in high prematurity rate but compares favorably with other immunosuppressive agents with regard to congenital malformations, birth weight, and neonatal problems
Antimetabolites		
Methotrexate	X	Teratogenic and embryotoxic in animals, resulting in chromosomal damage and miscarriage
		Used as an abortifacient in tubal pregnancies
		Should be avoided

*New.
IBD, inflammatory bowel disease.

should be used only when clinically indicated (see Table 14–10).[114,130-134]

Azathioprine and 6-Mercaptopurine

Azathioprine and 6-mercaptopurine are purine analogs that interfere with nucleic acid biosynthesis and are active against human leukemias. Azathioprine is a prodrug of 6-mercaptopurine and is rapidly converted to 6-mercaptopurine in vivo. These medications are rated in pregnancy category D. This rating is based on early human reports that revealed increased abortion rates.[135,136] Animal studies evaluating high doses in rats, mice, and rabbits reported increased incidences of congenital malformations, prematurity, low birth weight, and chromosomal abnormalities. However, in animal studies evaluating dosages similar to those recommended in humans (1.5 mg/kg for 6-mercaptopurine and 2.5 mg/kg for azathioprine), the only adverse outcomes were decreased fertility rates and low birth weight.[137-139]

Most of the human experience with these medications in pregnancy is found in the rheumatology and transplantation literature,[140-149] which shows azathioprine to be safe in these populations. Infants of renal transplant recipients had an increased rate of low birth weight; however, this was believed to be more likely secondary to the underlying renal function than to the use of these medications.

The literature covering azathioprine/6-mercaptopurine use in pregnancy is much less extensive (see Table 14–10).[150-152] Azathioprine and 6-mercaptopurine appear safe for use in pregnancy. Patients should generally not stop medication before they conceive. Once pregnant, the patient can stop her medication if the disease has been under good control for a prolonged period. Alternatively, the patient may elect to remain on the drug if the disease was chronic, active, and difficult to control before she started medication.

Cyclosporine

Cyclosporine is indicated for moderate to severe UC as either a steroid-sparing agent or as means of avoiding surgery in severe steroid-refractory cases.[153] It is also effective in treating fistulizing CD.[154,155] The indications in the pregnant patient are no different. The drug's usefulness in pregnant patients with steroid-refractory disease cannot be overstressed, inasmuch as surgery in this setting carries a high risk of fetal mortality.[156]

Like other immunosuppressive agents, most of the safety data in pregnancy come from the transplantation and rheumatology literature.[149,157-161] In these studies, cyclosporine did not demonstrate teratogenicity. There was a higher rate of prematurity and low birth weight; however, the survival rate was high.

Again, the IBD literature is much less extensive (see Table 14–10).[156,162] Cyclosporine appears safe for use in pregnancy if clinically indicated. As is true for all medicines, the risks of use should be weighed against the risks of the underlying disease.

Tacrolimus

Tacrolimus is a macrolide antibiotic, which acts by a mechanism similar to that of cyclosporine, although it differs structurally. It is 100 times as potent as cyclosporine and is absorbed independently from bile flow. It has been shown to be effective in the treatment of complicated or fistulous CD as well as colitis (UC and CC).[163,164] It is used predominantly in a steroid-sparing role or for steroid-refractory disease, as a "bridge" to other medications, such as azathioprine/6-mercaptopurine or methotrexate.[165,166]

Data on the safety of this drug during pregnancy are very limited. The transplantation literature shows that it appears to be safe (see Table 14–10).[167-171]

Methotrexate

Methotrexate is a folic acid antagonist. Feagan and colleagues first described this antimetabolite's role as an inductive agent in the management of CD.[172] The drug is used as an alternative to azathioprine/6-mercaptopurine in the management of steroid-dependent or steroid-resistant CD. Animal studies have shown methotrexate to be both teratogenic and embryotoxic, resulting in chromosomal damage and miscarriage.[142,149] Indeed, the drug's negative effects on fetal viability are utilized therapeutically as an abortifacient in high doses for tubal pregnancies.[173]

Although normal pregnancies have been reported during methotrexate treatment,[142,174] the risks are too great. Methotrexate is therefore contraindicated for use during pregnancy and is rated in category X by the FDA. Couples, either of whom is taking methotrexate, should be informed to use reliable contraception. The prospective father should remain off methotrexate for at least 3 months (time required for spermatogenesis), and the prospective mother, for 1 month. If conception should accidentally occur, therapeutic abortion should be discussed. If abortion is not an acceptable option for the parents, the high risks of spontaneous abortion and congenital abnormalities should be clearly discussed and documented. The mother should be instructed to stop methotrexate immediately and begin high-dose folic acid replacement.[175]

Infliximab

Infliximab (Remicade) is a chimeric monoclonal antibody directed against TNF-α and is indicated for the treatment and maintenance of moderate to severe refractory or fistulizing CD.[176-179] The literature reporting on its safety in humans during pregnancy is limited (see Table 14–10).[180] The infliximab postmarketing safety database demonstrates pregnancy results that are similar to those in healthy controls.

Thalidomide

Thalidomide has been shown to be effective in the treatment of inflammatory and fistulizing CD.[181,182] The mechanisms of action of thalidomide are not fully understood; however, its TNF-α suppression is thought to play a major role in its effectiveness in the management of CD. Use of this agent has been associated with major human fetal abnormalities. Furthermore, mortality at or shortly after birth has been reported in approximately 40% of cases.[183,184] For these reasons, thalidomide has been rated category X by the FDA. In women and men of childbearing age, it should be used only when all other viable options have failed and only after the patient has been properly counseled with regard to prevention of pregnancy and risks of use during pregnancy (see Table 14–10).

Total Parenteral Nutrition and Surgery

Total parenteral nutrition for IBD is considered safe to use during pregnancy,[185,186] despite concerns that fat emulsions may lead to fat embolization to the placenta. Surgery is indicated for severe disease not responsive to medical treatment, as well as for complications, such as obstruction, unremitting bleeding, and toxic megacolon. Although emergency surgery during pregnancy is rarely needed, it should be done without delay when indicated. Surgery during pregnancy is associated with a high (approximately 50%) complication rate (stillbirths and spontaneous abortions). In view of the high complication rate, it is prudent for the clinician to be aggressive with medical therapy if surgery can be delayed or even prevented.

Fertility and Inflammatory Bowel Disease

In general, infertility rates in patients with IBD are similar to those in the general population.[128] The rate in the general population is approximately 8% to 10%.[187] It was initially thought that fertility rates were lower in patients with IBD.[188] Indeed, patients with IBD do have fewer children than would be expected for the general population.[189] However, studies have shown that this decrease may be secondary to voluntary reasons, such as fear of disease transmission to offspring,[128] relationship difficulties (fear of intimacy or dyspareunia), body image problems,[190] or inappropriate medical advice.[191,192]

There are certain situations in which infertility is, indeed, increased. Although women with UC have normal fertility, infertility appears to be increased after ileal pouch–anal anastomosis (IPAA).[193-197] The reasons are not clear. Ravid and associates attempted to identify possible factors that may contribute to infertility, defined as the inability to conceive within 1 year.[198] These include age at diagnosis of UC, age at surgery, utilization of a two-stage procedure, postoperative complications, weight changes, smoking status, number of hospitalizations or transfusions, medications used, and comorbid medical problems. None of these factors appeared to be implicated in post-IPAA infertility. In this study, women who reported infertility were eventually able to conceive at a rate similar to that in the fertile group, but they more frequently required medications or surgery to achieve a successful pregnancy. Dyspareunia appears to be increased after IPAA; the frequency is reported to be as high as 22% to 38%.[128,193] Interestingly, sexual satisfaction was found to be increased after IPAA, probably because of improved general health.[193,199] In men, the incidence of sexual dysfunction after IPAA has been observed to be low, between 2% and 4%, and is therefore generally not a significant issue.[193,199]

Inactive CD does not appear to affect fertility; however, active disease does affect fertility.[191,200] Inflammation or adhesions involving the fallopian tubes or ovaries are believed to be responsible. Fertility seems to normalize when disease remission is achieved.

Medications utilized to treat IBD essentially have no effect on fertility except for the well-described effect of sulfasalazine on male fertility. Sulfasalazine causes a reversible, dose-related decrease in sperm count and motility. Of all men on the drug, up to 60% report impairment in fertility.[201-204] When sulfasalazine is substituted by another 5-ASA product, sperm function improves.[205] The negative effect of sulfasalazine is reversed 2 months after the drug is discontinued.

Effect of Inflammatory Bowel Disease on Pregnancy

There appears to exist a misconception among patients and many primary care physicians that pregnant women with IBD should avoid medications during pregnancy. When advising patients and referring physicians, it is important for primary care physicians to convey the risks of active IBD itself versus the risks of treated, controlled disease on the developing fetus.

Most studies show that UC, when inactive, has little effect on the course of pregnancy with regard to congenital abnormalities, spontaneous abortions, and stillbirths, in comparison with non-IBD controls.[206,207] The incidence of premature delivery is not likely to be substantially affected; however, some studies do show this adverse event to be increased.[191,208] It is therefore prudent to advise close obstetric follow-up during the third trimester.

The data on the effects of active UC on pregnancy are somewhat vague. Active UC during pregnancy persists in one third of the cases and worsens in another third of the patients. The poor course inevitably leads to poor maternal health, resulting in prematurity and low birth weight.[119] Indeed, there appears to be an increased risk of preterm birth when the birth occurs after the mother's first hospitalization, especially when the hospitalization takes place during the pregnancy.[209] One study suggests that active UC may be associated with increased reporting of congenital malformations.[210] As the disease becomes more active, there is a greater threat posed to both the mother and the fetus. Active, nonfulminant UC carries a combined abortion/stillbirth rate of 18% to 40%,[211,212] whereas severe or fulminant UC necessitating surgery carries a corresponding rate of up to 60%.[213]

Like UC, quiescent CD has minimal effects on the course and outcome of pregnancy.[200,206,207] As in UC, close follow-up is advised during the third trimester.[191,208] Active CD, either at the time of conception or during the pregnancy, has been shown to increase the incidence of fetal loss, stillbirths, preterm delivery, low birth weight, and developmental defects. The risks appear to be related to the disease activity rather than to the medications used to treat the disease.[206,214-216] In the most severe cases, surgery may be required. In these cases, maternal and fetal mortality rates are very high (up to 60%).[188,217] Thus, in CD, as in UC, there is every reason to strive for clinical remission before conception and to aggressively treat flares medically in order to prevent complications.

Effect of Pregnancy on Inflammatory Bowel Disease

The course of UC during pregnancy tends to be similar to that in the nonpregnant state if conception occurs at a time of disease inactivity. That is, approximately one third of affected patients experience relapse during the pregnancy or puerperium.[214] If a relapse occurs, it is likely to do so during the first trimester.[132] However, if the disease is active at the time of conception, disease activity persists or worsens in approximately two thirds of affected patients.[200,212,218] Physicians should therefore strongly advise a woman contemplating pregnancy to attempt to conceive only when the disease is in remission.

CD exhibits a similar trend. When conception occurs during a period of disease quiescence, approximately one third of affected patients experience relapse during the pregnancy; this rate would be expected in the nonpregnant population.[214] If conception occurs at a time of active disease, two thirds of affected patients have persistent activity, and, of these, about half experience deterioration during the pregnancy.[187,200,219] Of interest, it has been noted that the course of CD appears to be altered by pregnancy. As parity increases, the need for surgical intervention decreases, and the interval between surgeries increases.[219]

Other autoimmune diseases such as lupus and rheumatoid arthritis exhibit a similar relationship to pregnancy. It has been shown that if both the human leucocyte antigen-DR and -DQ alleles are disparate in a mother and her child, her disease remains stable or improves, whereas if the two are disparate at only one allele, the disease worsens.[220] It is theorized that as disparity increases, the more the mother's immune system must be suppressed to prevent rejection of the pregnancy.

Inflammatory Bowel Disease and Breast-Feeding

Breast-feeding while being treated with oral 5-ASA products or corticosteroids is generally safe. These drugs are poorly secreted in the breast milk. Topical mesalamine is probably safe during breast-feeding. There are no data about the safety of azathioprine/6-mercaptopurine, ciprofloxacin, or metronidazole in breast-feeding mothers. However, methotrexate and cyclosporine are contraindicated during breast-feeding.[119]

ACUTE PANCREATITIS

Acute pancreatitis rarely complicates pregnancy, and pregnancy does not directly predispose a patient to development of pancreatitis. The incidence has been reported to range from 1 per 1066 to 1 per 4000 pregnancies.[221-224] The most common causes of acute pancreatitis in pregnant patients are gallstones and hyperlipidemia. Pregnancy predisposes to gallstone formation and, in this way, may indirectly predispose to gallstone pancreatitis. Hyperlipidemia is more commonly seen than in nonpregnant women because lipids and lipoproteins increase during pregnancy.[225,226] Such hyperlipidemia of pregnancy may be exacerbated in patients with familial hyperlipidemia. Of course, as in the nonpregnant patient, other causes of acute pancreatitis, such as medications or trauma, are possible.

Although acute pancreatitis can occur at any time during pregnancy, it occurs most commonly in the third trimester, when the rise in serum triglyceride levels is greatest.[222,226,227] If acute pancreatitis occurs in the first trimester, it usually results from gallstones.[223] It is important to differentiate acute pancreatitis from hyperemesis gravidarum, which is more common than acute pancreatitis in the first trimester. Acute pancreatitis has the potential of being more progressive, relapsing, and dangerous if the diagnosis is missed. Knowledge of the diagnosis of acute pancreatitis can allow for better counseling to the patient and better fetal monitoring over time, if necessary. There does not appear to be an association between acute pancreatitis and pregnancy status.[222,224]

Clinically, acute pancreatitis is characterized by pain and tenderness in the epigastrium, which can be mild to incapacitating, and is accompanied by nausea, vomiting, and abdominal distention. The pain may radiate to the back, can be exacerbated by meals or lying down, and can be relieved by leaning forward. Associated signs include low-grade fever, tachycardia, and hypotension. Serum amylase levels are usually elevated; however, the severity of disease does not correlate with the degree of amylase elevation. Other conditions can lead to amylase elevations, and the serum lipase activity can be helpful in increasing diagnostic yield. Leukocytosis is usually present but may not be informative, in view of the normal leukocytosis of pregnancy. The serum bilirubin and aminotransferase levels may be elevated if local inflammation and edema are sufficient to affect the adjacent bile duct. Hypocalcemia can be present in up to 25% of cases.[228] Various prognostic factors can be predictive of severity; these include respiratory failure, shock, need for massive colloid replacement, hypocalcemia with measurements of less than 8 mg/dL, or hemorrhagic fluid identified by paracentesis. Indeed, if three of the first four are present, the survival rate is only 30%. In general, acute pancreatitis of pregnancy is more dangerous to the fetus than to the mother. The prognosis depends on the severity of the disease and the degree of complications. Preterm labor can occur in as many as 60% of patients with acute pancreatitis late in pregnancy, and gestational age is a primary determinant of perinatal outcome.[229] Prostaglandin elevation occurs in pancreatitis, and this may be the cause of increased preterm labor.[230] Preeclampsia is another complication of acute pancreatitis in pregnancy.[221,231]

The diagnosis of acute pancreatitis is based on the clinical history, physical examination findings, and elevations of serum amylase and lipase levels. These criteria are usually sufficient for diagnosis; however, in difficult cases, abdominal ultrasonography may be helpful in delineating a swollen, boggy pancreas. In addition, ultrasonography helps determine whether gallstones are implicated. As reviewed earlier, ultrasonography is safe during pregnancy and may be readily undertaken. Abdominal CT would also help to define the anatomy of the pancreas; however, it is best to avoid CT, if possible, because of the radiation exposure involved.

Supportive management is the cornerstone of treatment of acute pancreatitis, regardless of pregnancy status. Patients should not take anything by mouth, to prevent further secretions of proteolytic enzymes and arrest the autodigestion process, and they should be well hydrated intravenously to prevent cardiovascular collapse from the third spacing of fluid. If oral nutrition cannot be started within a week, parenteral nutrition should be started because this has been proven to sustain fetal growth, prevent the recurrence of pancreatitis, and aid in the management of lipoprotein disorders.[232,233] All medications that may be implicated in the causation of acute pancreatitis should be discontinued. The inflammation is usually self-limited and resolves within 5 to 7 days. In more severe cases, other interventions may be necessary. Lipoprotein apheresis and plasmapheresis have been found to decrease triglyceride levels and provide rapid relief of acute pancreatitis during pregnancy.[234] If gallstones are implicated, surgery can be performed during the second trimester or early postpartum period.[235] ERCP has been found to be safe during pregnancy.[12,13] It is indicated for fulminant gallstone pancreatitis, as an alternative to surgical cholecystectomy; surgery is reserved for the postpartum period.[236] Cholecystectomy can be performed safely either "open" or laparoscopically during pregnancy, if indicated, as for cholecystitis.[237]

APPENDICITIS

Appendicitis has been estimated to occur in approximately 1 per 1500 pregnancies.[238-241] It is the most common extrauterine surgical emergency encountered during pregnancy.[242] During pregnancy, the physical changes that take place, including the enlarging uterus, distended abdomen, and the migration of the appendiceal location, make the diagnosis of appendicitis challenging. It is, therefore, important for the clinician to have a thorough understanding of these anatomic changes, as well as the presentation of appendicitis, so that an accurate diagnosis can be made quickly. Because the ultimate decision to operate is usually based on clinical grounds, sound knowledge of the disorder should limit the morbidity caused by delaying necessary surgery, while also minimizing any unnecessary surgery.

Typically, appendicitis manifests as a colicky epigastric or periumbilical pain that eventually localizes to the right lower quadrant, where it remains and intensifies. In pregnant women, the appendix migrates up the right side of the abdomen after the third month and reaches the level of the iliac crest by the sixth month. After birth, the appendix returns to its original location by the 10th postpartum day.[243] Because of these changes, the pain may migrate not exactly to the right lower quadrant but to some other location on the right side, depending on the location of the appendix. Anorexia may accompany the disease; however, this is common in pregnancy and, therefore, not specific.[244-246]

Rebound tenderness is also not specific in the pregnant patient.[244,247] The temperature is usually less than 38°C, unless perforation has occurred.[246,248] Patients with appendicitis typically have an elevated white blood cell count. Because the white blood cell count in normal pregnancy can range from 6 to 16,000 cells/mm^3 during the first and second trimesters and from 20 to 30,000 cells/mm^3 during labor, an elevated white blood cell count in pregnancy may not be informative.[242] Ultrasound imaging is effective in making the diagnosis in the nonpregnant patient with a sensitivity of 75% to 90%, a specificity of 86% to 100%, and a positive predictive value of 89% to 93% for the diagnosis of acute appendicitis.[249-251] Ultrasonography is also somewhat successful in the pregnant patient.[252] CT is the most accurate radiologic test for appendicitis in the nonpregnant patient, with a sensitivity of 98%, specificity of 98%, and a positive predictive value of 98%.[253] In view of the significant radiation exposure to the fetus, it is not unreasonable to reserve the CT as the last-resort radiologic test in the pregnant patient suspected of having appendicitis. Ultimately, the decision to perform laparotomy is based on the clinical setting and on a high level of suspicion on the part of the physician, and it must be understood that a higher negative laparotomy rate is expected and acceptable in this population to minimize fetal and maternal mortality.[238] Most large series report a false-positive laparotomy rate of approximately 20% to 35% for appendicitis in pregnancy.[239,254]

Appendicitis increases the likelihood of preterm labor or abortion, particularly when peritonitis occurs.[228] The rate of fetal loss is as high as 36% if perforation occurs, and the rate is as low as 1.5% in the absence of perforation.[239] Such data demonstrate the importance of having a high level of suspicion and an early diagnosis. The perforation rate is highest in the third trimester, when the rate is double that in the second trimester.[255] Maternal mortality is a rarity. It is highest in the third trimester, approaching a rate of 5%. Furthermore, maternal mortality increases when the diagnosis is delayed.[238,256,257]

References

1. Brent RL: The effect of embryonic and fetal exposure to x-ray, microwaves, and ultrasound: Counseling the pregnant and nonpregnant patient about these risks. Semin Oncol 1989;16:347.
2. Hall EJ: Scientific view of low-level radiation risks. Radiographics 1991;11:509.
3. Toppenberg KS, Hill DA, Miller DP: Safety of radiographic imaging during pregnancy. Am Fam Physician 1999;59:1813.
4. Moore MM, Shearer DR: Fetal dose estimates for CT pelvimetry. Radiology 1989;171:265.
5. Brent RL, Meistrich M, Paul M: Ionizing and nonionizing radiations. In Paul M (ed): Occupational and Environmental Reproductive Hazards: A Guide for Clinicians. Baltimore, Williams & Wilkins, 1993, pp 165-189.
6. Adelstein SJ: Administered radionuclides in pregnancy. Teratology 1999;59:236.
7. Nicklas AH, Baker ME: Imaging strategies in the pregnant cancer patient. Semin Oncol 2000;27:623.
8. Garden AS, Griffiths RD, Weindling AM, Martin PA: Fast-scan magnetic resonance imaging in fetal visualization. Am J Obstet Gynecol 1991;164:1190.
9. Cappell MS, Sidhom O: Multicenter, multiyear study of safety and efficacy of flexible sigmoidoscopy during pregnancy in 24 females with follow-up of fetal outcome. Dig Dis Sci 1995;40:472.
10. Cappell MS, Colon VJ, Sidhom O: A study at 10 medical centers of the safety and efficacy of 48 flexible sigmoidoscopies and 8 colonoscopies during pregnancy with follow-up of fetal outcome and with comparison to control groups. Dig Dis Sci 1996;41:2353.
11. Cappell MS, Colon VJ, Sidhom O: A study of eight medical centers of the safety and clinical efficacy of esophagogastroduodenoscopy in 83 pregnant females with follow-up of fetal outcome and comparison to control groups. Dig Dis Sci 1996;91:348.
12. Jamidar PA, Beck GJ, Hoffman BJ, et al: Endoscopic retrograde cholangiopancreatography in pregnancy. Am J Gastroenterol 1995;90:1263.
13. Tham TCK, Vandervoort J, Wong RCK, et al: Safety of ERCP during pregnancy. Am J Gastroenterol 2003;98:308.
14. Physicians' Desk Reference, 57th ed. Oradell, N.J., Medical Economics Company, 2003, p 3551.
15. Rayburn WF, Rathke A, Leuschen MP, et al: Fentanyl citrate analgesia during labor. Am J Obstet Gynecol 1989;161:202.
16. Rayburn WF, Smith CV, Parriott JE, Woods RE: Randomized comparison of meperidine and fentanyl during labor. Obstet Gynecol 1989;74:604.
17. McElhatton PR: The effects of benzodiazepine use during pregnancy and lactation. Reprod Toxicol 1994;8:461.
18. Faigel DO, Baron TH, Goldstein JL, et al: Guidelines for the use of deep sedation and anesthesia for GI endoscopy. Gastrointest Endosc 2002;56:613.
19. Cappell MS: The fetal safety and clinical efficacy of gastrointestinal endoscopy during pregnancy. Gastroenterol Clin North Am 2003;32:123.
20. Klebanoff MA, Koslowe PA, Kaslow R, Rhoads GG: Epidemiology of vomiting in early pregnancy. Obstet Gynecol 1985;66:612.
21. Jarnefelte-Samsioe A, Samsioe G, Velinder G: Nausea and vomiting in pregnancy: A contribution to its epidemiology. Gynecol Obstet Invest 1983;16:221.
22. O'Brian B, Zhou Q: Variables related to nausea and vomiting during pregnancy. Birth 1995;22:93.

23. Baron TH, Ramirez B, Richter JE: Gastrointestinal motility disorders during pregnancy. Ann Intern Med 1993;118:366.

24. Deuchar N: Nausea and vomiting in pregnancy: A review of the problem with particular regard to psychological and social aspects. Br J Obstet Gynaecol 1995;102:6.

25. Samsioe G, Crona N, Enk L, Jarnefelte-Samsioe A: Does position and size of corpus luteum have any effect on nausea of pregnancy? Acta Obstet Gynecol Scand 1986;64:427.

26. Gadsby R, Barnie-Adshead AM, Jagger C: Pregnancy nausea related to women's obstetric and personal histories. Gynecol Obstet Invest 1997;43:108.

27. Lagiou P, Tamimi R, Mucci LA, et al: Nausea and vomiting in pregnancy in relation to prolactin, estrogens, and progesterone: A prospective study. Obstet Gynecol 2003;101:639.

28. Klebanoff MA, Mills JL: Is vomiting during pregnancy teratogenic? BMJ 1986;292:724.

29. Depue RH, Bernstein L, Ross RK, et al: Hyperemesis gravidarum in relation to estradiol levels, pregnancy outcome, and other maternal factors: A seroepidemiologic study. Am J Obstet Gynecol 1987;156:1137.

30. Schulman PK: Hyperemesis gravidarum: An approach to the nutritional aspects of care. J Am Diet Assoc 1982;80:577.

31. Kousen M: Treatment of nausea and vomiting in pregnancy. Am Fam Physician 1993;48:1280.

32. Kallen B: Hyperemesis during pregnancy and delivery outcome: A registry study. Eur J Obstet Gynecol Reprod Biol 1987;26:291.

33. Levine MG, Esser G: Total parenteral nutrition for treatment of severe hyperemesis gravidarum: Maternal nutritional effects and fetal outcome. Obstet Gynecol 1988;72:102.

34. Abell TL, Reilly CA: Hyperemesis gravidarum. Gastroenterol Clin North Am 1992;21:835.

35. Tsang IS, Katz VL, Wells SD: Maternal and fetal outcomes in hyperemesis gravidarum. Int J Gynecol Obstet 1996;55:231.

36. Gross S, Librach C, Cecutti A: Maternal weight loss associated with hyperemesis gravidarum: A predictor of fetal outcome. Am J Obstet Gynecol 1989;160:906.

37. Chin RKH, Lao TT: Low birth weight and hyperemesis gravidarum. Eur J Obstet Gynecol Reprod Biol 1988;28:179.

38. Godsey RK, Newman RB: Hyperemesis gravidarum: A comparison of single and multiple admissions. J Reprod Med 1991;36:287.

39. Weigel MM, Weigel R: Nausea and vomiting of early pregnancy and pregnancy outcome: An epidemiologic study. Br J Obstet and Gynaecol 1989;96:1304.

40. Masson GM, Anthony F, Chau E: Serum chorionic gonadotropin (hCG), schwangerschaftsprotein 1 (SP1), progesterone and oestradiol levels in patient with nausea and vomiting in early pregnancy. Br J Obstet Gynaecol 1985;92:211.

41. Jarvinen PA, Pesonen S, Vaananen P: Fractional determinations of urinary 17-ketosteroids in hyperemesis gravidarum. Acta Endocrinol 1962;41:123.

42. Hutson WR, Roehkasse RL, Wald A: Influence of gender and menopause in gastric emptying and motility. Gastroenterology 1989;96:11.

43. Datz FL, Christian PE, Moore J: Gender-related differences in gastric emptying. J Nucl Med 1987;28:1204.

44. Koch KL, Stern RM, Vasey M, et al: Gastric dysrhythmias and nausea of pregnancy. Dig Dis Sci 1990;35:961.

45. Shirin H, Sadan O, Shevah O, et al: Positive serology for *Helicobacter pylori* and vomiting in pregnancy. Arch Gynecol Obstet May 20, 2003. [Abstract accessed January 15, 2004, at *http://www.springer-link.com/app/home/contribution.asp?wasp=g4lgnwvhxnw6d4v5pn5u&re ferrer=parent&backto=searcharticlesresults,1,1;journal,1,1;linkingpublica-tionresults,id:100399,1*]

46. Bagis T, Gumurdulu Y, Kayaselcuk F, et al: Endoscopy in hyperemesis gravidarum and Helicobacter pylori infection. Int J Gynecol Obstet 2002;79:105.

47. Kazerooni T, Taallom M, Ghaderi AA: *Helicobacter pylori* seropositivity in patients with hyperemesis gravidarum. Int J Gynecol Obstet 2002;79:217.

48. Sahakian V, Rouse D, Sipes S, et al: Vitamin B$_6$ is effective therapy for nausea and vomiting of pregnancy: A randomized, double-blind placebo-controlled study. Obstet Gynecol 1991;78:33.

49. Reilly JG, Ayis SA, Ferrier IN, et al: QTc-interval abnormalities and psychotropic drug therapy in psychiatric patients. Lancet 2000;25:1048.

50. Nageotte MP, Briggs GG, Towers CV, Asrat T: Droperidol and diphenhydramine in the management of hyperemesis gravidarum. Am J Obstet Gynecol 1996;174:1801.

51. Albibi R, McCallum RW: Metoclopramide: pharmacology and clinical application. Ann Intern Med 1983;98:86.

52. Harrington RA, Hamilton CW, Brogden RN, et al: Metoclopramide. An updated review of its pharmacological properties and clinical use. Drugs 1983;25:451.

53. Buttino L, Coleman SK, Bergauer NK, et al: Home subcutaneous metoclopramide therapy for hyperemesis gravidarum. J Perinatol 2000;20:359.

54. Siu SS, Yip SK, Cheung CW, Lau TK: Treatment of intractable hyperemesis gravidarum by ondansetron. Eur J Gynecol Reprod Biol 2002;10:73.

55. Tincello DG, Johnstone MJ: Treatment of hyperemesis gravidarum with the 5-HT$_3$ antagonist ondansetron (Zofran). Postgrad Med J 1996;72:688.

56. Sullivan CA, Johnson CA, Roach H, et al: A pilot study of intravenous ondansetron for hyperemesis gravidarum. Am J Obstet Gynecol 1996;174:1565.

57. MacMahon B: More on Bendectin [Editorial]. JAMA 1981;246: 371.

58. Lee M: Nausea and vomiting. In Feldman M, Friedman LS, Sleisinger MH (eds): Sleisinger & Fordtran's Gastrointestinal and Liver Diseases: Pathophysiology, Diagnosis, Management, 7th ed. Philadelphia, Saunders, 2002, pp 119-130.

59. Baron TH, Richter JE: Gastroesophageal reflux disease in pregnancy. Gastroenterol Clin North Am 1992;21:777.

60. Olans IB, Wolf JL: Gastroesophageal reflux disease in pregnancy. Gastrointest Endosc Clin North Am 1994;4:699.

61. Larson JD, Patatanian E, Miner PB, Jr., et al: Double-blind, placebo-controlled study of ranitidine for gastroesophageal reflux symptoms during pregnancy. Obstet Gynecol 1997;90:83.

62. Steinlauf AF, Traube M: Esophageal reflux and anesthetic risk: Role of proton pump inhibitors and other new agents. Anesth Clin North Am: Annu Anesth Pharmacol 1998;2:17.

63. Al Amri SM: Twenty-four hour pH monitoring during pregnancy and at postpartum: A preliminary study. Eur J Obstet Gynecol Reprod Biol 2002;102:127.

64. Broussard CN, Richter JE: Treating gastro-oesophageal reflux disease during pregnancy and lactation: What are the safest therapy options? Drug Safety 1998;19:327.

65. Nikfar S, Abdollahi M, Moretti ME, et al: Use of proton pump inhibitors during pregnancy and rates of major malformations: A meta-analysis. Dig Dis Sci 2002;47:1526.

66. Brunner G, Meyer H, Athmann C: Omeprazole for peptic ulcer disease in pregnancy. Digestion 1998;59:651.

67. Wildeman RA: Focus on misoprostol: Review of worldwide safety data. Clin Invest Med 1987;10:243.

68. Magee LA, Inocencion G, Kamboj L, et al: Safety of first trimester exposure to histamine H$_2$ blockers. A prospective cohort study. Dig Dis Sci 1996;41:1145.

69. Levy N, Lemberg E, Sharf M: Bowel habits in pregnancy. Digestion 1977;4:216.

70. Greenhalf JO, Leonard HS: Laxatives in the treatment of constipation in pregnant and breast-feeding mothers. Practitioner 1973;210:259.

71. Anderson AS: Constipation during pregnancy: Incidence and methods used in its treatment in a group of Cambridgeshire women. Health Visitor 1984;12:363.

72. Christofides ND, Ghatei MA, Bloom SR, et al: Decreased plasma motilin concentrations in pregnancy. BMJ (Clin Res Ed) 1982; 285:1453.

73. Jewell DJ, Young G: Interventions for treating constipation in pregnancy. Cochrane Database Syst Rev 2001;2:CD001142.

74. Pashankar DS, Loening-Baucke V, Bishop WP: Safety of polyethylene glycol 3350 for the treatment of chronic constipation in children. Arch Pediatr Adolesc Med 2003;157:661.

75. Muller-Lissner SA, Fumagalli I, Bardhan KD, et al: Tegaserod, a 5-HT(4) receptor partial agonist, relieves symptoms in irritable bowel syndrome patients with abdominal pain, bloating and constipation. Aliment Pharmacol Ther 2001;15:1655.

76. Nelson MM, Forfar JO: Association between drugs administered during pregnancy and congenital abnormalities of the fetus. BMJ 1971;1:1453.

77. Heinonen OP, Slone D, Shapiro S: Birth Defects and Drugs in Pregnancy. Littleton, Mass., Publishing Sciences Group, 1977.

78. Isenberg JI, McQuaid KR, Laine L, Walsh JH: Acid-peptic disorders. In Yamada T (ed): Textbook of Gastroenterology, 2nd ed. Philadelphia, JB Lippincott, 1995, pp 1347-1430.

79. Bardhan KD, Thompson M, Bose K, et al: Combined antimuscarinic and H$_2$ receptor blockade in the healing of refractory duodenal ulcer. A double blind study. Gut 1987;28:1505.

80. Sarner A, Babyatsky MW: Peptic ulcer disease: Paradigms lost. Mt Sinai J Med 1996;63:387.

81. Semble EL, Wu WC: Antiinflammatory drugs and gastric mucosal damage. Semin Arthritis Rheum 1987;16:271.

82. Fries JF, Williams CA, Bloch DA, Michel BA: Nonsteroidal anti-inflammatory drug-associated gastropathy: Incidence and risk factor models. Am J Med 1991;91:213.

83. Lacy ER, Cowart KS, Hund P 3rd: Effects of chronic superficial injury on the rat gastric mucosa. Gastroenterology 1992;103:1179.

84. Larkai EN, Smith JL, Lidsky MD, Graham DY: Gastroduodenal mucosa and dyspeptic symptoms in arthritic patients during chronic nonsteroidal anti-inflammatory drug use. Am J Gastroenterol 1987;82:1153.

85. Hollander D: Gastrointestinal complications of nonsteroidal anti-inflammatory drugs: Prophylactic and therapeutic strategies. Am J Med 1994;96:274.

86. Bjarnason I, Hayllar J, MacPherson AJ, Russell AS: Side effects of nonsteroidal anti-inflammatory drugs on the small and large intestine in humans. Gastroenterology 1993;104:1832.

87. Taylor DN, Blaser MJ: The epidemiology of *Helicobacter pylori* infection. Epidemiol Rev 1991;13:42.

88. Bayerdorffer E, Lehn N, Hatz R, et al: Difference in expression of *Helicobacter pylori* gastritis in antrum and body. Gastroenterology 1992;102:1575.

89. Alam K, Schubert TT, Bologna SD, Ma CK: Increased density of *Helicobacter pylori* on antral biopsy is associated with severity of acute and chronic inflammation and likelihood of duodenal ulceration. Am J Gastroenterol 1992;87:424.

90. Graham DY, Go MF: *Helicobacter pylori*: Current status. Gastroenterology 1993;105:279.

91. Kuipers EJ, Thijs JC, Festen HP: The prevalence of *Helicobacter pylori* in peptic ulcer disease. Aliment Pharmacol Ther 1995;9(Suppl 2):59.

92. Vaira D, Miglioli M, Mule P, et al: Prevalence of peptic ulcer in *Helicobacter pylori* positive blood donors. Gut 1994;35:309.

93. Oderda G, Figura N, Bayeli PF, et al: Serologic IgG recognition of *Helicobacter pylori* cytotoxin associated protein, peptic ulcer and gastroduodenal pathology in childhood. Eur J Gastroenterol Hepatol 1993;5:695.

94. Martin DF, Montgomery E, Dobek AS, et al: *Campylobacter pylori*, NSAIDs, and smoking: Risk factors for peptic ulcer disease. Am J Gastroenterol 1989;84:1268.

95. Malaty HM, Engstrand L, Pedersen NL, Graham DY: *Helicobacter pylori* infection: Genetic and environmental influences. A study of twins. Ann Intern Med 1994;120:982.

96. Riccardi VM, Rotter JI: Familial *Helicobacter pylori* infection: Societal factors, human genetics, and bacterial genetics. Ann Intern Med 1994;120:1043.

97. Azuma T, Konishi J, Tanaka Y, et al: Contribution of HLA-DQA gene to host's response against *Helicobacter pylori*. Lancet 1994;343:542.

98. Calam J: *Helicobacter pylori*, acid and gastrin. Eur J Gastroenterol Hepatol 1995;7:310.

99. Graham DY, Lew GM, Lechago J: Antral G-cell and D-cell numbers in *Helicobacter pylori* infection: Effect of *H. pylori* eradication. Gastroenterology 1993;104:1655.

100. Isenberg JI, Selling JA, Hogan DL, Koss MA: Impaired proximal duodenal mucosal bicarbonate secretion in patients with duodenal ulcer. N Engl J Med 1987;316:374.

101. Jones PF, McEwan AB, Bernard RM: Haemorrhage and perforation complicating peptic ulcer in pregnancy. Lancet 1969;2:350.

102. Vessey MP, Villard-Mackintosh L, Painter R: Oral contraceptives and pregnancy in relation to peptic ulcer. Contraception 1992;46:349.

103. Warzech Z, Dembinski A, Ceranowicz P, et al: The influence of pregnancy on the healing of chronic gastric and duodenal ulcers: The role of endogenous EGF [Abstract]. Gastroenterology 1997;112:A326.

104. Atlay RD, Weeks ARL: The treatment of gastrointestinal disease in pregnancy. Clin Obstet Gynecol 1986;13:335.

105. Michaletz-Onody O: Peptic ulcer disease in pregnancy. Gastroenterol Clin North Am 1992;21:1992.

106. Nopdonrattakoon L: A comparison between intravaginal and oral misoprostol for labor induction: A randomized controlled trial. J Obstet Gynaecol 2003;29:87.

107. Sartor RB: Pathogenesis and immune mechanisms of chronic inflammatory bowel diseases. Am J Gastroenterol 1997;92:5S.

108. Van Kruiningen HJ: On the use of antibiotics in Crohn's disease. J Clin Gastroenterol 1995;20:310.

109. Hanan IM: Inflammatory bowel disease in the pregnant woman. Compr Ther 1998;24:409.

110. Connell W, Miller A: Treating inflammatory bowel disease during pregnancy: Risks and safety of drug therapy. Drug Saf 1999;21:311.

111. Singleton JW, Hanauer SB, Gitnick GL, et al: Mesalamine capsules for the treatment of active Crohn's disease: Results of a 16-week trial. Pentasa Crohn's Disease Study Group. Gastroenterology 1993;104:1293.

112. Jarnerot G, Into-Malmberg MB: Sulphasalazine treatment during breast feeding. Scand J Gastroenterol 1979;14:869.

113. Khan AK, Truelove SC: Placental and mammary transfer of sulphasalazine. BMJ 1979;2:1553.

114. Mogadam M, Dobbins WO 3rd, Korelitz BI, Ahmed SW: Pregnancy in inflammatory bowel disease: Effect of sulfasalazine and corticosteroids on fetal outcome. Gastroenterology 1981;80:72.

115. Habal FM, Hui G, Greenberg GR: Oral 5-aminosalicylic acid for inflammatory bowel disease in pregnancy: Safety and clinical course. Gastroenterology 1993;105:1057.

116. Esbjorner E, Jarnerot G, Wranne L: Sulphasalazine and sulphapyridine serum levels in children to mothers treated with sulphasalazine during pregnancy and lactation. Acta Paediatr Scand 1987;76:137.

117. Trallori G, d'Albasio G, Bardazzi G, et al: 5-Aminosalicylic acid in pregnancy: Clinical report. Ital J Gastroenterol 1994;26:75.

118. Present DH: How to do without steroids in inflammatory bowel disease. Inflamm Bowel Dis 2000;6:48.

119. Present DH: Pregnancy and inflammatory bowel disease. In Bayless TM, Hanauer SB (eds): Advanced Therapy of Inflammatory Bowel Disease. Hamilton, Ontario, Canada, BC Decker, 2001, pp 613-618.

120. Burtin P, Taddio A, Ariburnu O, et al: Safety of metronidazole in pregnancy: A meta-analysis. Am J Obstet Gynecol 1995;172:525.

121. Rosa FW, Baum C, Shaw M: Pregnancy outcomes after first-trimester vaginitis drug therapy. Obstet Gynecol 1987;69:751.

122. Piper JM, Mitchel EF, Ray WA: Prenatal use of metronidazole and birth defects: No association. Obstet Gynecol 1993;82:348.

123. Diav-Citrin O, Shechtman S, Gotteiner T, et al: Pregnancy outcome after gestational exposure to metronidazole: A prospective controlled cohort study. Teratology 2001;63:186.

124. Friedman J, Polifka J: Teratogenic effects of drugs: a resource for clinicians (TERIS). Baltimore, Md., Johns Hopkins University Press, 2000, pp 149-195.

125. Schaefer C, Amoura-Elefant E, Vial T, et al: Pregnancy outcome after prenatal quinolone exposure. Evaluation of a case registry of the European Network of Teratology Information Services (ENTIS). Eur J Obstet Gynecol Reprod Biol 1996;69:83.

126. Loebstein R, Addis A, Ho E, et al: Pregnancy outcome following gestational exposure to fluoroquinolones: A multicenter prospective controlled study. Antimicrob Agents Chemother 1998;42:1336.

127. Berkovitch M, Pastuszak A, Gazarian M, et al: Safety of the new quinolones in pregnancy. Obstet Gynecol 1994;84:535.

128. Kane SV: Managing pregnancy in IBD. Inflamm Bowel Dis Monit 2002;4:2.

129. Blanford AT, Murphy BP: In vitro metabolism of prednisone, dexamethasone, and cortisol by the human placenta. Am J Obstet Gynecol 1977;127:264.

130. Koren G, Pastuszak A, Ito S: Drugs in pregnancy. N Engl J Med 1998;338:1128.

131. DeCosta EJ, Abelman MA: Cortisone and pregnancy: An experimental and clinical study of the effects of cortisone on gestation. Am J Obstet Gynecol 1952;64:746.

132. Ferrero S, Ragni N: Inflammatory bowel disease: Management issues during pregnancy. Arch Gynecol Obstet April 30, 2003. [Abstract accessed January 15, 2004, at *http://www.springerlink.com/app/home/contribution.asp?wasp=9e2751k1pl0jpm5a5r8x&referrer=parent&backto=searcharticlesresults,2,2;journal,1,1;linkingpublicationresults,id:100399,1*]

133. Kallen B, Rydhstroem H, Aberg A: Congenital malformations after the use of inhaled budesonide in early pregnancy. Obstet Gynecol 1999;93:392.

134. Norjavaara E, de Verdier MG: Normal pregnancy outcomes in a population-based study including 2,968 pregnant women exposed to budesonide. J Allergy Clin Immunol 2003;111:736.

135. Blatt J, Mulvihill JJ, Ziegler JL, et al: Pregnancy outcome following cancer chemotherapy. Am J Med 1980;69:828.

136. Nicholson HO: Cytotoxic drugs in pregnancy. Review of reported cases. J Obstet Gynaecol Br Commonw 1968;75:307.

137. Platzek T, Bochert G: Dose-response relationship of teratogenicity and prenatal-toxic risk estimation of 6-mercaptopurine riboside in mice. Teratog Carcinog Mutagen 1996;16:169.

138. Voogd CE: Azathioprine, a genotoxic agent to be considered non-genotoxic in man. Mutat Res 1989;221:133.

139. Mosesso P, Palitti F: The genetic toxicology of 6-mercaptopurine. Mutat Res 1993;296:279.

140. Meehan RT, Dorsey JK: Pregnancy among patients with systemic lupus erythematosus receiving immunosuppressive therapy. J Rheumatol 1987;14:252.

141. Scantlebury V, Gordon R, Tzakis A, et al: Childbearing after liver transplantation. Transplantation 1990;49:317.

142. Roubenoff R, Hoyt J, Petri M, et al: Effects of antiinflammatory and immunosuppressive drugs on pregnancy and fertility. Semin Arthritis Rheum 1988;18:88.

143. Williamson RA, Karp LE: Azathioprine teratogenicity: Review of the literature and case report. Obstet Gynecol 1981;58:247.

144. Rayburn WF: Connective tissue disorders and pregnancy. Recommendations for prescribing. J Reprod Med 1998;43:341.

145. Hou S: Pregnancy in women with chronic renal disease. N Engl J Med 1985;312:836.

146. Hou S: Pregnancy in chronic renal insufficiency and end-stage renal disease. Am J Kidney Dis 1999;33:235.

147. Willis FR, Findlay CA, Gorrie MJ, et al: Children of renal transplant recipient mothers. J Paediatr Child Health 2000;36:230.

148. Ghandour FZ, Knauss TC, Hricik DE: Immunosuppressive drugs in pregnancy. Adv Ren Replace Ther 1998;5:31.

149. Bermas BL, Hill JA: Effects of immunosuppressive drugs during pregnancy. Arthritis Rheum 1995;38:1722.

150. Alstead EM, Ritchie JK, Lennard-Jones JE, et al: Safety of azathioprine in pregnancy in inflammatory bowel disease. Gastroenterology 1990;99:443.

151. Rajapakse RO, Korelitz BI, Zlatanic J, et al: Outcome of pregnancies when fathers are treated with 6-mercaptopurine for inflammatory bowel disease. Am J Gastroenterol 2000;95:684.

152. Francella A, Dyan A, Bodian C, et al: The safety of 6-mercaptopurine for childbearing patients with inflammatory bowel disease: A retrospective cohort study. Gastroenterology 2003; 124:9.

153. Lichtiger S, Present DH, Kornbluth A, et al: Cyclosporine in severe ulcerative colitis refractory to steroid therapy. N Engl J Med 1994;330:1841.

154. Egan LJ, Sandborn WJ; Tremaine WJ: Clinical outcome following treatment of refractory inflammatory and fistulizing Crohn's disease with intravenous cyclosporine. Am J Gastroenterol 1998; 93:442.

155. Hanauer SB, Shulman MI: New therapeutic approaches. Gastroenterol Clin North Am 1995;24:523.

156. Bertschinger P, Himmelmann A, Risti B, Follath F: Cyclosporine treatment of severe ulcerative colitis during pregnancy. Am J Gastroenterol 1995;90:330.

157. Armenti VT, Ahlswede KM, Ahlswede BA, et al: National Transplantation Pregnancy Registry—outcomes of 154 pregnancies in cyclosporine-treated female kidney transplant recipients. Transplantation 1994;57:502.

158. Armenti VT, Jarrell BE, Radomski JS, et al: National Transplantation Pregnancy Registry (NTPR): Cyclosporine dosing and pregnancy outcome in female renal transplant recipients. Transplant Proc 1996;28:2111.

159. Radomski JS, Ahlswede BA, Jarrell BE, et al: Outcomes of 500 pregnancies in 335 female kidney, liver, and heart transplant recipients. Transplant Proc 1995;27:1089.

160. Bar Oz B, Hackman R, Einarson T, Koren G: Pregnancy outcome after cyclosporine therapy during pregnancy: A meta-analysis. Transplantation 2001;71:1051.

161. al-Khader AA, Absy M, al-Hasani MK, et al: Successful pregnancy in renal transplant recipients treated with cyclosporine. Transplantation 1988;45:987.

162. Marion JF, Rubin PH, Lichtiger S, et al: Cyclosporine is safe for severe colitis complicating pregnancy [Abstract]. Am J Gastroenterol 1996;91:1975.

163. Bousvaros A, Kirschner BS, Werlin SL, et al: Oral tacrolimus treatment of severe colitis in children. J Pediatr 2000;137:794.

164. Sandborn WJ: Preliminary report on the use of oral tacrolimus (FK506) in the treatment of complicated proximal small bowel and fistulizing Crohn's disease. Am J Gastroenterol 1997;92:876.

165. Lowry PW, Weaver AL, Tremaine WJ, Sandborn WJ: Combination therapy with oral tacrolimus (FK506) and azathioprine or 6-mercaptopurine for treatment-refractory Crohn's disease perianal fistulae. Inflamm Bowel Dis 1999;5:239.

166. Fellermann K, Herrlinger KR, Witthoeft T, et al: Tacrolimus: A new immunosuppressant for steroid refractory inflammatory bowel disease. Transplant Proc 2001;33:2247.

167. Jain A, Venkataramanan R, Lever J, et al: FK506 and pregnancy in liver transplant patients. Transplantation 1993;56:1588.

168. Winkler ME, Niesert S, Ringe B, Pichlmayr R: Successful pregnancy in a patient after liver transplantation maintained on FK 506. Transplantation 1993;56:1589.

169. Jain A, Venkataramanan R, Fung JJ, et al: Pregnancy after liver transplantation under tacrolimus. Transplantation 1997;64:559.

170. Armenti VT, Moritz MJ, Davison JM: Drug safety issues in pregnancy following transplantation and immunosuppression: Effects and outcomes. Drug Saf 1998;19:219.

171. Kainz A, Harabacz I, Cowlrick IS, et al: Review of the course and outcome of 100 pregnancies in 84 women treated with tacrolimus. Transplantation 2000;70:1718.

172. Feagan BG, Rochon J, Fedorak RN, et al: Methotrexate for the treatment of Crohn's disease. The North American Crohn's Study Group Investigators. N Engl J Med 1995;332:292.

173. Goldenberg M, Bider D, Admon D, et al: Methotrexate therapy of tubal pregnancy. Hum Reprod 1993;8:660.

174. Kozlowski RD, Steinbrunner JV, MacKenzie AH, et al: Outcome of first-trimester exposure to low-dose methotrexate in eight patients with rheumatic disease. Am J Med 1990;88:589.

175. Alstead EM, Nelson-Piercy C: Inflammatory bowel disease in pregnancy. Gut 2003;52:159.

176. Targan SR, Hanauer SB, van Deventer SJ, et al: A short-term study of chimeric monoclonal antibody cA2 to tumor necrosis factor alpha for Crohn's disease. Crohn's Disease cA2 Study Group. N Engl J Med 1997;337:1029.

177. Present DH, Rutgeerts P, Targan S, et al: Infliximab for the treatment of fistulas in patients with Crohn's disease. N Engl J Med 1999;340:1398.

178. Rutgeerts P, D'Haens G, Targan S, et al: Efficacy and safety of retreatment with anti-tumor necrosis factor antibody (infliximab) to maintain remission in Crohn's disease. Gastroenterology 1999;117:761.

179. Hanauer SB, Feagan BG, Lichtenstein GR, et al: Maintenance infliximab for Crohn's disease: The ACCENT I randomised trial. Lancet 2002;359:1541.

180. Katz JA, Lichtenstein GR, Keenan GF, et al: Outcome of pregnancy in women receiving Remicade (infliximab) for the treatment of Crohn's disease or rheumatoid arthritis. Gastroenterology 2001;120:A69.

181. Vasiliauskas EA, Kam LY, Abreu-Martin MT, et al: An open-label pilot study of low-dose thalidomide in chronically active, steroid-dependent Crohn's disease. Gastroenterology 1999;117: 1278.

182. Ehrenpreis ED, Kane SV, Cohen LB, et al: Thalidomide therapy for patients with refractory Crohn's disease: An open-label trial. Gastroenterology 1999;117:1271.

183. Manson JM: Teratogenicity. In Klaassen CD, Amdur MO, Doull J (eds): Cassarett and Doull's Toxicology: The Basic Science of Poisons, 3rd ed. New York, MacMillan, 1986, pp 195-220.

184. Smithells RW, Newman CG: Recognition of thalidomide defects. J Med Genet 1992;29:716.

185. Gineston JL, Capron JP, Delcenserie R, et al: Prolonged total parenteral nutrition in a pregnant woman with acute pancreatitis. J Clin Gastroenterol 1984;6:249.

186. Hew LR, Deitel M: Total parenteral nutrition in gynecology and obstetrics. Obstet Gynecol 1980;55:464.

187. Alstead EM: Inflammatory bowel disease in pregnancy. Postgrad Med J 2002;78:23.

188. Korelitz BI: Inflammatory bowel disease and pregnancy. Gastroenterol Clin North Am 1998;27:213.

189. Moody GA, Probert C, Jayanthi V, Mayberry JF: The effects of chronic ill health and treatment with sulphasalazine on fertility amongst men and women with inflammatory bowel disease in Leicestershire. Int J Colorectal Dis 1997;12:220.

190. Moody G, Probert CS, Srivastava EM, et al: Sexual dysfunction amongst women with Crohn's disease: A hidden problem. Digestion 1992;52:179.

191. Baird DD, Narendranathan M, Sandler RS: Increased risk of preterm birth for women with inflammatory bowel disease. Gastroenterology 1990;99:987.

192. Mayberry JF, Weterman IT: European survey of fertility and pregnancy in women with Crohn's disease: A case control study by European collaborative group. Gut 1986;27:821.

193. Tiainen J, Matikainen M, Hiltunen KM: Ileal J-pouch–anal anastomosis, sexual dysfunction, and fertility. Scand J Gastroenterol 1999;34:185.

194. Wikland M, Jansson I, Asztely M, et al: Gynaecological problems related to anatomical changes after conventional proctocolectomy and ileostomy. Int J Colorectal Dis 1990;5:49.

195. Ravid A, Richard CS, Spencer LM, et al: Pregnancy, delivery, and pouch function after ileal pouch–anal anastomosis for ulcerative colitis. Dis Colon Rectum 2002;45:1283.

196. Ording Olsen K, Juul S, Berndtsson I, et al: Ulcerative colitis: Female fecundity before diagnosis, during disease, and after surgery compared with a population sample. Gastroenterology 2002;122:15.

197. Hudson M, Flett G, Sinclair TS, et al: Fertility and pregnancy in inflammatory bowel disease. Int J Gynaecol Obstet 1997;58:229.

198. Ravid A, Richard C, O'Connor BI, et al: Fertility after ileal pouch–anal anastomosis in women with ulcerative colitis [Abstract]. Gastroenterology 2001;120(Suppl 1):2417.

199. Damgaard B, Wettergren A, Kirkegaard P: Social and sexual function following ileal pouch–anal anastomosis. Dis Colon Rectum 1995;38:286.

200. Khosla R, Willoughby CP, Jewell DP: Crohn's disease and pregnancy. Gut 1984;25:52.

201. Narendranathan M, Sandler RS, Suchindran CM, Savitz DA: Male infertility in inflammatory bowel disease. J Clin Gastroenterol 1989;11:403.

202. Birnie GG, McLeod TI, Watkinson G: Incidence of sulphasalazine-induced male infertility. Gut 1981;22:452.

203. Levi AJ, Fisher AM, Hughes L, Hendry WF: Male infertility due to sulphasalazine. Lancet 1979;2:276.

204. Toth A: Reversible toxic effect of salicylazosulfapyridine on semen quality. Fertil Steril 1979;31:538.

205. Chatzinoff M, Guarino JM, Corson SL, et al: Sulfasalazine-induced abnormal sperm penetration assay reversed on changing to 5-aminosalicylic acid enemas. Dig Dis Sci 1988;33:108.

206. Baiocco PJ, Korelitz BI: The influence of inflammatory bowel disease and its treatment on pregnancy and fetal outcome. J Clin Gastroenterol 1984;6:211.

207. Hanan IM, Kirsner JB: Inflammatory bowel disease in the pregnant woman. Clin Perinatol 1985;12:669.

208. Fedorkow DM, Persaud D, Nimrod CA: Inflammatory bowel disease: A controlled study of late pregnancy outcome. Am J Obstet Gynecol 1989;160:998.

209. Norgard B, Fonager K, Sorensen HT, Olsen J: Birth outcomes of women with ulcerative colitis: A nationwide Danish cohort study. Am J Gastroenterol 2000;95:3165.

210. Dominitz JA, Young JC, Boyko EJ: Outcomes of infants born to mothers with inflammatory bowel disease: A population-based cohort study. Am J Gastroenterol 2002;97:641.

211. Nielsen OH, Andreasson B, Bondesen S, Jarnum S: Pregnancy in ulcerative colitis. Scand J Gastroenterol 1983;18:735.

212. Willoughby CP, Truelove SC: Ulcerative colitis and pregnancy. Gut 1980;21:469.

213. Anderson JB, Turner GM, Williamson RC: Fulminant ulcerative colitis in late pregnancy and the puerperium. J R Soc Med 1987;80:492.

214. Miller JP: Inflammatory bowel disease in pregnancy: A review. J R Soc Med 1986;79:221.

215. Larzilliere I, Beau P: Chronic inflammatory bowel disease and pregnancy. Case control study [in French]. Gastroenterol Clin Biol 1998;22:1056.

216. Fonager K, Sorensen HT, Olsen J, et al: Pregnancy outcome for women with Crohn's disease: A follow-up study based on linkage between national registries. Am J Gastroenterol 1998;93:2426.

217. Nielsen OH, Andreasson B, Bondesen S, et al: Pregnancy in Crohn's disease. Scand J Gastroenterol 1984;19:724.

218. Porter RJ, Stirrat GM: The effects of inflammatory bowel disease on pregnancy: A case-controlled retrospective analysis. Br J Obstet Gynaecol 1986;93:1124.

219. Nwokolo CU, Tan WC, Andrews HA, Allan RN: Surgical resections in parous patients with distal ileal and colonic Crohn's disease. Gut 1994;35:220.

220. Kane S: HLS disparity determines disease activity through pregnancy in women with IBD. Gastroenterology 1998;114:A1006.

221. Wilkinson EJ: Acute pancreatitis in pregnancy: A review of 98 cases and a report of 8 new cases. Obstet Gynecol Surv 1973;28:281.

222. Corlett RC Jr, Mishell DR Jr: Pancreatitis in pregnancy. Am J Obstet Gynecol 1972;113:281.

223. Legro RS, Laifer SA: First-trimester pancreatitis: Maternal and neonatal outcome. J Reprod Med 1995;40:689.

224. Chen CP, Wang KG, Su TH, Yang YC: Acute pancreatitis in pregnancy. Acta Obstet Gynecol Scand 1995;74:607.

225. Read G, Braganza JM, Howat HT: Pancreatitis—a retrospective study. Gut 1976;17:945.

226. Desoye G, Schweditsch MO, Pfeiffer KP, et al: Correlation of hormones with lipid and lipoprotein levels during normal pregnancy and postpartum. J Clin Endocrinol Metab 1987;64:704.

227. De Chalain TM, Michell WL, Berger GM: Hyperlipidemia, pregnancy and pancreatitis. Surg Gynecol Obstet 1988;167:469.

228. Cunningham FG, Gant NF, Leveno KJ, et al: Gastrointestinal disorders. In Cunningham F, McDonald P, Gant N (eds): Williams Obstetrics, 21st ed. New York, McGraw Hill, 2001, pp 1273-1306.

229. Young KR: Acute pancreatitis in pregnancy: Two case reports. Obstet Gynecol 1982;60:653.

230. Glazer G, Bennett A: Prostaglandin release in canine acute haemorrhagic pancreatitis. Gut 1976;17:22.

231. Koff RS: Case records of the Massachusetts General Hospital. N Engl J Med 1981;304:216.

232. Rivera-Alsina ME, Saldana LR, Stringer CA: Fetal growth sustained by parenteral nutrition in pregnancy. Obstet Gynecol 1984;64:138.

233. Weinberg RB, Sitrin MD, Adkins GM, Lin CC: Treatment of hyperlipidemic pancreatitis in pregnancy with total parenteral nutrition. Gastroenterology 1982;83:1300.

234. Achard JM, Westeel PF, Moriniere P, et al: Pancreatitis related to severe acute hypertriglyceridemia during pregnancy: Treatment with lipoprotein apheresis. Intensive Care Med 1991;17:236.

235. Block P, Kelly TR: Management of gallstone pancreatitis during pregnancy and the postpartum period. Surg Gynecol Obstet 1989;168:426.

236. Baillie J, Cairns SR, Putman WS, Cotton PB: Endoscopic management of choledocholithiasis during pregnancy. Surg Gynecol Obstet 1990;171:1.

237. Ramin KD, Ramsey PS: Disease of the gallbladder and pancreas in pregnancy. Obstet Gynecol Clin North Am 2001;28:571.

238. Sharp HT: Gastrointestinal surgical conditions during pregnancy. Clin Obstet Gynecol 1994;37:306.

239. Babaknia A, Parsa H, Woodruff JD: Appendicitis during pregnancy. Obstet Gynecol 1977;50:40.

240. Mazze RI, Kallen B: Appendectomy during pregnancy: A Swedish registry study of 778 cases. Obstet Gynecol 1991;77:835.

241. Black WP: Acute appendicitis in pregnancy. BMJ 1960;5190:1938.

242. Cozar RA, Roslyn JL: The Appendix. In Schwartz S (ed): Principles of Surgery, 7th ed. New York, McGraw-Hill, 1999, pp 1383-1394.

243. Baer JL, Reis RA, Arens RA: Appendicitis of pregnancy with changes in position and axis of the normal appendix in pregnancy. JAMA 1932;98:1359.

244. Bailey LE, Finley RK, Miller SF, Jones LM: Acute appendicitis during pregnancy. Am Surg 1986;52:218.

245. Tamir IL, Bongard FS, Klein SR: Acute appendicitis in the pregnant patient. Am J Surg 1990;160:571.

246. Masters K, Levine BA, Gaskill HV, Sirinek KR: Diagnosing appendicitis during pregnancy. Am J Surg 1984;148:768.

247. Richards C, Daya S: Diagnosis of acute appendicitis in pregnancy. Can J Surg 1989;32:358.

248. Dobberneck RC: Appendectomy during pregnancy. Am Surg 1985; 51:265.

249. Paulson EK, Kalady MF, Pappas TN: Acute appendicitis. N Engl J Med 2003;348:236.

250. Chesbrough RM, Burkhard TK, Balsara ZN, et al: Self-localization in US of appendicitis: An addition to graded compression. Radiology 1993;187:349.

251. Puylaert JB, Rutgers PH, Lalisang RI, et al: A prospective study of ultrasonography in the diagnosis of appendicitis. N Engl J Med 1987;317:666.

252. Landwehr JG, Leonardi MR, Bryant DR, et al: Graded compression ultrasound (GCUS) for early recognition of appendicitis in pregnancy [Abstract]. Am J Obstet Gynecol 1996;174:388.

253. Rao PM, Rhea JT, Novelline RA, et al: Effect of computed tomography of the appendix on treatment of patients and use of hospital resources. N Engl J Med 1998;338:141.

254. Sarson EL, Bauman S: Acute appendicitis in pregnancy: Difficulties in diagnosis. Obstet Gynecol 1963;22:382.

255. Weingold AB: Appendicitis in pregnancy. Clin Obstet Gynecol 1983;26:801.

256. Horowitz MD, Gomez GA, Santiesteban R, Burkett G: Acute appendicitis during pregnancy. Diagnosis and management. Arch Surg 1985;120:1362.

257. Cunningham FG, McCubbin JH: Appendicitis complicating pregnancy. Obstet Gynecol 1975;45:415.

15

LIVER DISEASES

Caroline A. Riely and Harold J. Fallon

THE EFFECTS OF PREGNANCY ON THE LIVER

Normal pregnancy can alter the results of so-called "liver function" tests. These changes are largely reversible but can present difficulty in the diagnosis of liver diseases during pregnancy.

Anatomic Changes

Liver weight increases during pregnancy in experimental animals, but a corresponding enlargement in humans has not been documented. Liver size is difficult to estimate in pregnancy, but autopsy records of women dying during pregnancy fail to show any substantial increase in liver weight in comparison with nonpregnant controls.[1] Therefore, detection of hepatomegaly is strong evidence for the presence of liver disease.

Minor histologic changes have been reported in the human liver during pregnancy. In a series of liver biopsies reported in 1945, variations in size and shape of the hepatocytes, occasional lymphocytic infiltration in the portal areas, and variable increases in glycogen and fat were noted.[2] These findings are nonspecific and may be seen in apparently healthy nonpregnant women. Administration of estrogens or oral contraceptives is also unaccompanied by significant histologic or electron microscopic alterations unless obvious clinical and laboratory evidence of cholestasis develops in response to these agents.

Physiology

Hepatic blood flow is maintained at a constant rate in pregnancy despite marked changes in the cardiovascular system. An increase in plasma and blood volume of 50% or more and a rise in cardiac output of up to 50% occur during pregnancy. These changes are maximal at the beginning of the third trimester. Blood flow increases to the kidneys and other organs, but hepatic blood flow is unaltered, which results in a decline of approximately 35% in the proportion of cardiac output delivered to the liver.[3]

Liver Function in Pregnancy

Proteins

Significant changes occur in the serum concentration of various plasma proteins during pregnancy. Virtually all serum proteins known to be synthesized in the liver are affected by pregnancy or by the administration of estrogens to nonpregnant women. The changes that arise during pregnancy may persist for several months after delivery.

The total serum protein concentration declines approximately 20% in midpregnancy, primarily a result of the substantial decline in serum albumin. There is a small increase in the α and β globulin fractions and a slight decline in γ globulin. A portion of the decrease in serum albumin may be attributed to simple dilution caused by the increase in total blood volume, although most other serum proteins either remain unchanged or increase in concentration. There is evidence of a reciprocal relationship between rising levels of α-fetoprotein and the fall in serum albumin.[4] The variable changes in the several globulin fractions remain unexplained. The hepatic parenchymal cell is not the site of globulin biosynthesis, and therefore other tissues are probably involved in the serum globulin alterations.

A significant rise in serum fibrinogen regularly accompanies pregnancy. Experimental evidence suggests that this is a consequence of increase fibrinogen synthesis.[5] Similarly, administration of estrogens or combined estrogen and progestin preparations to human beings induces a rise in serum fibrinogen levels. Other coagulation proteins, including factors VII, VIII, IX, and X, may be increased during pregnancy or after estrogen treatment.

The prothrombin time is normal in pregnancy, but fibrinolytic activity is slightly reduced.

Other serum proteins synthesized in liver may be altered by pregnancy. Ceruloplasmin levels gradually increase, reaching a maximum at term. Estrogens stimulate a similar increase in serum ceruloplasmin concentrations. In some pregnant patients with Wilson's disease, the level of ceruloplasmin may increase to nearly normal values. Transferrin levels are increased in the last trimester but are not affected by estrogen administration. An increase in serum binding capacity for thyroxine, vitamin D, folate, corticosteroid, and testosterone also occurs in pregnancy, altering the serum concentration of these hormones. These changes are attributed to increased levels of the specific binding proteins and have been reported after estrogen administration to nonpregnant women. Serum haptoglobin levels are decreased after estrogen administration, and this possibly accounts for the higher concentration of haptoglobin in men. Pregnancy does not alter haptoglobin concentration.

Liver Function Tests

The results of so-called liver function tests in normal pregnant women in all three trimesters have been compared with those of controls.[6] Most studies have failed to document significant bilirubin elevation in the absence of specific cause during normal pregnancy.[3] Therefore, an increased serum bilirubin level in pregnancy should be considered presumptive evidence for the presence of liver or hematologic disease. There is evidence that elevated maternal unconjugated bilirubin from whatever cause may be transferred to the fetus and cause neurologic complications in the infant.[7,8]

The total serum alkaline phosphatase level is elevated during the third trimester of normal pregnancy. The major source of this elevation during pregnancy appears to be the placenta, as established by differential inhibition studies, gel electrophoresis, heat stability determination, and immunochemical techniques. The portion of total serum alkaline phosphatase derived from placenta increases from less than 10% in the first month of pregnancy to more than 50% at the time of delivery. The placental alkaline phosphatase concentration decreases rapidly after delivery, usually reaching normal levels about 20 days post partum.[9] A pattern of rapidly decreasing placental alkaline phosphatase during the last trimester has been associated with fetal death in utero.[10] A rise in bone alkaline phosphatase has also been reported during pregnancy, although this increase is modest.

Serum alkaline phosphatase levels may be increased in nonpregnant women by administration of exogenous estrogens. It is obvious that the phosphatase under these conditions is not of placental origin; it is probably derived from the liver. The major sources of serum alkaline phosphatase in nonpregnant persons are the liver, bone, and the intestine.[11] Liver alkaline phosphatase production is stimulated by a variety of injuries to the canalicular membrane, including mechanical bile duct obstruction and intrahepatic cholestasis. Estrogens may produce the latter type of injury.[12] This possibility is supported by observations that serum 5′-nucleotidase, a more specific indicator

of canalicular membrane disturbance, is also increased in some women receiving estrogens.[13]

The serum γ-glutamyl-transpeptidase (GGTP) is an enzyme whose level is regularly but not invariably elevated in cholestasis and hepatocellular injury. It is normal in a very few cholestatic disorders, such as Byler's syndrome, now recognized as progressive familial intrahepatic cholestasis (PFIC) type 1.[14] It is reported to be normal or decreased during the third trimester of normal pregnancy.[6] Serum bile acid level is quite helpful in any form of cholestasis. The serum level is normal in normal pregnancy. Serum lactate dehydrogenase and ornithine transcarbamylase are increased near term.

Levels of serum aminotransferase—aspartate aminotransferase (AST) and alanine aminotransferase (ALT)—are normal in normal pregnancy. Therefore, these two serum enzyme determinations remain sensitive indicators of liver damage during pregnancy. The ALT is especially useful, because significant elevation of this enzyme does not occur with injury to tissues other than liver.

Serum Lipids

A substantial increase in the serum concentration of the major lipid classes occurs during pregnancy and is most marked at term. Inhibition of postheparin esterase activity and lipoprotein lipase occurs in late pregnancy, with a rapid return to normal after delivery.[15] These effects may be attributable to estrogenic compounds, which are known to reduce lipoprotein lipase activity in nonpregnant women. In addition, there is evidence that estrogens accelerate hepatic triglyceride biosynthesis.

Although the elevation in serum triglyceride levels may be quantitatively the most marked serum lipid change, the rise in serum cholesterol may cause the greatest confusion in the differential diagnosis of suspected liver disease. The upper limit of normal for cholesterol during the last trimester of pregnancy is approximately double the normal limit for nonpregnant women of the same age. Therefore, hypercholesterolemia in this range cannot be taken as evidence of cholestasis during pregnancy. The changes in serum lipid constituents are a consequence of corresponding increases in serum low-density lipoproteins and very-low-density lipoproteins.

Porphyrins

There are minor changes in porphyrin metabolism during pregnancy. Total urine coproporphyrin excretion may be increased slightly, but there is a marked decrease in urinary excretion of the coproporphyrin III isomer and a relative increase in the coproporphyrin I isomer. Porphobilinogen excretion is normal, but δ-aminolevulinic acid excretion is increased in about half of normal pregnancies.[16] A summary of the major biochemical changes in liver function during pregnancy is shown in Table 15-1.

Effects of Female Sex Hormones on Liver Function

Several authors have reviewed the effects of anabolic steroids, estrogens, progestins, and oral contraceptives on

TABLE 15–1   Liver Function Test Results in Normal Pregnancy

Test	Effect	Trimester of Maximum Change
Albumin	↓ 20%-50%	Second
γ Globulin	Normal to slight ↓	Third
α Globulin	Slight ↑	Third
β Globulin	Slight ↑	Third
Fibrinogen	↑ 50%	Second
Ceruloplasmin	↑	Third
Transferrin	↑	Third
Prothrombin time	None	—
Bilirubin	None	—
Alkaline phosphatase	Twofold to fourfold ↑	Third
GGTP	None	—
Bile acids	None	—
Lactate dehydrogenase	Slight ↑	Third
Serum AST	None	—
Serum ALT	None	—
Cholesterol	Twofold	Third
Triglyceride	Twofold to threefold ↑	Third

ALT, alanine aminotransferase; AST, aspartate aminotransferase; GGTP, γ-glutamyl-transpeptidase.
↑, increase; ↓, decrease.

liver structure and function.[12,17] Each of these classes of agents has significant and somewhat different effects on the liver. However, their role in mediating the physiologic and biochemical alterations associated with normal pregnancy or in mediating the liver diseases specifically related to pregnancy is not clear. This is because the liver is the major site of estrogen metabolism and contains estrogen receptors.[18]

Many natural and synthetic sex hormones produce variable degrees of cholestasis. Cholestasis is defined as centrilobular bile stasis associated with dilation of the canaliculi and loss of the normal microvillus structure of the canaliculus as seen by electron microscopy. The biochemical changes of cholestasis are extremely variable. The most reliable and sensitive test of cholestasis is the serum bile acid level. Other useful indices include the serum level of alkaline phosphatase, 5′-nucleotidase, GGTP, and, on occasion, bilirubin.

The anabolic steroids most likely to cause significant cholestasis are those containing a methyl or ethyl group in the C-17 position. Many of these compounds cause a small rise in AST without histologic evidence of hepatocellular injury. Much less commonly, alkaline phosphatase, lactate dehydrogenase, and serum bilirubin concentrations may be elevated. Intrahepatic cholestasis with anatomic changes limited to the canalicular membrane and sparing of most of the intracellular organelles is characteristic of this class of drugs. On occasion, hepatocellular necrosis is also reported.

The estrogens increase hepatic rough endoplasmic reticulum and accelerate synthesis of some hepatic proteins. Progesterone, in contrast, causes proliferation of the smooth endoplasmic reticulum and an increase in cytochrome P-450 in rats. The rise in mixed function oxidase activity is preceded by an increase in δ-aminolevulinic acid synthetase.

It is possible that hormones play a role in the production of cholestatic jaundice of pregnancy and other forms of liver injury in pregnancy.

LIVER DISEASES SPECIFICALLY RELATED TO PREGNANCY

Intrahepatic Cholestasis of Pregnancy

The syndrome of intrahepatic cholestasis of pregnancy (ICP) was first recognized in the 19th century, but adequate descriptions did not appear until the comprehensive studies of the disease in Swedish women in the 1950s.[19] The syndrome has been variously called recurrent jaundice of pregnancy, cholestatic jaundice of pregnancy, jaundice of late pregnancy, and hepatosis of pregnancy. ICP, however, is the preferred term, because jaundice is inconstant in any type of cholestatic disorder. The frequency of ICP is clearly higher among certain ethnic groups, including Scandinavians and Chileans. In the latter group, ICP may appear in 2.4% or more of pregnancies, the highest reported incidence in the world.[20,21] The incidence is quite high (20.9%) in twin pregnancies.[22]

Several studies have demonstrated a familial predisposition to the syndrome in Sweden, Chile, and the United States.[23,24] In one study of the disease in three generations, a mendelian dominant mode of transmission was suggested. Other studies suggest that incomplete penetrance and variable expression may occur with a dominant gene defect. It is likely that environmental or polygenic factors influence the occurrence and severity of the disease, and there may be more than one genetic disorder that results in a similar phenotypic expression.[23] The proposed genetic predisposition and precipitating factors result in an enhanced cholestatic response to physiologic estrogen levels during pregnancy.[13,25] Studies have shown that in some affected women, ICP may result from the heterozygous form of the gene associated with one of the PFIC syndromes.[26]

Clinical Description

Pruritus is the initial symptom and appears in the third trimester in more than 70% of cases. Most of the remaining patients date their onset of symptoms to the second trimester, although cases have appeared during early pregnancy.[20] Many patients report the appearance of dark urine without frank jaundice shortly after the onset of pruritus. Only a minority of patients develop obvious jaundice, and this is usually mild, although a marked elevation of bilirubin level has been reported in at least one case.[27]

Pruritus is the dominant and most disturbing clinical feature of ICP. The symptom may become very severe and usually involves the trunk and the extremities, including the palms and the soles of the feet. As a result of the pruritus, insomnia, fatigue, and even mental disturbances have been reported. It is notable that abdominal pain, biliary colic, fever, anorexia, nausea, vomiting, and arthralgias are absent. The physical findings are usually limited to evidence of scratching and, in rare cases, mild and slightly tender hepatomegaly.

The duration and severity of the syndrome varies with the time of onset during pregnancy. Early onset is reported to be associated with more severe symptoms and a higher incidence of fetal distress.[28] The improvement in both pruritus and jaundice begins to occur quite promptly after delivery, most often within 24 hours. However, jaundice may continue for several days after delivery, and some of the abnormal chemistry profiles persist for as long as several months.

Subsequent pregnancies are frequently accompanied by recurrences of the syndrome.[23,29] However, the syndrome may be quite mild or, on occasion, even absent in later pregnancies.[30]

Biochemical Changes

The most frequent biochemical abnormalities noted in ICP are shown in Table 15–2. The earliest and most consistent change is a rise in serum bile acid concentrations. This includes a 10- to 100-fold rise in the serum cholic acid level. There is also a rise in chenodeoxycholic acid, but the increase is usually less, and the ratio of cholic acid to chenodeoxycholic acid increases above 1.[31]

The rise in serum bile acid levels is frequently followed by increases in serum transaminase values.[32] The ALT is elevated in approximately 65% of cases and the AST in approximately 60% of cases.[31] Although the elevation in serum transaminase values is usually mild, it occasionally reaches 500 IU/L or higher. Alkaline phosphatase elevations are common, and levels are increased above the elevations noted in normal pregnancy. The rise in alkaline phosphatase in this disease is accompanied by an elevation in 5′-nucleotidase, which indicates a hepatic source for the increased alkaline phosphatase. Bilirubin elevations occur in approximately 20% of patients, and the increased bilirubin is almost exclusively direct reacting. Although bilirubin is usually in the range of 2 to 5 mg/dL, values as high as 35 mg/dL have been reported in the absence of hemolysis.[27] The serum levels of GGTP are normal in most cases of ICP.[32] The minority of affected patients who have elevations in GGTP may be those carrying a defect in the multidrug resistance gene 3 (MDR3), the gene associated with PFIC type 3.[33-35]

Other laboratory changes that are commonly observed include a rise in serum cholesterol, triglyceride, phospholipid, and lipoprotein levels, including low-density lipoprotein X. There is usually a decrease in the high-density lipoprotein fraction.[36,37]

Prothrombin time is usually normal in this syndrome unless there is significant malabsorption. When malabsorption is worsened by cholestyramine administration, significant prothrombin time prolongation may occur. In these cases, the prothrombin time responds quickly to parenteral administration of vitamin K. There is often a demonstrable increase in fecal fat excretion if the disorder lasts 3 weeks or more.[20] Other biochemical changes include a rise in coproporphyrin excretion in the urine.[38] Alterations in estrogen metabolism, including a depression in the excretion of urinary estriol glucuronide and a rise in estriol sulfate excretion, also occur. These changes result from a marked decline in the biliary excretion of estriol, which may exceed 95%.[39]

Diagnosis

The diagnosis of ICP is usually based on the clinical symptoms of severe pruritus that appear in the second or third trimester of pregnancy, accompanied by a rise in serum bile acids, transaminases, and, on occasion, bilirubin. Dark urine and light color stools may also be present. It is important to exclude alternative diagnoses, such as viral hepatitis, mechanical biliary tract obstruction, or underlying chronic liver disease. This may require additional laboratory studies, including evaluation of hepatitis markers, a review of drug intake, abdominal ultrasonography and, in rare cases, liver biopsy.

In areas of high endemic incidence, ICP may account for 50% of the patients with abnormal liver studies in the last trimester[3]; however, in the United States, ICP is less common.

Histologic Features

Histologic study of the liver in ICP usually reveals only simple cholestasis. There is dilatation of the centrilobular bile canaliculi, and many of these contain bile plugs. Electron microscopic study shows swelling, distortion, and atrophy of the canalicular microvilli. There are mild changes elsewhere in the liver, but all of these are nonspecific. The picture is indistinguishable from that of intrahepatic cholestasis of other causes. Follow-up studies after delivery and resolution of the clinical syndrome reveal no abnormalities.[40]

Mechanism

The mechanism of ICP is uncertain. Current evidence suggests that it is an inherited phenomenon caused by more than one genetic abnormality.[20,23] There exists strong evidence that several defects in MDR3 can result in ICP.[34,35,41] The fact that a similar syndrome may be produced in normal women by administration of oral contraceptives suggests that hormones may play a role in its pathogenesis. This hypothesis is strengthened by the observation that women with a history of ICP also

TABLE 15–2	Intrahepatic Cholestasis of Pregnancy	
Clinical Features	**Biochemical Changes**	
Pruritus	Serum bile acids	10- to 100-fold
Jaundice*	Alkaline phosphatase	7- to 10-fold ↑
No anorexia or malaise	5′-Nucleotidase	Twofold ↑
Second or third trimester onset*	GGTP	Normal to slight ↑
Recurrent*	Bilirubin (total)	Normal to 5 mg/dL
Familial*	AST/ALT	↑↑
	Prothrombin time	Normal to twofold ↑
	Cholesterol	Twofold to fourfold ↑
	Triglyceride	Normal to twofold ↑

*These clinical features are not invariably present.
ALT, alanine aminotransferase; AST, aspartate aminotransferase; GGTP, γ-glutamyl-transpeptidase.
↑, increase.

had a high incidence of oral contraceptive–induced cholestasis on the early high-dose regimens.[13,20] Also, there is an increased incidence in twin pregnancies, which are associated with higher estrogen levels.[29] Studies have shown that abnormalities in serum bile acid levels may be produced by administration of estrogens to women with a history of ICP. In some cases, men, who may transmit the defect to their daughters, also show such abnormalities. Thus, the evidence suggests that predisposed individuals have an exaggerated liver response to estrogens.[42] Reports suggest that progesterone may play a role.[32,43]

Despite this strong evidence, there are some difficulties with the hypothesis. First, not all patients who have ICP respond with a recurrence of chemical abnormalities or symptoms with estrogen administration after delivery.[44] Also, occasional patients develop the syndrome early in the first trimester, when hormonal levels are normal. In addition, some improve before delivery, when estrogen levels are highest. Furthermore, symptoms may persist in some patients for as long as 8 weeks after delivery. Moreover, not all affected women have a recurrence in subsequent pregnancies. These variations on the syndrome are unexplained and suggest that factors in addition to hereditary hepatic sensitivity to estrogens play a role in the clinical disorder. A drop in the prevalence of ICP in Chile suggests the influence of unknown environmental factors.[45]

Effects on the Mother

Although earlier reports suggested that the only effect of ICP on the mother was related to the discomfort of pruritus, more recent studies have suggested more serious complications. These include an increased risk of postpartum hemorrhage, especially in those given cholestyramine, and an increased risk for the development of gallstones after pregnancy.[20]

Effects on the Fetus

The implications of ICP for the fetus are considerably more ominous. An increased incidence of prematurity and fetal death has been reported in several studies.[45-47] Fetal distress is reported in one third of patients, leading to cesarean section in 30% to 60% of cases and prematurity in over 50% in some series.[20] Stillbirths are recorded in more than 9%. These outcomes are more likely if the disorder begins earlier in pregnancy.[28] Thus, ICP very clearly increases the risks to the fetus. Diagnosis of the disease requires that the patient be observed closely, with early delivery by cesarean section if fetal distress appears.

Treatment

Therapy is directed at alleviating pruritus in the mother. Ursodeoxycholic acid has been used successfully in the treatment of cholestasis in other settings, most prominently primary biliary cirrhosis. Improvement in both liver function test results and the symptom of pruritus has been documented in women with ICP treated with

a standard 15-mg/kg/day dosage.[43,48,49] A larger dosage, 20 to 25 mg/kg/day has been shown to be effective with no adverse affects on either mother or baby.[50] The safety of ursodeoxycholic acid for either mother or fetus during pregnancy has not been clearly established.

Other older treatments are well established but less effective. Phenobarbital in a dosage of 100 mg/day has been reported to be effective in approximately 50% of patients.[51] Cholestyramine may be somewhat effective and is usually given in a dosage of 4 g four or five times per day. Cholestyramine must not be given in conjunction with other medications because of its nonspecific anion-binding capacity. Although cholestyramine reduces pruritus in more than 50% of patients, side effects are common; these include mild nausea, anorexia, bloating, and occasionally constipation. In addition, the cholestyramine may worsen the malabsorption of fats and fat-soluble vitamins. Therefore, the prothrombin time must be monitored in patients treated with this regimen, and parenteral vitamin K should be given before delivery.

More recently, intravenous or oral S-adenosyl-L-methionine has been reported to lead to a significant improvement in pruritus and in serum transaminase and bilirubin levels, perhaps by reducing the negative effects of estrogens on bile secretion.[38,52] These clinical observations have revealed both clinical improvement in mother and reduced fetal prematurity. In contrast, Chilean investigations found no improvement with this agent in a double-blind study.[28] Whether this indicates differences in trial design or differences in the mechanisms of the disease between the two groups is unknown.

Although induction of labor is not routinely recommended for all patients with ICP, the high frequency of fetal distress and premature delivery mandates close observation. Some investigators recommend elective induction at 38 weeks or as early as 36 weeks if the fetus's lungs have matured.[45] It is also advisable for patients with this syndrome to be aware of the possible recurrence of symptoms in association with oral contraceptives or subsequent pregnancies.

Preeclamptic Liver Disease

Several clinically distinct syndromes of liver involvement occur in patients with preeclampsia and, presumably, are related etiologically to it. These conditions—HELLP syndrome, hepatic hematoma with rupture, and hepatic infarction—can be grouped together under the rubric of preeclamptic liver disease. Acute fatty liver of pregnancy (AFLP) often, perhaps even usually, occurs in patients with preeclampsia. However, it is a clinically and histologically distinct disease, one that traditionally is categorized separately.

Preeclampsia is a common but poorly understood disorder unique to humans, complicating 5% to 10% of pregnancies.[53,54] It is a multisystem disorder, best known by its effects on the cardiovascular system, which lead to hypertension, and on the kidneys, which lead to proteinuria and hyperuricemia. Involvement of the central nervous system can occur, and eclampsia is defined by the complication of seizures. These and other signs and symptoms result from some generalized underlying pathologic process that still eludes definition. What is known is that implantation of the trophoblast is abnormal, leading to restricted blood flow to the fetal-placental unit. An increase in systemic vascular resistant results, leading to hypoperfusion of various organs.[55]

The uncertainty about the origin of this disorder is reflected in the imprecision of its name. It was previously known as *toxemia of pregnancy*. More recently, it has been termed *pregnancy-induced hypertension*, although this term fails to highlight the multisystemic nature of the disorder. More precision in terminology and in diagnosis will have to await discovery of the underlying pathogenesis. Until such time, we must be content with the diagnostic uncertainty typical of other such clinically defined syndromes.

HELLP Syndrome

This term, coined in 1982, is an acronym for several clinical findings that, when they occur together, signify potentially serious involvement of the liver in the preeclamptic patient.[56] These findings are *h*emolysis (usually modest with bizarrely shaped red blood cells on peripheral smear), *e*levated *l*iver test results (primarily aminotransferases), and *l*ow *p*latelets (<100,000/m). Although the name and the collection of findings are awkward, the term is very evocative of the syndrome and has gained widespread acceptance among practitioners. It is not rare; it was diagnosed in 437 (20%) of 2331 women with severe preeclampsia.[57] As part of the syndrome of preeclampsia, its occurrence is limited to the latter half of pregnancy, usually the third trimester. It may have its onset, or be recognized clinically, after delivery in up to 30% of cases.

Prominent among the clinical characteristics of this syndrome (Table 15–3) is a chief complaint at presentation of pain, which may be quite variable, including pain in the right upper quadrant, the lower chest, or midepigastrium. Almost one third of affected patients have no symptoms other than the hypertension and proteinuria typical of preeclampsia. Indeed, not all patients who subsequently receive this diagnosis have hypertension or proteinuria at presentation. As much as 30% of patients with HELLP present after delivery.[57]

As the words of the acronym suggest, the diagnosis rests on laboratory test demonstration of liver involvement associated with thrombocytopenia. The liver test abnormalities are hepatocellular, in contrast with cholestatic, with elevations in AST and ALT. These elevations can be modest, as low as 70 U, or can be high enough to suggest viral hepatitis, up to several thousand. As a rule, true hepatic failure is not present, and liver function is normal, with a normal prothrombin time and fibrinogen level, unless the course is complicated by disseminated intravascular coagulation. Thrombocytopenia is present, usually below 100,000/m. Platelet levels late in normal pregnancy can be as low as 100,000 to 125,000/m, as a result of the hemodilution present late in pregnancy. The hemolysis usually is subclinical, signified only by microangiopathic changes on the peripheral blood smear. Bilirubin elevations are modest, usually below that which causes jaundice. The lactate dehydrogenase levels are often elevated, presumably because of the ongoing hemolysis or the sequestration of red blood cells in areas of hemorrhage within the liver.

Findings on liver biopsy in HELLP syndrome are unique.[58,59] Nevertheless, biopsy is not needed to confirm this disorder, which is defined by laboratory findings in a specific setting. Furthermore, biopsy carries potential risk in these patients and should be undertaken only with care. The histologic features of HELLP syndrome are those previously described in preeclampsia: namely, periportal hemorrhage and fibrin deposition (Fig. 15–1). The pathologic process is centered on the portal triad (zone 1), although in severe cases the areas of hemorrhage may extend well into the midzone. There are peliotic collections of red blood cells, with disruption of the hepatocytes and necrosis. These areas may also show fibrin deposition. There may be infiltration of neutrophils adjacent to the areas of hemorrhage. This lesion is unique, not reported in other disorders in either humans or experimental animals. Not all affected patients have these abnormalities, and the biopsy findings may be normal, which suggests that the involvement is spotty. Interestingly, there is no statistical correlation between the severity of the histologic involvement and the degree of abnormality in either aminotransferases or platelet count.[60] Thus, the clinician cannot safely predict the severity of the liver involvement on the basis of the laboratory findings.

The biopsy specimen in patients with HELLP syndrome may also demonstrate steatosis.[60,61] This may be either as large- or small-droplet fat. When present, the fatty infiltration is modest and not centered on the central veins. It is not superimposable on the microvesicular infiltration typical of AFLP and the other microvesicular fat disorders, including tetracycline toxicity and Reye's syndrome.[62]

The liver in preeclampsia also demonstrates deposition of fibrinogen along the sinusoids, even in the absence of detectable liver injury.[63] This is best seen with special stains, such as that used in immunofluorescence assays, and is similar to the glomerular deposition of fibrinogen documented in preeclampsia. It is also not specific, having been demonstrated in patients with AFLP.[64]

The course of HELLP syndrome is that of the underlying preeclampsia. Delivery is indicated for reasons

TABLE 15–3   HELLP Syndrome

Clinical Features	Laboratory Changes	
Pain		
Right upper quadrant	Bilirubin	Slight ↑, normal
Midepigastrium, right chest	AST/ALT	↑, 70-1500 U
Preeclampsia	Prothrombin time	Normal
Second half of gestation;	Uric acid	↑
postpartum onset possible		
Nausea, vomiting; post-	LDH	↑
partum onset possible	Fibrinogen	Normal
	Platelets	<100,000/m³

ALT; alanine aminotransferase; AST, aspartate aminotransferase; HELLP, hemolysis, elevated liver test results, and low platelets; LDH, lactate dehydrogenase.
↑, increase.

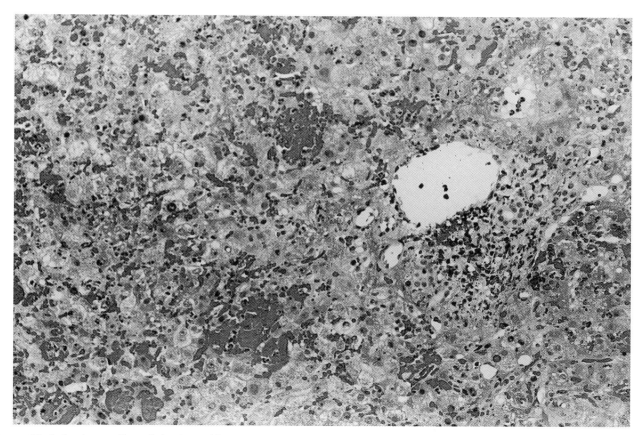

Figure 15–1. Syndrome of hemolysis, elevated liver enzymes, and low platelets (HELLP) as shown on liver biopsy specimen. The portal triad is surrounded by areas of hemorrhage with peliotic collections of red blood cells. There is a mixed cellular infiltrate. An area of fibrin deposition is seen adjacent to the portal triad in the upper right corner of the illustration. (From Gitnick G: Principles and Practice of Gastroenterology and Hepatology, 2nd ed. Norwalk, Conn, Appleton & Lange, 1994.)

involving both mother and fetus. Once delivered, most affected mothers have an uneventful recovery, with return of the platelet count to normal within 7 days. Failure to deliver the patient may lead to eclampsia or to extension of the liver disease to hepatic hematoma or rupture.[57] Occasional patients can be "tided over" on bed rest and antihypertensive treatment, with transient improvement in both the aminotransferase levels and the thrombocytopenia.[65] Corticosteroids can be used to delay delivery.[66,67] In such patients, serial monitoring of the fetus often demonstrates lack of intrauterine growth, which suggests that the preeclamptic process persists. Infants of affected mothers do not have HELLP syndrome, and thrombocytopenia in the newborn is rare in this setting.[68,69] They may, however, show results typical of preeclampsia, including intrauterine growth restriction and prematurity.

The differential diagnosis in patients with this disorder can be challenging. The gastroenterologist/hepatologist first considers other disorders leading to elevated aminotransferases, including viral hepatitis. Hepatitis serologic profiles are useful but often require more time to determine than is allowed by the urgency of the clinical setting. A history of risk factors, such as a new sexual partner within the preceding 4 months, which is suggestive of

hepatitis B, can be helpful. The primary hepatotropic viruses (hepatitis A, B, C, or D) do not result in disease that is more likely to manifest late in pregnancy, at the time typical for preeclampsia. On the other hand, both herpes simplex virus and hepatitis E are exacerbated by pregnancy and may manifest as severe hepatitis, with or without hepatic failure, at term.[70,71] No form of hepatitis is associated with hypertension, however. More troublesome to exclude is the diagnosis of AFLP, which is often associated with preeclampsia and may overlap with HELLP syndrome.[64] Unlike patients with HELLP syndrome, those with AFLP have true hepatic failure, with a prolonged prothrombin time, decreased fibrinogen, and, in severe cases, encephalopathy and hypoglycemia.

The differential diagnosis of thrombocytopenia in pregnancy is long.[68] Particularly problematic is the distinction of HELLP syndrome from thrombotic thrombocytopenic purpura (TTP). Although the microangiopathy and central nervous system and renal involvement typical of TTP may mimic those of preeclampsia, patients with TTP are not hypertensive, and fever is not a sign of HELLP syndrome. Also, TTP is not improved by delivery. Idiopathic thrombocytopenic purpura can also present a problem in differential diagnosis, but it is not associated with preeclampsia and usually has a benign outcome in pregnancy. Thrombocytopenia also occurs in patients with an antiphospholipid antibody, with or without systemic lupus erythematosus. Finally, as many as 75% to 80% of pregnant women with thrombocytopenia have a benign condition termed *gestational thrombocytopenia,* isolated thrombocytopenia as low as 70,000/m without associated preeclampsia or morbidity for the mother or infant.

Hepatic Hematoma and Rupture

Spontaneous rupture of the liver in pregnancy is a catastrophic event leading to fetal and maternal mortality in a large number of cases.[72-74] Although the precise disease progression is unclear, it can be presumed that this is the severe extreme of the spectrum of HELLP syndrome, and hematoma with rupture has been reported to occur in 1% of patients with HELLP syndrome.[57] Hepatic rupture occurs in patients with preeclampsia, although hypertension is often absent, at least when patients present in shock. Affected patients are more likely to be multigravida and to be older than 30 years. The initial symptoms are usually related to stretch or irritation of the liver capsule, with pain in the right upper quadrant or right lower chest. Initially, there is hemorrhage beneath the intact liver capsule, leading to a contained hematoma that lifts the capsule away from the surface of the liver.[75] If the capsule ruptures, then free hemorrhage develops from the exposed surface of the liver into the peritoneum, and the patient presents with abdominal distention, shock, and profound anemia. After resuscitation, the hypertension typical of the underlying preeclampsia may become evident.

The diagnosis of hematoma of the liver requires imaging of the abdomen.[76] Ultrasonography may demonstrate the collection of blood, but more complete information can be gained from computed tomographic (CT) scan, with and without contrast, or magnetic resonance imaging. Affected patients have the thrombocytopenia and elevated aminotransferases typical of HELLP syndrome. Liver biopsy is contraindicated in this setting; it should never be performed if hepatic hematoma is under consideration, but, if performed, it should be done in HELLP syndrome with only the utmost care. To avoid problems, it seems prudent to perform CT scanning before biopsy in this setting. When available, the histologic study shows that the region adjacent to a rupture has microscopic hemorrhage and fibrin deposits, with a neutrophilic infiltrate, similar to the findings typical of HELLP syndrome. After rupture of the liver, hemoperitoneum can be confirmed by peritoneal aspiration, which yields unclotted blood. Affected patients often have an associated consumptive coagulopathy, with prolongation of the prothrombin time and low fibrinogen levels.

Management of hepatic hematoma or rupture should be aggressive; if the patient survives, the liver will return to normal when the preeclampsia resolves. Toward this end, the patient should be delivered on an emergency basis. If the patient has a hematoma alone, without free rupture, then conservative management with observation and maximal support in an intensive care unit can be chosen. If the capsule has ruptured, then immediate surgery is the treatment of choice, preferably with the help of surgeons experienced in the management of trauma to the liver, the most comparable situation.[77] At operation, the liver surface is seen to be exposed with multiple bleeding points. An omental patch can be constructed, or the liver can be packed with Gelfoam with the intent of reoperating in several days. If the rupture is limited, a lobectomy can be undertaken.

Hepatic rupture is not common, and there exist no studies comparing possible modes of therapy. Some authors have suggested radiologic embolization or surgical ligation of the hepatic artery.[78] When called for, the liver can be removed and the patient held anhepatic until a donor for liver transplantation can be found; this is a rather radical approach to a problem that can resolve with maximal supportive care.[79,80] Recurrence of hepatic hematoma with rupture has been reported, and affected patients should be informed of this possibility.[81]

Hepatic Infarction

Another clinical scenario associated with preeclampsia, and presumably with HELLP syndrome, is hepatic infarction: large geographic infarctions in the liver.[82,83] Affected patients present with abdominal pain and fever. Laboratory tests demonstrate thrombocytopenia and massive elevations in aminotransferase, in the range of 5000 to 8000 U. Except in the most severe cases, hepatic failure is not present. CT scanning confirms the diagnosis and demonstrates punched-out, poorly vascularized areas, often in more than one lobe of the liver. Aspiration of these areas has been undertaken, particularly because of the attendant fever, and yields only necrotic debris. Histologic study shows hemorrhage with neutrophilic infiltration in areas adjacent to the infarction. Presumably, this disorder results when adjacent areas within the liver are affected with the periportal hemorrhage typical of HELLP syndrome, and these areas coalesce to form a geographic infarction. Despite the impressive elevations in aminotransferases and the alarming images, affected patients have few symptoms and recover with no therapy. As is true of the other preeclampsia-related syndromes, prompt delivery is indicated.

Acute Fatty Liver of Pregnancy

This rare liver disorder unique to pregnancy is justifiably feared.[64,83-85] Reports of probable cases were published almost a century and a half ago. Sheehan, who is perhaps now better known for his description of postpartum pituitary necrosis, first recognized this disorder as a distinct syndrome in 1940.[86] He named it *acute yellow atrophy,* but it is now more commonly known as *acute fatty liver of pregnancy.* The fact that the name of this disorder has remained essentially unchanged, and universally used, testifies to the fact that, unlike the preeclamptic liver disorders, this is a distinct clinical disease, not merely a syndrome or collection of signs and symptoms. AFLP is rare, encountered in a tertiary maternity hospital approximately once a year, with a reported incidence of 1 in 13,000 to 1 in 16,000 deliveries.[87,88] Despite its distinct clinical hallmarks and biopsy appearance, its underlying pathogenesis remains elusive. Preeclampsia is present in 50% or more of cases of AFLP and may play a role in its origin. Reports of occasional recurrent cases and an association with a deficiency of long-chain 3-hydroxyacyl-coenzyme A (CoA) dehydrogenase, raise the interesting notion that, at least in some instances, this disease results from an inborn error of metabolism.[89-95]

Clinical Characteristics

AFLP occurs in the latter half of pregnancy, usually close to term (Table 15-4). As with HELLP syndrome, affected patients may present after delivery.[96] It is reported to occur more commonly in a first pregnancy and in the presence of multiple pregnancy, both factors also prevalent in preeclampsia.[85] There are reports of an association between AFLP and gestation of a male fetus.[68,92] Affected women have nonspecific symptoms, including, prominently, nausea and vomiting, malaise and fatigue, jaundice, thirst, headache, and altered mental status. These can be signs and symptoms of acute hepatic failure. Such severe disease is not universal at presentation, however, and many reports of asymptomatic patients, who have a very mild clinical course, exist. In these cases, the diagnosis was based on liver biopsy performed in evaluation of abnormal liver function tests at term.[64] In severe cases that go untreated, there is progression over hours or days to fulminant hepatic failure, with hepatic coma, hypoglycemia, severe coagulopathy with hemorrhage from the gastrointestinal tract or the uterus, and death. Most affected women have signs of coexistent preeclampsia, including modest elevations in blood pressure, hyperuricemia, and proteinuria. Very high blood pressures are not usual in the setting of AFLP, because hepatic failure leads to diminished systemic vascular resistance and relative hypotension. The symptom of abdominal or substernal pain can often be elicited, but rarely is it a major symptom volunteered by the patient at presentation.

Laboratory tests confirm involvement of the liver, with elevations in aminotransferases, in cholestatic enzymes such as GGTP, and in bilirubin. The aminotransferase elevations are usually modest, below 1000 U, and normal aminotransferase values have been reported in confirmed cases.[64,85] More striking are the abnormalities in the true liver function tests, especially the prothrombin time and fibrinogen. There may be a marked reduction in antithrombin III levels.[97] As is the case in other forms of hepatic failure, the ammonia level may be high and the blood glucose level low. The platelet count may be low, because of attendant disseminated intravascular coagulation, leading to overlap with HELLP syndrome in some cases.[64,85] Many affected patients are also found to have leukocytosis, with elevations of white blood cell count above the high range expected during normal pregnancy.

The histologic features of this disease are distinctive but can be misleading.[64,85,98] The classic lesion of AFLP is microvesicular fatty infiltration, most prominently involving the pericentral region, zone 3 of the liver lobule (Fig. 15-2). The fat droplets are small, resulting in a picture of pallor and cell vacuolization in affected areas, rather than the empty cell with the asymmetric nucleus seen in large-droplet fat. This change can easily be overlooked or misinterpreted on histologic material handled in the routine way with paraffin embedding, which causes the fat to dissolve. Indeed, the biopsy appearance of AFLP can easily be interpreted as resulting from viral hepatitis, with ballooning of cells and cytolysis. In order to predictably detect the fatty change, the biopsy material must be processed in a special way. In the past, the technique used was frozen section, followed by staining with oil red O. This technique has its faults: The stain intensity is poorly reproducible, and it is difficult to interpret frozen material, particularly as the droplets can be smeared away from the affected areas to cover the whole specimen. A better technique is to handle the tissue as if for electron microscopy, with glutaraldehyde fixation and embedding in Epon. The microvesicular fat can be seen clearly by examining toluidine blue-stained sections under the light microscopy or by electron microscopy. The picture at the electron microscopic level is a nonspecific one, which includes non–membrane-bound fat droplets and mitochondrial changes.[85,99] As is true of the other microvesicular diseases, the fatty change is evanescent and resolves in several days. Therefore, the most typical histologic appearance is found early in the course. Involvement of other organs with microvesicular fatty change has been reported.[100]

Course and Management

Patients with undiagnosed AFLP are at risk for progression, with an unpredictable but often short time course, to fulminant hepatic failure and death for both mother and fetus. As recently as the 1960s, the conventional wisdom was that if the patient survived, the diagnosis could not have been AFLP. More recent reports give a much improved outlook in this disease, and now it is rare for a patient to die, with appropriate diagnosis and aggressive management.[64,85,88,101,102] Similarly, the outlook for the fetus of the affected pregnancy has also improved, although it remains worse than that of the mother.

Like Reye's syndrome, AFLP is well defined clinically, and histologic confirmation is not needed except in special circumstances. Usually, the diagnosis rests on finding

TABLE 15-4	**Acute Fatty Liver of Pregnancy**	
Clinical Features	**Laboratory Changes**	
Nausea, vomiting	Bilirubin	Slight ↑, normal
Malaise, fatigue	AST/ALT	↑, normal to 1000 U
Jaundice	GGTP	Slight ↑
Abdominal pain	Prothrombin time	↑↑
Preeclampsia	Fibrinogen	↓↓
Coma	Uric acid	↑
Bleeding	Ammonia	↑
Onset in second half of gestation; postpartum onset possible	Glucose	↓
	Leukocytes	↑
	Platelets	↔, ↑

ALT, alanine aminotransferase; AST, aspartate aminotransferase; GGTP, γ-glutamyl-transpeptidase.
↑, increased; ↓, decrease; ↔, no change from normal.

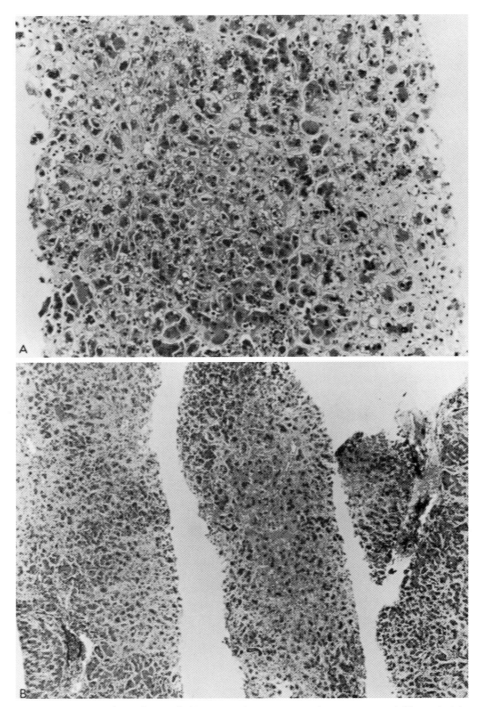

Figure 15–2. Fatty liver of pregnancy as shown by needle biopsy specimen. **A,** Many hepatocytes are infiltrated with small droplets of fat. These droplets stain positively with a Sudan stain for lipid. **B,** The predominance of the infiltration in pericentral areas is shown. There is relative sparing of the middle zone and periportal areas of the lobule. (Courtesy of The Klatskin Library, Yale University.)

hepatic failure at term in the absence of any risk factors, physical findings (such as vesicular rash in herpes simplex hepatitis), or serologic profiles suggestive of viral hepatitis.[103] Most patients have signs of preeclampsia, albeit subtle at times. Imaging may be useful; fat in the liver has been demonstrated in AFLP with ultrasonography and CT scanning.[89,104,105] These changes are modest, however,

and are best proven by comparing the CT scan during illness with that obtained several months later, after resolution of the disease. Thus, imaging may help confirm the diagnosis in retrospect but may not be helpful in the acute situation. The presence of a normal liver on CT scan certainly does not exclude AFLP. The liver biopsy is diagnostic, if the specimen is processed appropriately.

Biopsy is necessary only in special circumstances of diagnostic confusion. For example, if delivery is being delayed, then a biopsy finding compatible with AFLP should prompt it. In this setting, biopsy should be performed with care, because the coagulopathy and the potential overlap with the preeclampsia syndromes, including HELLP and rupture. The differentiation between HELLP syndrome and AFLP is of little immediate clinical relevance, because both are treated identically: namely, by delivery of the fetus.

Treatment of AFLP begins with delivery. The route should be guided by obstetric indications. Cesarean section is not always necessary; vaginal delivery can be accomplished. With delivery, repair of the liver disease begins, the initial sign of improvement being a fall in prothrombin time elevation. In severely ill patients, recovery may be lengthy, and complications such as gastrointestinal bleeding, adult respiratory distress syndrome, and pancreatitis with metastatic fat necrosis have been reported.[106] Diabetes insipidus has been reported in several patients with AFLP.[107] Diuresis in affected patients should not be assumed to result simply from normal postpartum shifts in volume. In this setting, the occurrence of diabetes insipidus should suggest that AFLP is the diagnosis, although it is not specific for this disease and has also been reported in patients with HELLP syndrome.[108] This interesting finding appears to result from abnormally high circulating levels of vasopressinase.[109] The management should include maximal support in an intensive care unit by a team that includes both obstetricians and hepatologists. Liver transplantation for AFLP has been reported.[110,111] Early diagnosis and delivery, with aggressive supportive management, should obviate the need for such herculean therapy, particularly as the disease is not chronic.

There are no residua after AFLP, and complete recovery of the affected patient should be expected. Cases of recurrent AFLP, as well as cases of nonketotic hypoglycemia in the offspring, have been reported and are discussed later. In view of this risk, mothers and the infants from affected pregnancies can be tested for the gene defect in long-chain 3-hydroxyacyl–CoA dehydrogenase.[94,112] In general, the risk to the mother in subsequent pregnancies is slim, although all patients with a history of AFLP should be managed by obstetricians expert in maternal-fetal medicine.

Cause and Pathogenesis

AFLP remains a disease of unclear origin. It appears to share some clinical hallmarks with the other disorders classified as microvesicular fatty liver diseases, including Reye's syndrome, Jamaican vomiting sickness, and the disorders of fatty acid metabolism, the most common of which is medium-chain acyl-CoA dehydrogenase deficiency.[62] These conditions share mitochondrial dysfunction as an underlying pathogenic mechanism. In Jamaican vomiting sickness, the toxin hypoglycin, present in the arils of unripe ackee fruit, poisons β oxidation in the mitochondrion, leading to a Reye's-like syndrome and the presence in the urine of abnormal organic acids.[113] Similarly, individuals with the inherited defect

medium-chain acyl-CoA dehydrogenase deficiency may have episodes during infancy and childhood, perhaps prompted by anorexia and stress such as a febrile illness, of hyperammonemia and nonketotic hypoglycemia suggestive of recurrent Reye's syndrome.[114] Most genotypically affected individuals never have clinical disease, however. Interestingly, tetracycline, which had previously been associated with an AFLP-like syndrome in both pregnant and nonpregnant patients receiving intravenous therapy, also affects mitochondrial function.[115,116] AFLP is not simply Reye's syndrome of pregnancy, and subtle differences can be detected on electron microscopy.[99]

The reports in the literature of recurrent AFLP suggest that perhaps this syndrome is also the result of an inborn error of metabolism. This postulate is supported by demonstrations that the offspring of AFLP pregnancies were affected with a defect in fatty acid oxidation, long-chain 3-hydroxyacyl–CoA dehydrogenase (LCHAD) deficiency.[91,92,95] These infants failed to thrive and died. Their mothers had either AFLP or HELLP during the pregnancy, although pregnancies that resulted in the birth of unaffected children were normal. Subsequent studies have shown that some but not all women with AFLP are heterozygous for LCHAD deficiency.[93,95] The molecular basis for this deficiency has been established, and DNA testing for it is available.[94] Genotyping should be carried out on both parents and the infant of the affected pregnancy. The implication is that disease in the fetus can affect the course of pregnancy for the mother, with the presumption that she is an otherwise phenotypically normal heterozygote. Other reports, however, fail to confirm the associations between LCHAD deficiency and AFLP.[117] These fascinating observations should prompt further investigation of affected patients, as well as of women with a history of AFLP.

The relationship of AFLP with preeclampsia is the subject of much debate. Half of reported cases of AFLP occur in women with preeclampsia, and the timing (at the end of pregnancy), the association with the primigravid state and with multiple gestation, and the improvement with delivery are all suggestive of underlying preeclampsia.[64,84] An overlap among the preeclamptic syndromes (HELLP, infarction, and rupture) has been reported.[106] Women with AFLP in association with LCHAD deficiency were more likely to have preeclampsia.[93] Nevertheless, at the bedside the problems are different and can usually be distinguished on purely clinical grounds. One group suggested that the fat found on biopsy in patients with preeclampsia or HELLP demonstrates that these conditions are one and the same.[61] However, the fatty change in HELLP syndrome is usually only modest in extent, may be both microvesicular and macrovesicular, and does not have the characteristic central location.[60] Furthermore, there are no reports of the occurrence of the histologic changes typical of HELLP (periportal hemorrhage and fibrin deposition) in patients with biopsy-documented AFLP. Therefore, until further explication, we surmise that preeclampsia is a permissive condition, a stress that brings out AFLP in susceptible individuals. Previous reports suggest that male gender in the fetus makes AFLP more likely.[85]

LIVER DISEASE DURING PREGNANCY

Common forms of liver disease occur during pregnancy, although the diagnosis, clinical course, and therapy for these diseases differ from those in nonpregnant persons. The major diseases of the liver are reviewed, with special emphasis on features relevant to pregnancy, including effects on the fetus.

Hepatitis

Hepatitis may be caused by a number of well-characterized viruses, as well as by drugs or autoimmune disease. Usually cytomegalovirus, measles, Epstein-Barr virus, and herpes simplex are not included as causes of "viral hepatitis," although each may cause hepatocellular necrosis and inflammation. Cytomegalovirus infection during pregnancy may cause hepatitis, even of the fulminant type, often with congenital infection in the newborn. Measles during pregnancy may cause maternal hepatitis and adverse outcomes for the infant, including prematurity, spontaneous abortion, and death.[118] Severe herpes simplex–related hepatitis in pregnancy has been successfully treated with acyclovir.[103,119]

The term *hepatitis* is conventionally reserved for viral infection caused by hepatitis A, hepatitis B, hepatitis C, δ hepatitis, and hepatitis E viruses. The characteristics of these forms of hepatitis are shown in Table 15-5. Advances in serologic identification of the hepatitis viruses have led to clearer separation of the clinical diseases caused by each of these infections. Although there is considerable overlap, the clinical course of each form of infection is somewhat different, and the complications of infection are substantially different. The latter differences are especially noteworthy during pregnancy because of variable implications for the subsequent health of both mother and infant.[120]

Hepatitis A

Hepatitis A virus (HAV) infection is common worldwide. It occurs more frequently in impoverished populations, in lower socioeconomic groups, and in developing nations, where poor hygienic conditions often exist. In Central America, Asia, and Africa, it is usually a disease of childhood or adolescence. In Western Europe and North America, it is a sporadic infection and usually affects adults. Localized epidemics occur.[121] In the remaining parts of the world, it is an epidemic disease of susceptible individuals of all ages. The overall incidence of positive serology for HAV infection in the United States averages approximately 30%. Evidence of prior infection is high among certain risk groups, including parenteral drug abusers, homosexual men, prostitutes, sexually promiscuous persons, and elderly persons. The disease is transmitted almost exclusively by the fecal-oral route. Contaminated food and water are the usual sources of epidemic HAV infection. In the United States, HAV infection is often reported in association with ingestion of contaminated shellfish. Another important source is exposure to diapered children in daycare settings.

The clinical syndrome of acute HAV infection consists of vague flu-like symptoms with fatigue, weakness, nausea, and loss of appetite. The onset is usually abrupt. A variety of extrahepatic manifestations, including myalgia, arthralgias, arthritis, and urticaria, may occur.[121] A small proportion of patients develop severe disease heralded by the onset of marked vomiting, abdominal pain, and fever. In a very small number, fulminant HAV infection with massive hepatocellular necrosis occurs, possibly leading to death. Other forms of HAV infection include cholestatic hepatitis, with a prolonged course marked by itching and jaundice, and relapsing hepatitis, with a relapse within 3 months of disease onset. In rare cases, HAV infection can precipitate autoimmune hepatitis, responsive to corticosteroids.[121] Most cases of hepatitis A, however, are subclinical.

TABLE 15–5 Forms of Viral Hepatitis

Characteristics	Hepatitis A	Hepatitis B	Hepatitis C
Older name	Infectious hepatitis	Serum hepatitis	Non-A, non-B hepatitis
Virus type	RNA	DNA	RNA
Virus size	27 nm	42 nm	30-60 nm
Incubation period	15-50 days	30-180 days	30-160 days
Transmission	Fecal-oral	Parenteral or body fluids	Parenteral, sporadic
Vertical transmission to fetus	Not observed	Common	Uncommon
Serologic diagnosis	Hepatitis A antibody IgM and IgG types	HBsAg, HBsAb; HBcAb, IgM, and IgG types HBeAg, Ab, hepatitis B virus DNA	Hepatitis C antibody RNA by PCR
Maximum infectivity	Prodrome	Prodrome or HbeAg positive	HIV co-infected
Carrier state	None	5%-10%	50%-85%
Acute clinical forms	Asymptomatic to fulminant	Asymptomatic to fulminant	Asymptomatic to severe; relapsing
Chronic clinical forms	None	Chronic persistent hepatitis Chronic active hepatitis Cirrhosis	Chronic persistent hepatitis Chronic active hepatitis Cirrhosis

HBsAb, hepatitis B surface-associated antibody; HBsAg, hepatitis B surface-associated antigen; HBcAb, hepatitis B core antibody; HBeAg, hepatitis B early antigen; HIV, human immunodeficiency virus; IgG, immunoglobulin G; IgM, immunoglobulin M; PCR, polymerase chain reaction.

Early in the onset of the disease, antibody to HAV appears in the serum. The antibody is of the immunoglobulin M (IgM) type during the acute illness and early recovery phase. Several months later, the antibody becomes predominantly immunoglobulin G in type. The latter antibody is protective and remains detectable for many years. Therefore, it is currently possible to confirm recent infection with HAV by the presence of IgM antibody. Because there exists no chronic carrier state for HAV, this is the only period in which HAV IgM antibody is present.

The characteristic changes in liver function test findings include marked elevations in AST and ALT. Most often, these reach levels of 1000 to 2000 U during the early part of the infection. Elevations in bilirubin and alkaline phosphatase also occur but are more unpredictable. The entire infection may be anicteric, but on occasion it is associated with severe jaundice, pruritus, and light-colored stools. The latter may be confused clinically with biliary obstruction. The acute illness usually lasts 10 to 15 days, and then gradual recovery begins. Most patients are free of symptoms by 1 to 2 months after the onset of the disease, although ill effects may linger longer in some. Except for fulminant HAV infection, there are no serious sequelae or chronic forms of this disease.

There is substantial evidence that pregnancy does not alter the course of HAV infection in the United States and Europe. However, a higher incidence of fulminant disease associated with acute HAV infection during pregnancy has been reported in developing nations, although the reason is uncertain. Concurrent malnutrition has been a suspected cause, but the evidence is conflicting. If the course of HAV infection is severe, it may precipitate premature labor in women in the third trimester of pregnancy.[121] There is no evidence that HAV causes birth defects,[122] and there is no evidence of maternal-fetal transmission.[123]

Clinical management of pregnant patients with HAV infection does not differ from that of those who are not pregnant. However, hospitalization may be indicated, especially during the last trimester and in the presence of severe anorexia, nausea, and vomiting. Under these circumstances, the differential diagnosis may be uncertain, and close observation indicated. On occasion, vomiting is so severe that parenteral administration of fluids is necessary.

HAV infection may be prevented in close household contacts by the administration of immune serum globulin. This is recommended for those at risk in the home. In rare circumstances in which the mother has acute HAV infection at the time of delivery, immune serum globulin may be administered to the infant. Even under these conditions, the risk of transmission to the infant seems very small.

Hepatitis B

Acute hepatitis B virus (HBV) infection has clinical similarities to HAV infection. However, the incubation period is longer (1 to 6 months), and the prodrome is more frequently associated with extrahepatic symptoms such as rash, arthralgias, myalgias, and occasionally frank arthritis. Jaundice may occur. In addition, 5% to 10% of patients enter a chronic phase of HBV infection, and almost half these patients develop chronic active hepatitis and cirrhosis. The 10% who become chronic HBV carriers also have a high incidence of hepatocellular carcinoma 10 to 25 years after initial infection.

The disease is worldwide in distribution but is most common in Asia and Africa, where transmission is frequently by the maternal-fetal route.[124] In North America, HBV is transmitted most commonly by heterosexual contact. However, maternal-fetal transmission is well recognized and presents a major problem for both obstetrician and pediatrician.

HBV infection is confirmed by the presence of specific serologic markers as listed in Table 15–6. Hepatitis B surface antigen (HBsAg), hepatitis B early antigen (HBeAg), and hepatitis B core antibody appear early in the disease, usually before the onset of clinical symptoms. Initially, this antibody is primarily of the IgM class, but late in normal recovery, a gradual transition to a predominant immunoglobulin G antibody occurs. The presence of IgM hepatitis B core antibody indicates acute infection. In those who do not become HBV carriers, hepatitis B surface antibody appears, and this antibody, as well as the hepatitis B core antibody, may persist for many years.

HBV infection accounts for approximately one third of sporadic cases of viral hepatitis in the general U.S. population. The incidence of the HBV carrier state among pregnant women is variable and depends on the patient group studied. The incidence of HBV carriers is considerably higher in populations in which drug abuse is commonplace or with a high incidence of sexual promiscuity. Also, Asian and African immigrants and some American Indian populations have a high incidence of the HBV carrier state. Evidence suggests that transmission of HBV to infants is common when mothers have acute infection in the third trimester or when they are chronic carriers of HBV infection and have positive results of serum tests for HBeAg or HBV DNA.[125]

Acute HBV infection during early pregnancy is usually accompanied by a normal course without significant implications for either the mother or the infant. In the past, hepatitis with a high acute mortality rate in certain areas of the world, including the Middle East, Africa, and India, was reported during pregnancy. This severe hepatitis in pregnancy has now been shown to be caused by infection with hepatitis E virus (HEV).[71]

Certainly, fulminant hepatitis that develops during the course of the acute infection in a small percentage of women in Western countries has a high mortality rate. However, the incidence of this severe form of viral hepatitis does not seem to be higher during pregnancy in the

TABLE 15–6 Hepatitis B Terminology	
Hepatitis B virus	Dane particle
Hepatitis B core antibody	HBcAb
Hepatitis B surface antigen	HBsAg
Hepatitis B surface antibody	HBsAb
Hepatitis Be antigen	HBeAg
Hepatitis Be antibody	HBeAb
Hyperimmune serum globulin	HBIG
Hepatitis B viral DNA	HBV DNA

TABLE 15–7   Management of Acute Viral Hepatitis in Pregnancy

Establish type by serologic test
Institute appropriate isolation and precautions
Determine need for contact prophylaxis with serum globulin preparation and/or vaccine
Activity: determined by tolerance
Diet: patient preference, parenteral if necessary
Antiemetics: phenothiazines may be used
Corticosteroids: not indicated
Immunoprophylaxis of infant: if hepatitis B is present

United States. For this reason, fulminant acute HBV infection is a relatively small factor in either maternal or fetal death in this country.

Clinical management of acute HBV during pregnancy should not be different from that in a nonpregnant individual (Table 15-7). However, when the infection occurs during the last trimester, there is a high risk of transmission of the disease to the infant.[126-128] The risk of transmission is highest in mothers who are HBeAg-positive at the time of delivery. The presence of HBeAg in serum is usually correlated with higher levels of serum HBV DNA. Thus, the presence of HBeAg in the mother is a measure of a high titer of virus in blood and, hence, increased risk of transmission to fetus and newborn. During acute viral hepatitis, HBeAg positivity is usually transient, and transmission in utero or to the newborn is much more likely when the mother has acute infection just before or at the time of delivery. It is estimated that approximately 5% of the infants may be infected with HBV at birth and have acquired the disease by the transplacental route.[128,129] Little can be done to prevent this kind of transmission to the fetus. In addition, other mothers who are incubating HBV at the time of delivery can infect their offspring before they become clinically ill. These two groups may account for a small number of infants who eventually become infected with HBV despite adequate therapy to prevent infection of the newborn after delivery.

The second group of mothers who may commonly transmit HBV to their infants are chronic carriers of HBV infection who are HBeAg-positive.[130] These mothers acquired acute infection with HBV months or years before the onset of pregnancy and continue to have intermittent viral replication. In most Western countries, fewer than 1% of the general population are HBsAg carriers. The rate is often higher in urban populations, especially among intravenous drug addicts. In parts of Asia and Africa, the incidence of HBV carriers may be as high as 30% to 40%. Among carriers, the risk of transmission of HBV infection to infants is largely dependent on HBeAg status. The rate of transmission is usually 90% or higher for those with HBeAg or high levels of HBV DNA in serum.[125,131] The rate is considerably lower and less consistent for those without HBeAg or in the presence of early antibody to hepatitis B.[127,130,131] This is not surprising, inasmuch as there is a correlation between HBeAg and the presence of circulating virus as measured by HBV DNA in serum. However, patients who are negative for HBeAg may have circulating viral particles; therefore, HBeAg status cannot be relied upon to determine the risk of infant transmission.

The administration of hyperimmune globulin and HBV vaccine protects 90% to 95% of infants from HBV infection. Therefore, it is appropriate to administer HBV vaccine and HBV hyperimmune globulin (HBIG) to infants of mothers who are HBsAg-positive regardless of the mother's HBeAg status.[130,132,133] This is both medically and economically effective in prevention of acute hepatitis, HBV carrier state, chronic hepatitis, cirrhosis, or hepatoma. It is recommended that 0.5 mL of HBIG be given at birth and that three doses of HBV vaccine be given beginning at birth according to manufacturers' recommendations for recombinant vaccines.[130] Variations in the timing of this regimen have also been highly effective, but both HBIG and HBV vaccine must be given for maximum effect.[126,129,134] HBIG and HBV vaccine may be given simultaneously without inhibiting the antibody production induced by HBV vaccine (Table 15-8). Complications of this regimen are rare and mild.[135]

TABLE 15–8   Transmission of Viral Hepatitis from Mother to Infant

	Hepatitis A		Hepatitis B		Hepatitis C
Maternal Infection	Acute Infection		Acute Infection	Carrier State	Acute and Chronic
Transmission risk to infant	Rare		First and second trimesters: <10% 3rd trimester: ~65%	HBeAg-positive: 85%-95% HBeAb-positive: <5% HBeAg-negative, HBeAb-negative: ≅50%	~10%
Infant disease	Rare clinical hepatitis (at 14-30 days of age) Passive antibody		Usually mild hepatitis, rarely severe hepatitis (at 30-120 days of age) Commonly become carriers	May have severe or fatal hepatitis (at 30-120 days of age) Commonly become carriers Cirrhosis or hepatoma (late complications 10-20 years later)	Acute hepatitis, also probable chronic hepatitis or carrier state
Recommended prophylaxis for infant	ISG: optional, for infant of mother with acute infection at birth		ISG: no HBIG at 24 hr, 1 mo, and 6 mo (20 mg each time) + hepatitis B vaccine	ISG: no HBIG at 24 hr, 1 mo, and 6 mo (20 mg each time) + hepatitis B vaccine	ISG ineffective

Combined HBIG and hepatitis B vaccine is 85-95% effective in preventing hepatitis B infection in infant.
HBeAb, hepatitis B early antibody; HBeAg, hepatitis B early antigen; HBIG, hyperimmune serum globulin; ISG, immune serum globulin.

Failures of this regimen may relate to transplacental infection before birth or incubating infection at the time of birth. It is also possible that some newborns acquire infection from household members other than the mother who are chronic HBsAg carriers (horizontal spread). This has been suggested as the cause of infection in infants born to hepatitis B early antibody–positive mothers when the infant did not receive prophylaxis.[136] It is a further argument for the use of HBIG and HBV vaccine in all situations in which the mother is identified as a carrier, because of the increased incidence of other HBsAg carriers in the family when the mother is a carrier. There have been reports of severe or fulminant hepatitis in infants of mothers with hepatitis B early antibody despite vaccination.[137-139] The presence of severe infection despite proper immunization of the infant has led to identification of a mutant virus with a single amino acid change in the precore region.[139] The frequency of this mutation and its possible transmission to other persons is not yet certain. Universal vaccination of all infants at birth for HBV is now the standard of care.[140] Vaccinations for all children previously not immunized is recommended as they enter puberty. In future generations, the specter of viral hepatitis B and its complications could be eliminated. Vaccine for pregnant women exposed to hepatitis B is safe.[141]

Hepatitis C

The genome of hepatitis C (HCV) was first reported in 1989.[142] This discovery led to the development of the enzyme-linked immunosorbent assays for detection of HCV antibody in serum now used clinically. Improvements in the initial serum tests have led to greater sensitivity and specificity for detecting evidence of HCV infection, including the development of polymer chain reaction–based assays for viral RNA. Clinical studies subsequently established that HCV was the major cause of non-A, non-B, post-transfusion hepatitis and also a cause of sporadic hepatitis in the United States and Western Europe. Evidence of HCV infection is higher among intravenous drug abusers, sexually promiscuous persons, and groups exposed to blood products (e.g., patients on hemodialysis, hemophiliac patients, health care workers). The relatively low levels of virus in blood in comparison with HBV infection probably explain the lower incidence of HCV person-to-person transmission. Sexual transmission has been recorded, but the risk is substantially lower than for HBV.[143] Despite these observations, HCV accounts for 40% to 50% of cases of hepatitis in the United States, with a prevalence of 1% to 5.4% in the population.[144] Moreover, as many as 50% to 85% of those infected become chronic carriers of HCV, and many carriers develop slowly progressing chronic active hepatitis and cirrhosis.[143] Therefore, the number of chronically infected individuals is high, and many have serious and often asymptomatic chronic liver disease. HCV was the subject of a recent National Institutes of Health–sponsored consensus development conference.[145]

The course of HCV infection in nonpregnant patients is unusual in comparison with those of other forms of hepatitis viruses. The acute phase is often asymptomatic and usually anicteric, although the disease is occasionally severe. More characteristic is the relapsing nature of abnormal liver function test findings and clinical symptoms over a period of many months or years after initial infection. This course may be accompanied by histologic changes in the liver that range from a mild form of hepatitis to severe chronic active hepatitis and cirrhosis.

HCV infection may cause acute hepatitis during pregnancy but may not be detected unless liver function tests and HCV antibody tests are obtained. It is important to note that development of a positive result of HCV antibody tests may be quite delayed after onset of infection, occasionally as long as several months. Thus, repetition of HCV antibody testing or the addition of tests for viral RNA during pregnancy in a suspected case may be necessary.

The course of chronic HCV infection during pregnancy is under debate. In a large study, the course was reported to not be different during pregnancy.[146] Other studies show either an improvement in ALT during pregnancy[147] or a worsening of histologic findings after pregnancy.[148] There are no reports of fetal or neonatal abnormalities in association with maternal HCV infection. Survival and prematurity rates are comparable, regardless of the mother's HCV antibody status.[144] However, there is evidence that acute or chronic infection during the third trimester may be accompanied by transmission to the fetus.[149-152] The rate of transmission may be higher in mothers co-infected with human immunodeficiency virus.[153] In other circumstances, the efficiency of vertical transmission is low, and the reasons for the variable results between studies are uncertain.[154,155] There is no known treatment to prevent vertical transmission of HCV infection, and routine screening of all mothers is currently unwarranted. Pregnant women at high risk for HCV infection can be offered antibody testing, and infants born to infected mothers observed for the development of hepatitis. Breast-feeding by infected mothers appears to be safe.[156] Testing the infant may yield misleading results, because a proportion who are HCV RNA–positive at birth eventually clear the virus. In a large Italian study, 13% of the infants born to HCV RNA–positive mothers were HCV RNA–positive at birth, but only 3% remained so at age 2 years.[157]

Severe chronic HCV infection has been successfully treated with interferon-α, although relapse is common after cessation of treatment.[143] Because interferon-α therapy is accompanied by frequent and sometimes severe side effects, and because the progression of chronic HCV infection is usually quite slow, it is unwise to use this agent during pregnancy. Moreover, effects of the interferons on fetal development and health in humans has not been well studied, and it should be considered contraindicated in pregnancy. Ribavirin has been teratogenic in animals and should not be used in pregnant women or in either men or women seeking pregnancy.

Hepatitis D

The hepatitis δ virus (HDV) is a defective RNA virus that replicates only in the presence of circulating HBV. Therefore, it is confined to patients with chronic HBV or to patients who become simultaneously co-infected with both HBV and HDV. Superinfection in a chronic HBV carrier by HDV may lead to serious deterioration or fulminant hepatic failure. The virus is most common in nations bordering the Mediterranean Sea. It is less common in the United States, where it is usually seen in intravenous drug abusers, in whom transmission of HBV and HDV may occur simultaneously or sequentially. HDV can be transmitted from mother to child at birth.[158]

Hepatitis E

The most recently described form of acute viral hepatitis, hepatitis E (caused by HEV), occurs most frequently in Asia, North Africa, South America, and Central America. It occurs in epidemics and resembles HAV in clinical manifestation and epidemiology. It is an RNA virus that is distinct from the others described. Antibody can be identified in serum.

In areas of the developing world that are endemic for HEV, a high incidence of fulminant HEV infection has been reported, especially among women in the third trimester of pregnancy.[159] The case fatality rate for hepatitis E is as high as 20% among women infected during the third trimester of pregnancy.[71,160] In the United States, hepatitis E occurs primarily in travelers from endemic areas. HEV can be transmitted to the fetus in utero and can cause acute hepatitis in the newborn.[161]

Atypical Forms of Hepatitis

Fulminant Viral Hepatitis A small percentage of patients with viral hepatitis, regardless of type, may present with fulminant disease. Fulminant hepatitis characteristically manifests with encephalopathy, jaundice, and marked aberrations in coagulation factors. The overall mortality rate is approximately 80%. The pathologic lesion in the liver reveals massive hepatocellular necrosis, in which virtually every hepatocyte is necrotic, or submassive necrosis, in which multilobular collapse and "bridging" necrosis alternate with areas of substantial hepatocyte preservation. Data suggest that the massive form is almost uniformly fatal, whereas some patients with submassive lesions survive. The differentiation of this disease from AFLP or severe preeclampsia may be difficult in patients during the third trimester. Most often, the transaminase and bilirubin elevations are higher in fulminant hepatitis, but overlap may occur. Coagulation abnormalities and disseminated intravascular coagulation may exist in either disease. The presence of serologic markers of acute HAV or HBV is helpful. If acute HCV is suspected, then testing for HCV RNA should be done, as antibodies now tested for HCV may not become detectable for several months. Liver biopsy is definitive but often difficult to obtain because of attendant coagulopathy. The major diseases with which fulminant hepatitis may be confused are AFLP and preeclampsia. Some of the differential features of these disorders are shown in Table 15–9.

Rapid delivery of the fetus is clearly indicated in AFLP and severe preeclampsia. It is desirable in fulminant hepatitis to spare the life of the infant. Therefore, rapid delivery is reasonable for either disease when the diagnosis is in doubt. The use of lactulose, prompt treatment of gastrointestinal bleeding, and supplementation of clotting factors with fresh-frozen plasma and platelets are imperative if patients and their infants are to be provided any opportunity for

TABLE 15–9   Liver Failure in Pregnancy

	Acute Fatty Liver of Pregnancy	Fulminant Viral Hepatitis	Preeclampsia and Eclampsia
Onset	Third trimester	Any time	Third trimester
Clinical symptoms	Nausea and vomiting, abdominal pain, coma	Nausea and vomiting, abdominal pain, hepatic encephalopathy	Nausea and vomiting, abdominal pain. May have convulsions
Other features	Hypertension, edema, proteinuria are common	May have hepatitis A or B serologic findings	Hypertension, edema, proteinuria
Laboratory findings			
AST	<1000	500-3000	Usually <2000
Bilirubin	2-10 mg/dL	20-30 mg/dL	1-6 mg/dL
Hemolysis	Occasional	Usual	Usual
Leukocytosis	90%-100%	Variable	Not found
Thrombocytopenia	Rare	~50%	90%-100%
FDP	Often	Occasional	Usual
Ammonia	Increased	Increased	Normal
Blood smear schistocytes	Occasional	Rare	Frequent
DIC	Common	Occasional	Usual
Hypoglycemia	Occurs	Rare	No
Diagnosis	Liver biopsy if coagulation studies permit	Hepatitis studies, biopsy if possible	Response to delivery, biopsy
Histology	Centrilobular microvesicular fat	Multilobular collapse and necrosis	Fibrin thrombi, periportal hemorrhage, peliosis
Treatment	Prompt delivery, fresh-frozen plasma	Delivery for fetal survival	Control preeclampsia and DIC, prompt delivery

AST, aspartate aminotransferase; DIC, disseminated intravascular coagulation; FDP, fibrin degradation products.

survival. Hepatic transplantation has been successfully accomplished in patients with fulminant hepatitis.

Chronic Hepatitis Pregnancy may occur in women with chronic hepatitis, most often in those with autoimmune disease that is responsive to corticosteroid therapy.[131,162] There is an increased risk of preeclampsia in mothers and prematurity in infants. Immunosuppressive therapy with corticosteroids and azathioprine should be continued during pregnancy in this group. Among those with chronic viral infection, many patients with mild or asymptomatic chronic active hepatitis C may sustain pregnancy. Similarly, chronic active hepatitis B that is mild or in spontaneous remission is compatible with pregnancy. The impact of pregnancy on the mother is dependent on the severity of the disease. Although congenital abnormalities are not increased in the infants of such patients, prematurity occurs with more severe maternal disease.[163-165] If the patient has cirrhosis and chronic hepatitis, early termination of pregnancy and perinatal mortality are clearly increased.[164] There is also an increased risk to the mother of esophageal bleeding, anemia, and toxemia. In one series, maternal complications occurred in 42% of patients. The relative reduction in hepatic blood flow and the increase in intravascular volume in pregnancy may account for reports of reduced hepatic function and increased risk of esophageal bleeding. Nonetheless, a patient with milder disease may proceed safely through pregnancy and deliver a normal infant. Careful observation of the mother during the pregnancy should include monthly measurement of liver function and control of weight gain and blood pressure.

Drug and Alcohol Reactions

Liver manifestations of drug reactions can be divided into two general classes: those that predominantly cause cholestasis and those that produce widespread hepatocellular injury. Many agents produce a mixed reaction. Although any of the drugs associated with hepatic injury in nonpregnant patients also may cause reactions during pregnancy, several agents are of special importance because of their frequent use in the treatment of complications of pregnancy. These include the antiemetic agents, especially chlorpromazine[166] and structurally related compounds; the antibiotics, especially tetracyclines[167] and the sulfonamides; anesthetics such as halothane[168]; tocolytics[169]; and other agents such as chlorothiazide, tranquilizers, and antidepressants. Other drugs associated commonly with hepatic injury include α-methyldopa, isoniazid, acetaminophen,[170] cimetidine, ranitidine, and penicillin.

Alcoholic liver disease may appear in pregnancy and is occasionally confused with other diseases that cause hepatic failure in pregnancy. Chronic alcoholism in the mother also may result in liver injury in the fetus.[171,172]

Diagnosis of hepatic injury related to drugs is difficult because liver function changes are variable and nonspecific, and even liver biopsy may yield inconclusive findings. Improvement with cessation of the drug or recurrence when treatment is resumed are the most convincing evidence of the cause. However, when the presumption is strong, the use of alternative therapy is indicated.

There are no unusual risks of hepatocellular or cholestatic drug reactions in the mother with the exception of intravenous tetracycline. However, confusion in diagnosis may cause difficulties in management. Cessation of treatment or substitution with a drug of different chemical structure usually results in clinical improvement, although recovery may be slow, lasting many weeks in some cases. The effects of drugs on fetal development are independent of their potential for causing hepatocellular or cholestatic reactions.

OTHER DISORDERS OF PREGNANCY AFFECTING THE LIVER

Hyperemesis Gravidarum

Hyperemesis gravidarum can be defined as excessive nausea and vomiting in pregnancy that result in dehydration and ketosis, severe enough to necessitate hospitalization. Although this is not primarily a liver disorder, it affects the liver in up to 50% of patients.[173,174] In modern times, this condition is almost invariably mild. In the pre–intravenous fluid era, this syndrome was known to result in jaundice and death.

Nausea is an extremely common accompaniment of early pregnancy, and "morning sickness" is often one of the first signs that a woman is pregnant. Hyperemesis gravidarum is considered to be the severe extreme of the spectrum of morning sickness. It is not rare, with rates reported from 3 per 1000 pregnancies to 1 per 100.[175]

Affected patients present in the first trimester, usually by weeks 10 to 12. They have persistent nausea and vomiting and experience weight loss, often of significant amounts. They also have ptyalism (excessive spitting). Factors thought to favor an increased risk for hyperemesis gravidarum include obesity, nulliparity, and twin gestation.[175,176] Laboratory testing demonstrates abnormal liver values in up to 50% of affected patients; the most sensitive test is the ALT, which may rise as high as 1000 U.[173] Severely affected patients also have elevations in bilirubin.[24] In some patients, laboratory testing may demonstrate either hyperthyroidism or hypercalcemia with hyperparathyroidism of unclear pathogenesis.[83,177-179] The electrogastrogram is abnormal in some patients in comparison with that of pregnant controls without hyperemesis gravidarum.[180,181] Liver biopsy, which is rarely indicated, shows very minimal abnormalities, primarily central cholestasis, and no inflammatory infiltrate.

Improvement in the nausea and vomiting and resolution of the liver test abnormalities occur when most affected patients are given intravenous fluids and put to gut rest. The syndrome resolves by week 20 in most, although rare patients have persistent vomiting and require enteral or total parenteral nutrition. Antiemetic therapy with drugs such as ondansetron[182] or droperidol[183] is helpful. Corticosteroid therapy has been reported with success.[184,185] Patients affected with hyperemesis gravidarum have no increased rate of prematurity, infants with low birth weight, or infants with birth defects.[186,187] The differential diagnosis includes viral hepatitis, especially in patients with high levels of aminotransferases, and gastroparesis (e.g., that caused by diabetes mellitus) is not associated with pregnancy. Hyperemesis gravidarum often recurs during subsequent pregnancies and has been reported to cause liver dysfunction in three successive pregnancies.[24]

The origin of the liver disease associated with hyperemesis gravidarum is unclear, as indeed is the syndrome itself. Not all affected patients have liver disease; therefore, the vomiting does not appear to be secondary to the liver involvement. Starvation alone does not seem to be an adequate explanation for the liver dysfunction, particularly inasmuch as biopsy in affected patients fails to show the fatty infiltration typical of starvation. It is tempting to think that this syndrome relates to the levels of gestational hormones, which are changing rapidly during this early part of pregnancy. However, a consistent relationship between hormone levels and the occurrence of hyperemesis gravidarum has not been established.[188]

Pyelonephritis

Pyelonephritis is not uncommon in pregnancy, and if it is untreated or is associated with preeclampsia, changes in liver function may occur.[189] Jaundice is rare, and the liver abnormalities respond when the infection is controlled by the proper use of antibiotics. Urinary infection has been reported with ICP and may play a role in precipitating this disorder.[190] It is important to recognize that some of the therapeutic agents used in treating urinary tract infections may also cause liver function changes.[167]

Cholelithiasis

Pregnancy does predispose to the formation of biliary sludge and gallstones, presumably because it slows biliary motility (the so-called sluggish gallbladder of pregnancy).[191] The sludge and gallstones that accumulate during pregnancy may resolve after delivery.[192,193] Indeed, the increased risk for gallstones reverts to normal 5 years after the last pregnancy.[194]

Surgical treatment for biliary colic may be associated in pregnancy with an increase in either maternal or fetal morbidity.[195,196] Treatment of common duct stones by endoscopic retrograde cholangiography and sphincterotomy has been reported in pregnancy. Lead shielding of the uterus resulted in minimal exposure of the infant to radiation.[197,198] Laparoscopic cholecystectomy can be used successfully,[199] although not without risk.[200] Many patients can be managed by conservative medical management.

Cirrhosis and Pregnancy

Pregnancy in patients with cirrhosis is unusual but is no longer considered rare.[165,201,202] Cirrhosis often leads to amenorrhea and infertility. However, therapy for certain forms of cirrhosis—for example, caused by autoimmune hepatitis or Wilson's disease—can result in improvement

in an increasing number of young women of childbearing age that is sufficient for them to conceive and have successful pregnancies.

Natural History

The natural history of 95 pregnancies in 78 patients with cirrhosis or chronic active hepatitis has been reported.[203] The majority of these patients had postnecrotic cirrhosis, although a few were diagnosed as having Laennec's cirrhosis, primary biliary cirrhosis, or chronic active hepatitis. In two thirds of the cases, there was no significant change in liver function during pregnancy. In the remaining patients, a deterioration of liver function appeared, and in some, jaundice occurred. Two patients improved during the pregnancy. Of 23 patients with demonstrated esophageal varices, 18 had gastrointestinal bleeding during the pregnancy. Six of the nine deaths in the series were a result of variceal bleeding. Several patients underwent successful portal decompressive surgical procedures during pregnancy. No adverse effects of the surgery on the mother or fetus were reported. The survival of the fetus was affected by the presence of maternal cirrhosis. There were 10 stillbirths, 7 spontaneous abortions, and 67 live births among the 78 patients with cirrhosis.

The results of another study are shown in Table 15–10. In this group, 70% of patients had postnecrotic cirrhosis or chronic active hepatitis, 20% had primary biliary cirrhosis, and 10% had Laennec's cirrhosis. The incidence of premature delivery and fetal mortality was high. The maternal complications included anemia, toxemia, postpartum hemorrhage, and bleeding from esophageal varices. The variceal bleeding occurred in 20% of patients and was associated with maternal death in approximately one third of the patients. The incidence of bleeding from esophageal varices during pregnancy may be less in those who have undergone portal decompressive surgery before pregnancy.[201]

These several studies indicate that pregnancy can occur in cirrhotic women and may result in a normal, healthy infant. However, the risk of complications, including deterioration in liver function and hemorrhage from varices, is high. Variceal hemorrhage accounts for most of the maternal deaths in cirrhotic patients. The risk of variceal bleeding in these patients is highest in the second and third trimesters, but the bleeding may occur shortly after delivery.[204] Prematurity and infant mortality are also increased. These risks, by themselves, are not sufficiently high to be considered absolute indications for interruption of the pregnancy. However, pregnant patients with

TABLE 15–10   Cirrhosis and Pregnancy

Outcome	%
Early termination (<20 weeks)	18
Prematurity (birth at 21-37 weeks)	20
Vaginal delivery	85
Perinatal mortality	18
Maternal complication	42

cirrhosis and varices should be aware of the substantial risk of variceal bleeding.

Problems in Therapy

Therapy for some chronic liver diseases presents specific problems during pregnancy. The effectiveness of immunosuppressive therapy in the treatment of severe chronic autoimmune hepatitis, with or without cirrhosis, has been established in several controlled studies.[162,205] The many undesirable side effects of long-term immunosuppressive therapy may appear during pregnancy and complicate management. In addition, there is, theoretically, a higher risk of congenital deformities in infants born to mothers receiving such therapy. However, serious deterioration in liver function during pregnancy in patients with autoimmune hepatitis poses an even greater risk to both mother and fetus. Therapy with the minimum effective dosages of corticosteroid and azathioprine is desirable. The dosages necessary to control the disease vary, but the lowest possible dosages should be used. One study documented the effect of pregnancy on autoimmune hepatitis. During pregnancy, the disease became less active, reflecting the relative immune suppression of pregnancy. After delivery, the disease flared, with ALT elevations.[206] This experience supports enhanced monitoring of patients with autoimmune hepatitis for several months after delivery.

Corticosteroids are not effective in HBV chronic hepatitis and should not be used in this setting. Treatment of chronic active HBV or HCV infections with interferon-α is contraindicated in pregnancy because of the numerous side effects and the uncertain effect on mother and fetus. Ribavirin therapy is contradicted in pregnancy.

Portal Hypertension

The presence of severe portal hypertension with esophageal varices is associated with an increased risk of hemorrhage during pregnancy. Patients previously treated with portacaval shunt for varices have become pregnant. Twenty-one pregnancies in 17 patients with portacaval shunts before pregnancy resulted in 17 live births, 2 neonatal deaths, 1 stillbirth, and 1 spontaneous abortion. No maternal deaths were recorded. Therefore, the presence of a portacaval shunt is not a contraindication to pregnancy and does not contribute an additional risk to that of the chronic liver disease alone.[207,208] In fact, it may reduce the risk of bleeding for the mother.[201]

The potential hazard of pregnancy for noncirrhotic patients with portal hypertension who have not had a prior shunt procedure is indicated by a report of two patients with extrahepatic portal hypertension.[209] Both patients had had previous multiple episodes of hematemesis, which were controlled by transthoracic ligation of varices. During pregnancy, both patients experienced bleeding, presumably because of increased portal hypertension resulting from the pregnancy. It is apparent that the risk of variceal hemorrhage is increased during pregnancy, regardless of the cause of the portal hypertension.

The use of sclerotherapy for bleeding varices during pregnancy may provide a safe alternative to portacaval anastomosis and has been reported to be effective.[210] Controlled trials have suggested efficacy in nonpregnant patients, and such treatment seems reasonable for the pregnant patient with bleeding esophageal varices.

Liver Transplantation

Women with chronic liver disease who undergo liver transplantation regain their fertility. Pregnancy in such women can be successful, although there is an increased risk of maternal complications such as hypertension, as well as prematurity.[211] Immunosuppression must be continued in such patients, and heightened monitoring of blood levels is indicated.[212] There is no reported teratogenicity of these drugs in this setting.[213] These pregnancies, like any in patients with preexisting liver disease, should be managed by experts in maternal-fetal medicine.

Liver transplantation has been performed successfully during pregnancy, although the risk to the fetus with this heroic therapy is high.[214-216] In choosing such treatment, the physician should bear in mind that many forms of liver disease in pregnancy, most notably AFLP and preeclamptic liver diseases, resolve after delivery, leaving the patient with no sequelae. Clearly, liver transplantation, with its risks and lifelong immunosuppression, should be reserved for only special situations.

Other Hepatic Disorders Occurring during Pregnancy

Wilson's Disease

Wilson's disease is a rare disorder characterized by cirrhosis, neurologic abnormalities, the Kayser-Fleischer corneal ring, and, less commonly, hematologic and renal dysfunction and osteopenia. The advent of effective therapy for this disease has increased the incidence of pregnancy but has also raised the issue of fetal injury produced by penicillamine. If therapy with penicillamine is started early in the disease, considerable improvement in all the manifestations of Wilson's disease results. The secondary amenorrhea is often corrected, and because many patients are in the childbearing period, successful pregnancies have ensued.[217-219]

Most patients given D-penicillamine or trientine for treatment of Wilson's disease during pregnancy have given birth to normal infants. Fifteen pregnancies studied in 10 mothers with Wilson's disease treated with penicillamine resulted in 15 normal births. However, one infant eventually died of prematurity. These studies provide evidence that pregnancy is possible and safe and that continued therapy with penicillamine or trientine seems to have no serious effects on either mother or infant.[220,221] Zinc therapy has also been shown to be effective and safe during gestation.[222] The danger of discontinuation of therapy for Wilson's disease during pregnancy has been shown by reports of fulminant hepatic failure and hemolysis occurring after delivery in a mother who stopped treatment during her third pregnancy.[223]

Sickle Cell Disease

Liver disease, primarily of a cholestatic type, has been reported in patients with sickle cell disease.[224] The disorder is associated with marked sickling of cells in the hepatic sinusoids and prominent swelling of the Kupffer cells, which are often seen engulfing the abnormal red blood cells. This process is exaggerated during sickle cell crisis and has also been associated with pregnancy. Marked jaundice, elevation in alkaline phosphatase, and a moderate increase in AST occur. The process subsides after delivery, and most authors recommend induction of labor in such patients.[3] The possible association of sickle cell trait with infarction of the liver during pregnancy has been noted.[225]

Budd-Chiari Syndrome

Budd-Chiari syndrome, or hepatic vein occlusion, is an uncommon disease that has been associated with both pregnancy and the use of oral contraceptives.[226,227] The disease may be of sudden onset and, when the major hepatic veins are involved, may result in death within several weeks to a few months. Alternatively, it may be more insidious, involve smaller intralobular veins, and be associated with prolonged survival. Unfortunately, the sudden-onset type has been most often recorded in association with pregnancy and may accompany preeclampsia.[228] Symptoms usually appear near term or, more commonly, within hours or days after delivery. Several reports suggested that Budd-Chiari syndrome in pregnancy is associated with the presence of an underlying procoagulant state, including antiphospholipid antibody,[229] anticardiolipin antibodies,[230] factor V Leiden mutation[231] or polycythemia rubra vera.[232]

Most often, pain in the upper abdomen is rapidly followed by abdominal distention and the development of ascites. Fever, vomiting, and jaundice may occur but are not constant. The ascitic fluid may show a high protein content (about 50% of cases). Liver biopsy reveals a characteristic centrilobular zonal congestion with hemorrhage and necrosis. Usually, sclerosis of the smaller central vein radicles is not seen, although venoocclusive disease also has been reported in pregnancy.[233] Hepatic vein wedge pressures, if possible to obtain, are elevated, and radiographic studies most often show blockage of the main hepatic veins, often with collateral circulation. In addition, inferior vena caval obstruction may occur. Hepatic scintigraphy often shows an unusual pattern, with hypertrophy and increased uptake in the caudate lobe, which has auxiliary drainage into the inferior vena cava. Magnetic resonance imaging may assist in diagnosis.[228]

The course of patients with major occlusion of hepatic veins is usually rapid deterioration, manifested by portal hypertension, bleeding varices, severe ascites, and hepatic failure. Direct surgical removal of the block is rarely successful. Side-to-side portacaval shunts have ameliorated portal hypertension and ascites and are recommended for patients with stable liver function. Because hepatic vein occlusion usually occurs after delivery, there are no direct effects on the fetus. In severe cases, liver transplantation may be necessary,[228] although most patients improve with conservative therapy, including anticoagulation. Recurrence when anticoagulants were stopped during pregnancy have been reported.[230]

AN APPROACH TO THE DIAGNOSIS OF LIVER DISEASE IN PREGNANCY

Symptoms

The appearance of jaundice or pruritus is often the first indication of liver disorder in pregnancy. It is important for the physician to be aware that significant liver disease may also be present in the absence of overt jaundice. Symptoms such as vague abdominal pain, fatigue, nausea, edema, and fever may be the earliest manifestations of liver dysfunction. Unless an obvious explanation exists for such complaints, careful physical examination and performance of liver function tests are indicated to evaluate the possibility of liver disease.

Physical Examination

The physical examination should include a careful search for icterus, spider angiomas, and palmar erythema. The latter two are common in uncomplicated pregnancy, appearing in approximately two thirds of normal pregnancies. However, if prominent in early pregnancy, they are more suggestive of antecedent liver disease. Estimation of the liver size in late pregnancy is difficult, but in early pregnancy, measurement by percussion is useful for determining liver size. Similarly, enlargement of the spleen may be exceedingly useful in directing attention to the possibility of long-standing liver disease with secondary portal hypertension. The relative sizes, consistencies, and tenderness of the two organs are of assistance to the clinician in suggesting various diagnostic possibilities. Other physical findings include evidence of ascites, edema, abdominal venous distention, and abdominal bruits or rubs.

Initial Laboratory Studies

Liver function studies for initial diagnostic purposes should include measurements of the major synthetic and excretory functions of the liver. Most often, these include determination of serum total protein, albumin, and globulin; direct and total bilirubin; alkaline phosphatase, 5'-nucleotidase, or GGTP; AST and ALT; cholesterol; and prothrombin time. Specific serologic tests may be useful as screening, including HBsAg and HCV antibody. If the physical findings or liver function test results suggest the possibility of liver disease, various clinical disorders must be considered and distinguished.

TABLE 15–11   Major Causes of Liver Function Abnormalities in Pregnancy

First Trimester	Second Trimester	Third Trimester
Viral hepatitis	Viral hepatitis	Cholestasis of pregnancy
Hyperemesis gravidarum	Gallstones	Viral hepatitis
Drug reaction	Pyelonephritis	Preeclampsia
	Cholestasis of pregnancy	Acute fatty liver of pregnancy
		Gallstones
		Pyelonephritis

Stage of Pregnancy

The stage of pregnancy at which liver disease first becomes clinically evident can often assist in delineating the major diagnostic possibilities. Certain diseases may be manifest in all three trimesters; however, others are restricted to the latter half of pregnancy.

The most common causes of major liver dysfunction in each trimester are indicated in Table 15–11. The incidence varies in different series and in various parts of the world; however, it is apparent that the number of disorders to be considered is highest in the third trimester. It is not surprising that episodes of anicteric hepatitis or mild cholestasis are frequently overlooked during the last trimester. Nevertheless, the importance of correct diagnosis is perhaps greatest during this stage of pregnancy because of the possible value of induced labor to the health and survival of mother and fetus.

Evaluation of the Liver Disease

The usual liver function changes for major forms of liver disease that occur in the third trimester are indicated in Table 15–12. None of these changes is diagnostic, and there is considerable overlap in the range of abnormalities. These studies are often useful in helping to suggest the clinical diagnosis and are important in evaluating the results of treatment. In many cases, the course of the changes is important; for example, a rapid improvement is seen after delivery in the preeclamptic patient, but this is not the case in patients with viral hepatitis.

Liver biopsy is only rarely indicated. It can be safely performed, despite the greater technical difficulties related to displacement of the liver by the enlarged uterus.

Clinical Course of the Disease

The clinical history is most useful in deciding among these various possibilities. For example, the abrupt onset of encephalopathy, bleeding, and labor should suggest AFLP, fulminant hepatitis, or preeclampsia (with or without hepatic rupture). Each is a life-threatening illness and is an indication for provision of an adequate airway, maintenance of normal blood pressure, and replacement of coagulation factors by intravenous infusion of fresh-frozen plasma or coagulation factors. In most patients, when vital signs have become stabilized, delivery of the infant is indicated. Immediate surgery is necessary for hepatic rupture that complicates preeclampsia. Final proof of diagnosis may require liver biopsy after stabilization of the clinical status. On the other hand, awareness of the typical clinical presentation and course often enables a reasonable presumptive diagnosis and quick identification of patients who require immediate obstetric or surgical intervention. Liver failure in pregnancy is a life-threatening event that must be treated promptly.

References

1. Combes B, Shibata H, Adams R, et al: Alterations in sulfobromophthalein sodium removal mechanisms from blood during normal pregnancy. J Clin Invest 1963;42:1431.
2. Ingerslev M, Teilum G: Biopsy studies on the liver in pregnancy. I. Normal histological features of the liver as seen on aspiration biopsy. Acta Obset Gynec Scand 1945;25:352.
3. Haemmerli U: Jaundice during pregnancy with special emphasis of recurrent jaundice during pregnancy and its differential diagnosis. Acta Med Scand 1967;44(Suppl):1.

TABLE 15–12   Diagnosis of Liver Disease in Third Trimester

Condition	Histologic Findings	Albumin, Percentage of Normal	AST	Bilirubin*	Alkaline Phosphatase*
Normal pregnancy	Normal	↓ 20	Normal	Normal	Twofold ↑
Viral hepatitis	Typical	↓ 20-40	500-2000	1-5 mg/dL	Twofold to threefold ↑
Cholestasis of pregnancy	Cholestasis	↓ 20	Normal to 1000	1-5 mg/dL	10-fold ↑
Preeclampsia	Sinusoidal fibrin	↓ 20	100-1500	Slight ↑	Twofold to threefold ↑
Acute fatty liver of pregnancy	Microvesicular fat	↓ 40	100-1000	1-10 mg/dL	Threefold ↑
Gallstone	Normal	↓ 20	Normal to slight ↑	Variable	Twofold to 10-fold ↑
Cirrhosis and chronic active hepatitis	Cirrhosis	↓ 20-40	50-150	1-5 mg/dL	Threefold ↑

*These values indicate the usual range for each condition.
AST, aspartate aminotransferase.
↑, increase; ↓, decrease.

4. Maher J, Goldenberg R, Tamura T, et al: Albumin levels in pregnancy: A hypothesis that decreased levels of albumin are related to increasing levels of alpha-seroprotein. Early Hum Devel 1993;34:209.

5. Regoeczi E, Hobbs K: Fibrinogen turnover in pregnancy. Scand J Haematol 1969;6:175.

6. Bacq Y, Zarka O, Brechot J-F, et al: Liver function tests in normal pregnancy: A prospective study of 103 pregnant women and 103 matched controls. Hepatology 1996;23:1030.

7. Lipsitz P, Flaxman L, Tartow L, et al: Maternal hyperbilirubinemia and the newborn. Am J Dis Child 1973;126:525.

8. Waffarn F, Carlisle S, Pena I, et al: Fetal exposure to maternal hyperbilirubinemia. Neonatal course and outcome. Am J Dis Child 1982;136:416.

9. Zuckerman H: Serum alkaline phosphatase in pregnancy and puerperium. Obstet Gynecol 1965;25:819.

10. Sussman H, Bowman M, Lewis J: Placental alkaline phosphatase in maternal serum during normal and abnormal pregnancy. Nature 1968;218:359.

11. Kaplan M: Alkaline phosphatase. Gastroenterology 1972;62:452.

12. Song C, Kappas A: The influence of estrogens, progestins and pregnancy on the liver. Vitam Horm 1968;26:147.

13. Kreek M, Weser E, Sleisenger M, et al: Idiopathic cholestasis of pregnancy. The response to challenge with the synthetic estrogen, ethinyl estradiol. N Engl J Med 1967;277:1391.

14. Maggiore G, Bernard O, Riely C, et al: Normal serum γ-glutamyl-transpeptidase activity identifies groups of infants with idiopathic cholestasis with poor prognosis. J Pediatr 1987;111:251.

15. Fabian E, Stork A, Kucerova L, et al: Plasma levels of free fatty acids, lipoprotein lipase, and postheparin esterase in pregnancy. Am J Obstet Gynecol 1968;100:904.

16. Koskelo P, Toivonen I: Urinary excretion of coproporphyrin isomeric 1 and 3 delta aminolaevulic acid in normal pregnancy and obstetric hepatosis. Acta Obstet Gynecol Scand 1968;47:292.

17. Aldercreutz H, Tenhunen R: Some aspects of the interaction between natural and synthetic female sex hormones and the liver. Am J Med 1970;49:630.

18. Iqbal M, Wilkinson M, Johnson P, et al: Sex steroid receptor proteins in fetal, adult and malignant liver tissue. Br J Cancer 1983;48:791.

19. Thorling L: Jaundice in pregnancy. Acta Med Scand (Suppl) 1955;302:1.

20. Reyes H: The enigma of intrahepatic cholestasis of pregnancy: lessons from Chile. Hepatology 1982;2:87.

21. Reyes H, Gonzalez M, Ribalta J, et al: Prevalence of intrahepatic cholestasis of pregnancy in Chile. Ann Intern Med 1978;88:487.

22. Gonzalez-Peralta R, Qian K, She J, et al: Clinical implications of viral quasispecies heterogeneity in chronic hepatitis C. J Med Virol 1996;49:242.

23. Holzbach R, Sivak D, Braun W: Familial recurrent intrahepatic cholestasis of pregnancy: A genetic study providing evidence for transmission of a sex-limited, dominant trait. Gastroenterology 1983;85:175.

24. Larrey D, Rueff B, Feldmann G, et al: Recurrent jaundice caused by recurrent hyperemesis gravidarum. Gut 1984;25:1414.

25. Reyes H, Ribalta J, Gonzalez M, et al: Sulfobromophthalein clearance tests before and after ethinyl estradiol administration, in women and men with familial history of intrahepatic cholestasis of pregnancy. Gastroenterology 1981;81:226.

26. Bacq Y: Intrahepatic cholestasis of pregnancy. Clin Liver Dis 1999;3:1.

27. Misra P, Evanov F, Wessely Z, et al: Idiopathic intrahepatic cholestasis of pregnancy. Am J Gastroenterol 1980;73:54.

28. Ribalta J, Reyes H, Gonzalez M, et al: S-adenosyl-L-methionine in the treatment of patients with intrahepatic cholestasis of pregnancy: A randomized, double-blind, placebo-controlled study with negative results. Hepatology 1991;13:1084.

29. Gonzalez M, Reyes H, Arrese M: Intrahepatic cholestasis of pregnancy in twin pregnancies. J Hepatol 1989;9:84.

30. Johnson P, Samsioe G, Gustafson A: Studies in cholestasis of pregnancy with special reference to clinical aspects and liver function tests. Acta Obstet Gynecol Scand 1975;54(Suppl):77.

31. Heikkinen J, Maentausta O, Ylostalo P, et al: Changes in serum bile acid concentrations during normal pregnancy, in patients with intrahepatic cholestasis of pregnancy and in pregnant women with itching. Br J Obstet Gynaecol 1981;88:240.

32. Bacq Y, Sapey T, Brechot M-C, et al: Intrahepatic cholestasis of pregnancy: A French prospective study. Hepatology 1997;26:358.

33. Jacquemin E, Cresteil D, Manouvrier S, et al: Heterozygous non-sense mutation of the MDR3 gene in familial intrahepatic cholestasis of pregnancy. Lancet 1999;353:210.

34. Gendrot C, Bacq Y, Brechot M, et al: A second heterozygous MDR3 nonsense mutation associated with intrahepatic cholestasis of pregnancy. J Med Genet 2003;40:E32.

35. Dixon P, Weerasekera N, Linton K, et al: Heterozygous MDR3 missense mutation associated with intrahepatic cholestasis of pregnancy: Evidence for a defect in protein trafficking. Hum Mol Genet 2000;9:1209.

36. Johnson P: Studies in cholestasis of pregnancy with special reference to lipids and lipoproteins. Acta Obstet Gynecol Scand Suppl 1973;27:1.

37. Johnson P, Samsioe G, Gustafson A: Studies in cholestasis of pregnancy. I. Clinical aspects and liver function tests. Acta Obstet Gynecol Scand 1975;54:77.

38. Frezza M, Pozzato G, Chiesa L, et al: Reversal of intrahepatic cholestasis of pregnancy in women after high dose S-adenosyl-L-methionine administration. Hepatology 1984;4:274.

39. Aldercreutz H, Tikkanen M, Wichmann K, et al: Recurrent jaundice in pregnancy. IV. Quantitative determination of urinary and biliary estrogens, including studies in pruritus gravidarum. J Clin Endocrinol Metab 1974;38:51.

40. Aldercreutz H, Svanborg A, Anberg A: Recurrent jaundice in pregnancy. I. A clinical and ultrastructural study. Am J Med 1967;42:335.

41. Jacquemin E, De Vree J, Cresteil D, et al: The wide spectrum of multidrug resistance 3 deficiency: From neonatal cholestasis to cirrhosis of adulthood. Gastroenterology 2001;120:1448.

42. Schorr-Lesnick B, Lebovics E, Dworkin B, et al: Liver diseases unique to pregnancy. Am J Gastroenterol 1991;86:659.

43. Meng L, Reyes H, Axelson M, et al: Progesterone metabolites and bile acids in serum of patients with intrahepatic cholestasis of pregnancy: Effect of ursodeoxycholic acid therapy. Hepatology 1997;26:1573.

44. Rannevik G, Jeppson S, Kullander S: Effect of oral contraceptives on the liver in women with recurrent cholestasis (hepatosis) during previous pregnancies. J Obstet Gynaecol Br Commonw 1972;79:1128.

45. Rioseco A, Ivankovic M, Manzur A, et al: Intrahepatic cholestasis of pregnancy: A retrospective case-control study of perinatal outcome. Am J Obstet Gynecol 1994;170:890.

46. Reyes H, Simon F: Intrahepatic cholestasis of pregnancy: An estrogen-related disease. Semin Liver Dis 1993;13:289-301.

47. Shaw D, Frohlich J, Wittmann BAK, et al: A prospective study of 18 patients with cholestasis of pregnancy. Am J Obstet Gynecol 1982;142:621.

48. Palma J, Reyes H, Ribalta J, et al: Effects of ursodeoxycholic acid in patients with intrahepatic cholestasis of pregnancy. Hepatology 1992;15:1043.

49. Palma J, Reyes H, Ribalta J, et al: Ursodeoxycholic acid in the treatment of cholestasis of pregnancy: A randomized, double-blind study controlled with placebo. J Hepatol 1997;27:1022.

50. Mazzella G, Nicola R, Francesco A, et al: Ursodeoxycholic acid administration in patients with cholestasis of pregnancy: Effects on primary bile acids in babies and mothers. Hepatology 2001;33:504.

51. Heikkinen J, Maentausta O, Ylostalo P, et al: Serum bile acid levels in intrahepatic cholestasis of pregnancy during treatment with phenobarbital or cholestyramine. Eur J Obstet Gynecol Reprod Biol 1982;14:153.

52. Stramentinoli G, Di Padova C, Gualano M, et al: Ethynylestradiol induced impairment of bile secretion in the rat: Protective effects of S-adenosyl-L-methionine and its implications in estrogen metabolism. Gastroenterology 1981;80:154.

53. Barron W: The syndrome of preeclampsia. Gastroenterol Clin North Am 1992;21:851.

54. Saftlas AF, Olson DR, Franks AL, et al: Epidemiology of preeclampsia and eclampsia in the United States, 1979-1986. Am J Obstet Gynecol 1990;162:460.

55. Redman CWG: Platelets and the beginnings of preeclampsia. N Engl J Med 1990;323:478.

56. Weinstein L: Syndrome of hemolysis, elevated liver enzymes, and low platelet count: A severe consequence of hypertension in pregnancy. Am J Obstet Gynecol 1982;142:159.

57. Sibai B, Ramadan M, Usta I, et al: Maternal morbidity and mortality in 442 pregnancies with hemolysis, elevated liver enzymes, and low platelets (HELLP syndrome). Am J Obstet Gynecol 1993;169:1000.

58. Barton J, Sibai B: Care of the pregnancy complicated by HELLP syndrome. Gastroenterol Clin North Am 1992;21:937.

59. Rolfes D, Ishak K: Liver disease in toxemia of pregnancy. Am J Gastroenterol 1986;81:1138.

60. Barton J, Riely C, Adamec T, et al: Hepatic histopathologic condition does not correlate with laboratory abnormalities in HELLP syndrome (hemolysis, elevated liver enzymes, and low platelet count). Am J Obstet Gynecol 1992;167:1538.

61. Minakami H, Oka N, Sato T, et al: Preeclampsia: A microvesicular fat disease of the liver. Am J Obstet Gynecol 1988;159:1043.

62. Sherlock S: Acute fatty liver of pregnancy and the microvesicular fat diseases. Gut 1983;24:265.

63. Arias F, Mancilla-Jimenez R: Hepatic fibrinogen deposits in preeclampsia. Immunofluorescent evidence. N Engl J Med 1976; 295:578.

64. Riely C, Latham P, Romero R, et al: Acute fatty liver of pregnancy: A reassessment based on observations in nine patients. Ann Intern Med 1987;106:703.

65. Visser W, Wallenburg H: Maternal and perinatal outcome of temporizing management in 254 consecutive patients with severe preeclampsia remote from term. Eur J Obstet Gynecol Reprod Biol 1995;63:147.

66. O'Brien J, Milligan D, Barton J: Impact of high-dose corticosteroid therapy for patients with HELLP (hemolysis, elevated liver enzymes, and low platelet count) syndrome. Am J Obstet Gynecol 2000; 183:921.

67. Tompkins M, Thiagarajah S: HELLP (hemolysis, elevated liver enzymes, and low platelet count) syndrome: The benefit of corticosteroids. Am J Obstet Gynecol 1999;181:304.

68. Burrows A, Kelton J: Fetal thrombocytopenia and its relation to maternal thrombocytopenia. N Engl J Med 1993;329:1467.

69. Harms K, Rath W, Herting E, et al: Maternal hemolysis, elevated liver enzymes, low platelet count, and neonatal outcome. Am J Perinatol 1995;12:1.

70. Klein N, Riely C: Liver disease. In Lee RV (ed): Current Obstetric Medicine. St. Louis, Mosby–Year Book, 1991, pp 99-124.

71. Hamid S, Jafri S, Khan H, et al: Fulminant hepatic failure in pregnant women: Acute fatty liver or acute viral hepatitis. J Hepatology 1996;25:20.

72. Bis K, Waxman B: Rupture of the liver associated with pregnancy: A review of the literature and report of 2 cases. Obstet Gynecol Surv 1976;31:763.

73. Hibbard L: Spontaneous rupture of the liver in pregnancy: A report of eight cases. Am J Obstet Gynecol 1976;126:334.

74. Nelson E, Archibald L, Albo D: Spontaneous hepatic rupture in pregnancy. Am J Surg 1977;134:817.

75. Manas K, Welsh J, Rankin R, et al: Hepatic hemorrhage without rupture in preeclampsia. N Engl J Med 1985;312:424.

76. Barton J, Sibai B: Hepatic imaging in HELLP syndrome (hemolysis, elevated liver enzymes, and low platelet count). Am J Obstet Gynecol 1996;174:1820.

77. Aziz S, Merrell R, Collins J: Spontaneous hepatic hemorrhage during pregnancy. Am J Surg 1982;146:680.

78. Herbert W, Brenner W: Improving survival with liver rupture complicating pregnancy. Am J Obstet Gynecol 1982;142:530.

79. Erhard J, Lange R, Niebel W, et al: Acute liver necrosis in the HELLP syndrome: Successful outcome after orthotopic liver transplantation. A case report. Transplant Int 1993;6:179.

80. Hunter S, Martin M, Benda J, et al: Liver transplant after massive spontaneous hepatic rupture in pregnancy complicated by preeclampsia. Liver Transplant 1995;85:819.

81. Greenstein D, Henderson J, Boyer T: Liver hemorrhage: Recurrent episodes during pregnancy complicated by preeclampsia. Gastroenterology 1994;106:1668.

82. Krueger K, Hoffman B, Lee W: Hepatic infarction associated with eclampsia. Am J Gastroenterol 1990;85:588.

83. Riely CA: Case studies in jaundice of pregnancy. Semin Liver Dis 1988;8:191.

84. Bacq Y, Riely C: Acute fatty liver of pregnancy: The hepatologist's view. Gastroenterologist 1993;1:257.

85. Burroughs A, Seong N, Dojcinov D, et al: Idiopathic acute fatty liver of pregnancy in 12 patients. Q J Med 1982;204:481.

86. Sheehan HL: The pathology of acute yellow atrophy and delayed chloroform poisoning. J Obstet Gynaecol Br Emp 1940;47:49.

87. Pockros P, Peters R, Reynolds T: Idiopathic fatty liver of pregnancy: Findings in ten cases. Medicine 1984;68:1.

88. Reyes H, Sandoval L, Wainstein A, et al: Acute fatty liver of pregnancy: A clinical study of 12 episodes in 11 patients. Gut 1994; 35:101.

89. Barton J, Sibai B, Mabie W, et al: Recurrent acute fatty liver of pregnancy. Am J Obstet Gynecol 1990;163:534.

90. Treem W, Rinaldo P, Hale D, et al: Acute fatty liver of pregnancy and long-chain 3-hydroxyacyl–coenzyme A hydrogenase deficiency. Hepatology 1994;19:339.

91. Schoeman MN, Batey RG, Wilcken B: Recurrent acute fatty liver of pregnancy associated with a fatty-acid oxidation defect in the offspring. Gastroenterology 1991;100:544.

92. Wilcken B, Leung K-C, Hammond J, et al: Pregnancy and fetal long-chain 3-hydroxyacyl coenzyme A hydrogenase deficiency. Lancet 1993;341:407.

93. Treem W, Shoup M, Hale D, et al: Acute fatty liver of pregnancy, hemolysis, elevated liver enzymes, and low platelets syndrome, and long chain 3-hydroxyacyl–coenzyme A dehydrogenase deficiency. Am J Gastroenterol 1996;91:2293.

94. Sims H, Brackett J, Powell C, et al: The molecular basis of pediatric long chain 3-hydroxyacyl–CoA dehydrogenase deficiency associated with maternal acute fatty liver of pregnancy. Proc Natl Acad Sci U S A 1995;92:841.

95. Ibdah J, Bennett M, Rinaldo P, et al: A fetal fatty-acid oxidation disorder as a cause of liver disease in pregnant women. N Engl J Med 1999;340:1723.

96. Rolfes DB, Ishak KG: Acute fatty liver of pregnancy: A clinicopathologic study of 35 cases. Hepatology 1985;5:1149.

97. Liebman H, McGehee W, Patch M, et al: Severe depression of antithrombin III associated with disseminated intravascular coagulation in women with fatty liver of pregnancy. Ann Intern Med 1983;98:330.

98. Rolfes D, Ishak K: Acute fatty liver of pregnancy: A clinicopathologic study of 35 cases. Hepatology 1985;5:1149.

99. Weber F, Snodgrass P, Powell D, et al: Abnormalities of hepatic mitochondrial urea-cycle enzyme activities and hepatic ultrastructure in acute fatty liver of pregnancy. J Lab Clin Med 1979;94:27.

100. Hatfield A, Stein J, Greenberger N, et al: Idiopathic acute fatty liver of pregnancy. Death from extrahepatic manifestations. Am J Dig Dis 1972;17:167.

101. Davies M, Wilkinson SP, Hanid MA, et al: Acute liver disease with encephalopathy and renal failure in late pregnancy and the early puerperium—a study of fourteen patients. Br J Obstet Gynaecol 1980;87:1005.

102. Usta I, Barton J, Amon E, et al: Acute fatty liver of pregnancy: An experience in the diagnosis and management of fourteen cases. Am J Obstet Gynecol 1994;171:1342.

103. Klein N, Mabie W, Shaver D, et al: Herpes simplex virus hepatitis in pregnancy. Gastroenterology 1991;100:239.

104. Mabie WC, Dacus JV, Sibai BM, et al: Computed tomography in acute fatty liver of pregnancy. Am J Obstet Gynecol 1988; 158:142.

105. Campillo B, Bernuau J, Witz M, et al: Ultrasonography in acute fatty liver of pregnancy. Ann Intern Med 1986;105:383.

106. Riely C: Acute fatty liver of pregnancy. Semin Liv Dis 1987;7:47.

107. Cammu H, Velkeniers B, Charels K, et al: Idiopathic acute fatty liver of pregnancy associated with transient diabetes insipidus. Case report. Br J Obstet Gynaecol 1987;94:173.

108. Combes C, Walker C, Matlock B, et al: Transient diabetes insipidus in pregnancy complicated by hypertension and seizures. Am J Perinatol 1990;7:287.

109. Durr J, Hoggard J, Hunt J, et al: Diabetes insipidus in pregnancy associated with abnormally high circulating vasopressinase activity. N Engl J Med 1987;316:1070.

110. Ockner SA, Brunt EM, Cohn SM, et al: Fulminant hepatic failure caused by acute fatty liver of pregnancy treated by orthotopic liver transplantation. Hepatology 1990;11:59.

111. Amon E, Allen S, Petrie R, et al: Acute fatty liver of pregnancy associated with preeclampsia: Management of hepatic failure with postpartum liver transplantation. Am J Perinatol 1991;8:278.

112. Ibdah J, Dasouki M, Strauss A: Long-chain 3-hydroxyacyl–CoA dehydrogenase deficiency: Variable expressivity of maternal illness during pregnancy and unusual presentation with infantile cholestasis and hypocalcaemia. J Inherit Metab Dis 1999;22:811.

113. Tanaka K, Kean E, Johnson B: Jamaican vomiting sickness. Biochemical investigation of two cases. N Engl J Med 1976;295:461.

114. Treem W, Witzleben C, Piccoli D, et al: Medium-chain and long-chain acyl CoA dehydrogenase deficiency: Clinical, pathologic and ultrastructural differentiation from Reye's syndrome. Hepatology 1986;6:1270.

115. Wenk R, Gebhardt F, Bhagavan B, et al: Tetracycline-associated fatty liver of pregnancy, including possible pregnancy risk after chronic dermatologic use of tetracycline. J Reprod Med 1981;26:135.

116. Kunelis C, Peters JL, Edmondson HA: Fatty liver of pregnancy and its relationship to tetracycline therapy. Am J Med 1965;38:359.

117. Mansouri A, Fromenty B, Durand F, et al: Assessment of the prevalence of genetic metabolic defects in acute fatty liver of pregnancy. J Hepatol 1996;25:781.

118. Atmar R, Englund J, Hammill H: Complications of measles during pregnancy. Clin Infect Dis 1992;14:217.

119. Jacques S, Qureshi F: Herpes simplex virus hepatitis in pregnancy: A clinical pathologic study of three cases. Hum Pathol 1992;23:183.

120. Adams R, Combes B: Viral hepatitis during pregnancy. JAMA 1965;192:195.

121. Willner I, Uhl M, Howard S, et al: Serious hepatitis A: An analysis of patients hospitalized during an urban epidemic in the United States. Ann Intern Med 1998;128:111.

122. Hieber J, Dalton D, Shorey J, et al: Hepatitis and pregnancy. J Pediatr 1977;91:545.

123. Zhang RL, Zeng JS, Zhang HZ: Survey of 34 pregnant women with hepatitis A and their neonates. Chin Med J (Engl) 1990;103:552.

124. Naggan L, Bar-Shany S, Shmuelewitz O, et al: Prevalence of hepatitis B markers (HBeAg and HBeAb) in women screened at time of delivery. Isr J Med Sci 1980;16:347.

125. Okada K, Kamiyama I, Inomata M, et al: e Antigen and anti-e in the serum of asymptomatic carrier mothers as indicators of positive and negative transmission of hepatitis B virus to their infants. N Engl J Med 1976;294:746.

126. Beasley R, Hwang L-Y, Stevens C, et al: Efficacy of hepatitis B immune globulin for prevention of perinatal transmission of hepatitis B virus carrier state: Final report of a randomized double-blind, placebo-controlled trial. Hepatology 1983;3:135.

127. Delaplane D, Yogev R, Crussi F, Shulman ST: Fatal hepatitis B in early infancy: The importance of identifying HBAg-positive pregnant women and providing immunoprophylaxis to their newborns. Pediatrics 1983;72:176.

128. Stevens C, Toy P, Taylor P, et al: Perinatal hepatitis B virus transmission in the United States. Prevention by passive-active immunization. JAMA 1985;253:1740.

129. Beasley R, Hwang L, Lee G, et al: Prevention of perinatally transmitted hepatitis B virus infections with hepatitis B immune globulin and hepatitis B vaccine. Lancet 1983;2:1099.

130. Sehgal A, Sehgal R, Gupta I, et al: Use of hepatitis B vaccine alone or in combination with hepatitis B immunoglobulin for immunoprophylaxis of perinatal hepatitis B infection. J Trop Pediatr 1992;38:247.

131. Stevens C, Neurath R, Beasley R, et al: HBeAg and anti-HBeAg and anti-HBe detection by radioimmunoassay: Correlation with vertical transmission of hepatitis B virus in Taiwan. J Med Virol 1979;3:237.

132. Brook M, Lever A, Kelly D, et al: Antenatal screening for hepatitis B is medically and economically effective in the prevention of vertical transmission: Three years' experience in a London hospital. Q J Med 1989;264:313.

133. Butterfield C, Shockley M, Miguel G, et al: Routine screening for hepatitis B in an obstetric population. Obstet Gynecol 1990;76:25.

134. Wong VC, Ip HM, Reesink HW, et al: Prevention of the HBsAg carrier state in newborn infants of mothers who are chronic carriers of HBsAg and HBeAg by administration of hepatitis-B vaccine and hepatitis-B immunoglobulin. Double-blind randomised placebo-controlled study. Lancet 1984;1:921.

135. Lee C, Huang L, Change M, et al: The protective efficacy of recombinant hepatitis B vaccine in newborn infant of hepatitis B e antigen–positive–hepatitis B surface antigen carrier mothers. Pediatr Infect Dis J 1991;10:299.

136. Nair PV, Weissman JY, Tong MJ, et al: Efficacy of hepatitis B immune globulin in prevention of perinatal transmission of the hepatitis B virus. Gastroenterology 1984;87:293.

137. Beath S, Boxall E, Watson R, et al: Fulminant hepatitis B in infants born to anti-HBe hepatitis B carrier mothers. BMJ 1992;304:1169.

138. Terazawa S, Kojima M, Yamanaka T, et al: Hepatitis B virus mutants with precore-region defects in two babies with fulminant hepatitis and their mothers positive for antibody to hepatitis B E antigen. Pediatr Res 1991;29:5.

139. Waters J, Kennedy M, Voet P, et al: Loss of the common "A" determinant of hepatitis B surface antigen by a vaccine-induced escape mutant. J Clin Invest 1992;90:2543.

140. Kane M: Implementing universal vaccination programmes: USA. Vaccine 1995;13:S75.

141. Levy M, Koren G: Hepatitis B vaccine in pregnancy: Maternal and fetal safety. Am J Perinatol 1991;8:227.

142. Choo Q, Kuo G, Weiner A, et al: Isolation of a cDNA clone derived from a blood-borne non-A, non-B viral hepatitis genome. Science 1989;244:359.

143. Alter M, Margolis H, Krawczynski K, et al: The natural history of community-acquired acute hepatitis C in the United States. N Engl J Med 1992;327:1899.

144. Bohman V, Stettler R, Little B, et al: Seroprevalence and risk factors for hepatitis C virus antibody in pregnant women. Obstet Gynecol 1992;36:315.

145. Seeff LB, Hoofnagle JH: National Institutes of Health Consensus Development Conference: Management of hepatitis C: 2002. Hepatology 2002;36(5, Suppl 1):S1.

146. Floreani A, Paternoster D, Zappala F, et al: Hepatitis C virus infection in pregnancy. Br J Obstet Gynaecol 1996;103:325.

147. Conte D, Fraquelli M, Prati D, et al: Prevalence and clinical course of chronic hepatitis C virus (HCV) infection and rate of HCV vertical transmission in a cohort of 15,250 pregnant women. Hepatology 2000;31:751.

148. Fontaine H, Nalpas B, Carnot F, et al: Effect of pregnancy on chronic hepatitis C: A case-control study. Lancet 2000;356:1328.

149. Inoue Y, Takeuchi K, Chou W, et al: Silent mother-to-child transmission of hepatitis C virus through two generations determined by comparative nucleotide sequence analysis of the viral cDNA. J Infect Dis 1992;166:1425.

150. Lynch-Salamon D, Combs C: Hepatitis C in obstetrics and gynecology. Obstet Gynecol 1992;79:621.

151. Ohto H, Terazawa S, Sasaki N, et al: Transmission of hepatitis C virus from mothers to infants. N Engl J Med 1994;330:744.

152. Sabatino G, Ramenghi LA, di Marzio M, et al: Vertical transmission of hepatitis C virus: An epidemiological study on 2,980 pregnant women in Italy. Eur J Epidemiol 1996;12:443.

153. Thaler M, Park C, Landers D, et al: Vertical transmission of hepatitis C virus. Lancet 1991;338:17.

154. Koff R: The low efficiency of maternal-neonatal transmission of hepatitis C virus: How certain are we? [Editorial]. Ann Intern Med 1992;117:967.

155. Reinus J, Leikin E, Alter H, et al: Failure to detect vertical transmission of hepatitis C virus. Ann Intern Med 1992;117:881.

156. Lin H, Kao J, JY J, et al: Absence of infection in breast-fed infants born to hepatitis C virus–infected mothers. J Pediatr 1995;126:589.

157. Ceci O, Margiotta M, Marello F, et al: Vertical transmission of hepatitis C virus in a cohort of 2,447 HIV-seronegative pregnant women: A 24-month prospective study. J Pediatr Gastroenterol Nutr 2001;33:570.

158. Deinhardt F, Gust I: Viral hepatitis. Bull World Health Organ 1982;60:661.

159. Asher L, Innis B, Shjrestha M, et al: Virus-like particles in the liver of a patient with fulminant hepatitis and antibody to hepatitis E virus. J Med Virol 1982;31:229.

160. Rab M, Bile M, Mubarik M, et al: Water-borne hepatitis E virus epidemic in Islamabad, Pakistan: A common source outbreak traced to the malfunction of a modern water treatment plant. Am J Trop Med Hyg 1997;57:151.

161. Khuroo M, Kamili S, Jameel S: Vertical transmission of hepatitis E virus. Lancet 1995;345:1025.

162. Cook G, Mulligan R, Sherlock S: Controlled prospective trial of corticosteroid therapy in active chronic hepatitis. Q J Med 1971;40:792.

163. Borhanmanesh F, Haghighi P: Pregnancy in patients with cirrhosis of the liver. Obstet Gynecol 1970;1970:315.

164. Cheng Y: Pregnancy in liver cirrhosis and/or portal hypertension. Am J Obstet Gynecol 1977;128:812.

165. Whelton MJ, Sherlock S: Pregnancy in patients with hepatic cirrhosis. Management and outcome. Lancet 1968;2:995.

166. Moradpour D, Altorfer J, Flury R, et al: Chlorpromazine-induced vanishing bile duct syndrome leading to biliary cirrhosis. Hepatology 1994;20:1437.

167. Schultz J, Adamson J, Workman W, et al: Fatal liver disease after intravenous administration of tetracycline in high dosage. N Engl J Med 1963;269:999.

168. Holden T, Sherline D: Hepatitis and hepatic failure in pregnancy. Obstet Gynecol 1972;40:586.

169. de Arcos F, Gratacos E, Palacio M, et al: Toxic hepatitis: A rare complication associated with the use of ritodrine during pregnancy. Acta Obstet Gynecol Scand 1996;75:340.

170. Wang P, Yang M, Lee W, et al: Acetaminophen poisoning in late pregnancy. A case report. J Reprod Med 1997;42:367.

171. Hubbick B, Casey R, Zaleski W, et al: Liver abnormalities in three patients with fetal alcohol syndrome. Lancet 1979;1:580.

172. Lefkowich J, Rushton A, Feng-Chen K: Hepatic fibrosis in fetal alcohol syndrome. Pathologic similarities to adult alcoholic liver disease. Gastroenterology 1983;85:951.

173. Abell T, Riely C: Hyperemesis gravidarum. Gastroenterol Clin North Am 1992;21:835.

174. Adams R, Gordon J, Combes B: Hyperemesis gravidarum: I. Evidence of hepatic dysfunction. Obstet Gynecol 1968;31:659.

175. Kallen B: Hyperemesis during pregnancy and delivery outcome: A registry study. Eur J Obstet Gynecol Reprod Biol 1987;26:292.

176. Klebanoff M, Koslowe P, Kaslow R, et al: Epidemiology of vomiting in early pregnancy. Obstet Gynecol 1985;66:612.

177. Bober S, McGill A, Tunbridge W: Thyroid function in hyperemesis gravidarum. Acta Endocrinologica 1986;111:404.

178. Bouillon R, Naesens M, VanAssche F, et al: Thyroid function in patients with hyperemesis gravidarum. Am J Obstet Gynecol 1982;143:922.

179. Budd D, Kumka M, Suda A, et al: Hyperparathyroidism masquerading as hyperemesis gravidarum. N J Med 1988;85:811.

180. Abell T: Nausea and vomiting of pregnancy and the electrogastrogram: Old disease, new technology. Am J Gastroenterol 1992;87:689.

181. Riezzo G, Pezzolla F, Darconza G, et al: Gastric myoelectrical activity in the first trimester of pregnancy: A cutaneous electrogastrographic study. Am J Gastroenterol 1992;87:702.

182. Sullivan CA, Johnson CA, Roach H, et al: A pilot study of intravenous ondansetron for hyperemesis gravidarum. Am J Obstet Gynecol 1996;174:1565.

183. Nageotte M, Briggs G, Towers C, et al: Droperidol and diphenhydramine in the management of hyperemesis gravidarum. Am J Obstet Gynecol 1996;174:1801.

184. Nelson-Piercy C, DeSwiet M: Corticosteroids for the treatment of hyperemesis gravidarum. Br J Obstet Gynaecol 1994;101:1013.

185. Taylor R: Successful management of hyperemesis gravidarum using steroid therapy. Q J Med 1996;89:103.

186. Hallak M, Tsalamandris K, Dombrowski M, et al: Hyperemesis gravidarum. Effects on fetal outcome. J Reprod Med 1996;41:871.

187. Tsang I, Katz V, Wells S: Maternal and fetal outcomes in hyperemesis gravidarum. Int J Gynecol Obstet 1996;55:231.

188. Depue R, Bernstein L, Ross R, et al: Hyperemesis gravidarum in relation to estradiol levels, pregnancy outcome, and other maternal factors. A seroepidemiologic study. Am J Obstet Gynecol 1987;156:1137.

189. Sworn M, Jones W: Peripartum hepatic dysfunction and xanthogranulomatous pyelonephritis. Br J Urol 1973;45:327.

190. Gonzales A, Mino M, Fontes J, et al: Colestasis gravidica intrahepatica. Implicaciones maternofetales. Rev Esp Enf Digest 1996;11:780.

191. Everson G: Gastrointestinal motility in pregnancy. Gastroenterol Clin North Am 1992;21:751.

192. Maringhini A, Marceno MP, Lanzarone F, et al: Sludge and stones in gallbladder after pregnancy. Prevalence and risk factors. J Hepatol 1987;5:218.

193. Tsimoyiannis E, Antoniou N, Tsaboulas C, et al: Cholelithiasis during pregnancy and lactation. Prospective study. Eur J Surg 1994;160:627.

194. Thijs C, Knipschild P, Leffers P: Pregnancy and gallstone disease: An empiric demonstration of the importance of specification of risk periods. Am J Epidemiol 1991;134:186.

195. Dixon N, Faddis D, Silberman H: Aggressive management of cholecystitis during pregnancy. Am J Surg 1987;154:292.

196. Swisher S, Hunt K, Schmit P, et al: Management of pancreatitis complicating pregnancy. Am Surg 1994;60:759.

197. Baillie J, Cairns S, Cotton P: Endoscopic management of choledocholithiasis during pregnancy. Surg Gynecol Obstet 1990;171:1.

198. Jamidar P, Beck G, Hoffman B, et al: Endoscopic retrograde cholangiopancreatography in pregnancy. Am J Gastroenterol 1995;90:1263.

199. Pucci RO, Seed RW: Case report of laparoscopic cholecystectomy in the third trimester of pregnancy. Am J Obstet Gynecol 1991;165:401.

200. Amos J, Schorr S, Norman P, et al: Laparoscopic surgery during pregnancy. Am J Surg 1996;171:435.

201. Schreyer P, Caspi E, El-Hindi J, et al: Cirrhosis-pregnancy and delivery: A review. Obstet Gynecol Surv 1982;37:304.

202. Varma R, Michelsohn N, Borkowf HI, Lewis JD: Pregnancy in cirrhotic and noncirrhotic portal hypertension. Obstet Gynecol 1977;50:217.

203. Huchzermeyer H: Pregnancy in patients with liver cirrhosis and chronic hepatitis. Acta Hepatosplenol (Stuttg) 1971;18:294.

204. Britton R: Pregnancy and esophageal varices. Am J Surg 1982;143:421.

205. Soloway R, Summerskill W, Baggenstoss A, et al: Clinical, biochemical and histological remission of severe chronic active liver disease. A controlled study of treatments and early prognosis. Gastroenterology 1972;63:820.

206. Buchel E, van Steenbergen W, Nevens F, et al: Improvement of autoimmune hepatitis during pregnancy but flare up following delivery. Am J Gastroenterol (in press).

207. Reisman T, O'Leary J: Portacaval shunt performed during pregnancy. A case report. Obstet Gynecol 1971;37:253.

208. Wilbanks G, Klinges K: Pregnancy after portacaval shunt. Report of 2 cases and review of the literature. Obstet Gynecol 1967;29:44.

209. Hermann R, Esselstyn C: The potential hazard of pregnancy in extrahepatic portal hypertension. Arch Surg 1967;95:956.

210. Pauzner D, Wolman I, Niv D, et al: Endoscopic sclerotherapy in extrahepatic portal hypertension in pregnancy. Am J Obstet Gynecol 1991;164:152.

211. Radomski J, Moritz M, Munoz S, et al: National transplantation pregnancy registry: Analysis of pregnancy outcomes in female liver transplant recipients. Liver Transpl Surg 1995;1:281.

212. Roberts M, Brown A, James O, et al: Interpretation of cyclosporin A levels in pregnancy following orthoptic liver transplantation. Br J Obstet Gynaecol 1995;102:570.

213. Jain A, Venkataramanan R, Fung J, et al: Pregnancy after liver transplantation under tacrolimus. Transplantation 1997;64:559.

214. Laifer S, Darby M, Scantlebury V, et al: Pregnancy and liver transplantation. Obstet Gynecol 1990;76:1083.

215. Merritt WT, Dickstein R, Beattie C, et al: Liver transplantation during pregnancy: Anesthesia for two procedures in the same patient with successful outcome of pregnancy. Transplant Proc 1991;23:1996.

216. Kato T, Nery J, Morcos J, et al: Successful living related liver transplantation in an adult with fulminant hepatic failure. Transplantation 1997;64:415.

217. Walshe JM: Pregnancy in Wilson's disease. Q J Med 1977;46:73.

218. Dupont P, Irion O, Beguin F: Pregnancy in a patient with treated Wilson's disease: A case report. Am J Obstet Gynecol 1990;163:1527.

219. Walshe J: The management of pregnancy in Wilson's disease treated with trientine. Q J Med 1986;58:81.

220. Fukuda K, Ishii A, Matsue Y, et al: Pregnancy and delivery in penicillamine treated patients with Wilson's disease. Tohoku J Exp Med 1977;123:279.

221. Toaff R, Toaff M, Peyser M, et al: Hepatolenticular degeneration (Wilson's disease) and pregnancy. Obstet Gynecol Surv 1977;32:497.

222. Brewer G, Johnson V, Dick R, et al: Treatment of Wilson's disease with zinc. XVII: Treatment during pregnancy. Hepatology 2000;31:531.

223. Shimono N, Ishibashi H, Ikematsu H, et al: Fulminant hepatic failure during perinatal period in a pregnant women with Wilson's disease. Gastroenterol Jpn 1991;26:69.

224. Rosenblate H, Einsenstein R, Holmes A: The liver in sickle cell anemia. Arch Pathol 1970;90:235.

225. Mengel C, Schauble JF, Hammond CB, Durham NC: Infarct-necrosis of the liver in a patient with SA hemoglobin. Arch Intern Med 1963;111:139.

226. Khuroo M, Datta D: Budd-Chiari syndrome following pregnancy. Report of 16 cases, roentgenologic, hemodynamic and histologic studies of the hepatic outflow tract. Am J Med 1980;68:113.

227. Maddrey W: Hepatic vein thrombosis (Budd-Chiari syndrome): Possible association with the use of oral contraceptives. Semin Liver Dis 1987;7:32.

228. Gordon S, Polson D, Shirkhoda A. Budd-Chiari syndrome complicating pre-eclampsia: Diagnosis by magnetic resonance imaging. J Clin Gastroenterol 1991;13:460.

229. Segal S, Shenhav S, Segal O, et al: Budd-Chiari syndrome complicating severe preeclampsia in a parturient with primary antiphospholipid syndrome. Eur J Obstet Gynecol Reprod Biol 1996;68:227.

230. Oewendijk R, Koster J, Wilson J, et al: Budd-Chiari syndrome in a young patient with anticardiolipin antibodies: Need for prolonged anticoagulant treatment. Gut 1994;35:1004.

231. Fickert P, Ramschak H, Kenner L, et al: Acute Budd-Chiari syndrome with fulminant hepatic failure in a pregnant woman with factor V Leiden mutation. Gastroenterology 1996;111:1670.

232. Valla D: Obstruction of the hepatic veins. Dig Dis 1990;8:226.

233. Hodkinson H, McKibbin J, Tim L, et al: Postpartum veno-occlusive disease treated with ascitic fluid reinfusion. S Afr Med J 1978;54:366.

BACTERIAL, FUNGAL, AND PARASITIC DISEASE

Maria C. Savoia

GENERAL CONSIDERATIONS

The Gravid State

Pregnancy both enhances the susceptibility to infection caused by certain microorganisms and increases the virulence of others. Many of the organisms causing infections in pregnant women require cell-mediated immunity for host defense. During pregnancy, the number of polymorphonuclear leukocytes increases, whereas the absolute number of lymphocytes in general falls. B cell numbers remain relatively constant,[1] whereas total T cell numbers decline.[1-3] Some authors have reported a diminution in the number of helper T cells and an increase in the number of suppressor cells[4]; others have reported that the helper/suppressor rate remains unchanged.[1] In vitro, lymphocyte proliferation in response to selected antigens, such as tuberculin,[5] cytomegalovirus,[6] and tetanus toxoid,[7] may be reduced. Natural killer cell activity has been reported to increase in the first trimester and early post partum and to decrease in the second and third trimesters.[8] Diminished natural killer cell activity and diminished lymphocyte proliferation may be the result of a progesterone-induced blocking factor, which depends on a specific progesterone suppressor-lymphocyte interaction.[9,10] The production of lymphokines such as interleukin-2, interleukin-6, and interferon-γ may also be diminished,[3,11-16] signaling a reduction in the type 2 immune response in pregnancy. The production of interleukin-4, interleukin-5, and interleukin-10—cytokines that strengthen humoral immunity—is not diminished.[13] Further complicating our understanding, murine studies have suggested that adequate levels of interferon-γ may be essential for successful pregnancy,[17] whereas other studies have demonstrated new unique immunosuppressive factors, such as pregnancy-specific glycoprotein-1α, in the serum of pregnant women.[15,18,19] Although levels of circulating immunoglobulin may be normal or increased, specific protective antibody production may be diminished, as demonstrated in a study of malaria in human pregnancy.[20] Some of the data on the immunologic change in pregnancy are contradictory, however, and much remains to be elucidated.

Most of the steroid hormones have been shown to be able to depress some aspect of cell-mediated immunity.[21,22] Estradiol, for example, can inhibit graft rejection in animal models and, together with human chorionic gonadotropins, can cause thymic involution.[9,22] The roles played by estrogen, progesterone, α-fetoprotein, and various trophoblastic factors in the modulation of immune function in pregnancy have not yet been clearly defined.[23] The hormonal changes associated with pregnancy may also predispose to infection by altering another host defense mechanism: the local mucosal barrier. High levels of estrogen, for example, have been associated with changes in genitourinary epithelial cells, changes that promote the adherence of pathogenic microorganisms.[24-26] Mammalian hormones may also directly stimulate the growth of pathogenic fungi such as *Coccidioides immitis*[27] and, perhaps, *Candida* species.[28]

Antimicrobial Therapy

Antibiotic use in pregnancy requires knowledge not only of the general principles of antimicrobial therapy but also of the altered physiology of pregnancy and potential effects of any drug on the fetus. The aim with any antimicrobial treatment is to achieve a level of drug in the affected tissue that exceeds the minimal inhibitory concentration of the infecting organism by as much as possible without incurring toxicity. Until the offending pathogen is identified, the choice of antibiotics should be based on knowledge of the usual organisms encountered in a particular clinical situation. The use of broad-spectrum agents may be required initially, especially when polymicrobial infections are suspected. On many occasions, however, an equally or more efficacious, safer, less expensive agent with a narrower spectrum may be substituted

305

for a broad-spectrum agent once culture and sensitivity results are available.

Pregnancy affects antibiotic levels through a variety of mechanisms. Decreased gastric motility and increased gastric acidity found in pregnancy may affect absorption of oral antibiotics. Plasma protein-binding capacity usually decreases in pregnancy, leading to increased active concentrations of some drugs. With pregnancy, the volume of distribution of drugs increases, and serum levels in general decrease. In addition, the increases in glomerular filtration and effective renal plasma flow found in pregnancy may lead to more rapid clearance of drugs by the kidney and lower serum and tissue levels. In complex clinical situations, monitoring serum drug concentrations may be necessary to ensure that treatment is adequate.

The choice of antibiotics in pregnancy may be affected by a requirement for adequate levels in fetal tissue (as in the treatment of maternal syphilis); conversely, the desire may be to limit fetal exposure. Antibiotics that are small, lipid soluble, and not protein bound diffuse most rapidly across the placenta. Any drug given to the mother does, however, cross the placenta to some extent and has the potential to affect the fetus adversely. As with any pharmacologic agent, antibiotics should be given only when the benefits to the mother outweigh the risks to the fetus.

The following is a brief discussion of selected common or new antibiotics and their use in pregnancy. Unfortunately, there have been few controlled clinical trials to provide guidance, and data are derived largely from animal studies and clinical practice. In 1979, using the data available, the U.S. Food and Drug Administration (FDA) established a classification system for drugs, including antibiotics, with regard to their potential for adverse fetal effects[29] (Table 16–1), and these ratings are included with the drugs discussed here, when available.

Penicillins

The penicillins are among the safest and most efficacious antibiotics in clinical use. They are bactericidal and act by inhibiting cell wall synthesis. Penicillin and ampicillin are active against the pneumococcus and most other streptococci, *Listeria* species, and non–β-lactamase–producing strains of *Haemophilus influenzae*. Methicillin, oxacillin, and nafcillin inhibit streptococci and *Staphylococcus aureus*. Carbenicillin, ticarcillin, piperacillin, azlocillin, and mezlocillin expand the spectrum of penicillin to inhibit more gram-negative rods, including many Enterobacteriaceae and some *Pseudomonas* species.

Much of the resistance to the penicillin family of antibiotics occurs because bacteria make β-lactamases. The combination of a β-lactam antibiotic with a β-lactamase inhibitor has been successful in overcoming this type of resistance. Clavulanic acid, sulbactam, and tazobactam are three such β-lactamase inhibitors. Currently available examples of this type of combination antibiotic include ampicillin-sulbactam (Unasyn), ticarcillin–clavulanic acid (Timentin), and piperacillin-tazobactam (Zosyn) for intravenous use, and ampicillin-clavulanic acid (Augmentin), an oral agent. Many strains of *S. aureus, H. influenzae, Escherichia coli, Neisseria gonorrhoeae,* and *Bacteroides fragilis* that are resistant to the penicillin base are susceptible to

TABLE 16–1	Fetal Risk Factors for Pharmaceuticals
Category A	Controlled studies in women fail to demonstrate a risk to the fetus in the first trimester (and there is no evidence of a risk in later trimesters), and the possibility of fetal harm appears remote.
Category B	Either animal reproduction studies have not demonstrated a fetal risk, but there are no controlled studies in pregnant women, or animal reproduction studies have shown an adverse effect (other than a decrease in fertility) that was not confirmed in controlled studies in women in the first trimester (and there is no evidence of a risk in later trimesters).
Category C	Either studies in animals have revealed adverse effects on the fetus (teratogenic or embryocidal or other) and there are no controlled studies in women, or studies in women and animals are not available. Drugs should be given only if the potential benefit justifies the potential risk to the fetus.
Category D	There is positive evidence of human fetal risk, but the benefits from use in pregnant women may be acceptable despite the risk (e.g., if the drug is needed in a life-threatening situation or for a serious disease for which safer drugs cannot be used or are ineffective).
Category X	Studies in animals or humans have demonstrated fetal abnormalities or there is evidence of fetal risk based on human experience, or both, and the risk of the use of the drug in pregnant women clearly outweighs any possible benefit. The drug is contraindicated in women who are or may become pregnant.

From the U.S. Food and Drug Administration: Federal Register 1980;44:37434.

these combination drugs. Isolates of *Streptococcus pneumoniae* that are intermediately susceptible or highly resistant to penicillin have become more common. This mechanism involves alterations in the organism's penicillin-binding proteins and is not reversed by β-lactamase inhibitors. Methicillin-resistant *S. aureus* isolates are also frequently encountered and necessitate treatment alternatives to the semisynthetic penicillins that used to be the mainstays of treatment.

Although controlled trials in pregnancy are lacking, the penicillins are widely used, and no evidence of adverse effects on the fetus has been demonstrated. All penicillins belong to FDA category B.

Cephalosporins

Like the penicillins, the cephalosporins possess a β-lactam ring, and they also bind to and inactivate enzymes that are necessary for the synthesis of the bacterial cell wall. Substitutions or modifications of the side chains of the six-member dihydrothiazine ring characteristic of the cephalosporins have resulted in a whole family of agents with different pharmacokinetic and antibacterial properties.

The cephalosporins are classified into generations, on the basis of their activity (Table 16–2). As a group, the first-generation cephalosporins, such as cefazolin, have excellent activity against staphylococci and streptococci. (However, methicillin-resistant staphylococci are resistant

TABLE 16–2   The Cephalosporin Family of Antibiotics

Generic Name	Proprietary Name	Route	Usual Adult Dosage and Range
First Generation			
Cefazolin	Ancef, Kefzol	IV	1 g q6-8h
Cephradine	Velosef, Anspor	Oral	250-500 mg q6h
		IV	1-2 g q6h
Cefadroxil	Duricef	Oral	1 g q.d.-b.i.d.
Cephalexin	Keflex	Oral	250-500 mg q6h
Second Generation			
Cefoxitin	Mefoxin	IV	1-2 g q6-8h
Cefotetan	Cefotan	IV	1-2 g b.i.d.
Cefamandole	Mandol	IV	500 mg to 1 g q4-8h
Cefonicid	Monocid	IV	1 g q.d.
Cefuroxime	Zinacef, Kefurox	IV	750 mg-1.5 g q8h
	Ceftin	Oral	250-500 mg b.i.d.
Cefaclor	Ceclor	Oral	250-500 mg q8h
Cefprozil	Cefzil	Oral	250-500 mg q12-24h
Third Generation			
Cefotaxime	Claforan	IV	1-2 g q4-12h
Ceftriaxone	Rocephin	IV	1-2 g q12-24h
Cefoperazone	Cefobid	IV	2-4 g q12h
Ceftazidime	Fortaz, Tazidime, Ceptaz, Tazicef, Pentacef	IV	1-2 g q8-12h
Ceftizoxime	Cefizox	IV	1-2 g q8-12h
Cefpodoxime	Vantin	Oral	100-400 mg q12h
Fourth Generation			
Cefepime	Maxipime	IV	500 mg to 2 g q8-12h

IV, intravenous.

to all cephalosporins. The enterococci also are not inhibited.) These agents are active against a limited number of gram-negative rods, including *E. coli, Klebsiella pneumoniae,* and some species of *Proteus.* The second-generation cephalosporins generally have greater gram-negative activity than do the first-generation agents. Some, such as cefoxitin and cefotetan, also have greater anaerobic activity, inhibiting approximately 75% of *B. fragilis* strains. The third-generation antibiotics have the broadest spectrum and the most potent activity against gram-negative rods, inhibiting most at levels far below 1 µg/mL.[30] Of the available third-generation cephalosporins, ceftazidime has the best and most reliable activity against *Pseudomonas aeruginosa.* Some anaerobes are inhibited by the third-generation agents, but activity against *B. fragilis,* for example, is not reliable. The tradeoff for enhanced gram-negative activity is poorer gram-positive coverage. Ceftazidime, for example, is 16 times less active than cefazolin against *S. aureus.*[31] Thus, these third-generation agents offer no advantage over the first-generation cephalosporins in the treatment of staphylococcal and streptococcal infections. Two of the third-generation cephalosporins (ceftriaxone and cefoperazone) are hepatically metabolized and excreted, achieving high concentrations in bile. Ceftriaxone's extended half-life allows once- or twice-daily intravenous administration, a convenience in outpatient therapy. Cefotaxime, ceftazidime, and ceftizoxime are excreted by the kidney, and dose adjustment is necessary in renal failure. Cefpodoxime has the greatest in vitro activity of any oral cephalosporin against the pneumococcus; its activity against *S. aureus* is in the moderate range.

Cefepime is the first fourth-generation cephalosporin. It has greater stability against chromosomal and plasmid-mediated β-lactamases than do third-generation agents, and it possesses no β-lactamase–inducing activity. This antibiotic possesses a gram-negative spectrum similar to that of ceftazidime and greater gram-positive activity. Gram-negative rods that are resistant to the third-generation cephalosporins may still be susceptible to cefepime. Its longer half-life allows for twice-daily dosing.[32]

Most cephalosporins readily cross the placenta, achieving cord blood levels 30% to 70% of those in serum, depending on the agent. Amniotic fluid levels are usually slightly lower.[33] Most cephalosporins are excreted in breast milk in low concentrations.

The first-generation cephalosporins are safe, inexpensive, effective drugs with a myriad of clinical uses. The second-generation cephalosporins are used in adult medicine primarily for preoperative prophylaxis in abdominal and pelvic surgery. They may also be useful in the treatment of "mixed" infections such as pelvic inflammatory disease (PID) or endometritis.[34,35] Most infections, especially those that are community acquired, do not necessitate treatment with third-generation cephalosporins because less expensive agents with a narrower spectrum of activity and equal efficacy are usually available. Third-generation cephalosporins have, however, been very useful in the treatment of gram-negative meningitis and in the treatment of complicated infections with resistant gram-negative rods, including penicillinase-producing *N. gonorrhoeae.* Cefepime should be reserved for the treatment of complicated mixed bacterial infections or when bacterial susceptibilities preclude treatment with other agents. Most patients who are allergic to penicillin can safely receive cephalosporins, but those with a history of anaphylaxis in response to penicillin must be carefully monitored. The cephalosporins are all FDA class B agents.

Monobactams

Aztreonam is the first member of a new class of antibiotics, the monobactams. It consists of a modified β-lactam ring structure with an acyl side chain at position 3. This antibiotic does not inhibit any gram-positive species, but it does penetrate through the outer wall of many gram-negative species (including some strains of *P. aeruginosa*), and it is not inhibited by most gram-negative β-lactamases. After infusion of 1 g of aztreonam intravenously, peak levels of 90 to 160 μg/mL are attained.[36] Most Enterobacteriaceae are inhibited at levels less than 1 μg/mL, but some (e.g., *Enterobacter, Serratia,* and *Pseudomonas* species) necessitate higher concentrations (≤16 μg/mL).[37] Aztreonam has no activity against anaerobes.

Aztreonam is cleared by the kidneys, and dose adjustment is required in patients with significant renal impairment. Few adverse effects have been noted with this agent, and there has been no evidence of mutagenicity or teratogenicity in extensive animal testing.[38] Aztreonam does not cross-react with the penicillins or cephalosporins, and it has been used safely in patients with severe penicillin allergy.[39]

Aztreonam is a safe and effective agent in the treatment of serious gram-negative infections. In the treatment of infections such as pyelonephritis, its limited spectrum has the advantage of leaving undisturbed the gram-positive and anaerobic flora of the body. Aztreonam has also been used successfully instead of gentamicin in combination therapy with clindamycin or metronidazole in the treatment of endometritis and PID.[40,41] Aztreonam is in FDA class B.

Carbapenems

Imipenem, the prototype drug of this class of compounds, is a novel antibiotic with a broad spectrum of activity. Although it is stereochemically different from the penicillins and cephalosporins, it binds to the penicillin-binding proteins of both gram-positive and gram-negative bacteria and causes rapid cell death. It has very good activity against most medically important bacteria, including *Enterococcus faecalis, P. aeruginosa, Serratia* species, and all *Bacteroides* species.[42] (It does not, however, inhibit *Pseudomonas maltophilia, Pseudomonas cepacia,* or some methicillin-resistant *S. aureus.*) Imipenem is not absorbed orally. Peak serum levels after 500 mg or 1 g of imipenem given intravenously are 33 and 52 μg/mL, respectively.[43] Imipenem is eliminated by the kidney, by both glomerular filtration and tubular secretion. It is not excreted in the bile and has no effect on the fecal flora. In the kidney, the drug by itself is rapidly metabolized to inactive forms.

To overcome this disadvantage, an inhibitor of the renal enzyme that inactivates imipenem was developed. This inhibitor, cilastatin, is included with imipenem in a 1:1 ratio in an available formulation, the brand name of which is Primaxin. Cilastatin and imipenem have similar pharmacokinetics. Cilastatin itself has no antibacterial properties and, like the β-lactamase inhibitors, does not interfere with the activity of imipenem or have any known adverse effects of its own. Cilastatin does have other properties that may be advantageous. Imipenem administered alone in high dosages to experimental animals is nephrotoxic. Cilastatin inhibits this nephrotoxicity,[42] and no nephrotoxicity has been observed with imipenem-cilastatin in humans. A second carbapenem, meropenem (Merrem) is more active than imipenem against gram-negative organisms and less active against gram-positive bacteria. It, too, possesses excellent anaerobic activity.[44] Some gram-negative organisms that are resistant to third-generation cephalosporins and to imipenem-cilastatin are sensitive to meropenem.[45] It is also stable against renal hydrolysis, and the coadministration of cilastatin is not required.[45] Like imipenem, it is renally excreted, and dose adjustment is necessary in renal failure.[46]

Adverse effects with imipenem include nausea and vomiting (which may be severe, especially at high dosages), neutropenia, thrombocytopenia, elevated liver enzymes, and seizures.[47] Meropenem is better tolerated than imipenem and may have reduced potential for causing seizures and other central nervous system toxic effects.[45] The carbapenems should be used with great caution in patients who display immediate sensitivity reactions to penicillin, because these drugs may cross-react.

Imipenem rapidly crosses the placenta and achieves levels in fetal tissues equal to or greater than 50% of those in serum. Levels in breast milk are comparable with those in serum.[48] In some species, treatment of pregnant animals caused emesis, diarrhea, weight loss, and death.[49] In animal studies, meropenem does not appear to impair fertility or cause fetal damage, but experience in pregnant women is quite limited. It is not known whether meropenem is excreted in breast milk, but, like imipenem, meropenem appears to penetrate well into most tissues.

Most infectious diseases specialists reserve the use of imipenem and meropenem for infections caused by otherwise resistant gram-negative organisms or serious polymicrobial infection. Imipenem has been used in the treatment of postpartum endometritis[50] and PID.[51] Imipenem is in FDA class C and should be used during pregnancy only when the potential benefits justify the potential risks. Meropenem compared favorably with clindamycin/gentamicin therapy in a prospective, randomized study of 515 patients with acute gynecologic and obstetric pelvic infections. Pregnant and nursing women were excluded from this study, however.[52] Meropenem is a drug in FDA category B.

Macrolides, Azalides, and Lincosamides

The macrolides, lincosamides, and azalides, although chemically unrelated, all bind to the 50s ribosome of bacteria and inhibit protein synthesis. Erythromycin and clarithromycin are macrolides; azithromycin's different structure properly classifies it as an azalide. Clindamycin is the only lincosamide commonly used today.

Erythromycin is a safe and effective antibiotic. It has been the drug of choice for the treatment of *Legionella* and *Mycoplasma* infections for a number of years. It is also the drug of choice for the treatment of chlamydial infections in pregnancy. Because of its spectrum of activity, erythromycin is also frequently prescribed for the treatment of respiratory tract infections and sinusitis. Erythromycin has traditionally been an alternative in the treatment of syphilis for patients with penicillin allergy, but its use for this purpose in pregnancy is no longer recommended because the concentration of drug in fetal tissues may be inadequate for eradication of the organism.[53-55] Erythromycin estolate causes cholestatic hepatitis more frequently than do other preparations[56] and should be avoided. Approximately 10% of women treated with erythromycin estolate in the second trimester had elevated liver function test values that returned to normal after therapy was discontinued.[57,58]

Two relatively new agents, clarithromycin and azithromycin, cause gastrointestinal distress less frequently than does erythromycin.[59] The three drugs are similar in spectrum. The newer drugs possess excellent activity against many of the atypical organisms responsible for respiratory tract infections, but, of note, (1) clarithromycin has greater activity against *H. influenzae* than does erythromycin, and (2) azithromycin, in general, has more gram-negative and less gram-positive activity than does erythromycin.[59-61] These agents penetrate well into tissues and concentrate in cells. Because of its long half-life, clarithromycin can be given twice daily. Azithromycin is especially noteworthy because of its long half-life and sustained high tissue levels[62]; 5-day courses of this antibiotic are comparable with 10-day courses of others. Azithromycin is given once daily. In clinical trials, clarithromycin and azithromycin appear approximately comparable with erythromycin in clinical efficacy in the treatment of sinus, skin and soft tissue, and respiratory tract infections.[63-66] Advantages in terms of side effect profiles, potential patient compliance, and pharmacokinetics with the two newer agents need be weighed against the disadvantage of increased cost (Table 16–3).

Ease of administration coupled with excellent clinical efficacy makes single-dose (1-g) azithromycin the drug of choice for the treatment of nongonococcal urethritis in

TABLE 16–3   Cost (in U.S. Dollars) of Common Oral Antibiotics

Agent	Oral Dosage	Pharmacy 1*	Pharmacy 2*
Sulfisoxazole	1 g q6h	16.00	14.00
	2 g q6h	25.00	22.00
Trimethoprim-sulfamethoxazole	2 SS b.i.d.	26.00	16.00
	1 DS b.i.d.	17.00	11.00
Amoxicillin	250 mg q8h	16.00	12.00
	500 mg q8h	15.00	17.00
Amoxicillin-clavulanic acid	250 mg q8h	79.00	83.00
	500 mg q8h	100.00	92.00
Dicloxacillin	250 mg q6h	20.00	21.00
	500 mg q6h	22.00	34.00
Cephalexin	250 mg q6h	30.00	16.00
	500 mg q6h	29.00	27.00
Cefaclor	250 mg q8h	30.00	27.00
	500 mg q8h	50.00	53.00
Cefuroxime	250 mg b.i.d.	59.00	56.00
	500 mg b.i.d.	131.00	103.00
Erythromycin	250 mg q6h	15.00	12.00
	500 mg q6h	16.00	16.00
Clarithromycin	250 mg b.i.d.	72.00	77.00
	500 mg b.i.d.	72.00	77.00
Azithromycin	500 mg × 1, then 250 mg × 5 days	60.00	63.00
Norfloxacin	400 mg b.i.d.	75.00	77.00
Ciprofloxacin	250 mg b.i.d.	81.00	79.00
	500 mg b.i.d.	94.00	94.00
	750 mg b.i.d.	98.00	98.00
Ofloxacin	200 mg b.i.d.	95.00	99.00
	300 mg b.i.d.	112.00	111.00
	400 mg b.i.d.	118.00	116.00
Gatifloxacin	200 mg po q.d. × 10 days	119.00	107.00
	400 mg po q.d. × 10 days	106.00	104.00
Lomefloxacin	400 mg q.d.	69.00	62.00
Levofloxacin	250 mg q.d.	63.00	85.00
	500 mg q.d.	79.00	94.00
Moxifloxacin	400 mg po q.d. × 10 days	123.00	111.00

*Data obtained in July 2003 from two San Diego, California, pharmacies belonging to different national chains. Costs given are those for a 7-day supply unless otherwise noted, with the least expensive formulation available, and have been rounded to the nearest dollar.
DS, double-strength; PO, orally; SS, single-strength.

patients who are not pregnant.[67,68] Both clarithromycin and azithromycin have been useful in the treatment of atypical mycobacterial infections.

Erythromycin (FDA category B) has a long history of efficacious use in pregnancy, and no major adverse effects on the fetus have been demonstrated. Because of teratogenicity in animal models, clarithromycin is in FDA category C. No such toxicity has been demonstrated with azithromycin,[69] which is in FDA category B.

Clindamycin has activity against streptococci, staphylococci, and both gram-positive and gram-negative anaerobes, including *B. fragilis*. It is available in both oral and intravenous forms. It is well distributed in most body fluids, including the reproductive tract, and achieves levels 30% to 50% of those of serum in the fetus. Most of the drug is metabolized by the liver and excreted in the bile. In the setting of combined renal and hepatic insufficiency, dose adjustment may be necessary.

Anaerobes often play a major role in pathogenesis of infection of the female genital tract, and clindamycin, usually in combination with another antibiotic, is frequently used in the treatment of postpartum endometritis, postoperative infection, and PID. Diarrhea is the major adverse side effect, and clindamycin is one of the most common antibiotics associated with pseudomembranous colitis. Clindamycin has not been associated with congenital defects and is in FDA category B.

Quinolones

The quinolones are another group of antibiotics that are in widespread use. They prevent bacterial replication by inhibiting DNA gyrase, an enzyme that coils and uncoils DNA. The quinolones are of interest because they are active against a wide variety of organisms and because they can be given orally. They penetrate well into tissues and achieve 30% to 50% of serum levels in amniotic fluid. Levels in breast milk equal or exceed those in serum.[70] Ciprofloxacin, one of the first agents marketed, achieves peak serum levels of 2 to 3 μg/mL after an oral dose of 500 mg.[71] Of all the available quinolones, ciprofloxacin has the greatest activity against gram-negative rods, inhibiting most strains (even *P. aeruginosa*) at no more than 1 μg/mL.[72] It is less active against gram-positive organisms, especially streptococci. Norfloxacin is, in general, less active than ciprofloxacin and achieves therapeutic concentrations only in urine. Enoxacin is less active than ciprofloxacin and offers no clear microbiologic or pharmacologic advantages. Ofloxacin is slightly more active than ciprofloxacin against gram-positive bacteria; it is slightly less active than ciprofloxacin against gram-negative organisms on a per-weight basis, but it is better absorbed (100% vs. 80%), and thus the two are approximately comparable. Most of the activity of ofloxacin resides in its S-(−)isomer, which has been marketed as levofloxacin. Levofloxacin, too, is virtually 100% absorbed when given orally, which is an advantage over ofloxacin, and it can be administered once daily. Gatifloxacin has a spectrum of activity very similar to that of levofloxacin, but it also has additional anaerobic coverage. Trovafloxacin has the broadest spectrum of any of these agents and possesses anaerobic activity, in addition to broad gram-positive and gram-negative coverage,[73] but rare cases of fulminant hepatic failure associated with its use has restricted its indications to severe, life-threatening infections. Lomefloxacin is not as active as either ciprofloxacin or ofloxacin, but it has a longer half-life, allowing for once-daily dosing for susceptible organisms.

Quinolones are frequently prescribed in the treatment of complicated urinary tract infections (UTIs) when the organism isolated is resistant to other, less expensive antibiotics. Ciprofloxacin has an excellent history in the treatment of bacillary dysentery and prostatitis. Therapy with a single dose of a number of the quinolones has been shown to be successful in eradicating penicillinase-producing *N. gonorrhoeae*, and they are useful in the treatment of many atypical organisms, such as *Legionella* and *Rickettsia* species.[74] The newer quinolones potentially offer considerable advantage as single oral agents useful in the treatment of serious polymicrobial infections if widespread, indiscriminate use does not limit their effectiveness.[75]

The quinolones are, in general, well tolerated, but nausea, anorexia, and central nervous system toxicity (headache, dizziness) and bad dreams may occur.[76,77] Sparfloxacin has been associated with prolongation of the QT interval, and 8% to 10% of patients taking it experience photosensitivity.[78] Absorption of all of the quinolones is reduced by concomitant administration of antacids containing divalent cations (Mg^{2+}, Ca^{2+}) and sucralfate. Of note, when administered to immature animals, all of the quinolones studied cause lesions in cartilage[79] and are therefore contraindicated in pregnant or lactating women. Their use in pregnancy should be considered only when alternatives are lacking and the benefits are thought to outweigh the risks to the fetus. The quinolones are in FDA category C.

BACTERIAL INFECTIONS

Major Clinical Syndromes

Urinary Tract Infection

UTI is the most common bacterial infection in pregnancy.[80] Three clinical syndromes are described: (1) asymptomatic bacteriuria, (2) acute cystitis, and (3) acute pyelonephritis. Asymptomatic bacteriuria is defined as the presence of at least 10^5 colony-forming units (CFUs) of bacteria per milliliter of clean, voided, midstream urine in specimens obtained on two separate occasions. Acute cystitis is symptomatic infection of the lower urinary tract. Signs of systemic toxicity, such as fever and leukocytosis, are usually absent. Symptoms include dysuria, frequency, urgency, and suprapubic tenderness, and urinalysis demonstrates pyuria and bacteriuria. Although for many years the "gold standard" for assessing the significance of bacteriuria in the setting of acute cystitis was also a colony count of at least 10^5 CFUs/mL, more recent evidence suggests that even low levels of bacteriuria (i.e., $\geq 10^2$ CFUs/mL), when accompanied by pyuria, are meaningful if patients have symptoms.

Pyelonephritis is infection of the kidney. The term *acute pyelonephritis* implies symptomatic infection, and patients have fever, chills, nausea, vomiting, and flank pain, often in addition to the symptoms of lower UTI. Leukocytosis is common. Significant pyuria (≥10 white blood cells per high-power field) and bacteriuria (≥10^5 CFUs/mL) are almost invariably present. The term *subclinical pyelonephritis* is used when infection of the kidney occurs in the absence of any signs of upper tract infection. Depending on the series, between 11% and 47% of cases of documented kidney infection fall into this category.[81] A significant number of women with symptoms of acute cystitis actually have subclinical pyelonephritis. Localization techniques such as ureteral catheterization, Fairley bladder washout,[82] and tests for antibody-coated bacteria[83] have demonstrated that subclinical pyelonephritis may also be the cause of asymptomatic bacteriuria. Thus, although symptoms are used to define the syndromes associated with UTI, their utility in predicting the anatomic site of infection is limited.

Cause and Pathogenesis

Although bacteria may infect the urinary tract by hematogenous or lymphatic routes, they most frequently ascend from the urethra. Periurethral colonization with facultative bowel flora such as *E. coli* commonly precedes ascending infection.[84,85] The ability to attach to uroepithelial cells is an important virulence factor for *E. coli*, the organism that causes more than 90% of community-acquired infections (Table 16-4). In the lower urinary tract, bacteria adhere to mannose receptors present on the surface of bladder epithelial cells. *E. coli* isolates recovered from patients with cystitis adhere to bladder uroepithelial cells in significantly higher numbers than do strains found in the fecal flora.[86] Attachment to different glycolipid receptors, found in high numbers in the upper urinary tract, may be important in the pathogenesis of pyelonephritis, inasmuch as preventing attachment to these receptors precludes pyelonephritis in animal models.[87] Normal women with a history of UTI express these glycolipid receptors in higher numbers than do uninfected control subjects.[88] *Staphylococcus saprophyticus,* the second most common agent causing acute cystitis in women, is also able to adhere to uroepithelial cells, whereas other species of staphylococci do not. In women, the short length of the urethra and sexual intercourse facilitate the ascent of bacteria into the bladder.[89-91] The use of diaphragms and spermicides also predisposes users to vaginal and periurethral colonization with *E. coli*. In pregnancy, there occur profound physiologic alterations that may also contribute to the development of symptomatic infection.

TABLE 16-4   Common Urinary Tract Isolates in Women

Escherichia coli
Klebsiella pneumoniae
Proteus species
Staphylococcus saprophyticus
Group B streptococci
Enterobacter cloacae
Citrobacter diversus
Group D streptococci

Mechanical and hormonal changes may lead to hydroureter, decreased ureteral peristalsis, bladder distention, and incomplete emptying, with subsequent vesicoureteral reflux and stasis.[92-94] Estrogens may also predispose to the development of renal infection in pregnancy through enhancement of growth of *E. coli*.[95-97] Supporting this line of evidence are data indicating that elderly women treated with estrogen[98] and young women taking oral contraceptives[99,100] also appear at increased risk for infection.

Asymptomatic Bacteriuria

Asymptomatic bacteriuria occurs in 2% to 11% of pregnancies; most related studies indicate a prevalence of 4% to 7%.[101,102] The frequency of bacteriuria increases with age, sexual activity, parity, and socioeconomic status. Certain subgroups have a higher incidence; for example, the incidences among diabetic patients and persons with a history of UTI are 12.5% and 18.5%, respectively.[103] Bacteriuria is twice as common in pregnant African American women with sickle cell trait than it is in African American women of the same socioeconomic status without sickle cell trait.[104] Rates among pregnant and non-pregnant sexually active women are similar, however, and there is no evidence that pregnancy predisposes to the acquisition of bacteriuria.

Bacteriuria in pregnancy is a clear predisposition to the development of acute pyelonephritis, which, in turn, poses significant risks to mother and fetus. Although acute pyelonephritis is rare in nonpregnant women with asymptomatic bacteriuria,[105,106] pyelonephritis develops in 13.5% to 65% of bacteriuric pregnant women.[102] Successful treatment of bacteriuria in pregnancy reduces the incidence of pyelonephritis to 2.9%.[102] Failure to eradicate bacteriuria after repeated courses of antibiotic therapy is associated with high rates of symptomatic infection.[107] The incidence of pyelonephritis during pregnancy in women without bacteriuria on initial screening is approximately 1.4%.[102]

Whether asymptomatic bacteriuria itself is a predictor of adverse maternal or fetal outcome has been a matter of debate.[108-111] A metaanalysis of the results of a number of studies showed that untreated asymptomatic bacteriuria during pregnancy significantly increased the rates of preterm delivery and low birth weight in infants. Antibiotic treatment significantly reduced these rates.[112,113]

Screening early in pregnancy with appropriate eradication of bacteriuria, if present, leads to the prevention of 70% to 80% of all cases of antenatal pyelonephritis.[102] Asymptomatic bacteriuria, if present, is found on the first prenatal visit in most women. Only 1% to 2% acquire bacteriuria later in pregnancy.[114] Screening women for asymptomatic bacteriuria on the first prenatal visit is a standard of obstetric care and has been demonstrated to be cost effective.[115] Several authors have advocated screening at the 16th week of gestation as optimal.[101,116] Urine cultures that initially yield positive results (defined as those with ≥10^5 CFUs/mL of urine) should be repeated, because 52% to 59% of women are found to have significant bacteriuria on a second clean-catch midstream specimen.[117,118] The screening method chosen should allow accurate quantification as well as identification of the organism isolated.

Because there is no imperative for immediate treatment in this asymptomatic population, the choice of antibiotic should be based on the results of sensitivity testing. Amoxicillin and sulfa preparations have a long history of efficacy and safety in pregnancy, but in many geographic locations, resistance to these agents is a problem. The combination of trimethoprim-sulfamethoxazole (Septra or Bactrim) is frequently first-line therapy for UTIs, but its use is generally not recommended in pregnancy because of fear of fetal abnormalities caused by trimethoprim. The use of sulfa drugs is not recommended near term because of the risk of kernicterus. Therapy with the combination agent amoxicillin-clavulanate (Augmentin) is successful in treatment of the Enterobacteriaceae (*E. coli, Klebsiella* species, *Proteus* species) that are resistant to amoxicillin alone. Oral cephalosporins may also be used, although their history of use in pregnancy is limited. The quinolones, which are especially useful as oral agents in the treatment of a complicated UTI, are generally not used in this setting in pregnancy because of the risk of fetal abnormalities.

The optimal duration of therapy for asymptomatic bacteriuria in pregnancy has not been established. To minimize toxicity to both the mother and fetus, therapy for asymptomatic bacteriuria should be for the shortest duration required for efficacy. Differences in study design, the small numbers of patients treated, and the use of different antibiotics make drawing conclusions from published trials difficult,[119] and this matter is one of considerable debate. Because of high recurrence rates, several authors initially recommended continuous therapy until term.[110,120] Continuous regimens were associated with adverse effects in the mother, however, and therapy with 7 to 10 days of antibiotics followed by a urine culture to monitor recurrence/reinfection became standard. Results of several studies comparing single-dose or short-course (3- to 5-day) therapy with 7- to 10-day regimens have generated some enthusiasm for single-dose or short-course regimens, because cure rates were comparable.[118,121] Enthusiasm for single-dose therapy in the treatment of uncomplicated cystitis in nonpregnant women, a group much easier to treat, has waned, however.[122-125] Analysis of 28 trials led Norrby to the conclusion that single-dose therapy was less efficacious than therapy for 3 days or more and that β-lactam antibiotics should be administered for a minimum of 5 days.[126] Of note, in most trials, oral cephalosporins have, in general, been less efficacious than amoxicillin or sulfa drugs and should not be used in abbreviated therapy.[127,128] For asymptomatic bacteriuria in pregnancy, most experts continue to recommend treatment for 7 to 10 days.[80,102,129,130]

Acute Cystitis

Symptomatic lower UTI occurs in 1.3% to 3.4% of pregnant women.[131] Urinary frequency, urgency, dysuria, and suprapubic pain define this syndrome. Although patients in whom pyelonephritis develops during pregnancy have frequently had preceding asymptomatic bacteriuria, those who present with cystitis often have not.[131] Likewise, detection and treatment of asymptomatic bacteriuria have decreased the incidence of acute pyelonephritis, but the incidence of acute cystitis has remained relatively constant.

Evidence in nonpregnant women suggests that the finding of even 100 CFUs/mL of bacteria in urine may be significant when urinary tract symptoms are accompanied by pyuria on urinalysis.[132] The presence of pyuria was a better predictor of response to treatment than was the number of bacteria isolated. Although this has not been studied specifically in pregnancy, lowering the threshold for "significant" bacteriuria in the presence of both symptoms and pyuria seems prudent in pregnant women as well. The organisms that cause cystitis are identical to those that cause asymptomatic bacteriuria and pyelonephritis. In pregnant women presenting with lower urinary tract symptoms, a urinalysis and urine culture should be performed.

Because many enteric organisms are resistant to ampicillin or sulfa alone, therapy should be initiated with amoxicillin-clavulanate or a cephalosporin. Older, more standard, less expensive agents can be substituted if the organisms are found to be susceptible. The optimal duration of treatment has not been established, but several factors persuade me to recommend treatment of both patients with asymptomatic bacteriuria and those with symptoms of cystitis for 7 to 10 days (see earlier discussion). In many of the treatment trials of acute uncomplicated cystitis, pregnant women and those with symptoms of more than 24 hours' duration were excluded. In addition, the absence of symptoms of an upper UTI is an imperfect predictor of disease localized to the bladder. As in the treatment of asymptomatic bacteriuria, a follow-up urine culture should be performed after therapy has been completed. If the same organism is again isolated, prolonged (6-week) or suppressive therapy should be considered. The rate of recurrence of acute cystitis is, however, quite low.[131]

Acute Pyelonephritis

Superficial bladder infection carries little morbidity and no mortality, but flank pain, nausea, vomiting, fever, and leukocytosis accompanying the signs and symptoms of a lower UTI indicate kidney involvement, which may have serious consequences for both the mother and the fetus. Pyelonephritis occurs in 1% to 2% of pregnant women,[80] usually in the second or third trimester. Maternal complications include septic shock in 1.3% to 3%[133,134]; adult respiratory distress syndrome is an uncommon complication.[135] Some authors have reported maternal anemia, toxemia, and chronic renal damage as consequences of pyelonephritis in pregnancy, but others disagree.[136] The association between pyelonephritis and preterm labor and delivery is well documented, however.[101,134]

Treatment of asymptomatic bacteriuria reduces the incidence of pyelonephritis.[110] Because pyelonephritis occurs predominantly in women who have had asymptomatic bacteriuria, screening for asymptomatic bacteriuria has become the standard of practice.

The organisms causing pyelonephritis are the same as those implicated in asymptomatic bacteriuria and acute cystitis (see Table 16–4), although in patients who have received prior antibiotic therapy, more resistant organisms may be encountered. Urine culture and sensitivity testing are imperative in the management of acute pyelonephritis. Patients with acute pyelonephritis during pregnancy should be hospitalized and treated with intravenous antibiotics. Third-generation cephalosporins, with or without an aminoglycoside (the latter indicated primarily until sensitivity testing is available), provide excellent broad coverage of most common etiologic organisms. Adjustment to less expensive, more familiar alternatives such as ampicillin, sulfa drugs, or first-generation cephalosporins can occur if the bacteria isolated are susceptible. Fever is common for the first 72 hours after the institution of antibiotic therapy, but the trend in the temperature should be downward. Fever that persists after 72 hours may indicate a complication, and investigation with repeat urine culture and ultrasound examination may be warranted.[137] Appropriate oral antibiotics may be substituted for intravenous therapy 72 hours after fever and leukocytosis have resolved and should be continued to complete a 14-day course.[138] Several analyses have failed to show superiority of any particular treatment regimen for symptomatic infection during pregnancy. Because of a high rate of recurrent pyelonephritis in the pregnant women successfully treated,[138,139] suppressive therapy until delivery[138] or close follow-up with repeated treatment if positive cultures develop[140] is warranted.

Pneumonia

Pneumonia is the second most common nonobstetric bacterial infection during pregnancy. Its incidence has varied widely in different surveys, ranging from 1 per 118 deliveries to 1 per 2288 deliveries.[141,142] Reports suggest an incidence of 1.5 to 2.5 per 1000 pregnancies.[143-145] Pneumonia may occur at any time during pregnancy but is most common in the second and third trimesters.[146] Even in severe cases, prompt antibiotic therapy and aggressive support have reduced maternal mortality rates substantially, from the 20% to 32% noted in the preantibiotic era to 0% to 4% noted currently.[141,143,147] The effects of maternal pneumonia on the fetus are difficult to assess. There is no evidence that congenital abnormalities result from pneumonia in pregnancy,[146] but maternal pneumonia can precipitate preterm labor.[148] In one series, mean birth weight for the children of mothers with antepartum pneumonia was reduced by 400 g, in comparison with a control group without pneumonia.[143]

Although pregnant women still have significant respiratory reserve, pregnancy renders women less capable of dealing with insults. Both defects in host immune response[3] and the increases in lung water noted in pregnancy may contribute to the pathogenesis of pneumonia in this setting. Mechanical factors may also decrease the ability of a pregnant woman to clear secretions. Underlying serious medical illnesses (including prior lung disease, anemia, and illicit drug use) and smoking are clear predispositions.[141-143]

The symptoms, signs, and causes of pneumonia do not differ substantially between pregnant and nonpregnant women. Pneumonia has frequently been divided into "typical" and "atypical" manifestations. In typical bacterial pneumonia, patients usually report the rather abrupt onset of fever, chills, and a cough production of purulent sputum. A history of a preceding upper respiratory tract infection is common. Leukocytosis is present, and chest radiographs classically reveal alveolar filling, usually in a lobar distribution. The bacterial pathogens most commonly isolated in this manifestation in pregnancy are those most common in pneumonia in nonpregnant people (i.e., S. pneumoniae and H. influenzae). In atypical pneumonia caused by Mycoplasma pneumoniae or Chlamydia pneumoniae, patients usually do not appear to be very ill. Their symptoms gradually increase in severity, and they note fever, headache, and a nonproductive, hacking cough. The white blood cell count is not impressive, and chest radiographs exhibit patchy or interstitial infiltrates.

Gram stain and culture of sputum are key to the diagnosis of the specific organism responsible for pneumonia, especially in typical manifestations. Lack of purulent sputum suggests infection by an atypical agent or a virus. The interpretation of sputum culture results in the absence of a Gram stain is fraught with difficulty because samples may be contaminated with organisms from the mouth.

The organisms that cause atypical pneumonia are not often easily isolated in the microbiology laboratory, and special media or prolonged incubation may be required. Diagnoses in these cases are often established with certainty only in retrospect, through comparison of acute and convalescent antibody titers.[149,150] In the setting of acute pneumonia in men and nonpregnant women, how vigorously a specific etiologic diagnosis is pursued often depends on the degree of illness of the patient, the clinical setting, and the confidence of the physician in establishing a clinical diagnosis. Once antibiotics are given, culture of the sputum has very limited usefulness.

The choice of agent for empirical treatment of community-acquired pneumonia depends on the patient's presentation, but penicillin or ampicillin (which inhibit the pneumococcus and non–β-lactamase–producing H. influenzae) or erythromycin (which inhibits the pneumococcus; some H. influenzae strains; and Mycoplasma, Chlamydia, and Legionella species) are still useful agents. At one time, all pneumococci were exquisitely sensitive to penicillin, but widespread use of antibiotics has resulted in the emergence of more resistant organisms. These organisms may be difficult to eradicate in anatomic sites where the concentration of penicillin may be low (e.g., the meninges or middle ear), but high doses of intravenous penicillin are still effective in treating most S. pneumoniae pulmonary infections. However, because of an increasing incidence of resistance of a number of respiratory pathogens, second- and third-generation cephalosporins are now commonly used as first-line empirical therapy, with the addition of a macrolide if the patient is quite ill and the cause is in doubt.[151,152]

Appendicitis

Acute appendicitis is the most common nongynecologic surgical emergency occurring during pregnancy.[153,154] It has an incidence of 1 per 1764 deliveries and is approximately twice as common in the second trimester as in the first and third trimesters.[155] The incidence of appendicitis does not appear to be increased in pregnant women, but diagnosis may be more difficult. In a review of 720 cases of acute appendicitis during pregnancy, perforation occurred in 25%, a rate more than twice that in the general population.[155] This high perforation rate generally reflects a delay in the time to operation. Early symptoms, such as nausea, vomiting, and abdominal pain, are frequently attributed to other, more common conditions in pregnancy. Right lower quadrant tenderness with rebound on examination may be more helpful diagnostically,[155] but guarding and rebound were absent in more than half of patients with appendicitis in the third trimester in one series.[156] As pregnancy progresses, diagnosis may become even more difficult as the appendix rotates cephalad,[155,157] because the disease then causes pain and tenderness in the right upper quadrant. Fever may also be low grade or absent. Leukocytosis with a left shift is common but must be distinguished from the relative leukocytosis of pregnancy.

The key to diagnosis remains a high index of suspicion. Ultrasonography may be helpful in excluding other diagnoses. The technique of ultrasonography with graded compression may visualize the diseased, distended appendix,[154,158,159] but its sensitivity in the presence of perforation is low,[160] and the old maxim "If in doubt, take it out" appears to apply. In the collected series reported by Mahmoodian, although the frequency of "normal appendices" at operation was 31%, a negative laparotomy was associated with low rates of fetal and maternal morbidity and mortality.[155] In contrast, in both this series and others, complications associated with perforation were substantial, with a rate of fetal loss of 17% to 20%.[153,161]

When there is a reasonable possibility that the patient has appendicitis, prompt surgical intervention is appropriate. Laparoscopic techniques are advocated by some authors and are becoming increasingly accepted.[162-164] Short-term, broad-spectrum antibiotics (most commonly ampicillin, an aminoglycoside, and clindamycin) are adjunctive. Antibiotics should be continued and adjusted on the basis of operative cultures if gross perforation has occurred.

Intraamniotic Infection

Bacterial infection of the amniotic cavity occurs in 0.5% to 1% of all pregnancies and causes both maternal morbidity and perinatal mortality.[165,166] Most infections occur after rupture of membranes and are caused by organisms in the cervical or vaginal flora. Risk factors in this setting include the number of vaginal examinations performed, the duration of ruptured membranes, the use of internal monitors, and the total duration of labor.[167] Charles and Edwards reported an increased incidence of intraamniotic infection (IAI) after cervical cerclage; chorioamnionitis developed in 9.6% of patients in the first 4 weeks of cerclage, and an additional 14.8% acquired this condition in the next 4 weeks.[168] Studies have identified meconium-stained amniotic fluid as an independent risk factor for the development of IAI and postpartum endometritis,[169-171] because meconium may enhance bacterial growth and render host defense mechanisms less effective.[172,173] Bacterial vaginosis (Fig. 16–1) has also been recognized as a risk factor for premature birth, IAI, and postcesarean endometritis.[174-176] Maternal bacteremia with organisms such as *Listeria monocytogenes* may also result in IAI, and it

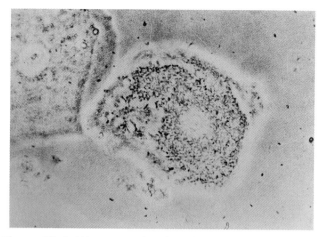

Figure 16–1. Wet mount of a "clue cell," a vaginal epithelial cell covered with bacteria and useful in the diagnosis of bacterial vaginosis.

is in this setting that the consequences to the fetus may be the most devastating.

Why some women acquire IAI after rupture of membranes and others do not probably reflects the interplay of host defense mechanisms, bacterial virulence, and inoculum size. Most infections are polymicrobial; *E. coli;* *Klebsiella* species; group B streptococci (GBS); and anaerobes such as *Bacteroides, Fusobacterium, Clostridium,* and *Peptococcus* species are common isolates.[177] Although both *Chlamydia* and *Mycoplasma* species have been cultured from amniotic fluid of women with clinical chorioamnionitis, their pathogenic potential is unclear.[178-180] Cervical colonization with *Chlamydia trachomatis,* has, however, been associated with adverse pregnancy outcomes (e.g., low birth weight, preterm delivery, and premature rupture of membranes), whereas colonization with the genital mycoplasmas in general has not.[181] Clinically evident IAI is often accompanied by preterm delivery. Subclinical chorioamnionitis, or histologic inflammation of the placenta, has also been associated with early labor.[182,183] *Fusobacterium, Mycoplasma,* and *Ureaplasma* species are the most common isolates in this setting. Although histologic chorioamnionitis is associated with prematurity and perinatal mortality, the correlation between the pathologic and clinical entities is poor,[184] and a metaanalysis failed to demonstrate a clear overall benefit of antibiotic therapy on neonatal outcomes[185] in patients with intact membranes. However, in those with premature rupture of membranes, antibiotic administration is associated with significant neonatal benefit.[186] An analysis of two trials involving 838 women revealed a statistically significant reduction in chorioamnionitis and endometritis in women who received antibiotics for prelabor rupture of membranes at or near term,[187] and a subsequent analysis of more than 6000 women also demonstrated a reduction in neonatal morbidity.[186] In several studies, treatment of bacterial vaginosis during the second trimester in the subset of women who had risk factors for premature delivery significantly reduced rates of preterm birth,[188-190] and a metaanalysis also suggested that treatment of bacterial vaginosis during pregnancy may reduce the risk of low birth weight and preterm prelabor rupture of membranes.[191] Screening for bacterial vaginosis should therefore be considered in patients with risk factors for prematurity.[181,192] Those with positive test results or symptoms of bacterial vaginosis should be treated with oral metronidazole.[192,193] The regimen of 500 mg orally twice daily for 7 days appears most effective.[194] Clindamycin, 300 mg orally twice daily for 7 days, is an alternative. (Although topical therapies may cure bacterial vaginosis, they do not appear to be effective in reducing preterm births.[193]) Making the diagnosis of IAI requires a high index of suspicion because clinical signs and symptoms are neither sensitive nor specific. Fever is the most common clinical finding and is present in 90% to 100% of patients. Maternal tachycardia and uterine tenderness are found in 20% to 80% and 13% to 25%, respectively.[195] The presence of malodorous amniotic fluid is uncommon but is suggestive of mixed aerobic-anaerobic infection. Leukocytosis is frequently present but is also seen in uncomplicated labor. Fetal tachycardia is common but also nonspecific. IAI should be considered in any febrile pregnant woman, especially if rupture of membranes has occurred.

Direct examination of the amniotic fluid may provide very useful information when IAI is suspected. Specimens may be obtained by aspiration through an intrauterine pressure catheter, if one is present, or by amniocentesis, before rupture of membranes. Fluid should be sent for culture, Gram stain, and cell count. A low amniotic fluid glucose level (≤5 to 25 mg/dL) is a good predictor of a positive culture result.[196] However, bacteria and leukocytes may be present in patients who are not clinically infected. In a study of patients with clinical IAI, Gibbs and colleagues found bacteria in 80.5% of patients with IAI, in comparison with 30.8% of control subjects. Infected patients had at least 10^2 CFUs/mL of bacteria, whereas control patients with positive cultures had low numbers of bacteria isolated. The results of Gram stains were positive in 67.4% of infected patients and 11.6% of control subjects. Samples from 80.8% of the infected patients had detectable leukocytes, in comparison with 28.8% of the control samples. In patients with clinical infection, virulent bacteria such as E. coli and GBS were more likely to be isolated, whereas nonpathogenic bacteria, such as lactobacilli and diphtheroids, were the predominant isolates in the uninfected.[177] With infection, amniotic fluid levels of inflammatory cytokines such as interleukin-8 and interleukin-6[196,197] are elevated, and high levels of interleukin-8 may also be present in the urine.[198,199] The clinical utility of such measurements is questionable, however.

Treatment of IAI should include both prompt administration of antibiotics and delivery. Delay in antibiotic therapy increases both maternal and neonatal morbidity. Several studies have demonstrated a significant decline in the incidence of neonatal sepsis when antibiotics are given during parturition versus post partum.[200-202] Gibbs and associates also demonstrated significant improvement in maternal outcome measures with intrapartum treatment,[200] although in one metaanalysis, the difference between giving antibiotics during parturition versus post partum did not achieve statistical significance.[203] There are few

controlled clinical trials to guide the choice of antibiotics in this setting. Traditionally, ampicillin (2 g intravenously every 4 to 6 hours) and gentamicin (1.5 to 2 mg/kg intravenously every 8 hours) have been used with generally good results. Some authors have advocated the addition of clindamycin if delivery is by cesarean section because of the importance of resistant Bacteroides species and the high failure rate of ampicillin-gentamicin alone in postcesarean endometritis.[165] However, in one study in which women were randomly assigned to receive therapy with either ampicillin-gentamicin or ampicillin-gentamicin-clindamycin, no significant differences in the incidence of endometritis or neonatal morbidity or mortality were found.[204] Infusion of larger doses of aminoglycosides once daily results in equal or superior efficacy and less cost and less toxicity than do regimens with infusions every 8 hours.[205] There are very few reports of the use of the new third-generation cephalosporins, extended-spectrum penicillins, or combination β-lactam/β-lactamase inhibitors in the treatment of chorioamnionitis.[206] These drugs usually have the appropriate spectrum of activity and a pharmacokinetic advantage over the aminoglycosides, however, and their use merits serious consideration.

Although studies in general do not indicate a critical time interval from the diagnosis of IAI to delivery, delivery should be prompt, usually within 12 hours of diagnosis.[166,200,207] Although chorioamnionitis is not an indication for cesarean section per se, the rates of cesarean delivery are increased in this population because of dysfunctional labor and fetal distress.[208,209]

In studies since the late 1970s, no maternal deaths from chorioamnionitis have been reported.[165,201,207,210] Postpartum infection is common, however, especially after cesarean delivery. Perinatal mortality rates are increased in IAI, especially in Listeria infection. Premature infants fare much more poorly than their full-term counterparts, and although they may not die of sepsis, infection causes their course to be more complicated. In a total of 371 full-term deliveries reported in two studies, no neonatal deaths occurred, although neonatal sepsis and pneumonia were complications.[201,207] Infants born after IAI may also be at increased risk for the development of cerebral palsy.[211]

Endometritis and Postpartum Infection

Endometritis is the most common infectious complication after parturition. It occurs in approximately 2% to 5% of women delivering vaginally and 15% to 20% of those undergoing cesarean section, although rates vary widely among studies.[212]

In the preantibiotic era, most postpartum infection was caused by group A streptococci, and mortality was significant.[213] Since that time, advances in the understanding of the pathogenesis and treatment of puerperal fever have led to a major decline in rates of morbidity and mortality. Today, nosocomially acquired group A streptococci are a rare cause of puerperal sepsis. Most patients are infected with organisms that are part of their own vaginal flora and respond promptly to antibiotic therapy. Septic shock, necrotizing fasciitis, septic thrombophlebitis, and abscess formation are rare but potentially serious complications.

Cesarean delivery is the major predisposition to post-partum pelvic infection, and infection in this group of patients is also more severe.[214-218] Operative technique may affect infection rates: There is evidence that manual placental removal and exteriorization of the uterus for repair of the surgical incision increase the incidence of endometritis in both the absence and the presence of prophylactic antibiotics.[219,220] Length of operation, not surprisingly, is also a positive correlate.[216,221] The duration of labor before abdominal delivery has been found to be the most significant factor related to infectious complications.[216,222,223] Other commonly cited risk factors include preterm birth and premature rupture of membranes,[224] duration of membrane rupture before delivery,[225-227] colonization of the vagina with virulent organisms, bacterial vaginosis, and high colony counts of bacteria in amniotic fluid.[228] Positive amniotic fluid cultures (collected without contamination at cesarean section) are strongly associated with puerperal infection.[227,229-231]

In indigent patients, regardless of race, puerperal infection rates are higher than those in patients of higher socioeconomic status.[230,232] Some studies have questioned whether the number of vaginal examinations correlated with an increase in the infection rate,[233,234] whereas others have reported an increase in infection with internal fetal monitoring.[235] Results vary among studies, however. The interrelated nature of many of these variables complicates analysis, and some authors question whether all of these factors are independent predictors of infection or simply part of a high-risk state.[236]

Endometritis occurring in the first 24 to 36 hours after delivery tends to be caused by a single organism, and GBS is most commonly identified.[237,238] Most cases of endometritis are polymicrobial, however, and occur 48 or more hours after delivery[227] (Table 16-5). "Ascending" infection with contamination of the uterine cavity by organisms present in the vagina is the most common route of infection. Endometritis may result from clinical or subclinical chorioamnionitis present before parturition or may occur solely as a consequence of delivery. Both host defense and the nature and virulence of the organisms in the vaginal flora play an important role in pathogenesis. The presence of bacterial vaginosis[213,239] or *Mycoplasma hominis*[217] is correlated with increased risk. The isolation of *C. trachomatis* was correlated with late-onset endometritis in one study[180] but was not correlated with infection in several others.[240,241] Colonization with group B streptococci also is a risk factor for postpartum endometritis; colonized

patients have an 80% greater likelihood of developing this infection.[242] Tissue trauma, hematoma formation, retained placental tissue, and the presence of any foreign material predispose the host to endometritis. Once the endometrium is involved, infection may spread to the myometrium, parametrium, and adnexal structures. In cesarean deliveries, wound infection may also occur. Infection becomes more serious as it progresses. Bacteremia accompanies endometritis in 8% to 20% of cases.[230] Three cases of endometritis caused by herpes simplex virus have been reported in the medical literature.[243,244]

The most common signs and symptoms of endometritis include fever, leukocytosis, lower abdominal pain, uterine tenderness, and purulent or foul-smelling lochia.[245] Although transient fever to 38° C (100.4° F) is found in approximately 20% of postpartum patients,[246] persistent fever is probably the most important hallmark of true infection. When virulent organisms such as the β-hemolytic streptococci, *S. aureus,* or *Clostridium perfringens* are involved, the patient may quickly become critically ill with chills, high fever, severe pain, and abdominal distention. With the β-hemolytic streptococci and *C. perfringens,* discharge may be serosanguineous rather than foul smelling or purulent, and a Gram stain of the lochia may reveal large numbers of gram-positive cocci or gram-positive rods, respectively. Most postpartum endometritis of polymicrobial origin is more insidious in onset. Intermittent low-grade fever may be the only clinical finding. Other causes of fever, such as atelectasis, UTI, or wound or episiotomy infection, should be sought, but postpartum pyrexia must be considered to be caused by endometritis until proven otherwise.[232]

When endometritis is suspected, both endometrial cultures and blood cultures should be obtained. Bacteremia occurs in 5% to 25% of women with endometritis. In one study, 1 (0.8%) of 126 patients with a temperature lower than 38.8° C had a positive blood culture, whereas 9 (21.4%) of 42 patients with a temperature higher than 38.8° C had documented bacteremia.[247] Although the utility of endometrial cultures is debated,[245] and anaerobic isolates may not even be fully identified by the time the patient is discharged, the isolation of facultative aerobic organisms is straightforward and may be useful in guiding therapy. Because of the risk of vaginal contamination of specimens with the transcervical approach, the use of protected catheters (double-lumen, triple-lumen, or brush)[248-250] and of transfundal needle aspiration[251] has been advocated, but no clear consensus on the optimal culture method exists.

Once endometritis is suspected and appropriate cultures have been obtained, broad-spectrum antibiotic coverage should be begun. For many years, standard therapy consisted of clindamycin plus gentamicin, although monotherapy has been shown to be equally efficacious with second-generation cephalosporins such as cefoxitin or cefotetan; extended-spectrum penicillins such as mezlocillin, piperacillin, and ticarcillin; and β-lactam/β-lactamase inhibitor combinations such as ticarcillin-clavulanate or ampicillin-sulbactam.[239,252-257] An analysis of 47 treatment trials suggested regimens with appropriate coverage for penicillin-resistant anaerobes were superior to those without such coverage.[258] Intravenous therapy

---

TABLE 16-5   Common Organisms Causing Endometritis

Escherichia coli
Klebsiella species
Group B streptococci
Group D streptococci (enterococci)
Gardnerella vaginalis
Peptostreptococci and peptococci
Bacteroides species
Clostridium species
Fusobacterium species

should be continued until the patient is afebrile for a minimum of 36 to 48 hours and clinical signs have abated. Cure rates of postpartum endometritis approach 95%, and additional outpatient oral antibiotic therapy does not appear to be necessary in most patients without bacteremia.[259,260] If fever persists 48 to 72 hours after the initiation of appropriate antibiotic therapy, wound infection, parametrial abscess formation necessitating draining, or septic thrombophlebitis may be present. Pelvic ultrasonography, computed tomography, or magnetic resonance imaging may be useful in this setting.[261] In critically ill or persistently febrile patients, drainage of any fluid collections and uterine curettage should be considered. Uterine gas formation may signal myonecrosis and the need for emergency hysterectomy, although nonsurgical management has been reported to be adequate for patients not seriously ill.[262,263] On occasion, a resistant organism not covered by the antibiotic regimen chosen (e.g., enterococci with clindamycin-gentamicin therapy) may be encountered, and appropriate adjustments in antibiotic treatment (e.g., the addition of penicillin or ampicillin) should be made.

Septic thrombophlebitis is a common complication of protracted pelvic infection and causes persistent fever despite appropriate antibiotic coverage. Patients may experience wide fluctuations in temperature but usually do not appear dangerously ill and have only vague abdominal discomfort. Septic embolus to the lungs is an infrequent but serious complication. Although it is commonly said that the institution of heparin therapy usually results in defervescence within 48 to 72 hours, one review noted a median of 5 days before patients became afebrile.[264] Anticoagulants should be continued for 10 days.

The incidence of postpartum endometritis has been greatly reduced through the use of prophylactic antibiotics after cesarean section.[212,265,266] A single dose of antibiotic may be given after cord clamping to avoid exposure of the fetus if no evidence of intrapartum infection is present. Many different antibiotics have been used as prophylaxis and are effective. First-generation cephalosporins, such as cefazolin (Ancef), appear to be as effective as newer agents in this case and are less expensive.[267]

Sexually Transmitted Diseases

Syphilis

Syphilis is caused by the spirochete *Treponema pallidum*, and the illness that results from this infection is typically one of stages. Primary syphilis occurs after spirochetal inoculation into a skin or mucous membrane site, which results in a characteristic painless, indurated ulcer called a *chancre*. The incubation period for primary syphilis varies, depending on the size of the inoculum, but averages approximately 21 days. Organisms are plentiful in the primary lesion, and painless inguinal adenopathy is frequently present. Even without treatment, chancres spontaneously heal, usually in approximately 6 weeks. The secondary stage of infection usually occurs after the chancre has healed and represents hematogenous dissemination with replication of the organism in multiple organs. This stage is characterized by fever, malaise, and a generalized maculopapular rash involving the palms and soles (Fig. 16–2). Mucous patches and condyloma lata represent proliferation of organisms in moist areas of the skin during the second stage of infection. Generalized lymphadenopathy may be present at this stage, and hepatitis is fairly common. Headache may be severe enough to warrant lumbar puncture; subsequent results are compatible with aseptic meningitis. The findings of secondary syphilis also spontaneously remit but may recur over the next several years. Syphilis then typically enters a latent phase in which patients are completely asymptomatic. In approximately one third of infected people, the disease progresses to the development of tertiary syphilis, which involves the central nervous system (e.g., tabes dorsalis, general paresis), cardiovascular system, or skin and musculoskeletal tissues. The latent period between secondary and tertiary syphilis is usually a decade or more; the course may be significantly shortened in patients infected with human immunodeficiency virus (HIV). On pathologic examination, an obliterative small vessel endarteritis is characteristic of syphilis in all stages.[268]

Syphilis is transmitted primarily through sexual contact or transplacentally. Accidental direct inoculation by health care workers through the handling of infected specimens is rare, as is transmission by blood transfusion.

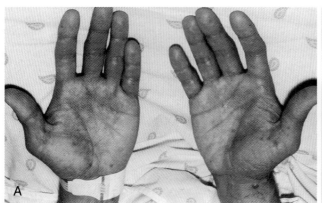 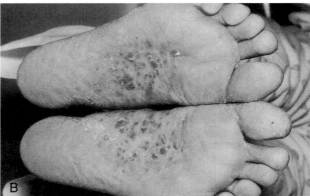

Figure 16–2. Secondary syphilis. Maculopapular skin lesions involving the palms (**A**) and soles (**B**).

Syphilis in pregnancy usually occurs in women who are young and unmarried and in those who receive little or no prenatal care.[269] In the early 1990s, the incidence of syphilis in women and cases of congenital syphilis nearly tripled; however, since the mid-1990s, a decline to previous levels has again been noted.[269] Although congenital syphilis is now rare in the United States, with 30 cases per 100,000 live births noted in 1996, it is still a major problem in sub-Saharan Africa and in countries of the former Soviet Union.[270,271]

The manifestations and clinical course of syphilis in pregnant women are no different than in women who are not pregnant. In women, chancres on the external genitalia may be easy to identify, but when present on the cervix or in the vagina, they may go undetected; when present in the mouth, chancres may be misidentified. In some people, especially those with prior infection, no primary lesion or only a small papule may develop.[272] Syphilis should be considered in the differential diagnosis of any genital lesion and any generalized rash, especially one involving the palms and soles.

The primary aim of screening programs in pregnancy is to prevent transmission to the fetus, which can occur as early as 6 weeks' gestation and can result in spontaneous abortion, stillbirth, nonimmune hydrops, intrauterine growth restriction, premature delivery, and perinatal death.[269,272-277] The risk of transmission is related to the stage of maternal infection and reflects the degree of maternal bloodstream infection. In a study reported by Fiumara and associates in 1952, half of the infants born to mothers with untreated primary or secondary syphilis were premature or stillborn or died soon after birth; congenital syphilis developed in the other 50%. Of the children delivered during the late latent stage in their mothers, 10% were stillborn and 10% had congenital infection.[278]

The manifestations of congenital syphilis are quite variable; however, most frequently, affected offspring initially appear normal.[268] In early congenital syphilis, which encompasses the period of the first 2 years of life, rhinitis (snuffles) may be the earliest sign. A diffuse, desquamative, maculopapular rash involving the palms and soles may follow. Osteochondritis and perichondritis are common. In severely infected infants, hepatosplenomegaly, jaundice, generalized lymphadenopathy, anemia, and thrombocytopenia may be present. Surviving infants may enter a latent period and may eventually manifest the signs of late congenital syphilis such as interstitial keratitis, eighth nerve deafness, abnormal notched teeth, frontal bossing, and saber shins.[268] In early congenital syphilis, spirochetes are plentiful in affected organs. As the disease progresses, more of the manifestations reflect scars induced by early lesions or reactions to persistent inflammation, and organisms are few.[279]

The approach to diagnosis of maternal syphilis depends on the stage of infection. Darkfield examination of primary or secondary stage skin lesions often reveals characteristic, coiled, motile spirochetes. Early in infection, serologic tests may be negative, but by the time secondary lesions are present, high titers of antibodies are found. Both primary and secondary lesions have characteristic pathologic processes. Silver stains and specific immunofluorescent or immunoperoxidase stains may demonstrate spirochetes in tissue samples, but biopsies are rarely necessary. Macroscopically, the placenta may be large, thick, and pale, and the umbilical cord may resemble a barber's pole. In necrotizing funisitis, the microscopic appearance of the umbilical cord is that of perivascular inflammation and obliterative endarteritis of the matrix; this appearance is pathognomonic of congenital infection.[268]

Most cases of syphilis in pregnancy are detected through screening serologic tests. Serologic testing should be performed at the time of the first prenatal visit. Some states require that all mothers be tested at the time of delivery; the Centers for Disease Control and Prevention (CDC) recommends testing twice during the third trimester in patients thought to be at high risk, with the second test at 28 weeks. The CDC also recommends testing all women who deliver a stillborn infant after 20 weeks' gestation.

There are two types of serologic tests used in the diagnosis of syphilis. Nontreponemal tests (e.g., the rapid plasma reagin and the Venereal Disease Research Laboratory test) measure antibodies to cardiolipin-cholesterol-lecithin. Infection with *T. pallidum* induces production of these antibodies, but they are also present in a variety of other clinical situations. These tests have the advantage of being rapid and inexpensive to perform, but false-positive results are common in settings in which there is a strong immunologic stimulus, in intravenous drug users, and in patients with rheumatologic disease.[268] Pregnancy itself may also result in false-positive nontreponemal tests. Specific treponemal tests (the fluorescent treponemal antibody absorption test, the *T. pallidum* hemagglutination test, and the microhemagglutination assay for *T. pallidum*), in which lyophilized *T. pallidum* or a lysate of pathogenic *T. pallidum* is used as the source of antigen, should be performed to confirm the diagnosis. The Venereal Disease Research Laboratory or rapid plasma reagin test usually yields positive results 4 to 8 weeks after acquisition of the organism, but up to one fourth of patients may have negative test results when a chancre is first present.[280] Titers usually parallel the course of infection. Quantitative rapid plasma reagin values should start to fall after therapy is initiated and should be negative 1 year after treatment of primary syphilis and 2 years after treatment of secondary syphilis.[268] Specific treponemal test results usually remain positive for life, although reversion to a nonreactive status has been documented in patients with HIV infection and in those treated very early in infection.[281,282]

The diagnosis of maternal syphilis is fairly straightforward. Determining whether a neonate is infected may be more problematic because many infants are asymptomatic at birth and the standard treponemal and nontreponemal antibody tests primarily measure immunoglobulin G (IgG), which crosses the placenta. Newer serologic tests (immunoglobulin M [IgM] enzyme-linked immunosorbent assay [ELISA], IgM and immunoglobulin A [IgA] immunoblotting) and the use of polymerase chain reaction (PCR) may be helpful in the future, but experience with these modalities is currently limited.[269]

Penicillin is the treatment of choice for all stages of syphilis, and there are no proven alternatives to penicillin for treatment of syphilis during pregnancy[270] (Table 16-6). Penicillin is effective in preventing transmission to the

TABLE 16–6   Treatment Regimens for Syphilis

Adult

Primary, secondary, or early latent* syphilis: Benzathine penicillin, 2.4 mU, in a single IM dose

Late latent syphilis or syphilis of unknown duration: Benzathine penicillin, 7.2 mU, administered as three doses of 2.4 million units IM each at 1-wk intervals

Tertiary syphilis (gummatous and cardiovascular): Benzathine penicillin, 7.2 mU, administered as three doses of 2.4 million units IM each at 1-wk intervals

Tertiary syphilis (neurosyphilis): Aqueous crystalline penicillin G, 18-24 mU/day, administered as 3-4 mU IV every 4 hr for 10-14 days, *or* procaine penicillin, 2.4 mU/day IM, plus probenecid, 500 mg orally q.i.d., both for 10 to 14 days

Congenital

Aqueous crystalline penicillin G, 100,000-150,000 U/kg/day, administered as 50,000 U/kg/dose IV every 12 hours during the first 7 days of life and every 8 hours thereafter for a total of 10 days, *or* procaine penicillin G, 50,000 U/kg IM as a single dose for 10 days

From Centers for Disease Control and Prevention: Guidelines for treatment of sexually transmitted diseases. MMWR Morb Mortal Wkly Rep 2002;51(RR-6):1.
*Syphilis acquired during the previous year (i.e., those with documented seroconversion within 1 year; those with unequivocal symptoms of primary or secondary syphilis during the past year; those with a sex partner with primary, secondary, or early latent syphilis within the past year). All others with positive serologic profiles in the absence of symptoms are assumed to have late latent syphilis. IM, intramuscularly; IV, intravenously.

fetus and in treating in utero infection. Women with a history of significant penicillin allergy should be desensitized and treated with penicillin. (For regimens for skin testing to confirm penicillin allergy and for desensitization protocols, readers are referred to the latest CDC monograph on the treatment of sexually transmitted diseases.[270]) Infants born to mothers with untreated syphilis at the time of delivery, mothers whose treatment occurred no more than 1 month before delivery, or mothers who were treated with regimens other than penicillin should receive penicillin therapy. In addition, infants born to mothers who experienced a fourfold rise in nontreponemal antibody titers during pregnancy (indicating reinfection or relapse) and those born to mothers treated early in pregnancy who fail to demonstrate a significant decline in antibody or whose serologic response was not documented should also be treated[270] (see Table 16–6).

Women with a history of syphilis during pregnancy are at high risk for delivering infants with congenital syphilis during subsequent pregnancies. McFarlin and Bottoms retrospectively reviewed the charts of 46 women with documented syphilis who had delivered at least two consecutive infants at their institution, and they found that 40% who delivered an infant with congenital syphilis during the first pregnancy delivered another infant with congenital syphilis during a second pregnancy. Of those whose first infants were free of infection, 42% transmitted syphilis to their second offspring. Lack of prenatal care, continued drug abuse, and failure to re-treat those with documented treatment during the first pregnancy appeared to be risk factors. McFarlin and Bottoms found that serologic titers were not clinically useful and urged caution in assuming that one-time treatment is adequate in patients with continued risk for reinfection.[283]

All women found to have syphilis in pregnancy should be screened for the presence of other sexually transmitted diseases, including HIV infection.

Gonorrhea

Approximately 600,000 new cases of gonorrhea occur each year in the United States, and many of these cases in women are asymptomatic.[270] The responsible organism, *N. gonorrhoeae*, is a nonmotile, gram-negative diplococcus that is shaped like a kidney bean. The gonococcus attaches to columnar or cuboidal epithelial cells lining mucosal surfaces and eventually penetrates into the submucosal tissues, causing neutrophil migration and microabscess formation. Although gonorrhea is primarily a mucosal infection (i.e., cervicitis, urethritis, proctitis, pharyngitis, and conjunctivitis), some strains are able to circumvent host defense mechanisms, enter the bloodstream, and cause disseminated gonococcal infection.[284]

Gonorrhea is transmitted primarily through sexual contact, although neonates may also acquire the disease in utero, during delivery, or in the postpartum period.[285] As is the case in most sexually transmitted diseases, the risk of transmission from men to women during sexual intercourse is greater than that from women to men[286,287] and exceeds 90% after three exposures.[288] In favorable conditions, *N. gonorrhoeae* can survive in the environment for up to 24 hours, but transmission through fomites is extremely uncommon.[289]

The incidence of gonorrhea in pregnancy ranges from less than 1% to 7.3%, depending on the population studied. Most infected women are asymptomatic. The endocervix is the major site of infection, and symptoms, when present, usually develop approximately 10 days after exposure. These include dysuria without other symptoms of UTI, increased vaginal discharge, and intermenstrual bleeding.[286,290,291] Up to 40% of infected women may also have positive rectal cultures, and the rectum may be the only infected site in approximately 5%.[286,291] Pharyngeal infection can be found in 10% to 20% of infected women, and one study suggests that the incidence is higher in infected pregnant women than in infected nonpregnant women.[286,292,293] Symptomatic proctitis and pharyngitis may be present, but, again, most infected patients are symptom free. Of note, those with symptomatic gonorrhea infection often also are infected with other sexually transmitted pathogens, such as *C. trachomatis.*

PID is a well-recognized complication of gonorrhea, but both PID and perihepatitis (the Fitz-Hugh–Curtis syndrome) are uncommon in pregnant women after the first trimester.[294] Pregnant women with gonorrhea have an increased incidence of spontaneous abortion, preterm labor, premature rupture of membranes, and perinatal infant mortality.[286,294,295] There is debate about whether disseminated gonococcal infection, which represents bacteremic gonococcal infection, is more common in pregnancy.[286,296-298] This syndrome, which usually occurs in persons who carry *N. gonorrhoeae* asymptomatically, consists of fever, malaise, arthralgia, multiple pustular skin lesions (Fig. 16–3), tenosynovitis, or septic arthritis, most commonly involving the knee, ankle, or wrist. The strains of *N. gonorrhoeae* that cause disseminated gonococcal infection have been found to share several characteristics: They are

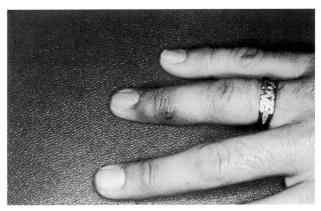

Figure 16–3. Disseminated gonococcal infection. Note the pustular skin lesion over the distal interphalangeal joint of the ring finger. (Photograph courtesy of Allen McCutcheon, MD, University of California, San Diego, School of Medicine.)

resistant to complement-mediated lysis, they share certain auxotypes and surface membrane protein serotypes, and they are exquisitely sensitive to penicillin. Disseminated gonococcal infection was fairly common in the 1970s, but the strains of *N. gonorrhoeae* that produced it have become less prevalent, and, thus, so has the syndrome.[286]

The most common manifestation of gonorrhea infection in the newborn is conjunctivitis, called *ophthalmia neonatorum*. Purulent conjunctival exudate affecting both eyes usually develops within 1 week after birth and may lead to permanent corneal scarring and blindness if left untreated. To establish the diagnosis, the organism can be seen on a Gram stain of the discharge, and it is easily cultured on appropriate media. Topical application of a 1% silver nitrate solution soon after delivery is highly effective prophylaxis, but the best prevention is to ensure that mothers have been appropriately screened and treated for infection, if present, before giving birth.

The CDC recommends screening for *N. gonorrhoeae* at the first prenatal visit for women at risk or for women living in areas where the prevalence of *N. gonorrhoeae* is high. A repeat test should be performed during the third trimester for those at continued risk.[270] Culture remains the diagnostic procedure of choice. If specimens are collected adequately and processed with reasonable speed (≤6 hours), a single culture with commercially available transport media and subsequently inoculated onto selective growth media has a sensitivity in women of 80% to 90%. In asymptomatic women, sampling endocervical secretions alone is recommended, but specimens from additional sites (e.g., oropharynx, rectum, blood) should be cultured, depending on the clinical history in those with symptoms. A number of new sensitive diagnostic tests for *N. gonorrhoeae* involving rapid antigen detection methods or amplification techniques, such as PCR or ligase chain reaction, have been developed and are useful in screening endocervical swabs (preferred) or urine when culture is not feasible.[299-301]

Cefixime, an oral third generation cephalosporin, was a widely used drug for the treatment of gonorrhea in pregnancy, but it is no longer manufactured. Studies with small numbers of women suggest that amoxicillin plus probenecid may be an acceptable oral alternative, but intramuscular regimens are the only ones currently recommended in this setting.[270,302] Pregnant women with uncomplicated gonococcal infections of the cervix, urethra, rectum, or oropharynx should be treated with ceftriaxone, 125 mg intramuscularly in a single dose. Those who cannot receive cephalosporin should be treated with 2 g of spectinomycin in a single intramuscular dose. Gonococcal infections of the oropharynx are more difficult to eradicate than urogenital or anorectal infections, and ceftriaxone, 125 mg intramuscularly in a single dose, is the only regimen recommended in pregnancy. Patients with disseminated gonococcal infection should usually be hospitalized and treated with ceftriaxone, 1 g intravenously or intramuscularly every 24 hours, for a 7-day course.

Chlamydial Infections

C. trachomatis probably causes more sexually transmitted infections in the United States than any other pathogen.[303] It is the major cause of nonspecific urethritis and postgonococcal urethritis in men. Although most women with chlamydial infection are asymptomatic, it may cause various clinical syndromes, and it is isolated in approximately 20% of women with PID; the range is approximately 5% to 51%, depending on the population studied.[304] Certain serovars or strains of *C. trachomatis* are responsible for lymphogranuloma venereum (LGV), a specific clinical syndrome endemic in Africa, Southeast Asia, India, and South America with sporadic cases elsewhere. Worldwide, *C. trachomatis*, the agent of ocular trachoma, is a leading cause of blindness. In the United States, it is a major cause of neonatal conjunctivitis and pneumonia during the first 6 months of life.

Chlamydiae are bacteria that have a complex, two-part life cycle. The extracellular form, called an elementary body, is metabolically inert and most closely resembles a spore. It attaches to specific receptors on host epithelial cells and subsequently becomes internalized, probably through receptor-mediated endocytosis. The elementary body then reorganizes into the replicative form, the reticulate body, which must rely on the host cell as its source of energy. The ability to survive within cells and inhibit phagolysosomal fusion is critical for establishing infection, and infected cells release multiple elementary bodies to continue the life cycle. Chlamydiae most closely resemble gram-negative bacteria. They contain lipopolysaccharide but lack peptidoglycan, which helps other bacteria maintain their rigid cell walls. Although all isolates of *C. trachomatis* share some common epitopes, the strains that cause LGV can be distinguished from those causing trachoma and those causing oculogenital disease in adults and children.

In the tropics, ocular trachoma is spread by person-to-person contact, through fomites, or through vectors such as flies that feed on the exudate from active conjunctivitis. LGV and the serovars responsible for urogenital infection in adults are spread through sexual contact. The risk of transmission with sexual intercourse has not been precisely quantified, but it appears to be less than that for gonorrhea.[305] Adolescents and adults with genital infection may acquire acute follicular conjunctivitis from autoinoculation. Spread between individuals through nonsexual contact with infected secretions also occurs.[306] Infants usually acquire infection by passage through an infected birth canal. Approximately 65% of infants born to infected mothers acquire the organism during vaginal delivery.[307]

Ocular trachoma is a chronic follicular conjunctivitis that causes conjunctival scarring and distortion of the eyelids, eventually resulting in corneal ulcerations and loss of vision. The L1, L2, and L3 serovars of *C. trachomatis* cause LGV, which begins as a small papule or painless ulceration at the site of inoculation, usually on the genital mucosa or adjacent skin. The incubation period ranges from 3 to 30 days, and the primary lesion heals spontaneously without treatment.[308,309] Days to weeks after the appearance of the primary lesion, the lymph nodes draining the area become painful, erythematous, and enlarged. Lymphadenopathy is unilateral in two thirds of patients.[308,309] Initially, the nodes may be discrete, but eventually they may become an inflammatory mass (bubo) that becomes fluctuant and ruptures in one third of those infected. In this stage of the illness, patients frequently experience fever, headache, and myalgias, which may improve as the buboes rupture and form sinus tracts. Relapses occur in approximately 20% of untreated patients.[310] The diagnosis is usually made through serologic testing or through isolation of the organism from infected tissue. LGV has a fairly characteristic histopathologic process that also can aid in establishing a diagnosis in the appropriate clinical setting.

The serovars of *C. trachomatis* that produce urogenital infection are less invasive than those causing LGV. Most women and up to 50% of men who are infected with these strains are asymptomatic.[303] When symptoms are present in women, they most frequently are mild and consist of vaginal discharge, lower abdominal pain, bleeding with intercourse, and dysuria. Vaginal discharge usually reflects endocervical rather than vaginal infection because the organism does not infect the squamous epithelium of the adult vagina. Chlamydiae are also a frequent cause of the acute urethral syndrome, which consists of dysuria and frequency in the absence of at least 10^5 CFUs/mL of bacteria in urine. In one study, approximately 25% of patients with the acute urethral syndrome and pyuria were infected with *C. trachomatis* and responded to appropriate antibiotics.[311] *C. trachomatis* infection can lead to clinical endometritis and salpingitis, and it is isolated from approximately 20% of patients with PID.[304] In comparison with PID caused by *N. gonorrhoeae*, the disease caused by *C. trachomatis* is generally more subacute but just as frequently results in tubal scarring and infertility. Recurrent infections are not uncommon. In men, chlamydiae are responsible for 30% to 50% of cases of symptomatic nongonococcal urethritis and are the most frequent cause of epididymitis in men aged 35 years or younger.[308,312,313]

The prevalence of *C. trachomatis* infection in pregnancy depends on the population studied and ranges from 2% to 35%.[179,303,314,315] Although there is controversy,[316-318] some studies have found an association between *C. trachomatis* infection and spontaneous abortion, premature rupture of membranes, preterm delivery, stillbirth, and neonatal death.[179,314,315,319-322]

Neonatal inclusion conjunctivitis usually develops 5 to 12 days after birth. From 15% to 44% of children born to infected mothers manifest overt findings, whereas serologic evidence of infection can be found in 60%.[323,324] Prophylaxis with silver nitrate or topical antibiotics does not appear to be effective. Pneumonia develops in 3% to 16%, usually 4 to 17 weeks after delivery.[324,325] This pneumonia may be subacute in onset. Frequently, the infants are afebrile or have only low-grade fever. Cough is a prominent feature. Of note, infection can result in subsequent pulmonary dysfunction.[326,327]

Inoculation into cell culture traditionally has been the "gold standard" for the detection of chlamydial infection, but it is expensive and time consuming, and many laboratories no longer use this technique. The sensitivity and specificity of all of the diagnostic tests for chlamydiae are directly related to the adequacy of the specimen obtained for testing.[303] In women, endocervical specimens containing columnar epithelial cells are required. Chlamydial urethritis in men is best diagnosed from urethral swabs obtained several hours after urination. For culture, specimens should be placed in a special transport medium and refrigerated immediately after collection at 2° to 8° C.[303] Antigen detection techniques such as direct fluorescent antibody, enzyme immunoassay, or DNA hybridization tests usually are quicker and easier to perform than culture but are not suitable for vaginal, rectal, nasopharyngeal, or female urethral specimens.[328] They also lack specificity in a low-prevalence population and may lack sensitivity in pregnancy and in women with disturbed vaginal lactobacillary flora.[300,301] However, DNA probe tests for *N. gonorrhoeae* and chlamydiae may be performed with a single specimen, which is an advantage.[329] Commercial PCR and ligase chain reaction kits for the detection of *C. trachomatis* are the most sensitive and specific tests available.[301,303,330] Both tests allow detection with urine specimens, a major advantage in screening programs. Direct cytologic examination with Giemsa staining of smears taken from newborns with conjunctivitis demonstrates typical intracellular chlamydial inclusions in more than 90%[331] but lacks sensitivity in other clinical situations. Serologic tests have little utility except in the diagnosis of LGV (in which a single or stable complement fixation titer of ≥1:64 is supportive) or pneumonitis in infants (detection of a titer of IgM antibodies of ≥1:32 by micro-immunofluorescence is diagnostic).[301]

The CDC recommends screening women younger than 25 years and those who have new or multiple sex partners for chlamydial infection during the third trimester of pregnancy.[270] In those who lack symptoms, a positive result on a nonculture screening test should be confirmed by culture or another nonculture test.[303,328]

Azithromycin, doxycycline, and ofloxacin are the preferred agents for treatment of uncomplicated chlamydial infections in adults who are not pregnant. Erythromycin, 500 mg orally four times a day for 7 days, has been the traditional treatment in pregnancy, but side effects (nausea, vomiting, diarrhea and abdominal pain) are frequent and limit its usefulness. Doxycycline and ofloxacin are not recommended in pregnancy because of their potential to harm the fetus. Although experience with azithromycin in pregnancy is not as extensive as that with erythromycin, it appears to be safe and is better tolerated. A single 1-g dose of azithromycin offers advantages in terms of compliance and efficacy.[332] Amoxicillin, 500 mg three times daily for 7 days, is now also considered first-line therapy and is preferable to erythromycin regimens.[332] Repeat testing, preferably by culture, is recommended 3 weeks after therapy is completed.[270] Sex partners should also be referred for evaluation and treatment. Patients should be counseled to refrain from intercourse for the 7 days of treatment or for 7 days after single-dose azithromycin.

Specific Etiologic Agents of Note

Group B Streptococcal Infections

The GBS, also known as *Streptococcus agalactiae*, was first described as a human pathogen in 1938 in a report by Fry of three cases of fatal puerperal sepsis.[333] This organism was estimated to cause approximately 7600 infections in infants in 1990, and it accounts for 10% to 20% of positive blood cultures in women admitted to obstetric services.[238,334-336] Despite advances in the treatment of critically ill newborns, GBS can cause significant neonatal morbidity and mortality.

Group B streptococci all share a common carbohydrate group antigen that is detected in the Lancefield grouping system. In addition, six type-specific polysaccharide capsular antigens (designated Ia, Ib, II, III, IV, and V) have been identified. Current serotype classification also depends on the presence or absence of another group of antigens called C proteins, which may be present in strains of any capsular polysaccharide type. Both the strain-specific capsular polysaccharides and the C proteins appear to be virulence factors for GBS by aiding the bacteria in evading opsonization and phagocytosis,[337,338] and antibody against either offers protection in animal models of infection.[339] The sialic acid residues present in the capsule appear to be important in virulence because capsule-deficient or desialylated isogenic transposon mutants of type III GBS are less virulent.[340] It has been suggested that the sialic acid residues prevent activation of the alternative complement pathway.[337] Of note, other bacteria with sialylated polysaccharide capsules, such as *E. coli* K_1 and *N. meningitidis* types B and C, are important etiologic agents in meningitis.

Women harbor GBS as part of the normal fecal and vaginal flora. Rates of asymptomatic carriage are estimated to be between 10% to 30%, but rates vary according to the culture technique used, the number of samples cultured, and the nature of the populations studied.[341-343] Risk factors for colonization include sexual intercourse, timing during the first half of the menstrual cycle, use of an intrauterine device, age younger than 20 years, and ethnicity.[343,344] Vaginal colonization may be transient, and only approximately one third of women have chronic persistent carriage throughout pregnancy.[345] When maternal colonization is present, transmission to the neonate is estimated to occur in approximately 60% of cases, and early-onset invasive disease develops in approximately 1% to 2%. This is in contrast to a group A streptococcal colonization rate of 0.03%.[346,347]

GBS is isolated in 2% to 29% of women with asymptomatic bacteriuria during pregnancy[346] and may be a cause of acute pyelonephritis. Subclinical GBS infection may be a cause of preterm labor,[342,348] and heavy colonization with GBS in the second trimester is associated with clinical chorioamnionitis.[242]

GBS causes approximately 20% of cases of postpartum endometritis, which is often associated with cesarean deliveries.[349] High fever usually develops rapidly after delivery, and uterine and adnexal tenderness may be marked. The lochia is usually sanguinous but not foul smelling. Bacteremia is common, and GBS may also cause bacteremia in the absence of focal signs and symptoms. Pass and colleagues estimated the attack rate for GBS-related puerperal sepsis to be 2 in 1000 deliveries.[350] The question of why some women who carry GBS acquire infection and others do not remains unresolved, but factors such as maternal immunity, length of time since rupture of membranes, invasive fetal and maternal monitoring, and preterm delivery[350] may play a role. GBS is also an important cause of postpartum wound infections, intrapartum chorioamnionitis, and both asymptomatic and symptomatic UTIs in pregnancy. Most affected women respond well to antibiotic therapy[351]; fatal complications include septic shock, adult respiratory distress syndrome, meningitis, and necrotizing fasciitis.[346]

Neonatal infection with GBS encompasses two fairly distinct syndromes that depend on the time of clinical presentation.[352] Early-onset disease, which accounts for most illness, occurs within the first 6 days after birth and usually reflects exposure to the organism in utero or in passage through a colonized birth canal. Infants are often ill at birth or become ill shortly thereafter. Between one half and two thirds of infants show symptoms within the first 12 hours of life; the mean age at onset is 20 hours.[335,353,354] Prematurity and low birth weight are risk factors, although most affected infants are full term. Additional risk factors include premature rupture of membranes, prolonged labor, maternal chorioamnionitis, multiple births, high GBS genital inoculum, maternal GBS bacteremia in pregnancy, and low levels of maternal type-specific capsular antibodies.[346] The signs of early-onset GBS infection in the newborn are nonspecific and include fever, lethargy, respiratory distress, jaundice, and hypotension. Bacteremia is almost always present, and may be manifested by neonatal sepsis without a definite focus of infection, pneumonia, or meningitis. The overall rate of mortality from early-onset GBS has declined from approximately 50% in 1977 to approximately 6% currently,[336] although infants of low birth weight are still at substantial risk.[355] Early-onset GBS disease has an incidence of 1.8 cases per 1000 live births[336] and is equally divided among capsular antigen types I, II, and III GBS (although 80% of early-onset meningitis is caused by type III).[356]

Late-onset GBS infection occurs in 0.5 to 1.8 cases per 1000 live births and carries a mortality rate of approximately 10%.[346] The mean age at onset is 24 days. The route of transmission to the neonate is less clear. Nosocomial, environmental, and maternal spread are all possible. The maternal obstetric history is usually unremarkable, and the birth is uncomplicated. Most infants affected are full term.

Meningitis occurs in 85%, but infants may also present with bacteremia without localizing findings.[357] Neurologic sequelae develop in approximately 50%.[358] Of note, approximately 90% of late-onset GBS infection is attributable to type III.[356]

The definitive diagnosis of GBS infection in the mother or child requires isolation of the organism from blood or other appropriate specimens. Several rapid methods for detection of GBS antigen are commercially available. These methods have the advantage of producing results within hours, but their overall sensitivity is low,[359,360] and GBS has developed in neonates born to mothers with a negative result of a rapid screening test.[361] A rapid PCR-based assay for GBS holds promise,[362] but isolation from culture is still recommended.

When GBS is suspected, broad-spectrum coverage should be initiated until results of the culture are known. Penicillin is the drug of choice for the treatment of documented GBS infection; the adult dosage is 12 million U intravenously every day in four to six divided doses, and higher doses (24 million U every day) are given if meningitis is present.

Most GBS infections could, in theory, be prevented, and GBS is high on the list of priorities for vaccine development.[363,364] Immunization of women with type-specific GBS vaccines could provide protection to the mother and protection to the infant both in utero and after birth through transfer of protective antibody. Capsular polysaccharide vaccines have undergone purification and testing in small numbers of women, but these vaccines are not highly immunogenic. Vaccines that couple the capsular polysaccharides with tetanus toxoid produce an antibody response that is greater than that of capsular polysaccharide alone and appear to be well tolerated in pregnant women.[365-367] Coupling of capsular polysaccharides with C proteins or other group B protein surface antigens show promise but have not undergone extensive testing in humans.[368-370]

Prevention of GBS infections is, however, partially attainable at present through intrapartum administration of antibiotics. In 1992, the American Academy of Pediatrics, on the basis of the results of a randomized, clinical trial[371] and other available data,[345] recommended screening all pregnant women for GBS at 26 to 28 weeks of pregnancy.[372] Treatment was advocated for those who subsequently had preterm labor, prolonged time since rupture of membranes, or intrapartum fever. Although this approach had merit, concerns were raised about the predictive value of cultures so far removed from the time of delivery,[373] logistics and communication issues, and the pressure on clinicians to treat before the intrapartum period, a strategy with very limited effectiveness.[342] The American College of Obstetricians and Gynecologists took a different approach, favoring treating with intrapartum chemoprophylaxis all women who had risk factors for GBS without any culture-based screening.[374] Neither strategy, however, addressed the 25% of all early-onset GBS cases that occur in GBS carriers without risk factors.

In 1996, these groups, in conjunction with representatives from the CDC and the American Academy of Family Physicians, issued another set of guidelines for the prevention of GBS infection in mothers and infants that were a modification of the previous approaches.[342] Both an approach based on screening and one based on risk factor assessment without screening were acceptable alternatives. Subsequent analysis of the results of these two strategies led to the conclusion that universal screening is over 50% more effective than the risk-based approach in preventing perinatal GBS disease.[376-380] On the basis of these data, the CDC, in consultation with multiple partners, issued new guidelines that are summarized in Figure 16-4. These guidelines advocate obtaining vaginal and rectal cultures from all

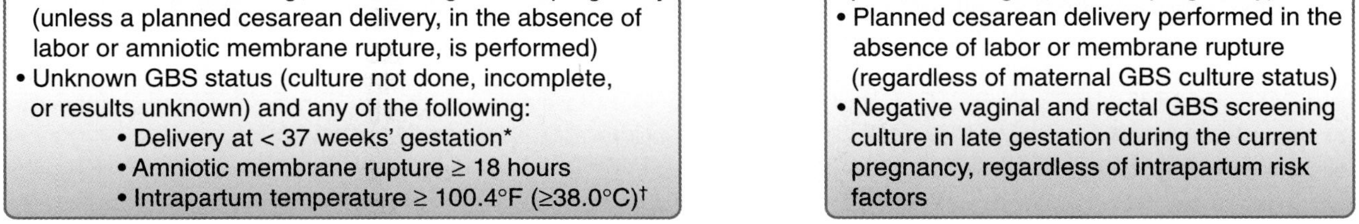

Figure 16–4. Indications for intrapartum antibiotic prophylaxis to prevent perinatal group B streptococcal (GBS) disease under a universal prenatal screening strategy based on combined vaginal and rectal cultures collected at 35 to 37 weeks' gestation from all pregnant women. (From Schrag SJ, Gorwitz R, Fulty-Butts K, Schuchat A: Prevention of perinatal group B streptococcal disease. Revised guidelines from CDC. MMWR Recomm Rep 2002;51[RR-11]:8.)
*If onset of labor or rupture of amniotic membranes occurs at less than 37 weeks' gestation and there is a significant risk for preterm delivery (as assessed by the clinician), a suggested algorithm for GBS prophylaxis management is provided (see Figure 16–5).
†If amnionitis is suspected, broad-spectrum antibiotic therapy that includes an agent known to be active against GBS should replace GBS prophylaxis.

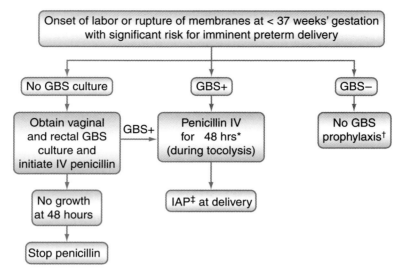

Figure 16–5. Sample algorithm for group B streptococcus prophylaxis for women with threatened preterm delivery. This algorithm is not an exclusive course of management. Variations that incorporate individual circumstances or institutional preferences may be appropriate. (From Schrag SJ, Gorwitz R, Fulty-Butts K, Schuchat A: Prevention of perinatal group B streptococcal disease. Revised guidelines from CDC. MMWR Recomm Rep 2002;51[RR-11]:12.)
*Penicillin should be continued for a total of at least 48 hours, unless delivery occurs sooner. At the physician's discretion, antibiotic prophylaxis may be continued beyond 48 hours in a GBS culture–positive woman if delivery has not yet occurred. For women in whom GBS cultures are positive, antibiotic prophylaxis should be reinitiated when labor likely to proceed to delivery occurs or recurs.
†If delivery has not occurred within 4 weeks, a vaginal and rectal GBS screening culture should be repeated, and the patient should be managed as described, according to the result of the repeat culture.
‡Intrapartum antibiotic prophylaxis.

pregnant women between 35 and 37 weeks of pregnancy. An algorithm for GBS prophylaxis in those at significant risk for preterm delivery is presented in Figure 16-5. Culture techniques that maximize the likelihood of GBS recovery should be used (Table 16-7). The recommended regimens for intrapartum prophylaxis are presented in Table 16-8.

Listeriosis

L. monocytogenes is a gram-positive bacillus that primarily infects pregnant women, immunosuppressed patients, and those at the extremes of age. Using data collected in Scotland between 1967 and 1988, Campbell calculated the annual incidence of listeriosis as 1 affected pregnancy per 3500 pregnant women,[381] whereas in Melbourne, Australia, Craig and associates found an incidence of 1 infection per 5000 pregnancies.[382] In a summary of 722 cases of human listeriosis in Great Britain from 1967 to 1985, 34% of cases were associated with pregnancy.[383] Although there was only one major maternal complication, 96% of fetuses were infected, and intrauterine death occurred in 19%. After birth, neonatal listeriosis was recognized in 54% within 2 days and 23% shortly after 2 days. Mortality rates were 38% and 25%, respectively, in these two groups.

Listeriosis is a zoonosis, causing abortions and "circling disease" (meningoencephalitis) in mammals. Animals may also harbor *Listeria* in the gastrointestinal tract, and the organism has been isolated from healthy cattle, pigs, sheep, chickens, turkeys, and ducks.[384] Most cases of human listeriosis lack animal contact, however, and *Listeria* is now recognized to be ubiquitous in the environment, in which it survives well. A number of large outbreaks of listeriosis have been traced to contaminated foods. The initial evidence for a foodborne source of this organism was revealed by the investigation of a high rate of neonatal listeriosis at a maternity hospital in Nova Scotia.[385] In a 6-month period, 7 adults and 34 neonates were infected; infection resulted in five spontaneous abortions, four stillbirths, and a mortality rate of 27% among the liveborn infants. The outbreak was eventually traced to ingestion of coleslaw that had been made from cabbage fertilized by sheep manure containing *Listeria*. The largest epidemic of listeriosis in North America occurred in Los Angeles in 1985 and affected primarily pregnant Hispanic women and their children.[386] The case fatality rate was 63% for early neonatal or fetal infections. This outbreak was eventually traced to the consumption of cheese that had been made in part from unpasteurized milk. In the Los Angeles outbreak, the incubation period for listeriosis ranged from 11 to 70 days, with a median of 31 days. Such a long incubation period is unusual in foodborne illness and complicates epidemiologic association.[384] It is certainly possible that many sporadic cases of listeriosis result from ingestion of contaminated foodstuffs as well. In various microbiologic surveys, *L. monocytogenes* was cultured from 15% to 80% of poultry samples and 30% of ready-to-eat meat products.[387] Of note, listeriosis has also been transmitted by inadequate hand washing, breaks in barrier nursing technique, and contamination of equipment in the hospital setting, usually after the birth of an infected infant.[388-390]

L. monocytogenes has been cultured from the feces of 1% to 12% of normal people. Higher rates have been noted in household contacts of infected people and slaughterhouse workers. The gastrointestinal tract is presumed to be the origin of most human infection, although colonization of the cervix may play a role in some cases of chorioamnionitis and spontaneous abortion.[391] Why some hosts tolerate colonization but infection develops in

TABLE 16–7   Procedures for Collecting and Processing Clinical Specimens for Group B Streptococcal Culture

Procedure for Collecting Clinical Specimens for Culture of Group B Streptococcus at 35-37 Weeks of Pregnancy

Swab the lower vagina (vaginal introitus), followed by the rectum (i.e., insert swab through the anal sphincter), using the same swab or two
  different swabs. Cultures should be collected in the outpatient setting by the health care provider or the patient herself, with appropriate
  instruction. Cervical cultures are not recommended, and a speculum should not be used for culture collection.
Place the swab(s) into a nonnutritive transport medium. Appropriate transport systems (e.g., Amies' or Stuart's medium without charcoal)
  are commercially available. If vaginal and rectal swabs were collected separately, both swabs can be placed into the same container of medium.
  Transport media will maintain GBS viability for up to 4 days at room temperature or under refrigeration.
Specimen labels should clearly identify specimens as being for group B streptococcal culture. If susceptibility testing is ordered for penicillin-
  allergic women (Table 16-8), specimen labels should also identify the patient as penicillin allergic and should specify that susceptibility testing
  for clindamycin and erythromycin should be performed if group B streptococcus is isolated.

Procedure for Processing Clinical Specimens for Culture of Group B Streptococcus

Remove swab(s) from transport medium.* Inoculate swab(s) into a recommended selective broth medium, such as Todd-Hewitt broth
  supplemented either with gentamicin (8 µg/mL) and nalidixic acid (15 µg/mL) or with colistin (10 µg/mL) and nalidixic acid (15 µg/mL).
  Examples of appropriate commercially available options include TransVag broth supplemented with 5% defibrinated sheep blood or
  LIM broth.†
Incubate inoculated selective broth for 18-24 hours at 35°-37° C in ambient air or 5% CO_2. Subculture the broth to a sheep blood agar plate
  (e.g., tryptic soy agar with 5% defibrinated sheep blood).
Inspect and identify organisms suggestive of group B streptococcus (i.e., narrow zone of β-hemolysis, gram-positive cocci, catalase negative).
  Note that hemolysis may be difficult to observe; therefore, typical colonies without hemolysis should also be further tested. If group B
  streptococcus is not identified after incubation for 18-24 hours, reincubate and inspect at 48 hours to identify suspected organisms.
Various streptococcus grouping latex agglutination tests or other tests for group B streptococcus antigen detection (e.g., generic probe) may be
  used for specific identification, or the CAMP test may be employed for presumptive identification.

Modified from Centers for Disease Control and Prevention: Prevention of Perinatal Group B Streptococcal Disease: Revised Guidelines from CDC. MMWR Morb Mortal
Wkly Rep 45(RR-11):4, 2002.
*Before inoculation strep, some laboratories may choose to roll swab(s) on a single sheep blood agar plate or CAN sheep blood agar plate. This should be done only in
addition to, and not instead of, inoculation into selective broth. The plate should be streaked for isolation, incubated at 35°-37° C in ambient air or 5% CO_2 for
18-24 hours and inspected for organisms suggestive of group B streptococcus as described. If suspected colonies are confirmed as group B streptococcus, the broth
can be discarded, thus shortening the time to obtaining culture results.
†Source: Fenton LJ, Harper MH: Evaluation of colistin and nalidixic acid in Todd-Hewitt broth for selective isolation of group B streptococci. J Clin Microbiol
1979;9:167-169. Although Trans-Vag medium is often available without sheep blood, direct comparison of medium with and without sheep blood has shown higher
yield when blood is added. LIM broth may also benefit from the addition of sheep blood, although the improvement in yield is smaller and sufficient data are not yet
available to support a recommendation.
CAMP, Christie, Atkins, and Munch-Peterson.

others is unclear. What is clear from data in experimental
animals and humans is that T lymphocytes and activated
macrophages are very important in host defense.[392] The
decreases in cell-mediated immunity associated with pregnancy may be a predisposition to this illness. Women with
multiple gestations may also be at increased risk.[393]

Although the mortality rate in immunocompro-
mised adults with listeriosis is substantial,[394,395] that in
pregnant women is virtually zero,[383,394,396-398] and meningoencephalitis, common in other patient populations, is
rare.[399] Pregnant women with listeriosis may exhibit only
a mild, flu-like illness (possibly representing maternal
bacteremia), which may resolve even without treatment,
or they may present with fever, malaise, abdominal pain,
and the premature onset of labor, usually associated with
signs of chorioamnionitis.[396] In Craig and colleagues'
series, premature labor was the most common presenting
symptom and occurred in 66%.[382] Three forms of
fetal/neonatal infection have been described:

1. Overwhelming intrauterine infection (granulomatosus
   infantisepticum), which has a characteristic pathologic
   process and usually results in fetal demise.[400]
2. Early-onset disease, also a result of intrauterine infection,
   in which clinical illness is apparent at birth or shortly
   thereafter. A septic picture is common. Meningitis is rare.
3. Late-onset disease, occurring several days to weeks after
   birth. Meningitis is very common in this presentation,
   as it is in late-onset GBS infection.

In a review of 222 cases of maternal listeriosis, details on
the outcome of the pregnancy were available in 178 cases.
In 36 (20.2%), pregnancy resulted in spontaneous abortions
or stillbirth. Among the remaining 142 liveborn infants,
68.3% were infected and 31.7% were not.[401]

Late-onset disease has a better prognosis than early-onset
disease.[383,402] Antibiotic therapy may prevent or ameliorate
adverse fetal outcome,[397,403-405] although uninfected infants
of even untreated mothers have been reported.[386,400,406]
Of note, in an epidemiologic investigation of listeriosis
reported by Cherubin and associates, the earlier the stage
of gestation in which infection occurred, the higher the
incidence of fetal demise.[396]

The diagnosis of maternal listeriosis is commonly
made from isolation of the organism from blood cultures,
placenta, or amniotic fluid. Because *Listeria* infection may
manifest as a nonspecific, flu-like illness inpregnancy,
blood cultures in this setting should be readily obtained.
Ampicillin and penicillin have excellent activity against
Listeria; addition of an aminoglycoside produces synergy,
and combination therapy is commonly used in severe
infections.[392] A common regimen consists of ampicillin,
2 g intravenously every 4 to 6 hours, and gentamicin,
2 mg/kg intravenously every 8 hours. The optimal duration of therapy has not been established. Although
2 weeks of therapy appear to be adequate in pregnancy,
recurrences in immunosuppressed patients have prompted
some authorities to advocate 3 to 6 weeks of treatment. In
the absence of fetal demise, or if the fetus is not mature,

TABLE 16–8   Recommended Regimens for Intrapartum Antimicrobial Prophylaxis for Perinatal Group B Streptococcal Disease*

For Patients Not Allergic to Penicillin	
Recommended	Penicillin G, 5 mU IV load, then 2.5 mU IV every 4 hr until delivery
Alternative	Ampicillin, 2 g IV load, then 1 g IV every 4 hr until delivery

For Patients Allergic to Penicillin†	
Patients not at high risk for anaphylaxis‡	Cefazolin, 2 g IV initial dose, then 1 g IV every 8 hours until delivery
Patients at high risk for anaphylaxis	
Group B streptococcus susceptible to clindamycin and erythromycin§	Clindamycin, 900 mg IV every 8 hr until delivery or Erythromycin, 500 mg IV every 6 hr until delivery
Group B streptococcus resistant to clindamycin or erythromycin or susceptibility unknown	Vancomycin,¶ 1 g IV every 12 hours until delivery

From Centers for Disease Control and Prevention: Prevention of Perinatal Group B Streptococcal Disease: A Public Health Perspective. MMWR Morb Mortal Wkly Rep 2002;51(RR-11):10.
*Broader spectrum agents, including an agent active against group B streptococci, may be necessary for treatment of chorioamnionitis.
†History of penicillin allergy should be assessed to determine whether a high risk for anaphylaxis is present. Penicillin-allergic patients at high risk for anaphylaxis are those who have experienced immediate hypersensitivity to penicillin, including a history of penicillin-related anaphylaxis; other high-risk patients are those with asthma or other diseases that would make anaphylaxis more dangerous or difficult to treat, such as persons being treated with β-adrenergic–blocking agents.
‡If laboratory facilities are adequate, clindamycin and erythromycin susceptibility testing (Table 16-7) should be performed on prenatal group B streptococcal isolates from penicillin-allergic women at high risk for anaphylaxis.
§Resistance to erythromycin is often but not always associated with clindamycin resistance. If a strain is resistant to erythromycin but appears susceptible to clindamycin, it may still have inducible resistance to clindamycin.
¶Cefazolin is preferred over vancomycin for women with a history of penicillin allergy other than immediate hypersensitivity reactions, and pharmacologic data suggest it achieves effective intraamniotic concentrations. Vancomycin should be reserved for penicillin-allergic women at high risk for anaphylaxis.

antibiotic management without immediate delivery may be successful.[404,407,408]

Guidelines for the prevention of listeriosis include the avoidance of unpasteurized milk or cheese, raw eggs, and undercooked meats. Vegetables and fruits should be thoroughly washed.

Borrelia burgdorferi *and Lyme Disease*

Lyme disease is caused by a thin, gram-negative spirochetal organism, *Borrelia burgdorferi,* and is transmitted by the bite of infected *Ixodes* ticks. This disease occurs in stages, and the skin, central nervous system, cardiovascular system, and musculoskeletal system are commonly affected. Because of similarities to another spirochetal organism, *T. pallidum,* the agent of syphilis, concerns about maternofetal transmission and the risk of congenital infection in infants born to mothers infected with *B. burgdorferi* have been raised. There are published case reports of infants born with congenital heart disease,[409,410] hyperbilirubinemia, blindness, and syndactyly[411]; miscarriages and stillbirths[412]; and neonatal demise with spirochetes seen in the brain at autopsy[413] in association with Lyme disease during pregnancy. However, prospective, controlled studies in endemic areas have failed to find evidence that intrauterine exposure to *B. burgdorferi* causes congenital anomalies or death. A survey of 2000 pregnant women concluded that maternal Lyme disease or an increased risk of exposure to Lyme disease was not associated with fetal death, decreased birth weight, or decreased length of gestation at delivery.[414] Tick bites or Lyme disease at the time of conception were not associated with congenital malformations.[415] In another serologic survey of 1416 mothers with 1434 offspring, one woman with clinically active, untreated Lyme disease gave birth to a child with a ventricular septal defect. The child never developed antibody to *B. burgdorferi,* however, and no serologic evidence of intrauterine infection was found in offspring born to women with elevated titers against *B. burgdorferi.*[416] It appears that vertical transmission of *B. burgdorferi* can occur but is probably uncommon.

Maternal Lyme disease appears to pose minimal risks to the fetus if the mother is appropriately and aggressively treated.[417-419] Women with limited local skin disease and no signs of systemic illness or disseminated infection can be treated safely with oral amoxicillin, 500 mg three times daily for 3 weeks. Similar therapy has been recommended as prophylaxis for tick bites in pregnancy.[420] In patients with more extensive disease, intravenous ceftriaxone therapy is recommended. Counseling patients to avoid heavily wooded areas and to wear protective clothing to prevent tick attachment may help prevent infection.

Mycobacterial Infections

From 1985 through 1992, the number of reported cases of tuberculosis in the United States increased 20%.[421] During 1985 to 1991, tuberculosis cases increased 44% among those aged 25 to 44 years and 27% among children younger than 15 years.[422] Although tuberculosis in pregnant women and their newborns used to be rare,[423,424] this incidence, unfortunately, also rose during this period. In two large, inner-city hospitals in New York, tuberculosis was diagnosed in 12.4 per 100,000 births from 1985 to 1990 and in 94.8 per 100,000 births during 1991 to 1992.[425] Poverty, drug abuse, and co-infection with HIV were important risk factors in this cohort. Other factors that contributed to the general increase in cases of tuberculosis included an increase in immigration from countries with a high prevalence of tuberculosis and the general decline both in public health services and in access to medical care in many communities.[424] This increased incidence, together with the emergence of multidrug-resistant tuberculosis, resulted in more stringent public health controls and greater vigilance on the part of physicians. Data again show a decline in cases, especially in inner-city areas where treatment programs have been directed. However, heightened awareness still is warranted, particularly among those who care for immigrants.[426-428]

Tuberculosis is acquired through inhalation. Primary infection usually occurs in the dependent portions of the lung. Asymptomatic hematogenous dissemination of organisms occurs before host defense (through cell-mediated immune mechanisms) intervenes and halts replication. Disease may develop at the time of primary infection if host defense is not adequate, or viable but contained organisms may reactivate and begin replication years later. The most common sites of reactivated infection are the upper lobes of the lung. Common sites of extrapulmonary infection arising from hematogenous dissemination include the lymph nodes, bone, meninges, and genitourinary tract.

Maternal tuberculosis does not appear to cause congenital malformations,[429] but it may lead to fetal infection. Infection in the neonate may be acquired congenitally or perinatally. Congenital infection arises from hematogenous dissemination from the mother or from aspiration of infected amniotic fluid arising from placental infection. The infant may also be infected at the time of birth through aspiration of infected material if the mother has tuberculous endometritis or through the traditional airborne route if persons in the infant's environment have pulmonary tuberculosis. Congenital or neonatal infection is uncommon but carries a high mortality rate. In a review of 390 women with tuberculin skin test conversion or culture-proven tuberculosis during pregnancy, only three cases of neonatal tuberculosis were found[430]; however, several studies of congenital tuberculosis reported mortality rates ranging from 30% to 46%.[430,431]

Hippocrates believed that pregnancy had a beneficial effect on the course of tuberculosis,[432] whereas physicians in the early 20th century believed that the consequences to the mother frequently warranted therapeutic abortion.[424] Neither of these views has withstood the test of time. In the 1940s and 1950s, studies appeared that did not substantiate the notion that tuberculous disease progression was greatly accelerated during pregnancy.[433,434] Although some studies found a higher-than-expected rate of relapse post partum,[434,435] others did not.[436,437] Most authorities now believe that pregnancy has little effect on the progression or reactivation of asymptomatic disease.[424]

The clinical manifestations of tuberculosis in pregnancy do not differ from those in the nonpregnant state. One half to two thirds of patients may be asymptomatic or have minimal symptoms early in disease.[438,439] Cough, weight loss, fever, malaise, and fatigue are the most common symptoms in pulmonary tuberculosis.[440] Extrapulmonary disease occurs in 5% to 10% of those without an underlying significant immunosuppressive disease,[439] a statistic not substantially different from that found in nonpregnant people. Extrapulmonary manifestations are quite common in persons with concomitant HIV infection, however.[421] Tuberculosis of the female reproductive tract can occur but is uncommon in pregnancy because sterility and menstrual abnormalities are common in women with tuberculous endometritis. Asymptomatic endometrial tuberculosis is frequently found in mothers of congenitally infected infants, however.[430,441] Tuberculosis mastitis appears to be very rare but occurs almost exclusively in young women.[442] Up to one third of women are lactating when the disease is diagnosed.[443] Miliary disease has been reported but is quite rare.[145] In some cases, maternal tuberculosis is suspected only after infection in the neonate becomes apparent.[431,444] The manifestation of tuberculosis in neonates is variable and depends on the timing of the infection (in utero, perinatal, or postnatal) and the infecting dose.[441] Symptoms may be present at birth and may mimic those of bacterial sepsis or other congenital infections. More commonly, clinical illness becomes apparent during the second or third week of life. Intrauterine growth restriction, respiratory distress, hepatosplenomegaly, fever, irritability, and poor feeding are important but nonspecific clinical features.[431] A high index of suspicion and a careful maternal and family history often provide the key to diagnosis.

Despite a generalized decrease in cell-mediated immunity, the tuberculin skin test result is frequently positive in pregnant women, and studies in which patients were their own controls have demonstrated no effect of pregnancy on cutaneous delayed hypersensitivity to tuberculin.[445,446] Screening of all pregnant women with a Mantoux skin test (which involves the intradermal injection of 0.1 mL of 5 tuberculin unit–strength purified protein derivative) identifies most of those with inactive, healed, or prior infection and those with true asymptomatic or symptomatic disease. Those with positive reactions should undergo further evaluation (Table 16–9). If symptoms suggestive of tuberculosis are present, a chest radiograph should be obtained as soon as possible. In the absence of symptoms, routine chest radiographs with proper shielding of the abdomen should be performed after the 12th week of pregnancy.[424] Review of systems, physical examination, and laboratory results should be done carefully and completely to rule out extrapulmonary tuberculosis. Approximately 10% of

TABLE 16–9   Interpretation of Skin Test Results for Tuberculosis*

Area of Induration (mm)	Reading
<5	Negative
≥5	Positive if the patient is a known TB contact, has abnormal chest radiograph, has clinical evidence of TB, or is HIV positive
≥10	Positive in any high-risk† or high-prevalence group
≥15	Positive

*Per recommendations of the American Thoracic Society and Centers for Disease Control and Prevention. (From American Thoracic Society: Diagnostic standards of classification of tuberculosis. Am Rev Respir Dis 1990;142:725.)
†High-risk groups include foreign-born people, health care workers, residents of nursing homes, the homeless, drug addicts, or those residing in an area of a high TB prevalence.
HIV, human immunodeficiency virus; TB, tuberculosis.

immunocompetent people and 40% of HIV-infected people with active tuberculosis have negative skin test results.[424,447] Therefore, symptoms suggestive of tuberculosis should be actively pursued even if the skin test result is negative.

The diagnosis of tuberculosis is confirmed by isolation of the organism from involved sites. Inoculation of specimens into the BACTEC culture system[448] has shortened the time required for isolation of *Mycobacterium hominis* by several weeks, and specific DNA probes now available have simplified identification.[449] Biopsies may reveal the caseating granulomas with acid-fast organisms typical of tuberculosis and should prompt therapy even in the absence of microbiologic confirmation. In HIV infection, granuloma formation may be absent, but acid-fast organisms are usually plentiful.

In the preantibiotic era, rates of mortality in mothers and children from untreated, advanced tuberculosis were between 30% and 40%.[438] Rates of miscarriage and prematurity were also substantial.[429,450] With the advent of chemotherapy, the prognosis of tuberculosis has been altered dramatically. More recent studies have found no adverse effects of pregnancy and the postpartum period on the course in women receiving chemotherapy.[451,452]

Initial treatment of active tuberculosis in pregnancy should consist of isoniazid (INH), ethambutol, and rifampin, and therapy should be continued for 9 months.[421,424] Pyrazinamide should be added if drug resistance is probable, and an infectious diseases specialist should be consulted. INH, rifampin, and ethambutol are generally considered safe during pregnancy.[424,432] There are no data on the use of pyrazinamide in pregnancy, but in the setting of drug resistance, benefits probably outweigh risks.[421,424] Unfortunately, streptomycin, a very useful first-line antitubercular agent, may cause significant eighth nerve damage in the fetus,[432] and this toxic effect limits its use. Pyridoxine should always be given with INH during pregnancy because pregnancy itself increases the requirements for this vitamin.[453]

In young, nonpregnant patients who have a positive skin test result but no evidence of active disease, treatment now usually consists of 6 to 9 months of INH therapy. If INH resistance is present, rifampin is given. Most authors advocate withholding prophylaxis for a positive skin test result during pregnancy until after delivery, because the risks of reactivation of infection are minimal unless it is likely that the mother has recently been infected.[424,454-456] In that case, INH should be started after the first trimester.[457] Reports of an increased incidence of INH-associated hepatitis among pregnant and early postpartum women reinforce the need for careful monitoring of this population if INH is given.[458]

Breast-feeding is not contraindicated in women receiving antitubercular medications, because no toxic effects have been reported and only low levels of drugs are found in breast milk.[455] Supplemental pyridoxine for the breast-feeding infant has been advocated.[424] If the infant is also receiving antitubercular medication, the potential for toxicity is greater. Discontinuation of breast-feeding or giving the mother medication after feeding and substituting formula for the next feeding has been recommended in this setting.[455]

Other Bacterial Infections

Any bacteria may infect women during pregnancy. In cases of maternal bacteremia or prepartum infection, consequences to the mother may be less significant than those to the fetus. Case reports and reviews of *Campylobacter fetus*,[459] *Salmonella* organisms,[460-462] *Pasteurella multocida*,[463] *H. influenzae*,[464] group C streptococci,[465] *S. pneumoniae*,[466] *S. aureus*,[467] and brucellosis[468] complicating pregnancy have been published. Separate discussion of all these organisms is beyond the scope of this chapter.

FUNGAL INFECTIONS

Candidal Infections

Candida species are isolated from the vagina of 15% to 21% of nonpregnant women and 30% of those who are pregnant,[469-471] and the incidence of symptomatic candidal vulvovaginitis is increased late in pregnancy.[469] Factors that may contribute to this predisposition include increased candidal adherence to vaginal epithelial cells in pregnancy, high glycogen levels in the vagina, increased candidal proliferation in the presence of high levels of estrogens, and depression in cell-mediated immunity.[472-474] *Candida* species have been implicated in chorioamnionitis complicating midtrimester cervical incompetence, but serious candidal infections in pregnancy are rare.[475-479] In a review of the English literature from 1956 to 1991, Potasman and associates found eight cases of candidal sepsis complicating pregnancy.[480] All patients treated with amphotericin survived, whereas three of four who went untreated died. Seven of eight patients had had prior antibiotic therapy or had a foreign body (i.e., an intrauterine device or intravenous catheter) in place.

Intense pruritus, vulvar burning, dysuria, and dyspareunia are the most frequent manifestations of vaginal yeast infections in both pregnant and nonpregnant women. *Candida albicans* is the most frequent isolate, and *Torulopsis glabrata* (formally *Candida glabrata*) accounts for approximately 10% to 15% of cases. Discharge is frequently thick and white and resembles cottage cheese. Examining the vaginal discharge under the microscope with 10% potassium hydroxide or the Gram stain technique reveals budding oval yeast forms and pseudohyphae, which establish the diagnosis. These organisms are easily cultured in the microbiology laboratory, and a culture may be indicated if there is clinical suspicion and a negative finding on potassium hydroxide preparation.

Local treatment of candidal vulvovaginitis is usually sufficient to ameliorate symptoms. The imidazole agents (miconazole or clotrimazole) appear to be more effective than nystatin in this setting.[481-483] In nonpregnant women, 3-day therapy with either fluconazole or itraconazole produces cure rates comparable with intravaginal treatment and is preferred by patients.[484,485] However, fluconazole is teratogenic in humans, and related compounds are likely to be teratogenic as well.[486,487] Although single-dose or short-course therapy with fluconazole has been administered to pregnant women without obvious effects in the fetus,[488] more prolonged administration has been associated with multiple craniofacial and skeletal congenital abnormalities.[487] The treatment for systemic or serious candidal infections remains amphotericin B.[489] After an intravenous test dose of 1 mg, dosages can be rapidly advanced to 0.3 to 0.5 mg/kg/day. The duration of treatment depends on the clinical situation. Removal of any foreign body (often the portal of entry of infection) is often the key to a successful cure.

Coccidioidomycosis

Coccidioides immitis is a dimorphic fungus present in the soil in the southwestern United States. Inhalation of fungal spores, called arthroconidia, results in localized respiratory infection that is often asymptomatic or may mimic "flu." Symptomatic disease is usually mild and self-limited, although severe pneumonia and progressive cavitary pulmonary disease infrequently occur. In approximately 0.1% to 0.2% of all *C. immitis* infections, the fungus disseminates to other organs, notably the meninges, skin, and joints. Disseminated disease may be rapidly fatal, especially in immunosuppressed patients, or may result in lifelong disability.

Pregnancy is a major predisposition to disseminated coccidioidomycosis, with rates in pregnant women 40 to 100 times those in the general population.[490] Pregnant African-American women and women of Filipino or Mexican ancestry appear to be at particular risk. Previously resolved, limited coccidioidal infection does not usually present a problem to women who become pregnant,[491,492] although "healed" disseminated disease may reactivate during pregnancy.[493,494]

The time of acquisition of infection during pregnancy significantly affects prognosis. The later in pregnancy the primary disease is acquired, the greater is the risk of dissemination and death.[490,491,494] In a review by Peterson and associates, 5 of 23 patients who acquired coccidioidomycosis in the first trimester went on to acquire disseminated disease, whereas 26 of 38 who had third-trimester infection did so.[490] Of note, in a review of the 109 published cases of coccidioidomycosis in pregnancy, there was no maternal mortality in the absence of disseminated disease, even though antifungal therapy was instituted in only 2 of 35.[494] As is the case with nonpregnant individuals, the presence of erythema nodosum is correlated with a positive outcome. In a review of 61 pregnant patients with coccidioidomycosis, none of the 30 patients with erythema nodosum developed disseminated disease, whereas 35% of the remaining 31 patients without erythema nodosum experienced dissemination.[495]

Mortality rates of 29% to 90% have been reported in pregnant women with dissemination,[491,496,497] although some authors believe that both the high rates of dissemination and mortality rates noted in earlier studies represent reporting bias. Advances in diagnosis, care, and treatment may also play a role in declining mortality rates. In an outbreak in Kern County, California, in the early 1990s, dissemination occurred in 9% of pregnant patients (vs. 2.9% of nonpregnant women in the same age range), and there were no maternal deaths.[498]

Transplacental spread to the fetus has not been reported in disseminated coccidioidomycosis,[490,499] although the placenta may be involved microscopically, and the risks of fetal loss and prematurity are substantial (43% and 29%, respectively, in one series of 15 patients reported by Smale and Waechter[500]). Of note, *C. immitis* has been grown from vaginal secretions of mothers with dissemination. Infection of neonates is quite uncommon but may occur during passage through an infected birth canal.[501,502]

Several factors may contribute to the increased rate of disseminated coccidioidomycosis in pregnancy. Decreases in cell-mediated immunity have long been thought to play a role.[503] Barbee and associates have demonstrated a decrease in tetanus-associated, coccidioidin spherulin (*Coccidioides* tissue phase) antigen blast transformation in pregnancy, whereas blast transformation to nonspecific mitogens was maintained.[504] In addition, Drutz and associates have noted that female sex hormones bind to *C. immitis*. The serum concentrations of progesterone and 17β-estradiol that are present during the latter half of pregnancy can stimulate the growth and maturation of this organism in vitro.[505]

Coccidioidomycosis should be considered in the differential diagnosis of respiratory tract infection in pregnant women who live in or have traveled through endemic areas. Pleuritic chest pain and hilar adenopathy are common features. Eosinophilia is an important clue to diagnosis. Erythema nodosum, if present, is a good prognostic sign. Patients may also present with fever and disseminated illness involving the joints, skin, and meninges that may rapidly progress to coma, respiratory insufficiency, and death.

The diagnosis of coccidioidomycosis can be made microbiologically, pathologically, or serologically. The organism grows easily from sputum, cerebrospinal fluid, or tissue, and growth is usually visible in 3 to 4 days on appropriate media. Very early in infection, *C. immitis* elicits a polymorphonuclear response. By the time of most biopsies, well-formed granulomas are present, and the typical tissue form of the organism, the spherule, which is pathognomonic, may be found (Fig. 16–6).

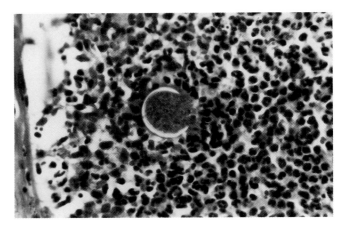

Figure 16–6. A ruptured spherule of *Coccidioides immitis* with surrounding acute inflammation.

Antibodies to *C. immitis* antigens may be measured by a number of different techniques. IgM precipitins occur early in primary infection and usually disappear within 4 months.[492] Titers of antibody measured by either immunodiffusion or complement fixation techniques appear to parallel the course of the disease and are very useful. A complement-fixing antibody titer of at least 1:16 is strongly suggestive of disseminated disease. The presence of antibody in the cerebrospinal fluid indicates meningeal involvement.

A positive result of a skin test for coccidioidin or spherulin antigens (derived from the form of the organism in nature or in tissue, respectively) indicates only that prior exposure to the organism has occurred. Because a positive skin test result is a measure of delayed hypersensitivity, it is a good prognostic sign. Skin tests for coccidioidomycosis frequently yield negative results in disseminated disease. Unfortunately, however, the antigens used for skin testing for coccidioidomycosis are no longer available.

The treatment of choice for disseminated coccidioidomycosis in both pregnant and nonpregnant people remains amphotericin B. With treatment, the prognosis of coccidioidomycosis in pregnancy improves substantially.[490] After a test dose of 1 mg, amphotericin B in dosages of 0.5 to 0.75 mg/kg/day should be instituted promptly. The duration of therapy should be based on the patient's clinical and serologic response; cumulative doses of 2 g or more are often necessary. Intrathecal therapy is also necessary to treat meningitis; doses are administered by lumbar puncture, beginning at 0.01 to 0.05 mg and increasing to 0.5 mg every other day.[492]

Because of the risks of dissemination, treatment of all pregnant women with active disease appears warranted. Dosages of 0.6 to 1.0 mg/kg of amphotericin B every other day to a cumulative dose of about 1 g are recommended.[506] No major fetal abnormalities or long-term toxicities have been noted with the use of this drug.[493] Although a number of nonpregnant patients with localized and stable disseminated coccidioidomycosis have been treated with ketoconazole, fluconazole, and itraconazole, their use in pregnancy has been extremely limited. Concerns about ketoconazole in pregnancy include potential hepatotoxicity in the mother and interference with fetal testosterone synthesis.[493] Although some women have received single-dose or short-term fluconazole therapy with no apparent ill effects to the fetus, fluconazole has been associated with congenital malformations in several reports.[486,487,507]

PARASITIC INFECTIONS

Toxoplasmosis

Toxoplasmosis is caused by the intracellular protozoan parasite *Toxoplasma gondii,* whose definitive host is felines. Ubiquitous in nature, *T. gondii* is found wherever cats are encountered, but its prevalence in humans varies widely by geographic location, which probably reflects both climatic conditions and eating habits. Colder regions have fewer human infections than warm, moist areas, where the parasite oocyst excreted in cat feces remains infectious

in the soil for up to a year.[508] In areas where the ingestion of partially cooked meat is common, such as France, infection is particularly frequent. In the United States, seroprevalence rates among pregnant women vary widely, from 22% in New York City[509] to 3% in Colorado[510] to 0.06% in Alabama.[511] The risk of seroconversion during pregnancy is estimated to be less than 0.1% in the United States.[512] The risk of fetal infection ranges from 1 per 1000 live births to 1 per 10,000 live births.[512,513]

T. gondii undergoes both sexual and asexual reproduction. There are three major forms of the organism important for understanding the infection in humans: (1) the oocyst, (2) the cyst, and (3) the trophozoite or tachyzoite. Cats excrete oocysts, the sexual form of the organism, in their feces, and sexual reproduction occurs only in felines. Once excreted, oocysts become infectious after a period of 1 to 5 days, and they then may be ingested by a number of intermediate hosts, including humans. Ingested oocysts develop in the intestinal epithelium into tachyzoites, which spread throughout the body, especially to the brain, heart, and skeletal muscle. With the development of immunity, tissue cysts are formed (Fig. 16–7). Intact cysts invoke little inflammatory response but contain large numbers of viable parasites for many years. Cats become infected when they ingest infected rodents or birds that contain tissue cysts, and the cycle is repeated.

Human infection is incidental in the life cycle of this parasite and occurs through ingestion of soil or foods that have been contaminated by cat feces or by ingestion of undercooked meat that contains viable cysts. (Of note, 10% to 70% of lamb, 25% of pork, and 10% of beef samples have been reported to contain *T. gondii* cysts.[514-516]) Transmission may also occur transplacentally when a woman acquires infection during pregnancy.

Infection in humans is often subclinical or mild and self-limited, although those who are immunosuppressed may have severe primary infection or secondary recurrences. In acquired immunodeficiency syndrome (AIDS), for example, encephalitis is common, and myocarditis, pneumonitis, and hepatitis are also reported. Infection in pregnant women is also often subclinical or may be mistaken for the flu. A mononucleosis-like syndrome with

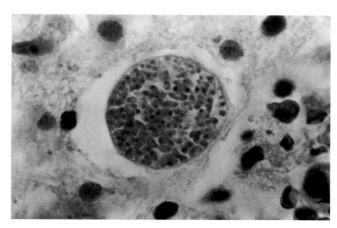

Figure 16–7. A tissue cyst of *Toxoplasma gondii* containing numerous tachyzoites.

fatigue, malaise, cervical lymphadenopathy, and atypical lymphocytosis may occur. Pregnancy does not appear to predispose to severe toxoplasmosis, although there exist case reports of severe primary infection,[517] and some report an increased incidence of complications in women who become infected.[518]

If a pregnant woman acquires toxoplasmosis during pregnancy, there is a 40% chance that her fetus will be infected.[519] The later in pregnancy that primary infection occurs, the more likely that transmission to the fetus will result; transmission rates of 17% in the first trimester and 65% in the third trimester have been reported.[520] Most infants with congenital toxoplasmosis are asymptomatic, but approximately 15% are severely affected.[518] Findings may include chorioretinitis, blindness, deafness, seizures, convulsions, hydrocephalus, microcephaly, fever, jaundice, hepatosplenomegaly, pneumonitis, and coagulopathy. The earlier in pregnancy transmission occurs, the more likely the fetus is to manifest severe illness. Most infected fetuses asymptomatic at birth eventually have chorioretinitis, which may lead to blindness in adolescence or adulthood.[521,522] Although it is not possible to predict outcome in those asymptomatic at birth, some data suggest that the children of women with high antibody titers (≥256) are at risk for eventual development of disease.[518] In a report by Couvreur, children who had chorioretinitis also had twice the IgG antibody titers at birth of those who did not.[523]

Serologic methods are the mainstay of diagnosis of toxoplasmosis in pregnancy and the newborn. IgG antibodies develop several weeks after infection and decline slowly over months to years. Infected persons remain seropositive for life. IgM antibodies appear earlier than IgG antibodies and usually signify acute infection. They increase rapidly and then usually disappear, although persistence of *T. gondii* IgM titers for years has been reported.[524,525] IgA and immunoglobulin E (IgE) levels also rise during acute infection. Five percent of people with acute toxoplasmosis fail to manifest detectable levels of IgA; however, in most, levels peak 2 months after initial infection.[526] Titers of IgE are usually measurable for only 4 months.[513,527] A number of methods of measuring both IgG and IgM antibodies are available. The Sabin-Feldman dye test, an immunofluorescent antibody test, and an agglutination test are commonly used to measure IgG. IgM antibodies are measured by immunofluorescent antibody test, ELISA, or an immunosorbent agglutination assay. IgA-ELISA kits are also commercially available.

Because most pregnant women with acute toxoplasmosis are asymptomatic, the diagnosis is unsuspected until an affected fetus is born. In France, screening of women for antibodies to *T. gondii* is mandatory. Because the incidence of congenital toxoplasmosis in the United States is relatively low (1 to 10 per 10,000 live births), the utility of widespread screening continues to be debated. Nevertheless, the demonstration of IgG antibody (positive serologic test result) to *T. gondii* in a woman before conception indicates that future pregnancies are at no risk, unless the woman becomes severely immunocompromised.[508] A negative serologic test result before or during pregnancy means that the woman is at risk, and preventive counseling should be undertaken. A single positive

IgG titer obtained during pregnancy is difficult to interpret, and serial IgM and IgG titers should then be obtained to establish a diagnosis (Table 16–10). In patients presenting with symptoms compatible with acute toxoplasmosis, both IgM and IgG antibodies should be measured as soon as possible. Commercially available kits for the measurement of *T. gondii* IgM antibodies vary greatly in specificity and reliability, however, and an FDA Public Health Advisory has warned against relying on any single test result as the sole determinant in diagnosing recently acquired infection.[528] In one study, 60% of patients with positive IgM antibodies in whom tests were performed in nonreference laboratories were probably not acutely infected.[529] If acute infection is suspected, sera should be sent to a reference laboratory for confirmation.[530]

Measurement of levels of IgG, IgM, IgA, and IgE[531] in combination on serial samples, together with the determination of acute phase–specific IgG antibodies (the differential agglutination [AC/HS] test,[532] which is not commercially available), is currently the most accurate diagnostic method. If maternal infection is confirmed, fetal ultrasonography should be performed to identify abnormalities of the intracranial sutures, hydrocephalus, aqueductal stenosis, intracerebral calcifications, or microcephaly.[533] Previously, if acute infection in the mother occurred before the 20th week of gestation, Couvreur and Desmonts recommended fetal blood sampling by ultrasonographically guided puncture of the umbilical cord and amniotic fluid sampling.[508] In a study of 746 women at risk who underwent these procedures, samples were inoculated into mice for isolation of the organism, and serologic and routine testing on fetal blood were performed. The authors were able to identify 93% of the infected fetuses in utero.[534] The availability of PCR testing of amniotic fluid specimens has made diagnosis of fetal infection simpler, safer, quicker, and more accurate, however,[535,536] and cordocentesis to obtain samples no longer appears necessary.[530] Amniocentesis for PCR testing is generally performed. After birth, infants suspected of having congenital toxoplasmosis should undergo serial serologic testing. IgM antibody signifies congenital infection,

---

TABLE 16–10   Interpretation of Toxoplasma Serologic Findings

Immunoglobulin M (IgM)	Immunoglobulin G (IgG)	Interpretation
+	−	Acute infection, early; IgG titers should be retested in several weeks
+	+	Acute infection, recent; IgM titers should fall over the next several months
−	+	Low titers of IgG with negative IgM signify remote infection
−	−	Patient at risk for infection

whereas declining IgG titers in the absence of IgM indicates only passive transfer of maternal antibody.

If maternal infection is established, treatment with spiramycin should be started, although there exists controversy about its benefits. In a study reported by Couvreur and Desmont in 1974, treatment with spiramycin, 3 g orally in two divided doses daily, throughout the remainder of the pregnancy was reported to reduce the incidence of congenital toxoplasmosis by approximately 60%.[519] Spiramycin is a macrolide antibiotic that has been widely used in Europe and is available in the United States through application to the FDA. Toxicity is minimal, but if transmission has occurred, disease in the fetus does not appear to be modified,[519] because spiramycin concentrates in the placenta but does not cross it. Whether the azalide drug azithromycin (FDA category B), which has been used to treat toxoplasmosis in AIDS, is useful in this setting remains to be determined.

The combination of pyrimethamine 25 mg orally every day, plus sulfadiazine, 1 g orally four times daily, acts synergistically in the killing of *T. gondii* and can both reduce the rate of transmission and prevent progressive fetopathy.[523] Although this combination is more toxic than spiramycin, it is also more effective. Because of the potential for teratogenicity, some authors recommend beginning pyrimethamine only after the 14th week of gestation. Folinic acid (6 mg orally 3 times weekly) should be given concurrently. Sulfonamides should be avoided close to term because of the risk of kernicterus. Using both spiramycin and pyrimethamine-sulfadiazine results in the greatest decrease in placental infection,[537] and 3 weeks of triple therapy alternating with 3 weeks of spiramycin alone is recommended for fetuses infected before the 28th week of gestation.[509,534] For those infected later in gestation, spiramycin alone has been advocated. Clindamycin has been successfully used in combination with pyrimethamine in the treatment of toxoplasmic encephalitis in AIDS,[538] but it has not been evaluated for therapy in pregnancy.

Treatment of overt congenital toxoplasmosis in the neonate involves 6 months of pyrimethamine plus sulfadiazine with folinic acid, and an additional 6 months of alternating monthly therapy with spiramycin. Couvreur and associates recommended 1 year of therapy with alternating 6-week cycles of pyrimethamine-sulfadiazine and spiramycin for infants infected but asymptomatic at birth.[523] Healthy infants suspected of having congenital toxoplasmosis can be treated with pyrimethaminesulfadiazine for 21 days, followed by spiramycin, until a definitive diagnosis is established.

Prevention of toxoplasmosis in seronegative women involves thorough cooking of meat, washing hands after handling raw meat, washing fruits and vegetables thoroughly, and avoiding contact with cat feces or cat litter boxes.[539]

Malaria

More than 100 million cases of malaria are estimated to occur yearly, with more than 1 million deaths per year

in Africa alone.[540] Since 1976, when the World Health Organization eradication program was declared a failure, malaria has become an increasing worldwide health problem because both the mosquito vectors have become resistant to pesticides and *Plasmodium falciparum* has become resistant to antimalarial agents.

Each year, approximately 100 cases of malaria are reported in the United States.[541] Most of these cases occur in people who have traveled to or immigrated from malarious areas,[542] although occasional transmission within the borders of the United States has been documented.

Human malaria is a protozoan infection caused by four species of *Plasmodium*, which are (in order of decreasing worldwide prevalence) *P. falciparum, Plasmodium vivax, Plasmodium malariae,* and *Plasmodium ovale.* Transmission most commonly occurs through the bite of an infected female *Anopheles* mosquito, but malaria can also be acquired through blood transfusion, through organ transplantation, through use of contaminated needles, or during parturition. After a bite from an infected mosquito, sporozoites rapidly enter hepatocytes, where they transform into hepatic exoerythrocytic forms. The exoerythrocytic stage is clinically silent. After a period of approximately a week, forms called merozoites are released from the liver and invade red blood cells, initiating the erythrocytic stage. Some merozoites undergo a process called schizogony within the red blood cell, which leads to replication of more merozoites and red blood cell rupture. Merozoites of *P. vivax* invade only young red blood cells, and *P. malariae* parasites invade only senescent red blood cells; however, *P. falciparum* infects red blood cells of any age, which results in much higher levels of parasitemia. The fever and chills characteristic of malarial infection are a consequence of the rupture of red blood cells. The periodicity of fever in malaria reflects the time required for schizogony of each species (48 hours for *P. vivax, P. ovale,* and *P. falciparum;* 72 hours for *P. malariae*). Merozoites in other red blood cells also may develop into male and female gametocytes that, when ingested by a mosquito during a blood meal, begin the cycle again. Merozoites never reinvade the liver, but the exoerythrocytic forms of *P. vivax* and *P. ovale* species may remain dormant in the liver for extended periods and can cause a relapse many months later.

The clinical manifestations of malaria commonly begin with a flu-like prodrome, followed by paroxysms of fever, rigors, nausea, abdominal pain, and severe headache. When fever abates, symptoms resolve, and patients usually feel well but exhausted. Early in infection or in severe *P. falciparum* infection, fever may be continuous. Hepatomegaly, splenomegaly, anemia, thrombocytopenia, and signs of intravascular hemolysis may be present. In *P. falciparum* malaria during pregnancy, infected erythrocytes are sequestered in the placenta, and blood flow may be disrupted.[543] Malaria may mimic other disorders more common in pregnancy,[544,545] and the ensuing delays in treatment may lead to significant morbidity and mortality for both the mother and child. Pregnancy increases susceptibility to malaria, and the complications of malaria are more frequent in this population. The factors responsible have not been completely elucidated but may reflect changes in both cell-mediated immunity[546] and antibody production.[20]

In countries where malaria is endemic, this disease is a particular problem in primigravidas, who appear to have higher rates of parasitemia and greater parasite burdens than either nonpregnant control subjects or multigravidas.[547,548] Malaria increases the risk of second trimester abortion and premature labor,[541,547] and maternal malarial infection is the most important infectious cause of low birth weight in tropical Africa[546,549-551]; offspring of primigravidas are most severely affected. Multiple factors, including maternal anemia and cytotrophoblastic thickening, probably contribute to the impairment in nutrient transport to the fetus. Malaria in nonimmune travelers to endemic areas may pose even greater health risks to mother and fetus.[552] Cerebral malaria, rare in adults except during pregnancy, may be present.[546] Almost all deaths from malaria in pregnancy are caused by severe *P. falciparum* infection. In addition to causing low birth weight and premature delivery, the consequences of malaria in the fetus also include a substantial decrease in the transfer of maternal antibodies,[543] such as those to respiratory syncytial virus, *S. pneumoniae, H. influenzae,* and tetanus.[553-556]

Diagnosis is made by detection of parasites on the peripheral blood smear. The different species of malaria have characteristic morphologic features. Thick blood smears (in which red blood cells are concentrated in a small area and then lysed) optimize the chances of detecting parasites but make species identification difficult. Thin smears, prepared identically to those for routine hematologic purposes, allow species identification and estimation of the magnitude of infection. Malarial parasites localize in the placenta, and placental blood films may be a better indicator of infection than are maternal peripheral smears.[546]

The reported incidence of congenital malaria ranges from 0.1% to 42% and probably reflects maternofetal transfusion during labor or parturition rather than transplacental spread.[557-560] Although most infants with congenital malaria are born to mothers with symptomatic infection, congenital malaria can occur without evidence of active malarial infection in the mother.[562,563] Neonates born to immune mothers may spontaneously clear the infection because of transplacental transfer of IgG, and clinical congenital malaria in this group is relatively uncommon. In infants of nonimmune mothers, rates as high as 10% have been reported.[560] Congenital malaria usually becomes symptomatic from 2 to 8 weeks after birth,[557] although symptoms may appear within a few hours and mimic neonatal sepsis.[560,561] Fever, hepatomegaly, splenomegaly, and anemia were noted in 84% to 93% of infants for whom data were available in Hulbert's review of congenital malaria in the United States.[557] Anorexia and lethargy may also be prominent. Unfortunately, all these findings are common in congenital infection, and a proper epidemiologic history and a high index of suspicion are necessary for establishing the diagnosis.

Once maternal malaria infection is confirmed, treatment should commence promptly. Chloroquine is the drug of choice for treatment of *P. vivax, P. malariae,* and *P. ovale* infections. Treatment with pyrimethamine is necessary in addition to chloroquine to eradicate the exoerythrocytic phase of *P. vivax* and *P. ovale* infections,

but pyrimethamine therapy should be delayed until after delivery because of a risk of hemolytic anemia in the fetus. Weekly doses of chloroquine may be given during pregnancy to prevent a relapse.[560] Chloroquine is generally considered safe during pregnancy.

Unfortunately, chloroquine-resistant *P. falciparum* is widespread.[564,565] Quinine has been the mainstay of therapy since 1961, when chloroquine resistance was first recognized. Although some quinine-resistant strains of *P. falciparum* have been reported, this drug remains very useful in the treatment of most chloroquine-resistant strains. Quinine may be given orally to patients who are not seriously ill. Some authorities recommend the addition of pyrimethamine-sulfadoxine (Fansidar) if the patient is not near term or clindamycin if *P. falciparum* malaria was acquired in Southeast Asia because of the multidrug resistance of some of these strains.[566-568] In critically ill patients and those unable to take oral medication, intravenous therapy should be instituted without delay. The CDC recommends intravenous quinidine for severe *P. falciparum* malaria because intravenous quinine is not available in the United States.[569] Hemodynamic parameters and the QT interval on the electrocardiogram should be monitored in patients receiving intravenous quinidine, and close monitoring of the blood glucose level in pregnant women receiving either quinine or quinidine is important, because significant and recurrent hypoglycemia has been reported in this population.[568,570] Exchange transfusion has been used successfully in addition to intravenous quinidine in severe malaria (>10% parasitized cells) in pregnancy.[571]

Neither quinine nor quinidine is free of potential serious adverse consequences to the fetus. When used in large doses as an abortifacient, quinine has been associated with a number of fetal malformations, most notably central nervous system anomalies and limb defects. Auditory and optic nerve damage have also been reported with dosages higher than those used to treat malaria.[57] Quinidine appears to be relatively safe, but neonatal thrombocytopenia after maternal use has been reported. In the setting of drug-resistant *P. falciparum* malaria, the risks to the mother and fetus are outweighed by treatment benefits. Quinine has been used extensively in the treatment of malaria during pregnancy[572] but is in FDA category D, and quinidine is in category C.[57] Pyrimethamine (FDA category C) and sulfadoxine (FDA category B) are considered safe during pregnancy, although folinic acid should also be administered with these agents to prevent folate deficiency.

The therapeutic armamentarium for the treatment of resistant *P. falciparum* malaria in pregnancy is otherwise quite limited.[573] Tetracyclines are active against chloroquine-resistant strains but are associated with maternal hepatotoxicity and with fetal dental discoloration and dysplasia. Mefloquine is a relatively new oral antimalarial agent that is active against both chloroquine-sensitive and multidrug-resistant *P. falciparum* strains. It has been used extensively as both prophylaxis and treatment in nonpregnant patients.[574] It has also been used successfully during pregnancy.[575,576] Although it has been associated with teratogenicity in laboratory animals and its use is not without some risk, a study of inadvertent exposure to mefloquine in female soldiers during their first trimester revealed no evidence of congenital malformations in offspring.[577] The World Health Organization concluded that evidence to date has not confirmed initial fears of embryotoxic or teratogenic effects, and mefloquine may be given with confidence during the second and third trimesters.

In areas of endemic malaria, chemoprophylaxis appears to be of limited utility in preventing placental malaria or in improving mean birth weight except in primigravidas or women with low parity.[578] In areas of unstable endemism, chemoprophylaxis may be more beneficial because morbidity in mothers and fetuses is more severe.[572,579] Chloroquine remains effective prophylaxis in areas where resistant *P. falciparum* is not prevalent. Most authorities recommend that pregnant women refrain from traveling to areas where multidrug-resistant *P. falciparum* is endemic.[560,580,581] If travel cannot be avoided, vigorous attempts to reduce exposure to mosquito bites through the use of protective clothing, mosquito repellent, and netting should be made. Because of the major risks of severe *P. falciparum* malaria during pregnancy, some authorities recommend prophylaxis with chloroquine and proguanil hydrochloride.[540,560] The CDC has stated that "Mefloquine may be considered for use by health care providers for prophylaxis in women who are pregnant or likely to become pregnant when exposure to chloroquine resistant *P. falciparum* is unavoidable." If the former regimen is used, travelers should be given a therapeutic dose of either pyrimethamine-sulfadoxine or mefloquine if a febrile illness develops and medical help is not available. Because of the importance of the appropriate prophylaxis and treatment of malaria and the difficulty in keeping abreast of changing resistance patterns, physicians are urged to call the CDC hotline at 404-332-4555 if questions arise. An international effort to develop a vaccine to prevent malaria in pregnancy is under way.[543]

Other Parasitic Infections

Pregnant women may become infected by numerous other parasitic infections. In addition to the malaria species and *T. gondii*, other common protozoa include *Entamoeba histolytica* (the agent of amebic dysentery) and *Giardia lamblia*. Amoebiasis is more frequently fatal in women at all stages of pregnancy than in nonpregnant women.[582] In two studies, 68% and 72% of the deaths from amoebiasis occurred in women who were pregnant.[583,584] In the United States, *G. lamblia* is the most commonly isolated intestinal parasite. It may cause epidemics in daycare centers; preschool children then may introduce this agent into the home environment. Giardiasis is also more severe during pregnancy, although its incidence is not increased.[585] Helminthic (worm or fluke) infections are very common worldwide, and many are still quite prevalent in the United States, especially in the southeastern states. In many experimental models, worm burdens are increased during pregnancy.[22] A detailed description of the multitude of parasitic infections is beyond the scope of this chapter. Specific issues relating to pregnancy in a number

TABLE 16–11 Important Parasitic Infections

Schistosomiasis[587-594]
Protozoal infections
Giardiasis[585,595-599]
Amoebiasis[582-584,597,600-602]
Trypanosomiasis[603]
Nematode (roundworm) infections
Ascariasis[604,605]
Hookworm[606-608]
Strongyloidiasis[606,608,609]
Trichinosis[610,611]
Trematode (fluke) infections
Cestode (tapeworm) infections[611]
Cysticercosis[612-614]
Echinococcosis[615-618]

of these illnesses are well covered in the text *Parasitic Infections in Pregnancy and Newborns*, edited by MacLeod.[586] General reviews are cited in Table 16–11. Readers are also referred for guidance to standard textbooks of infectious diseases.

References

General Considerations

The Gravid State

1. Scott JR: T- and B-cell distribution in pregnancy. JAMA 1978;239:2769.
2. MacLean MA, Wilson R, Thomson JA, et al: Changes in immunologic parameters in normal pregnancy and spontaneous abortion. Am J Obstet Gynecol 1991;165:890.
3. Lederman MM: Cell mediated immunity pregnancy. Chest 1984;86(3 Suppl):6S.
4. Sumiyoshi Y, Gorai I, Hirahara F, et al: Cellular immunity in normal pregnancy and abortion: Subpopulations of T lymphocytes bearing Fc receptors for IgG and IgM. Am J Reprod Immunol 1981;1:145.
5. Anderson FD, Ushijima RN, Larson CL: Recurrent herpes genitalis: Treatment with Mycobacterium bovis (BCG). Obstet Gynecol 1974;43:797.
6. Gehrz RC, Christianson WR, Linner KM, et al: Cytomegalovirus-specific humoral and cellular immune responses in human pregnancy. J Infect Dis 1981;143:391.
7. Gehrz RC, Christianson WR, Linner KM, et al: A longitudinal analysis of lymphocyte proliferative responses to mitogens and antigens during human pregnancy. Am J Obstet Gynecol 1981;140:665.
8. Hidaka Y, Amino N, Iwatani Y, et al: Changes in natural killer cell activity in normal pregnant and postpartum women: Increases in the first trimester and postpartum period and decrease in late pregnancy. J Reprod Immunol 1991;20:73.
9. Pope RM: Immunoregulatory mechanisms present in the maternal circulation during pregnancy. Baillieres Clin Rheumatol 1990;4:33.
10. Szekeres-Bartho J, Autran B, Debre P, et al: Immunoregulatory effects of a suppressor factor from healthy pregnant women's lymphocytes after progesterone induction. Cell Immunol 1989;122:281.
11. Drutz DH, Huppert M, Sun SH, et al: Human sex hormones stimulate the growth and maturation of *Coccidioides immitis*. Infect Immun 1981;32:897.
12. Shirahata T, Muroya N, Ohta C, et al: Correlation between increased susceptibility to primary *Toxoplasma gondii* infection and depressed production of gamma interferon in pregnant mice. Microbiol Immunol 1992;36:81.
13. Luppi P: How immune mechanisms are affected by pregnancy. Vaccine 2003;21:3352.
14. Luppi P, Haluszczak C, Betters D, et al: Monocytes are progressively activated in the circulation of pregnant women. J Leukoc Biol 2002;72:874.

15. Matthiesen L, Berg G, Ernerudh J, Hakansson L: Lymphocyte subsets and mitogen stimulation of blood lymphocytes in normal pregnancy. Am J Reprod Immunol 1996;35:70.

16. Sabahi F, Rola-Plesczcynski M, O'Connell S, Frenkel LD: Qualitative and quantitative analysis of T lymphocytes during normal pregnancy. Am J Reprod Immunol 1995;33:381.

17. Ashkar AA, Di Santo JP, Croy BA: Interferon gamma contributes to initiation of uterine vascular modifications, decidual integrity and uterine natural killer cell maturation during murine pregnancy. J Exp Med 2000;192:259.

18. Langer-Gould A, Garren H, Slansky A, et al: Late pregnancy suppresses relapses in experimental autoimmune encephalomyelitis: Evidence for a suppressive pregnancy related serum factor. J Immunol 2002;169:1084.

19. Motran CC, Diaz FL, Gruppi A, et al. Human pregnancy-specific glycoprotein 1a (PSG1a) induces alternative activation in human and mouse monocytes and suppresses the accessory cell-dependent T-cell proliferation. J Leukoc Biol 2002;72:512.

20. Mvondo JL, James MA, Suler AJ, et al: Malaria and pregnancy in Cameroonian women: Naturally acquired antibody responses to asexual blood-stage antigens and the circumsporozoite protein of *Plasmodium falciparum.* Trans R Soc Trop Med Hyg 1992;86:486.

21. Rocklin RE, Kitzmiller JL, Kaye MD: Immunobiology of the maternal-fetal relationship. Annu Rev Med 1979;30:375.

22. Weinberg ED: Pregnancy-associated depression of cell-mediated immunity. Rev Infect Dis 1984;6:814.

23. Styrt B, Sugarman B: Estrogens and infection. Rev Infect Dis 1991; 13:1139.

24. Sharma S, Madhur BS, Singh R, et al: Effect of contraceptives on the adhesion of *Escherichia coli* to uroepithelial cells. J Infect Dis 1987; 156:490.

25. Sobel JD, Schneider J, Kaye D, et al: Adherence of bacteria to vaginal epithelial cells at various times in the menstrual cycle. Infect Immun 1981;32:194.

26. Sugarman B, Mummaw N: The effect of hormones on *Trichomonas vaginalis.* J Gen Microbiol 1988;134:1623.

27. Dudley DJ, Chen CL, Mitchell MD, et al: Adaptive immune responses during murine pregnancy: Pregnancy-induced regulation of lymphokine production by activated T lymphocytes. Am J Obstet Gynecol 1993;168:1155.

28. Braun PC: Influence of corticosterone and estradiol on the metabolic activities of *Candida albicans* [Abstract F104]. In Abstracts of the Annual Meeting of the American Society for Microbiology. Washington, DC, American Society for Microbiology, 1989.

Antimicrobial Therapy

29. U.S. Food and Drug Administration: Pregnancy categories for prescription drugs. FDA Drug Bull Sept. 1979.

30. Thornsberry C: Review of in vitro activity of third-generation cephalosporins and other newer β-lactam antibiotics against clinically important bacteria: Symposium on Advances in Cephalosporins. Am J Med 1985;79(Suppl 2A):14.

31. Donowitz GR, Mandell GL: Cephalosporins. In Mandell GL, Douglas RG, Bennett JE (eds): The Principles and Practice of Infectious Diseases, 3rd ed. New York, Churchill Livingstone, 1990, p 246.

32. Cunha BA, Gill MV: Cefepime. Med Clin North Am 1995;79:721.

33. Neu HC: In vitro activity of a new broad spectrum, β-lactamase-stable oral cephalosporin, cefixime. Pediatr Infect Dis J 1987;6:958.

34. Herman G, Cohen AW, Talbot GH, et al: Cefoxitin versus clindamycin and gentamicin in the treatment of the postcesarean section infections. Obstet Gynecol 1986;67:371.

35. Sweet RL, Schachter J, Landers DV, et al: Treatment of hospitalized patients with acute pelvic inflammatory disease: Comparison of cefotetan plus doxycycline and cefoxitin plus doxycycline. Am J Obstet Gynecol 1988;158:736.

36. Scully BE, Swabb EA, Neu HC: Pharmacology of aztreonam after intravenous infusion. Antimicrob Agents Chemother 1983; 24:18.

37. Kucers A, Bennet NMcK: The Use of Antibiotics: A Comprehensive Review with Clinical Emphasis, 4th ed. Philadelphia, JB Lippincott, 1988, p 543.

38. Keim GR, Sibley PL, Hines FA, et al: Parenteral toxicological profile of the monocyclic β-lactam antibiotic SQ 26,776 in mice, rats and dogs. J Antimicrob Chemother 1981;8(Suppl E):141.

39. Adkinson NF, Saxon A, Spence MR, Swabb EA: Cross-allergenicity and immunogenicity of aztreonam. Rev Infect Dis 1985;7(Suppl): S613.

40. Dodson MG: Optimum therapy for acute pelvic inflammatory disease. Drugs 1990;39:511.

41. Neu HC: Aztreonam activity, pharmacology, and clinical uses. Am J Med 1990;88(Suppl 3C):2S.

42. Birnbaum J, Kahan FM, Kropp H, MacDonald JS: Carbapenems: A new class of β-lactam antibiotics. Am J Med 1985;78(Suppl 6A):3.

43. Drusano GL, Standiford HC: Pharmacokinetic profile of imipenem/cilastatin in normal volunteers. Am J Med 1985;78(Suppl 6A):47.

44. Pfaller MA, Jones RN: A review of the in vitro activity of meropenem and comparative antimicrobial agents tested against 30,254 aerobic and anaerobic pathogens isolated world wide. Diagn Microbiol Infect Dis 1997;28:157.

45. Fish DN, Singletary TJ: Meropenem, a new carbapenem antibiotic. Pharmacotherapy 1997;17:644.

46. Craig WA: The pharmacology of meropenem, a new carbapenem antibiotic. Clin Infect Dis 1997;24(Suppl 2):S266.

47. Zajac BA, Fisher MA, Gibson GA, MacGregor RR: Safety and efficacy of high-dose treatment with imipenem-cilastatin in seriously ill patients. Antimicrob Agents Chemother 1985;27:745.

48. Clissold ST, Todd PA, Campoli-Richards DM: Imipenem-cilastatin: A review of its antibacterial activity, pharmacokinetic properties and therapeutic efficacy. Drugs 1987;33:183.

49. Physicians' Desk Reference, 52nd ed. Montvale, N.J., Medical Economics, 1998.

50. Gonik B: Postpartum endometritis: Efficacy and tolerability of two antibiotic regimens. Clin Ther 1992;14:83.

51. McGregor JA, Christensen FB, French JI: Intramuscular imipenem/cilastatin treatment of upper reproductive tract infection in women: Efficacy and use characteristics. Chemotherapy 1991; 37(Suppl 2):31.

52. Hemsell DL, Martens MG, Faro S, et al: A multicenter study comparing intravenous meropenem with clindamycin plus gentamicin for the treatment of acute gynecologic and obstetric pelvic infections in hospitalized women. Clin Infect Dis 1997; 24(Suppl 2):S222.

53. Fenton LJ, Light LJ: Congenital syphilis after maternal treatment with erythromycin. Obstet Gynecol 1976;47:492.

54. Kiefer L, Rubin A, McCoy JB, et al: The placental transfer of erythromycin. Am J Obstet Gynecol 1955;69:174.

55. Philipson A, Sabath LD, Charles D: Transplacental transfer of erythromycin and clindamycin. N Engl J Med 1973;288:1219.

56. Braun P: Hepatotoxicity of erythromycin. J Infect Dis 1969;119:300.

57. Briggs GG, Freeman RK, Yaffe SJ (eds): Drugs in Pregnancy and Lactation, 2nd ed. Baltimore, Williams & Wilkins, 1983.

58. McCormack WM, George H, Donner A, et al: Hepatotoxicity of erythromycin estolate during pregnancy. Antimicrob Agents Chemother 1977;12:630.

59. Piscitelli SC, Danziger LH, Rodvold KA: Clarithromycin and azithromycin: New macrolide antibiotics. Clin Pharm 1992;11:137.

60. Neu HC: Clinical microbiology of azithromycin. Am J Med 1991; 91(Suppl 3A):12S.

61. Peters DH, Clissold SP: Clarithromycin: A review of its antimicrobial activity, pharmacokinetic properties and therapeutic potential. Drugs 1992;44:117.

62. Krohn K: Gynaecological tissue levels of azithromycin. Eur J Clin Microbiol Infect Dis 1991;10:864.

63. Chien SM, Pichotta P, Siepman N, et al: Treatment of community-acquired pneumonia: A multicenter, double-blind, randomized study comparing clarithromycin with erythromycin: Canada-Sweden Clarithromycin-Pneumonia Study Group. Chest 1993; 103:697.

64. Peters DH, Friedel HA, McTavish D: Azithromycin: A review of its antimicrobial activity, pharmacokinetic properties and clinical efficacy. Drugs 1992;44:750.

65. Schonwald S, Gunjaca M, Kolacny-Babic L, et al: Comparison of azithromycin and erythromycin in the treatment of atypical pneumonias. J Antimicrob Chemother 1990;25(Suppl A):123.

66. Sturgill MG, Rapp RP: Clarithromycin: Review of a new macrolide antibiotic with improved microbiologic spectrum and favorable pharmacokinetic and adverse effect profiles. Ann Pharmacother 1992;26:1099.

67. Johnson RB: The role of azalide antibiotics in the treatment of *Chlamydia.* Am J Obstet Gynecol 1991;164:1794.

68. Martin DH, Mroczkowski TF, Dalu ZA, et al: A controlled trial of a single dose of azithromycin for the treatment of chlamydial urethritis and cervicitis: The Azithromycin for Chlamydial Infections Study Group. N Engl J Med 1992;327:921.

69. Amacher DE, Ellis JH, Joyce AJ, et al: Preclinical toxicology studies with azithromycin: Genetic toxicology evaluation. Mutat Res 1993;300:79.

70. Giamarellou H, Kolokythas E, Petrikkos G, et al: Pharmacokinetics of three newer quinolones in pregnant and lactating women. Am J Med 1989;87(Suppl 5A):49S.

71. Bergan T, Thorsteinsson SB, Solberg R, et al: Pharmacokinetics of ciprofloxacin: Intravenous and increasing oral doses. Am J Med 1987;82(Suppl 4A):97.

72. Sanders CC, Sanders WE Jr, Goering RV: Overview of preclinical studies with ciprofloxacin. Am J Med 1987;82(Suppl 4A):2.

73. Ernst ME, Ernst EJ, Klepser ME: Levofloxacin and trovafloxacin: The next generation of fluoroquinolones? Am J Health Syst Pharm 1997;54:2569.

74. Chan ASC: Results of treatment with quinolones of sexually transmitted diseases in the Far East: A brief summary. Rev Infect Dis 1989;11(Suppl 5):S1305.

75. Hendershot EF: Fluoroquinolones. Infect Dis Clin North Am 1995; 9:715.

76. Andriole VT: Quinolones. In Mandell GL, Douglas RG, Bennett JE (eds): Principles and Practice of Infectious Diseases, 3rd ed. New York, Churchill Livingstone, 1990, p 334.

77. Ball P, Tillotson G: Tolerability of fluoroquinolone antibiotics: Past, present and future. Drug Saf 1995;13:343.

78. Just PM: Overview of the fluoroquinolone antibiotics. Pharmacotherapy 1993;13:4S.

79. Christ W, Lehnert T, Ulbrich B. Specific toxicologic aspect of the quinolones. Rev Infect Dis 1988;10(Suppl 1):S141.

Bacterial Infections

Urinary Tract Infections

80. McNeeley SG: Treatment of urinary tract infections during pregnancy. Clin Obstet Gynecol 1988;31:480.

81. Sheldon CA, Gonzalez R: Differentiation of upper and lower urinary tract infections: How and when? Med Clin North Am 1984;68:321.

82. Fairley KF, Bond AG, Brown RB, et al: Simple test to determine the site of urinary tract infection. Lancet 1967;1:427.

83. Jones SR, Smith JW, Sanford JP: Localization of urinary tract infections by detection of antibody-coated bacteria in urine sediment. N Engl J Med 1974;290:591.

84. Sobel JD, Kaye D: Host factors in the pathogenesis of urinary tract infections. Am J Med 1984;76(5A):122.

85. Stamey TA: The role of introital colonization in recurrent urinary infections. J Urol 1973;109:467.

86. Svanborg-Edén C, Hanson LA, Jodal U, et al: Variable adherence to normal human urinary tract epithelial cells of Escherichia coli strains associated with various forms of urinary tract infections. Lancet 1976;1:490.

87. O'Hanley P, Lark D, Falkow S, et al: Molecular basis of Escherichia coli colonization of the upper urinary tract in BALB/c mice. J Clin Invest 1985;75:347.

88. Lomberg H, Hanson LÅA, Jacobsson B, et al: Correlation of P blood group, vesicoureteral reflux, and bacterial attachment in patients with recurrent pyelonephritis. N Engl J Med 1983;308:1189.

89. Bran JL, Levison ME, Kaye D: Entrance of bacteria into the female urinary bladder. N Engl J Med 1972;286:626.

90. Buckley RM, McGuckin M, MacGregor RR: Urine bacterial counts following sexual intercourse. N Engl J Med 1978;298:321.

91. Nicolle LE, Harding GK, Preiksaitis J, et al: The association of urinary tract infection with sexual intercourse. J Infect Dis 1982; 146:579.

92. Andriole VT: Urinary tract infections in pregnancy. Urol Clin North Am 1975;2:485.

93. Fainstat T: Urethral dilatation in pregnancy: A review. Obstet Gynecol Surv 1963;18:845.

94. Lindheimer MD, Katz AI: The kidney in pregnancy. N Engl J Med 1970;283:1095.

95. Andriole VT, Cohn GL: The effect of diethylstilbestrol on the susceptibility of rats to hematogenous pyelonephritis. J Clin Invest 1964;43:1136.

96. Harle EMJ, Bullen JJ, Thompson DA: Influence of estrogen on experimental pyelonephritis caused by Escherichia coli. Lancet 1975;2:283.

97. MacLaren DM: Pyelonephritis and coliform infections of the urinary tract. Lancet 1975;2:556.

98. Orlander JD, Jick SS, Dean AD, et al: Urinary tract infections and estrogen use in older women. J Am Geriatr Soc 1992;40:817.

99. Guyer PB, Delaney D: Urinary tract dilatation and oral contraceptives. BMJ 1970;4:588.

100. Takahashi M, Loveland CM: Bacteriuria and oral contraceptives. JAMA 1974;227:762.

101. Andriole VT, Patterson TF: Epidemiology, natural history, and management of urinary tract infections in pregnancy. Med Clin North Am 1991;75:359.

102. Sweet RL: Bacteriuria and pyelonephritis during pregnancy. Semin Perinatol 1977;1:25.

103. Golan A, Wexler S, Amit A, et al: Asymptomatic bacteriuria in normal and high risk pregnancy. Eur J Obstet Gynecol Reprod Biol 1989;33:101.

104. Whalley PJ, Marlin F, Peters P: Significance of asymptomatic bacteriuria detected during pregnancy. JAMA 1965;193:879.

105. Gaymans R, Valkenberg HA, Haverkorn MJ, et al: A prospective study of urinary tract infection in a Dutch general practice. Lancet 1976;2:674.

106. Sussman M, Asscher AW, Waters WE, et al: Asymptomatic significant bacteriuria in the non-pregnant woman: I. Description of a population. BMJ 1969;1:799.

107. Condie AP, Williams JD, Reeves DS, et al: Complications of bacteriuria in pregnancy. In O'Grady F, Brumfelt W (eds): Urinary Tract Infection. London, Oxford University Press, 1968, p 148.

108. Brumfelt W: The effects of bacteriuria in pregnancy on maternal and fetal health. Kidney Int 1975;8(Suppl):113.

109. Gilstrap LC, Leveno KJ, Cunningham FG, et al: Renal infection and pregnancy outcome. Am J Obstet Gynecol 1981;141:709.

110. Kass EH: Bacteriuria and pyelonephritis of pregnancy. Arch Intern Med 1960;105:194.

111. Stuart KL, Cummins GT, Chin WA: Bacteriuria, prematurity and hypertensive disorders of pregnancy. BMJ 1965;1:554.

112. Romero R, Oyarzun E, Mazor M, et al: Meta-analysis of the relationship between asymptomatic bacteriuria and preterm delivery/low birth weight. Obstet Gynecol 1989;73:576.

113. Smaill F: Antibiotics for asymptomatic bacteriuria in pregnancy. Cochrane Database Syst Rev 2001;(2):CD000490.

114. Nordern CW, Kass EH: Bacteriuria of pregnancy: A critical approach. Annu Rev Med 1968;19:431.

115. Wadland WC, Plante DA: Screening for asymptomatic bacteriuria in pregnancy: A decision and cost analysis. J Fam Pract 1989; 29:372.

116. Stenqvist K, Dahlen-Nilsson I, Linden-Janson G, et al: Bacteriuria in pregnancy. Am J Epidemiol 1989;129:372.

117. McFadyen R, Campbell-Brown M, Stephenson M, et al: Single dose treatment of bacteriuria in pregnancy. Eur Urol 1987; 13(Suppl 1):22.

118. Olsen L, Nielsen IK, Zachariassen A, et al: Single-dose versus six-day therapy with sulfamethizole for asymptomatic bacteriuria during pregnancy. Dan Med Bull 1989;36:486.

119. Rubin RH, Beam TR, Stamm WE: An approach to evaluating antibacterial agents in the treatment of urinary tract infection. Clin Infect Dis 1992;14(Suppl 2):S246.

120. Whalley PJ, Cunningham FG: Short-term versus continuous antimicrobial therapy for asymptomatic bacteriuria in pregnancy. Obstet Gynecol 1977;49:262.

121. Gerstner GJ, Muller G, Nahler G: Amoxicillin in the treatment of asymptomatic bacteriuria in pregnancy: A single dose of 3 g amoxicillin versus a 4-day course of 3 doses 750 mg amoxicillin. Gynecol Obstet Invest 1989;27:84.

122. Fihn SD: Lower urinary tract infection in women. Curr Opin Obstet Gynecol 1992;4:571.

123. Fihn SD, Stamm WE: Interpretation and comparison of treatment studies for uncomplicated urinary tract infections in women. Rev Infect Dis 1985;7:468.

124. Hooton TM, Stamm WE: Management of acute uncomplicated urinary tract infection in adults. Med Clin North Am 1991;75:339.

125. Philbrick JT, Bracikowski JP: Single-dose antibiotic treatment for uncomplicated urinary tract infections. Arch Intern Med 1985; 145:1672.

126. Norrby SR: Short-term treatment of uncomplicated lower urinary tract infections in women. Rev Infect Dis 1990;12:458.

127. Greenberg RN, Reilly PM, Luppen KL, et al: Randomized study of single-dose, three-day, and seven-day treatment of cystitis in women. J Infect Dis 1986;153:277.

128. Souney P, Polk BF: Single-dose antimicrobial therapy for urinary tract infections in women. Rev Infect Dis 1982;4:29.

129. Krieger JN: Complications and treatment of urinary tract infections during pregnancy. Urol Clin North Am 1986;13:685.

130. Thomas S, Bhatia NN: New approaches in the treatment of urinary tract infections. Obstet Gynecol Clin North Am 1989;16:897.

131. Harris RE, Gilstrap LC: Cystitis during pregnancy: A distinct clinical entity. Obstet Gynecol 1981;198:578.

132. Stamm WE, Counts GW, Running KR, et al: Diagnosis of coliform infection in acutely dysuric women. N Engl J Med 1982;307:463.

133. Cunningham FG, Morris GB, Mickal A: Acute pyelonephritis of pregnancy: A clinical review. Obstet Gynecol 1973;42:112.

134. Duff P: Pyelonephritis in pregnancy. Clin Obstet Gynecol 1984;27:17.

135. Gurman G, Schlaeffer F, Kopernic G: Adult respiratory distress syndrome as a complication of acute pyelonephritis during pregnancy. Eur J Obstet Gynecol Reprod Biol 1990;36:75.

136. Martens MG: Pyelonephritis. Obstet Gynecol Clin North Am 1989;16:305.

137. Savoia MC: Complications of pyelonephritis: A clinical review. Infect Urol 1990;3:166.

138. Faro S, Pastorek JG, Plauche WC, et al: Short-course parenteral antibiotic therapy for pyelonephritis in pregnancy. South Med J 1984;77:455.

139. Harris RE, Gilstrap LC: Prevention of recurrent pyelonephritis during pregnancy. Obstet Gynecol 1974;44:637.

140. Lenke RR, VanDorsten JP, Schifrin BS: Pyelonephritis in pregnancy: A prospective randomized trial to prevent recurrent disease evaluating suppressive therapy with nitrofurantoin and close surveillance. Am J Obstet Gynecol 1983;146:953.

Pneumonia

141. Benedetti TJ, Valle R, Ledger WJ: Antepartum pneumonia in pregnancy. Am J Obstet Gynecol 1982;144:413.

142. Hopwood HG: Pneumonia in pregnancy. Obstet Gynecol 1965;25:875.

143. Berkowitz K, LaSala A: Risk factors associated with the increasing prevalence of pneumonia during pregnancy. Am J Obstet Gynecol 1990;163:981.

144. Rickey SD, Roberts SW, Ramin KD, et al: Pneumonia complicating pregnancy. Obstet Gynecol 1994;84:525.

145. Riley L: Pneumonia and tuberculosis in pregnancy. Infect Dis Clin North Am 1997;11:119.

146. Rodrigues J, Niederman MS: Pneumonia complicating pregnancy. Clin Chest Med 1992;13:679.

147. Madinger NE, Greenspoon JS, Ellrodt AG: Pneumonia during pregnancy: Has modern technology improved maternal and fetal outcome? Am J Obstet Gynecol 1989;161:657.

148. Ramsey PS, Ramin KD: Pneumonia in pregnancy. Obstet Gynecol Clin North Am 2001;28:553.

149. Eisenberg VH, Eidelman LA, Arbel R, et al: Legionnaire's disease during pregnancy: A case presentation and review of the literature. Eur J Obstet Gynecol Reprod Biol 1997;72:15.

150. Gherman RB, Leventis LL, Miller RC: Chlamydial psittacosis during pregnancy: A case report. Obstet Gynecol 1995;86:648.

151. Rigby FR, Pastorek JG: Pneumonia during pregnancy. Clin Obstet Gynecol 1996;39:107.

152. Mandell LA, Bartlett JG, Dowell SF, et al: Update of practice guidelines for the management of community acquired pneumonia in immunocompetent adults. Clin Infect Dis 2003;37:1405.

Appendicitis

153. Al-Mulhim AA: Acute appendicitis in pregnancy: A review of 52 cases. Int Surg 1996;81:295.

154. Puylaert JBCM: Acute appendicitis: Ultrasound evaluation using graded compression. Radiology 1986;158:355.

155. Mahmoodian S: Appendicitis complicating pregnancy. South Med J 1992;85:19.

156. Weingold AB: Appendicitis in pregnancy. Clin Obstet Gynecol 1983;26:801.

157. Baer JL, Reis RA, Arens RA: Appendicitis in pregnancy with changes in position and axis of normal appendix in pregnancy. JAMA 1932;98:1359.

158. Barloon TJ, Brown BP, Abu-Yousef MM, et al: Sonography of acute appendicitis in pregnancy. Abdom Imaging 1995;20:149.

159. Moore L, Wilson SR: Ultrasonography in obstetric and gynecologic emergencies. Radiol Clin North Am 1994;32:1005.

160. Richards C, Daya S: Diagnosis of acute appendicitis in pregnancy. Can J Surg 1989;32:358.

161. McGee TM: Acute appendicitis in pregnancy. Aust N Z J Obstet Gynaecol 1989;29:378.

162. Al-Fozan H, Tulandi T: Safety and risks of laparoscopy in pregnancy. Curr Open Obstet Gynecol 2002:14:375.

163. Bisharah M, Tulandi T: Laparoscopic surgery in pregnancy. Clin Obstet Gynecol 2003;46:92.

164. Rollins MD, Chan KJ, Price RR: Laparoscopy for appendicitis and cholelithiasis during pregnancy: A new standard of care. Surg Endosc 2003:Dec. 29, PM ID 14691706.

Intraamniotic Infection

165. Gibbs RS, Duff P: Progress in pathogenesis and management of clinical intraamniotic infection. Am J Obstet Gynecol 1991;164:1317.

166. Yoder PR, Gibbs RS, Blanco JD, et al: A prospective controlled study of maternal and perinatal outcome after intra-amniotic infection at term. Am J Obstet Gynecol 1983;145:695.

167. Soper DE, Mayhall CG, Dalton HP: Risk factors for intraamniotic infection: A prospective epidemiologic study. Am J Obstet Gynecol 1989;161:562.

168. Charles D, Edwards WR: Infectious complications of cervical cerclage. Am J Obstet Gynecol 1981;141:1065.

169. Adair CD, Ernest JM, Sanchez-Ramos L, et al: Meconium stained amniotic fluid–associated infectious morbidity: A randomized double blind trial of ampicillin-sulbactam prophylaxis. Obstet Gynecol 1996;88:216.

170. Chapman S, Duff P: Incidence of chorioamnionitis in patients with meconium-stained fluid. Infect Dis Obstet Gynecol 1995;2:210.

171. Wen TS, Eriksen NL, Blanco JD, et al: Association of clinical intra-amniotic infection and meconium. Am J Perinatol 1993;10:438.

172. Clark P, Duff P: Inhibition of neutrophil oxidative burst and phagocytosis by meconium. Am J Obstet Gynecol 1995;173:1301.

173. Florman AL, Teubner D: Enhancement of bacterial growth in amniotic fluid by meconium. J Pediatr 1969;74:111.

174. Goldenberg RL, Thom E, Moawad AH, et al: The preterm prediction study: Fetal fibronectin, bacterial vaginosis, and peripartum infection. Obstet Gynecol 1996;87:656.

175. Hillier SL, Nugent RP, Eschenbach DA, et al: Association between bacterial vaginosis and preterm delivery of a low-birth-weight infant. N Engl J Med 1995;333:1737.

176. Newton ER, Piper J, Peairs W: Bacterial vaginosis and intraamniotic infection. Am J Obstet Gynecol 1997;176:672.

177. Gibbs RS, Blanco JD, St Clair PJ, et al: Quantitative bacteriology of amniotic fluid from women with clinical intraamniotic infection at term. J Infect Dis 1982;145:1.

178. Blanco JD, Gibbs RS, Malherbe H, et al: A controlled study of genital mycoplasmas in amniotic fluid from patients with intra-amniotic infection. J Infect Dis 1983;147:650.

179. Sweet RL, Landers DV, Walker C, Schachter J: *Chlamydia trachomatis* infection and pregnancy outcome. Am J Obstet Gynecol 1987;156:824.

180. Wager GP, Martin DH, Koutsky L, et al: Puerperal infectious morbidity: Relationship to route of delivery and antepartum *Chlamydia trachomatis* infection. Am J Obstet Gynecol 1980;138:1028.

181. Gibbs RS, Eschenbach DA: Use of antibiotics to prevent preterm birth. Am J Obstet Gynecol 1997;177:375.

182. Gibbs RS, Romero R, Hillier SL, et al: A review of premature birth and subclinical infection. Am J Obstet Gynecol 1992;166:1515.

183. Romero R, Sirtori M, Oyarzun E, et al: Infection and labor: Prevalence, microbiology, and clinical significance of intraamniotic infection in women with preterm labor and intact membranes. Am J Obstet Gynecol 1989;161:817.

184. Driscoll SG: The placenta and membranes. In Charles D, Finland M (eds): Obstetric and Perinatal Infections. Philadelphia, Lea & Febiger, 1973, p 529.

185. King J, Flenady V: Prophylactic antibiotics for inhibiting preterm labour with intact membranes. Cochrane Database Syst Rev 2002;(4):CD000246.

186. Kenyon S, Bouvain M, Neilson J: Antibiotics for preterm premature rupture of membranes. Cochrane Database Syst Rev 2001;(3): CD001058.

187. Flenady V, King J: Antibiotics for prelabour rupture of membranes at or near term. Cochrane Database Syst Rev 2002;(3):CD001807.

188. Hauth JC, Goldenberg RL, Andrews WW, et al: Reduced incidence of preterm delivery with metronidazole and erythromycin in women with bacterial vaginosis. N Engl J Med 1995;333:1732.

189. McDonald HM, O'Loughlin JA, Vigneswaran R, et al: Impact of metronidazole therapy on preterm birth in women with bacterial vaginosis flora (*Gardnerella vaginalis*): A randomised, placebo controlled trial. Br J Obstet Gynaecol 1997;104:1391.

190. Morales WJ, Schorr S, Albritton J: Effect of metronidazole in patients with preterm birth in preceding pregnancy and bacterial vaginosis: A placebo-controlled, double-blind study. Am J Obstet Gynecol 1994;171:345.

191. McDonald H, Brocklehurst P, Parsons J, Vigneswaran R: Antibiotics for treating bacterial vaginosis in pregnancy. Cochrane Database Syst Rev 2003;(2):CD000262.

192. Bacterial Vaginosis Screening for Prevention of Preterm Delivery. Committee Opinion No. 198. Washington, D.C., American College of Obstetricians and Gynecologists, February 1998.

193. Joesoef MR, Hillier SL, Wiknjosastro G, et al: Intravaginal clindamycin treatment for bacterial vaginosis: Effects on preterm delivery and low birth weight. Am J Obstet Gynecol 1995;173:1527.

194. Joesoef MR, Schmide GP: Bacterial vaginosis: Review of treatment options and potential clinical indications for therapy. Clin Infect Dis 1995;20(Suppl 1):S72.

195. Gilstrap LC, Cox SM: Acute chorioamnionitis. Obstet Gynecol Clin North Am 1989;16:373.

196. Romero R, Yoon BH, Mazor M, et al: The diagnostic and prognostic value of amniotic fluid white blood cell count, glucose, interleukin-6, and gram stain in patients with preterm labor and intact membranes. Am J Obstet Gyecol 1993;169:805.

197. Yoon BH, Romero R, Kem CJ, et al: Amniotic fluid interleukin-6: A sensitive test for antenatal diagnosis of acute inflammatory lesions of the preterm placenta and prediction of perinatal morbidity. Am J Obstet Gynecol 1995;172:960.

198. Romero R, Mazor M, Avila C, et al: Neutrophil activating peptide-1/interleukin-8 and intra-amniotic infection. Am J Obstet Gynecol 1991;165:813.

199. Stiemer B, Buschmann A, Bisson S, et al: Interleukin-8 in urine: A new diagnostic parameter for intra-amniotic infection after premature rupture of the membranes. Br J Obstet Gynaecol 1997;104:499.

200. Gibbs RS, Castillo MS, Rodgers PJ: Management of acute chorioamnionitis. Am J Obstet Gynecol 1980;136:709.

201. Gilstrap LC, Leveno KJ, Cox SM, et al: Intrapartum treatment of acute chorioamnionitis: Impact on neonatal sepsis. Am J Obstet Gynecol 1988;159:579.

202. Sperling RS, Ramamurthy RS, Gibbs RS: A comparison of intrapartum versus immediate postpartum treatment of intra-amniotic infection. Obstet Gynecol 1987;70:861.

203. Hopkins L, Smaill F: Antibiotic regimens for management of intraamniotic infection. Cochrane Database Syst Rev 2002;(3): CD003254.

204. Maberry MC, Gilstrap LC, Bawdon R, et al: Anaerobic coverage for intra-amnionic infection: Maternal and perinatal impact. Am J Perinatol 1991;8:338.

205. Mitra AG, Whitten MK, Laurent SL, Anderson WE: A randomized, prospective study comparing once-daily gentamicin versus thrice-daily gentamicin in the treatment of puerperal infection. Am J Obstet Gynecol 1997;177:786.

206. Bourget P, Fernandez H, Quinquis V, Delouis C: Pharmacokinetics and protein binding of ceftriaxone during pregnancy. Antimicrob Agents Chemother 1993;37:54.

207. Hauth JC, Gilstrap LC, Hankins GDV, et al: Term maternal and neonatal complications of acute chorioamnionitis. Obstet Gynecol 1985;66:59.

208. Duff P, Sanders R, Gibbs RS: The course of labor in term patients with chorioamnionitis. Am J Obstet Gynecol 1983;147:391.

209. Silver RK, Gibbs RS, Castillo M: Effect of amniotic fluid bacteria on the course of labor in nulliparous women at term. Obstet Gynecol 1986;68:587.

210. Koh KS, Chan FH, Monfared AH, et al: The changing perinatal and maternal outcome in chorioamnionitis. Obstet Gynecol 1979; 53:730.

211. Grether JK, Nelson KB: Maternal infection and cerebral palsy in infants of normal birth weight. JAMA 1997;278:207.

Endometritis and Postpartum Infection

212. Chaim W, Bashiri A, Bar-David J, et al: Prevalence and clinical significance of postpartum endometritis and wound infection. Infect Dis Obstet Gynecol 2000;8:77.

213. Eschenbach DA, Rosene K, Tompkins LS, et al: Endometrial cultures obtained by a triple lumen method from afebrile and febrile postpartum women. J Infect Dis 1986;153:1038.

214. Blanco JD, Gibbs RS: Infections following classical cesarean section. Obstet Gynecol 1980;55:167.

215. Gibbs RS, Jones PM, Wilder CJ: Antibiotic therapy of endometritis following cesarean section: Treatment successes and failures. Obstet Gynecol 1978;52:31.

216. Gibbs RS, Rodgers PJ, Castaneda YS, et al: Endometritis following vaginal delivery. Obstet Gynecol 1980;56:555.

217. Newton ER, Prihoda TJ, Gibbs RS: A clinical and microbiologic analysis and risk factors for puerperal endometritis. Obstet Gynecol 1990;75:402.

218. Sweet RL, Ledger WJ: Puerperal infectious morbidity. Am J Obstet Gynecol 1973;117:1093.

219. Lasley DS, Eblen A, Yancey MK, et al: The effect of placental removal method on the incidence of postcesarean infections. Am J Obstet Gynecol 1997;176:1250.

220. Magann EF, Dodson MK, Harris RL, et al: Does method of placental removal or site of uterine repair after endometritis alter cesarean delivery? Infect Dis Obstet Gynecol 1993;177:389.

221. Magann EF, Washburne JF, Harris RL, et al: Infectious morbidity, operative blood loss, and length of the operative procedure after cesarean delivery by method of placental removal and site of uterine repair. J Am Coll Surg 1995;181:517.

222. D'Angelo LJ, Sokol RJ: Time-related peripartum determinants of postpartum morbidity. Obstet Gynecol 1980;55:319.

223. Gibbs RS, Listwa HM, Read JA: The effect of internal fetal monitoring on maternal infection following cesarean section. Obstet Gynecol 1976;48:653.

224. Seo K, McGregor JA, French JI: Preterm birth is associated with increased risk of maternal and neonatal infection Obstet Gynecol 1992;79:75.

225. Bobitt JR, Ledger WJ: Amniotic fluid analysis: Its role in maternal and neonatal infection. Obstet Gynecol 1978;51:56.

226. Gibbs RS: Clinical risk factors for puerperal infection. Obstet Gynecol 1980;55:178.

227. Gilstrap LC, Cunningham FG: The bacterial pathogenesis of infection following cesarean section. Obstet Gynecol 1979;53:545.

228. Blanco JD, Gibbs RS, Castaneda YS, et al: Correlation of quantitative amniotic fluid cultures with endometritis after cesarean section. Am J Obstet Gynecol 1982;143:897.

229. Awadalla SG, Perkins RP, Mercer LJ: Significance of endometrial cultures performed at cesarean section. Obstet Gynecol 1986;68:220.

230. Gibbs RS: Severe infections in pregnancy. Med Clin North Am 1989;73:713.

231. Williams CK, Okada DM, Marshall JR, et al: Clinical and microbiologic risk evaluation for post-cesarean section endometritis by multivariate discriminant analysis: Role of intraoperative mycoplasma, aerobes, and anaerobes. Am J Obstet Gynecol 1987; 156:967.

232. Charles J, Charles D: Postpartum infection. In Charles D (ed): Obstetric and Perinatal Infections. St. Louis, Mosby–Year Book, 1993, p 60.

233. Hawrylyshyn PA, Bernstein P, Papsin FR: Risk factors associated with infection following cesarean section. Am J Obstet Gynecol 1981;139:294.

234. Rehu M, Nilsson CG: Risk factors for febrile morbidity associated with cesarean section. Obstet Gynecol 1980;56:269.

235. Larsen JW, Goldbrand JW, Hanson TM, et al: Intrauterine infection on an obstetric service. Obstet Gynecol 1974;43:838.

236. Gibbs RS, Jones PM, Wilder CJY: Internal fetal monitoring and maternal infection following cesarean section: A prospective study. Obstet Gynecol 1978;52:193.

237. Faro S, Phillips LE, Martens MG: Perspectives on the bacteriology of postoperative obstetric and gynecologic infections. Am J Obstet Gynecol 1988;158:694.

238. Faro S: Group B β-hemolytic streptococci and puerperal infections. Am J Obstet Gynecol 1981;139:686.

239. Watts DW, Krohn M, Hillier SL, et al: Bacterial vaginosis as a risk factor for post-cesarean endometritis. Obstet Gynecol 1990;75:52.

240. Blanco JD, Diaz KC, Lipscomb KA, et al: *Chlamydia trachomatis* isolation in patients with endometritis after cesarean section. Am J Obstet Gynecol 1985;152:278.

241. Ismail MA, Pridjian G, Hibbard JU, et al: Significance of positive cervical cultures for *Chlamydia trachomatis* in patients with preterm premature rupture of membranes. Am J Perinatol 1992;9:368.

242. Krohn MA, Hillier SL, Baker CJ: Maternal peripartum complications associated with vaginal group B streptococcal colonization. J Infect Dis 1999;179:1410.

243. Hollier LM, Scott LL, Murphree SS, et al: Postpartum endometritis caused by herpes simplex virus. Obstet Gynecol 1997;89:836.

244. Remadi S, Finci V, Ismail A, et al: Herpetic endometritis after pregnancy. Pathol Res Pract 1995;191:31.

245. Cox SM, Gilstrap LC: Postpartum endometritis. Obstet Gynecol Clin North Am 1989;16:363.

246. Filker R, Monif GRG: The significance of temperature during the first 24 hours postpartum. Obstet Gynecol 1979;53:358.

247. Spandorfer SD, Graham E, Forouzan I: Postcesarean endometritis: Clinical risk factors predictive of positive blood cultures. J Reprod Med 1996;41:797.

248. Duff P, Gibbs RS, Blanco JD, et al: Endometrial culture techniques in puerperal patients. Obstet Gynecol 1983;61:217.

249. Eschenbach DA: Bacterial vaginosis and anaerobes in obstetric-gynecologic infection. Clin Infect Dis 1993;16(Suppl 4):S282.

250. Knuppel RA, Scarbo JC, Mitchell GW, et al: Quantitative transcervical uterine cultures with a new device. Obstet Gynecol 1981;57:243.

251. Ledger WJ, Gee C, Pollin PA: A new approach to patients with suspected anaerobic postpartum infections: Transabdominal uterine aspiration for culture and metronidazole for treatment. Am J Obstet Gynecol 1976;126:1.

252. Bracero LA: Ampicillin/sulbactam versus cefotetan for the prevention of infection following cesarean delivery in high-risk patients: A randomized double-blind trial. Gynecol Obstet Invest 1997;44:21.

253. Casey BM, Cox SM: Chorioamnionitis and endometritis. Infect Dis Clin North Am 1997;11:203.

254. McGregor JA, Crombleholme WR, Newton E, et al: Randomized comparison of ampicillin-sulbactam to cefoxitin and doxycycline or clindamycin and gentamicin in the treatment of pelvic inflammatory disease or endometritis. Obstet Gynecol 1994;83:998.

255. Pastorek JG, Miller JM: Postcesarean section infection. Infect Surg 1987;6:532.

256. Resnik E, Harger JH, Kuller JA: Early postpartum endometritis: Randomized comparison of ampicillin/sulbactam vs. ampicillin, gentamicin and clindamycin. J Reprod Med 1994;39:467.

257. Sweet RL, Roy S, Faro S, et al: Piperacillin and tazobactam versus clindamycin and gentamicin in the treatment of hospitalized women with pelvic infection: The Piperacillin/Tazobactam Study Group. Obstet Gynecol 1994;83:280.

258. French LM, Smaill FM: Antibiotic regimens for endometritis after delivery. Cochrane Database Syst Rev 2002;(1):CD001067.

259. Dismoor MJ, Newton ER, Gibbs RS: A randomized, double-blinded, placebo-controlled trial of oral antibiotics following intravenous antibiotic therapy for postpartum endometritis. Obstet Gynecol 1991;77:60.

260. Soper DE, Kemmer CT, Conover WB: Abbreviated antibiotic therapy for the treatment of postpartum endometritis. Obstet Gynecol 1987;69:127.

261. Zuckerman J, Levine D, McNicholas MM, et al: Imaging on pelvic postpartum complications. AJR Am J Roentgenol 1997;168:663.

262. Dylewski J, Wiesenfeld H, Latour A: Postpartum uterine infection with *Clostridium perfringens*. Rev Infect Dis 1989;11:470.

263. Ebright JR, Moldenhauer J, Gonik B: Non-surgical management of post-cesarean endometritis associated with myometrial gas formation. Infect Dis Obstet Gynecol 2000;8:181.

264. Witlin AG, Mercer BM, Sibai BM: Septic pelvic thrombophlebitis on refractory postpartum fever of undetermined etiology. J Matern Fetal Med 1996;5:355.

265. Smaill F, Hofmeyr GJ: Antibiotic prophylaxis for cesarean section. Cochrane Database Syst Rev 2002;(2):CD000933.

266. Sweet RL, Gibbs RS: Infectious Diseases of the Female Genital Tract. Baltimore, Williams & Wilkins, 1990, pp 356, 460.

267. Probst JR, Benrubi GI, Sanchez-Ramos L, et al: Comparison of one dose cefazolin versus one dose cefotetan for cesarean section prophylaxis. J Fla Med Assoc 1989;76:1027.

Sexually Transmitted Diseases

Syphilis

268. Tramont EC: Spirochetes: *Treponema pallidum* (syphilis). In Mandell GL, Bennett JE, Dolin R (eds): Principles and Practice of Infectious Diseases, vol 2, 4th ed. New York, Churchill Livingstone, 1995, p 2117.

269. Sanchez PJ, Wendel GD: Syphilis in pregnancy. Clin Perinatol 1997;24:71.

270. Genc M, Ledger WJ: Syphilis is pregnancy. Sex Transm Infect 2000;76:73.

271. Magnuson HJ, Thomas EW, Olansky S, et al: Inoculation syphilis in human volunteers. Medicine (Baltimore) 1956;35:33.

272. Baton JR, Thorpe EM, Shaver DC, et al: Nonimmune hydrops fetalis associated with maternal infection with syphilis. Am J Obstet Gynecol 1992;167:56.

273. Harter CA, Benirschke K: Fetal syphilis in the first trimester. Am J Obstet Gynecol 1976;124:705.

274. Lee WK, Schwartz DA, Rice RJ, et al: Syphilitic endometritis causing first trimester abortion: A potential infectious cause of fetal morbidity in early gestation. South Med J 1994;87:1259.

275. McFarlin BL, Bottoms SF, Dock BS, et al: Epidemic syphilis: Maternal factors associated with congenital infection. Am J Obstet Gynecol 1994;170:535.

276. Ricci JM, Fojaco RM, O'Sullivan MJ: Congenital syphilis: The University of Miami/Jackson Memorial Medical Center Experience 1986-88. Obstet Gynecol 1989;74:687.

277. Fiumara NJ, Fleming WL, Downing JG, et al: The incidence of prenatal syphilis at the Boston City Hospital. N Engl J Med 1952;247:48.

278. Ingall D, Sanchez PJ, Musher D: Syphilis. In Remington JS, Klein JD (eds): Infectious Diseases: The Fetus and Newborn, 4th ed. Philadelphia, WB Saunders, 1994, p 529.

279. Larsen SA, Steiner BM, Rudolph AH: Laboratory diagnosis and interpretation of tests for syphilis. Clin Microbiol Rev 1995;8:1.

280. Gowievitch MN, Selwyn PA, Davenny K, et al: Effects of HIV infection on the serologic manifestations and response to treatment of syphilis in intravenous drug users. Ann Intern Med 1995;118:350.

281. Romanowski B, Sutherland R, Fick GH, et al: Serologic response to treatment of infectious syphilis. Ann Intern Med 1991;114:1005.

282. Sexually transmitted diseases treatment guidelines 2002. Centers for Disease Control and Prevention. MMWR Morb Mortal Wkly Rep 2002;51(RR-6):1.

283. McFarlin BL, Bottoms SF: Maternal syphilis: The next pregnancy. Am J Perinatol 1996;13:513.

Gonorrhea

284. Handsfield HH: Disseminated gonococcal infection. Clin Obstet Gynecol 1975;18:131.

285. Alexander ER: Gonorrhea in the newborn. Ann N Y Acad Sci 1988;549:180.

286. Handsfield HH, Sparling PF: *Neisseria gonorrhoeae*. In Mandell GL, Bennett JE, Dolin R (eds): Principles and Practice of Infectious Diseases, vol 2, 4th ed. New York, Churchill Livingstone, 1995, p 1909.

287. Judson FN: Gonorrhea. Med Clin North Am 1990;74:1353.

288. Thin RNT, Williams IA, Nicol CS: Direct and delayed methods of immunofluorescent diagnosis of gonorrhea in women. Br J Vener Dis 1971;47:27.

289. Elmros T, Larsson PA: Survival of gonococci outside the body. BMJ 1972;2:403.

290. Brunham RC, Paavonen J, Stevens CE, et al: Mucopurulent cervicitis: The ignored counterpart in women of urethritis in men. N Engl J Med 1984;311:1.

291. McCormack WM, Stumacher RJ, Johnson K, et al: Clinical spectrum of gonococcal infections in women. Lancet 1977;1:1182.

292. Corman LC, Levinson ME, Knight R, et al: The high frequency of pharyngeal gonococcal infection in a prenatal clinic population. JAMA 1974;230:568.
293. Weisner PJ, Tronca E, Bonin P, et al: Clinical spectrum of pharyngeal gonococcal infections. N Engl J Med 1973;288:181.
294. Edwards LE, Barrada MMI, Harmann AA, et al: Gonorrhea in pregnancy. Am J Obstet Gynecol 1978;132:637.
295. Handsfield HH, Hodson WA, Holmes KK: Neonatal gonococcal infection: I. Orogastric contamination with Neisseria gonorrhoeae. JAMA 1973;225:697.
296. Holmes KK, Counts GW, Beaty HN: Disseminated gonococcal infection. Ann Intern Med 1971;74:979.
297. Kerle KK, Mascola JR, Miller TA: Disseminated gonococcal infection. Am Fam Physician 1992;45:209.
298. O'Brien JA, Goldenberg DL, Rice PA: Disseminated gonococcal infection: A prospective analysis of 49 patients and a review of pathophysiology and immune mechanisms. Medicine (Baltimore) 1983;62:395.
299. Livengood CH, Wrenn JW: Evaluation of COBAS AMPLICOR (Roche): Accuracy in detection of Chlamydia trachomatis and Neisseria gonorrhoeae by coamplification of endocervical specimens. J Clin Microbiol 2001;39:2928.
300. Koumans EH, Johnson RE, Knapp JS, St. Louis ME: Laboratory testing for Neisseria gonorrhoeae by recently introduced nonculture tests: A performance review with clinical and public health considerations. Clin Infect Dis 1998;27:1171.
301. Centers for Disease Control and Prevention: Screening tests to detect Chlamydia trachomatis and Neisseria gonorrhoeae infections—2002. MMWR 2002;51:1.
302. Brocklehurst P: Antibiotics for gonorrhoea in pregnancy. Cochrane Database Syst Rev 2002;(2):CD000098.

Chlamydial Infections

303. Black CM: Current methods of laboratory diagnosis of Chlamydia trachomatis infections. Clin Microbiol Rev 1997;10:160.
304. Cates WJ, Wasserhect JN: Genital chlamydial infections: Epidemiology and reproductive sequelae. Am J Obstet Gynecol 1991;164:1771.
305. Lycke E, Lowhagen G-B, Hallhagen G, et al: The risk of transmission of genital Chlamydia trachomatis infection is less than that of genital Neisseria gonorrhoeae infection. Sex Transm Dis 1980;7:6.
306. Stenberg K, Mardh PA: Genital infection with Chlamydia trachomatis in patients with chlamydial conjunctivitis: Unexplained results. Sex Transm Dis 1991;18:1.
307. Schachter J, Grossman M, Sweet RL, et al: Prospective study of perinatal transmission of Chlamydia trachomatis. JAMA 1986;255:3374.
308. Jones RB: Chlamydia trachomatis (trachoma, perinatal infections, lymphogranuloma venereum, and other genital infections). In Mandell GL, Bennett JE, Dolin R (eds): Principles and Practice of Infectious Diseases, vol 2, 4th ed. New York, Churchill Livingstone, 1995, p 1679.
309. Schachter J: Chlamydial infections. N Engl J Med 1978;298:428.
310. Perine PL, Osoba AD: Lymphogranuloma venereum. In Holmes KK, Mardh PA, Spraling PF, et al (eds): Sexually Transmitted Diseases, 2nd ed. New York, McGraw-Hill, 1990, p 195.
311. Stamm WE, Wagner KF, Amsel R, et al: Causes of the acute urethral syndrome in women. N Engl J Med 1980;303:409.
312. Berger RE, Alexander ER, Harnisch JP, et al: Etiology, manifestations and therapy of acute epididymitis. J Urol 1979;121:750.
313. Bowil WR, Alexander ER, Holmes KR: Etiologies of postgonococcal urethritis in homosexual and heterosexual men: Roles of Chlamydia trachomatis and Ureaplasma urealyticum. Sex Transm Dis 1978;5:151.
314. Martin DH, Koutsky L, Eschenbach DA, et al: Prematurity and perinatal mortality in pregnancies complicated by maternal Chlamydia trachomatis infection. JAMA 1982;247:1585.
315. Ryan GT, Abdella TN, McNeeley SG, et al: Chlamydia trachomatis infection in pregnancy and the effect of treatment on pregnancy outcome. Am J Obstet Gynecol 1990;162:34.
316. Hardy PH, Hardy JB, Nell EE, et al: Prevalence of sexually transmitted disease agents among pregnant inner city adolescents and pregnancy outcome. Lancet 1984;2:333.
317. Harrison HR, Costin M, Meder JB, et al: Cervical Chlamydia trachomatis and Mycoplasma infection in pregnancy: Epidemiology and outcomes. JAMA 1983;250:1721.
318. McGregor JA, French JI: Chlamydia trachomatis infection during pregnancy. Am J Obstet Gynecol 1991;164:1782.

319. Cohen I, Viella JC, Calkins BM: Improved pregnancy outcome following successful treatment of chlamydial infection. JAMA 1990;263:3160.
320. Gravett MG, Nelson HP, De Rouen T, et al: Independent associations of bacterial vaginosis and Chlamydia trachomatis infection with adverse pregnancy outcome. JAMA 1986;256:1899.
321. Martins J, Krohn MA, Hillier SL, et al: Relationship of vaginal Lactobacillus species, cervical Chlamydia trachomatis and bacterial vaginosis to preterm birth. Obstet Gynecol 1988;71:89.
322. Witkins SS, Ledger WJ: Antibodies to Chlamydia trachomatis in sera with recurrent spontaneous abortion. Am J Obstet Gynecol 1992; 167:135.
323. Harrison HR, Alexander ER: Chlamydial infections in infants and children. In Holmes KK, Mardh PA, Sparling PF, et al (eds): Sexually Transmitted Diseases, 2nd ed. New York, McGraw-Hill, 1990, p 811.
324. Preece PM, Anderson JM, Thompson RG: Chlamydia trachomatis infection in infants: A prospective study. Arch Dis Child 1989; 64:525.
325. Claesson BA, Trollfors B, Brolin I, et al: Etiology of community acquired pneumonia in children based on antibody responses to bacterial and viral antigens. Pediatr Infect Dis 1989;8:856.
326. Weirs SG, Newcomb RW, Beem MD: Pulmonary assessment of children after chlamydial infection in infancy. J Pediatr 1986;108:659.
327. Mardh, PA: Influence of infection with Chlamydia trachomatis on pregnancy outcome, infant health and life-long sequelae in infected offspring. Best Prac Res Clin Obstet Gynecol 2002;16:847.
328. Centers for Disease Control and Prevention: Recommendations for the prevention and management of Chlamydia trachomatis infections. MMWR Morb Mortal Wkly Rep 1993;42(RR-12):1.
329. Limberger RJ, Biega R, Evancoe A, et al: Evaluation of culture and the Gen-Probe PACE2 assay for detection of Neisseria gonorrhoeae and Chlamydia trachomatis in endocervical specimens transported to a state health laboratory. J Clin Microbiol 1992;30:1162.
330. Watson EJ, Templeton A, Russell I, et al. The accuracy and efficacy of screening tests for Chlamydia trachomatis: A systematic review. J Med Microbiol 2002;51:1021.
331. Schachter J, Stamm WE: Chlamydia. In Murray PR, Pfaller MA, Tenover FC, et al (eds): Manual of Clinical Microbiology. Washington, DC, American Society for Microbiology, 1995, p 669.
332. Genc MR: Treatment of genital Chlamydia trachomatis infection in pregnancy. Best Pract Res Clin Obstet Cynecol 2002;16(6):913.

Specific Etiologic Agents of Note

Group B Streptococcal Infections

333. Fry RM: Fatal infections caused by haemolytic streptococcus group B. Lancet 1938;1:199.
334. Ledger WJ, Norman J, Gee C, et al: Bacteremia on an obstetric-gynecology service. Am J Obstet Gynecol 1975;121:205.
335. Schuchat A, Oxtoky M, Cochi S, et al: Population based risk factors for neonatal group B streptococcal disease: Results of a cohort study in metropolitan Atlanta. J Infect Dis 1990;162:672.
336. Zangwill KM, Schuchat A, Wenger JD: Group B streptococcal disease in the United States, 1990: Report from a multistate active surveillance system. MMWR CDC Surveill Summ 1992;41:25.
337. Edwards MS, Nicholson-Weller A, Baker CJ, et al: The role of specific antibody in alternative complement pathway–mediated opsonophagocytosis of type III, group B Streptococcus. J Exp Med 1980;151:1275.
338. Madoff LC, Hori S, Michel JL, et al: Phenotypic diversity in the alpha C protein of group B streptococcus. Infect Immun 1991; 59:2638.
339. Lancefield RC, McCarty M, Everly WN: Multiple mouse-protective antibodies directed against group B streptococci: Special reference to antibodies effective against protein antigens. J Exp Med 1975; 142:165.
340. Wessels MR, Rubens CE, Benedi VJ, et al: Definition of a bacterial virulence factor: Sialylation of the group B streptococcal capsule. Proc Natl Acad Sci U S A 1989;86:8983.
341. Boyer KM, Gadzala CA, Kelly PD, et al: Selective intrapartum chemoprophylaxis of neonatal group B streptococcal early onset disease. II: Predictive value of prenatal cultures. J Infect Dis 1983; 148:802.
342. Centers for Disease Control and Prevention: Prevention of perinatal group B streptococcal disease: A public health perspective. MMWR Morb Mortal Wkly Rep 1996;45(RR-7):1.

343. Regan JA, Klebanoff MA, Nugent RP: The epidemiology of group B streptococcal infections in pregnancy: Vaginal infections and prematurity study group. Obstet Gynecol 1991;77:604.

344. Baker CJ, Goroff DK, Alpert S, et al: Vaginal colonization with group B streptococcus: A study in college women. J Infect Dis 1977;135:392.

345. Noya FJ, Baker CJ: Prevention of group B streptococcal infection. Infect Dis Clin North Am 1992;6:41.

346. Baker CJ, Edwards MS: Group B streptococcal infections. In Remington JS, Klein JO (eds): Infectious Diseases of the Fetus and Newborn Infant, 4th ed. Philadelphia, WB Saunders, 1995, p 980.

347. Mead PB, Winn WC: Vaginal-rectal colonization with group A streptococci in late pregnancy. Infect Dis Obstet Gynecol 2000;8:217.

348. Regan JA, Klebanoff MA, Nugent RP, et al: Colonization with group B streptococci in pregnancy and adverse outcome: VIP study group. Am J Obstet Gynecol 1996;174:1354.

349. Pass MA, Gray BM, Dillon HJ: Puerperal and perinatal infections with group B streptococci. Am J Obstet Gynecol 1982;143:147.

350. Jacobs MR, Koornhof HJ, Stein H: Group B streptococcal infections in infants and neonates. S Afr Med J 1978;54:154.

351. Blanco JD, Gibbs RS, Castaneda YS: Bacteremia in obstetrics: Clinical course. Obstet Gynecol 1981;58:621.

352. Baker CJ, Barrett FF, Gordon RC, et al: Suppurative meningitis due to streptococci of Lancefield group B: A study of 33 infants. J Pediatr 1973;82:724.

353. Boyer KM, Gadzala CA, Burd LI, et al: Selective intrapartum chemoprophylaxis of neonatal group B streptococcal early onset disease. I: Epidemiologic rationale. J Infect Dis 1983;148:795.

354. Pyati SP, Pildes RS, Jacobs NM, et al: Penicillin in infants weighing two kilograms or less with early onset group B streptococcal disease. N Engl J Med 1983;308:1383.

355. Pyati SP, Pildes RS, Ramamurthy RS, et al: Decreasing mortality in neonates with early onset group B streptococcal infection: Reality or artifact. J Pediatr 1981;98:625.

356. Madoff LC, Kasper DL: Group B streptococcal disease. In Charles D (ed): Obstetric and Perinatal Infections. St. Louis, Mosby–Year Book, 1993, p 210.

357. Dillon HC, Khare S, Gray BM: Group B streptococcal carriage and disease: A six year prospective study. J Pediatr 1987;110:31.

358. Edwards MS, Rench MA, Haffar AA, et al: Long term sequelae of group B streptococcal meningitis in infants. J Pediatr 1985;106:717.

359. Walker CK, Crombleholme WR, Ohm-Smith MJ, et al: Comparison of rapid tests for detection of group B streptococcal colonization. Am J Perinatol 1992;9:304.

360. Yancey MK, Armer T, Clark P, Duff P: Assessment of rapid identification tests for genital carriage of group B streptococci. Obstet Gynecol 1992;80:1038.

361. Armer T, Clark P, Duff P, et al: Rapid intrapartum detection of group B streptococcal colonization with the enzyme immunoassay. Am J Obstet Gynecol 1993;168:39.

362. Bergeron MG, Ke D, Menarc C, et al: Rapid detection of group B streptococci in pregnant women at delivery. N Engl J Med 2000;343:175.

363. Institute of Medicine, National Academy of Sciences: New Vaccine Development: Establishing Priorities, vol 1: Diseases of Importance in the United States. Washington, D.C., National Academy Press, 1985, p 242, Appendix P.

364. Mohle-Boetani JC, Schuchat A, Plikaytis BD, et al: Comparison of prevention strategies for neonatal group B streptococcal infection: A population-based economic analysis. JAMA 1993;270:1442.

365. Kasper DL, Paoletti LC, Wessels MR, et al: Immuno response to type III group B streptococcal polysaccharide–tetanus toxoid conjugate vaccine. J Clin Invest 1996;98:2308.

366. Baker CJ, Paoletti LC, Wessels MR, et al: Safety and immunogenicity of capsular polysaccharide–tetanus toxoid conjugate vaccines for group B streptococcal types Ia and Ib. J Infect Dis 1999;179:142.

367. Baker CJ, Paoletti LC, Pench MA, et al: Use of capsular polysaccharide–tetanus toxoid conjugate vaccine for type II group B streptococcus in healthy women. J Infect Dis 2000;182:1129.

368. Madoff LC, Paoletti LC, Tai JY, Kasser DL: Maternal immunization of mice with group B streptococcal type III polysaccharide–beta C protein conjugate elicits protective antibody to multiple serotypes. J Clin Invest 1994;94:286.

369. Cheng Q, Carlson B, Pillai S, et al: Antibody against surface bound C5a peptidase is opsonic and initiates macrophage killing of group B streptococci. Infect Immun 2001;69:2302.

370. Brodeur BR, Boyer M, Charlebois I, et al: Identification of group B streptococcal Sip protein, which elicits cross-protective immunity. Infect Immun 2001;69:2302.

371. Boyer KM, Gotoff SP: Prevention of early onset neonatal group B streptococcal disease with selection intrapartum chemoprophylaxis. N Engl J Med 1986;314:1665.

372. American Academy of Pediatrics, Committee on Infectious Diseases and Committee on Fetus and Newborn: Guidelines for prevention of group B streptococcal infection by chemoprophylaxis. Pediatrics 1992;90:775.

373. Yancey MK, Schuchat A, Brown LK, et al: The accuracy of late antenatal screening cultures in predicting genital group B streptococcal colonization at delivery. Obstet Gynecol 1996;88:811.

374. American College of Obstetricians and Gynecologists: Universal antepartum screening for maternal GBS not recommended. Am Coll Obstet Gynecol Newsl January 1993, Section 1-2.

375. Schrag SJ, Zell ER, Lynfield R, et al: A population-based comparison of strategies to prevent early-onset group B streptococcal disease in neonates. N Engl J Med 2002;347:233.

376. Schrag SJ, Gorwitz R, Fulty-Butts K, Schuchat A: Prevention of perinatal group B streptococcal disease. Revised guidelines from CDC. MMWR Recomm Rep 2002;51(RR-11):1.

377. Locksmith GJ, Clark P, Duff P: Maternal and neonatal infection rates with three different protocols for prevention of group B streptococcal disease. Am J Obstet Gynecol 1999;7:210.

378. Gilson GJ, Christensen F, Bekes K, et al: Prevention of group B streptococcus early-onset neonatal sepsis: Comparison of the Centers for Disease Control and Prevention screening-based protocol to a risk-based protocol in infants at greater than 37 weeks gestation. J Perinatol 2000;20:491.

379. Hafner E, Sterniste W, Rosen A, et al: Group B streptococci during pregnancy: A comparison of two screening and treatment protocols. Am J Obstet Gynecol 1998;179:677.

380. Main EK, Slagle T: Prevention of early-onset invasive neonatal group B streptococcal disease in a private hospital setting: The superiority of culture-based protocols. Am J Obstet Gynecol 2000;182:1344.

Listeriosis

381. Campbell DM: Human listeriosis in Scotland 1967-1988. J Infect 1990;20:241.

382. Craig S, Permezel M, Doyle L, et al: Perinatal infection with *Listeria monocytogenes*. Aust N Z J Obstet Gynecol 1996;36:286.

383. McLauchlin J: Human listeriosis in Britain, 1967-85, a summary of 722 cases. I: Listeriosis during pregnancy and in the newborn. Epidemiol Infect 1990;104:181.

384. Schuchat A, Swaminathan B, Broome CV: Epidemiology of human listeriosis. Clin Microbiol Rev 1991;4:169.

385. Schlech WF, Lavigne PM, Bortolussi RA, et al: Epidemic listeriosis: Evidence for transmission by food. N Engl J Med 1983;308:203.

386. Linnan MJ, Mascola L, Lou XD, et al: Epidemic listeriosis associated with Mexican-style cheese. N Engl J Med 1988;319:823.

387. World Health Organization: Report of the informal working group on food-borne listeriosis. Bull World Health Organ 1988;66:421.

388. Campbell AN, Sill PR, Wardle JK: *Listeria* meningitis acquired by cross infection in a delivery suite. Lancet 1981;2:752.

389. Nelson KE, Warren D, Tomasi AM, et al: Transmission of neonatal listeriosis in a delivery room. Am J Dis Child 1985;139:903.

390. Simmons MD, Cochcroft PM, Okurbadejo OA: Neonatal listeriosis due to cross infection in an obstetric theatre. J Infect 1986;13:235.

391. Rappaport F, Rabinowitz M, Toaff R, et al: Genital listeriosis as a cause of repeated abortion. Lancet 1960;1:1273.

392. Armstrong D: *Listeria monocytogenes*. In Mandell GL, Douglas RG, Bennett JE (eds): Principles and Practice of Infectious Diseases, 3rd ed. New York, Churchill Livingstone, 1990, p 1587.

393. Mascola L, Ewert D, Eller A: Listeriosis: A previously unreported medical complication in women with multiple gestations. Am J Obstet Gynecol 1994;170:1328.

394. Samuelsson S, Rothgardt NP, Carvajal A, et al: Human listeriosis in Denmark 1981-1987 including an outbreak November 1985–March 1987. J Infect 1990;20:251.

395. Skogberg K, Syrjänen J, Jahkola M, et al: Clinical presentation and outcome of listeriosis in patients with and without immunosuppressive therapy. Clin Infect Dis 1992;14:812.

396. Cherubin CE, Appleman MD, Heseltine PN, et al: Epidemiological spectrum and current treatment of listeriosis. Rev Infect Dis 1991; 13:1108.

397. Frederiksen B: Maternal septicemia with *Listeria monocytogenes* in second trimester without infection of the fetus. Acta Obstet Gynecol Scand 1992;71:313.

398. Mascola L, Sorvillo F, Neal J, et al: Surveillance of listeriosis in Los Angeles County, 1985-1986. Arch Intern Med 1989;149:1569.

399. Sirry HW, George RH, Whittle MJ: Meningo-encephalitis due to *Listeria monocytogenes* in pregnancy. Br J Obstet Gynaecol 1994; 101:1083.

400. Lallemand AV, Gaillard DA, Paradia PH, et al: Fetal listeriosis during the second trimester of gestation. Pediatr Pathol 1992;12:655.

401. Mylonakis E, Paliou M, Hohmann E, et al: Listeriosis during pregnancy. Medicine 2002;81:260.

402. Frederiksen B, Samuelsson S: Feto-maternal listeriosis in Denmark 1981-1988. J Infect 1992;24:277.

403. Boucher M, Youkera L: Perinatal listeriosis (early onset): Correlation of antenatal manifestations and neonatal outcome. Obstet Gynecol 1986;68:593.

404. Cruikshank DP, Warenski JC: First-trimester maternal *Listeria monocytogenes* sepsis and chorioamnionitis with normal neonatal outcome. Obstet Gynecol 1989;73:469.

405. MacGowan AP, Cartlidge PHT, MacLeod F, et al: Maternal listeriosis in pregnancy without fetal or neonatal infection. J Infect 1991; 22:53.

406. Hume OS: Maternal *Listeria monocytogenes* septicemia with sparing of the fetus. Obstet Gynecol 1976;48(Suppl):335.

407. Kalstone C: Successful antepartum treatment of listeriosis. Am J Obstet Gynecol 1991;164:57.

408. Katz VL, Weinstein L: Antepartum treatment of *Listeria monocytogenes* septicemia. South Med J 1982;75:1353.

Borrelia burgdorferi and Lyme Disease

409. MacDonald AB, Benach JL, Burgdorfer W: Stillbirth following maternal Lyme disease. N Y State J Med 1987;87:615.

410. Schlesinger PA, Duray PH, Burke BA, et al: Maternal-fetal transmission of the Lyme disease spirochete, *Borrelia burgdorferi*. Ann Intern Med 1985;103:67.

411. Markowitz LE, Steere AC, Benach JL, et al: Lyme disease during pregnancy. JAMA 1986;255:3394.

412. MacDonald AB: Gestational Lyme borreliosis: Implications for the fetus. Rheum Dis Clin North Am 1989;15:657.

413. Weber K, Bratzke HJ, Neubert U, et al: *Borrelia burgdorferi* in a newborn despite oral penicillin for Lyme borreliosis during pregnancy. Pediatr Infect Dis J 1988;7:286.

414. Williams CL, Benach JL, Curran AS, et al: Lyme disease during pregnancy: A cord blood serosurvey. Ann N Y Acad Sci 1988; 539:504.

415. Strobino BA, Williams CL, Abid S, et al: Lyme disease and pregnancy outcomes: A prospective study of two thousand prenatal patients. Am J Obstet Gynecol 1993;169:367.

416. Nadal D, Hunziker UA, Bucher HU, et al: Infants born to mothers with antibodies against *Borrelia burgdorferi* at delivery. Eur J Pediatr 1989;148:426.

417. Cooke WD, Dattwyler RJ: Complications of Lyme borreliosis. Annu Rev Med 1992;43:93.

418. Rahn DW, Malawista SE: Lyme disease: Recommendations for diagnosis and treatment. Ann Intern Med 1991;114:472.

419. Sigal LH: Current recommendations for the treatment of Lyme disease. Drugs 1992;43:683.

420. Lyme disease during pregnancy. ACOG Committee Opinion: Committee on Obstetrics: Maternal and fetal medicine. Number 99— November 1991. Int J Gynaecol Obstet 1992;39:59.

Mycobacterial Infections

421. Initial therapy for tuberculosis in the era of multidrug resistance: Recommendations of the Advisory Council for the Elimination of Tuberculosis. MMWR Recomm Rep 1993;42(RR-7):1. [Published erratum appears in MMWR Morb Mortal Wkly Rep 1993:42:536.]

422. Prevention and control of tuberculosis in U.S. communities with at-risk minority populations. Recommendations of the Advisory Council for the Elimination of Tuberculosis. MMWR Recomm Rep 1992;41(RR-5):1.

423. Smith MHD, Teele DW: Tuberculosis. In Remington JS, Klein JO (eds): Infectious Diseases of the Fetus and Newborn, 3rd ed. Philadelphia, WB Saunders, 1990, p 834.

424. Vallejo JG, Starke JR: Tuberculosis and pregnancy. Clin Chest Med 1992;13:693.

425. Tuberculosis among pregnant women: New York City, 1985-1992. MMWR Morb Mortal Wkly Rep 1993;42(31):605.

426. Banerji S, Bellomy AL, Yu ES, et al: Tuberculosis in San Diego County: A border community perspective. Public Health Rep 1996; 111:431.

427. McCray E, Weinbaum CM, Braden CR, Onorato IM: The epidemiology of tuberculosis in the United States. Clin Chest Med 1997; 18:99.

428. Nolan TE, Espinosa TL, Pastorek JG II: Tuberculosis skin testing in pregnancy: Trends in a population. J Perinatol 1997;17:199.

429. Bjerkedal T, Bahna SL, Lehmann EH: Course and outcome of pregnancy in women with pulmonary tuberculosis. Scand J Respir Dis 1975;56:245.

430. Machin GA, Honoré LH, Fanning EA, et al: Perinatally acquired neonatal tuberculosis: Report of two cases. Pediatr Pathol 1992; 12:707.

431. Hageman J, Shulman S, Schreiber M, et al: Congenital tuberculosis: Critical reappraisal of clinical findings and diagnostic procedures. Pediatrics 1980;66:980.

432. Snider DE: Pregnancy and tuberculosis. Chest 1984;86:115.

433. Cohen RC: Effect of pregnancy and parturition on pulmonary tuberculosis. BMJ 1943;2:775.

434. Hedvall E: Pregnancy and tuberculosis. Acta Med Scand 1953; 147(Suppl 286):1.

435. Crombie JB: Pregnancy and pulmonary tuberculosis. Br J Tuberc 1954;48:97.

436. Edge JR: Pulmonary tuberculosis and pregnancy. BMJ 1952;2:845.

437. Rosenbach LM, Gangemi CR: Tuberculosis and pregnancy. JAMA 1956;161:1035.

438. Schaefer G, Zervoudakis IA, Fuchs FF, et al: Pregnancy and pulmonary tuberculosis. Obstet Gynecol 1975;46:706.

439. Wilson EA, Thelin TJ, Dilts PV: Tuberculosis complicated by pregnancy. Am J Obstet Gynecol 1972;115:526.

440. Good JT, Iseman MD, Davison PT, et al: Tuberculosis in association with pregnancy. Am J Obstet Gynecol 1981;140:492.

441. Göğüş S, Ümer H, Akócören Z, et al: Neonatal tuberculosis. Pediatr Pathol 1993;13:299.

442. Banneryee SM, Anathakkrishman MS, Mehta RB, et al: Tuberculous mastitis: A continuing problem. World J Surg 1989; 11:105.

443. Jacobs RF, Abernathy RS: Management of tuberculosis in pregnancy and the newborn. Clin Perinatol 1988;15:305.

444. Starke JR: Tuberculosis: An old disease but a new threat to the mother, fetus, and neonate. Clin Perinatol 1997;24:107.

445. Montgomery WP, Young RC, Allen MP, et al: The tuberculin test in pregnancy. Am J Obstet Gynecol 1968;100:829.

446. Present PA, Comstock GW: Tuberculin sensitivity in pregnancy. Am Rev Respir Dis 1975;112:413.

447. Purified protein derivative (PPD)–tuberculin anergy and HIV infection: Guidelines for anergy testing and management of anergic persons at risk of tuberculosis. MMWR Recomm Rep 1991; 40(RR-5):27.

448. Anargyros P, Astill DS, Lim IS: Comparison of improved BACTEC and Lowenstein-Jensen media for culture of mycobacteria from clinical specimens. J Clin Microbiol 1990;28:1288.

449. Lebrun L, Espinasse F, Poveda JD, et al: Evaluation of nonradioactive DNA probes for identification of mycobacteria. J Clin Microbiol 1992;30:2476.

450. Ratner B, Rostler AE, Salgado PS: Care, feeding and fate of premature and full-term infants born of tuberculosis mothers. Am J Dis Child 1951;81:471.

451. DeMarch P: Tuberculosis and pregnancy. Chest 1975;68:800.

452. Mehta BR: Pregnancy and tuberculosis. Dis Chest 1961;39:505.

453. Atkins JN: Maternal plasma concentrations of pyridoxal phosphate during pregnancy: Adequacy of B6 supplementation during isoniazid therapy. Am Rev Respir Dis 1982;126:714.

454. American Thoracic Society: Treatment of tuberculosis and tuberculosis infection in adults and children. Am Rev Respir Dis 1986; 134:355.

455. Hamadeh MA, Glassroth J: Tuberculosis and pregnancy. Chest 1992;101:1114.

456. Maccato ML: Pneumonia and pulmonary tuberculosis in pregnancy. Obstet Gynecol Clin North Am 1989;16:417.

457. Brost BC, Newman RB: The maternal and fetal effects of tuberculosis therapy. Obstet Gynecol Clin North Am 1997;24:659.

458. Franks AL, Binkin NJ, Snider DE, et al: Isoniazid hepatitis among pregnant and postpartum Hispanic patients. Public Health Rep 1989;104:151.

Other Bacterial Infections

459. Wong S, Tam AY, Yuen K: *Campylobacter* infection in the neonate: Case report and review of the literature. Pediatr Infect Dis J 1990;9:665.

460. Dildy GA, Martens MG, Faro S, et al: Typhoid fever in pregnancy: A case report. J Reprod Med 1990;35:273.

461. Grandien M, Sterner G, Kalin M, et al: Management of pregnant women with diarrhoea at term and of healthy carriers of infectious agents in stools at delivery. Scand J Infect Dis Suppl 1990;71:9.

462. Scialli AR, Rarick TL: *Salmonella* sepsis and second-trimester pregnancy loss. Obstet Gynecol 1992;79:820.

463. Waldor M, Roberts D, Kazanjian P: In utero infection due to *Pasteurella multocida* in the first trimester of pregnancy: Case report and review. Clin Infect Dis 1992;14:497.

464. Farley MM, Stephens DS, Brachman PS, et al: Invasive *Haemophilus influenzae* disease in adults: A prospective, population-based surveillance. Ann Intern Med 1992;116:806.

465. Salata RA, Lerner PI, Shlaes DM, et al: Infections due to Lancefield group C streptococci. Medicine (Baltimore) 1989;68:225.

466. Westh H, Skibsted L, Korner B: *Streptococcus pneumoniae* infections of the female genital tract and in the newborn child. Rev Infect Dis 1990;12:416.

467. Glock JL, Morales WJ: Acute epiglottitis during pregnancy. South Med J 1993;86:836.

468. Sharif A, Reyes Z, Thomassen P: Screening for brucellosis in pregnant women. J Trop Med Hyg 1990;93:42.

Fungal Infections

Candidal Infections

469. Carroll CJ, Hurley R, Stanley VC: Criteria for diagnosis of *Candida* vulvovaginitis in pregnant women. J Obstet Gynaecol Br Commonw 1973;80:258.

470. Gillespie HL, Immon WB, Slater V: Incidence of *Candida* in the vagina during pregnancy. Obstet Gynecol 1960;16:185.

471. Goldacre MJ, Watt B, Loudon N, et al: Vaginal microbial flora in normal young women. BMJ 1979;1:1450.

472. Kalo-Klein A, Witkin SS: *Candida albicans:* Cellular immune system interactions during different stages of the menstrual cycle. Am J Obstet Gynecol 1989;161:1132.

473. Powell BL, Frey CL, Drutz DJ: Identification of a 17-estradiol binding protein in *Candida albicans* and *Candida (torolopsis) glabrata.* Exp Mycol 1984;8:304.

474. Sobel JD, Myers PD, Kaye D, et al: Adherence of *Candida albicans* to human vaginal and buccal epithelial cells. J Infect Dis 1981; 143:76.

475. Berry DL, Olson GL, Wen TS, et al: *Candida* chorioamnionitis: A report of two cases. J Matern Fetal Med 1997;6:151.

476. Nichols A, Khong TY, Crowther CA: *Candida tropicalis* chorioamnionitis. Am J Obstet Gynecol 1995;172:1045.

477. Romero R, Gonzalez R, Sepulveda W, et al: Microbial invasion of the amniotic cavity in patients with suspected cervical incompetence: Prevalence and clinical significance. Am J Obstet Gynecol 1992; 167:1086.

478. Shalev E, Battino S, Romano S, et al: Intraamniotic infection with *Candida albicans* successfully treated with transcervical amnioinfusion of amphotericin. Am J Obstet Gynecol 1994;170:1271.

479. Van Winter JT, Ney JA, Ogburn PL, et al: Preterm labor and congenital candidiasis: A case report. J Reprod Med 1994;39:987.

480. Potasman I, Leibovitz Z, Sharf M: *Candida* sepsis in pregnancy and the postpartum period. Rev Infect Dis 1991;13:146.

481. Fleury FJ: Adult vaginitis. Clin Obstet Gynecol 1981;24:407.

482. McNellis D, McLeod M, Lawson J, et al: Treatment of vulvovaginal candidiasis in pregnancy: A comparative study. Obstet Gynecol 1977;50:674.

483. Wallenburg HCS, Wladimiroff JW: Recurrence of vulvovaginal candidiasis during pregnancy: Comparison of miconazole versus nystatin treatment. Obstet Gynecol 1976;48:491.

484. Stein GE, Christensen S, Mummaw W: Comparative study of fluconazole and clotrimazole in the treatment of vulvovaginal candidiasis. DICP 1991;25:582.

485. Stein GE, Mummaw W: Placebo-controlled trial of itraconazole for treatment of acute vaginal candidiasis. Antimicrob Agents Chemother 1993;37:89.

486. Lind J: Limb malformations in a case of hydrops fetalis with ketoconazole use during pregnancy [Abstract]. Arch Gynecol 1985; 237(Suppl):398.

487. Pursley TJ, Blomquist IK, Abraham J, et al: Fluconazole-induced congenital anomalies in three infants. Clin Infect Dis 1996;22:336.

488. Inman W, Pearce G, Wilton L: Safety of fluconazole in the treatment of vaginal candidiasis. Eur J Clin Pharmacol 1994;46:115.

489. Dean JL, Wolf JE, Ranzini AC, Laughlin MA: Use of amphotericin B during pregnancy: Case report and review. Clin Infect Dis 1994; 18:364.

Coccidioidomycosis

490. Peterson CM, Schuppert K, Kelly PC, et al: Coccidioidomycosis and pregnancy. Obstet Gynecol Surv 1993;48:149.

491. Harris RE: Coccidioidomycosis complicating pregnancy. Obstet Gynecol 1966;28:401.

492. Stevens DA: *Coccidioides immitis.* In Mandell GL, Douglas RG, Bennett JE (eds): Principles and Practice of Infectious Diseases, 3rd ed. New York, Churchill Livingstone, 1990, p 2008.

493. Peterson CM, Johnson SL, Kelly JV, et al: Coccidioidal meningitis and pregnancy: A case report. Obstet Gynecol 1989;73:835.

494. Walker MPR, Brody CZ, Resnik R: Reactivation of coccidioidomycosis in pregnancy. Obstet Gynecol 1992;79:815.

495. Arsura EL, Kilgore WB, Ratnayake SN: Erythema nodosum in pregnant patients with coccidioidomycosis. Clin Infect Dis. 1998; 27:1201.

496. Deresinski SA, Steven DA: Coccidioidomycosis in compromised hosts. Medicine (Baltimore) 1974;54:377.

497. Pappagianis D: Epidemiology of coccidioidomycosis. In Stevens DA (ed): Coccidioidomycosis: A Text. New York, Plenum, 1980, p 80.

498. Caldwell JW, Arsura EL, Kilgore WB, et al: Coccidioidomycosis in pregnancy during an epidemic in California. Obstet Gynecol 2000; 95:236.

499. Spark RP: Does transplacental spread of coccidioidomycosis occur? Report of a neonatal fatality and review of the literature. Arch Pathol Lab Med 1981;105:347.

500. Smale LE, Waechter KG: Dissemination of coccidioidomycosis in pregnancy. Am J Obstet Gynecol 1970;107:356.

501. Bernstein DI, Tipton JR, Schott SF, et al: Coccidioidomycosis in a neonate, maternal infant transmission. J Pediatr 1981;110:752.

502. Van Bergen WS, Fleury FJ, Cheatle EL: Fatal maternal disseminated coccidioidomycosis in a non-endemic area. Am J Obstet Gynecol 1974;124:661.

503. Mendenhall JC, Black WC, Pottz GE: Progressive (disseminated) coccidioidomycosis during pregnancy. Rocky Mt Med J 1948; 45:472.

504. Barbee RA, Hicks MJ, Grosso D, et al: The maternal immune response in coccidioidomycosis: Is pregnancy a risk factor for serious infection? Chest 1991;100:709.

505. Drutz DJ, Huppert M: Coccidioidomycosis: Factors affecting the host-parasite infection. J Infect Dis 1983;147:372.

506. Stamm AM, Dismukes WE: Infections caused by fungi and higher bacteria. In Gleicher N (ed): Principles of Medical Therapy in Pregnancy. E. Norwalk, Conn, Appleton & Lange, 1985, p 519.

507. Lee BE, Feinberg M, Abraham JJ, et al: Congenital malformations in an infant born to a woman treated with fluconazole. Pediatr Infect Dis 1992;11:1062.

Parasitic Infections

Toxoplasmosis

508. Couvreur J, Desmonts G: Toxoplasmosis. In MacLeod C (ed): Parasitic Infections in Pregnancy and the Newborn. New York, Oxford University Press, 1988, p 112.

509. Shay-Pederson B, Lorentzen-Styr A: Uterine *Toxoplasma* infections and repeated abortion. Am J Obstet Gynecol 1977;128:716.

510. Hershey DW, McGregor JA: Low prevalence of *Toxoplasma* infection in a Rocky Mountain prenatal population. Obstet Gynecol 1987; 70:900.
511. Hunter K, Stagnos S, Capps E, et al: Prenatal screening of pregnant women for infections caused by cytomegalovirus, Epstein-Barr virus, herpes virus, rubella and *Toxoplasma gondii*. Am J Obstet Gynecol 1983;145:269.
512. Guerina NG, Hsu HW, Meissner HC, et al: Neonatal serologic screening and early treatment for congenital *Toxoplasma gondii* infection. N Engl J Med 1994;330:1858.
513. Wong SY, Remington JS: Toxoplasmosis in pregnancy. Clin Infect Dis 1994;18:853.
514. Calar G, Bergendi L, Holkova R: Isolation of *Toxoplasma gondii* from swine and cattle. J Parasitol 1969;55:952.
515. Jacobs L, Remington JS, Melton M: A survey of meat samples from swine, cattle and sheep for the presence of encysted *Toxoplasma*. J Parasitol 1960;46:11.
516. Work K: Isolation of *Toxoplasma gondii* from the flesh of sheep, swine and cattle. Acta Pathol Microbiol Scand 1967;71:296.
517. Candolfi E, de Blay F, Rey D, et al: A parasitologically proven case of *Toxoplasma* pneumonia in an immunocompetent pregnant woman. J Infect 1993;26:79.
518. Sever J, Elleberg J, Ley A, et al: Toxoplasmosis: Maternal and pediatric findings in 23,000 pregnancies. Pediatrics 1988;82:181.
519. Desmonts G, Couvreur J: Congenital toxoplasmosis: A prospective study of 378 pregnancies. N Engl J Med 1974;290:1110.
520. Desmonts G, Couvreur J: Toxoplasmosis in pregnancy and its transmission to the fetus. Bull N Y Acad Med 1974;50:146.
521. Koppe JG, Kloosterman GJ, deRoever-Bonnet H, et al: Toxoplasmosis and pregnancy, with long term follow up of children. Eur J Obstet Gynecol Reprod Biol 1974;4:101.
522. Koppe JG, Loewer-Sieger DH, deRoever-Bonnet H: Results of 20 year follow up of congenital toxoplasmosis. Lancet 1986;1:254-256.
523. Couvreur J, Thulliez P, Daffos F: Toxoplasmosis. In Charles D (ed): Obstetric and Perinatal Infections. St. Louis, Mosby–Year Book, 1993, p 158.
524. Bobic B, Sibalic D, Djurkovic-Djakovic O: High levels of IgM antibodies specific for *Toxoplasma gondii* in pregnancy 12 years after primary *Toxoplasma* infection. Gynecol Obstet Invest 1991;31:182.
525. Fung JC, Tilton RC: TORCH serologies and specific IgM antibody determination in acquired and congenital infections. Am Clin Lab Sci 1985;15:204.
526. Bessieres MH, Roques C, Berrebi A, et al: IgA antibody response during acquired and congenital toxoplasmosis. J Clin Pathol 1992;45:605.
527. Pinon JM, Toubas D, Marx C, et al: Detection of specific immunoglobulin E in patients with toxoplasmosis. J Clin Microbiol 1990;28:1739.
528. U.S. Food and Drug Administration: FDA Public Health Advisory: Limitations of *Toxoplasma* IgM Commercial Test Kits. Washington, D.C., U.S. Food and Drug Administration, July 25, 1997. Available at *http://www.fda.gov/cdrh/toxopha.html*.
529. Liesenfeld O, Montoya JG, Tathineri NJ, et al: Confirmatory serologic testing for acute toxoplasmosis and rate of induced abortions among women reported to have positive *Toxoplasma* immunoglobin M antibody titers. Am J Obstet Gynecol 2001;184:140.
530. Alger LS: Toxoplasmosis and parvovirus B19. Infect Dis Clin North Am 1997;11:55.
531. Wong S, Hadju M, Ramirez R, et al: Role of specific immunoglobulin E in diagnosis of acute *Toxoplasma* infection and toxoplasmosis. J Clin Microbiol 1993;31:2952.
532. Dannemann B, Vaughan WC, Thulliez P, et al: Differential agglutination test for diagnosis of recently acquired infection with *Toxoplasma gondii*. J Clin Microbiol 1990;28:1928.
533. Romero R: Prenatal Diagnosis of Congenital Anomalies. E. Norwalk, Conn, Appleton & Lange, 1988, pp 23, 25, 67.
534. Daffos F, Forestier F, Capella-Pavlovsky M, et al: Prenatal management of 746 pregnancies at risk for congenital toxoplasmosis. N Engl J Med 1988;318:271.
535. Grover CM, Thulliez P, Remington JS, et al: Rapid prenatal diagnosis of congenital *Toxoplasma* infection by using polymerase chain reaction and amniotic fluid. J Clin Microbiol 1990;28:2297.
536. Hohlfeld P, Daffos F, Costa JM, et al: Prenatal diagnosis of congenital toxoplasmosis with a polymerase-chain-reaction test on amniotic fluid. N Engl J Med 1994;331:695.
537. Couvreur JU, Desmonts G, Thulliez P: Prophylaxis of congenital toxoplasmosis: Effects of spiramycin on placental infection. J Antimicrob Chemother 1988;22:193.
538. Dannemann B, McCutchan JA, Israelski D, et al: Treatment of toxoplasmic encephalitis in patients with AIDS: A randomized trial comparing pyrimethamine plus clindamycin to pyrimethamine plus sulfadiazine: The California Collaborative Treatment Group. Ann Intern Med 1992;116:33.
539. Wilson CB, Remington JS: What can be done to prevent congenital toxoplasmosis? Am J Obstet Gynecol 1980;138:357.

Malaria

540. Wyler DJ: *Plasmodium* species (malaria). In Mandell GL, Douglas RG, Bennett JE (eds): Principles and Practice of Infectious Diseases, 3rd ed. New York, Churchill Livingstone, 1990, p 2056.
541. Wyler DJ: Malaria: Overview and update. Clin Infect Dis 1993; 16:449.
542. Froude JR, Weiss LM, Tanowitz HB, et al: Imported malaria in the Bronx: Review of 51 cases from 1986 to 1991. Clin Infect Dis 1992; 15:774.
543. Duffy PE: Maternal immunization and malaria in pregnancy. Vaccine 2003;21:3358.
544. Endeshaw Y: Malaria in pregnancy: Clinical features and outcome of treatment. Ethiop Med J 1991;29:103.
545. Prien-Larsen JC, Stjernquist M: Malaria in pregnancy: A master of masquerade. Acta Obstet Gynecol Scand 1993;72:496.
546. MacLeod CL: Malaria. In MacLeod C (ed): Parasitic Infections in Pregnancy and the Newborn. New York, Oxford University Press, 1988, p 8.
547. Luzzi GA, Peto TE: Risk factors of malaria infection during pregnancy in Burkina Faso: Suggestion of a genetic influence. Am J Trop Med Hyg 1993;48:358.
548. Mvondo JL, James MA, Campbell CC: Malaria and pregnancy in Cameroonian women: Effect of pregnancy on *Plasmodium falciparum* parasitemia and the response to chloroquine. Trop Med Parasitol 1992;43:1.
549. Meuris S, Piko BB, Eerens P, et al: Gestational malaria: Assessment of its consequences on fetal growth. Am J Trop Med Hyg 1993; 48:603.
550. Nyirjesy P, Kavasya T, Axelrod P, et al: Malaria during pregnancy: Neonatal morbidity and mortality and the efficacy of chloroquine chemoprophylaxis. Clin Infect Dis 1993;16:127.
551. Taha T, Gray RH, Mohamedani AA: Malaria and low birth weight in central Sudan. Am J Epidemiol 1993;138:318.
552. Warrell DM: Treatment of severe malaria. J R Soc Med 1989; 82(Suppl 17):45.
553. Brair ME, Brabin BJ, Milligan P, et al: Reduced transfer of tetanus antibodies with placental malaria. Lancet 1994;343:208.
554. Okoko BJ, Wesumperuma LH, Hart AC: Materno-foetal transfer of *H. influenzae* and pneumoccocal antibodies is influenced by prematurity and low birthweight: Implications for conjugate vaccine trials. Vaccine 2001;20:647.
555. Okoko BJ, Wesumperuma LH, Ota MO, et al: The influence of placental malaria infection and maternal hypergammaglobulinemia on placental transfer of antibodies and IgG subclasses in a rural West African population. J Infect Dis 2001;184:627.
556. Wesumperuma LH, Perera AJ, Pharoah PO, Hart CA: The influence of prematurity and low birthweight on transplacental antibody transfer in Sri Lanka. Ann Trop Med Parasital 1999;93(2):169.
557. Hulbert TV: Congenital malaria in the United States: Report of a case and review. Clin Infect Dis 1992;14:922.
558. Kaushik A, Sharma VK, Sadhna, et al: Malarial placental infection and low birth weight babies. Mater Med Pol 1992;24:109.
559. Larkin GL, Thuma PE: Congenital malaria in a hyperendemic area. Am J Trop Med Hyg 1991;45:587.
560. Subramanian D, Moise KJ, White AC: Imported malaria in pregnancy: Report of four cases and review of management. Clin Infect Dis 1992;15:408.
561. Ibhanesebhor SE, Okolo AA: Malaria parasitaemia in neonates with predisposing risk factors for neonatal sepsis: Report of six cases. Ann Trop Pediatr 1992;12:297.
562. Davies HD, Keystone J, Lester ML, et al: Congenital malaria in infants of asymptomatic women. CMAJ 1992;146:1755.
563. Harvey B, Remington JS, Sulzer AJ: IgM malaria antibodies in a case of congenital malaria in the United States. Lancet 1969;1:333.

564. Centers for Disease Control and Prevention: Malaria. In Health Information for International Travel. Atlanta, MMWR Morb Mortal Wkly Rep 1997, p 128.

565. Rukaria RM, Ojwang SB, Oyieke JB, et al: In vivo and in vitro response of *Plasmodium falciparum* to chloroquine in pregnant women in Kilifi district, Kenya. East Afr Med J 1992;69:306.

566. Panisko DM, Keystone JS: Treatment of malaria—1990. Drugs 1990;39:160.

567. Rolfe M: Multiple drug resistant *Plasmodium falciparum* malaria in a pregnant indigenous Zambian woman. Trans R Soc Trop Med Hyg 1988;82:554.

568. Saeed BO, Atabani GS, Nawwaf A, et al: Hypoglycemia in pregnant women and malaria. Trans R Soc Trop Med Hyg 1990;84:349.

569. Treatment of severe *Plasmodium falciparum* malaria with quinidine gluconate: Discontinuation of parenteral quinine from CDC drug service. MMWR Recomm Rep 1991;40(14):240.

570. White NJ, Warrell DA, Chanthavanich P, et al: Severe hypoglycemia and hyperinsulinemia in *falciparum* malaria. N Engl J Med 1983;309:61.

571. Wong RD, Murthy AR, Mathisen GE, et al: Treatment of severe *falciparum* malaria during pregnancy with quinidine and exchange transfusion. Am J Med 1992;92:561.

572. Silver H: Malarial infection during pregnancy. Infect Dis Clin North Am 1997;11:99.

573. Nathwani D, Currie PF, Douglas JG, et al: *Plasmodium falciparum* malaria in pregnancy: A review. Br J Obstet Gynaecol 1992;99:118.

574. From the Centers for Disease Control and Prevention. Recommendations for the prevention of malaria among travelers. JAMA 1990;263:2729.

575. Collignon P, Hehir J, Mitchell D: Successful treatment of falciparum malaria in pregnancy with mefloquine. Lancet 1989;1:967.

576. Nosten F, Karbwang J, White NJ, et al: Mefloquine antimalarial prophylaxis in pregnancy: Dose finding and pharmacokinetic study. Br J Clin Pharm 1990;30:79.

577. Smoak BL, Writer JV, Keep LW, et al: The effects of inadvertent exposure of mefloquine chemoprophylaxis on pregnancy outcomes and infants of US Army servicewomen. J Infect Dis 1997;176:831.

578. Garner P, Gulmezoglu AM: Drugs for preventing malaria-related illness in pregnant women and death in the newborn. Cochrane Database Syst Rev 2003;(1):CD000169.

579. Garner P, Brabin B: A review of randomized controlled trials of routine antimalaric drug prophylaxis during pregnancy in endemic malaria areas. Bull World Health Organ 1994;72:89.

580. Bia FJ: Medical considerations for the pregnant traveler. Infect Dis Clin North Am 1992;6:371.

581. Currier JS, Maguire JH: Problems in the management of *falciparum* malaria. Rev Infect Dis 1989;11:988.

Other Parasitic Infections

582. Reinhardt MC: Effects of parasitic infections in pregnant women. Ciba Found Symp 1980;77:149.

583. Abioye AA: Fatal amoebic colitis in pregnancy and puerperium: A new clinico-pathological entity. J Trop Med Hyg 1973;76:977.

584. Armon PJ: Amoebiasis in pregnancy and the puerperium. Br J Obstet Gynaecol 1978;85:264.

585. Kreutner AK, Del Bene VE, Amstey MS: Giardiasis in pregnancy. Am J Obstet Gynecol 1981;140:895.

586. MacLeod C: Parasitic Infections in Pregnancy and the Newborn. New York, Oxford University Press, 1993.

587. Dias JC: Tropical diseases and the gender approach. Bull Pan Am Health Org 1996;30:242.

588. El-Sahn F, Darwish O, Soliman N: Socio-cultural and nutritional risk factors of adolescents and young pregnant women in an endemic area of schistosomiasis. J Egypt Public Health Assoc 1992;67:311.

589. Helling-Giese G, Kjetland EF, Gundersen SG, et al: Schistosomiasis in women: Manifestations in the upper reproductive tract. Acta Trop 1996;62:225.

590. Michelson EH: Adam's rib awry? Women and schistosomiasis. Soc Sci Med 1993;37:493.

591. Montero R, Ostrosky P: Genotoxic activity of praziquantel. Mutat Res 1997;387:123.

592. Moore GR, Smith CV: Schistosomiasis associated with rupture of the appendix in pregnancy. Obstet Gynecol 1989;74:446.

593. Siegrist D, Siegrist-Obimpeh P: *Schistosoma haematobium* infection in pregnancy. Acta Trop 1992;50:317.

594. Ville Y, Leruez M, Picaud A, et al: Tubal schistosomiasis as a cause of ectopic pregnancy in endemic areas? A report of three cases. Eur J Obstet Gynecol Reprod Biol 1991;42:77.

595. Farthing MJ: *Giardia* comes of age: Progress in epidemiology, immunology and chemotherapy. J Antimicrob Chemother 1992;30:563.

596. Flanagan PA: *Giardia:* Diagnosis, clinical course and epidemiology: A review. Epidemiol Infect 1992;109:1.

597. Levine GI: Sexually transmitted parasitic diseases. Prim Care 1991;18:101.

598. Ortega YR, Adam RD: *Giardia:* Overview and update. Clin Infect Dis 1997;25:545.

599. Wolfe MS: Giardiasis. Clin Microbiol Rev 1992;5:93.

600. Bruckner DA: Amebiasis. Clin Microbiol Rev 1992;5:356.

601. Reitano M, Masci JR, Bottone EJ: Amebiasis: Clinical and laboratory perspectives. Crit Rev Clin Lab Sci 1991;28:357.

602. Wagner VP, Smale LE, Lischke JH: Amebic abscess of the liver and spleen in pregnancy and the puerperium. Obstet Gynecol 1975;45:562.

603. Tietze PE, Jones JE: Parasites during pregnancy. Prim Care 1991;18:75.

604. Asrat T, Rogers N: Acute pancreatitis caused by biliary *Ascaris* in pregnancy. J Perinatol 1995;15:330.

605. Villar J, Klebanoff M, Kestler E: The effect on fetal growth of protozoan and helminthic infection during pregnancy. Obstet Gynecol 1989;74:915.

606. Evans AC, Stephenson LS: Not by drugs alone: The fight against parasitic helminths. World Health Forum 1995;16:258.

607. Stoltzfus RJ, Dreyfuss ML, Chwaya HM, Albonico M: Hookworm control as a strategy to prevent iron deficiency. Nutr Rev 1997;55:223.

608. Walden J: Parasitic diseases: Other roundworms: Trichuris, hookworm, and *Strongyloides*. Prim Care 1991;18:53.

609. Young RL, Zund G, Mason BA, et al: Pelvic inflammatory disease complicated by massive helminthic hyperinfection. Obstet Gynecol 1989;74:484.

610. Bailey TM, Schantz PM: Trends in the incidence and transmission patterns of trichinosis in humans in the United States: Comparisons of the periods 1975-1981 and 1982-1986. Rev Infect Dis 1990;12:5.

611. Schantz PM, McAuley J: Current status of food-borne parasitic zoonoses in the United States. Southeast Asian J Trop Med Public Health 1991;22(Suppl):65.

612. Aggarwal SK: Diagnosis and management of neurocysticercosis. Hosp Pract (Off Ed) 1993;28:106.

613. Bandres JC, White AC, Samo T, et al: Extraparenchymal neurocysticercosis: Report of five cases and review of management. Clin Infect Dis 1992;15:799.

614. Couldwell WT, Apuzzo ML: Cysticercosis cerebri. Neurosurg Clin North Am 1992;3:471.

615. Crow JP, Larry M, Vento EG, Prinz RA: Echinococcal disease of the liver in pregnancy. HPB Surg 1990;2:115.

616. Jasper P, Peedicayil A, Nair S, et al: Hydatid cyst obstructing labour: A case report. J Trop Med Hyg 1989;92:393.

617. Krogstad DJ: Echinococcal disease. Curr Clin Top Infect Dis 1991;11:52.

618. Munzer D: New perspectives in the diagnosis of *Echinococcus* disease. J Clin Gastroenterol 1991;13:415.

17

VIRAL INFECTIONS

Marie Louise Landry

Viral infections occur frequently throughout life, and most are of little consequence. However, some viral infections can be more severe during pregnancy, and even infections that are mild or subclinical in the mother can have damaging effects on the fetus or newborn. Infection can occur in utero, at birth, or in the neonatal period, with very different outcomes (Table 17–1). Intrauterine or congenital viral infections usually result from maternal viremia that infects the placenta and, subsequently, the fetus.

In 1941, Sir Norman Gregg first definitively established that viruses could cause congenital defects when he reported cataracts and other abnormalities in the children of mothers who contracted rubella during pregnancy.[1] These observations were later confirmed by investigators around the world. Since Gregg's observations, many factors have contributed to changes in the incidence and epidemiology of viral infections in pregnancy, such as the introduction and wider usage of vaccines, the increase in sexually transmitted viral infections, the appearance of new viruses such as human immunodeficiency virus (HIV), the shift in acquisition of some infections from childhood to childbearing years, and the increasing use of daycare facilities by women of higher socioeconomic groups. A number of antiviral agents are also now available but have not been carefully investigated in pregnancy and must be used with caution (Table 17–2).

Although the proportion of viral infections adversely affecting the mother or child may be small, the opportunities for prevention and treatment are increasing. It is critical that clinicians recognize and seize those opportunities. Various diagnostic tests are available through local and reference laboratories. As a cautionary note, the use of highly sensitive tests leads to the recognition of more subclinical infections, and the prognostic implications of a positive result are thus altered. In all cases, infection must be distinguished from disease. Furthermore, some newer methods, such as polymerase chain reaction (PCR), are exquisitely sensitive but are generally not standardized. Thus, results can vary tremendously among laboratories.

A number of viruses, including some covered in this chapter, have been implicated over the years, on the basis of case reports, as causes of congenital defects. Sporadic association with a particular virus infection is not sufficient to distinguish causation from coincidence. Large prospective studies are needed to show consistent patterns of disease and to document a correlation with defects. Such studies are often either lacking or give conflicting results.

This chapter focuses on viral infections commonly of concern to clinicians and their patients (Table 17–3). The hepatitis viruses are discussed in Chapter 15. The reader is also referred to several excellent textbooks[2-4] and is reminded that it is essential to keep abreast of the most recent developments, especially in HIV therapy.

CYTOMEGALOVIRUS

From its first recognition, cytomegalovirus (CMV) has been appreciated as a cause of congenital infection.[5] When acquired after birth in the normal host, CMV infection

TABLE 17–1 Possible Outcomes of Viral Infection of the Fetus or Neonate

Congenital Infection	Perinatal Infection
Resorption of embryo	Acute illness resulting in
Abortion	Complete recovery
Stillbirth	Long-term sequelae
Prematurity	Death
Intrauterine growth restriction	Persistent infection, clinical
Clinical disease at birth	or subclinical, with late
Congenital malformation or defect	sequelae
Death in infancy	Subclinical infection
Asymptomatic infection	
Late-onset congenital disease or defect	
Normal infant	

TABLE 17–2   Risk Categories for Antiviral Drugs in Pregnancy

Category	Definition	Antiviral Drugs
A	Adequate and well-controlled studies of pregnant women fail to demonstrate a risk to the fetus in the first trimester, and no evidence exists of risk during later trimesters	—
B	Animal reproduction studies fail to demonstrate a risk to the fetus, but adequate and well-controlled studies of pregnant women have not been conducted	Acyclovir (ACV) Didanosine (ddI), ritonavir, saquinavir, nelfinavir, tenofovir
C	Safety in human pregnancy has not been determined; animal studies are either positive for fetal risk or have not been conducted, and the drug should not be used unless the potential benefit outweighs the potential risk to the fetus	Ganciclovir (GCV), foscarnet Zidovudine (AZT), zalcitabine (ddC), stavudine (d4T), lamivudine (3TC), delavirdine, nevirapine, indinavir, abacavir, amprenavir, lopinavir, efavirenz Amantadine, rimantadine, zanamivir, oseltamivir
D	Positive evidence of human fetal risk that is based on adverse reaction data from investigational or marketing experience, but the potential benefits from the use of the drug among pregnant women might be acceptable despite its potential risks (e.g., in a life-threatening situation)	—
X	Studies among animals or reports of adverse reactions have indicated that the risk associated with the use of the drug for pregnant women clearly outweighs any possible benefit	—

TABLE 17–3   Viral Infections in Pregnancy

Virus	Manifestations of Maternal Infection	Transmission to Fetus/Neonate	Clinical Manifestations in Fetus/Neonate	Long-Term Sequelae	Preventive Measures against Maternal or Neonatal Infection
Cytomegalovirus	Subclinical Fever, mononucleosis	Maternal viremia Contact with infected genital secretions at birth Breast milk	Cytomegalic inclusion disease (hepatosplenomegaly, jaundice, petechial rash, microcephaly, chorioretinitis, and cerebral calcifications)	Deafness Neurologic damage	Good hygiene, especially when changing diapers Seronegative or filtered blood products
Herpes simplex	Subclinical Genital herpes	Maternal viremia (rare) Contact with genital lesions or infected secretions at birth Contact with skin lesions of caregivers	Microcephaly, vesicular skin lesions Disseminated infection; localized infection of skin, eyes and mouth; encephalitis	Neurologic damage Recurrent skin lesions	Cesarean section within 4-6 hr of ruptured membranes ACV in late pregnancy to reduce reactivations Prophylactic ACV in neonates exposed to herpes simplex virus at birth
HIV-1	Subclinical Fatigue, lymphadenopathy, opportunistic infections, AIDS	Maternal viremia Contact with infected blood and body fluids at birth Breast milk	None at birth	AIDS	AZT given to mother during pregnancy and delivery and to infant for 6 wk after birth Cesarean section if maternal viral load >1,000 copies/mL Avoidance of breast-feeding
Parvovirus B19	Subclinical Fifth disease, arthralgias	Maternal viremia	Hydrops fetalis Congenital anemia	Chronic anemia and persistent infection	None recommended
Rubella	Subclinical Rash, adenopathy, arthralgias	Maternal viremia	Congenital rubella syndrome (cataracts, heart disease, deafness) Purpura	Cataracts Heart defects Deafness Neurologic sequelae Diabetes mellitus	Vaccination (before pregnancy)

TABLE 17–3   Viral Infections in Pregnancy—cont'd

Virus	Manifestations of Maternal Infection	Transmission to Fetus/Neonate	Clinical Manifestations in Fetus/Neonate	Long-Term Sequelae	Preventive Measures against Maternal or Neonatal Infection
Varicella-zoster	Chickenpox Pneumonia Respiratory insufficiency	Maternal viremia	Fetal varicella syndrome Neonatal varicella Zoster in infancy	Limb hypoplasia Cutaneous scarring ("cicatrices") Microcephaly Psychomotor retardation	Vaccination (before pregnancy) VZIG to ameliorate or prevent maternal and neonatal infection*
Entero-viruses	Subclinical Febrile illness, abdominal pain	Maternal viremia Contact with blood, body fluids, or stool at birth	Febrile illness Myocarditis Meningoencephalitis	Congenital heart disease?	Good hygiene Standard precautions in newborn nurseries
Influenza	Influenza syndrome Pneumonia, myocarditis, pericarditis, myositis, encephalopathy	Respiratory droplets or contact with respiratory secretions	Asymptomatic Upper respiratory symptoms, poor feeding, abdominal distention, fever, respiratory distress, apnea	None	Vaccination with inactivated vaccine
HTLV-I	Subclinical Tropical spastic paraparesis	Breast milk Contact with blood and body fluids at birth	None	HAM/TSP, ATL in later life	Avoidance of breast-feeding
Papilloma-virus	Subclinical Condyloma acuminatum Flat genital warts Abnormal cervical cytologic findings	Contact with infected genital tissues during birth	None	Laryngeal or respiratory papillomatosis	None recommended
Measles	Fever, rash, cough, and conjunctivitis Pneumonia	Maternal viremia	Neonatal measles	Unknown	Vaccination (before pregnancy) Immune globulin for exposed pregnant women and neonates of mothers with measles
Mumps	Subclinical Parotitis, meningitis	Maternal viremia	Nonspecific respiratory illness	Endocardial elastosis?	Vaccination (before pregnancy)

Note: Hepatitis is covered in Chapter 15.
*VZIG has not been shown to prevent congenital infection.
ACV, acyclovir; AIDS, acquired immunodeficiency syndrome; ATL, adult T cell leukemia; AZT, zidovudine; HAM/TSP, HTLV-associated myelopathy/tropical spastic paraparesis; HIV-1, human immunodeficiency virus type 1; HTLV-I, human T-cell leukemia virus type I; VZIG, varicella-zoster immune globulin.

is usually subclinical and self-limited; symptoms, when present, are generally mild and nonspecific. Clinical manifestations, such as a mononucleosis syndrome, hepatitis, pneumonia, or Guillain-Barré syndrome, occur in far fewer than 1% of infections. However, in the fetus, premature infant, and immunocompromised host, CMV is a more serious pathogen.

Transmission

Primary infection with CMV results from initial exposure to the virus, when the host lacks specific antibody. The incubation period for acquired CMV ranges from 3 weeks to 4 months. The virus is present in blood leukocytes and is shed for prolonged periods after primary infection in oropharyngeal secretions, urine, tears, feces, cervical and vaginal secretions, semen, and breast milk. Latent infection

is established, and the virus can subsequently reactivate spontaneously or in association with immunosuppression or pregnancy.

Transmission of CMV requires close or even intimate contact. The closer the contact, the higher is the rate of infection. In addition, CMV can be transmitted by blood transfusion and organ or tissue transplantation from seropositive donors. Although CMV infection can be acquired at any time, two periods of greatest risk have been recognized: (1) early in life, from exposure to maternal infection either in utero, during the birth process, or after birth, and (2) after puberty, when sexual activity begins.[6] The infection is acquired at a younger age in lower socioeconomic groups, and by young adulthood, seroprevalence varies from 35% to 80% in different populations within the United States.[7,8] Thus, many women of childbearing age, particularly in higher socioeconomic groups, are susceptible to primary infection.

Daycare centers have been recognized as fertile ground for CMV transmission.[9] Especially among toddlers, transmission is very high, presumably caused by the sharing of saliva-contaminated objects.[10] Studies have found that 80% of toddlers in daycare centers become infected with CMV, in comparison with 20% of toddlers who are cared for at home.[11] This has important implications for the children's nonimmune mothers and female caregivers if they become pregnant.[12,13]

Maternal Infection during Pregnancy

The risk of fetal infection and damage is associated almost exclusively with primary CMV infection in the mother.[14] Although fetal damage can occur throughout pregnancy, the effects on the fetus are most severe in the first two trimesters. The seroconversion rate during pregnancy is the same as that for nonpregnant women, approximately 2% per year.[15] There is no evidence for increased severity of symptoms in pregnant women, and, in fact, most primary infections are silent.

In seropositive women, CMV reactivation increases late in pregnancy and is virtually always asymptomatic in the normal host. At the time of delivery, the virus may be shed from the cervix, in urine, or in saliva, and, post partum, in breast milk.[16,17]

Reinfection in seropositive pregnant women with a different strain of CMV has been linked to symptomatic congenital infection.[17a] Reinfection is most likely to occur in poor, young, unmarried women.

Congenital Infection

Transplacental infection of the fetus occurs in 35% to 50% of primary infections and about 1% of reactivation infections.[8,14,18] The titer of the viremia, the virulence of the virus strain, and the protective effect of transplacental antibody all affect the outcome of fetal infection. In reactivation infection, viremia is less common and of lower titer, and maternal antibody is available to prevent or modify infection in the fetus. Thus, CMV reactivation is rarely associated with symptomatic disease or sequelae in congenitally infected infants; however, severe congenital infection after recurrent CMV was documented in the fetus of an immunocompromised mother.[19]

CMV is the most common congenital viral infection in humans. In the United States, 0.2% to 2.2% of all births, or 40,000 infants per year, are infected in utero with CMV.[8,14-16,18] Approximately 10% of these infected neonates are symptomatic at birth. Manifestations of congenital CMV include petechiae, thrombocytopenia, hepatomegaly, splenomegaly, hyperbilirubinemia, intracranial calcifications, chorioretinitis, deafness, and microcephaly. Severe organ dysfunction can lead to death.

The changes in liver, spleen, and bone marrow resolve over time. Neurologic damage, however, is permanent and is the major source of long-term morbidity. Many symptomatic and some asymptomatic neonates suffer long-term sequelae, including psychomotor retardation, microcephaly, chorioretinitis, and, most common, sensorineural

hearing loss. The proportion of infants with sequelae varies according to the methods used to identify congenitally infected infants. In an infant identified on the basis of clinical symptoms or elevated immunoglobulin M (IgM) levels in cord blood, there is a greater likelihood of sequelae. If more sensitive methods, such as virus isolation from urine or PCR, are used to diagnose congenital infections, the proportion of infants with sequelae decreases as a result of the enhanced detection of mild infections.

Infants infected in utero shed virus from the nasopharynx and in urine at birth and for years thereafter. They can serve as a significant source of CMV for uninfected caregivers and family members.

Perinatal or Acquired Infection

Infants who have escaped intrauterine infection may be infected at the time of birth from contact with infected cervical secretions or in the first few months after birth from breast milk.[17] In fact, breast milk transmission may be the most common mode of CMV transmission worldwide.

When infection is acquired at or after birth, the virus is not shed until the end of a 3- to 4-week incubation period. Although most infants infected in the neonatal period are asymptomatic, as many as one third have symptoms that coincide with their first positive urine culture, including interstitial pneumonia, lymphadenopathy, maculopapular rash, hepatosplenomegaly, and atypical lymphocytosis.[7,16] Transplacental antibody from seropositive mothers, which crosses the placenta late in pregnancy, undoubtedly ameliorates infection in these babies. Despite shedding virus for years, these infants develop normally.

In contrast, CMV infection of preterm infants, especially of infants of very low birth weight, can have both acute and long-term sequelae.[20] CMV infection acquired from transfusion was once a serious problem but is now rare because of the use of seronegative or leukocyte-reduced blood products.[21] However, transmission of CMV via breast milk from seropositive mothers to their infants remains a problem.[22] Although freezing milk at −20°C reduces CMV titers in the milk, viable CMV has been recovered from milk after 10 days at −20°C. Short-term pasteurization by heating at 72°C for 10 seconds inactivates virus while preserving nutritional and immunologic constituents of milk; however, the means to accomplish this are not readily available in general.[22]

Diagnosis

Because CMV infection is not clinically unique and is most often present without symptoms, laboratory diagnosis is essential.[23] In immunocompetent adults, viral shedding in urine and saliva even in primary infection can be intermittent and does not distinguish primary from recurrent infection. Primary infection in the mother is best documented by seroconversion. A sensitive method, such as enzyme-linked immunosorbent assay (ELISA) or latex agglutination, should be used and not the complement fixation test. Detection of IgM may precede seroconversion and provide supporting information but should not be relied on as the sole source of diagnosis. Interference by rheumatoid factor, heterologous rises of IgM caused by infection with other herpesviruses, and detection of IgM with reactivation infection are all potential problems.[24] Anti-CMV immunoglobulin G (IgG) avidity assays can be useful in the first trimester to assess whether maternal infection is recent. Low-avidity IgG indicates a recent infection, whereas high-avidity IgG indicates that infection occurred more than 3 months earlier, i.e., prior to pregnancy, and therefore of no risk to the fetus.[25]

Prenatal documentation of fetal infection can be attempted by testing amniotic fluid for infectious virus or DNA or by testing umbilical vein blood for IgM.[26,27] Positive results are not synonymous with fetal damage, and negative results do not guarantee absence of infection, especially because the quality of testing may vary.[8] However, when primary infection in the mother has been documented, a combination of tests performed on amniotic fluid and fetal blood after 21 weeks' gestation, together with abnormal findings on ultrasonography (e.g., hydrocephaly, periventricular brain or liver lesions, hydrops fetalis, severe oligohydramnios) can help identify the infected fetus with an unfavorable prognosis.[26,27] Quantification of CMV DNA has been proposed as a predictor of fetal outcome; however, it is also dependent on other factors such as gestational age and time elapsed since maternal infection.[28]

Congenital infection in the neonate is best diagnosed from culture of urine at birth. It is important to recognize that samples must be obtained as soon as possible after birth. If laboratory diagnosis is not attempted until the infant is 3 to 4 weeks old, it will not be possible to confirm congenital infection, because perinatally infected babies begin shedding virus at this time. Rapid shell vial centrifugation culture provides results in 1 to 2 days, whereas conventional tube cultures may require 1 to 3 weeks. DNA amplification methods, such as PCR, may be more sensitive than culture, especially if the sample is transported to a distant laboratory. An IgM antibody test at birth may detect only 20% of cases in infants found to be shedding CMV in urine[24,29] and can yield false-positive results. If the result of the urine culture is positive, there is no need to confirm the diagnosis with an IgM test. However, a positive IgM result may indicate a more serious prognosis. Maternal IgG masks seroconversion in the baby, but IgG persists in the infected infant beyond the 6 to 12 months expected for transplacentally acquired antibody.

Perinatal or postnatal infection can be diagnosed from culture of urine, saliva, or nasopharyngeal swabs, but viral shedding does not occur until 3 to 6 weeks after the infant acquires the infection.

Treatment

Serious CMV infections in immunocompromised hosts are treated with intravenous ganciclovir or foscarnet. Ganciclovir is associated with neutropenia and foscarnet with renal insufficiency and electrolyte imbalances. Cidofovir and oral valganciclovir are effective in treatment of retinitis in immunocompromised adults but have not been studied in children.[30] There is a paucity of information about therapy in the normal host, and little information is available on the effects of these drugs on the fetus. It is not known whether therapy in the mother prevents fetal infection and, if so, how long treatment should be continued. Ganciclovir has appeared to be beneficial in the treatment of congenitally infected infants with central nervous system (CNS) manifestations at birth, but data for routine recommendations in other settings are insufficient.[30,31]

Furthermore, because 90% of congenitally infected infants have no apparent sequelae, there is currently no recommendation for termination of pregnancy in primary maternal CMV.

Prevention

No data currently exist to support the use of CMV immune globulin to prevent or ameliorate infection of the fetus. In addition, most maternal infections are not recognized until after congenital infection is diagnosed in the newborn.

Serologic testing can be used to identify nonimmune individuals.[26,32] Seronegative mothers should be educated about modes of CMV transmission. In caring for young children, the importance of good hygiene and hand washing, especially after changing diapers, should be emphasized.

Transmission of CMV by blood transfusion to preterm infants and pregnant women can be prevented by the use of seronegative or filtered blood products.

Vaccination of seronegative women before pregnancy has received much attention as a strategy to prevent congenital infection,[33,34] and the Institute of Medicine listed development of a CMV vaccine as a high priority. Several CMV vaccines, including a recombinant glycoprotein B vaccine, are in clinical trials.

HERPES SIMPLEX VIRUS

Herpes simplex virus (HSV) infections are common and, once contracted, lifelong. HSV type 1 (HSV-1) is most commonly associated with herpes labialis, and HSV type 2 (HSV-2), with genital herpes. Infections of the eye, other areas of the skin, and, in rare cases, the brain and the viscera can also occur.[35] Approximately 70% to 90% of oral and 75% of genital herpes infections are asymptomatic. Furthermore, clinical lesions may not appear until years after an initial subclinical infection.

In the United States, the majority of children of lower socioeconomic status are infected with HSV-1 in childhood, whereas in more affluent groups, infection is delayed until adulthood in 50% to 70% of cases.[35,36] HSV-2 is spread by sexual contact; therefore, seroconversion begins with onset of sexual activity and increases with the number of sexual partners.[37] Since the early 1970s, the seroprevalence of HSV-2 has risen in the United States to approximately 20% of young adults.[38] Genital HSV-1 infections are also increasing.[39] This has increased concerns about genital herpes in pregnancy. Furthermore, genital ulcer disease has been linked to an increased susceptibility to infection with HIV.[40]

Transmission and Pathogenesis

Transmission of HSV is by contact with infected oral or genital secretions. The incubation period is 2 to 12 days, with an average of 4 days. The virus infects the epithelium at the site of entry and is then transported via sensory nerves to dorsal root ganglia, where a latent infection is established. Periodic reactivation results in recurrent lesions and viral shedding.

Primary infection, which occurs when the host lacks specific antibody, is more severe than reactivation, because of higher virus titers, longer duration of virus shedding, and more frequent complications. Prior infection with the heterologous HSV type can ameliorate symptoms.

Although vesicular lesions harbor the highest titers of the virus, HSV can be shed and transmitted before lesions occur and even in the absence of lesions.[41] Viremia has been reported in infected neonates and immunocompromised hosts but rarely occurs in normal hosts[42]; in the absence of viremia, the potential for transplacental transmission is limited.

Genital Herpes in Pregnancy

Two percent or more of susceptible women acquire HSV infection during pregnancy.[43] Primary genital herpes in pregnancy has been associated with a more severe course, an increase in miscarriage in first trimester infections, and premature delivery in third trimester infections in some studies but not others.[44-47] All studies, however, have found that the risk of transmission to the fetus is greatest when primary genital herpes occurs at term and ranges from 30% to 50% for infants delivered vaginally.[37,47]

Recurrent HSV is much more common than primary infection during pregnancy. A fetus exposed to recurrent herpes at the time of delivery has only a 3% to 5% chance of being infected,[48] because of lower virus titers and the protective effect of transplacental maternal antibody. Transmission is much more likely if a lesion is present; in recurrent infection, asymptomatic shedding carries an extremely low risk of transmission to the fetus.[48,49]

Nevertheless, because most mothers with obvious genital herpes lesions undergo cesarean section, infants who ultimately contract neonatal herpes are usually born to mothers without symptoms at term. A Centers for Disease Control and Prevention (CDC) study of neonatal herpes found that only 22% of mothers had a history of genital herpes and only 9% had recognized lesions at delivery.[50] Surveys in the United States have detected HSV shedding from the cervix in 0.01% to 0.39% of women at term, regardless of history.[47-49] Factors affecting the transmission of HSV to the fetus include high virus titers, lack of transplacental antibody, rupture of membranes more than 6 hours before delivery, and trauma to fetal skin.[51-54]

Congenital Infection

Congenital infection with HSV has been documented but is rare.[55] It is usually associated with transplacental transmission of primary genital herpes early in gestation and is characterized by intrauterine growth restriction, CNS involvement (microcephaly, hydranencephaly), vesicular skin lesions or skin scarring, eye findings (chorioretinitis, microphthalmia), and, in a small number of affected patients, enlargement of liver and spleen. With the exception of skin scarring, these manifestations have also been identified in infants with congenital toxoplasmosis, rubella, CMV, and syphilis.

In addition, intrauterine HSV infections can be acquired in the intrapartum period from ascending infection after prolonged rupture of the membranes. Skin lesions may be present at birth. To document intrauterine infection, samples must be collected within 48 hours of birth. The clinical manifestations are described in the following section.

Neonatal Infection

The incidence of neonatal HSV infection varies in different parts of the world for unclear reasons and is quite rare in some populations, despite a high incidence of HSV-2 infections. In the United States, neonatal HSV has increased in affluent populations, perhaps because of a lower prevalence of HSV-1 antibody when sexual activity begins and, thus, a higher risk of seroconversion in pregnancy.[38,39] Despite an HSV-2 seroprevalence of 20% in the United States, the incidence of neonatal herpes is 1 per 3000 to 1 per 10,000 deliveries per year.[55a,56]

HSV-2 accounts for about 70% of neonatal herpes and is acquired from genital infection in the mother. Sources of neonatal HSV-1 infections include maternal genital herpes and skin lesions, oral herpes, or herpetic whitlow in relatives or hospital personnel.[57-59] Because of the greater neurovirulence of HSV-2, the outcome for HSV 2–infected neonates appears to be worse than for HSV-1.[49]

The portal of entry of neonatal HSV includes the umbilical cord, eye, oral and nasal orifices, and traumatized skin. HSV in the neonate is rarely subclinical. For therapeutic and prognostic purposes, the clinical picture has been classified as follows.[60]

Disseminated Infection

Disseminated infection in the neonate has the worst prognosis. Involvement of multiple organs, especially the brain, liver, lungs, and adrenal glands, is characteristic. Vesicular skin lesions occur in 80% of affected neonates, but their appearance may be delayed. In the absence of skin lesions, HSV may not be recognized. Death is often caused by disseminated intravascular coagulation and pneumonitis; survivors suffer severe sequelae. In the past, because of delay in diagnosis and treatment, this condition was the most common manifestation. With earlier recognition, disseminated HSV infection is now diagnosed in only about 23% of cases.

Encephalitis

Encephalitis may occur alone, as part of a disseminated infection, or together with skin, eye, and mouth involvement. In disseminated infection, HSV reaches the CNS by viremia. However, isolated encephalitis is presumably contracted from retrograde axonal transport to the CNS and is often associated with reactivation, rather than primary, infection in the mother. Thus, infants with isolated encephalitis are likely to have received transplacental antibody, which results in a longer incubation period. Skin vesicles occur in 60% and their appearance may be delayed. Cerebrospinal fluid (CSF) cultures are positive in only 25% to 40%; thus, PCR is the preferred test. Survivors suffer severe sequelae.

Skin, Eyes, and Mouth

Neonates with HSV infection localized to the skin, eyes, or mouth have the most favorable prognosis. Nevertheless, approximately 10% have long-term neurologic sequelae.

Disseminated infections commonly manifest at 9 to 10 days of age; encephalitis, at 16 to 17 days of age; and localized skin, eye, or mouth infections, at 10 to 11 days of age. Consequently, neonates do not usually become ill until after they are discharged from the hospital.

Postnatal Infection

Postnatal transmission of HSV to neonates can also occur from another HSV-infected neonate in the neonatal nursery, from orolabial HSV or herpetic whitlow of family members or staff, and from skin lesions on the breast of a nursing mother.[57-59] Most postnatal infections are HSV-1.

Diagnosis

A rapid, sensitive, and specific test for HSV, available 24 hours a day and obtained at the onset of labor, is needed but is not yet available. Thus, clinical management at delivery still relies on examination of the mother's genital tract for lesions.

The laboratory method in most hospitals for routine detection of active HSV infection is virus isolation. Culture can detect HSV in skin lesions, as well as asymptomatic shedding from the cervix and vagina at the time of delivery and during the incubation period in neonatal herpes. Swabs and tissues should be placed in viral transport media, body fluids should be put in sterile containers, and both should be transported promptly to the laboratory. If any delay is necessary, samples should be kept at 4°C. Results are available in 1 to 5 days, depending on the amount of virus in the sample. Restriction endonuclease mapping of isolates has helped trace the source of neonatal HSV infections.[58]

PCR is more rapid and more sensitive than culture for detection of HSV, is the test of choice for CSF, and may become the test of choice for all sample types.[60,61] Assays are currently available primarily in reference laboratories and vary in sensitivity. Cross-contamination with false-positive results remains a concern.[62]

Direct fluorescent antibody (DFA) staining of HSV-infected cells from skin lesions can provide sensitive detection with same-day results.[63] A good quality sample must be collected by vigorously swabbing fresh lesions.

Tzanck smears are neither sensitive nor specific for HSV, and their use is not encouraged.

Serologic testing is generally not helpful. Standardized, reliable HSV IgM assays are lacking; furthermore, IgM levels rise very late in the course of illness or not at all. Most antibody tests also do not reliably distinguish between HSV-1 and HSV-2, and the presence of antibody to HSV-1 can mask seroconversion to HSV-2. Several type-specific serologic tests based on HSV glycoprotein D have been approved by the U.S. Food and Drug Administration (FDA). These include POCkit HSV-2 (Diagnology), HerpeSelect-1 ELISA IgG, HerpeSelect-2 ELISA IgG, and HerpeSelect 1 and 2 Immunoblot (Focus Technology, Inc.). The sensitivities of these tests for HSV-2 antibody vary from 80% to 98%, and the specificities are higher than 96%.[64]

Treatment

Maternal HSV infections during pregnancy are self-limited and generally resolve without ill effects on the fetus. Oral acyclovir treatment is currently recommended for a first episode of genital herpes or severe recurrent herpes, and intravenous therapy is recommended for severe or complicated maternal infections. In more than 1000 cases reported to the Acyclovir Pregnancy Registry at GlaxoWellcome, adverse effects on the fetus have not been described.[65]

High-dose intravenous acyclovir should be administered to all infants with neonatal HSV infection.[60,66] Because most infants are not recognized to be at risk for HSV, and skin lesions may be delayed or even absent, a high index of suspicion is necessary for detection. Acyclovir therapy should be administered empirically for clinically compatible illnesses if severe sequelae and viral dissemination are to be reduced.[67] Treatment of mucocutaneous HSV prevents progression to more serious infection in more than 90% of cases. Despite antiviral therapy, disseminated HSV still carries a mortality rate of more than 50%. Although the rate of mortality from encephalitis is reduced to less than 15% with treatment, 70% of survivors have serious psychomotor retardation.

Prevention of Neonatal Herpes

All women should be questioned during a prenatal visit and during labor for a history of genital herpes or genital lesions in themselves or their sexual partners. At the time of delivery, all women should be carefully examined for external genital lesions, and those with a history of genital herpes should have a cervical examination. If no lesions are present, the fetus can be delivered vaginally. If any lesion is present, cesarean section should be performed over intact membranes. If rupture of membranes has occurred, cesarean section should be performed, ideally within 6 hours, to prevent transmission of herpes to the fetus. Opinion is divided as to whether cesarean section is still of benefit if membranes were ruptured more than 6 hours before delivery. Fetal scalp monitors should be avoided, if possible, when the mother has a history of genital herpes.[45,68] Weekly cervicovaginal cultures in late pregnancy or culture at delivery, as previously recommended, have not proved useful in identifying infants at high risk of infection.[69] Several studies have suggested that acyclovir given late in pregnancy may prevent recurrences at term in women known to have genital herpes and thus reduce the need for cesarean section.[45,70] Some specialists now recommend such treatment.

If an infant has been exposed to HSV lesions during delivery and is asymptomatic, the decision to treat the infant empirically with intravenous acyclovir is controversial. When risk of HSV transmission is high, as in primary genital infection, premature delivery, or trauma to fetal skin, some authorities would initiate treatment at birth after cultures of the mouth, nasopharynx, eyes, urine, stool or rectum, and CSF are obtained. Others would obtain cultures 24 to 48 hours after delivery (to distinguish true infection from contamination at birth) and treat only if cultures are positive for HSV, if CSF is abnormal, or if symptoms develop.

When risk of transmission is low, as in infants exposed to recurrent herpes lesions or those delivered by cesarean section, most experts would not treat empirically without culture confirmation or evidence of clinical disease. In such infants, cultures should also be obtained 24 to 48 hours after birth, and the infants should then be observed carefully for signs of infection.

Breakthrough infection has occurred despite prophylactic treatment of neonates, and further study has been recommended before such a protocol is accepted as routine.[71] The role of prophylactic immune globulin therapy remains unclear. However, an antibody against HSV glycoprotein D is in development for clinical investigation.[60]

Because asymptomatic infants are discharged untreated, parents and caregivers must be thoroughly educated in the signs and symptoms of neonatal herpes and should seek medical attention promptly if symptoms appear.

Preterm rupture of the membranes in the presence of active genital lesions presents a difficult management dilemma when the fetus is immature. Although the risks and benefits of intravenous acyclovir in this situation have not been defined, many specialists would recommend its use.

To prevent postnatal HSV infection, parents, family members, and hospital staff must be educated on the risks of transmission in the neonatal period. Masks should be worn when cold sores are present to prevent inadvertent touching; skin lesions should be covered; and hand washing should be reinforced. Personnel with herpetic whitlow should not be allowed to work with neonates, because gloves are not sufficient protection.

Strategies to prevent acquisition of primary genital HSV in pregnancy include screening for HSV-2–specific antibodies in all pregnant women and their sexual partners; HSV-2–negative women with HSV-2–positive partners could then be counseled to avoid transmission by using condoms or by abstinence.[45,64] Such a screening policy is controversial because of its cost. Furthermore, such a policy does not prevent the 30% of neonatal HSV-1 infections or infections arising from contacts with multiple sexual partners. Thus, current recommendations are that pregnant women without known genital herpes avoid intercourse during the third trimester with partners with a history suggestive of genital herpes. Pregnant women

without a history of orolabial herpes, who potentially lack HSV-1 antibody, should be advised to avoid oral-genital sex during the third trimester, to avoid acquiring a primary genital HSV-1 infection.

Although considerable effort has been expended on developing and testing vaccines for genital HSV-2 infections, an effective vaccine is not yet available.[72]

HUMAN IMMUNODEFICIENCY VIRUS TYPE 1

HIV type 1 (HIV-1) infection, with rare exception, causes a slow but relentless destruction of the immune system that ultimately results in acquired immunodeficiency syndrome (AIDS).[73] HIV type 2 (HIV-2) infection has a more variable and benign course.[74] HIV-2 has remained largely confined to West Africa, whereas HIV-1 strains are causing increasing epidemics around the world.

HIV is a retrovirus that is acquired through direct contact with infected body fluids, including blood, blood products, semen, vaginal and cervical secretions, amniotic fluid, and breast milk. Transmission most commonly occurs from (1) sexual contact that involves exchange of semen, genital secretions, or blood; (2) parenteral inoculation via transfusion or injection drug use; and (3) infection of a child by an infected mother during pregnancy, birth, or breast-feeding.

HIV-1 primarily targets CD4+ T lymphocytes; however, dendritic cells and monocyte-macrophages are also infected. A DNA copy (provirus) of HIV RNA is stably integrated into the chromosomes of infected cells; infectious virus is continuously produced and can be detected free in the plasma. Within 6 weeks to 6 months, HIV-specific antibody appears in the blood, and virus titers decrease. Eventually, the progressive destruction and decline in CD4+ T cells in lymphoid tissue, accompanied by an increase in HIV in the blood, lead to the immunodeficiency and opportunistic infections that are the hallmarks of AIDS.

HIV-1 infection is an increasing problem among women of childbearing age, and HIV has become a leading cause of death for young children in many parts of the world. Without identification of HIV-infected mothers and use of preventive therapy, 20% to 30% of these children will become infected with HIV.[75]

Antiretroviral Therapy in Nonpregnant Patients

An increasing array of highly active antiretroviral therapeutic agents are available, and direct measurement of HIV RNA, or viral load, in plasma is used to monitor response to treatment. Drug toxicities and interactions, the development of drug resistance, the introduction of new drugs, and changing recommendations have all made the management of HIV-infected patients increasingly complex. Thus, it is essential that an HIV/AIDS specialist participate in the care of all patients found to be infected with HIV and that clinicians consult the latest guidelines issued by the United States Public Health Service and by expert National Institutes of Health panels.[76] The most recent information is available at *www.aidsinfo.nih.gov.*

As of 2003, 16 antiretroviral agents have been licensed: 6 protease inhibitors and 10 reverse transcriptase inhibitors (7 nucleoside and 3 nonnucleoside), and combination therapy, or highly active anti-retroviral therapy (HAART), has become the standard of care. All patients with symptomatic HIV disease should be treated. However, initiation of therapy in asymptomatic chronic HIV infection can be delayed with careful monitoring of plasma viral load and CD4+ T cell counts. Most experts agree on initiating therapy when CD4+ counts are less than 350 cells/μL or plasma HIV RNA levels are higher than 55,000 copies/mL.[75,76] Some physicians and patients may choose to initiate therapy earlier than the official guidelines. The goal of therapy is suppression of HIV to undetectable levels to prevent loss of immune function and emergence of resistant strains.

Human Immunodeficiency Virus Type 1 Infection in Pregnancy

When caring for the pregnant woman, the clinician is faced with the dual responsibility of optimizing therapy for the mother and reducing transmission of HIV from the mother to the child. Current recommendations stipulate that treatment directed at HIV and opportunistic infections not be withheld from women during pregnancy, unless there are known adverse effects that outweigh the benefits of therapy. Pregnant women should be evaluated and offered prophylaxis and treatment similar to that given to nonpregnant patients,[75,77,78] including new regimens as they become available. Women who do not meet the current guidelines for treatment of nonpregnant patients should also be offered antiretroviral therapy. Viral load in the blood generally correlates with transmission to the fetus[79,80]; thus, it is prudent to reduce it to as low a level as possible. Treatment that reduces plasma HIV-1 RNA levels to less than 1000 copies/mL significantly lowers the risk for perinatal transmission and reduces the need to consider elective cesarean delivery.[81] Nevertheless, the virus can still be present in the genital tract, despite undetectable levels in the plasma.[82,83]

Information concerning the effects of antiretroviral drugs on the fetus is minimal.[75] The current FDA-approved drugs are in pregnancy category B or C (see Table 17-2). New agents should be used if they offer a clear advantage over therapies for which there is greater evidence of safety.

Many drugs traverse the placenta, and the first 6 to 12 weeks of gestation is the period of greatest teratogenic risk. In particular, treatment with efavirenz and hydroxyurea should be avoided in the first trimester because of teratogenic effects.[75] Women who are not taking antiretroviral therapy might wish to delay initiating therapy until after the 10th to 12th weeks of gestation. In general, if the mother is already receiving therapy, treatment should continue. However, some women may want to interrupt therapy in the first trimester; in such cases, it is recommended that all drugs be stopped simultaneously and then restarted simultaneously to reduce risk of resistance.

When combination antiretroviral therapy is administered during pregnancy, zidovudine (AZT) should be included whenever possible to prevent vertical transmission (see later discussion).

In addition, clinicians should be aware that HIV-infected pregnant women are more likely to have serious vaginal candidiasis, venereal warts, cervical dysplasia, carcinoma in situ, and overt cervical carcinoma than are uninfected women. They are also more likely to shed HSV-2 asymptomatically from the vulva and the cervix.[84-86]

Vertical Transmission

HIV can be transmitted from mother to child (1) transplacentally, (2) during labor and delivery, and (3) through breast milk. The percentage of infections transmitted during each of these periods is not precisely known. Half or more may occur near or during birth, and another 10% to 20% from breast-feeding.

Increased risk of transmission has been associated with low CD4+ T lymphocyte counts, high viral titers, advanced HIV disease, detectable HIV p24 antigen in serum, placental membrane inflammation, events that increase exposure of the fetus to maternal blood, breast-feeding, low vitamin A levels, premature rupture of the membranes, and premature delivery.[87-93] The overall risk of transmission, in the absence of antiretroviral therapy, ranges from 13% to 40%; differences are attributed to the prevalence of these risk factors.

Prevention of Vertical Transmission

Antiretroviral Treatment

In 1994, Pediatric AIDS Clinical Trials Group (PACTG) Protocol 076 demonstrated that AZT administered to a selected group of HIV-infected pregnant women and their infants reduced the risk of transmission by approximately two thirds, from 25.5% in the placebo recipients to 8.3% among those receiving AZT.[94] There was an inverse relationship between CD4+ T cell concentration and risk of transmission, but subjects at all levels benefited. The mechanism for the reduction in transmission by AZT is not simply reduction in maternal viral load and is not fully understood. The regimen consisted of oral AZT beginning at 14 to 34 weeks of pregnancy and continuing throughout pregnancy, intravenous AZT during labor and delivery, and, finally, administration of AZT syrup to the newborn, beginning 8 to 12 hours after birth and continuing for 6 weeks. The only adverse effect among infants was a transient mild anemia. The initial trial used 100 mg of AZT five times per day. Comparable clinical response has been observed with AZT, 200 mg three times per day and 300 mg two times per day, and the less frequent schedule is acceptable.[76]

In Thailand, a study in collaboration with the CDC evaluated a short-term AZT regimen, which consisted of oral AZT beginning at 36 weeks of pregnancy and continuing through labor until delivery, with no infant component. This short-term regimen has been found to decrease transmission by 51%.[95] Infants were not breast-fed. However, in the United States, identification of women as early as possible during pregnancy and the use of the full three-part AZT regimen is recommended. If HIV infection is not diagnosed until delivery, or if for other reasons an infected mother was not given AZT during pregnancy or labor, the infant should nonetheless be treated with AZT, beginning as soon as possible after birth.

Transmission that occurs despite drug therapy may be a result of resistance to the drug, noncompliance, anomalies in transplacental transport, fetal infection occurring before initiation of therapy, and other unknown factors. The contributions of intrapartum, parenteral, and neonatal AZT to the reduced transmission rate have not been elucidated.[96,97] Because there are insufficient data at present to recommend substituting another drug, AZT must be included in any regimen aimed at prevention of transmission from the mother to the child. AZT may be unique in that it is metabolized into active triphosphate within the placenta, which may enhance its protective effect.[98]

Although AZT monotherapy is no longer considered the standard of care, AZT alone can be used to prevent transmission to the fetus in asymptomatic women who would not otherwise be treated. There is some concern, however, that AZT monotherapy could reduce the efficacy of subsequent antiretroviral regimens.

Pregnant women should be informed of the known benefits of treatment to their babies and that the long-term risks are thought to be minimal but are unknown. It is ultimately the woman's decision to accept all or part of a treatment protocol or to consider termination of the pregnancy.

Avoidance of Breast-Feeding

HIV, both cell free and cell associated, has been found in breast milk samples, and women infected after delivery by blood transfusion have transmitted HIV to their babies.[99] In industrialized countries, adequate alternatives to breast milk exist, and breast-feeding should be avoided by HIV-infected women. In underdeveloped parts of the world, such a directive is more problematic; breast milk provides significant protection against life-threatening gastrointestinal and respiratory tract infections. Thus, decision to avoid breast-feeding can also have serious and even fatal consequences.

Cesarean Section

Cesarean section has been proposed as an additional means to reduce transmission at birth. Cesarean sections, performed electively before both onset of labor and rupture of membranes, showed a 55% to 80% reduction in vertical transmission.[100,101] However, these studies were performed before HAART and routine viral load monitoring; thus, the benefit for women receiving HAART or with very low or undetectable viral load is not known. Current recommendations from the American College of Obstetricians and Gynecologists support cesarean section when viral load is higher than 1000 copies/mL. The benefit when membranes have been ruptured, especially for more than 4 hours, is not known.[102]

Monitoring Therapy in the Mother and the Child

All prenatal exposures to antiretroviral drugs should be reported to the Antiretroviral Pregnancy Registry, at (800) 258-4263 (www.apregistry.com). HIV-infected pregnant women should be monitored for drug toxicity according to the guidelines for each agent used.[75,76] Clinicians should be alert for lactic acidosis and hepatic steatosis that results from antiretroviral-associated mitochondrial toxicity, especially in association with the combination of stavudine and didanosine. These latter two drugs should be avoided if possible. Hepatic enzymes and electrolytes should be assessed more frequently during the last trimester of pregnancy and any new symptoms evaluated carefully. Maternal HIV-1 RNA levels should be monitored every 3 to 4 months and again shortly before delivery to allow for appropriate planning for delivery. HIV resistance testing should be considered in pregnant women with acute HIV infection, those with virologic failure despite treatment, and those likely, on the basis of epidemiologic factors, to have resistant virus.

Maternal CD4+ T-cell counts should be monitored, and *Pneumocystis carinii* prophylaxis should be initiated if CD4 cell counts fall to less than 200 cells/μL.[75,103] However, cotrimoxazole should be discontinued for a few weeks during the peripartum period, as with other sulfa drugs.

Fetal monitoring should be performed only if clinically indicated. Infants should be monitored for anemia and for HIV infection. *P. carinii* prophylaxis and antiretroviral therapy should be initiated in accordance with published recommendations and in consultation with a pediatric AIDS specialist.[104]

Diagnosis of Human Immunodeficiency Virus Infection

To prevent transmission of HIV from a mother to her child, it is essential that all HIV-infected pregnant women be identified.[105] The U.S. Public Health Service has issued recommendations for HIV counseling and voluntary testing of pregnant women.[106] Testing must be offered to all pregnant women, not just to those who report risk factors; otherwise, 50% to 70% of infected women will be missed. Testing should be performed early in pregnancy and again in the third trimester for patients with ongoing risk factors.

In the mother, HIV-1 infection is routinely diagnosed through antibody testing. The HIV-1 test algorithm recommended by the U.S. Public Health Service should be followed, whereby initial screening with an FDA-licensed ELISA is followed by confirmatory testing of repeatedly reactive ELISAs with an FDA-licensed supplemental test (e.g., Western blot or immunofluorescence assay). Rapid HIV tests can provide initial screening results within 30 minutes; however, confirmatory testing is still needed and usually requires several days or more. Indeterminate Western blot results can occur when HIV-infected persons have been infected recently, are seroconverting, or have end-stage HIV disease. False-positive ELISA results and indeterminate Western blot results can occur for uninfected persons and have been observed more frequently in pregnant or parous women.

A second serum sample should be tested from all patients with positive results to exclude sample handling or testing errors. Second samples submitted from patients with previous indeterminate results may detect seroconversion and confirm HIV infection. To resolve repeated Western blot–indeterminate samples, a sensitive test to detect virus in blood directly, such as PCR, can be used. Of note, falsely low-positive HIV RNA results have been reported. Thus, test results should be interpreted in view of risk factors, additional virologic and immunologic test results, and clinical follow-up findings. HIV RNA in plasma should be quantitated if HIV infection is confirmed. Of note, recently infected patients may be HIV antibody-negative, but have high levels of HIV RNA in plasma.

Maternal transplacental antibody, which can be detected in all infants born to HIV-infected mothers for up to 18 months, complicates the diagnosis of HIV-infected infants. PCR to detect proviral DNA in peripheral blood mononuclear cells (PBMCs) is very sensitive in infants older than 2 weeks of age, and almost all infected infants are seropositive by 1 month of age. Infants born to HIV-infected women should be tested with PCR for HIV DNA within 48 hours of birth, at 1 to 2 months of age, and at 3 to 6 months of age. A positive result must be confirmed by testing a second blood sample. Cord blood should not be used for the initial PCR screen because it may be contaminated with maternal blood. PCR is more sensitive than virus isolation and HIV p24 antigen, and these latter tests are not recommended.

Blood for HIV DNA should be collected in ethylenediaminetetraacetic acid (EDTA) (lavender) tubes or acid-citrate-dextrose (yellow) tubes and PBMCs separated by Ficoll-hypaque gradient or sent by overnight mail to the testing laboratory. Although PCR to detect proviral DNA in PBMCs is the standard protocol, there is some evidence that the plasma HIV RNA test is more sensitive in young infants.[107] For HIV RNA testing, plasma must be separated within 6 hours of collection but can then be stored at room temperature up to a day, at 2° to 8°C for up to 5 days, or frozen at −20° to −80°C for longer periods. Heparin inhibits PCR, and green-top tubes should thus not be used. Other sensitive tests such as nucleic acid sequence–based amplification (NASBA) can also be used.

PARVOVIRUS B19

In 1975, blood donor serum number B19, used as a negative control in an assay for hepatitis B virus, gave a false-positive reaction. When the serum was examined by electron microscopy, parvovirus virions were visualized.[108] Parvovirus B19 was subsequently found to be the cause of erythema infectiosum, or fifth disease, a benign exanthematous illness of childhood, as well as the cause of transient aplastic crisis in patients with chronic hemolytic anemias.[109,110] In 1984, adverse effects of parvovirus B19 on the human fetus, which include miscarriage, hydrops fetalis, and stillbirth, were first reported.[111]

Parvovirus B19 replicates only in mitotically active cells and results in a productive lytic infection of erythroid precursor cells in the bone marrow.[109] The resultant transient absence of reticulocytes is followed by a drop in hemoglobin, which is of little consequence in the normal host but is potentially life-threatening in individuals with hemolytic anemias. Failure to mount a neutralizing antibody response can result in persistent infections in immunocompromised hosts, including infants infected in utero.[112-114] Manifestations include pure red blood cell aplasia, which may remit and then recur. Other cells, such as megakaryocytes, placental cells, fetal liver cells, and myocardial cells also possess P antigen or globoside, the receptor for parvovirus B19; these cells can be infected but are not thought to produce infectious virus.

Parvovirus B19 infection is common, with greater activity in late winter, spring, and summer. Transmission is via respiratory secretions but may involve close contact, fomites, and droplets rather than aerosols. Although the risk is low, parvovirus B19 can also be transmitted in blood products, especially pooled coagulation factor concentrates.[115]

Parvovirus B19 infection has two phases. The first phase is characterized by viral replication in bone marrow, viremia, and viral shedding in the throat. The second phase, associated with rash and arthralgias, is coincident with the immune response and the presence of antigen-antibody complexes. Fifth disease, or erythema infectiosum, is recognized in the second phase by the characteristic "slapped cheek" erythematous facial rash accompanied by a lacy, reticular rash on the trunk and upper extremities that waxes and wanes over a period of days or weeks. However, infection is often subclinical or associated with nonspecific flu-like symptoms. In adults, symmetric joint pain, swelling, and stiffness, commonly involving hands, knees, and ankles, often occur in the absence of rash. Parvovirus B19 can thus be mistaken for Lyme disease, rheumatoid arthritis, or systemic lupus erythematosus.[116] Transient detection of rheumatoid factor or antinuclear antibodies further confuses the diagnosis. Simultaneous manifestation of acute parvovirus B19 infection and systemic lupus erythematosus has also been described.[117]

Maternal Parvovirus B19 Infection

About 50% of adults have antibody to parvovirus B19, and the annual seroconversion rate is estimated at 1.5%.[110,118] Pregnant women neither are more susceptible to infection nor suffer more severe disease than other patients.[119] In epidemics, 20% to 30% of susceptible adults in school and daycare settings become infected.[120] School-aged children are also a major source of infection for family members, including mothers. In addition, pregnant health care workers may be exposed to patients with transient aplastic crisis who shed high titers of virus.

In approximately 30% of maternal infections, virus is transmitted to the fetus. Intrauterine infection usually terminates uneventfully when maternal antibody crosses the placenta. However, spontaneous abortion may occur in the first half of pregnancy and hydrops fetalis in the second half. Nonhydropic intrauterine fetal death occurring late in gestation has also been linked to parvovirus B19.[121] The overall risk of fetal death from maternal B19 infection has been estimated at 1.66%[122] to 6.5%[123]; fetal demise usually occurs 3 to 6 weeks after maternal infection.

Hydrops Fetalis

Parvovirus B19 causes approximately 10% to 15% of non-immune hydrops fetalis.[124,125] The main mechanism appears to be parvovirus B19–induced severe anemia with resultant congestive heart failure. However, parvovirus B19–associated hydrops has been reported even with mild anemia,[126] and parvovirus B19–associated viral myocarditis with impaired cardiac function has been implicated.[127-129] Spontaneous resolution of hydrops fetalis has been documented.[126,127,130,131] Risk of a fatal outcome is highest in the first two trimesters.

Congenital Defects

Congenital malformations have been reported after parvovirus B19 infection,[132,133] but the rate is no higher than the baseline risk in the general population. However, persistent infection at birth has been documented, with chronic anemia, susceptibility to frequent infections, and low levels of viral replication.[111,114] At autopsy, virus has been detected in many organs, including the liver, heart, and brain.[134,135]

Laboratory Diagnosis

Accurate laboratory diagnosis is important in pregnant women because the symptoms of parvovirus B19 can be confused with rubella, measles, nonpolio enteroviruses, Lyme disease, rheumatoid arthritis, and systemic lupus erythematosus.[136,137]

Because the rash and arthralgias coincide with termination of viremia and appearance of the immune response, antibodies are usually present when the patient seeks medical attention. Thus, diagnosis of fifth disease is by detection of parvovirus B19 IgM and IgG antibodies in serum.[109] False-positive IgM results caused by cross-reacting antibodies and rheumatoid factor can be a problem. The most reliable method is the class capture ELISA.[138,139]

To diagnose fetal infection, tests to detect virus in fetal serum, ascitic fluid, or tissues should be used. Viral culture for parvovirus B19 is too specialized for routine use[140]; therefore, detection of virus is most often accomplished by DNA hybridization or PCR of tissues, cells, serum, or bone marrow.[129,134,135,141,142] Likewise, PCR should be used for immunocompromised hosts in whom antibodies do not develop. In infants with persistent congenital infection, virus does not circulate in the blood but is present in low levels in the bone marrow and can be detected by PCR.[114]

Histopathologic examination may reveal typical viral cytopathic effects and intranuclear inclusions in erythroblasts in fetal liver.[134] In bone marrow, viral cytopathic effect is manifested by giant pronormoblasts[113] or, if these cells have already been lysed, by absence of red blood cell precursors.

Treatment

No specific therapy is available, and in the normal host, the infection is usually mild and self-limited. In the immunocompromised host with chronic infection, administration of immune globulin containing neutralizing antibody has been associated with improvement, but repeated therapy may be needed.[113,143]

The patient with transient aplastic crisis requires red blood cell support until the immune response terminates the infection and red blood cells are again produced.

The optimal management of the infected fetus is controversial.[123,144] If seroconversion in the mother is detected during pregnancy, termination of pregnancy is not indicated, because the incidence of congenital malformations is not increased; rather, the fetus should be monitored by ultrasonography weekly for 12 weeks. If mild hydrops is detected, a conservative approach is recommended. For worsening hydrops or fetal distress, diagnostic cordocentesis and intrauterine red blood cell transfusion should be considered.[123,145] Great care must be taken to optimize the volume of blood transfused and to counter possible bleeding from thrombocytopenia. Because the fetus can recover without treatment and intrauterine blood transfusion can cause fetal death, further study is needed to better define the risks and benefits for this treatment. The use of Doppler sonography of the middle cerebral artery peak systolic velocity for early noninvasive detection of anemia may be a helpful adjunct to management.[146]

A single case of fetal recovery after treatment of the mother with high-dose intravenous immune globulin has been reported.[147] Treatment of chronic persistent congenital infections with intravenous immune globulin has not produced encouraging results.[114]

Prevention

Prevention of parvovirus B19 infection is difficult. It is an annual problem, especially in schools, daycare centers, and households with school-aged children. Many infections are subclinical, and when the rash appears, the individual is no longer infectious. Transmission may be lessened by routine hygienic practices such as hand washing. Pregnant health care workers should avoid caring for patients with transient aplastic crisis or immunocompromised hosts with parvovirus B19 infection, since these patients may be highly contagious. A vaccine with recombinant capsid proteins is under development but is not yet available.[148]

RUBELLA

For more than 100 years after it was first recognized as a distinct entity, rubella was considered a mild childhood illness characterized by a morbilliform rash and lymphadenopathy. In 1941, however, an Australian ophthalmologist noted a surprising number of children with cataracts, often accompanied by serious congenital defects, after a large rubella epidemic.[1] After some initial skepticism, it was confirmed that rubella infection during pregnancy can have devastating consequences for the fetus.[149]

Postnatal rubella is spread by direct contact or respiratory droplets.[150] Virus then replicates in the respiratory tract and lymph nodes. After 7 to 9 days, viremia ensues, accompanied by lymphadenopathy and virus shedding in nasopharynx, stool, and urine. A maculopapular rash appears about 16 to 21 days after infection, accompanied by suboccipital, postauricular, and cervical adenopathy, and coincides with the appearance of serum antibodies. The virus is shed in the nasopharynx for an additional week. Acute arthralgia or arthritis is a common feature of rubella in adolescent girls and in women. Joint symptoms most frequently involve the fingers and knees and usually resolve within weeks but may last for years. Approximately half of all infections are asymptomatic.

Before introduction of the vaccine, rubella epidemics occurred every 6 to 9 years with a peak in the spring months in temperate zones. The last major epidemic in the United States in 1964 left 20,000 infants with permanent damage. Since the introduction of rubella vaccine in 1969, the incidence of rubella in the United States has been reduced by more than 99%. In the 1990s, a median of 232 rubella cases were reported annually.[151,152]

Because most countries of the world do not require rubella vaccination, congenital rubella syndrome (CRS) remains an international problem, and 100,000 to 200,000 cases of CRS occur annually in the world. In the United States, there remain pockets of unvaccinated and susceptible women, many of them poor or immigrants, particularly of Hispanic origin. From 1997 through 1999, a total of 24 infants with CRS were born in the United States, most of them to Hispanic and/or foreign-born mothers.[151-153] Indigenous rubella and CRS had been targeted for elimination in the United States by the year 2000, and significant progress was made. However, prevention of imported cases requires other countries to implement national rubella vaccination policies as well.[151-154]

Maternal Rubella

There is no evidence that rubella is more severe in pregnant women than in other patients, and at least half of infections are subclinical. Maternal viremia leads to infection of the placenta; once the placenta is infected, the virus can disseminate to the fetus. Primary rubella in the first trimester of pregnancy results in abortions, miscarriages, stillbirths, and fetal malformations. Reinfections occur in rare cases and usually result in a boost in antibody but no risk to the fetus. Nevertheless, several cases of CRS after reinfection have been reported.[155,156]

Congenital Rubella Syndrome

Fetal infection can occur throughout pregnancy, but the risk is highest in the first trimester and rises again near term.[157-159] CRS is largely confined to infants infected in the first trimester and is rare among those infected after 16 weeks' gestation. Maternal infection during the first 10 weeks of pregnancy almost always results in fetal infection, and CRS occurs in about 90% of those infected. With infection occurring between 11 and 12 weeks of gestation,

the risk of CRS drops to 50%, and with infection occurring between 13 and 16 weeks of gestation, it drops to 33%. With infections occurring after the 12th week, deafness is usually the sole manifestation of CRS,[160] and with infections occurring after 17 to 18 weeks, defects attributable to rubella are rare.

Although fetal loss can occur very early in gestation, most fetuses are carried to term. Anomalies associated with CRS include hearing loss, congenital heart defects, cataracts or glaucoma, chorioretinitis, and neurologic disorders. In addition, intrauterine growth restriction, hepatosplenomegaly, and thrombocytopenic purpura are common. Radiolucent bone disease is less frequent. Infection may be disseminated, may involve a single organ, or may be subclinical. Some manifestations, particularly hearing loss, may not be evident for several years.[159-161] Infants with multiple abnormalities at birth have a poor prognosis, and in such infants, the rate of mortality during the first year of life is high.

Infants with CRS shed high titers of virus in nasopharyngeal secretions and urine at birth and should be considered contagious for at least a year, unless the results of cultures are repeatedly negative.[162]

Differences in the clinical manifestations of CRS have been reported and may be attributed to strain differences. For example, in Japan, CRS is less frequent, for unclear reasons, and in Iceland, the epidemic of 1963 to 1964 resulted in congenital infections characterized by severe hearing loss but no cataracts or heart disease.[163]

Diagnosis

It is critical to establish an accurate laboratory diagnosis. The symptoms of rubella (rash, low-grade fever, lymphadenopathy) can be confused with drug-related eruptions or a number of other infections, including measles, scarlet fever, roseola, fifth disease, enterovirus, adenovirus, and dengue.

Nasopharyngeal and throat swabs or washes collected at onset of rash can be used for viral culture, but the virus is labile, and conventional culture methods are slow. Reverse transcriptase PCR (RT-PCR) is useful, but assays vary in sensitivity.[164,165] Detection of rubella IgM is useful in detecting postnatal and congenital infections, but false-positive and false-negative results occur.[136,137,166-168] Only about 50% of patients are seropositive for rubella IgM on the day of rash onset. However, by 7 days after rash onset, most patients will be IgM seropositive. Because of the impact of the diagnosis in the first trimester of pregnancy, testing of multiple specimen types for rubella and for other viruses that cause similar clinical disease should be performed.

The most reliable method for diagnosing postnatal rubella is to document seroconversion. Acute-stage and convalescent-stage serum samples, the latter collected 3 weeks after the former sample, should be submitted. The widely used hemagglutination inhibition rubella antibody test has been replaced by more convenient and equally sensitive assays, such as ELISA, latex agglutination, and immunofluorescence assay.[164] When a pregnant woman of unknown immune status is exposed to rubella, a serum sample should be obtained and tested for rubella IgG as soon as possible. If antibody is detected, the patient is considered immune. If antibody is not detected, an aliquot should be frozen and retested in parallel with a second sample obtained 3 to 4 weeks after exposure. If the second sample is also negative, a third sample should be obtained 6 weeks after exposure and tested in parallel with the first sample. The presence of antibody in the second or third samples, but not in the first, indicates seroconversion and thus recent infection.

Diagnosis of CRS requires virus isolation from the nasopharynx, urine, CSF, or tissues; demonstration of rubella-virus IgM in cord blood or neonatal serum; or persistence of rubella virus IgG in the infant's serum at 1 year or after maternal antibody has waned. In CRS, virus is shed in high titers for months, thus facilitating virus isolation. However, as rubella infections become uncommon in the United States, routine diagnostic laboratories may not maintain the cell cultures and expertise necessary for rubella virus isolation. Before isolation is attempted, the laboratory should be notified and, if necessary, arrangements should be made for specimen transport to a specialized laboratory. All cases of suspected CRS should be thoroughly investigated and reported through local or state health departments to the CDC.

PCR has also been used to detect rubella virus prenatally, but it does not always correctly predict fetal rubella viral infection.[164,165]

Treatment

Treatment of acquired rubella is supportive. There are no reports of successful antiviral therapy in congenitally infected infants.

Prevention

The routine use of immune globulin to prevent infection or CRS in pregnant contacts of patients with rubella is not recommended. Although clinical manifestations may be reduced in the mother, CRS may still occur in the fetus. Administration of immune globulin should be considered only if termination of pregnancy is not an option.[169,170]

A live attenuated rubella vaccine is available, and two doses are now recommended in accordance with the two-dose measles immunization schedule. Thus, emphasis should be placed on immunization of all individuals who lack a vaccination history or serologic evidence of immunity; a clinical history alone is unreliable. More than half of CRS cases in outbreaks since the 1990s could have been prevented if mothers had received postpartum immunization after previous pregnancies as recommended.[157,171] Vaccination results in transient arthritis and arthralgias in 10% to 25% of vaccinated postpubertal females, but the incidence is lower after vaccination than after natural infection.[172]

Pregnant women should not receive rubella vaccine, and postpubertal females should be warned to avoid pregnancy for 28 days after receiving rubella vaccine.[173] Despite a theoretical risk of 1.6% for CRS after first-trimester vaccination,[4] no infants delivered to mothers inadvertently vaccinated in the first trimester have had signs of CRS. This suggests that vaccine strains are not teratogenic, despite their ability to infect the placenta and fetus. Susceptible women should be given rubella vaccine in the immediate postpartum period before hospital discharge.[171]

Subunit vaccines designed to protect against viremia without the side effects of live attenuated virus vaccines are being developed.

VARICELLA-ZOSTER VIRUS

Varicella-zoster virus (VZV) derives its name from the two diseases it causes: varicella (chickenpox) and zoster (shingles). Varicella is acquired by the nonimmune host via the respiratory route from aerosol, droplet, or direct contact with vesicular skin lesions. Subsequent viremia carries the virus to the skin and internal organs. The incubation period is 10 to 21 days and is followed by the appearance of vesicular rash, fever, and malaise. After primary infection, a latent infection is established in dorsal root ganglia, from which virus can reactivate, usually causing zoster, a rash in a dermatomal distribution. In temperate zones, more than 95% of individuals are infected in childhood, and most adults without a history of varicella are immune when tested. In contrast, only 50% of adults in the tropics are immune.[174] Thus, Hispanic Americans and persons who are natives of tropical countries should be considered susceptible unless vaccination or serologic immunity have been documented.

When acquired in childhood, varicella is usually a benign illness. When infection is delayed until adulthood, the mortality rate is higher, usually as a result of pneumonia and disseminated intravascular coagulation. Although fewer than 5% of varicella cases occur in adults older than 20 years, more than 55% of varicella-related deaths occur in this age group.[175-177] Susceptible persons with HIV infection or malignancies, those receiving steroid therapy, and pregnant women are at increased risk for severe varicella and complications.

Maternal Varicella

Only 0.05% to 0.07% of pregnancies in the United States, or 7000 to 10,000 cases annually, are complicated by varicella.[178,179] With the upward shift in the age distribution of varicella cases observed in the United States and United Kingdom, this statistic could increase.[180] Pulmonary involvement occurs in about 10% of pregnant women with varicella, which is not more frequent than in nonpregnant adults.[181,182] Risk factors for varicella-related pneumonia include smoking and presence of more than 100 skin lesions.[182] The onset is often insidious, with cough, dyspnea, and chest pain developing 1 to 7 days after the appearance of the rash; chest radiograph results may be normal initially. Although most cases of pneumonitis resolve within 1 week, death may occur as a result of pulmonary insufficiency, bacterial superinfection, or progressive pulmonary fibrosis. Onset during the third trimester is a risk factor for a fatal outcome. Maternal hypoxemia is potentially damaging to the fetus, and severe maternal infections can result in fetal demise.[179] Thus, prompt recognition and treatment are essential.

Even in the absence of complications in the mother, viremia associated with primary VZV infection can result in infection of the fetus. Intrauterine VZV infection may result in congenital varicella syndrome, varicella in the neonatal period, or zoster during infancy or early childhood.[179,182] The consequences to the fetus are of greatest concern early in pregnancy and near the time of delivery.

Congenital Varicella Syndrome

Infection with VZV during the first 20 weeks of gestation can produce an embryopathy characterized by limb hypoplasia, cutaneous scarring, and eye and brain damage.[183-185] Data combined from several prospective studies in the United States indicate that the risk of congenital varicella syndrome is 0.7% to 1.2% during the first trimester of pregnancy.[186-188] In one prospective study, the risk of fetal damage was greater during the 13th to 20th weeks of gestation (2%) than when infection occurred in the first 12 weeks of gestation (0.4%).[186]

Fetal infection that occurs between 20 weeks of gestation and 5 days before delivery is usually associated with a benign outcome; however, affected infants have a risk of developing zoster during infancy or early childhood.[179] One case of zoster present at birth has been reported.[189] In a few cases, infants infected in utero may have VZV IgM antibody in the neonatal period.[186] A more reliable marker is VZV IgG immunity that persists after 1 year of age, when maternal transplacental antibody has waned.

There is no credible evidence that maternal zoster causes congenital defects.[179,186]

Neonatal Varicella

When the onset of maternal varicella rash occurs 4 days before to 2 days after delivery, severe varicella infection can occur in the neonate.[190] In these cases, the fetus is infected through maternal viremia but is delivered before sufficient transplacental antibody is available to lessen the severity of the disease.[191] A mortality rate of 31% among infants whose mothers experienced onset of rash up to 4 days before birth has been estimated on the basis of a limited retrospective analysis of the literature; however, this rate is probably falsely high because of selective reporting.[179,192]

Diagnosis

The most rapid and sensitive routine test for detection of VZV in vesicular skin lesions is DFA staining of cell scrapings with VZV-specific monoclonal antibody. DFA provides results within hours and is more sensitive than culture.[193] Tzanck stains lack both sensitivity and specificity and have little, if any, use in current diagnosis.

Virus can be isolated from lesion swabs, vesicular fluid, bronchoalveolar lavage, CSF, and tissue samples. In contrast, throat swabs rarely yield positive results for varicella and should not be submitted. Shell vial centrifugation cultures for VZV provide results in 2 to 5 days and yield more positive findings than do conventional cell cultures, which require 3 to 14 days for a positive result.[193] PCR is more sensitive than DFA or culture but is largely confined to reference laboratories. Improved methods and instrumentation should lead to wider availability in the future.

Susceptibility and seroconversion to VZV can be determined by ELISA or latex agglutination tests.[194] Complement fixation tests are not sufficiently sensitive for determining immune status.

The diagnosis of congenital varicella is usually made by identifying classic anomalies in the fetus, within the context of a history of maternal varicella during pregnancy. IgM antibody tests may have a role in supporting the diagnosis of congenital varicella when active skin lesions are not present at birth. The diagnosis must be confirmed by documenting the persistence of VZV-specific IgG in the infant after 1 year of age, when maternal antibody has waned. Due to both sensitivity and specificity problems, IgM assays should never be the sole basis for laboratory diagnosis.[186,195] PCR has been used on chorionic villus tissue and amniotic fluid for prenatal diagnosis of congenital infection, but results may not correlate with fetal disease.[183,195-197]

Treatment

The safety of systemic acyclovir among pregnant women has not been established by controlled trials. However, analysis of more than 1000 cases of acyclovir administration to pregnant women, reported to the Acyclovir in Pregnancy Registry at GlaxoWellcome, has revealed a frequency of birth defects no different from baseline risk in the general population.

Oral acyclovir has not been recommended for routine treatment of uncomplicated varicella in pregnant women, because the risks and benefits to the mother and fetus are unknown. Nevertheless, some experts would consider its use, especially in the third trimester. Intravenous acyclovir is recommended in pregnancy for serious complications, such as pneumonia.[198,199]

Intravenous acyclovir should also be considered for treatment of neonatal varicella.

Prevention

Varicella-zoster immune globulin (VZIG) is prepared from plasma of blood donors with high antibody titers to VZV and is useful in preventing or modifying illness caused by VZV infection if given intramuscularly as early as possible but within 72 to 96 hours of exposure.[176] A new intravenous VZIG has been reported to confer higher levels of VZV antibodies and is comparable in safety.[200]

VZIG is administered when the patient is susceptible to VZV, has had an exposure likely to result in infection,[176] and is at greater risk for complications than is the general population. Continuous exposure to household members with varicella constitutes the greatest risk (approximately 90% chance of contracting varicella). Susceptible pregnant women should be strongly considered for VZIG to prevent complications of maternal varicella, such as pneumonia.[201] VZIG has not been proved to prevent viremia or infection of the fetus. Neonates should also receive VZIG if the mother received VZIG prophylaxis in the 5 days before delivery, because it is unlikely that sufficient antibody will cross the placenta in this period. Neonates who are born to mothers with varicella rash onset from 5 days before to 2 days after delivery should receive VZIG; many such neonates nonetheless contract varicella, but infection is milder. Some authors have argued that this time period should be extended from 5 days to 7 days before delivery.[192]

A live attenuated varicella virus vaccine is available for use in susceptible children and adults.[176,177,202] Individuals over 12 are given two doses 4 to 8 weeks apart. The susceptibility of all adolescents and adults without a history of varicella should be determined and vaccination encouraged. The effects of varicella virus vaccine on the fetus are unknown; therefore, pregnant women should not receive the vaccine, and nonpregnant women should avoid becoming pregnant for 1 month after each injection. A pregnant mother is not a contraindication for vaccination of a child; however, some experts would defer immunization of the child until the third trimester or after delivery. Transmission of vaccine virus from a healthy child to his pregnant mother has been reported.[203]

Reports of mistaken administration of vaccine instead of VZIG to pregnant women with household exposure to varicella underscore the need for health care providers to understand the indications for each of these products and to read labels carefully before administration.[204] Inadvertent vaccination during pregnancy should be reported to the VARIVAX Pregnancy Registry (800-986-8999).[205]

ENTEROVIRUSES

The enteroviruses constitute a genus of the *Picornaviridae* family that includes polioviruses, group A Coxsackie viruses, group B Coxsackie viruses, echoviruses, and numbered enterovirus serotypes. Enteroviruses are named after their propensity to replicate in the enteric tract.

Poliovirus vaccination has led to the elimination of indigenous poliovirus circulation in the Americas and to the hope of eradicating polio worldwide.[206] In contrast, nonpolio enterovirus infections are very common worldwide; they occur throughout life and circulate predominantly in the summer and fall in temperate zones. The majority of all enterovirus infections, polio and nonpolio, are subclinical. Nevertheless, various clinical syndromes have been associated with nonpolio enteroviruses, including summer colds, pneumonia, meningitis, encephalitis, paralysis, myocarditis, pericarditis, pleurodynia, hepatitis, hand-foot-and-mouth disease, herpangina, and a variety of rashes.[207]

Transmission and Pathogenesis

Enteroviruses are transmitted postnatally predominantly by the fecal-oral route, but respiratory transmission is also possible. The incubation period is usually 3 to 6 days. A viremia seeds target organs, and virus is shed from throat, urine, stool, and cervix.

Transmission to the fetus or newborn may occur transplacentally, but the majority of infections are probably acquired either during the birth process or after birth.[208] Ascending infection may also occur presumably from an infected cervix.[209] Enteroviruses have been recovered from amniotic fluid in association with chorioamnionitis and fetal demise.[210]

Nonpolio Enterovirus Infections in Pregnancy

Nonpolio enterovirus infections have been detected frequently in pregnant women in a number of studies.[211,212] Although severe illness has been reported,[213] virus shedding is usually associated with minimal or no symptoms.

Congenital Infection

A number of case reports have implicated nonpolio enteroviruses as causes of spontaneous abortion, stillbirth, and fetal loss in the second and third trimesters.[214-216] However, population-based studies of past enterovirus epidemics have not shown an association with an increase in risk for these complications.[217,218] In retrospective analyses of pregnancies with adverse outcomes or neurodevelopmental delay in newborns, enteroviruses were detected by PCR in amniotic fluids in some cases.[219,220] In utero and postnatal enterovirus infections have also been linked to juvenile-onset diabetes.[221]

Whether nonpolio enteroviruses can cause congenital defects is unresolved. One group of investigators reported that a rise in maternal antibody titers to certain enteroviruses was associated with specific abnormalities, such as fetal cardiovascular abnormalities with Coxsackie B3 and B4 serotypes and gastrointestinal anomalies with Coxsackie A9 serotype.[211] Surprisingly, the antibody rises did not follow a typical enterovirus seasonal pattern (i.e., summer and fall). In a number of large studies,[217,218,222] the rate of congenital anomalies was the same in pregnancies complicated by enterovirus infection as in those without infection. Furthermore, epidemics of enterovirus infections have not been followed by an increase in congenital defects.[208,223]

Perinatal Infection

Transplacental transmission late in gestation can occur, and neonatal enterovirus infections have been documented after cesarean section.[209,224,225] Infections contracted in utero during maximal maternal viremia, with delivery before maternal antibody development, tend to be the most severe.[208,226] Onset of neonatal illness is within 3 days of birth. Postnatal transmission of the same virus type results in milder illness.[208] Fortunately, in the majority of infected newborns, the infection is acquired either during the birth process or postnatally from exposure to infected maternal blood, feces, or oropharyngeal secretions. Neutralizing antibody acquired from the mother may prevent or ameliorate clinical disease but does not always prevent infection.

Although most infected newborns are asymptomatic, undifferentiated fevers, sepsis, meningoencephalitis, hepatitis, myocarditis, and even skin lesions can occur.[227] Most patients recover uneventfully, but some infants have severe disease, and the clinical course may be biphasic. Death is most often a result of severe hepatitis in echovirus infections or myocarditis in Coxsackie B virus infections. Mortality rates of 10% have been reported.[208]

One half to two thirds of infected mothers report viral symptoms in the week before delivery; and some mothers complain of abdominal pain mimicking a so-called acute abdomen.[208,226]

Postnatal Infection

In addition to the mother, infected family members and hospital personnel have also been implicated in neonatal enterovirus infection.[226] Nosocomial infection in hospital nurseries has been well documented and has resulted in respiratory, hepatic, gastrointestinal, cardiac, or neurologic disease. Neonates infected vertically have served as source patients, with virus transmitted to other infants by hospital staff.[225] Low birth weight and prematurity are risk factors for disease.

Diagnosis

Enteroviruses are routinely diagnosed by virus isolation in cell culture. A selection of susceptible cell types is needed for optimal results, and detection of many Coxsackie group A serotypes requires inoculation of newborn mice. RNA amplification methods, such as RT-PCR and NASBA, have become the tests of choice for detection of enterovirus RNA in CSF[228,229] and can be performed on other samples as well but are often available only in reference laboratories.

Enteroviruses can be recovered from throat, nasopharynx, stool, and urine. Because enteroviruses replicate in high titer in the enteric tract, the stool provides the highest yield of isolates. Virus can be isolated from the blood of newborns who present during the viremic phase with fever and lethargy. Virus can be cultured from CSF in approximately half of CNS infections; use of RT-PCR or NASBA increases the detection rate.[229] Isolation of virus from stool alone may not be indicative of acute infection in older children and adults, because virus may be shed for weeks or even months after infection. In neonates, however, this is not an issue.

Antibody titers to selected enterovirus types can be determined by a neutralization test. However, this is very labor intensive and is not generally available. The complement fixation test is more widely available, but cross reactions and the presence of antibodies from prior infections make test results difficult to interpret.

Treatment and Prevention

Specific antiviral therapy is not currently available for enterovirus infections. Intravenous immune globulin therapy may have some benefit if high titers of type-specific neutralizing antibody are present in the preparation. Immune globulin has been administered to exposed infants in nursery outbreaks[230] and has been used to treat severe infections.[231] Passive immunization of newborns of mothers diagnosed with enterovirus infection within a few days before birth has also been suggested, but its value remains untested.[224]

Careful attention to hand washing, especially when changing diapers, should be emphasized. When an enterovirus epidemic has occurred in the hospital, closing newborn units, restricting visitors, and enforcing contact precautions are indicated.

INFLUENZA VIRUS

Influenza virus types A and B cause annual epidemics of varying severity during the winter months in temperate zones.[232,233] Influenza viruses continually undergo minor antigenic changes of their surface proteins, hemagglutinin and neuraminidase, and thus evade the host's immunity. Influenza type A, but not influenza type B, can undergo major antigenic changes with emergence of a new subtype as a result of reassortment with animal influenza A viruses. The appearance of a new subtype of influenza A can result in a worldwide pandemic that is associated with substantial mortality. During the 20th century, new subtypes of influenza A appeared and led to pandemics in 1918 (H1N1), 1957 (H2N2), and 1968 (H3N2).

Transmission occurs via airborne droplets, and the incubation period is 1 to 5 days. The typical influenza syndrome consists of sudden onset of fever, myalgia, headache, photophobia, cough, and prostration. Influenza causes a tracheobronchitis, and complications include primary viral pneumonia, combined viral-bacterial pneumonia, secondary bacterial pneumonia, myocarditis, pericarditis, myositis, toxic shock syndrome, encephalopathy, and postinfluenzal encephalitis.[233] Reye's syndrome, characterized by encephalopathy and fatty infiltration of the liver, is a disease of children and adolescents that follows infection with respiratory viruses, including influenza, as well as VZV and gastrointestinal infections. Use of salicylates is a risk factor for development of Reye's syndrome and is contraindicated in patients with influenza infection.

During a nonpandemic year, influenza-associated mortality is primarily confined to the very young, the elderly, and persons with chronic cardiopulmonary or metabolic disorders. Although the influenza mortality rate is low, the number of deaths is significant because so many persons are infected. In the 1990s in the United States, approximately 36,000 deaths per year have been attributed to influenza.[232]

Maternal Infection

Excess deaths among pregnant women were documented during the pandemics of 1918 and 1957.[234,235] In interpandemic years, pregnancy has also been associated with an increased risk of serious medical complications.[236-238] Reasons for this increased risk for predominantly cardiorespiratory complications include pregnancy-associated increases in heart rate, stroke volume, and oxygen consumption; decreased lung volume; and changes in immunologic function. Hospitalization occurs predominantly in the third trimester and has been estimated to be needed for 250 per 100,000 pregnant women.[239]

Congenital Infection

Influenza virus infection is generally confined to the respiratory tract, and viremia, if it occurs, is very low grade. In fatal cases of maternal influenza, virus is usually not recovered from the fetus, and the virus itself has not been found to cause congenital defects.[240,241] Although congenital anomalies and hematologic malignancies have been reported after influenza infection in pregnancy, no consistent association has been determined.[240-244] Schizophrenia and autism have also been linked to influenza and other viral infections during pregnancy,[245] but findings have not been not conclusive.

Neonatal Infection

Influenza infection of neonates, including nosocomial outbreaks, have been reported, and infants with lower birth weight are more severely affected.[246-248] Clinical manifestations include rhinorrhea, cough, sneezing, poor feeding, vomiting, abdominal distention, fever, respiratory distress, and apnea. However, many cases are mild, and infections may also be asymptomatic.

Diagnosis

Influenza can be diagnosed by virus isolation in cell culture or by a number of rapid assays, some of which can be performed in doctors' offices. Rapid nonculture tests, such as ELISA, have a sensitivity of only 50% to 90%; optimal sample collection increases the detection rate. DFA of respiratory epithelial cells can provide rapid and sensitive results in experienced laboratories and can detect infection with other respiratory viruses as well.[232,233,249]

Upper respiratory samples should be collected during the first 24 to 48 hours of illness, when viral shedding is maximal. Either a nasopharyngeal swab and an oropharyngeal swab or two nasopharyngeal swabs, combined in a single tube, increase the amount of virus and improve the sensitivity of the results. Nasopharyngeal washes or aspirates, endotracheal aspirates, and bronchoalveolar lavage specimens are also excellent samples.

Serologic tests to detect a rise in influenza antibodies provide a retrospective diagnosis, because serum samples must be collected both during the acute stage and 2 to 3 weeks into convalescence.

RT-PCR is also available in some reference laboratories.[249]

Prevention and Treatment

Women whose pregnancies will be in the second or third trimester during influenza season should be vaccinated.

To avoid coincidental association with spontaneous abortion in the first trimester, clinicians may prefer to wait until the end of the first trimester to vaccinate women who are otherwise at low risk.[232] However, women who have medical conditions that increase their risk for influenza-related complications should be vaccinated before influenza season, regardless of the stage of pregnancy.

Inactivated influenza vaccine contains the three influenza strains likely to be circulating in the upcoming winter: two influenza A subtypes (H3N2 and H1N1) and an influenza B virus. Because the vaccine viruses are grown in embryonated hens' eggs, persons allergic to eggs should not receive the vaccine. Inactivated influenza vaccines also contain a low level of thimerosal, a mercury-containing compound, as a preservative. Although no evidence of harm from thimerosal in vaccines has been reported,[250] a limited number of preservation-free or reduced-thimerosal influenza vaccine doses are available from the manufacturers. The benefits of standard or reduced-thimerosal influenza vaccine far outweigh any theoretical risk from thimerosal. Breast-feeding is not a contraindication to influenza vaccination. Many obstetricians, however, fail to offer influenza vaccine to their patients.[251,252]

A live attenuated, intranasally administered influenza vaccine has been approved by the FDA but is not for use in pregnant women. Four antiviral drugs—amantadine, rimantadine, zanamivir, and oseltamivir—are available in the United States as adjuncts to vaccination.[232] Two cases of treatment of pregnant women with amantadine have been reported.[253,254] No clinical studies have been conducted in pregnant women, and amantadine and rimantadine have been shown to be teratogenic and embryotoxic in high doses in animal studies. Thus, these drugs should be used in pregnancy only if the potential benefit justifies the risk.

EPSTEIN-BARR VIRUS

Epstein-Barr virus (EBV) is the causative agent of heterophil-positive infectious mononucleosis, a disease of adolescents and young adults. In early childhood, however, infection is most often subclinical. EBV has also been linked to African Burkitt's lymphoma, poorly differentiated nasopharyngeal carcinoma, post-transplantation lymphoproliferative disease, hairy leukoplakia in patients with AIDS, and Hodgkin's disease.

EBV is transmitted in saliva by close or intimate contact. After primary infection, the virus establishes a persistent infection in epithelial cells of the nasopharynx and in B lymphocytes and may be shed intermittently or at a chronic low level in saliva. Infection occurs at a young age in persons in lower socioeconomic groups but is delayed until puberty in a significant proportion of persons in higher socioeconomic groups. Eventually, most people acquire infection.

About 3% to 4% of pregnant women are susceptible to EBV.[255,256] Despite isolated reports,[257] there is no convincing evidence that primary EBV infection in pregnancy causes congenital defects. Some investigators have explored the frequency of congenital infection by culturing cord blood lymphocytes of neonates. Only 1 infant of 696 was infected, and this infant was normal on follow-up.[258]

In another study, one infant shedding EBV in saliva had transient hepatomegaly but was otherwise normal.[259]

In a different approach, primary infections in pregnant women were identified by serologic tests. Pregnancy outcome was monitored, but convincing evidence of fetal defects or disease was not found.[256] Reactivation of EBV in pregnancy, as determined by increases in antibody to EBV early antigen, was also investigated, with conflicting results.[256,260] PCR has been applied to the detection of EBV transmission in pregnancy, and several cases of possible vertical transmission were identified.[261] However, the outcome of the affected infants was not reported.

Diagnosis

Primary EBV infection is diagnosed by heterophil and EBV-specific antibodies.[262] Heterophil antibodies are positive in fewer than 50% of young children with primary EBV, but 85% to 90% of older children and adults have a positive result. For a more specific diagnosis, a panel of EBV antibodies can be tested, preferably by immunofluorescence. ELISA tests have yielded unreliable results in the past but are improving. Both IgG and IgM antibodies to EBV viral capsid antigen should be elevated in primary infection. Test findings for antibody to EBV nuclear antigen are negative during primary infection, rise in convalescence, and remain positive for life.

Virus isolation requires transformation of human umbilical cord blood lymphocytes and is confined to the research laboratory. Virus can be detected by PCR in saliva, blood, CSF, and tissue samples, but assays are, in general, available only in reference laboratories.

HUMAN T CELL LYMPHOTROPIC VIRUS TYPE I

Human T cell lymphotropic virus type I (HTLV-I) is a retrovirus associated with adult T cell leukemia/lymphoma (ATL) and with myelopathy (HTLV-associated myelopathy [HAM]), which is also called tropical spastic paraparesis (TSP).[263] ATL is a malignancy of HTLV-I–infected CD4+ T lymphocytes that occurs in 2% to 4% of infected persons, after a latent period of decades. Most cases of ATL occur in 40- to 60-year-old patients. HAM/TSP is a chronic, progressive demyelinating disease that mainly affects the spinal cord. It occurs in fewer than 1% of HTLV-I–infected persons with a latency period that is shorter than that of ATL. It is characterized by progressive lower extremity weakness, spasticity, hyperreflexia, sensory disturbances, and urinary incontinence.

HTLV-I infection is endemic in the Caribbean basin, parts of Africa, Melanesia, and southwestern Japan. Seroprevalence rates as high as 15% have been reported in endemic areas; rates are highest in older age groups and in women.[264] HTLV type II (HTLV-II) is a related virus prevalent among intravenous drug users in the United States, Europe, and among some Native American populations. It has not been clearly linked to any disease. In the United States, donated blood is routinely screened for HTLV-I and HTLV-II; approximately 0.016% of blood donors are infected, half with HTLV-I and half with HTLV-II. HTLV-I–infected individuals either are from endemic areas or have had sexual contact with people from those areas. A small number have a history of intravenous drug use or blood transfusion.

HTLV-I is transmitted from mother to child, by sexual contact, by blood transfusion, or by contaminated needles. Mother-to-child transmission occurs primarily as a result of breast-feeding.[265] In endemic areas, about 25% of breast-fed infants of infected mothers become infected. Intrauterine or perinatal transmission occurs in about 5% of infants who are not breast-fed. Infections early in life carry the greatest risk of ATL.

Diagnosis

Most HTLV-I–infected patients of childbearing age are asymptomatic. Infection may be first recognized when the patient gives blood. If the patient is from an endemic area, serologic testing in pregnancy should be considered.[266] If results are positive, breast-feeding should be avoided.

The diagnosis is by two-step serologic testing. A positive ELISA screening test must be confirmed by Western blot. If Western blot results are indeterminate, PCR to detect HTLV-I in PBMCs can be performed. Whole blood in EDTA should be sent by overnight delivery to a competent reference laboratory.

HTLV-I infection cannot be distinguished from HTLV-II infection by ELISA. However, commercial Western blot preparations have been spiked with type-specific envelope glycoproteins (gp46-I and gp46-II) to differentiate HTLV-I and HTLV-II infections.[267]

Prevention

Infection of the newborn can be reduced significantly by avoidance of breast-feeding. Short-term breast-feeding, for 6 months or less, was reported to reduce the infection rate from 20% to about 4%.[268] It was hypothesized that maternal antibody may protect babies from infection through breast milk during the first 6 months.

Sexual transmission, which is most efficient from infected men to women, can be reduced by use of condoms. A vaccine is not yet available.[269]

Treatment

Acute ATL is treated with standard chemotherapy but with poor results. HAM/TSP has been treated with corticosteroids or danazol with some benefit.[263]

PAPILLOMAVIRUS

Human papillomaviruses (HPV) cause warts, which are benign, proliferative lesions that undergo spontaneous regression after a variable period of time. Despite variations in appearance and location, warts can be recognized by characteristic histologic features. Infection is confined to the epithelium, results from contact of virus particles with susceptible skin or mucous membranes, and is facilitated by minor trauma to the epithelium.[270] Transmission is by direct contact with infected tissue or by contact with contaminated objects. Warts are found on the skin, in the genital tract, in the oral cavity, and in the respiratory tract. More than 90 genotypes have been identified.

The course of HPV infection is determined by the immune response. Spontaneous regression within 2 years is common, presumably as a result of cell-mediated immunity. Conditions associated with depression of T cell function, such as pregnancy, transplantation, HIV infection, and immunosuppressive drug ingestion, have been associated with increases in the prevalence, size, and number of warts. Likewise, warts regress when the immunosuppressive condition improves or resolves.

Papillomaviruses in both humans and animals have been associated with cancers. However, only some types appear to be oncogenic. The interval between infection and malignancy is often long, and cofactors are required for malignant transformation.

Genital Warts

Papillomavirus infection of the genital tract has been increasing in incidence in the United States, and HPV is now considered the most common sexually transmitted viral pathogen. Condyloma acuminata are exophytic warts on the external genitalia and have been recognized for centuries. Flat and subclinical warts involving the cervix and vagina are now recognized to be more common. When sensitive DNA amplification methods are used, almost half of college-aged women are found to be infected. Most of these women have no clinical manifestations and have normal cervical cytologic profiles, and many clear the infection.[271] During pregnancy, clearance of HPV appears to be slowed during the first and second trimesters but accelerates in the postpartum period.[272]

More than 25 HPV types infect the genital tract. HPV types 6 and 11 are responsible for the large majority of exophytic condylomata. HPV has been strongly linked to the pathogenesis of squamous cell carcinoma of the cervix. Consequently, genital HPV types have been classified by risk of progression to cervical cancer into low risk (e.g., types 6 and 11), intermediate risk, and high risk (types 16 and 18). Fortunately, cancer is a rare outcome.

Genital Warts in Pregnancy

The effect of pregnancy on genital HPV infections has been the subject of several studies, with conflicting results.[273] However, there is some evidence that condyloma acuminata can grow more rapidly during pregnancy. These warts can be located throughout the lower genital tract and perianal region and can grow so large as to prevent vaginal delivery. Furthermore, disruption of these lesions during delivery can lead to substantial maternal blood loss. Therefore, many specialists advocate their removal during pregnancy.[274] Cesarean delivery may be indicated in cases of pelvic outlet obstruction or if vaginal delivery would result in excessive bleeding.

Respiratory Papillomavirus

Laryngeal papillomas or recurrent respiratory papillomatosis are believed to be transmitted by aspiration of HPV-infected secretions during vaginal delivery.[275-277] Most laryngeal papillomas are caused by genital tract HPV types 6 and 11. The most common presenting symptom is a voice change or abnormal cry, caused by involvement of the larynx; the trachea, lungs, nose, and oral cavity can also be involved. Respiratory papillomatosis may occur at any age, but children younger than 5 years are at the highest risk. Conjunctival papillomas in infants have also been reported.[278] These complications are rare despite the frequency of genital HPV.[279]

Diagnosis

Warts are diagnosed by clinical examination. Histologic examination can be performed when the diagnosis is in doubt. Papanicolaou smears may detect characteristic koilocytes. Subclinical lesions necessitate colposcopic examination and staining with 3% acetic acid or iodine for visualization of affected areas.

HPV DNA testing can also be performed with commercially available reagents on cervical swabs or biopsies. DNA probes are available to distinguish common high- and low-risk HPV types. However, because treatment is based on clinical disease and histopathologic findings, HPV-specific diagnosis is currently limited to management of women whose cervical cytologic profile shows atypical squamous cells of undetermined significance.[280] In these cases, repeat cytologic testing, colposcopy or DNA testing for high-risk HPV types are all acceptable approaches.

Treatment

Treatment of visible genital warts is directed at symptomatic relief, and multiple applications and modalities are often necessary. The warts may initially disappear after treatment, but recurrences are common. There is no evidence that treatment affects the natural history of HPV infection or the development of cervical cancer.

Podophyllin, podofilox, and imiquimod are contraindicated in pregnancy.[279] Trichloroacetic acid, cryosurgery, electrocautery, laser therapy, and surgical excision may be used.

Laryngeal papillomas pose a difficult problem. Use of interferon has met with limited or transient success.[281] CO_2 laser surgery remains the mainstay of treatment when papillomas compromise the airway. However, scarring may occur because surgery may be needed every year or even more frequently. Progression to cancer has occurred when lesions have been treated with radiation.

Prevention

Condoms provide some protection against sexual transmission. Laryngeal papillomas may be prevented by cesarean section, but because of the rarity of transmission, no such preventive measures have been recommended.[282] An HPV-16 vaccine has been shown to reduce the incidence of both HPV-16 infection and HPV-16–related cervical intraepithelial neoplasia and may eventually reduce the incidence of cervical cancer.[283]

MEASLES

Measles is a highly contagious infection of childhood characterized by cough, coryza, and conjunctivitis followed by an erythematous maculopapular rash. Complications include giant cell pneumonia, encephalitis, and bacterial superinfections. Malnutrition and vitamin A deficiency greatly increase the associated morbidity and mortality. As vaccination has become more widely used, the annual deaths from measles worldwide have decreased from almost 6 million in 1980 to approximately 800,000 in 2000.[164,284]

A universal measles vaccination policy and the introduction of a two-dose vaccination schedule have led to the reduction in measles cases from 500,000 per year in the United States to a record low of 86 cases in 2000.[285] Endemic transmission of measles was probably interrupted in 1993, and subsequent cases have been linked to importations from Europe and Asia.

Measles in Pregnancy

Measles is rare in pregnancy. However, it has been associated with an increased risk of pneumonia in the third trimester and puerperium, as well as an increase in mortality from heart failure and pulmonary edema.[286,287] Measles during pregnancy has also been implicated in an increase in premature deliveries and in first trimester spontaneous abortions.

Congenital Measles

Measles has not been implicated in congenital defects. Congenital infection from transplacental transmission near term can manifest at birth or during the first 10 days after birth. Infection can be mild or rapidly fatal, especially in premature infants or in infants who fail to develop the rash. The overall mortality rate is 30% in the absence of immune globulin prophylaxis. Previous reports suggesting that measles virus infection in utero may be a risk factor for Crohn's disease have not been confirmed.[288]

Diagnosis

Virus isolation should be attempted because isolates are useful in public health efforts to trace the origin and spread of outbreaks. If testing is not available locally, arrangements can often be made to send samples to a reference laboratory. Nasal washes or nasopharyngeal aspirates, throat swabs, and urine should be collected within 1 to 3 days of onset of rash and be submitted for culture. RT-PCR can also be useful, especially for tissue specimens.[164]

In addition, an acute-stage serum sample should be obtained as soon as possible, followed by a convalescent-stage serum sample 2 to 4 weeks later. Serum samples should be tested in parallel to document seroconversion or a significant rise in IgG antibody. Measles-specific IgM can be detected beginning 3 to 7 days after the onset of the rash.[164,289] However, false-negative and false-positive results occur.

Treatment

No specific antiviral therapy is available. However, the World Health Organization recommends the administration of high doses of vitamin A to all children with acute measles to reduce morbidity and mortality in countries where the fatality rate is 1% or more.

Prevention

Immune globulin can be given to prevent or modify measles in susceptible persons within 6 days of exposure. Earlier administration confers better protection. Immune globulin is indicated for susceptible pregnant women and for newborns delivered from mothers who have measles during the last week of pregnancy.

Measles vaccine is a live attenuated vaccine and is contraindicated in pregnancy, on the basis of theoretical risk of fetal infection.[241] Rubella susceptibility is predictive of measles susceptibility.[290] Hence measles-mumps-rubella (MMR) vaccine, instead of rubella vaccine, should be given to susceptible women, as currently recommended by the Advisory Committee on Immunization Practices.[291]

Of note, the World Health Organization, the Pan American Health Organization, and the CDC have adopted the goal of global eradication of measles by 2005 to 2010.

MUMPS

Mumps is a highly contagious and usually benign childhood infection characterized by fever and parotitis. It has also been associated with meningitis, orchitis (in postpubertal boys), oophoritis, pancreatitis, and myocarditis. Mumps is spread by respiratory droplets and has an incubation period of 16 to 18 days. Up to 30% of infections are asymptomatic. Although the widespread use of vaccination has led to a marked decline in the incidence of mumps, vaccination is not universal, and a number of states in the United States still do not require mumps vaccination.[292,293] There has been a rise in the average age at the time of disease, and young adults are at risk of acquiring infection in the workplace or during travel because mumps is still endemic throughout the world.

Infection is no more severe in pregnant women than in nonpregnant adults.[294] However, maternal mumps in the first trimester may cause spontaneous abortion or intrauterine death as a result of placental or fetal infection.[295-297] Infection in the second and third trimester is usually uncomplicated.

Mumps virus can be transmitted by viremia to the fetus near term and is shed in breast milk.[298] Nevertheless, perinatal infection of the neonate, which can manifest as upper respiratory symptoms (without parotitis), pneumonia, fever (with splenomegaly), and thrombocytopenia,[299] is uncommon.

There does not appear to be an increase in congenital malformations after maternal mumps. Some studies have found a higher prevalence of mumps infection during pregnancy in infants with endocardial fibroelastosis, but this link has not been proved.[300,301]

Diagnosis

Isolation of the virus is the test of choice; mumps virus can be isolated from throat swabs, saliva, urine, and CSF for up to 5 days after onset of symptoms. To ensure that the appropriate tests are performed, the laboratory should be notified when mumps is suspected.

Serologic assays can also be helpful in diagnosing primary infection, but heterologous rises to parainfluenza viruses can occur. In the acute and convalescent stages, serum should be tested in parallel. Immunity is assessed by testing a single serum sample by ELISA or hemagglutination inhibition testing; the complement fixation test is not sufficiently sensitive.[302]

Treatment

There is no specific treatment.

Prevention

Immune globulin is not beneficial. A live attenuated vaccine is available but should not be given in pregnancy. The requirement for a second dose of MMR vaccine has helped reduce the incidence of mumps in the United States. However, because the use of MMR vaccine is restricted to affluent countries, mumps is expected to remain a common infection worldwide.

MOLLUSCUM CONTAGIOSUM

Molluscum contagiosum is caused by a poxvirus of the same name, and humans are the only host.[303,304] Infection is worldwide and most common in children, although people of all ages can be affected. Transmission is by direct person-to-person contact or through fomites. In the United States, infection has become more common and can be a marker for more serious sexually transmitted infections.

The skin lesions of molluscum contagiosum are characterized by multiple small papular skin lesions, 2 mm to 1 cm in size, with an expressible core of degenerating epidermal cells and keratin. In children, skin lesions are scattered over the body, whereas in immunocompetent adults, lesions are usually found in the genital and perianal regions as well as on the upper thighs. Lesions often occur in crops in localized areas, probably a result of

mechanical spread or multiple initial infections. There is no evidence of viremia.

Skin lesions are notable for lack of inflammatory response, and reinfections are fairly common. Lesions persist for weeks to several years and then regress. The condition is a trivial infection in normal hosts, but in immunocompromised hosts, widespread and recurrent lesions may occur. This has been an increasing problem in immunocompromised hosts, especially patients with AIDS.

Molluscum Infection during Pregnancy

Molluscum is not a particular problem during pregnancy.

Diagnosis

The diagnosis is made clinically on the basis of the appearance of lesions and, if needed, can be confirmed by biopsy. Solitary lesions on the face can be mistaken for basal cell carcinomas. Histologic examination reveals a characteristic large acidophilic cytoplasmic mass or "molluscum body." Electron microscopy reveals characteristic poxvirus particles. The virus has not yet been propagated in culture.

Treatment

Lesions can be removed simply by curettage.[305] Cryotherapy can also be used. Caustic agents such as podophyllin are contraindicated in pregnancy.

References

1. Gregg NM: Congenital cataract following German measles in the mother. Trans Ophthalmol Soc Aust 1941;3:34.
2. Evans AS, Kaslow RA (eds): Viral Infections of Humans, 4th ed. New York, Plenum Medical Books, 1997.
3. Richman DD, Whitley RJ, Hayden FG (eds): Clinical Virology, 2nd ed. Washington, D.C., ASM Press, 2002.
4. Pickering L (ed): Red Book: 2003 Report of the Committee on Infectious Diseases, 26th ed. Elk Grove Village, Ill, American Academy of Pediatrics, 2003.

Cytomegalovirus

5. Farber S, Wolback SB: Intranuclear and cytoplasmic inclusions ("protozoan-like bodies") in salivary glands and other organs of infants. Am J Pathol 1932;8:123.
6. Ho M: Epidemiology of cytomegalovirus infections. Rev Infect Dis 1990;12(Suppl):701.
7. Nankervis GA, Kumar ML, Cox EE, et al: A prospective study of maternal cytomegalovirus infection and its effect on the fetus. Am J Obstet Gynecol 1984;149:435.
8. Stagno S, Pass R, Cloud G, et al: Primary cytomegalovirus infection in pregnancy: Incidence, transmission to fetus, and clinical outcome. JAMA 1986;256:1904.
9. Stagno S, Cloud GA: Working parents: The impact of day care and breast-feeding on cytomegalovirus infections in offspring. Proc Natl Acad Sci U S A 1994;91:2384.
10. Hutto C, Little A, Ricks R, et al: Isolation of CMV from toys and hands in a day care center. J Infect Dis 1986;154:527.
11. Pass RF, Hutto C, Reynolds DW, Polhill RB: Increased frequency of cytomegalovirus in children in group day care. Pediatrics 1984;74:121.
12. Pass RF, Little EA, Stagno S, et al: Young children as a probable source of maternal and congenital cytomegalovirus infection. N Engl J Med 1987;316:1366.

13. Adler SP: Cytomegalovirus transmission among children in day care, their mothers and caretakers. Pediatr Infect Dis J 1988;7:279.

14. Fowler KB, Stagno S, Pass RF: Maternal immunity and prevention of congenital cytomegalovirus infection. JAMA 2003;289:1008.

15. Dworsky M, Welch K, Cassady G, et al: Occupational risk for primary cytomegalovirus infection among pediatric health-care workers. N Engl J Med 1983;309:950.

16. Reynolds DW, Stagno S, Hosty TS, et al: Maternal cytomegalovirus excretion and perinatal infection. N Engl J Med 1973;289:1.

17. Dworsky M, Yow M, Stagno S, et al: Cytomegalovirus infection of breast milk and transmission in infancy. Pediatrics 1983; 72:295.

17a. Boppana SB, Rivera LB, Fowler KB, et al. Intrauterine transmission of cytomegalovirus to infants of women with preconceptual immunity. N Engl J Med 344: 1366, 2001.

18. Demmler GJ: Congenital cytomegalovirus infection and disease. Adv Pediatr Infect Dis 1996;11:135.

19. Blau EB, Gross JR: Congenital cytomegalovirus infection after recurrent infection in a mother with a renal transplant. Pediatr Nephrol 1997;11:361.

20. Maschmann J, Hamprecht K, Dietz K, et al: Cytomegalovirus infection of extremely low–birth weight infants via breast milk. Clin Infect Dis 2001;33:1998.

21. Roback JD: CMV and blood transfusions. Rev Med Virol 2002;12:211.

22. Vochem M, Hamprecht K, Jahn G, Speer CP: Transmission of cytomegalovirus to preterm infants through breast milk. Pediatr Infect Dis J 1998;17:53.

23. Ehrnst A: The clinical relevance of different laboratory tests in CMV diagnosis. Scand J Infect Dis Suppl 1996;100:64.

24. Lazzarotto T, Brojanac S, Maine GT, Landini MP: Search for cytomegalovirus-specific immunoglobulin M: Comparison between a new Western blot, conventional Western blot, and nine commercially available assays. Clin Diagn Lab Immunol 1997;4:483.

25. Ruellan-Eugene G, Barjot P, Campet M, et al: Evaluation of virological procedures to detect fetal human cytomegalovirus infection: Avidity of IgG antibodies, virus detection in amniotic fluid and maternal serum. J Med Virol 1996;50:9.

26. Lipitz S, Yagel S, Shaleve E, et al: Prenatal diagnosis of fetal primary cytomegalovirus infection. Obstet Gynecol 1997;89:763.

27. Lazzarotto T, Varani S, Guerra B, et al: Prenatal indicators of congenital cytomegalovirus infection. J Pediatr 2000;137:90.

28. Gouarin S, Gault E, Vabret A, et al: Real-time PCR quantification of human cytomegalovirus DNA in amniotic fluid samples from mothers with primary infection. J Clin Microbiol 2002;40:1767.

29. Nelson CT, Istas AS, Wilkerson MK, Demmler GJ: PCR detection of cytomegalovirus DNA in serum as a diagnostic test for congenital cytomegalovirus infection. J Clin Microbiol 1995;33:3317.

30. Griffiths PD: The treatment of cytomegalovirus infections. J Antimicrob Chemother 2002;49:243.

31. Whitley RJ, Kimberlin DW: Treatment of viral infections during pregnancy and the neonatal period. Clin Perinatol 1997;24:267.

32. Adler SP, Finney JW, Manganello AM, et al: Prevention of child-to-mother transmission of cytomegalovirus by changing behaviors: A randomized controlled trial. Pediatr Infect Dis J 1996;15:240.

33. Griffiths PD: Strategies to prevent CMV infection in the neonate. Semin Neonatol 2002;7:293.

34. Pass RF, Burke RL: Development of cytomegalovirus vaccines: Prospects for prevention of congenital CMV infection. Semin Pediatr Infect Dis 2002;13:196.

Herpes Simplex Virus

35. Corey L, Spear PG: Infections with herpes simplex viruses. N Engl J Med 1986;314:686.

36. Gibson JJ, Hornung CA, Alexander GR, et al: A cross-sectional study of herpes simplex virus types 1 and 2 in college students: Occurrence and determinants of infection. J Infect Dis 1990;162:306.

37. Corey L, Adams H, Brown A, Holmes K: Genital herpes simplex virus infections: Clinical manifestations, course, and complications. Ann Intern Med 1983;98:958.

38. Corey L: Challenges in genital herpes simplex virus management. J Infect Dis 2002;186(Suppl 1):S29.

39. Engelberg R, Carrell D, Krantz E, et al: Natural history of genital herpes simplex virus type 1 infection. Sex Transm Dis 2003; 30:174.

40. Hook E, Cannon R, Nahmias AJ, et al: Herpes simplex virus infection as a risk factor for human immunodeficiency virus infection in heterosexuals. J Infect Dis 1992;165:251.

41. Mertz GJ, Schmidt O, Jourden JL, et al: Frequency of acquisition of first-episode genital infection with simplex virus from symptomatic and asymptomatic source contacts. Sex Transm Dis 1985;12:133.

42. Stanberry LR, Floyd-Reising SA, Connelly BL, et al: Herpes simplex viremia: Report of eight pediatric cases and review of the literature. Clin Infect Dis 1994;18:401.

43. Brown ZA, Selke S, Zeh J, et al: The acquisition of herpes simplex virus during pregnancy: Its frequency and impact on pregnancy outcome. N Engl J Med 1997;337:509.

44. Frederick DM, Bland D, Gollin Y: Fatal disseminated herpes simplex virus infection in a previously healthy pregnant woman. A case report. J Reprod Med 2002;47:591.

45. Sexually transmitted disease treatment guidelines 2002. Centers for Disease Control and Prevention. MMWR Morb Mortal Wkly Rep 2002;51(RR-6):1.

46. Prober CG, Corey L, Brown ZAS, et al: The management of pregnancies complicated by genital infections with herpes simplex virus. Clin Infect Dis 1992;15:1031.

47. Brown ZA, Vontver LA, Benedetti J, et al: Effects on infants of a first episode of genital herpes during pregnancy. N Engl J Med 1987;317:1246.

48. Prober CG, Sullender WM, Yasukawa LL, et al: Low risk of herpes simplex virus infections in neonates exposed to the virus at the time of vaginal delivery to mothers with recurrent genital herpes simplex virus infections. N Engl J Med 1987;316:240.

49. Brown ZA, Benedetti J, Ashley R, et al: Neonatal herpes simplex virus infection in relation to asymptomatic maternal infection at the time of labor. N Engl J Med 1991;324:1247.

50. Stone KM, Brooks CA, Guinan ME, Alexander ER: National surveillance for neonatal herpes simplex virus infections. Sex Transm Dis 1989;16:152.

51. Yeager AS, Arvin AM, Urbani LJ, Kemp JA III: Relationship of antibody to outcome in neonatal herpes simplex infections. Infect Immun 1980;29:532.

52. Ashley RL, Dalessio J, Burchett S, et al: Herpes simplex virus–2 (HSV-2) type-specific antibody correlates of protection in infants exposed to HSV-2 at birth. J Clin Invest 1992;90:511.

53. Whitley RJ, Arvin A, Prober C, et al: Predictors of morbidity and mortality in neonates with herpes simplex virus infections. N Engl J Med 1991;324:450.

54. Kaye EM, Dooling EC: Neonatal herpes simplex meningoencephalitis associated with fetal monitor scalp electrodes. Neurology 1981;31:1045.

55. Hutto C, Arvin A, Jacobs R, et al: Intrauterine herpes simplex virus infections. J Pediatr 1987;110:97.

55a. Gutierrez KM, Falkovitz Halpern MS, Maldonado Y, Arvin AM: Epidemiology of neonatal herpes simplex virus infections in California from 1985 to 1995. J Infect Dis 1999;180:199.

56. Brown ZA, Wald A, Morrow RA, et al: Effect of serologic status and cesarean delivery on transmission rates of herpes simplex virus from mother to infant. JAMA 2003;289:203.

57. Hammerberg O, Watts J, Chernesky M, et al: An outbreak of herpes simplex virus type 1 in an intensive care nursery. Pediatr Infect Dis J 1983;2:290.

58. Linnemann CC Jr, Buchman TG, Light IJ, et al: Transmission of herpes simplex virus type-1 in a nursery for the newborn: Identification of viral species isolated by DNA fingerprinting. Lancet 1978;1:964.

59. Sullivan-Bolyai JZ, Fife KH, Jacobs RF, et al: Disseminated neonatal herpes simplex virus type 1 from maternal breast lesion. Pediatrics 1983;71:455.

60. Kimberlin DW: Advances in the treatment of neonatal herpes simplex infections. Rev Med Virol 2001;11:157.

61. Kimura H, Futamura M, Kito H, et al: Detection of viral DNA in neonatal herpes simplex virus infections: Frequent and prolonged presence in serum and cerebrospinal fluid. J Infect Dis 1991;164:289.

62. Landry ML: False-positive polymerase chain reaction results in the diagnosis of herpes simplex encephalitis. J Infect Dis 1995;172:1641.

63. Landry ML, Ferguson D, Wlochowski J: Detection of herpes simplex virus in clinical specimens by cytospin-enhanced direct immunofluorescence. J Clin Microbiol 1997;35:302.

64. Wald A, Ashley-Morrow R: Serological testing for herpes simplex virus (HSV)-1 and HSV-2 infection. Clin Infect Dis 2002;35(Suppl 2):S173.

65. Reiff-Eldridge RA, Heffner CR, Ephross SA, et al: Monitoring pregnancy outcomes after prenatal drug exposure through prospective pregnancy registries: A pharmaceutical company commitment. Am J Obstet Gynecol 2000;182:159.

66. Kimberlin DW, Lin CY, Jacobs RF, et al: National Institute of Allergy and Infectious Diseases Collaborative Antiviral Study Group: Safety and efficacy of high-dose intravenous acyclovir in the management of neonatal herpes simplex virus infections. Pediatrics 2001;108:230.

67. Kimberlin DW, Lin CY, Jacobs RF, et al: National Institute of Allergy and Infectious Diseases Collaborative Antiviral Study Group: Natural history of neonatal herpes simplex virus infections in the acyclovir era. Pediatrics 2001;108:223.

68. American College of Obstetricians and Gynecologists. Management of herpes in pregnancy. Washington, D.C., American College of Obstetricians and Gynecologists, 1999.

69. Arvin AM, Hensleigh PA, Prober CG, et al: Failure of antepartum maternal cultures to predict the infant's risk of exposure to herpes simplex virus at delivery. N Engl J Med 1986;315:796.

70. Watts DH, Brown ZA, Money D, et al: A double-blind, randomized, placebo-controlled trial of acyclovir in late pregnancy for the reduction of herpes simplex virus shedding and cesarean delivery. Am J Obstet Gynecol 2003;188:836.

71. Guttman LT, Wilfert CM, Eppes S: Herpes simplex virus encephalitis in children: Analysis of cerebrospinal fluid and progressive neurodevelopmental deterioration. J Infect Dis 1986;154:415.

72. Koelle DM, Corey L: Recent progress in herpes simplex virus immunobiology and vaccine research. Clin Microbiol Rev 2003;16:96.

Human Immunodeficiency Virus Type 1

73. Guatelli JC, Siliciano RF, Kuritzkes D, Richman D: Human immunodeficiency virus. In Richman DD, Whitley RJ, Hayden FG (eds): Clinical Virology, 2nd ed. Washington, D.C., ASM Press, 2002, pp 685-729.

74. Clavel F, Guetard D, Brun-Vezinet F, et al: Isolation of a new human retrovirus from West African patients with AIDS. Science 1986;233:343.

75. Mofenson LM, Centers for Disease Control and Prevention, U.S. Public Health Service Task Force: U.S. Public Health Service Task Force recommendations for the use of antiretroviral drugs in pregnant HIV-1–infected women for maternal health and interventions to reduce perinatal HIV-1 transmission in the United States. MMWR Morb Mortal Wkly Rep 2002;51(RR-18):1.

76. Dybul M, Fauci AS, Bartlett JG, et al: Guidelines for using antiretroviral agents among HIV-infected adults and adolescents. Recommendations of the Panel on Clinical Practices for Treatment of HIV. MMWR Recomm Rep 2002;51(RR-7):1.

77. Andiman WA: Medical management of the pregnant woman infected with human immunodeficiency virus type 1 and her child. Semin Perinatol 1998;22:72.

78. Minkoff H: Human immunodeficiency virus infection in pregnancy. Obstet Gynecol 2003;101:797.

79. Weiser F, Nachman S, Tropper P, et al: Quantitation of human immunodeficiency virus type 1 during pregnancy: Relationship of viral titer to mother-to-child transmission and stability of viral load. Proc Natl Acad Sci U S A 1994;91:8037.

80. Garcia PM, Kalish LA, Pitt J, et al: Maternal levels of plasma human immunodeficiency virus type 1 RNA and the risk of perinatal transmission. Women and Infants Transmission Study Group. N Engl J Med 1999;341:394.

81. Ioannidis JP, Abrams EJ, Ammann A, et al: Perinatal transmission of human immunodeficiency virus type 1 by pregnant women with RNA virus loads <1000 copies/mL. J Infect Dis 2001;183:539.

82. Rasheed S, Li Z, Xu D, et al: Presence of cell-free human immunodeficiency virus in cervicovaginal secretions is independent of viral load in the blood of human immunodeficiency virus–infected women. Am J Obstet Gynecol 1996;175:122.

83. Tuomala RE, O'Driscoll PT, Bremer JW, et al: Women and Infants Transmission Study: Cell-associated genital tract virus and vertical transmission of human immunodeficiency virus type 1 in antiretroviral-experienced women. J Infect Dis 2003;187:375.

84. Chirgwin KD, Feldman J, Augenbraun M, et al: Incidence of venereal warts in human immunodeficiency virus–infected and uninfected women. J Infect Dis 1995;172:235.

85. Vermund SH, Kelley KF, Klein RS, et al: High risk of human papillomavirus infection and cervical squamous intraepithelial lesions among women with symptomatic human immunodeficiency virus infection. Am J Obstet Gynecol 1991;165:392.

86. Augenbraun M, Feldman J, Chirgwin K, et al: Increased genital shedding of herpes simplex virus type 2 in HIV-seropositive women. Ann Intern Med 1995;123:845.

87. Gabiano C, Tovo PA, de Martino M, et al: Mother-to-child transmission of human immunodeficiency virus type 1: Risk of infection and correlates of transmission. Pediatrics 1992;90:369.

88. Goedert JJ, Duliege A, Amos CL, et al: High risk of HIV-1 infection for first-born twins. Lancet 1991;338:1471.

89. Landesman SH, Kalish LA, Burns DN, et al: Obstetrical factors and the transmission of human immunodeficiency virus type 1 from mother to child. N Engl J Med 1996;334:1617.

90. Luzuriaga K, Sullivan JL: Pathogenesis of vertical HIV-1 infection: Implications for intervention and management. Pediatr Ann 1994;23:159.

91. Minkoff H, Burns DN, Landesman S, et al: The relationship of the duration of ruptured membranes to vertical transmission of human immunodeficiency virus. Am J Obstet Gynecol 1995;173:585.

92. Minkoff H, Mofenson LM: The role of obstetric interventions in the prevention of pediatric human immunodeficiency virus infection. Am J Obstet Gynecol 1994;171:1167.

93. Scarlatti G, Hodara V, Rossi P: Transmission of human immunodeficiency virus type 1 (HIV-1) from mother to child correlates with viral phenotype. Virology 1993;197:624.

94. Connor EM, Sperling RS, Gelber R, et al: Reduction of maternal-infant transmission of human immunodeficiency virus type 1 with zidovudine treatment. N Engl J Med 1994;33:1173.

95. Shaffer N, Chuachoowong R, Mock PA, et al: Short-course zidovudine for perinatal HIV-1 transmission in Bangkok, Thailand: A randomized controlled trial. Lancet 1999;353:773.

96. Frenkel LM, Cowles MK, Shapiro DE, et al: Analysis of the maternal components of the AIDS Clinical Trials Group 076 zidovudine regimen in the prevention of mother-to-infant transmission of human immunodeficiency virus type 1. J Infect Dis 1997;175:971.

97. Mofenson LM: Interaction between timing of perinatal human immunodeficiency virus infection and the design of preventive and therapeutic interventions. Acta Paediatr Suppl 1997;491:1.

98. Qian M, Bui T, Ho RJY, et al: Metabolism of 3′-azido-3′-deoxythymidine (AZT) in human placental trophoblasts and Hofbauer cells. Biochem Pharmacol 1994;48:383.

99. Bertolli J, St. Louis ME, Simonds RJ, et al: Estimating mother-to-child transmission of human immunodeficiency virus in a breast-feeding population in Kinshasa, Zaire. J Infect Dis 1996;174:722.

100. The International Perinatal HIV Group: The mode of delivery and the risk of vertical transmission of human immunodeficiency virus type 1. A meta-analysis from 15 prospective cohort studies. N Engl J Med 1999;340:977.

101. The European Mode of Delivery Collaboration: Elective cesarean-section versus vaginal delivery in prevention of vertical HIV-1 transmission: A randomized clinical trial. Lancet 1999;353:1035.

102. The International Perinatal HIV Group: Duration of ruptured membranes and vertical transmission of HIV-1: A meta-analysis from 15 prospective cohort studies. AIDS 2001;15:357.

103. Rich KC, Siegel JN, Jennings C, et al: CD4+ lymphocytes in perinatal human immunodeficiency virus (HIV) infection: Evidence for pregnancy-induced immune depression in uninfected and HIV-infected women. J Infect Dis 1995;172:1221.

104. Guidelines for the use of antiretroviral agents in pediatric HIV infection. Centers for Disease Control and Prevention. MMWR Recomm Rep1998;47(RR-4):1.

105. Peters V, Liu KL, Dominguez K, et al: Missed opportunities for perinatal HIV prevention among HIV-exposed infants born 1996-2000, pediatric spectrum of HIV disease cohort. Pediatrics 2003;111:1186.

106. Centers for Disease Control and Prevention: Revised guidelines for HIV counseling, testing and referral and revised recommendations for HIV screening of pregnant women. MMWR Recomm Rep 2001;50(RR-19):1.

107. Steketee RW, Abrams EJ, Thea DM, et al: Early detection of perinatal human immunodeficiency virus (HIV) type 1 infection using HIV RNA amplification and detection. J Infect Dis 1997; 175:707.

Parvovirus B19

108. Cossart YE, Field AM, Cant B, et al: Parvovirus-like particles in human sera. Lancet 1975;1:72.
109. Brown KE, Young NS: Parvovirus B19 in human disease. Annu Rev Med 1997;48:59.
110. Heegaard ED, Brown KE: Human parvovirus B19. Clin Microbiol Rev 2002;15:485.
111. Brown TA, Anand A, Ritchie LD, et al: Intrauterine parvovirus infection during pregnancy. Lancet 1984;2:1033.
112. Belloy M, Morinet F, Blondin G, et al: Erythroid hypoplasia due to chronic infection with parvovirus B19. N Engl J Med 1990;322:633.
113. Frickhofen N, Abkowitz J, Safford M, et al: Persistent parvovirus B19 infection in patients infected with human immunodeficiency virus type 1 (HIV-1): A treatable cause of anemia in AIDS. Ann Intern Med 1990;113:926.
114. Brown KE, Green S, Antunez-de-Mayolo J, et al: Congenital anemia following transplacental B19 parvovirus infection. Lancet 1994;343:895.
115. Brown KE, Young NS, Alving BM, Barbosa LH: Parvovirus B19: Implications for transfusion medicine. Summary of a workshop. Transfusion 2001;41:130.
116. Nesher G, Osborn TG, Moore TL: Parvovirus infection mimicking systemic lupus erythematosus. Arthritis Rheum 1995;24:297.
117. Cope AP, Jones A, Brozovic M, et al: Possible induction of systemic lupus erythematosus by human parvovirus. Ann Rheum Dis 1992;51:803.
118. Koch WC, Adler SP: Human parvovirus B19 infections in women of childbearing age and within families. Pediatr Infect Dis J 1989;8:83.
119. Hall SM, Cohen BJ, Mortimer PP, et al: Prospective study of human parvovirus (B19) infection in pregnancy. BMJ 1990;300:1166.
120. Gillespie SM, Cartter ML, Asch S, et al: Occupational risk of human parvovirus B19 infection for school and day care personnel during an outbreak of erythema infectiosum. JAMA 1990;263:2061.
121. Norbeck O, Papadogiannakis N, Petersson K, et al: Revised clinical presentation of parvovirus B19–associated intrauterine fetal death. Clin Infect Dis 2002;35:1032.
122. Gratacos E, Torres PJ, Vidal J, et al: The incidence of human parvovirus B19 infection during pregnancy and its impact on perinatal outcome. J Infect Dis 1995;171:1360.
123. Levy R, Weissman A, Blomberg G, et al: Infection by parvovirus B19 during pregnancy: A review. Obstet Gynecol Surv 1997;52:254.
124. Warsof SL, Nicolaides KH, Rodeck C: Immune and nonimmune hydrops. Clin Obstet Gynecol 1986;29:533.
125. Jordan JA: Identification of human parvovirus B19 infection in idiopathic nonimmune hydrops fetalis. Am J Obstet Gynecol 1996;174:37.
126. Pryde PG, Nugent CE, Pridjian G, et al: Spontaneous resolution of nonimmune hydrops fetalis secondary to human parvovirus B19 infection. Obstet Gynecol 1992;79:859.
127. Morey AL, Nicolini U, Welch CR, et al: Parvovirus B19 infection and transient fetal hydrops. Lancet 1991;1:496.
128. Porter HJ, Quantrill AM, Fleming KA: B19 parvovirus infection of myocardial cells. Lancet 1988;1:535.
129. Toroc TJ, Wang QY, Gary GW: Prenatal diagnosis of intrauterine infection with parvovirus B19 by the polymerase chain reaction technique. J Infect Dis 1992;14:149.
130. Petrikovsky BM, Baker D, Schneider E: Fetal hydrops secondary to human parvovirus infection in early pregnancy. Prenat Diagn 1996;16:342.
131. Humphrey W, Magoon M, O'Shaughnessy R: Severe nonimmune hydrops secondary to parvovirus B-19 infection: Spontaneous reversal in utero and survival of a term infant. Obstet Gynecol 1991;78:900.
132. Katz VL, McCoy MC, Kuller JA, Hansen WF: An association between fetal parvovirus B19 infection and fetal anomalies: A report of two cases. Am J Perinatol 1996;13:43.
133. Tiessen RG, vanElsacker-Niele AMW, Vermeij-Keers CHR, et al: A fetus with a parvovirus B19 infection and congenital anomalies. Prenat Diagn 1994;14:173.
134. Clewley JP, Cohen BJ, Field AM: Detection of parvovirus B19 DNA, antigen, and particles in the human fetus. J Med Virol 1987;23:367.
135. Schwartz TF, Nerlich A, Hottentragen B, et al: Parvovirus B19 infection of the fetus: Histology and in situ hybridization. Am J Clin Pathol 1991;96:121.
136. Kurtz JB, Anderson MJ: Cross-reactions in rubella and parvovirus specific IgM tests. Lancet 1985;2:1356.
137. Thomas HI, Barrett E, Hesketh LM, et al: Simultaneous IgM reactivity by EIA against more than one virus in measles, parvovirus B19 and rubella infection. J Clin Virol 1999;14:107.
138. Andersen LJ, Tsou C, Parker RA, et al: Detection of antibodies and antigens of human parvovirus B19 by enzyme-linked immunosorbent assay. J Clin Microbiol 1986;24:522.
139. Bruu AL, Nordbo SA: Evaluation of five commercial tests for detection of immunoglobulin M antibodies to human parvovirus B19. J Clin Microbiol 1995;33:1363.
140. Ozawa K, Kurtzman G, Young NS: Replication of the B19 parvovirus in human bone marrow cultures. Science 1986;233:883.
141. Knoll A, Louwen F, Kochanowski B, et al: Parvovirus B19 infection in pregnancy: Quantitative viral DNA analysis using a kinetic fluorescence detection system (TaqMan PCR). J Med Virol 2002;67:259.
142. Zerbini M, Musiani M, Gentilomi G, et al: Comparative evaluation of virological and serological methods in prenatal diagnosis of parvovirus B19 fetal hydrops. J Clin Microbiol 1996;34:603.
143. Kurtzman G, Frickhofen N, Kimball J, et al: Pure red-cell aplasia of 10 years' duration due to persistent parvovirus B19 infection and its cure with immunoglobulin therapy. N Engl J Med 1989;321:519.
144. Smoleniec JS, Pillai M: Management of fetal hydrops associated with parvovirus B19 infection. Br J Obstet Gynaecol 1994;101:1079.
145. Peters MT, Nicolaides KH: Cordocentesis for the diagnosis and treatment of human fetal parvovirus infection. Obstet Gynecol 1990;75:501.
146. Cosmi E, Mari G, DelleChiaie L, et al: Noninvasive diagnosis by Doppler ultrasonography of fetal anemia resulting from parvovirus infection. Am J Obstet Gynecol 2002;187:1290.
147. Selbing A, Josefsson A, Dahlo LO, Lindgren R: Parvovirus B19 infection during pregnancy treated with high-dose intravenous gamma globulin. Lancet 1995;345:660.
148. Ballou WR, Reed JL, Noble W, et al: Safety and immunogenicity of a recombinant parvovirus B19 vaccine formulate with MF59C.1. J Infect Dis 2003;187:675.

Rubella

149. Lee JY, Bowden DS: Rubella virus replication and links to teratogenicity. Clin Microbiol Rev 2000;13:571.
150. Holmes SJ, Orenstein WA: Rubella. In Evans AS, Kaslow RA (eds): Viral Infections of Humans, 4th ed. New York, Plenum Medical Books, 1997, pp 839-860.
151. Reef SE, Frey TK, Theall K, et al: The changing epidemiology of rubella in the 1990s: On the verge of elimination and new challenges for control and prevention. JAMA 2000;287:464.
152. Control and prevention of rubella: Evaluation and management of suspected outbreaks, rubella in pregnant women, and surveillance for congenital rubella syndrome. MMWR Morb Mortal Wkly Rep 2001;50(RR-12):1.
153. Danovaro-Holliday MC, LeBaron CW, Allensworth C, et al: A large rubella outbreak with spread from the workplace to the community. JAMA 2000;284:2733.
154. Plotkin SA: Rubella eradication. Vaccine 2001;19:3311.
155. Aboudy Y, Fogel A, Barnea B, et al: Subclinical rubella reinfection during pregnancy followed by transmission of virus to the fetus. J Infect 1997;34:273.
156. Robinson J, Lemay M, Vaudry WL: Congenital rubella after anticipated maternal immunity: Two cases and a review of the literature. Pediatr Infect Dis J 1994;13:812.
157. Mellinger AK, Cragan JD, Atkinson WL, et al: High incidence of congenital rubella syndrome after a rubella outbreak. Pediatr Infect Dis J 1995;14:573.
158. Miller E, Cradock-Watson JE, Pollock TM: Consequences of confirmed maternal rubella at successive stages of pregnancy. Lancet 1982;2:781.
159. Peckham CS: Clinical and laboratory study of children exposed in utero to maternal rubella. Arch Dis Child 1972;47:571.
160. Munro ND, Sheppard S, Smithells RW, et al: Temporal relations between maternal rubella and congenital defects. Lancet 1987;2:201.

161. Sever JL, South MA, Shaver KA: Delayed manifestations of congenital rubella. Rev Infect Dis 1985;7:S164.

162. Rawls WE, Phillips CA, Melnick JL, et al: Persistent virus infection in congenital rubella. Arch Ophthalmol 1967;77:430.

163. Ueda K, Nonaka S, Yoshikawa K, et al: Seroepidemiologic studies of rubella in Fukuoka in Southern Japan during 1965-1981: Rubella epidemic pattern, endemicity, and immunity gap. Int J Epidemiol 1983;12:450.

164. Bellini WJ, Icenogle JP: Measles and rubella viruses. In Murray PR, Baron EJ, Jorgensen JH, et al (eds): Manual of Clinical Microbiology, 8th ed. Washington, D.C., ASM Press, 2003, pp 1389-1403.

165. Bosma TJ, Corbett KM, Eckstein MB, et al: Use of PCR for prenatal and postnatal diagnosis of congenital rubella. J Clin Microbiol 1995;33:2881.

166. Meegan JM, Evans BK, Horstmann DM: Comparison of the latex agglutination test with the hemagglutination test, enzyme-linked immunosorbent assay, and neutralization test for detection of antibodies to rubella virus. J Clin Microbiol 1982;16:644.

167. Matter L, Gorgievski-Hrisoho M, Germann D: Comparison of four enzyme immunoassays for detection of immunoglobulin M antibodies against rubella virus. J Clin Microbiol 32:2134, 1994.

168. Best JM, O'Shea S, Tipples G, et al: Interpretation of rubella serology in pregnancy—pitfalls and problems. BMJ 2002;325:147.

169. Public Health Laboratory Service Working Party on Rubella: Studies of the effect of immunoglobulin on rubella in pregnancy. BMJ 1970;2:497.

170. Doege TC, Kim KSW: Studies of rubella and its prevention with immune globulin. JAMA 1967;200:104.

171. Bath SK, Singleton JA, Strikas RA, et al: Performance of US hospitals on recommended screening and immunization practices for pregnant and postpartum women. Am J Infect Control 2000; 28:327.

172. Polk BF, Modlin JF, White JA, De Girolami PC: A controlled comparison of joint reactions among women receiving one of two rubella vaccines. Am J Epidemiol 1982;115:19.

173. Revised ACIP recommendation for avoiding pregnancy after receiving a rubella-containing vaccine. MMWR Morb Mortal Wkly Rep 2001;50:1117.

Varicella-Zoster Virus

174. Longfield JN, Winn RE, Gibson RL, et al: Varicella outbreak in army recruits from Puerto Rico: Varicella susceptibility in a population from the tropics. Arch Intern Med 1990;150:970.

175. Preblud SR: Age-specific risks of varicella complications. Pediatrics 1981;68:14.

176. Centers for Disease Control and Prevention: Prevention of varicella: Recommendations of the Advisory Committee on Immunization Practices (ACIP). MMWR Recomm Rep 1996;45(RR-11):1-36.

177. Varicella-related deaths among adults—United States, 1997. MMWR Morb Mortal Wkly Rep 1997;46:409.

178. Chapman SJ: Varicella in pregnancy. Semin Perinatol 1998;22:339.

179. Brunell PA: Varicella in pregnancy, the fetus, and the newborn: Problems in management. J Infect Dis 1992;166(Suppl 1):S42.

180. Fairley CK, Miller E: Varicella-zoster virus epidemiology—a changing scene? J Infect Dis 1996;174(Suppl 3):S314.

181. Prober CG, Gershon AA, Grose C, et al: Consensus: Varicella-zoster infections in pregnancy and the perinatal period. Pediatr Infect Dis J 1990;9:865.

182. Harger JH, Ernest JM, Thurnau GR, et al: Risk factors and outcome of varicella-zoster virus pneumonia in pregnant women. J Infect Dis 2002;185:422.

183. Sauerbrei A, Wutzler P: The congenital varicella syndrome. J Perinatol 2000;20:548.

184. Laforet EG, Lynch CL Jr: Multiple congenital defects following maternal varicella: Report of a case. N Engl J Med 1947;236:534.

185. Higa K, Dan K, Manabe H: Varicella-zoster virus infections during pregnancy: Hypothesis concerning the mechanisms of congenital malformations. Obstet Gynecol 1987;69:214.

186. Enders G, Miller M, Cradock-Watson J, et al: Consequences of varicella and herpes zoster in pregnancy: Prospective study of 1739 cases. Lancet 1994;343:1548.

187. Balducci J, Rodis JF, Rosengren S, et al: Pregnancy outcome following first-trimester varicella infection. Obstet Gynecol 1992;79:5.

188. Pastuszak AL, Levy M, Schick B, et al: Outcome after maternal varicella infection in the first 20 weeks of pregnancy. N Engl J Med 1994;330:901.

189. Mogami S, Muto M, Mogami K, et al: Congenitally acquired herpes zoster infection in a newborn. Dermatology 1997;194:276.

190. Meyers JD: Congenital varicella in term infants: Risk reconsidered. J Infect Dis 1974;129:215.

191. van Der Zwet WC, Vandenbroucke-Grauls CM, van Elburg RM, et al: Neonatal antibody titers against varicella-zoster virus in relation to gestational age, birth weight, and maternal titer. Pediatrics 2002;109:79.

192. Miller E, Cradock-Watson JE, Ridehalgh MKS: Outcome in newborn babies given anti–varicella-zoster immunoglobulin after perinatal maternal infection with varicella-zoster virus. Lancet 1989;2:371.

193. Perez JL, Garcia A, Niubo J, et al: Comparison of techniques and evaluation of three commercial monoclonal antibodies for laboratory diagnosis of varicella-zoster virus in mucocutaneous specimens. J Clin Microbiol 1994;32:1610.

194. Landry ML, Ferguson D: Comparison of a latex agglutination test with enzyme-linked immunosorbent assay for detection of antibody to varicella-zoster virus. J Clin Microbiol 1993;31:3031.

195. Kustermann A, Zoppini C, Tassis B, et al: Prenatal diagnosis of congenital varicella infection. Prenat Diagn 1996;16:71.

196. Isada NB, Paar DP, Johnson MP, et al: In utero diagnosis of congenital varicella zoster virus infection by chorionic villus sampling and polymerase chain reaction. Am J Obstet Gynecol 1991;165:1727.

197. Mouly F, Mirlesse V, Meritet JF, et al: Prenatal diagnosis of fetal varicella-zoster virus infection with polymerase chain reaction of amniotic fluid in 107 cases. Am J Obstet Gynecol 1997;177:894.

198. Haake DA, Zakowski PR, Haake DL, et al: Early treatment of acyclovir for varicella pneumonia in otherwise healthy adults: Retrospective controlled study and review. Rev Infect Dis 1990;112:788.

199. Smego RA, Asperilla MO: Use of acyclovir for varicella pneumonia during pregnancy. Obstet Gynecol 1991;78:1112.

200. Koren G, Money D, Boucher M, et al: Serum concentrations, efficacy, and safety of a new, intravenously administered varicella zoster immune globulin in pregnant women. J Clin Pharmacol 2002;42:267.

201. Rouse DJ, Gardner M, Allen SJ, Goldenberg RL: Management of the presumed susceptible varicella (chickenpox)—exposed gravida: A cost-effectiveness/cost-benefit analysis. Obstet Gynecol 1996;87:932.

202. Gershon AA, Steinberg SP: National Institute of Allergy and Infectious Diseases Varicella Vaccine Collaborative Study Group. Live attenuated varicella vaccine: Protection in healthy adults compared with leukemic children. J Infect Dis 1990;161:661.

203. Salzman MB, Sharrar RG, Steinberg S, LaRussa P: Transmission of varicella-vaccine virus from a healthy 12-month-old child to his pregnant mother. J Pediatr 1997;131:151.

204. Unintentional administration of varicella virus vaccine—United States, 1996. MMWR Morb Mortal Wkly Rep 1996;45:1017.

205. Establishment of VARIVAX pregnancy registry. MMWR Morb Mortal Wkly Rep 1996;45:239.

Enteroviruses

206. Progress toward global poliomyelitis eradication, 1999. MMWR Morb Mortal Wkly Rep 2000;49:349.

207. Rotbart HA: Enteroviruses. In Richman DD, Whitley RJ, Hayden FG (eds): Clinical Virology, 2nd ed. Washington, D.C., ASM Press, 2002; pp 971-994.

208. Modlin JF: Perinatal echovirus infection: Insights from a literature review of 61 cases of serious infection and 16 outbreaks in nurseries. Rev Infect Dis 1986;8:918.

209. Reyes MP, Zalenski D, Smith F, et al: Coxsackievirus-positive cervices in women with febrile illnesses during the third trimester in pregnancy. Am J Obstet Gynecol 1986;155:159.

210. Nielsen JL, Berryman GK, Hankins GDV: Intrauterine fetal death and the isolation of echovirus 27 from amniotic fluid. J Infect Dis 1988;158:501.

211. Brown GC, Karunas RS: Relationship of congenital anomalies and maternal infection with selected enteroviruses. Am J Epidemiol 1971;95:207.

212. Sever JL, Huebner RJ, Costellano GA: Serologic diagnosis "en masse" with multiple antigens. Am Rev Respir Dis 1963;88:342.

213. Archer JS: Acute liver failure in pregnancy. A case report. J Reprod Med 2001;46:137.

214. Basso NGS, Fonseca MEF, Garcia AGP, et al: Enterovirus isolation from fetal and placental tissues. Acta Virol 1990;34:49.

215. Brady WK, Purdon A: Intrauterine fetal demise associated with enterovirus infection. South Med J 1986;79:770.

216. Chow KC, Lee CC, Lin TY, et al: Congenital enterovirus 71 infection: A case study with virology and immunohistochemistry. Clin Infect Dis 2000;31:509.

217. Landsman JB, Grist NR, Ross CAC: Echo 9 virus infection and congenital malformations. Br J Prev Soc Med 1964;18:152.

218. Rantasalo I, Penttinen K, Saxen L, Ojala A: Echo 9 virus antibody status after an epidemic period and the possible teratogenic effect of the infection. Ann Paediatr Fenn 1960;6:175.

219. Van den Veyver IB, Ni J, Bowles N, et al: Detection of intrauterine viral infection using the polymerase chain reaction. Mol Genet Metab 1998;63:85.

220. Euscher E, Davis J, Holzman I, Nuovo GJ: Coxsackie virus infection of the placenta associated with neurodevelopmental delays in the newborn. Obstet Gynecol 2001;98:1019.

221. Dahlquist GG, Ivarsson S, Lindberg B, Forsgren M: Maternal enteroviral infection during pregnancy as a risk factor for childhood IDDM. A population-based case-control study. Diabetes 1995;44:408.

222. Kleinman H, Prince JT, Mathey WE, et al: ECHO 9 virus infection and congenital abnormalities: A negative report. Pediatrics 1962;29:261.

223. Overall JC: Intrauterine virus infections and congenital heart disease. Am Heart J 1972;84:823.

224. Spector SA, Straube RC: Protean manifestations of perinatal enterovirus infections. West J Med 1983;138:847.

225. Nagington J, Wreghitt TG, Gandy G, et al: Fatal echovirus 11 infections in outbreak in special-care baby unit. Lancet 1978;2:725.

226. Abzug MJ, Levin MJ, Rotbart HA: Profile of enterovirus disease in the first two weeks of life. Pediatr Infect Dis J 1993;12:820.

227. Sauerbrei A, Gluck B, Jung K, et al: Congenital skin lesions caused by intrauterine infection with coxsackievirus B3. Infection 2000;28:326.

228. Rotbart HA, Kinsella JP, Wasserman RL: Persistent enterovirus infection in culture-negative meningoencephalitis—demonstration by enzymatic RNA amplification. J Infect Dis 1990;161:787.

229. Landry ML, Garner R, Ferguson D: Rapid enterovirus RNA detection in clinical specimens using nucleic acid sequence based amplification (NASBA). J Clin Microbiol 2003;41:346.

230. Pasic S, Jankovic B, Abinun M, et al: Intravenous immunoglobulin prophylaxis in an echovirus 6 and echovirus 4 nursery outbreak. Pediatr Infect Dis 1997;16:718.

231. Valduss D, Murray DL, Karna P, et al: Use of intravenous immunoglobulin in twin neonates with disseminated Coxsackie B1 infection. Clin Pediatr 1993;32:561.

Influenza Virus

232. Bridges CB, Harper SA, Fukuda K, et al: Prevention and control of influenza. Recommendations of the Advisory Committee on Immunization Practices (ACIP). MMWR Morb Mortal Wkly Rep 2003;52(RR-8):1.

233. Hayden FG, Palese P: Influenza virus. In Richman DD, Whitley RJ, Hayden FG (eds): Clinical Virology, 2nd ed. Washington, D.C., ASM Press, 2002, pp 891-920.

234. Harris JW: Influenza occurring in pregnant women: A statistical study of thirteen hundred and fifty cases. JAMA 1919;72:978.

235. Freeman DW, Barno A: Deaths from Asian influenza associated with pregnancy. Am J Obstet Gynecol 1959;78:1172.

236. Griffiths PD, Ronalds CJ, Heath RB: A prospective study of influenza infections during pregnancy. J Epidemiol Community Health 1980;34:124.

237. Ie S, Rubio ER, Alper B, Szerlip HM: Respiratory complications of pregnancy. Obstet Gynecol Surv 2002;57:39.

238. Irving WL, James DK, Stephenson T, et al: Influenza virus infection in the second and third trimesters of pregnancy: A clinical and seroepidemiological study. BJOG 2000;107:1282.

239. Neuzil KM, Reed GW, Mitchel EF, et al: Impact of influenza on acute cardiopulmonary hospitalizations in pregnant women. Am J Epidemiol 1998;148:1094.

240. Karkinen-Jaaskelainen M, Saxen L: Maternal influenza, drug consumption, and congenital defects of the central nervous system. Am J Obstet Gynecol 1974;118:815.

241. Monif GR, Sowards DL, Eitzman DV: Serologic and immunologic evaluation of neonates following maternal influenza infection during the second and third trimesters of gestation. Am J Obstet Gynecol 1972;114:239.

242. Hakosalo J, Saxen L: Influenza epidemic and congenital defects. Lancet 1971;2:1346.

243. Austin DF, Karp S, Dworsky R, et al: Excess leukemia in cohorts of children born following influenza epidemics. Am J Epidemiol 1975;101:77.

244. Randolph VL, Heath CW Jr: Influenza during pregnancy in relation to subsequent childhood leukemia and lymphoma. Am J Epidemiol 1974;100:399.

245. Brown AS, Susser ES: In utero infection and adult schizophrenia. Ment Retard Dev Disabil Res Rev 2002;8:51.

246. Sagrera X, Ginovart G, Raspall F, et al: Outbreaks of influenza A virus infection in neonatal intensive care units. Pediatr Infect Dis J 2002;21:196.

247. Steininger C, Holzmann H, Zwiauer KF, Popow-Kraupp T: Influenza A virus infection and cardiac arrhythmia during the neonatal period. Scand J Infect Dis 2002;34:782.

248. Cunney RJ, Bialachowski A, Thornley D, et al: An outbreak of influenza A in a neonatal intensive care unit. Infect Control Hosp Epidemiol 2000;21:449.

249. Habib-Bein NF, Beckwith WH III, Mayo D, Landry ML: Comparison of SmartCycler real-time reverse transcription–PCR assay in a public health laboratory with direct immunofluorescence and cell culture assays in a medical center for detection of influenza A virus. J Clin Microbiol 2003;41:3597.

250. Summary of the joint statement on thimerosal in vaccines. American Academy of Family Physicians, American Academy of Pediatrics, Advisory Committee on Immunization Practices, Public Health Service. MMWR Morb Mortal Wkly Rep 2000; 49:622.

251. Yeager DP, Toy EC, Baker B 3rd: Influenza vaccination in pregnancy. Am J Perinatol 1999;16:283.

252. Schrag SJ, Fiore AE, Gonik B, et al: Vaccination and perinatal infection prevention practices among obstetrician-gynecologists. Obstet Gynecol 2003;101:704.

253. Kirshon B, Faro S, Zurawin RK, et al: Favorable outcome after treatment with amantadine and ribavirin in a pregnancy complicated by influenza pneumonia: A case report. J Reprod Med 1988;33:399.

254. Kort BA, Cefalo RC, Baker VV: Fatal influenza A pneumonia in pregnancy. Am J Perinatol 1986;3:179.

Epstein-Barr Virus

255. Le CT, Chang S, Lipson MH: Epstein-Barr virus infections during pregnancy. Am J Dis Child 1983;137:466.

256. Fleischer GR, Bolognese R: Seroepidemiology of Epstein-Barr virus in pregnant women. J Infect Dis 1982;245:537.

257. Goldberg G, Fulginti V, Ray G: In utero Epstein-Barr virus (infectious mononucleosis) infection. JAMA 1981;246:1579.

258. Chang RS, Blankenship W: Spontaneous in vitro transformation of leukocytes from a neonate. Proc Soc Exp Biol Med 1973; 144:337.

259. Visintine AM, Gerber P, Nahmias AJ: Leukocyte transforming agent (Epstein-Barr virus) in newborn infants and older individuals. J Pediatr 1976;89:571.

260. Cart J, Didier J: Infections due to Epstein-Barr virus during pregnancy. J Infect Dis 1981;143:499.

261. Meyohas MC, Marechal V, Desire N, et al: Study of mother-to-child Epstein-Barr virus transmission by means of nested PCRs. J Virol 1996;70:6816.

262. Andiman WA: Epstein-Barr virus. In Schmidt NJ, Emmons RW (eds): Diagnostic Procedures for Viral, Rickettsial and Chlamydial Infections, 6th ed. Washington, D.C., American Public Health Association, 1989, pp 407-452.

Human T Cell Lymphotropic Virus Type I

263. Hollsberg P, Hafler DA: Pathogenesis of diseases induced by human lymphotropic virus type I infection. N Engl J Med 1993;328:1173.

264. Recommendations for counseling persons infected with human T-lymphotrophic virus, types I and II. Centers for Disease Control and Prevention and U.S. Public Health Service Working Group. MMWR Morb Mortal Wkly Rep 1993;42(RR-9):1.

265. Kusuhara K, Sonoda S, Takahashi K, et al: Mother-to-child transmission of human T-cell leukemia virus type I (HTLV-I): A fifteen year follow-up study in Okinawa, Japan. Int J Cancer 1987;40:755.
266. Otigbah C, Kelly A, Aitken C, et al: Is HTLV-I status another antenatal screening test that we need? Br J Obstet Gynaecol 1997;104:258.
267. Wiktor SZ, Alexander SS, Shaw GM, et al: Distinguishing between HTLV-I and HTLV-II by Western blot. Lancet 1990;335:153.
268. Takezaki T, Tajima K, Ito M, et al: Short-term breast-feeding may reduce the risk of vertical transmission of HTLV-I. Leukemia 1997;11(Suppl 3):60.
269. de The G, Bomford R: An HTLV-I vaccine: Why, how, for whom? AIDS Res Hum Retroviruses 1993;9:381.

Papillomavirus

270. Bonnez W: Papillomavirus. In Richman DD, Whitley RJ, Hayden FG (eds): Clinical Virology, 2nd ed. Washington, D.C., ASM Press, 2002, pp 557-596.
271. Ho GYF, Bierman R, Beardsley L, et al: Natural history of cervicovaginal papillomavirus infection in young women. N Engl J Med 1998;338:423.
272. Nobbenhuis MA, Helmerhorst TJ, van den Brule AJ, et al: High-risk human papillomavirus clearance in pregnant women: Trends for lower clearance during pregnancy with a catch-up postpartum. Br J Cancer 2002;87:75.
273. Chang-Claude J, Schneider A, Smith E, et al: Longitudinal study of the effects of pregnancy and other factors on detection of HPV. Gynecol Oncol 1996;60:355.
274. Human papillomavirus infection. In: Sexually transmitted diseases treatment guidelines 2002. Centers for Disease Control and Prevention. MMWR Morb Mortal Wkly Rep 2002;51(RR-6):53.
275. Puranen MH, Yliskoski MH, Saarikoski SV, et al: Vertical transmission of human papillomavirus from infected mothers to their newborn babies and persistence of the virus in childhood. Am J Obstet Gynecol 1996;174:694.
276. Puranen MH, Yliskoski MH, Saarikoski SV, et al: Exposure of an infant to cervical human papillomavirus infection of the mother is common. Am J Obstet Gynecol 1997;176:1039.
277. Shah K, Kashima H, Polk BF, et al: Rarity of cesarean delivery in cases of juvenile-onset respiratory papillomatosis. Obstet Gynecol 1986;68:795.
278. Egbert JE, Kersten RC: Female genital tract papillomavirus in conjunctival papillomas of infancy. Am J Ophthalmol 1997;123:551.
279. Watts DH, Koutsky LA, Holmes KK, et al: Low risk of perinatal transmission of human papillomavirus: Results from a prospective cohort study. Am J Obstet Gynecol 1998;178:365.
280. Wright TC Jr, Cox JT, Massad LS, et al: 2001 Consensus Guidelines for the management of women with cervical cytological abnormalities. JAMA 2002;287:2120.
281. Derkay CS: Task force on recurrent respiratory papillomatosis: A preliminary report. Arch Otolaryngol Head Neck Surg 1995;121:1386.
282. Kosko JR, Derkay CS: Role of cesarean section in prevention of recurrent respiratory papillomatosis—is there one? Int J Pediatr Otorhinolaryngol 1996;35:31.
283. Koutsky LA, Ault KA, Wheeler CM, et al: A controlled trial of a human papillomavirus type 16 vaccine. N Engl J Med. 347:1645, 2002.

Measles

284. Muller CP: Measles elimination: Old and new challenges? Vaccine 2001;19:2258.

285. Measles—United States, 2000. MMWR Morb Mortal Wkly Rep 2002;51:120.
286. Kamaci M, Zorlu CG, Belhan A: Measles in pregnancy. Acta Obstet Gynecol Scand 1996;75:307.
287. Eberhart-Phillips JE, Frederick PD, Baron RC, et al: Measles in pregnancy: A descriptive study of 58 cases. Obstet Gynecol 1993;82:797.
288. Lawrenson R, Farmer R: Measles, measles vaccination, and Crohn's disease. Age specific prevalences do not suggest association with in utero exposure. BMJ 1998;316:1746.
289. Helfand RF, Heath JL, Anderson LJ, et al: Diagnosis of measles with an IgM capture EIA: The optimal timing of specimen collection after rash onset. J Infect Dis 1997;175:195.
290. Libman MD, Behr MA, Martel N, Ward BJ: Rubella susceptibility predicts measles susceptibility: Implications for postpartum immunization. Clin Infect Dis 2000;31:1501.
291. Watson JC, Hadler SC, Dykewicz CA, et al: Measles, mumps, and rubella—vaccine use and strategies for elimination of measles, rubella, and congenital rubella syndrome and control of mumps: Recommendations of the Advisory Committee on Immunization Practices (ACIP). MMWR Recomm Rep 1998;47(RR-8):1.

Mumps

292. van Loon FP, Holmes SJ, Sirotkin BI, et al: Mumps surveillance—United States, 1988-1993. MMWR CDC Surveill Summ 1995;44(SS-3):1.
293. Mumps outbreaks in university campuses—Illinois, Wisconsin, South Dakota. MMWR Morb Mortal Wkly Rep 1987;36:496.
294. Ylinen O, Jarvinen PA: Parotitis during pregnancy. Acta Obstet Gynecol 1953;32:121.
295. Siegel M, Fuerst HT, Peress NS: Comparative fetal mortality in maternal virus diseases: A prospective study on rubella, measles, mumps, chickenpox and hepatitis. N Engl J Med 1966;274:768.
296. Garcia AG, Pereira JM, Vidigal N, et al: Intrauterine infection with mumps virus. Obstet Gynecol 1980;56:756.
297. Kurtz JB, Tomlinson AH, Pearson J: Mumps virus isolated from a fetus. BMJ 1982;284:471.
298. Kilham L: Mumps virus in human milk and in milk of infected monkey. JAMA 1951;78:1231.
299. Lacour M, Maherzi M, Vienny H, et al: Thrombocytopenia in a case of neonatal mumps infection: Evidence for further clinical presentations. Eur J Pediatr 1993;152:739.
300. Gersony WM, Katz SL, Nadas AS: Endocardial fibroelastosis and the mumps virus. Pediatrics 1966;37:430.
301. St. Geme JW, Noren GR, Adams P: Proposed embryopathic relation between mumps virus and primary endocardial fibroelastosis. N Engl J Med 1966;275:339.
302. Linde GA, Granstrom M, Orvell C: Immunoglobulin class and immunoglobulin G subclass enzyme-linked immunosorbent assays compared with microneutralization assay for serodiagnosis of mumps infection and determination of immunity. J Clin Microbiol 1987;25:1653.

Molluscum Contagiosum

303. Epstein WL: Molluscum contagiosum. Semin Dermatol 1992;11:184.
304. Smith MA, Singer C: Sexually transmitted viruses other than HIV and papillomaviruses. Urol Clin North Am 1992;19:47.
305. National guideline for the management of molluscum contagiosum. Clinical Effectiveness Group (Association of Genitourinary Medicine and the Medical Society for the Study of Venereal Diseases) Sex Transm Infect 1999;75(Suppl 1):S80.

18

PULMONARY DISEASES

Jess Mandel and Steven E. Weinberger

Pregnancy is associated with both mechanical and biochemical changes that may affect maternal respiratory function and gas exchange. Although it is clear that dyspnea may result from these changes even in women without prior lung disease, it does not automatically follow that women with preexisting lung disease are adversely affected by pregnancy or that the fetus necessarily suffers as a result of maternal lung disease. Consequently, the goal of this chapter is to analyze the effects of pregnancy on respiratory function and disease, as well as the effects of lung disease on pregnancy and the fetus. In addition, the potential adverse effects of drugs used to treat lung disease and of maternal cigarette smoking are discussed.

PHYSIOLOGIC CHANGES IN PREGNANCY AFFECTING THE RESPIRATORY SYSTEM

Mechanical and biochemical factors interact in the pregnant woman to produce the observed changes in respiratory function and gas exchange that are described subsequently. The most prominent of these factors appear to be the mechanical effect of the enlarging abdomen on diaphragmatic position and the effect of increased levels of circulating progesterone on ventilation. Other factors such as alterations in maternal corticosteroid and prostaglandin levels may also be important, particularly in women with underlying lung disease, but their role remains speculative at present.

Mechanical Changes

The enlarging uterus, which produces obvious changes in abdominal shape and size, also alters the resting position of the diaphragm and the configuration of the thorax.[1] In one early study of the mechanical changes during pregnancy, the diaphragm at rest rose to a level up to 4 cm above its usual resting position, and the chest enlarged in transverse diameter by up to 2.1 cm. Simultaneously, the subcostal angle progressively increased from an average of 68.5 degrees in early pregnancy to 103.5 degrees during the latter part of pregnancy.[2] However, the increase in uterine size could not entirely explain the observed changes in chest wall configuration, because the increase in subcostal angle occurred before it could be satisfactorily accounted for by mechanical pressure from the enlarging uterus. Abdominal enlargement and the high resting position of the diaphragm apparently do not impair diaphragmatic motion, which consistently has been increased in several studies quantifying diaphragmatic excursion with tidal breathing during pregnancy.[3-5,12]

Biochemical Changes

Progesterone and Estrogen

It is well established that serum progesterone levels rise gradually through the course of pregnancy, from approximately 25 ng/mL at 6 weeks to 150 ng/mL at term.[6,7] There is also a corresponding increase in urinary excretion of pregnanediol, the major metabolite of progesterone found in maternal urine.

The possibility that elevated progesterone levels in pregnancy influence ventilation was suggested by workers who first demonstrated that intramuscular administration of progesterone to normal subjects resulted in increased minute ventilation.[8] The subjects also exhibited a heightened ventilatory response to hypercapnia, which suggested that progesterone enhanced the sensitivity of the respiratory center to carbon dioxide. Pregnant women tested under the same conditions but without receiving exogenous progesterone demonstrated a similar increase in sensitivity to carbon dioxide inhalation, and the investigators concluded that their increased circulating level of progesterone was responsible for increased respiratory center sensitivity to carbon dioxide.

The mechanism of action of progesterone on ventilation is not entirely clear, although it appears that the effect is not mediated through either an increase in basal temperature or an increase in metabolic rate.[9] Together, several studies suggest that progesterone acts in a receptor-mediated manner to directly stimulate the central respiratory center, rather than by only altering its sensitivity to existing stimuli, as was previously believed.[10,11]

Although a role for progesterone in modulating the ventilatory changes in pregnancy has been well established since the 1940s, the contribution of estrogen to this response has been documented more recently. Early studies suggested that estrogen increased the "irritability" of the respiratory center to stimulation by progesterone, but the results were not consistently reproducible, and the mechanism by which this might occur was unclear. More recent data from studies with cats imply that estrogen acts through an estrogen receptor–mediated mechanism to induce increased central expression of progesterone receptors; this effect, when coupled with increased progesterone levels, results in a significantly increased ventilatory drive.[10,13]

Corticosteroids

Pregnancy is associated with a rise in plasma cortisol concentration, partly because of the increased corticosteroid-binding globulin levels observed during pregnancy. However, there is also an increase in metabolically active cortisol, as demonstrated by the twofold to threefold elevation of unbound cortisol levels over those found in nonpregnant women.[14-16] This normal hypercortisolism of pregnancy is related at least in part to the production of corticotropin-releasing hormone by the placenta.[17]

Presumably, the increase in endogenous corticosteroids has no clinically observable respiratory effects in normal women during pregnancy. However, it has been hypothesized that the alteration in corticosteroid concentrations may be responsible for the improvement in steroid-responsive pulmonary disease that is sometimes associated with pregnancy and for the exacerbations of autoimmune phenomena that are frequently observed as cortisol production decreases in the postpartum period.[18]

PULMONARY FUNCTION AND GAS EXCHANGE DURING PREGNANCY

Changes in the respiratory system during pregnancy can best be described by measurements of pulmonary function and gas exchange and by quantitation of ventilation.[19] Such data are available primarily from women without underlying lung disease, and the following discussion refers specifically to women without known respiratory disease. In situations in which data for specific lung diseases during pregnancy are available, they are discussed under the individual disease entities.

Lung Volumes

Lung volumes are routinely measured by a combination of spirometry and either inert gas dilution or body plethysmography.[20] Total lung capacity (TLC) is the total volume of gas present in the respiratory tract at the end of a maximal inspiration. When the patient exhales as completely as possible from TLC, the expired volume is the vital capacity (VC), and the volume remaining in the lungs after a maximal expiration is the residual volume (RV). At the resting position of the thorax (i.e., the position at the end of a normal expiration), the volume of gas within the lungs is called the functional residual capacity (FRC). If the patient then exhales from FRC down to RV, the volume that has been expired is called the expiratory reserve volume (ERV). A diagrammatic representation of these volumes is shown in Figure 18–1.

During pregnancy, the major factors that alter lung volumes appear to be the changes in diaphragmatic position and configuration of the chest wall. As mentioned previously, although the diaphragm during pregnancy is elevated in its resting position, diaphragmatic motion with respiration is unimpaired. In accordance with these roentgenographic observations, a decreased volume in the lungs would be expected at their resting position (FRC), whereas VC should be relatively preserved because

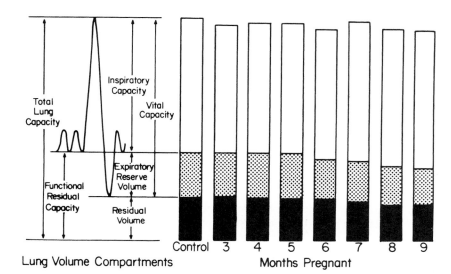

Figure 18–1. Serial measurements of lung volume compartments during pregnancy. (From Prowse CM, Gaensler EA: Respiratory and acid-base changes during pregnancy. Anesthesiology 1965;26:381.)

of normal movement of the diaphragm and thoracic musculature.

Measurements of lung volumes in a number of studies have generally confirmed these predictions, even though some variation may be found from study to study. In an extensive evaluation of pulmonary function in 19 normal women during pregnancy, lung volumes were found to be unchanged until the latter half of pregnancy, at which time a decrease in ERV and RV combined to produce an 18% mean decrease in FRC.[21] VC was unchanged, and therefore TLC (the sum of RV and VC) was slightly diminished at term.

Other studies have found a similar decrease in ERV in late pregnancy, with a range of values between 8% and 40% less than in nonpregnant control subjects. RV at term was also decreased by 7% to 22%, and thus the net effect of lower RV and ERV was a 9.5% to 25% diminution in FRC. Although minor changes in both directions have been observed for TLC and VC, the magnitude of these changes was sufficiently small to suggest they are probably of no clinical significance (see Fig. 18-1). In studies in which pulmonary function was monitored serially during pregnancy, the observed changes in RV and ERV were apparent after the fifth to sixth months of pregnancy and were progressive throughout the remainder of pregnancy.[21,22]

The decrease in FRC during pregnancy has the potential to adversely affect ventilation at the lung bases. As lung volume decreases during exhalation, small airways near the lung bases are subject to closure. In the healthy nonpregnant person, airway closure at the lung bases normally occurs between RV and FRC and is therefore not a problem during tidal breathing, when FRC is the smallest volume reached. However, if FRC decreases and no longer exceeds the closing capacity (the lung volume at which airways start to close), airway closure at the lung bases theoretically occurs during part of each respiratory cycle (i.e., whenever the volume in the lungs falls below closing capacity). Under these circumstances, ventilation to the lung bases decreases, ventilation/perfusion ratios in affected areas decrease, and arterial hypoxemia results.

Most studies agree that airway closure frequently occurs above FRC near the end of pregnancy,[23,24] which suggests that airway closure may occur during normal tidal breathing. Positioning of the subject is an important additional consideration. Because the diaphragm is higher when the subject is supine rather than sitting, FRC is lower, and airway closure is more likely to occur above FRC in the supine position than in the sitting position.[24]

In summary, because ERV and thus FRC decrease during pregnancy, airway closure during late pregnancy occurs either above FRC or closer to FRC than it does in the nonpregnant state. Although the significance of such changes has not been clearly proved, it has been suggested that airway closure near or above FRC can lower arterial oxygen tension as the result of a decrease in ventilation at the lung bases, and hence ventilation/perfusion ratios, in involved areas of lung. In addition, this tendency toward airway closure can complicate the clinical measurement of lung volumes by interfering with the uniform distribution of helium that gas dilution techniques require; for this reason, plethysmographic techniques should preferentially be used when lung volume measurements are indicated during the third trimester.[25]

Airway Function and Mechanics

Airway function is most commonly assessed by spirometry, with the absolute values and the ratio between the volume exhaled in the first second and the total volume exhaled on a forced expiratory breath from TLC to RV; this is expressed as forced expiratory volume in 1 second (FEV_1)/FVC. In numerous studies that have investigated forced expiratory flow rates during pregnancy, FEV_1 and FEV_1/FVC have been unchanged from values in nonpregnant subjects, which suggests that airway function is preserved during pregnancy.[21,22,26,27] Similarly, another measurement of airway function, the peak expiratory flow rate (PEFR), which is commonly used for monitoring asthmatic patients, does not change in normal women throughout pregnancy.[28]

Measurement of airway resistance is another method for assessing airway function, but the technique requires a body plethysmograph and is less readily available. The available studies of respiratory resistance performed during pregnancy have demonstrated either a decrease in airway resistance and the expected increase in its reciprocal, airway conductance,[29,30] or no change in airway conductance.[31] In an early study of pulmonary resistance, it was suggested that relaxation of airway smooth muscle occurs during pregnancy, possibly as a result of hormonal changes, but no direct proof is available for this theory.[32]

Lung compliance, a measurement of the "stiffness" of the lungs, can be determined by correlating changes in pleural pressure, measured indirectly by an esophageal balloon, with the associated changes in lung volume. In one study of 10 normal women during pregnancy, postpartum lung compliance was unchanged from that measured during the last trimester of pregnancy.[30] However, because of pressure exerted on the diaphragm by the enlarging uterus, chest wall compliance does decrease during pregnancy, leading to a decrease in overall respiratory system compliance (which reflects the combination of the lungs and the chest wall) late in pregnancy.[19]

Respiratory muscle function during pregnancy but before labor also appears to be unchanged, according to the finding that maximal inspiratory and expiratory pressures are not altered.[33] During labor, however, the strong expulsive efforts are associated with a subsequent decrease in maximal inspiratory pressure and an alteration in the electromyographic power spectrum of the diaphragm, which is suggestive of the development of transient acute diaphragmatic fatigue.[34] These studies of respiratory muscle function are potentially confounded by changes in diaphragmatic position and configuration during pregnancy and by difficulty obtaining reproducible effort immediately after delivery.

Diffusing Capacity

The diffusing capacity of the lung for carbon monoxide (DLCO) is a nonspecific test that measures the ability of carbon monoxide to diffuse from the alveolus into pulmonary capillary blood, where it combines with hemoglobin in the circulating red blood cells. The DLCO may be partitioned into its two separate determinants—a membrane component and a pulmonary capillary blood volume component—and abnormalities in the DLCO can generally be attributed to qualitative or quantitative changes in either the alveolar-capillary interface or pulmonary capillary blood volume. Some of the major disease categories in which DLCO is abnormal include emphysema, interstitial lung disease, and pulmonary vascular disease.

Early studies investigating DLCO in pregnancy found no change from values in nonpregnant women, and there was an appropriate increase in DLCO with exercise (over resting levels) in pregnant subjects.[35,36] When DLCO was partitioned into membrane and pulmonary capillary blood volume components, either no change or a slight decrease was found in the membrane component, whereas pulmonary capillary blood volume remained unaltered.[37] Again, there was no significant net effect on overall DLCO.

In a more extensive study in which serial changes were evaluated throughout pregnancy, an increase was found in single-breath DLCO during the first trimester.[39] This was followed by a decrease until approximately the 24th to 27th weeks, after which it remained constant until delivery. The postpartum DLCO was slightly but significantly greater than the value measured between 36 weeks and term. There is no apparent explanation for these minor changes, which appear to be of little clinical significance. The changes could not be attributed to any alterations in hemoglobin concentration, alveolar volume, or plasma 17β-estradiol levels during pregnancy.

In summary, DLCO during early pregnancy is generally unchanged or increased over control values in the same patients. Subsequently, there is a frequent decrease to a plateau during the latter half of pregnancy that is equivalent to or slightly less than the control value. The relative roles of alterations in membrane DLCO or pulmonary capillary blood volume in producing these changes are not entirely clear.

Ventilation, Oxygen Consumption, and Carbon Dioxide Production

In the early 1900s, several investigators observed that resting ventilation increases during pregnancy, and this finding has since been the most consistently demonstrated physiologic change in maternal respiration. Although oxygen consumption, carbon dioxide production, and basal metabolic rate are elevated during pregnancy, most studies indicate that the increment in minute ventilation is out of proportion to any increment in measures of maternal metabolism.[40] In one specific series, minute ventilation at term increased by 48% over the control level, whereas oxygen consumption and basal metabolic rate were augmented by only 21% and 14%, respectively (Fig. 18–2).[9] Subsequent studies confirmed that minute ventilation increases approximately 30% to 50% during pregnancy, with a corresponding 50% to 70% increase in alveolar ventilation.[19,40-44] The progressive rise in minute ventilation appears to start as early as 8 weeks of pregnancy.[9,19,45] An increase in tidal volume appears to be the major factor accounting for the increase in minute ventilation, whereas respiratory rate remains essentially unchanged throughout the course of pregnancy.[9,21,40,44]

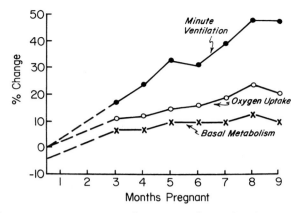

Figure 18–2. Time course of percentage changes in minute ventilation, oxygen uptake, and basal metabolism during pregnancy. (From Prowse CM, Gaensler EA: Respiratory and acid-base changes during pregnancy. Anesthesiology 1965;26:381.)

That the increase in minute ventilation usually exceeds that of oxygen consumption, carbon dioxide production, or metabolic rate suggests an additional factor must contribute to the genesis of hyperventilation in pregnancy. The currently accepted theory is based on the well-described stimulatory effect of progesterone on ventilatory drive, discussed in a previous section of this chapter. According to this theory, the elevated progesterone levels during pregnancy are responsible for the maternal hyperpnea that exceeds the change that can be attributed to increased metabolic rate.

Several investigators have also accumulated data on the physiologic response of minute ventilation and oxygen consumption to exercise during pregnancy,[46] and there is a similar augmentation of the ventilatory response in comparison with postpartum results.[47] During exercise, pregnant subjects increased ventilation and oxygen consumption by 38% and 15%, respectively, above the comparable levels with postpartum exercise.[42,43] Because the increment in minute ventilation exceeded the increase in oxygen consumption, the ventilatory equivalent, which is the ratio of minute ventilation to oxygen consumption, was significantly higher with antepartum than postpartum exercise.[41,48]

In summary, both at rest and with exercise, minute ventilation and, to a lesser extent, oxygen consumption and carbon dioxide production are increased during pregnancy over the nonpregnant control values. Although the increase in oxygen consumption and carbon dioxide production may account for part of the rise in minute ventilation, the respiratory stimulating effect of progesterone is probably the major factor explaining the disproportionate increase in minute ventilation over oxygen consumption observed during pregnancy.

Arterial Blood Gases and Acid-Base Status

A fall in arterial partial pressure of carbon dioxide (PCO_2) during pregnancy is a well-documented finding and is a consequence of the progesterone-induced increase in alveolar ventilation. Numerous studies have consistently demonstrated that maternal arterial P_{CO_2} generally falls to a plateau of 27 to 32 mm Hg,[1,49-54] but there is no general agreement about the time course of this change. Some investigators have observed a progressive serial decrease in alveolar and arterial P_{CO_2} starting early in pregnancy,[53-55] whereas others have noted that arterial P_{CO_2} remains at a low but constant level throughout pregnancy.[49,56] During labor, there is a further transient fall in arterial P_{CO_2} with each contraction; by the time that the cervix is fully dilated, the decrease in P_{CO_2} persists, even between contractions.[57]

As a consequence of the hyperventilation and respiratory alkalosis of pregnancy, renal excretion of bicarbonate secondarily increases, and the overall pH remains relatively intact. The loss of bicarbonate appears to be a compensatory phenomenon, and attempts to document a primary metabolic acidosis have been unsuccessful.[58] In most studies, the pH resulting from the respiratory alkalosis and metabolic compensation has been approximately 7.40 to 7.45,[49,51,56,58] although one series of 37 pregnant women reported a mean pH as high as 7.47.[53] Corresponding serum bicarbonate levels have decreased to 18 to 21 mEq/L, resulting in a base deficit of approximately 3 to 4 mEq/L.[49,52,53,56]

In studies in which maternal oxygenation has been monitored serially throughout pregnancy, mean values of arterial partial pressure of oxygen (P_{O_2}) have generally been increased, ranging from 106 to 108 mm Hg in the first trimester to 101 to 104 mm Hg in the third trimester.[49,56] It is important to note that interpretation of arterial P_{O_2} during pregnancy must include evaluation of arterial P_{CO_2}, because changes in arterial and alveolar P_{CO_2} are accompanied by changes in alveolar and hence arterial P_{O_2}. During pregnancy, low arterial P_{CO_2} is associated with a low alveolar P_{CO_2}, and the corresponding increase in alveolar P_{O_2} should thus result in an elevation of arterial P_{O_2}.

In order to evaluate whether maternal oxygenation is deranged during pregnancy, a more meaningful value than the arterial P_{O_2} is the alveolar-arterial P_{O_2} gradient. This gradient takes into account the effect of P_{CO_2} changes on arterial P_{O_2}, and any alterations in the gradient therefore truly reflect maternal gas exchange by the respiratory system. The alveolar-arterial P_{O_2} gradient has been reported as either unchanged[56] or slightly increased[59] during pregnancy. An increase in the gradient might be explained by hypothesizing that a decrease in FRC in late pregnancy contributes to airway closure, and thus a decreased P_{O_2}, as closing capacity approaches FRC.

Postural effects also appear to influence measured arterial P_{O_2} and the alveolar-arterial gradient during pregnancy. One group demonstrated a 13–mm Hg decrease in capillary P_{O_2} near term on changing from the sitting to supine position,[60] whereas another group noted an increase in the alveolar-arterial oxygen gradient from 14.3 to 20 mm Hg under similar conditions.[59] Although augmented effects of diaphragmatic pressure in the supine position may contribute to airway closure, it is not clear whether an additional role is played by caval compression and hemodynamic alterations.

Summary

Alterations in respiratory physiology occur during normal pregnancy, not only because of the obvious increase in abdominal girth but also because of the changing hormonal milieu that accompanies pregnancy. Although there may be some variability in pulmonary function tests from person to person, a distinct pattern of changes during pregnancy has emerged. The most apparent change in lung volumes is a decrease in FRC, the resting position of the lungs at the end of a normal expiration, caused primarily by elevation of the diaphragm by pressure from the enlarging uterus. This decrease in FRC, which occurs during the second half of pregnancy, is the net result of a decreased ERV and a lesser decrease in RV. Despite the alteration in resting diaphragmatic position, diaphragm excursion is unaffected, so that VC is preserved. TLC is generally either unchanged or decreased by a minor amount.

Airway function appears to be normal during pregnancy, as reflected by normal FEV_1 and FEV_1/FVC, normal PEFR, and by normal or even increased specific conductance. Respiratory muscle function is preserved during pregnancy, although transient acute diaphragmatic fatigue can follow the strong expulsive efforts of labor. DL_{CO} is frequently unchanged; however, an increase early in pregnancy and a decrease late in pregnancy have been observed in some patients.

Ventilatory changes are perhaps the most apparent alterations in respiratory physiology during pregnancy; resting minute ventilation increases by approximately 50% over postpartum control values. This hyperventilation, which is in excess of the observed changes in oxygen consumption or carbon dioxide production, is presumed to be a result of the respiratory stimulant effect of progesterone and is expressed primarily as an increased tidal volume with an unchanged respiratory frequency. As a result of the hyperventilation, arterial P_{CO_2} decreases during pregnancy, but metabolic compensation by renal excretion of bicarbonate partially offsets the expected pH change. Therefore, the net effect of the respiratory alkalosis and metabolic compensation is a slightly alkalotic pH in arterial blood.

As a result of the increased ventilation, not only does arterial (and hence alveolar) P_{CO_2} decrease but also alveolar (and therefore arterial) P_{O_2} increases. However, even though arterial P_{O_2} is generally elevated, the alveolar-arterial P_{O_2} gradient may be increased, especially near term, and may partially offset the increase in arterial P_{O_2} expected from hyperventilation. There is a further decrease in arterial P_{O_2} and an increase in the alveolar-arterial P_{O_2} gradient in the supine position, in comparison with the sitting position, in late pregnancy. Nevertheless, in patients without underlying pulmonary disease, these changes in arterial P_{O_2} appear to have little clinical significance.

EFFECTS OF ABNORMAL ARTERIAL BLOOD GASES ON THE FETUS

Because most pulmonary disorders affecting the pregnant woman can disturb maternal gas exchange (i.e., oxygenation and carbon dioxide elimination), it is important to consider the impact of altered maternal arterial blood gases on the fetus. According to theoretical models, an acute decrease in maternal arterial P_{O_2} to 70 mm Hg has relatively little effect on fetal gas exchange, whereas more significant maternal hypoxemia (to 50 mm Hg or less) can have significant effects on fetal P_{O_2}.[61] In one study involving very brief (10-minute) maternal exposure to 10% inspired oxygen during the third trimester, there were no detectable physiologic changes in the fetus, despite a mean decrease in oxygen saturation to 82%.[62]

A long-term decrease in maternal P_{O_2} to approximately 70 to 75 mm Hg, as seen at moderate altitude, is not associated with a significant decrease in fetal umbilical venous P_{O_2}.[63] However, a number of studies have indicated that birth weight is reduced in infants born to mothers at high altitude, which is suggestive of an effect of low maternal P_{O_2} on fetal growth.[64,65] On the basis of the data currently available, it seems reasonable to aim for a maternal P_{O_2} above 70 mm Hg to maintain a normal fetal umbilical venous P_{O_2}.

According to experimental data obtained in animals, alterations in maternal P_{CO_2} (probably acting by changing maternal pH) appear to have an effect on fetal oxygenation. Changes in uterine blood flow and a leftward shift of the maternal oxyhemoglobin dissociation curve are potential mechanisms by which these changes may be seen. In pigs, acute elevation of maternal P_{CO_2} decreases uterine vascular resistance, increases uterine blood flow, and increases the P_{O_2} of fetal umbilical venous blood.[66] Conversely, acute lowering of maternal P_{CO_2} in sheep is associated with decreased fetal umbilical venous P_{O_2}.[67,68] A similar relationship between maternal P_{CO_2} and fetal umbilical venous P_{O_2} has also been demonstrated in humans.[69] Consequently, acute respiratory disorders during pregnancy have the potential for adverse effects on fetal oxygenation not only because of a decrease in maternal P_{O_2} but also because of a respiratory alkalosis beyond that normally seen during pregnancy.

DYSPNEA OF PREGNANCY

It is well established that women often have dyspnea at some time during a normal pregnancy.[70] Consequently, dyspnea may erroneously suggest the development of lung disease, even when it is merely a result of the normal physiologic changes of pregnancy.

It has been stated that dyspnea may be expressed at some time during the course of pregnancy by as many as 60% to 70% of pregnant women.[9] In a 1953 series, the development of dyspnea was not correlated with changes in a number of pulmonary function tests, including maximal breathing capacity, VC, resting ventilation, breathing reserve, oxygen uptake, and subdivisions of TLC.[21]

When dyspnea occurs, it commonly commences during the first or second trimester,[71,72] before any significant increase in abdominal girth. In one study of dyspnea during normal pregnancy, it was found that the frequency increased from 15% in the first trimester to approximately 50% by 19 weeks and 75% by 31 weeks (Fig. 18-3).[73] By the last trimester, the severity of dyspnea was generally stable.

Although several mechanisms have been postulated to explain the dyspnea of pregnancy, the underlying pathophysiologic mechanism is still not entirely clear. The frequent onset in the first or second trimester suggests that mechanical factors do not play a significant role in its genesis, inasmuch as abdominal girth is often not yet appreciably increased. It has been postulated that dyspnea might be caused by a decrease in DL_{CO}, according to a finding that DL_{CO} differed between women who experienced dyspnea and those who did not.[74] However, the observed changes were small and are unlikely to serve as an adequate explanation for the symptom.

The most generally accepted theories to explain dyspnea of pregnancy are based on an unusual awareness of the hyperventilation that occurs with pregnancy.[70,75] It was suggested in 1953 that the newness of the sensation of hyperventilation might result in dyspnea, and a gradual acclimatization might explain the frequent improvement of the symptom as pregnancy progresses.[21] In a later study, the presence of dyspnea was correlated with a low P_{CO_2} during pregnancy, but the women most likely to experience dyspnea were those who had relatively high nonpregnant values for P_{CO_2}.[72] These investigations therefore suggested that the marked change in P_{CO_2} to a particularly unfamiliar low level might account for the observed symptoms. Other studies have shown that patients who experienced dyspnea appeared to have a greater

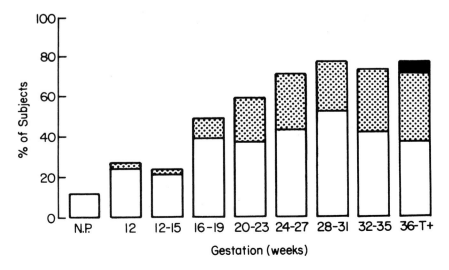

Figure 18-3. Incidence, time course, and severity of dyspnea during normal pregnancy. *White areas* denote dyspnea present on climbing hills or more than one flight of stairs; *dotted areas* denote dyspnea present on climbing one flight of stairs, walking at an even pace on level ground, or during routine performance of housework; *black areas* denote dyspnea on slightest exertion or at rest. N.P., not pregnant. (From Milne JA: The respiratory response to pregnancy. Postgrad Med J 1979;55:318.)

ventilatory response to inhaled carbon dioxide[71,76] and to hypoxia[77] than did those who did not experience dyspnea. Therefore, a number of studies point to a relationship between dyspnea of pregnancy and increased ventilation, decreased PCO_2, and increased ventilatory responsiveness, which perhaps suggests that dyspnea of pregnancy is caused by increased ventilatory drive and a level of ventilation that is inappropriately high for the demand.[78]

Dyspnea of pregnancy is a diagnosis of exclusion. Dyspnea that is acute and severe, is progressive and intractable, or leads to curtailment of daily activities is generally more likely to be secondary to demonstrable cardiac or pulmonary disease.[70]

SPECIFIC DISEASES

Asthma

Definition and Cause

Asthma is one of several specific disease entities included in the general category of obstructive lung disease, which is characterized by limitation of airflow that is generally more marked during expiration than inspiration. In asthma, the obstruction is a reversible process caused by airway inflammation and increased responsiveness of the airways to a variety of stimuli. The airway response to these stimuli includes contraction of bronchial smooth muscle, mucus hypersecretion, and mucosal edema, all of which contribute to the pathophysiologic process of reversible airway obstruction characteristic of this disease.

Although reversible airway narrowing is the final common pathway in patients with asthma, it is still not clear what underlying abnormality distinguishes the asthmatic patient from his or her normal counterpart. For a number of years, interest has focused on airway inflammation as a primary feature in the pathogenesis of asthma. Inflammation, release of inflammatory mediators, and disruption of the epithelial barrier on the mucosal surface of the airway are now thought to be important factors underlying airway hyperresponsiveness and episodic smooth muscle constriction. This emphasis on airway inflammation has important implications for the current approach to asthma therapy.

The well-recognized and common association of asthma with a history of atopy and elevated immunoglobulin E (IgE) levels also suggests a link between asthma and allergic factors. In such cases, particularly when there is a strong personal or family history of allergies, the patient has been sensitized to specific allergens and has corresponding antibodies of the IgE class. Exposure to the allergen then results in an antigen-antibody complex bound primarily to mast cells, inducing airway inflammation and release of a variety of humoral mediators, including histamine, leukotrienes, eosinophil chemotactic factor of anaphylaxis, and platelet-activating factor. These and other humoral mediators have several adverse effects, including stimulation of irritant receptors, constriction of bronchial smooth muscle, recruitment of more inflammatory cells, and an increase in vascular permeability.

Disease in the Nonpregnant State

Asthma is a relatively common disorder that affects approximately 3% to 5% of the population. Although the onset is most commonly in childhood, the disease can occur at any age, and it is therefore a common problem in women of childbearing age.

The classic symptoms during an exacerbation of asthma are dyspnea, cough, and wheezing. Although specific inciting events, such as allergen exposure or a respiratory tract infection, may be identified for a particular exacerbation, it is common for the patient to present with symptoms but no clear precipitating factor. It has also been recognized that cough may be the sole presenting feature of asthma,[79] and the diagnosis may be missed in such patients if investigation for reversible airway obstruction is not specifically pursued.

Common physical findings during an exacerbation include diffuse wheezing and evidence of hyperinflation, such as increased anteroposterior diameter and hyperresonance of the thorax to percussion. The presence of a pulsus paradoxus and the use of accessory muscles of respiration indicate severe airflow obstruction, whereas the amount of wheezing is not correlated with the severity of an exacerbation. In fact, wheezing may sometimes diminish with worsening airflow obstruction if airway diameter is critically reduced and there is insufficient airflow to generate a wheeze.

Pulmonary function tests during an exacerbation demonstrate abnormal expiratory flow rates, including depressed FEV_1, FVC, and FEV_1/FVC ratio. Arterial blood gases most frequently reveal hypoxemia (decreased PO_2) and respiratory alkalosis (decreased PCO_2 with increased pH). Normalization or elevation of the PCO_2 is an ominous finding, generally indicative of severe obstruction and an FEV_1 less than 20% of the predicted value. Even when the patient improves with treatment of an asthmatic exacerbation, the disappearance of symptoms and even signs is not a sensitive indicator of clinical status, because pulmonary function abnormalities are still frequently present at this stage.

Asthma in Pregnancy

In view of the frequency of asthma in the general population, it is probably the most common form of lung disease encountered during pregnancy.[80-84] Several studies have investigated the natural history of asthma in pregnancy, and although there are minor differences in the results, most data suggest that the course of asthma during pregnancy is variable. In a review of more than 1000 cases reported in nine studies, maternal asthma during pregnancy was found to be unchanged in 49%, improved in 29%, and worse in 22%.[84] In a more recent study of 366 pregnancies monitored prospectively in 330 asthmatic women, asthma worsened during pregnancy in 35%, improved in 28%, and was unchanged in 33% of women; 4% of women were uncertain about a change.[85] Further analysis from this study provided several additional conclusions: (1) In general, asthma was less frequent and less severe during the last 4 weeks of pregnancy than during other periods of the pregnancy; (2) when asthma improved during pregnancy, improvement was gradual as the pregnancy progressed; (3) when asthma worsened during pregnancy, symptoms increased primarily in the period between the 29th and 36th weeks; (4) the course of asthma in an individual patient tends to be similar during successive pregnancies; and (5) labor and delivery are not associated with worsening of asthma.

In a prospective study of asthmatic women of childbearing age who became pregnant, airway responsiveness to methacholine, which is a measure of airway hyperresponsiveness, improved during pregnancy.[86] Although the investigators thought that this decrease in airway smooth muscle contractility might be caused by progesterone, they were unable to correlate changes in responsiveness with levels of progesterone.

It has been suggested that the severity of asthma is an important factor predictive of the likelihood of deterioration during pregnancy,[87,88] but other data to refute this association have also been presented.[89] In one study of 210 patients, those with mild asthma were unlikely to have further problems during pregnancy, whereas 44% of those with severe asthma experienced worsening of the disease during pregnancy.[88] In another study of 47 patients during pregnancy, the patients were divided into categories by severity, although objective measurements were not made.[87] Overall, the condition in 43% of the patients remained unchanged, whereas in 43% it was worse and in 14% better. In general, patients with severe asthma before pregnancy were more likely to experience worsening, whereas those with mild asthma tended to experience no change. Preliminary data from this study suggested that patients with increased or unchanged IgE levels during pregnancy tended to have exacerbations of their disease, whereas those with a decrease in IgE levels frequently experienced improvement. In contrast to the aforementioned studies, Schatz and Hoffman[89] found that the prepregnancy severity of asthma was not reliably predictive of the course of asthma during pregnancy. They also found no relationship between the course of asthma and IgE levels during pregnancy.

Several interacting factors have been postulated to account for changes in the course of asthma during pregnancy, although the relative importance of any of these factors is unclear.[87,89] An increase in circulating free cortisol, a decrease in plasma histamine, and a decrease in bronchomotor tone and airway resistance (possibly caused by progesterone) could each contribute to improvement in the frequency and severity of asthma exacerbations during pregnancy. Conversely, increased levels of progesterone and mineralocorticoids, which compete for glucocorticoid receptors, an increased incidence of viral respiratory infections or bacterial sinusitis, increased levels of prostaglandin F_{2a}, increased gastroesophageal reflux, and hyperventilation could provoke exacerbations or an increase in symptoms. The unpredictable course of asthma during pregnancy makes it especially difficult to quantitate the role of these or other factors in any given patient.

One study found that asthma exacerbations occurring during pregnancy were not uniformly distributed over time throughout the duration of pregnancy but rather were most common between 17 and 24 weeks of pregnancy.[90] In the same study, failure to use inhaled antiinflammatory therapy during pregnancy was strongly associated with an increased likelihood of an acute asthmatic exacerbation. Of asthmatic women receiving inhaled antiinflammatory therapy from the start of pregnancy, only 4% subsequently experienced an acute asthma exacerbation, in comparison with 17% of those women not initially taking inhaled corticosteroids.

The effect of asthma on the outcome of pregnancy has also been examined in some of the previously mentioned studies as well as others. No significant increase in prematurity or spontaneous abortion, in comparison with control subjects, was documented in a 1961 series[91]; the few patients who had severe asthmatic exacerbations during pregnancy did not go into premature labor. In a 1970 study, complications and fetal morbidity or mortality in 277 pregnancies were assessed in asthmatic women in comparison with a control group with more than 30,000 deliveries.[92] These investigators found an approximately twofold (5.9% vs. 3.2%) increase in incidence of perinatal mortality in infants born to asthmatic mothers in comparison with control subjects, although no significantly increased risk of prematurity was observed. Fetal morbidity and mortality were problems, especially when maternal asthma was severe; in this latter group, there was a particularly high incidence of perinatal mortality or neurologic abnormality at 1 year of age.

More recently, analysis of large databases from Sweden, New Jersey, and Canada has suggested that pregnancies of asthmatic women continue to carry a small but significantly higher risk of complications such as perinatal mortality, preeclampsia, preterm birth, low birth weight outcomes, and congenital anomalies.[93-96] These risks should be discussed frankly with the asthmatic woman who is planning pregnancy, but it should also be emphasized that perinatal outcomes are uncomplicated in most cases and that good control of asthma during pregnancy is thought to ameliorate some of the risk.[97]

Several studies have investigated the relationship between the outcome of pregnancy and the severity of asthma. In one study investigating perinatal outcome in women with asthma, preterm delivery, premature rupture of membranes, and low birth weight were all found more frequently with pregnancy complicated by asthma than in a control population.[98] When the asthmatic patients were separated into steroid-dependent and non–steroid-dependent groups (as a way to distinguish patients with more severe asthma from those with less severe asthma, respectively), all these differences were observed for each subgroup in comparison with a control group. In addition, the steroid-dependent subgroup had a higher frequency of preterm delivery and infants with low birth weight than did the non–steroid-dependent subgroup, which was suggestive of a possible correlation of these complications with asthma severity. Another study[99] similarly found a small but statistically significant correlation between infant birth weight and maternal FEV_1, which was also suggestive of a relationship between asthma severity and infant birth weight.

Three other studies that investigated the use of oral and inhaled corticosteroids found no increase in fetal or maternal morbidity and mortality associated with relatively severe maternal asthma.[80,100,101] In one of these studies,[100] the mean birth weight of infants was approximately

500 g less when the mothers required hospitalization for status asthmaticus than when no emergency therapy for asthma was required during pregnancy. In a total of 171 pregnancies in 146 patients in these three series, no fetal or maternal deaths attributable to asthma were reported. It is now generally accepted that adequate therapy and good control of asthma during pregnancy, including use of corticosteroids when necessary, are critical for minimizing complications during pregnancy.

In summary, there is no predictable effect of pregnancy on asthma, because individual patients may experience improvement, no change, or worsening. However, as a general rule, the course of asthma in a particular individual tends to be similar with successive pregnancies. In older studies, the major documented effect of asthma on the course of pregnancy was an approximately twofold increase in perinatal mortality, particularly when maternal asthma was severe. On the basis of the most recent studies, in which corticosteroid therapy was used for severe asthma, it is now accepted that adequate control of asthma during pregnancy reduces the increase in mortality reported in

earlier studies.[82,89] Other suggested complications, such as increased frequencies of prematurity and low birth weight, may also be reduced by adequate asthma control.

Treatment

The treatment of asthma has been discussed in detail in several reviews,[102,103] and specific drugs are summarized in Table 18–1. Although bronchodilators were for many years the primary form of therapy for asthma, emphasis has shifted to the earlier use of antiinflammatory agents such as inhaled corticosteroids and cromolyn. For outpatient treatment of occasional mild asthma exacerbations, inhaled β agonists are often sufficient and remain the mainstay of therapy. These agents activate adenylyl cyclase and therefore increase intracellular cyclic adenosine monophosphate (cAMP), which has a bronchodilator effect through action on airway smooth muscle cells and an inhibitory effect on release of mediators from mast cells.

The inhaled β agonists used most frequently on an as-needed basis are those that are β_2 selective and whose

TABLE 18–1 | **Drug Therapy for Asthma**

Category	Specific Examples	Dosage	Pregnancy Class	Comments
Bronchodilators				
β agonists inhaled				Preferred form of administration of β-agonists
Short-acting (rescue)	Albuterol	2 puffs q4-6h PRN	C	
	Metaproterenol	2 puffs q4-6h PRN	C	
	Terbutaline	2 puffs q4-6h PRN	B	
	Pirbuterol	2 puffs q4-6h PRN	C	
Long-acting (maintenance)	Salmeterol	2 puffs b.i.d. (metered-dose inhaler) or 1 puff b.i.d. (diskus)	C	Should not be used PRN
Subcutaneous	Epinephrine	0.3 mL, 1:1000 SC	C	Alternative to inhaled administration for acute therapy; epinephrine should ideally be avoided during pregnancy
	Terbutaline	0.25 mL, SC	B	Same as for epinephrine
Oral	Albuterol	2-4 mg PO t.i.d.	C	Infrequently used because of systemic side effects
	Terbutaline	2.5-5 mg PO t.i.d.	B	Same as for albuterol
Xanthines	Theophylline (slow-release)	Variable (200-500 mg b.i.d.)	C	Dosage adjusted to maintain serum level 5-15 µg/mL
Antiinflammatory agents				
Corticosteroids		Variable, dependent on preparation (divided b.i.d.-q.i.d.)		Rinse and gargle after use to decrease risk of oral candidiasis
Inhaled	Beclomethasone		C	
	Triamcinolone		C	
	Flunisolide		C	
	Fluticasone		C	
	Budesonide		B	
Oral	Prednisone	Variable (taper from initial dose of 40-60 mg)	B	
Mast cell stabilizers	Cromolyn	2 puffs q.i.d.	B	
	Nedocromil	2 puffs q.i.d.	B	
Agents affecting leukotrienes				
LTD₄ receptor blocker	Zafirlukast	20 mg b.i.d.	B	Must be taken 1 hr before or 2 hr after meals
	Montelukast	10 mg q.d.	B	Dose is given in the evening
5-Lipoxygenase inhibitor	Zileuton	600 mg q.i.d.	C	Can cause abnormal liver function test results

LTD$_4$, leukotriene D$_4$; PO, per os (orally); PRN, pro re nata (as needed); SC, subcutaneously.

actions last for several hours, such as albuterol. Salmeterol and formoterol, which have a duration of action of approximately 12 hours, can be used twice a day on a regular basis or at night for control of nocturnal asthma, but their slower onset and longer duration of action make them inappropriate for use on an as-needed basis.

Because adequate delivery of the medication is dependent on proper use of the inhaler, the technique of inhalation should be demonstrated to the patient. For patients who have difficulty with the proper coordination of inspiration and actuation of the inhaler, use of a spacer (e.g., Inspirease, Aerochamber) or a dry powder drug preparation may be helpful. In the acute setting, subcutaneous epinephrine or terbutaline can be given, particularly to patients unable to use an inhaled form of β agonist effectively.

Patients whose asthma cannot be controlled adequately with infrequent (several times per week) use of a β agonist inhaler should generally be started on an inhaled antiinflammatory agent (either an inhaled corticosteroid or a mast cell stabilizer) or a drug affecting leukotriene metabolism. These agents do not have bronchodilator activity and are not useful for treatment of acute exacerbations. Rather, they are used on a regular basis as preventive agents and can then be supplemented with inhaled β agonists on an as-needed basis. Inhaled corticosteroids such as beclomethasone, triamcinoline, flunisolide, budesonide, and fluticasone are used to suppress airway inflammation and have now become first-line therapy for patients with moderate or severe asthma. Potential side effects include oropharyngeal candidiasis and hoarseness. Systemic side effects are absent or minimal except at very high dosages.

Inhaled cromolyn and nedocromil are also used for their antiinflammatory effect, which generally has been ascribed to inhibition of mediator release from mast cells. Either agent is most useful on a regular basis for patients whose asthma is triggered by exposure to inhaled allergens, but both are also often effective for prophylactic use before exercise in patients with exercise-induced asthma.

The newest groups of antiinflammatory agents in asthma are those targeted toward blocking the synthesis or action of leukotrienes.[104] Currently available agents include zafirlukast and montelukast (leukotriene D_4 antagonists) and zileuton (an inhibitor of the enzyme 5-lipoxygenase). Although these agents are typically used for mild to moderate asthma, their role in comparison with that of inhaled corticosteroids is not entirely clear. Their efficacy is generally less than that of inhaled corticosteroids, but this may be outweighed by improved compliance with therapy in patients who are unable or unwilling to use inhaled corticosteroids regularly.[105]

Xanthine bronchodilators such as theophylline have traditionally been thought to act by inhibition of phosphodiesterase leading to increased cAMP, but this mechanism has now been questioned. Theophylline is now used less frequently as a primary agent in asthma; instead, patients whose asthma is not adequately controlled with infrequent inhaled β agonists are preferentially treated with inhaled corticosteroids. However, the slowest release preparations of theophylline, when taken in the evening, are often useful for managing nocturnal asthma. The major side effects of xanthines are gastrointestinal symptoms

(nausea, vomiting, diarrhea) or nervousness, and toxic levels may result in cardiac arrhythmias or seizures.

For severe exacerbations or for patients not responding rapidly to acute bronchodilator therapy, a course of oral (or parenteral) corticosteroids is indicated. As the dosage of systemic steroids is tapered, treatment is often converted to inhaled steroids for maintenance outpatient therapy. For patients with refractory disease, oral steroids may need to be maintained at a low to moderate daily or alternate-day dose, although the toxic effects of the drug make this an option of last resort.

Management in Pregnancy

Management of the asthmatic patient during pregnancy has been discussed in several review articles[80,97,103,106] and in the Report of the Working Group on Asthma and Pregnancy of the National Asthma Education Program.[83] Objective measurements of lung function should be monitored during pregnancy as a guide to the need for and the effectiveness of therapy. Although measurement of FEV_1 by spirometry is useful during office visits, measurement of PEFR with a portable peak flow meter has the advantage of allowing ongoing home monitoring during pregnancy. Worsening of PEFR from baseline indicates that the therapeutic regimen may need to be intensified.

Because of the absence of potentially deleterious side effects, nonpharmacologic regimens—avoidance of allergic and nonallergic triggering factors—should be the first form of therapy for asthma during pregnancy.[107] Depending on a given patient's triggering factors, measures such as cockroach elimination; removal of pets; or the use of barriers, heat treatment, or regulation of humidity to decrease dust mite exposure may be indicated.

Fortunately, medications currently used for asthma are generally well tolerated during pregnancy and appear to be safe for the fetus; therefore, the management of asthma in the pregnant woman differs little from management in the nonpregnant patient.[108,109] It is also widely accepted that the risk to the fetus is higher as a result of poorly controlled asthma than as a result of any of the drugs that are necessary to gain optimal control. Nevertheless, it is important to be aware of available data regarding use of each of these drugs in the pregnant woman. The overall approach to chronic asthma therapy during pregnancy, stratified according to the severity of asthma, is summarized in Figures 18-4 to 18-6, taken from the Report of the Working Group on Asthma and Pregnancy of the National Asthma Education Program.[83]

β Agonist bronchodilators appear to be relatively safe during pregnancy, although some potential effects on the uterus and fetus must be considered. Several studies have examined how systemic administration of sympathomimetic drugs affects uterine blood flow. A radiographic study in monkeys has shown vasoconstrictive effects of epinephrine on the uteroplacental circulation,[110] but the intraarterial mode of administration in that study makes it difficult to attribute any clinical applicability to this finding. On the other hand, uterine blood flow appears to be preserved or even enhanced after administration of terbutaline.[111,112] Intravenous infusion of albuterol initially causes a decrease in uteroplacental blood flow,[113]

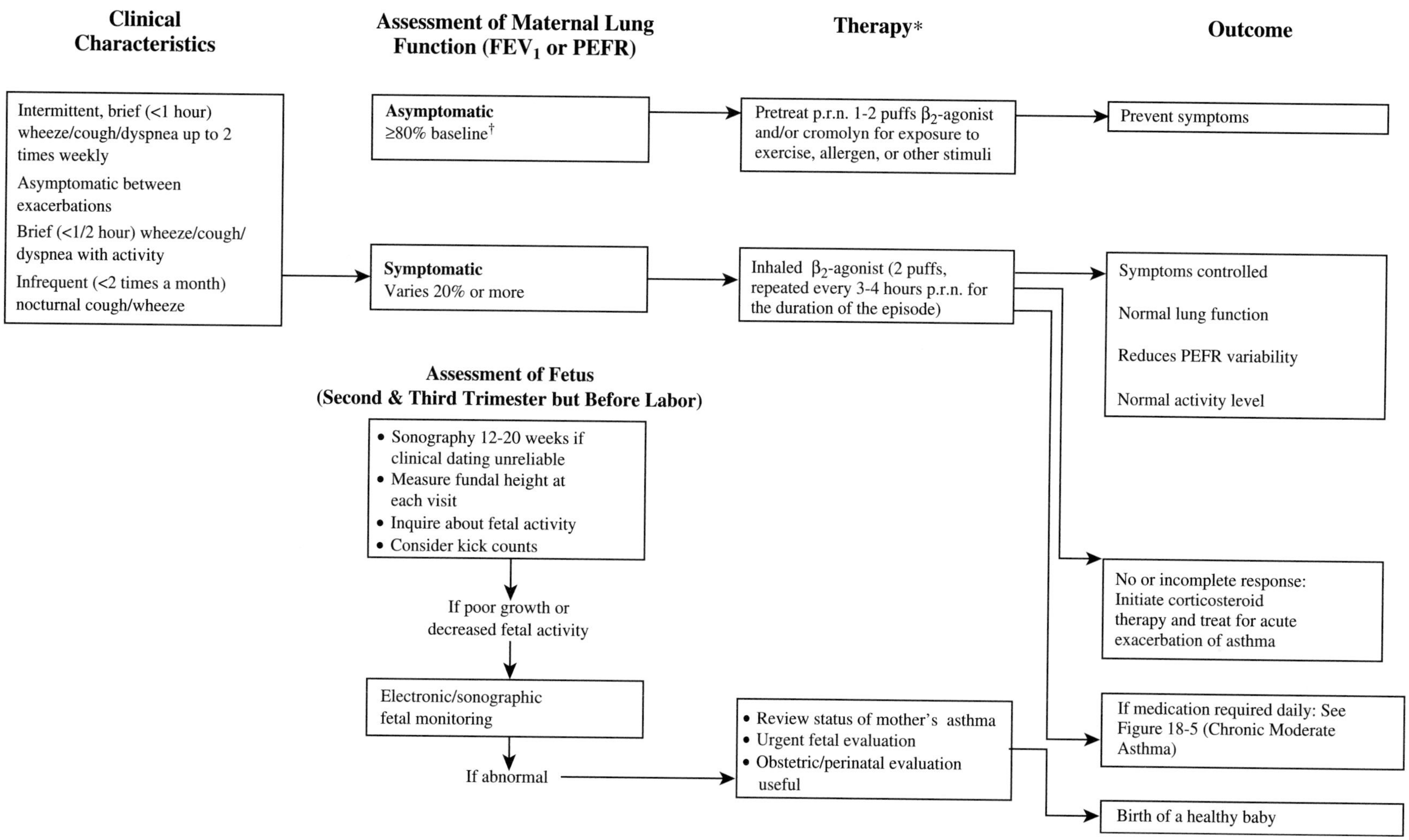
Clinical Characteristics
Assessment of Maternal Lung Function (FEV_1 or PEFR)
Therapy*
Outcome
Intermittent, brief (<1 hour) wheeze/cough/dyspnea up to 2 times weekly
Asymptomatic between exacerbations
Brief (<1/2 hour) wheeze/cough/dyspnea with activity
Infrequent (<2 times a month) nocturnal cough/wheeze
Asymptomatic
≥80% baseline†
Pretreat p.r.n. 1-2 puffs β_2-agonist and/or cromolyn for exposure to exercise, allergen, or other stimuli
Prevent symptoms
Symptomatic
Varies 20% or more
Inhaled β_2-agonist (2 puffs, repeated every 3-4 hours p.r.n. for the duration of the episode)
Symptoms controlled
Normal lung function
Reduces PEFR variability
Normal activity level
No or incomplete response: Initiate corticosteroid therapy and treat for acute exacerbation of asthma
If medication required daily: See Figure 18-5 (Chronic Moderate Asthma)
Assessment of Fetus
(Second & Third Trimester but Before Labor)
• Sonography 12-20 weeks if clinical dating unreliable
• Measure fundal height at each visit
• Inquire about fetal activity
• Consider kick counts
If poor growth or decreased fetal activity
Electronic/sonographic fetal monitoring
If abnormal
• Review status of mother's asthma
• Urgent fetal evaluation
• Obstetric/perinatal evaluation useful
Birth of a healthy baby

* All therapy must include patient education about prevention (including environmental control as appropriate) as well as control of symptoms.

† PEFR percent baseline refers to the norm for the individual, established by the clinician. This may be percent predicted based on standardized norms or percent of patient's personal best.

Figure 18–4. Flowchart outlining management of patients with chronic mild asthma during pregnancy. FEV_1, forced expiratory volume in 1 second; PEFR, peak expiratory flow rate; p.r.n., according to circumstances. (From National Asthma Education Program: Report of the Working Group on Asthma and Pregnancy. Management of asthma during pregnancy [NIH publication no. 93-3279A]. Bethesda, Md., National Institutes of Health, 1993.)

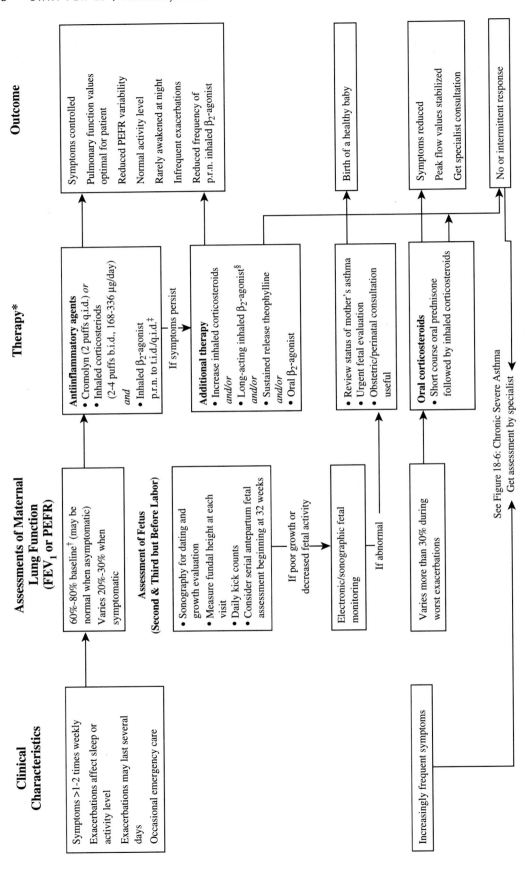

Clinical Characteristics

Symptoms >1-2 times weekly

Exacerbations affect sleep or activity level

Exacerbations may last several days

Occasional emergency care

Increasingly frequent symptoms

Assessments of Maternal Lung Function (FEV₁ or PEFR)

60%-80% baseline† (may be normal when asymptomatic)
Varies 20%-30% when symptomatic

Assessment of Fetus (Second & Third but Before Labor)

• Sonography for dating and growth evaluation
• Measure fundal height at each visit
• Daily kick counts
• Consider serial antepartum fetal assessment beginning at 32 weeks

If poor growth or decreased fetal activity

Electronic/sonographic fetal monitoring

If abnormal

Varies more than 30% during worst exacerbations

See Figure 18-6: Chronic Severe Asthma
Get assessment by specialist

Therapy*

Antinflammatory agents
• Cromolyn (2 puffs q.i.d.) *or*
• Inhaled corticosteroids (2-4 puffs b.i.d., 168-336 µg/day)
and
• Inhaled β₂-agonist p.r.n. to t.i.d./q.i.d.‡

If symptoms persist

Additional therapy
• Increase inhaled corticosteroids
and/or
• Long-acting inhaled β₂-agonist§
and/or
• Sustained release theophylline
and/or
• Oral β₂-agonist

• Review status of mother's asthma
• Urgent fetal evaluation
• Obstetric/perinatal consultation useful

Oral corticosteroids
• Short course oral prednisone followed by inhaled corticosteroids

Outcome

Symptoms controlled
Pulmonary function values optimal for patient
Reduced PEFR variability
Normal activity level
Rarely awakened at night
Infrequent exacerbations
Reduced frequency of p.r.n. inhaled β₂-agonist

Birth of a healthy baby

Symptoms reduced
Peak flow values stabilized
Get specialist consultation

No or intermittent response

*All therapy must include patient education about prevention (including environmental control as appropriate) as well as control of symptoms.
†PEFR percent baseline refers to norm for the individual, established by the clinician. This may be percent predicted based on standardized norms or percent of patient's personal best.
‡If exceed 3-4 doses a day, consider additional therapy other than inhaled β₂-agonist.
§Added by authors to original flow chart.

Figure 18–5. Flowchart outlining management of patients with chronic moderate asthma during pregnancy. FEV₁, forced expiratory volume in 1 second; PEFR, peak expiratory flow rate; p.r.n., according to circumstances. (Modified from National Asthma Education Program: Report of the Working Group on Asthma and Pregnancy. Management of asthma during pregnancy [NIH publication no. 93-3279A]. Bethesda, Md., National Institutes of Health, 1993.)

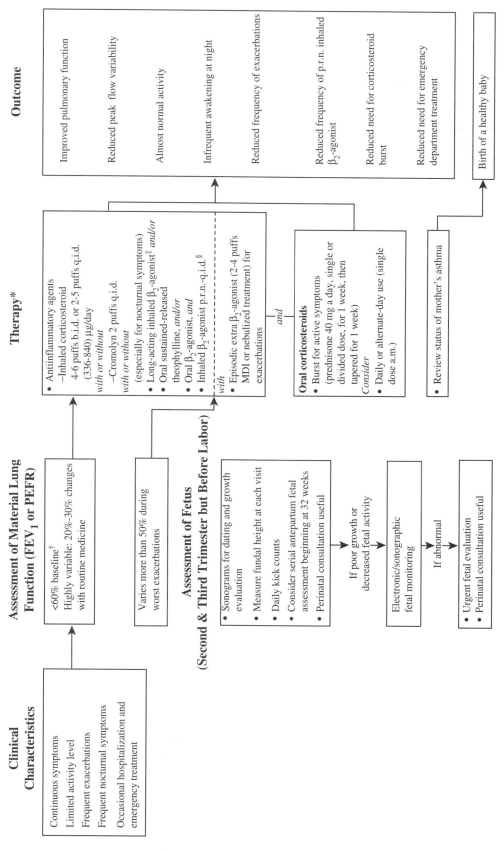

Figure 18–6. Flowchart outlining management of patients with chronic severe asthma during pregnancy. FEV₁, forced expiratory volume in 1 second; MDI, metered-dose inhaler; PEFR, peak expiratory flow rate; p.r.n., according to circumstances. (Modified from National Asthma Education Program: Report of the Working Group on Asthma and Pregnancy. Management of asthma during pregnancy [NIH publication no. 93-3279A]. Bethesda, Md., National Institutes of Health, 1993.)

Note: Individuals with severe asthma should be evaluated by an asthma specialist.

*All therapy must include patient education about prevention (including environmental control as appropriate) as well as control of symptoms.

†PEFR percent baseline refers to the norm for the individual, established by the clinican. This may be percent predicted based on standardized norms or percent of patient's personal best.

‡Added by authors to original flow chart.

§If exceed 3-4 doses a day, consider additional therapy other than inhaled β₂-agonist.

but in a sheep model, the initial reduction is followed by an increase above the basal value.[114] For all of these studies, any relevance to patients receiving sympathomimetic agents for management of asthma has not been documented.[115] Lack of comparability of dose and route of administration makes it impossible to extrapolate the findings of these studies to the clinical setting of the pregnant asthmatic patient.

No teratogenicity has been documented for ephedrine in humans or for metaproterenol in animals, but a slightly increased incidence of malformations over the expected number was found by the Collaborative Perinatal Project in infants of women given epinephrine during pregnancy.[116,117] In a study of 259 pregnant asthmatic women using inhaled β agonist bronchodilators (primarily metaproterenol), no adverse effects on the fetus were noted in comparison with control subjects.[118] Although there are no human studies specifically concerning other inhaled β agonists such as albuterol, these agents have been used frequently by clinicians treating pregnant asthmatic patients, and to date, no consistent problems with malformations have been reported.

By virtue of their stimulation of uterine β receptors, sympathomimetics inhibit uterine contractility at term and are useful in the management of premature labor.[119] This effect has been documented for intravenous administration of metaproterenol, terbutaline, and albuterol.[120-122] Oral terbutaline has a similar action on uterine contractility and has therefore also been used for inhibition of premature labor.[123] However, a number of cases of pulmonary edema have been reported after sympathomimetic therapy used in this setting; no cases have been reported after the use of sympathomimetics for management of the pregnant asthmatic patient.[124-126] The problem of sympathomimetic-induced pulmonary edema is discussed in more detail in the section "Pulmonary Edema Associated with Sympathomimetic Therapy" later in this chapter.

Disodium cromoglycate appears to be safe during pregnancy. In a French study of 296 pregnant women, there was no documented increased risk of malformations,[127] and no other adverse effects on the fetus have been reported.

Xanthine bronchodilators also appear to be safe for the fetus.[84,128] Although there is some evidence of digital malformations in laboratory animals given large doses of aminophylline parenterally,[129] no teratogenic effect has been demonstrated in human studies.[117] Despite animal data suggestive of an increased risk of stillbirth with theophylline, its use in human pregnancy is not associated with an increased risk of stillbirth.[130] In nonpregnant women, aminophylline can inhibit and, in some cases, abolish uterine motility, presumably by an inhibitory effect of increased cAMP on uterine smooth muscle.[131] Whether aminophylline alters uterine contractility at the time of labor has not been well studied, but it is reasonable to expect that an inhibitory effect is possible. When theophylline is used during pregnancy, serum concentrations should be monitored closely, because clearance of the drug has been reported to decrease during the third trimester.[132,133] Xanthines are transferred across the placenta, and theophylline concentrations in neonatal and cord blood are similar to those in maternal blood.[134,135] In one study, mean neonatal heart rate and Apgar scores were apparently unaffected by maternal administration of theophylline.[135] However, transient tachycardia and myocardial irritability have been reported in some neonates of mothers receiving xanthine agents, presumably as a direct effect of the drug.

Agents affecting leukotriene synthesis or action are relatively new, and there is little information about their use in human pregnancy. However, animal data on zafirlukast and montelukast have shown no teratogenicity at oral doses more than 150 times the maximum human daily oral dose on a milligram-per-square-meter basis. According to a position statement by the American College of Obstetrics and Gynecology and the American College of Allergy, Asthma, and Immunology, zafirlukast and montelukast "can be considered for use in pregnant women who have shown a uniquely favorable response before pregnancy."[136] In contrast, zileuton has proven teratogenic in some animal models and generally should not be used in this setting.

Numerous studies have been reported concerning use of corticosteroids during pregnancy.[137] Any potential risk appears to be small, and it is generally agreed that corticosteroids should not be withheld in this setting if they are clinically indicated. The main potential problems fall into the following three categories: (1) congenital malformations, mainly cleft palate; (2) placental insufficiency, prematurity, and fetal or neonatal death; and (3) neonatal adrenal insufficiency. Each is discussed in turn.

In animals, it has been demonstrated that maternal administration of corticosteroids may be associated with cleft palate in the offspring.[138] In human studies, a few cases of cleft palate have been reported in offspring of women receiving corticosteroids during pregnancy,[139] but a causal relationship has been difficult to prove. Because closure of the palatal processes is usually complete by the 12th week, administration of steroids beyond the first trimester should not be associated with any risk of cleft palate. On the basis of several studies, any risk for cleft palate associated with first-trimester administration of steroids is likely to be relatively small.[101,117,140] It is reasonable to approach steroid use during the first trimester with caution, but corticosteroids should not be withheld when their use is clearly indicated.

An increased incidence of placental insufficiency and resulting low birth weight or stillbirth has been suggested to be associated with maternal steroid use. One group noted a high frequency of stillbirth or placental insufficiency among mothers receiving prednisolone during pregnancy, and they speculated that prednisolone had a deleterious effect on placental function.[141] Others have found an apparently high rate of fetal loss and perinatal mortality,[142,143] but because a control population was not examined in either study, it is difficult to assess the contribution of steroids in comparison with that of the underlying disease.[144] Another study found that use of prednisone, 10 mg/day, throughout the duration of pregnancy was associated with a significantly lower birth weight in offspring, unassociated with any change in the length of gestation.[145] This finding was confirmed by a parallel experimental study in mice, in which it was clear that reduction in birth weight was attributable to steroid exposure and not to other maternal disease. The authors speculated that the effect of steroids could result either from placental transfer of the hormone and a direct inhibition of fetal growth or from indirect effects on the placenta or other aspects of maternal physiology.

Several studies specifically concerning the use of systemic steroids for management of asthma during pregnancy have been performed. In one study, there was no increase in the risk of abortion, stillbirth, or neonatal death when mothers received prednisone in an average daily dosage of 8.2 mg.[101] A slightly increased frequency of prematurity was noted (14%, in comparison with 9.3% in a historical control population), but whether this increase was caused by steroids, asthma, or other factors is unknown. The other study reported the outcome of 56 pregnancies in 51 women with severe asthma who required oral or inhaled steroids.[100] Although there were no malformations or neonatal deaths, the incidence of prematurity and low birth weight was slightly higher than expected on the basis of data from a historical control group. However, these complications appeared to be associated more with the severity of asthma during pregnancy than with the use of steroids. Overall, although it is still remotely possible that steroids contribute to prematurity or to retardation of intrauterine growth, it is more likely that the severe underlying disease being treated is the more important factor for both of these complications.

A potential risk of fetal adrenal suppression after maternal administration of corticosteroids has been suggested, and cases of fetal adrenal atrophy documented in pathologic studies have been reported.[143,144] However, clinical evidence of adrenal insufficiency in the newborn in such circumstances is unusual. In one series, there was no evidence of neonatal adrenal insufficiency in any of 71 infants born to mothers receiving an average daily dosage of 8.2 mg of prednisone for variable periods of time during pregnancy.[101] In another study, adrenal cortical reserve, as assessed by an adrenocorticotropic hormone stimulation test, was normal in each of six neonates exposed in utero to prolonged maternal administration of prednisone.[146] Although neonates born to mothers receiving prolonged steroids during pregnancy should be observed for signs of adrenal insufficiency, this complication is distinctly unusual. However, of importance is that the use of steroids during pregnancy does suppress maternal adrenal function, and supplemental corticosteroids for the mother at the time of labor and delivery may be required.

The inhaled steroid budesonide does not appear to be associated with an increased risk of congenital malformations when used early in pregnancy, according to a report from Sweden of more than 2000 pregnancies.[147] As a result, inhaled budesonide has recently been reclassified by the U.S. Food and Drug Administration from pregnancy category C (in which all other inhaled steroids are listed) to pregnancy category B. To date, the inhaled steroid preparations beclomethasone and triamcinolone also appear to be safe during pregnancy, but information is more limited. In a study of 45 pregnancies in 40 women, no complications attributable to beclomethasone were found.[148] Cardiac malformations in one infant in this study were more likely to have resulted from the mother's underlying medical problems and complicated pregnancy rather than from beclomethasone. Preliminary experience with triamcinolone in 15 pregnant women demonstrated no statistically significant difference in birth weight in comparison with infants of pregnant women treated with inhaled beclomethasone or oral theophylline.[149] Use of these and other asthma and allergy medications during pregnancy has been reviewed.[150]

Finally, several cases have been reported in which life-threatening status asthmaticus during pregnancy could not be controlled by intensive medical therapy.[151] In these cases, termination of pregnancy by cesarean section was followed by dramatic improvement in the patient's otherwise uncontrolled asthma.

Other Forms of Obstructive Lung Disease

Chronic Obstructive Lung Disease

Because chronic bronchitis and emphysema are unusual in women of childbearing age, information regarding interactions between pregnancy and chronic obstructive lung disease is available only in case report form. Several pregnancies in women with α_1-antitrypsin deficiency, a genetic disease associated with the early onset of panacinar emphysema, have been reported.[152-156] Uneventful maternal and fetal courses have been noted in most of these reports, although elective cesarean section was performed at 37 weeks in one patient because of worsening dyspnea and deteriorating spirometry ($FEV_1 = 0.6$ L).[153] An unresolved issue is whether intravenous supplementation of α_1-antitrypsin (Prolastin) should be discontinued during pregnancy. Animal reproduction studies have not been undertaken with the drug, and it is not known whether the drug can cause fetal harm or adversely affect fertility.

Pregnancy in patients with α_1-antitrypsin deficiency–unrelated chronic obstructive pulmonary disease has rarely been reported. In one such case, the patient developed respiratory distress and delivered prematurely at 32 weeks.[157] The severity of her disease was demonstrated by chronic hypercapnia and an FEV_1 of approximately 0.7 L (<25% of predicted value). Although she required intubation and mechanical ventilation in the postpartum period, the patient recovered, and her child was entirely normal.

Finally, there was a report of a patient with severe combined obstructive and restrictive lung disease, a relatively uncomplicated pregnancy, and delivery of a healthy infant at approximately 36 weeks.[158] Her disease, which was apparently a combination of chronic obstructive lung disease from previous heavy smoking and interstitial disease related to fibrosis from a prior episode of acute respiratory distress syndrome (ARDS), was associated with an FEV_1 of approximately 1 L (35% of predicted value).

Bronchiectasis

Bronchiectasis, an irreversible dilatation of bronchi often associated with chronic cough, sputum production, and recurrent infections, is occasionally found in women of childbearing age. It is often the result of prior bronchial injury caused by various types of infection, particularly necrotizing viral or bacterial pneumonia in childhood.[159]

One author reported a total of 44 pregnancies in 21 patients with bronchiectasis[160]; in only one instance could difficulty during pregnancy or the postpartum period be attributed to bronchiectasis. In another study,[161] little change was found in pulmonary function, degree of dyspnea, or volume of sputum production in each of three pregnant women with bronchiectasis, and no evidence of intrauterine growth retardation was observed. However, there have been two individual case reports of patients with bronchiectasis who experienced deterioration during pregnancy or whose fetuses had complications. In one, a patient with bronchiectasis and a prior lobectomy had pregnancies resulting in an infant of low birth weight and an intrauterine fetal death at 38 weeks.[162] In the other, the patient's respiratory status deteriorated during pregnancy, and fetal development was complicated by intrauterine growth restriction.[163]

Cystic Fibrosis

Altered epithelial electrolyte transport and abnormal exocrine gland secretions characterize cystic fibrosis, the most common lethal genetic disorder in white persons. Abnormally viscous mucus results in pancreatic disease, with ductal obstruction and pancreatic insufficiency, and in lung disease, with airway plugging, inflammation, bronchiectasis, and recurrent bronchopulmonary infections. The diagnosis is confirmed by the finding of an elevated sweat chloride concentration obtained by pilocarpine iontophoresis on two or more occasions, by identification of mutations known to cause cystic fibrosis in each *CFTR* gene, or by in vivo demonstration of characteristic abnormalities in ion transport across the nasal epithelium.[164] The pulmonary pathologic process that occurs with cystic fibrosis generally does not produce a pure obstructive physiologic pattern but rather a mixed picture of obstructive and restrictive disease.

The initial description of pregnancy in a woman with cystic fibrosis was published in 1960.[165] Since then, numerous other cases have been reported, particularly as increasing numbers of children with the disease are surviving into adulthood.[166] In addition, initial diagnoses are now more commonly made in late adolescence and early adulthood than they were in the past, and cases have even been reported in which the diagnosis was first made during pregnancy.[167] Although almost all men with cystic fibrosis are infertile because of absence of the vas deferens, many affected women are capable of bearing children. It is generally believed that fertility is decreased in women with cystic fibrosis, presumably because of thick cervical mucus providing a mechanical hindrance to sperm penetration.[168,169] However, there are few published studies of fertility in women with this disease in comparison with a control population.[170,171]

In a landmark 1980 survey of cystic fibrosis centers in the United States and Canada, 129 pregnancies were identified in women with the disease.[170] This study found a high rate of two complications of pregnancy: congestive heart failure in 13% and low maternal weight gain in 41% of patients. Although spontaneous abortions were not increased, there was a higher frequency of prematurity (27%) and perinatal deaths (11%) than expected on the basis of data from a control population. Mortality rates over a 2-year period after delivery were high (18%) but not increased over those expected for age-matched nonpregnant women with cystic fibrosis. No congenital anomalies were found, even though antibiotics were used frequently during the course of pregnancy.

Most subsequent studies have produced similar results.[172] Overall, 70% to 80% of pregnancies in mothers with cystic fibrosis result in a delivery of a healthy infant after an uncomplicated maternal course. Predictors of maternal and fetal complications include exocrine pancreatic insufficiency, poor weight gain, more severely affected pulmonary function, and the presence of diabetes mellitus.[111,173-175]

The effect of pregnancy on the long-term course of cystic fibrosis has also been examined.[176-180] Overall, no deleterious effect of pregnancy on the long-term prognosis of maternal cystic fibrosis has been documented. For example, one study of more than 300 women with cystic fibrosis who became pregnant and more than 1000 nulliparous controls with cystic fibrosis found no significant differences in the rates of FEV_1 decline, pneumothorax, hemoptysis, or infectious exacerbations during pregnancy or the 2 years after delivery.[178] A history of pregnancy was not an independent risk factor for death, and survival rates in both groups were worse among patients with poor pulmonary function, diabetes mellitus, or poor nutritional status.

Counseling a woman with cystic fibrosis about pregnancy often poses a difficult problem, and there are no universally accepted guidelines.[181] With severe disease, characterized by marked airflow obstruction (FEV_1 <50% of predicted value, or rapidly progressing disease), pulmonary hypertension, cor pulmonale, significant hypoxemia, or poor nutritional status, pregnancy may not be advisable.[168,171] In contrast, patients with mild disease generally do well during pregnancy. In those with disease of intermediate severity, potential health risks to the mother, shortened maternal life expectancy, and decreased ability to provide day-to-day child care because of limited exercise tolerance must all be weighed in the decision about whether to have children.[166,170,175] Genetic counseling should be offered, and issues regarding genetic screening should be discussed.[182] According to the autosomal recessive nature of the disease and the known frequency of the gene, the general risk of bearing a child with cystic fibrosis is up to 2.5%, although all children are at least carriers of the abnormal gene.

Interstitial Lung Disease

Interstitial inflammation and fibrosis can occur in many conditions and are characterized by reduced lung volumes and often an increase in the FEV_1/FVC ratio. In many cases, the onset of physiologically significant disease occurs after menopause; therefore, it is relatively unusual to confront a pregnant woman with these disorders. Data regarding the maternal and fetal outcomes of pregnancy in the setting of interstitial lung disease are sparse, although a number of successfully managed cases have been reported.[183,184]

However, two types of interstitial lung disease, sarcoidosis and lymphangioleiomyomatosis (LAM), can occur in younger women. Consequently, there is greater clinical experience with pregnancy in these conditions; therefore, more definitive conclusions regarding the advisability and management of pregnancy can be drawn.

Sarcoidosis

Definition

Sarcoidosis is a multisystem granulomatous disease of unknown cause that manifests frequently in young adults.[185,186] It most commonly affects the lungs; however, other organs or systems, including lymph nodes, skin, eyes, heart, and liver, can be involved. The characteristic pathologic finding in affected tissues is the noncaseating granuloma, but no specific etiologic agent initiating the granuloma formation has yet been identified. Immunologic abnormalities—namely, impaired delayed hypersensitivity and excessive immunoglobulin production—are well described as frequent accompaniments of the disease, and current theories of pathogenesis rely heavily on immunologic mechanisms.

Disease in the Nonpregnant State

The pulmonary abnormalities that may occur in sarcoidosis include bilateral hilar adenopathy or interstitial lung disease. These may or may not be accompanied by extrathoracic involvement or systemic symptoms. The most common manifestations of the disease are respiratory symptoms, especially dyspnea and nonproductive cough, or an abnormal chest radiograph but no symptoms.

Definitive diagnosis is made in the appropriate clinical setting by the finding of noncaseating granulomas in affected tissues, particularly the lungs. Techniques for obtaining involved tissue within the chest include transbronchial biopsy via fiberoptic bronchoscopy, mediastinoscopy, and thoracoscopic lung biopsy. The first of these procedures is the most popular method for diagnosing sarcoidosis because it is relatively noninvasive and has a high yield of diagnostic findings, even when the chest radiograph does not show parenchymal disease.

Although the course of the disease is variable, in approximately two thirds of patients, the manifestations of disease improve or clear within 2 to 3 years, leaving minor or no residual chest radiographic abnormalities and no active extrathoracic disease. Of the remaining one third of patients, most have a smoldering course over years.

Disease in Pregnancy

Several series investigating the effects of pregnancy on sarcoidosis have produced generally consistent results. One report described 16 pregnancies in 10 patients with sarcoidosis and found that pregnancy frequently ameliorated the patient's underlying disease.[187] In 8 of the 10 patients, improvement in at least some of the manifestations of sarcoidosis occurred during the antenatal period; the condition of the other 2 patients remained unchanged. However, the abnormal findings returned within several months of delivery in approximately half of the patients, and some had new manifestations of sarcoidosis not previously noted.

Another author monitored 10 patients with sarcoidosis through 17 pregnancies, concluded that pregnancy had no consistent effect on the course of the disease,[188] and subsequently reported two patients who had successful pregnancies despite severe restrictive lung disease caused by sarcoidosis.[189] Several other studies each suggested that pregnancy does not adversely affect the course of sarcoidosis, because almost all patients experience improvement or no change.[184,190-194] A few patients seem to get worse during the antepartum period,[190] and maternal death with severe sarcoidosis has been reported.[195]

Scadding perhaps best summarized the overall effects of pregnancy on sarcoidosis and described characteristic patterns in different categories of patients.[196] When a woman's chest radiograph showed resolution to normal or inactive fibrotic residua before pregnancy, it remained unchanged throughout pregnancy. When the radiograph showed continuing resolution before pregnancy, the disease generally continued on the course of resolution throughout the prenatal period. Finally, patients with active disease tended to have partial or complete resolution of their radiographic changes during pregnancy, although most patients in this group experienced an exacerbation of their disease within 3 to 6 months after delivery.

Because corticosteroids suppress the manifestations of sarcoidosis (see the following section on treatment), it has been suggested that the elevated circulating levels of both free and total cortisol during pregnancy may explain the frequent tendency for improvement at this time. Although this seems to be a reasonable explanation, there is no definite proof that changes in circulating corticosteroid levels are responsible. In fact, because sarcoidosis improves spontaneously in many patients, it is likely that improvement in some patients is coincident with but not caused by their pregnancy.

There is no current evidence for any adverse effect of sarcoidosis on either fertility or the course of pregnancy.[196] Although a few patients have been described with either miscarriages or congenital abnormalities,[187,188] the incidence of such problems with pregnancy or the fetus does not appear to be increased over that in mothers without sarcoidosis.[193,196] It is also of interest that histologic examination of placental tissue has shown no evidence of granulomatous disease.[189,197] In the single reported case of antepartum death in a patient with sarcoidosis,[197] the patient also had preeclampsia, and the contribution of the patient's pulmonary disease to her death is therefore not clear.

Treatment

Corticosteroids are the treatment of choice for patients with sarcoidosis. However, even though steroids clearly suppress many of the manifestations of the disease, it has not been definitely shown that they alter its overall course. Treatment decisions are further complicated by the fact that sarcoidosis often follows a course of spontaneous improvement and radiographic resolution, even without any therapy.[185]

Well-accepted indications for treatment include significant disease affecting a vital organ, especially with myocardial, ocular, or central nervous system involvement. Pulmonary involvement should not be treated on the basis of radiographic manifestations alone, because those findings may not be correlated with functional impairment and may also spontaneously improve. Corticosteroid treatment for pulmonary sarcoidosis should instead be based on pulmonary functional impairment and respiratory symptoms; if available, information about the course of a patient's disease, by observation over at least two times, may also be useful in deciding whom and when to treat.

When therapy is begun, the starting dosage is often prednisone, 40 to 60 mg/day. It is usually continued for at least a 6-month period but is generally tapered during this time to a lower maintenance dose, administered on either a daily or an every-other-day basis.

Treatment in Pregnancy

Use of corticosteroids for treatment of sarcoidosis during pregnancy generally follows the same guidelines as treatment in the nonpregnant patient. Because it is unusual for sarcoidosis to develop or become worse during pregnancy, indications for treatment rarely develop de novo during pregnancy. In women who are already receiving steroids for sarcoidosis, the dose should be kept constant or decreased because of the frequent amelioration of the disease during pregnancy.

Potential complications of steroid use during pregnancy have been discussed in detail in previous sections of this chapter and are not repeated here.

Lymphangioleiomyomatosis

Pulmonary LAM is a rare lung disease that afflicts young women of childbearing age and is histopathologically characterized by the proliferation of atypical pulmonary interstitial smooth muscle cells.[198] The disease generally manifests both obstructive and restrictive physiology, and may manifest clinically with dyspnea, pneumothorax, hemoptysis, or chylothorax and may progress to respiratory failure and death. The radiographic appearance of innumerable small pulmonary cysts is so characteristic of the disease that tissue confirmation is sometimes not necessary.[199] The course of the disease is variable, although progression is common.

The pathogenesis of LAM remains incompletely understood, although most data suggest that the loss of a functional tumor suppressor locus may play a role and that the disease may share important genetic characteristics with tuberous sclerosis.[198] However, LAM is distinct from other interstitial lung disorders and the phakomatoses in that estrogen appears to play a role in promoting disease progression. LAM rarely occurs before menarche or after menopause, and oophorectomy has resulted in long-term remissions.[200] Both estrogen and progesterone receptors have been documented in the abnormal smooth muscle cells that characterize the disease.[201]

As might be inferred from the preceding discussion, pregnancy is generally contraindicated in LAM because of the belief that the hormonal changes that accompany pregnancy exacerbate the disease. For example, one study concluded that complications of LAM, such as chylous effusions or pneumothorax, were 11 times more frequent during pregnancy than at other times.[202] Counseling of women with LAM should include a discussion of the dangers of pregnancy to maternal health and of the potential impact of shortened maternal life expectancy on the child. Unfortunately, no trials have addressed the optimal management of LAM during pregnancy should it occur.

Tuberculosis

Since 1980, concern about tuberculosis has increased considerably, as has recognition that this disease is again a major public health problem. Two factors are responsible for this resurgence of concern: (1) a transient increase in the incidence of tuberculosis beginning in 1985, related in large part to human immunodeficiency virus (HIV) infection, and (2) an increasing frequency of drug-resistant organisms, including strains resistant to multiple drugs.[203] Tuberculosis is classified as active when symptoms and signs of disease are present, such as fever, cough, hemoptysis, weight loss, or auscultatory or radiographic abnormalities. When a purified protein derivative skin test result is positive in an untreated patient without any evidence of active disease, a state of latent tuberculosis infection is present.

Active Tuberculosis

The acid-fast bacillus *Mycobacterium tuberculosis* can cause either pulmonary or extrapulmonary infection. Although the lung remains the major site of involvement, 38% of patients with HIV infection have disseminated disease.[204] Atypical manifestations of both pulmonary and extrapulmonary disease now force the clinician to consider the diagnosis in many more clinical settings than was the case before 1990.

When there is reactivation of old infection, frequently in elderly or debilitated patients, disease often appears on chest radiograph as upper lobe infiltrates with or without cavitation. Patients may be asymptomatic or may present with constitutional symptoms (low-grade fever, weight loss, malaise, anorexia, night sweats) or respiratory symptoms (cough, sputum production, hemoptysis).

Primary tuberculosis infection, although formerly considered mainly a childhood problem, is not uncommon in the adult population, particularly as the frequency of previous exposure during childhood has declined considerably. Patients are frequently asymptomatic at the time of infection and are often recognized only by conversion of the tuberculin skin test. Primary infection may also result in (1) nonspecific symptoms of pneumonia (fever and cough, often nonproductive), with radiographic findings of parenchymal infiltrates or adenopathy; (2) pleural effusion, with symptoms of pleuritic chest pain, fever, and cough; and (3) extrapulmonary or disseminated disease, especially in patients immunocompromised by HIV infection. Patients occasionally present with direct progression to upper lobe disease, similar to the classic "reactivation" pattern.

Diagnosis in Pregnancy

In the hope of detecting cases of active or inactive tuberculosis that might necessitate therapeutic intervention, many clinicians in the past advised routine prenatal chest radiographs.[205-207] However, this practice is no longer justified, because a positive history, positive physical examination findings, or a positive tuberculin skin test result generally suggests the need for a radiograph in patients eventually found to have an abnormality.[208,209] Thus, radiography should be reserved for patients with a history or findings suggestive of pulmonary disease or tuberculosis or for those with a positive tuberculin skin test result.

If a chest radiograph is clinically indicated, pregnancy should not be considered a contraindication to the study. The exposure to radiation from a chest radiograph is approximately 50 mrad to the chest and 2.5 to 5 mrad to the gonads.[208,210,211] In a detailed analysis of prenatal radiation exposure and subsequent occurrence of malformations or cancer, an overall risk has been estimated of 0 to 1 case per 1000 patients who received 1 rad in utero during the first 4 months of pregnancy.[212] Because the radiation exposure from a chest radiograph is much smaller than the 1-rad dose used to calculate that risk, there appears to be no measurable risk associated with a chest radiograph during pregnancy.[208,210] When indicated, however, the radiograph should be performed with abdominal shielding and preferably after the first trimester to avoid even this small amount of exposure to rapidly dividing and differentiating fetal tissues.

Definitive diagnostic proof of tuberculosis in both pregnant and nonpregnant patients is dependent on demonstration of *M. tuberculosis* by culture, especially of sputum. If a spontaneous sputum specimen cannot be obtained, sputum can frequently be induced by chest physiotherapy and inhalation of an aerosol effective in generating a productive cough (e.g., hypertonic saline). If necessary, specimens can be obtained with washings and brushings with a fiberoptic bronchoscope. In many cases, a provisional diagnosis of tuberculosis can be made by demonstration of acid-fast bacilli on an appropriately stained smear, but culture should always be performed, in addition, for definitive identification and for determination of drug sensitivity.

In patients who present with a tuberculous pleural effusion, acid-fast organisms are rarely found on a smear of pleural fluid, and culture of the fluid is positive in only 30% of affected patients. In such cases, a strong clinical suspicion of tuberculous effusion can be based on an unexplained exudative effusion with predominantly lymphocytes in a patient with a positive tuberculin skin test result. Diagnostic yield is greatest by combining culture of pleural fluid with culture and histologic examination of a pleural biopsy; the combined procedures document a tuberculous cause in approximately 80% of cases. In the setting of a strong clinical suspicion of tuberculosis, however, it is generally advisable to begin therapy while awaiting culture results.[213]

Course in Pregnancy

Medical opinion about the interaction between pregnancy and tuberculosis has changed several times since antiquity.[214-217] From the time of Hippocrates until the middle of the 19th century, it was thought that pregnancy had an overall beneficial effect on tuberculosis. A diametrically opposite view was taken from 1850 until the 1940s,

and therapeutic abortion was frequently recommended to avert the presumed deleterious effect of pregnancy. An intermediate view was taken in 1953 by Hedvall,[218] who reached the conclusion, on the basis of experience with a large number of patients, that pregnancy and labor seldom have a harmful effect on women with tuberculosis. A comparison of the course of tuberculosis in 22 pregnant and 40 nonpregnant women of the same age also yielded no differences between the two groups.[219] Three criteria were used for comparison: rate of stabilization of disease, conversion of sputum and gastric washings, and cavity closure. There was no significant difference between the two groups in any of these three criteria.

Even though pregnancy itself may have little effect on the natural history of tuberculous infection, several studies in the prechemotherapeutic era found an increased rate of deterioration or progressive disease during the first postpartum year. In one series of 276 women whose tuberculosis remained stable throughout the course of pregnancy, 37 (13.4%) showed deterioration during the first postpartum year.[218] In another study of 930 women with pulmonary tuberculosis, progression of disease occurred in 90 cases within the first 6 weeks after delivery, even though the antenatal course was favorable in 70 of the 90 patients.[220] Several theories have been proposed to explain this phenomenon, including rapid hormonal changes, postpartum descent of the diaphragm, the nutritional strain of lactation, and insufficient sleep because of the time-consuming demands of a newborn. However, it is not universally accepted that an increased risk of progression exists in the first postpartum year, in comparison with the potential for deterioration that exists in any untreated patient over a 1-year period.[206]

Any unsettled controversy about the effect of pregnancy or the postpartum period on tuberculosis became unimportant after the advent of effective chemotherapy. With adequate treatment for active tuberculosis, pregnant women appear to have the same excellent prognosis as their nonpregnant counterparts. In one series,[206] all 72 pregnant women with active tuberculosis showed regression and control of disease with treatment. Women with inactive latent tuberculosis given prophylactic isoniazid similarly had a stable course without reactivation during pregnancy and the postpartum period. Of 444 such patients with inactive disease, 442 remained stable and had no evidence of activation; 2 had some progression of disease despite isoniazid prophylaxis. These latter patients required more intensive therapy in order to control the disease.

Several more studies confirmed the excellent prognosis of treated tuberculosis in pregnant women. A 1975 review of the course of 149 pregnancies in 100 women with tuberculosis showed no adverse effect of pregnancy, birth, the postpartum period, or lactation.[221] There was no risk of relapse when the lung disease was adequately treated, even in patients with active disease or those with persistence of a postchemotherapy cavity. The experience at New York Lying-In Hospital in 1565 patients monitored between 1933 and 1972 was also reviewed.[222] After 1965, the incidence of tuberculosis diagnosed during pregnancy was in the range of 0.6% to 1%. Among patients seen between 1957 and 1972 and therefore treated with antituberculosis drugs, progression of disease occurred in fewer than 1%. The comparable progression rate from 1933 to 1956 was 3% to 4%.

Most series investigating the effect of tuberculosis on the course of pregnancy and on the newborn have concluded that pregnancy is not altered by tuberculosis in the mother. In one large series, 600 of 616 pregnancies resulted in the birth of 602 normal live infants.[206] There were seven cases of early, spontaneous abortion and nine cases of antepartum or intrapartum fetal death. The authors did not note an effect of tuberculosis on the duration of pregnancy. One group reported no increase in prematurity and no cases of congenital tuberculosis in the 1588 infants delivered in their series.[222]

However, such findings have not been universal. A carefully controlled series investigating the course and outcome of pregnancy in women with pulmonary tuberculosis was reported from Norway[223]; in a comparison of pregnancies in 542 women with pulmonary tuberculosis and 112,530 women without tuberculosis, the authors found an excessive occurrence of pregnancy complications, miscarriage, and difficult labor in women with tuberculosis. Among antepartum complications, the study population had a statistically significant higher frequency of toxemia (7.4% vs. 4.7%) and vaginal hemorrhage (4.1% vs. 2.2%), whereas the incidence of hyperemesis was not significantly increased. Labor was induced more often in the study group than in control subjects (14.6% vs. 9.1%) and was more often complicated (15.1% vs. 9.6%), and interventions during labor were required more frequently (12.6% vs. 7.7%). However, the most striking difference between the two groups was in the risk of miscarriage, defined in this study as fetal death between 16 and 28 weeks' gestation. The frequency of miscarriage was approximately ninefold higher (20.1 per 1000 vs. 2.3 per 1000) in the patients with tuberculosis than in controls. No differences were found in numbers of multiple births or congenital malformations. Comparison of live births revealed no differences in the mean gestation period, percentage of premature infants, percentage of infants with low birth weights, or mean birth weight. In interpreting this study, however, it is difficult to define which factors contributed to the greater frequency of miscarriage and pregnancy complications. In particular, because tuberculosis is more common in lower socioeconomic groups, the potential role of social or economic factors, rather than tuberculosis, must be considered.

Because of the generally excellent prognosis for treated tuberculosis in pregnant women, the recommendation for therapeutic abortion that was commonly given for these patients has long since been abandoned. Nevertheless, the development of chemotherapy has not entirely eradicated the complicated management problems that can occur in pregnancy. Even in the more recent literature, there are reports of women who have been quite ill from meningeal,[224,225] miliary,[225] and peritoneal[226] involvement with tuberculosis during pregnancy. Similarly, there are still case reports of infants with congenital tuberculosis, occurring especially as a complication of maternal miliary tuberculosis with endometrial involvement.[216,227,228] In a study of 27 patients with tuberculosis during pregnancy or the postpartum period, maternal outcome was worse and fetal complications were more frequent with drug-resistant disease than with drug-sensitive disease.[229]

Treatment

The treatment of active tuberculosis is based on the principles that (1) more than one drug must be used in order to prevent selection and growth of resistant organisms and (2) therapy must be prolonged. Within this framework, newer regimens have been devised to simplify treatment and reduce the duration of drug administration, and these regimens are accepted as routine therapy in many instances. However, at the same time, increasing concern for drug resistance has generally prompted the use of additional initial therapy until the results of drug susceptibility studies are available. Detailed guidelines for treatment have been published by the American Thoracic Society and the Centers for Disease Control and Prevention[213] and have been reviewed.[230]

Short-course chemotherapy is now considered to be the preferred therapeutic regimen for management of tuberculosis.[213,230,231] Therapy is started on a daily basis, but after the initial 1 to 2 months of therapy, an alternative to daily therapy is twice-weekly therapy (ideally administered as directly observed therapy) with adjusted dosages of the drugs.[213] The standard regimen for treatment of active tuberculosis in the nonpregnant patient is isoniazid and rifampin given daily for 6 months, supplemented by pyrazinamide for the first 2 months. In addition, unless the patient has a very low (<4%) risk of having a drug-resistant organism, ethambutol should be added until the results of drug susceptibility studies become available.

Although there had initially been concern about giving pyrazinamide during pregnancy because of relatively little information about its use in this setting, subsequent experience suggests that it can be used without adverse consequences.[232,233] As a result, the initial regimen that is often preferred for the pregnant woman is isoniazid (300 mg/day), rifampin (600 mg/day), and pyrazinamide (25 mg/kg/day); ethambutol (15 to 25 mg/kg/day) is added initially unless drug resistance is extremely unlikely. Pyrazinamide is given for the first 2 months, and ethambutol can be discontinued if the organism is found to be sensitive to both isoniazid and rifampin. Pyridoxine should be given with isoniazid to the pregnant woman to satisfy the increased requirement for this vitamin during pregnancy.[234]

Of note, the 1994 recommendation from the American Thoracic Society does not include the initial use of pyrazinamide,[213] whereas other international organizations do recommend its use during pregnancy.[231,233] If pyrazinamide is not used, then the duration of isoniazid and rifampin therapy must be extended to 9 months (rather than 6 months).

Identical initial regimens are used for tuberculosis regardless of whether HIV co-infection is present.[213] Despite the immunocompromise associated with HIV infection, patients seem to respond as well to therapy for tuberculosis as their counterparts without HIV infection.[235]

The major potential side effects of isoniazid are hepatitis, hypersensitivity reactions, and peripheral neuropathy. Transient elevation of serum aspartate aminotransferase (AST) levels, occurring in 10% to 20% of patients, is not necessarily an indication for discontinuing therapy; serious hepatotoxicity resembles viral hepatitis, and its incidence increases with advancing age. According to data from a large study,[236] serious hepatotoxicity seems to be avoidable if AST and symptoms are routinely monitored on a monthly basis, and isoniazid is discontinued if AST elevation is more than five times normal levels.

Because of the age of pregnant women, they had been considered to be at low risk for isoniazid-associated hepatotoxicity. However, a number of deaths from isoniazid-associated hepatitis in women of childbearing age (in some cases, post partum) have suggested that the risk may be higher than previously expected.[237,238] For incompletely understood reasons, pregnant and postpartum Hispanic women may be at particularly high risk of isoniazid-associated hepatitis, but the actual risk needs to be defined further.[239]

In patients with symptoms suggestive of toxicity accompanied by elevation of AST levels, it is uniformly accepted that isoniazid should be stopped. Peripheral neuropathy with isoniazid can be prevented by supplemental administration of pyridoxine, 25 to 100 mg/day; although pyridoxine is not necessary in the normal well-nourished patient, it is generally recommended for the pregnant woman receiving isoniazid to prevent any potential neurotoxicity in the mother or the fetus.[213,240,241] Hypersensitivity reactions to isoniazid may include fever, rash, and a lupus-like syndrome, often with a positive result of a test for antinuclear antibodies.

Although optic neuritis has been well described as a potential complication of ethambutol therapy, it is quite rare with a dose of 15 mg/kg/day. Rifampin may cause hepatitis, hypersensitivity reactions, and occasional hematologic toxicity. Patients should be forewarned to expect orange discoloration of urine, sweat, tears, and saliva. When given intermittently, rifampin has occasionally been described to cause a "flu syndrome," abdominal pain, acute renal failure, or thrombocytopenia. Although these potential reactions were initially a cause of concern over the use of rifampin in intermittent chemotherapy, more recent studies have not shown a clinically important frequency of these effects.

Effect of Treatment on Pregnancy and the Fetus

Indications for chemotherapy of proved or suspected active tuberculosis and the principles of management are similar in the pregnant woman and the nonpregnant patient. A substantial amount of data about use of four antituberculosis drugs during pregnancy—isoniazid, ethambutol, rifampin, and streptomycin—has been tabulated.[232,242] This experience is most helpful in guiding the clinician with regard to safety and choice of therapy during pregnancy.

Extensive experience with isoniazid in pregnancy has been accumulated,[242] and it appears to be the safest agent for use in this setting.[243,244] Even though isoniazid crosses the placenta, its use is not contraindicated during pregnancy.

Although the ability of rifampin to inhibit DNA-dependent RNA polymerase led to some concern about its use during pregnancy, adverse fetal effects of rifampin have not been definitively demonstrated. A risk of limb reduction has been suggested (1 per 150 pregnancies vs. 1 per 435 pregnancies in healthy women), but this difference was not statistically significant.[242] An association between maternal rifampin use and hemorrhagic disease of the newborn has been suggested, and prophylactic vitamin K administration to the newborn is recommended.[232] Overall, given rifampin's efficacy as an antituberculosis agent and the absence of proven adverse fetal effects, it remains an important part of antituberculosis therapy during pregnancy.[214,217]

Pyrazinamide now has an important place in certain short-course regimens used in nonpregnant patients. As mentioned earlier, increasing experience with this drug in pregnancy has allayed initial concerns about absence of objective data regarding adverse effects during pregnancy.[232,233]

Use of ethambutol during pregnancy has been reported in several series; the drug does not appear to be contraindicated during pregnancy.[244-246] No relationship has been established between use of ethambutol during pregnancy and subsequent fetal abnormalities, and overall experience has not suggested any other adverse maternal or fetal effects in this setting.[242]

Streptomycin used to be given frequently for treatment of tuberculosis during pregnancy, but an unacceptable 17% risk of fetal ototoxicity has made other first-line drugs far preferable.[247] Although the most frequently observed effects in offspring of treated mothers are minor vestibular impairment, auditory impairment, or both,[248] cases of severe and bilateral hearing loss and marked vestibular abnormalities have been reported.[249] Unlike the effect of most teratogens, streptomycin ototoxicity can occur at any time during pregnancy, and the hazard is therefore not limited to critical periods in the first trimester.[242]

Little is also known about the specific effects in pregnancy of the second-line, much less commonly used antituberculosis drugs. Their usefulness is clearly limited, more by the potential side effects on the mother than by documented adverse effects on the fetus. For example, because of the gastrointestinal effects of *para*–aminosalicylic acid and the central nervous system effects of cycloserine, their use during pregnancy is undesirable. A teratogenic effect has been attributed to ethionamide, and its use is therefore relatively contraindicated in pregnancy.[250]

In patients who are likely to have contracted their disease in areas where drug-resistant organisms are common, and in patients who may have secondary drug resistance related to previous inadequate chemotherapy, treatment must be altered accordingly. Discussion of the management of drug-resistant tuberculosis is beyond the scope of this chapter; further information can be obtained from other sources.[213,251,252]

Neonatal Management

Management of the infant born to a mother with tuberculosis generally involves preventing or treating early infection contracted in the neonatal period. Congenital infection, presumably transmitted either by a hematogenous route or by aspiration of infected amniotic fluid, is uncommon, and most infection is by postpartum maternal contact.[253-256] As mentioned earlier, when congenital tuberculosis does occur, it is often associated with endometrial involvement in the mother and the disease commonly disseminates. Further discussion of the management of the neonate born to a mother with tuberculosis is beyond the scope of this chapter but can be found in detail in published articles.[214,217,257]

Latent Tuberculosis

It must be recognized that a positive skin test result indicates only tuberculous infection and not necessarily active disease. Furthermore, patients with active tuberculosis do not necessarily have a positive skin test result, mainly as a result of anergy caused by immunocompromise. Although there had been concern in the past that pregnancy might suppress positive skin test reactions,[258] it is now generally accepted that tuberculin skin test results are unchanged and valid through the course of pregnancy.[240,259-261]

The tuberculin skin test is currently an important screening test for tuberculosis but should not be performed indiscriminately in all pregnant women.[240] A tuberculin skin test should be placed only on individuals who are considered to be at high risk for contracting and/or failing to contain tuberculosis infection. Conditions and circumstances that should prompt tuberculin skin testing are listed in Table 18–2, as are the criteria for a positive result in a specific group.

If a tuberculin skin test reaction is positive, a search for active disease should be undertaken with a thorough history, physical examination, and chest radiograph with appropriate shielding as discussed previously. If only latent tuberculosis infection is documented, treatment with isoniazid should be undertaken for a total of 9 months. There is less clinical experience with alternative regimens of either 4 months of rifampin monotherapy or 2 months of rifampin plus pyrazinamide; episodes of severe liver injury have been associated with the latter.[240,262]

However, although there is near universal agreement on the advisability of the eventual treatment of latent tuberculosis infection discovered in the setting of pregnancy, there is less agreement on when this therapy should commence. Because pregnancy is not believed to increase the risk of reactivation of latent infection[263] and several studies have suggested an increased risk for hepatotoxicity when antituberculosis medications are used during pregnancy or the immediate postpartum period, a number of experts have suggested that therapy for latent tuberculosis infection should be postponed until well after delivery.[240] In contrast, others have suggested that the absence of demonstrated teratogenic effects of isoniazid supports the strategy that all patients with latent tuberculosis should begin treatment at the time of diagnosis.[240,264] Most practitioners have adopted a middle ground, delaying the initiation of isoniazid until after the first trimester, except in cases of HIV infection or recent close contact with an infectious patient, in which case the risk of developing active disease that can endanger both the mother and baby is thought to outweigh risks of the early institution of therapy.

As stated previously, pyridoxine supplementation should be administered routinely to all pregnant women receiving isoniazid. Baseline and monthly measurements of serum AST and bilirubin are recommended, as are monthly clinical examinations to evaluate for signs and symptoms of drug toxicity.[240]

Other Infectious Diseases of the Lung

Apart from tuberculosis, the major infectious agents that affect the lung during pregnancy are the same ones that usually cause community-acquired pneumonia in nonpregnant adults of childbearing age. These include typical bacterial pathogens (especially *Streptococcus pneumoniae*, *Mycoplasma pneumoniae*, *Chlamydia pneumoniae*) and viruses. Fungal infections are an additional consideration in the pregnant patient residing in or visiting an endemic area, and coccidioidomycosis is of particular concern because of a possible predisposition to dissemination during pregnancy, as is discussed in the section on fungal infections.

Community-Acquired Pneumonia

Community-acquired pneumonia must be considered in the otherwise healthy patient who presents with relatively acute symptoms of fever and cough (either productive or nonproductive) and infiltrates on chest radiograph. The cause of community-acquired pneumonia is never identified in a high proportion of patients, perhaps as high as 50%. In one series of 71 cases of pneumonia complicating pregnancy, a diagnosis was obtained in only 27% of patients, but in many of these cases, diagnostic specimens were not collected.[265]

Community-acquired pneumonia remains a significant cause of nonobstetric maternal mortality in the United States.[266] The overall frequency of pneumonia during pregnancy ranges from approximately 1 per 400 to 1 per 1200.[267,268] Significant risk factors for development of pneumonia during pregnancy include cocaine use,

---

TABLE 18–2   Tuberculin Skin Testing: Indications and Criteria for Positivity

Indication	Size of Induration Indicating Positive Test Result
HIV seropositivity	5 mm
Recent contact with patients who have active tuberculosis	5 mm
Fibrotic change on chest radiograph consistent with prior tuberculosis	5 mm
Organ transplantation or other immunosuppression-related condition necessitating >15 mg/day of prednisone or the equivalent	5 mm
Recent (<5 years) immigration from an area of high tuberculosis prevalence	10 mm
Injection drug users	10 mm
Residents and employees of high-risk congregate settings, such as prisons, nursing homes, hospitals, homeless shelters	10 mm

HIV, human immunodeficiency virus.

infection with HIV, underlying medical illness, and smoking.[267,269,270] Maternal mortality may be higher when pneumonia occurs during the third trimester or in immunocompromised patients.[266]

Although the relative frequencies of bacterial, mycoplasmal, chlamydial, and viral pneumonia during pregnancy are not well established, it appears that *S. pneumoniae* is the most common bacterial cause of pneumonia in this population. For example, in one series, *S. pneumoniae* was responsible for 13 of 21 cases of culture-proven bacterial pneumonia during pregnancy.[271] In patients who are smokers or those with acquired immunodeficiency syndrome, *Haemophilus influenzae* is the other organism that is relatively common.

Other types of bacterial pneumonia are less common in this age group, unless the pneumonia is acquired in the hospital rather than in the community. It is also important to note that viral infections, particularly influenza, may sometimes be complicated by development of a superimposed bacterial pneumonia. In these cases, the pneumococcus is still a common pathogen, but additional considerations include pneumonias caused by other streptococci, staphylococci, and *H. influenzae*. Pneumonia caused by *Legionella pneumophila* has been reported in pregnancy[272] and should be sought in the particularly ill patient with an atypical presentation or with nondiagnostic sputum examination findings.

A number of publications have addressed the general diagnostic and therapeutic approach to the patient with community-acquired pneumonia.[273,274] Although it is difficult to establish with certainty the frequencies of various causes of community-acquired pneumonia, it is believed that the presence of a coexisting disease and the severity of the illness at initial presentation affect the likelihood of particular etiologic agents. As a result, these factors should affect the initial choice of antimicrobial therapy. Although is not known whether pregnancy affects the likelihood of different causes of pneumonia or the response to treatment, it seems reasonable at present to apply the same guidelines to community-acquired pneumonia in the pregnant woman, albeit with particular care to select antibiotics with acceptable safety profiles in this setting.

Although a general guiding principle for managing infectious disease is to obtain specimens before use of antimicrobial therapy, guidelines from the American Thoracic Society propose that outpatients with community-acquired pneumonia be treated empirically.[273] Patients are categorized into one of four groups, on the basis of specific risk factors for mortality or a complicated course of pneumonia. In patients who have no coexisting cardiopulmonary disease, do not require hospitalization, and have no risk factors for drug-resistant *S. pneumoniae*, the most common pathogens include *S. pneumoniae*, *M. pneumoniae*, respiratory viruses, *C. pneumoniae*, and *H. influenzae*. The preferred therapeutic regimen is a macrolide antibiotic, particularly azithromycin. In patients who have coexisting illness but can still be treated in an outpatient setting, *S. pneumoniae* (including drug-resistant strains), *M. pneumoniae*, *H. influenzae*, and aerobic gram-negative bacilli remain important. Recommended regimens include a second-generation cephalosporin plus azithromycin.

The third and fourth groups differ from the first two on the basis of the severity of the pneumonia. The third group is defined by a need for hospitalization, whereas the fourth group includes patients who have the most severe disease and who require admission to an intensive care unit. Gram-negative bacilli and *Legionella* organisms become of significant concern in these groups of patients, and therapy is adjusted accordingly. A second-generation cephalosporin plus azithromycin is appropriate for hospitalized patients not requiring intensive care, and a fluoroquinolone or aminoglycoside may need to be added to this regimen in critically ill patients with risk factors for *Pseudomonas aeruginosa*,[273] although both classes of medications have potentially deleterious effects on the fetus.

The course and potential complications of pneumonia in pregnant women have been examined in a number of studies since the mid-1960s.[267-269,271] In several studies comprising 161 patients with presumed pneumonia, there was one maternal death.[265,267,268,271] In one of these studies, however, a number of maternal complications were observed, including bacteremia, empyema, and the need for mechanical ventilation.[268] Fetal outcome was generally excellent, except for cases in which the mother had additional complicating medical problems. In one study reporting a high frequency of maternal complications, preterm labor was seen in 44% of cases and perinatal death occurred in 12% of cases.[268] Pregnancy itself does not appear to affect adversely the response to antibiotic therapy, but the choice of antibiotics must take into account possible adverse effects on the fetus (see Chapter 15).

Viral Pneumonia

The viral pathogens that can cause pneumonia in the pregnant woman are presumably similar to those that cause pneumonia in the nonpregnant patient, influenza being particularly common (see Chapter 16). Influenza virus does not appear to cross the placenta or result in the production of harmful autoantibodies, but severely affected patients have a higher rate of pregnancy complications.[275] Influenza vaccination, with the standard inactivated virus preparation, is recommended for all women who will be in the second or third trimester of pregnancy during influenza season.[276]

The safety of the antiviral drugs amantadine, rimantadine, zanamivir, and oseltamivir has not been adequately established during pregnancy, and these medications should be employed only if the potential benefit is thought to outweigh the potential risks to the fetus. In view of the relatively small clinical benefits that have been demonstrated with their use, it is difficult to justify prescription of these drugs in the setting of pregnancy. Both amantadine and rimantadine have proven teratogenic at high doses in animals; human case reports have suggested a link between first trimester amantadine use and congenital anomalies, although this association remains unproven.[276,277]

Another viral infection that has been well described during pregnancy is that of varicella.[278-285] In the older literature, the maternal mortality rate from varicella pneumonia was approximately 35% to 45%, in comparison with the 15% to 20% mortality rate described among nonpregnant patients. In addition to the high maternal mortality rate, only approximately one of six pregnancies was free of neonatal complications, including abortion, in utero death associated with maternal death, prematurity, or neonatal varicella.[281] It is presumed that maternal hypoxia caused by extensive pneumonia is the primary factor resulting in maternal and fetal complications when the infection occurs in later pregnancy.[284] Infection in the first trimester may result in congenital varicella syndrome, with anomalies such as cutaneous scars, limb hypoplasia, muscle atrophy, malformed digits, psychomotor retardation, microcephaly, cortical atrophy, cataracts, chorioretinitis, and microophthalmia.[279]

Nonimmune pregnant women with a significant exposure history to varicella-zoster virus should be considered for prophylactic treatment with varicella-zoster immune globulin.[283] Most authors suggest that if chickenpox develops in the mother, oral acyclovir should be implemented within 24 hours of the first skin eruptions in an attempt to ameliorate the severity of maternal infection. Although clinical experience suggests that acyclovir is safe in this setting, its true risk to the fetus is not precisely known, and thorough informed consent must be obtained from the mother. In the case of varicella pneumonia, hospitalization and treatment with intravenous acyclovir are generally indicated because of the significant risk posed to maternal and therefore fetal health.[283] On the basis of a reported mortality rate of 14% in treated cases, acyclovir appears to reduce the high rate of maternal mortality associated with varicella pneumonia during pregnancy.[278,285]

Fungal Infections

A detailed analysis of the clinical aspects and diagnosis of the various fungal disorders of the lung is beyond the scope of this discussion but can be found in a number of review articles.[286-290]

Of the various fungal infections encountered during pregnancy, coccidioidomycosis has generated the most interest, primarily because of its reported tendency to disseminate during pregnancy.[291] Of the 50 cases of coccidioidomycosis either reported or reviewed by Harris,[292] 22 became disseminated. In patients in whom the onset of coccidioidomycosis occurred before pregnancy, the risk of dissemination increased to 20% from the 0.2% risk expected for dissemination in the nonpregnant patient. The risk was even higher in patients who contracted the infection during pregnancy, particularly in the second or third trimester.[292] Reactivation of coccidioidomycosis during pregnancy has also been reported in a woman successfully treated 4 to 5 years earlier and disease-free in the interim.[293]

Two major theories have been proposed to explain an increased risk of dissemination during pregnancy. One of these is based on studies showing an increased rate of growth of *Coccidioides immitis,* as well as an increased rate of release of endospores in the presence of 17β-estradiol and progesterone.[293a] In addition, binding proteins for progesterone and estradiol were identified in the cytosol of the fungus, whereas little or no binding was found in a variety of other fungal organisms.[294] These studies suggested a mechanism by which nanomolar concentrations of sex hormones during pregnancy could bind to the fungus and stimulate growth and release of endospores. The other theory proposes that decreased cell-mediated immunity during pregnancy could predispose to dissemination. Support for this theory was provided by demonstration of impaired lymphocyte blast transformation in response to spherulin antigen during pregnancy.[295]

Despite the past interest in and acceptance of an increased risk of coccidioidal dissemination and mortality during pregnancy, Catanzaro[296] suggested that the risk has been substantially overestimated. On the basis of a survey of physicians in endemic areas, he thought that there is much less dissemination and mortality from maternal coccidioidomycosis than have been reported in the literature. However, the data on which this statement is based were obtained from an informal survey subject to inaccuracies of sampling and recall rather than from a formal epidemiologic study. In the most recent large study of coccidioidomycosis during pregnancy, only 10 cases were found among more than 47,000 pregnancies in an endemic area. All patients with disease diagnosed during the first or second trimester did well, although two of three patients in whom coccidioidomycosis was diagnosed during the first 10 days post partum developed disseminated disease.[297]

When coccidioidomycosis remains in its benign, nondisseminated form, there appears to be no particular hazard for either the mother or the fetus. Early literature found that the maternal mortality rate for untreated disseminated coccidioidomycosis was almost 100%, in comparison with a 50% mortality rate among untreated nonpregnant patients with disseminated disease.[292] However, it has been reported that amphotericin B therapy in pregnant women with disseminated disease saves a significant proportion of patients.[298]

Various other fungi have been reported in pregnant women, but except for coccidioidomycosis, involvement appears to occur primarily in women who are immunosuppressed.[288,299]

Amphotericin B, despite its multiple potential maternal side effects and the fact that it crosses the placenta, is considered the drug of choice for treating serious fungal infections in the pregnant patient because of its established efficacy.[300,301] Furthermore, although extensive data regarding its effect on the fetus are not available, amphotericin appears not to have any common detrimental effects on the fetal or the neonatal course.[302-304] At least one case of amphotericin use during the first trimester has been reported, and no adverse effects on the fetus were observed.[302] There is less experience with the newer liposomal forms of amphotericin, but most practitioners consider these forms also to be suitable for use in pregnant patients.[300,301]

The azole class of antifungal agents has been used far less during pregnancy, and therefore, despite their lesser maternal toxicity and ease of oral administration, they are best avoided in pregnant women. Although a number of studies have shown no excess risk of congenital malformations with low doses of fluconazole,[305-307] a number of infants with multiple skeletal abnormalities have been delivered to mothers who received 400 to 800 mg of the drug per day.[300,308] There are fewer data regarding the teratogenic potential of itraconazole and voriconazole, but the use of these drugs in pregnancy should be restricted to cases of life-threatening fungal infections in which no other treatment options are available.[301,309]

Pulmonary Hypertension

The most common pulmonary vascular disease encountered during and after pregnancy is thromboembolic disease. The problems of peripheral venous thrombosis, pulmonary embolism, and anticoagulation are discussed in detail in Chapter 5. Another pulmonary vascular condition encountered in women of childbearing age, pulmonary hypertension, is discussed in this section. Amniotic fluid embolism, although it involves the pulmonary vasculature, is discussed in the following section, "Acute Respiratory Distress Syndrome in Pregnancy."

Pulmonary hypertension is currently defined as a pulmonary artery systolic pressure higher than 40 mm Hg.[310] This condition can occur as a result of more than 30 different diseases or associations. Pulmonary hypertension affecting women of childbearing age in industrialized nations is most commonly caused by primary pulmonary hypertension, connective tissue disease such as progressive systemic sclerosis (scleroderma), or Eisenmenger's syndrome resulting from an uncorrected congenital cardiac defect.[311]

Pathologic changes in the walls of small pulmonary arteries and arterioles lead to narrowing and sometimes to obliteration of the lumen of these vessels. Pulmonary resistance and pulmonary arterial pressures increase, and right ventricular hypertrophy ensues. Symptoms in patients with pulmonary hypertension include dyspnea, limited exercise tolerance, chest pain, and syncope; the hemodynamic stresses of pregnancy may markedly intensify the symptoms in previously well-compensated individuals.[312] The presence of elevated pulmonary arterial pressures may be suggested by findings on cardiac examination, electrocardiogram, or chest radiograph, and transthoracic echocardiography can be strongly suggestive of the diagnosis and estimate its severity.

It is well recognized that pregnancy poses a serious and often life-threatening risk to patients with pulmonary hypertension. In a review of 23 pregnancies in 16 patients with primary pulmonary hypertension, 9 patients died during pregnancy or the postpartum period.[313] Although the time of death was variable, death was often sudden and most frequently occurred during the last 2 months of pregnancy or in the postpartum period. Several patients died during or just after labor from apparent cardiovascular collapse.

Pulmonary hypertension of any cause interferes with normal cardiac adaptations to pregnancy, and the increase of 30% to 50% in cardiac output that normally occurs may not be possible because of a high, fixed pulmonary vascular resistance. The result is a mortality rate as high as 30% to 50% among patients with severe pulmonary hypertension.[311,313-316] An additional problem during labor may be the substantial increase in pulmonary blood volume that occurs with each contraction.

The high risk of sudden death in the postpartum period is probably related to elevation of cardiac output

and pulmonary blood volume after evacuation of the uterus. Once the uterus contracts, an augmentation in venous return produces the postpartum increase in cardiac output and pulmonary blood volume.[313] In addition, release of pressure of the gravid uterus on the inferior vena cava after delivery may further contribute to a sudden increase in venous return.[317] With markedly increased pulmonary vascular resistance, a volume shift to the lungs may acutely elevate pulmonary arterial and right-sided heart pressures, leading to acute right ventricular failure and cardiovascular collapse.

Because of the high risk of death during pregnancy in such patients, it is reasonable to consider pulmonary hypertension a contraindication to pregnancy. When such a patient does become pregnant and does not desire a therapeutic abortion, management is quite difficult, particularly during labor and the postpartum period. Placement of a pulmonary artery (Swan-Ganz) catheter in preparation for labor and delivery may be helpful in assessing the hemodynamic status of these patients.[317] With a pulmonary artery catheter in place, vasodilators such as inhaled nitric oxide may also be used if necessary and their effect closely monitored to judge efficacy. Keeping patients in the lateral position during labor and delivery may also be helpful, at least on a theoretical basis. With the patient in the lateral position, sudden alterations in venous return after delivery may be minimized when caval flow is released from the pressure of the uterus.[317]

Pregnancy has important ramifications for the longer term medical management of pulmonary hypertension. Bosentan (Tracleer), an orally active endothelin-1 receptor antagonist that was approved by the U.S. Food and Drug Administration in 2001, is contraindicated in pregnancy because of its high teratogenic activity in animal models.[318] Likewise, warfarin, which may slow the progression of the pulmonary hypertension, also cannot be safely employed. Continuous intravenous epoprostenol (Flolan, prostacyclin) and inhaled nitric oxide have been used both acutely and chronically in pregnant patients with pulmonary hypertension without reported adverse fetal effects, although their precise risk profile is unknown.[319-323] Nonetheless, because of the high maternal mortality rate, their use in this setting must be judicious.[311]

Acute Respiratory Distress Syndrome in Pregnancy

ARDS is a syndrome of noncardiogenic pulmonary edema characterized by diffuse injury to alveolar epithelial and capillary endothelial cells in the lung. As a result of the injury, which can be produced in many settings and by many different etiologic agents, fluid leaks out of pulmonary capillaries and into the alveolar interstitium and the alveolar spaces.[324-326]

Although ARDS can be initiated in many diverse ways, the clinical syndrome that develops has certain characteristic features independent of the underlying cause. These include dyspnea, hypoxemia, "stiff lungs," and diffuse infiltrates poorly compliant on chest radiograph. Patients frequently develop refractory hypoxemia and respiratory failure, which necessitate use of mechanical ventilation.

Of the causes of ARDS that are common in nonpregnant patients, infection (either sepsis or primary pulmonary infection) is the most common seen during pregnancy.[327,328] In addition, amniotic fluid embolism and pulmonary edema associated with tocolytic therapy are causes of ARDS that are unique to pregnancy, whereas ARDS caused by aspiration of gastric contents is an important additional concern during pregnancy.

Mechanical ventilation, institution of positive end-expiratory pressure (PEEP), other supportive measures, and treatment of the underlying cause of the condition form the cornerstones of management. Hypocapnia should be avoided because it may compromise uteroplacental perfusion,[329] and a mechanical ventilation strategy of tidal volumes of 6 mL/kg and plateau pressures less than 30 cm H_2O should be pursued unless otherwise contraindicated.[330] Because spontaneous tidal volumes in pregnancy may exceed 6 mL/kg, a high respiratory rate may need to be set on the ventilator to maintain adequate alveolar ventilation if a low tidal volume has been selected; such patients require close monitoring for the development of intrinsic PEEP.[331] Many patients develop multisystem organ failure, which is often responsible for death. The management of ARDS is further detailed in other sources.[325,326,331]

Amniotic Fluid Embolism

Amniotic fluid embolism is one cause of ARDS that is uniquely associated with pregnancy.[332] Although it is not a common disorder (occurring in 1 per 8000 to 1 per 80,000 pregnancies), its high mortality rate renders it accountable for up to 15% of maternal deaths.[333,334] At present, there is no way to predict which patients will develop amniotic fluid embolism, and there is no therapy to prevent it.[335]

In this disorder, amniotic fluid enters the maternal circulation during or after labor, with resulting embolization to the pulmonary vasculature. The material that embolizes includes not only amniotic fluid but also fetal squamae, lanugo hairs, meconium, fat, mucin, and bile.[336,337]

This syndrome does not appear to be caused by embolization of amniotic fluid itself, because intravenous infusion of fresh, autologous amniotic fluid into pregnant rabbits or rhesus monkeys is innocuous.[338,339] Rather, one of many contaminants, of either fetal or placental origin, is presumably responsible for initiating the clinical syndrome. Although the major precipitating feature of the disorder is unknown, speculation has centered on several theories: (1) mechanical occlusion of the pulmonary vasculature by particulate material in the amniotic fluid, (2) hypersensitivity or an anaphylactoid reaction to fetal antigens or particulate matter, (3) left ventricular failure,[340] and (4) alveolar-capillary leakage secondary to microvascular injury from extensive amniotic fluid embolism.[332,340,341] The last of these theories is the most popular and puts amniotic fluid embolism into the broad category of diffuse alveolar-capillary injury with ARDS.

There have been several postulated sites for entry of amniotic fluid into the maternal venous circulation, including (1) endocervical veins, which are lacerated even during normal labor; (2) the placental site, especially with placenta previa, uterine rupture, premature separation of the placenta, or cesarean section with an incision involving the placental implantation site; and (3) uterine veins, at sites of uterine trauma.[336] Several risk factors have been postulated to predispose the mother to development of amniotic fluid embolism: (1) tumultuous labor, (2) use of uterine stimulants, (3) meconium in the amniotic fluid, (4) advanced maternal age, (5) multiparity, and (6) intrauterine death.[120,336,342] It has been suggested that the association with intrauterine fetal death may be related to increased permeability and friability of fetal membranes.[343]

However, the role of uterine stimulants and exceptionally strong uterine contractions has been questioned.[333] A temporal association in some patients between artificial rupture of the membranes, placement of an intrauterine pressure catheter, or cesarean section and development of the syndrome suggests that high pressure is not related to entry of amniotic fluid into the maternal circulation. Rather, under the proper but yet undefined conditions, simple exposure of the maternal circulation to even small amounts of amniotic fluid may initiate the syndrome.[333]

Clark and coworkers suggested that the pathogenesis of amniotic fluid embolism may be analogous to both septic shock and anaphylaxis, perhaps with a variety of mediators being released in response to foreign material or substances entering the circulation.[333] Such mediators could include leukotrienes, histamine, bradykinin, and prostaglandins. These authors believed that the syndrome is therefore not contingent on embolism of amniotic fluid, and they proposed that the term *amniotic fluid embolism* be discarded in favor of the term *anaphylactoid syndrome of pregnancy*.

The clinical picture of amniotic fluid embolism consists of respiratory distress, cardiovascular collapse, and disseminated intravascular coagulation associated with or occurring after labor and delivery. However, because the course of the illness is frequently catastrophic, the full clinical syndrome may not have time to develop. Presenting features may include dyspnea, cyanosis, profound shock, seizures, cardiac arrest, or fetal bradycardia.[333,341,342,344] In some cases, symptoms may not appear until many hours after delivery.[332] Heavy bleeding is not a sole presenting feature but rather occurs along with or after other manifestations of the disorder. Pulmonary edema, bronchospasm, and pulmonary hypertension are frequently clinically apparent; pathologic examination of the lungs demonstrates pulmonary edema in addition to amniotic fluid debris in the pulmonary vasculature.[342]

A national registry of patients with amniotic fluid embolism accumulated 46 cases.[333] Embolism occurred during labor in 70%, after vaginal delivery in 11%, and during cesarean section after delivery of the infant in 19%. The maternal mortality rate was 61%; only 15% of the women both survived and were neurologically intact. Survival among fetuses in utero at the time of the event was only 39%.

Diagnosis of amniotic fluid embolism has generally been made clinically, on the basis of the constellation of findings just discussed. In particular, the dramatic appearance of dyspnea, hypoxemia, and hypotension in the early postpartum period is suggestive of the diagnosis.[345] Pulmonary thromboembolism may manifest with similar findings, but the presence of disseminated intravascular coagulation (see Chapter 4) is suggestive of amniotic fluid embolism rather than thromboembolic disease. Diagnosis has been made by cytologic examination and demonstration of squamous cells and cellular debris in blood drawn from a wedged pulmonary artery (Swan-Ganz) catheter.[345,346] This technique has been called *pulmonary microvascular cytology*.[346] However, the presence of fetal squamous cells in the pulmonary circulation of women who died of other causes suggests that this finding is not specific.[333]

The maternal mortality rate exceeds 60% to 80% in amniotic fluid embolism, with death often occurring immediately or within the first several hours of onset.[333,336] Treatment revolves primarily around circulatory and respiratory support. During the acute episode, intubation is commonly necessary for ventilatory support; addition of PEEP may also be necessary to decrease the intrapulmonary shunt and assist oxygenation. Decisions about use of vasopressors, volume expansion, or diuresis are made on an individual basis and often guided by hemodynamic measurements made with a pulmonary artery catheter. One case report has suggested benefit from administration of cryoprecipitate, given with the rationale of repleting fibronectin.[347] Fibronectin, an opsonic protein, may protect the integrity of the reticuloendothelial system and allow it to remove debris and particulate material, such as that generated by amniotic fluid embolism. Although the patient in the case report improved after cryoprecipitate administration, additional cases need to be reported before this can be considered a valuable form of therapy. The use of high doses of corticosteroids has also been proposed, but there are no data to support or refute this mode of therapy.[333,348] Extracorporeal membrane oxygenation in conjunction with aortic balloon counterpulsation also has been employed, although it unclear whether the intervention was responsible for the successful outcome reported.[349]

Pulmonary Edema Associated with Sympathomimetic Therapy

As mentioned in the section on asthma, a number of cases of pulmonary edema during or after sympathomimetic therapy for inhibition of premature labor have been reported.[124-126,350,351] This complication of tocolytic therapy is rare; one study of 8709 women receiving terbutaline noted that it occurred in 28 patients (0.32%).[352] A variety of sympathomimetic agents have been implicated (e.g., ritodrine, terbutaline, albuterol), generally when administered by intravenous infusion. In most cases, a corticosteroid preparation was given simultaneously, but because cases without concomitant steroid use have also been described, steroids are not crucial to the development of pulmonary edema.[126,350] Additional proposed risk factors are twin births[351] and the presence of coexistent maternal infection, perhaps related to infection that contributes to a pulmonary capillary permeability defect.[353,354]

The mean duration of tocolytic therapy in patients developing this syndrome is 54 hours. Although most patients develop pulmonary edema while receiving therapy, approximately 25% developed symptoms after the sympathomimetic agent was discontinued. In almost all of the latter cases, symptoms occurred within 12 hours of a cesarean section performed after tocolytic agents failed to arrest labor.[351]

The mechanism of pulmonary edema associated with tocolytic therapy remains uncertain. Invasive hemodynamic monitoring in several cases demonstrated normal pulmonary capillary wedge pressures, which suggests that the pulmonary edema was not cardiogenic in origin but rather caused by increased pulmonary capillary permeability (i.e., ARDS).[124,126] In another case, elevated pulmonary capillary wedge pressure in the setting of normal left ventricular function shown by echocardiography suggested that volume overload may sometimes contribute to or be primarily responsible for pulmonary edema.[355] In their review of 58 cases reported through 1988, Pisani and Rosenow[351] concluded that hypotonic fluid overload, exacerbated by increased secretion of antidiuretic hormone and decreased secretion of serum albumin induced by tocolytic agents, is responsible for pulmonary edema.

Fortunately, pulmonary edema in most of these patients has been transient and self-limited, but there have also been case reports of maternal death from tocolytic-induced pulmonary edema.[356] Therapy involves discontinuation of the sympathomimetic agent and support of oxygenation, with supplemental oxygen and sometimes mechanical ventilation with PEEP.[126] Diuretics are generally indicated and are helpful in reducing interstitial and alveolar edema. In patients with complications or who are particularly ill, a pulmonary artery (Swan-Ganz) catheter may be helpful in guiding fluid management and diuretic therapy.

Aspiration of Gastric Contents

Aspiration of gastric contents into the lungs is a well-recognized cause of ARDS in both pregnant and nonpregnant patients.[357] During pregnancy, aspiration is a problem primarily at the time of labor and delivery. It has been suggested that pregnant women may be particularly susceptible to aspiration, and the following mechanisms have been proposed[358,359]: (1) elevation of intragastric pressure as a result of compression of abdominal contents by the gravid uterus, (2) relaxation of the gastroesophageal sphincter mechanism by progesterone, (3) delayed gastric emptying secondary to depressed motilin release, and (4) use of medications such as narcotics of which emesis is a common side effect. In addition, it is not uncommon for the stomach to be full at the time of labor, and any complication of labor necessitating general anesthesia may be associated with vomiting and aspiration at the time of induction. Although maternal aspiration appears to be a relatively uncommon problem, it has been estimated that approximately 2% of maternal deaths result from aspiration.[360]

Two major types of aspiration can be seen at the time of labor and delivery. In the first, inhalation of liquid gastric contents (with a pH < 2.5) into the lungs can induce a chemical pneumonitis; in the second, there is airway obstruction caused by aspiration of particulate material. These syndromes were originally described in 1946 in a classic paper by Mendelson.[361] Of the 66 obstetric patients with aspiration reported in this series, 5 had acute obstructive reactions from aspiration of food particles, and 61 aspirated liquid gastric contents.

In the syndrome caused by inhalation of acid gastric contents, aspiration is soon followed by tachypnea, cyanosis, tachycardia, and hypotension. An inflammatory pneumonitis ensues, and the clinical picture of ARDS may result, with leakage of fluid into the alveoli and dyspnea, hypoxemia, and noncompliant lungs. On chest radiograph, there are fluffy infiltrates conforming to an alveolar filling pattern; they may be generalized or may correspond to the dependent areas at the time of aspiration. Treatment is mainly supportive, with maintenance of adequate oxygenation by supplemental oxygen and, if necessary, intubation and positive-pressure ventilation. Although corticosteroids were commonly used in the past, there is no clear evidence that they are beneficial. In fact, one study suggested no difference in mortality but an increase in gram-negative bacterial superinfection in patients treated with steroids.[362]

Aspiration of food particles, the other major aspiration syndrome seen in obstetric patients, may cause variable amounts of airway obstruction, depending on the size and consistency of the particles. If the particulate material is sufficiently large, the patients may actually asphyxiate. Supportive measures are again essential, with maintenance of adequate oxygenation as just described. Suctioning should be done to remove particles from the larger airways, and bronchoscopy may be necessary to further localize and remove aspirated food.

Because definitive treatment of aspiration pneumonitis is problematic, attempts should be made to lower the risk of aspiration. The most important measure is limitation of oral intake during labor; H_2 antagonists and dopamine antagonists are also employed prophylactically before obstetric surgery in some centers.[359]

Pleural Effusion

The development of a significant pleural effusion during pregnancy presents an important diagnostic problem similar to that in the nonpregnant patient. To our knowledge, no studies have specifically examined the frequency or causes of pleural effusion developing during pregnancy. In view of the age of the patients, the most likely causes are pulmonary embolism, tuberculosis, and pneumonia with an adjacent (i.e., parapneumonic) effusion. One review has also summarized some of the rarer causes of pregnancy-associated effusions.[363] Thoracentesis and analysis of the fluid are often extremely helpful in the diagnostic workup of these patients. Further discussion of the differential diagnosis and diagnostic evaluation of pleural effusion is beyond the scope of this chapter but can be found in other sources.[364,365]

According to posteroanterior and lateral chest radiographs, asymptomatic pleural effusions, usually small and bilateral, are quite common in the first 24 hours after delivery. In two studies, approximately 25% to 50% of patients had effusions documented by radiography or ultrasonography in the absence of any evidence of symptoms or cardiopulmonary disease.[366,367] However, another study with ultrasonography found that postpartum effusions were less frequent, occurring in only 1 of 50 patients examined within 45 hours of delivery.[368]

Despite the uncertainty about the incidence of postpartum pleural effusions, potential contributing factors include increased blood volume and decreased oncotic pressure, which are normal occurrences during pregnancy, complicated by repeated Valsalva maneuvers during labor that impair lymphatic drainage from the pleural space.[363] When these effusions do occur, they are clinically unimportant and do not necessitate any diagnostic evaluation or intervention unless they are moderate to large or are accompanied by clinical signs or symptoms.

Pneumomediastinum and Pneumothorax

Pneumomediastinum, the presence of free air in the mediastinal space, is an uncommon complication of pregnancy, generally occurring at the time of labor. The pathogenesis is believed to involve rupture of marginally situated alveoli into perivascular tissue planes, with tracking of air toward the hilum and into the mediastinum.[369] Under most circumstances, air subsequently dissects through fascial planes in the neck to result in subcutaneous emphysema. This escape of air from the mediastinum into the subcutaneous tissues prevents buildup of pressure within the mediastinum, which might otherwise impede venous return to the intrathoracic veins.

Spontaneous pneumomediastinum often occurs in the setting of high intraalveolar pressure, especially with coughing, vomiting, or a Valsalva maneuver. During labor, the intense Valsalva maneuver associated with "bearing down" induces transient marked elevations in intraalveolar pressure, occasionally resulting in alveolar rupture and the sequence of events outlined previously.[370]

Although approximately 200 cases of pneumomediastinum or subcutaneous emphysema associated with pregnancy have been reported to date, very few are in the most recent medical literature.[371-374] Almost all the cases have occurred during labor, but a few have been reported at other times during pregnancy.

The main symptom of spontaneous pneumomediastinum is substernal chest pain of abrupt onset, often accompanied by dyspnea. The pain commonly radiates to the shoulders and both arms and is generally aggravated by coughing, deep inspiration, and swallowing. On physical examination, subcutaneous emphysema is found most commonly in the neck and over the face and chest wall; however, it may require hours for a large amount of subcutaneous crepitation to develop. On auscultation, Hamman's sign, a crunching or crackling sound synchronous with the heartbeat, may be heard over the precordium, particularly at the cardiac apex with the patient in the left lateral position.

Free mediastinal air on posteroanterior chest radiographs appears as a radiolucent stripe outlining the heart border, most prominently along the left; there may also be a longitudinal air shadow adjacent to the thoracic aorta. On the lateral projection, there is frequently retrosternal air, and the posterior mediastinal structures, particularly the aorta, may be much more clearly defined than usual.

In spontaneous pneumomediastinum, there is usually resorption of air over the course of several days. Resorption can be accelerated if necessary by the administration of supplemental oxygen. Although tension pneumomediastinum with death has been reported, it is quite rare, and the development of subcutaneous emphysema almost uniformly relieves the buildup of pressure before any significant hemodynamic sequelae.

Pneumothorax, the presence of free air in the pleural space, has also been reported during pregnancy; most cases appear during labor or shortly after delivery[363] or, less commonly, as a consequence of hyperemesis gravidarum.[375,376] Although some patients have had underlying lung diseases known to predispose to pneumothorax, others probably have rupture of previously unrecognized subpleural blebs. The frequent association with labor and delivery suggests that high intrathoracic pressure from repeated Valsalva maneuvers causes rupture of the blebs and release of air into the pleural space.

If the pneumothorax is large, poorly tolerated, or associated with significant hypoxemia, drainage with a pleural catheter or a chest tube is indicated.[377] If a pneumothorax develops near term but before labor, consideration should be given to inducing labor while a chest tube is in place because of the potential for recurrence or worsening during labor. Thoracoscopy or thoracotomy during pregnancy for resection of blebs and pleurodesis has also been reported because of the concern for recurrence and/or problems with labor.[377-379]

Pregnancy in the Woman with Chronic Respiratory Insufficiency

Women with limited respiratory reserve who wish to become pregnant are not encountered frequently, because the disorders associated with chronic respiratory insufficiency generally occur in an older age group. However, occasionally the obstetrician or internist is faced with a patient with limited reserve as a result of pulmonary fibrosis, cystic fibrosis, or neuromuscular or chest wall disease. These cases are particularly challenging, because the paucity of available data makes it difficult to predict the outcome of pregnancy. Unfortunately, decisions to recommend abortion are therefore more often based on subjective feelings of the physician rather than on hard data regarding contraindications to pregnancy. We review the limited data available, but we stress that no reliable cutoff points regarding pulmonary function have been established.

The course of pregnancy in patients with pulmonary insufficiency was first systematically investigated in a series of seven women with 40% to 75% of VC as a result of lung resection or operative collapse.[380] The patients all tolerated pregnancy well, without any diminution in ventilatory capacity; subjective dyspnea was notably infrequent in these patients. The ones with more severe impairment met the greater ventilatory requirements of pregnancy by increasing respiratory rate rather than tidal volume. It is difficult, however, to extrapolate the course in these patients with surgically induced limitation of function to patients with severe obstructive disease or to those with restriction caused by diffuse parenchymal fibrosis.

Nevertheless, it was suggested that an impaired respiratory system is better able to cope with the additional respiratory demands of pregnancy than is the damaged heart with the increased circulatory demands.

It is difficult to quantitate the actual VC necessary to sustain a patient during pregnancy. Because normal women have little change in VC with pregnancy, an unchanged VC in patients with lung disease might be expected to be sufficient to sustain them during pregnancy. Unfortunately, patients with the most severe disease may frequently experience deterioration of pulmonary function during the course of pregnancy. Although it has been said that a VC of 1 L is the minimum functional requirement necessary to maintain a successful pregnancy,[381] there is little objective support for this particular value, and successful pregnancy has been reported with a VC as low as 800 mL.[382] Pulmonary artery catheterization has been useful in some of these patients to allow better monitoring of their cardiopulmonary status and management during labor and delivery.[383]

Theoretically, patients with baseline carbon dioxide retention or pulmonary hypertension might not be expected to handle the added ventilatory or circulatory demands of pregnancy, respectively. Although insufficient data regarding carbon dioxide retention are available, there exists some information regarding pulmonary hypertension, mainly in patients with primary pulmonary hypertension. As mentioned earlier in this chapter, the maternal mortality rate in this disorder has been reported as greater than 50%,[313] but the degree of pulmonary hypertension seen as a result of chronic lung disease is generally much less than in primary pulmonary hypertension.

There is also relatively little information regarding the effect of abnormal maternal gas exchange on the fetus. This topic is discussed in the earlier "Effects of Abnormal Arterial Blood Gases on the Fetus" section of this chapter. Whether the fetus becomes hypoxic is also dependent on numerous factors other than maternal Po_2, including uterine and placental compensatory mechanisms.[381] Any possible effect of maternal hypercapnia on the fetus is unknown. It has been suggested that premature labor is one potential effect of hypoxemia and hypercapnia, but this hypothesis is as yet unproved.[381]

As is evident from this discussion, knowledge about pregnancy in the woman with borderline respiratory function and limited reserve is inadequate for the development of useful recommendations. Each case must clearly be considered individually, and all the relevant information, including the natural history of the patient's disease during pregnancy, must be collated and then evaluated. Results of spirometry, arterial blood gas analysis, and clinical assessment for pulmonary hypertension all form an important part of the database, but, unfortunately, the relative weight that should be attached to each factor has not yet been defined.

SMOKING AND PREGNANCY

Although all physicians are aware of the major role played by cigarette smoking in the production of cancer, coronary artery disease, and chronic obstructive lung disease, the impact of cigarette smoking on the health and viability of the fetus and the newborn is not as well recognized. Since the publication of previous editions of this book, there has been a virtual explosion in research on the effects of cigarette smoking and pregnancy. The prevalence of cigarette smoking among married women aged 20 and over decreased between 1967 and 1980, from 40% to 25% of white persons and 33% to 23% of black persons.[384] Current estimates are that between 15% and 29% of women smoke during pregnancy.[385] Predictors of smoking cessation during pregnancy include younger age, marital status, higher education, smoking less than one pack per day, and Hispanic race.[386] However, the indirect effects of smoking on the fetus and the rarity of cigarette-induced disease in young mothers deflect clinical attention from this extremely important problem. Maternal cigarette smoking has important health consequences in five areas: (1) fetal and infant mortality, (2) birth defects, (3) birth weight, (4) lactation and breast-feeding, and (5) childhood disease.

Fetal and Infant Mortality

Perinatal mortality rates are higher among offspring of women who smoke than among offspring of their non-smoking counterparts.[387] However, there exists controversy about the magnitude of the increase in risk in relation to other important patient characteristics associated with fetal loss, such as race, low socioeconomic status, increased age and parity, and anemia. The most definitive study on this question is the work of Kleinman and coworkers.[388] These investigators used a large database (covering all Missouri residents during 1979 through 1983 and including 360,000 births, 2500 fetal deaths, and 3800 infant deaths) to assess the impact of smoking on fetal and infant mortality. The investigators controlled for the effects of age, parity, education, marital status, and race in examining the effects of maternal smoking on total mortality (infant and fetal deaths). They found a difference between primiparous and multiparous women in terms of the effects of cigarette smoking. Primiparous women who smoked less than one pack per day had a 25% greater risk of fetal and infant mortality than did non-smoking primiparous women. Those who smoked one or more packs per day had a 56% greater risk. Among multiparous women, fetal and infant mortality rates were 30% higher among smokers than among nonsmokers, with no difference by amount smoked. These authors also noted that racial differences in fetal and infant mortality could not be explained by differences in smoking, nor did adjustment for social class or other covariates greatly influence the results. They estimated that if all pregnant women stopped smoking, the number of fetal and infant deaths would decrease by 10%.

The underlying mechanisms by which cigarette smoke increases fetal and infant mortality are unknown and likely to be multifactorial. When causes of fetal death are studied, no differences have been noted between offspring of smokers and nonsmokers. Data from the Ontario Perinatal Mortality Study suggest that maternal problems specifically related to the placenta are important, because

abruptio placentae, placenta previa, bleeding during pregnancy, and premature rupture of the membranes all exhibited a significant dose-response relationship with levels of cigarette smoking.[389] Maternal complications of toxemia and preeclampsia are not increased among cigarette smokers, which suggests that these clinical problems do not play a significant role.

Prematurity is another important aspect of mortality. Although preterm births account for a small percentage of total births, they account for a disproportionate number of deaths. Some studies have noted an increase in preterm birth among cigarette smokers, and approximately 10% of such births can be attributed to this risk factor alone.[390] The frequency of preterm births rises with increased levels of cigarette smoking, thus confirming a dose-response effect. Data from a study in Denmark suggested that the preterm birth effect is limited to women who are also heavy users of caffeine (>4 cups of coffee per day).[391] Spontaneous abortion is also more common in cigarette smokers than in nonsmokers.[392] Case ascertainment of this condition is difficult, but in one carefully done study, an 80% excess of spontaneous abortions was noted in smokers versus nonsmokers.[393]

The increase in prematurity, spontaneous abortion, and placental problems suggests that the effects of cigarette smoking on infant mortality may be indirectly mediated by placental malfunction or malformation or by changes in uterine and placental oxygenation or blood flow. Physiologic studies have directly documented such effects.[394] In studies of the acute effect of smoking one cigarette, it was found that smoking caused a direct increase in vascular resistance of the placenta from the fetal side. This increased resistance may impair oxygen exchange across the placenta and contribute to the increased perinatal mortality associated with smoking. A corollary of decreased placental function is depressed Apgar scores at both 1 minute and 5 minutes in infants born to smoking mothers.[395] Nicotine is known to cross the placenta of humans, leading to a reflex increase in blood pressure and respiratory rate in the fetus. However, the role of nicotine in altering human uterine and placental blood flow is unknown.

More data on the effects of carbon monoxide are available.[396,397] Carbon monoxide binds avidly to hemoglobin, thus making less hemoglobin available to carry oxygen. The net effect is a decrease in the amount of oxygen carried to the fetus and other body tissues, which produces a functional anemia. Oxygen consumption is increased in pregnancy, and the high carbon monoxide level can effectively diminish oxygen delivered to the fetus for its metabolic needs. In addition, carbon monoxide shifts the maternal oxyhemoglobin dissociation curve to the left, leading to less release of oxygen to the fetus. Carbon monoxide levels in the fetus are in equilibrium with maternal levels and after 5 to 6 hours are comparable. A 10% concentration of carboxyhemoglobin, achieved in women smoking two packs of cigarettes per day, is equivalent to a 60% decrease in fetal blood flow. Placentas of smoking women are also often larger than those of nonsmokers and are abnormal histologically.[398] Whether these changes are related solely to hypoxia or other effects of cigarette smoke is unknown.

It is now firmly established that maternal cigarette smoking is an important cause of the sudden infant death syndrome (SIDS).[399,400] Mothers of infants who die of SIDS are more likely to smoke heavily and smoke during pregnancy than are mothers whose infants do not die of SIDS. The maternal smoking–SIDS relationship is independent of other SIDS risk factors, including low birth weight, gestational age, and gender. There seems to be a dose-response effect.[401]

Although available human studies cannot differentiate whether prenatal or postnatal exposure is more important, studies in a rat model show that maternal nicotine administration during pregnancy is associated with abnormalities of the fetal rat brain stem, which is suggestive of an important role for prenatal exposure.[38] Paradoxically, the risk for neonatal respiratory distress syndrome is reduced in infants of mothers who smoke. This is because lung maturity, as measured by amniotic fluid lecithin-sphingomyelin ratio, is increased, perhaps as a result of fetal hypoxia or by increased cortisol production.[402]

Birth Defects

The effect of maternal cigarette smoking during pregnancy on birth defects has been controversial. Evidence suggests that there is an association with at least three common birth defects: (1) cleft lip/palate, (2) terminal transverse limb deficiency (absence of the distal structures of a limb), and (3) urinary tract anomalies.

Czeizel and colleagues examined data from the Hungarian birth registry: 1,575,904 births between 1975 and 1984. Using a case-control design of 537 case-control pairs, they found a 48% increase in transverse limb deficiency that they attributed to vascular disruption.[403] Wyszynski and associates performed a metaanalysis of studies on the effect of maternal smoking on nonsyndromic oral cleft lip and palate.[404] They examined a total of 11 studies, and they observed an overall increase in oral clefts of 30% that was statistically significant. Li and colleagues performed a case-control study of congenital urinary tract anomalies and maternal smoking during pregnancy. A total of 118 cases and 369 control subjects were studied. There was a 230% increase in urinary tract anomalies among children of smoking mothers, and an inverse dose-response relationship (greater effect in light smokers) was observed.[405]

It is likely that the birth defects relationship with maternal smoking is biased by increased fetal death, and thus the risk is underestimated.

Birth Weight

Cigarette smoking leads to an average reduction in birth weight of approximately 200 g that is independent of other factors influencing birth weight. This effect is related to the number of cigarettes smoked (i.e., the greater the number of cigarettes smoked, the lower the birth weight).[406] It is also independent of gestational age, which suggests that there is a growth-retardant effect of cigarette smoking. Findings have suggested that more than one mechanism might be operative: one that operates at low levels of exposure and one that is linear and dose dependent.[407]

Besides a direct effect of smoking on birth weight, studies suggest that maternal cigarette smoking may be correlated with a variety of nutritional deficiencies that exacerbate or enhance this effect on birth weight. Nonsmokers tend to have higher intakes of almost all nutrients during pregnancy than do smokers, and their diets are nutritionally healthier.[408] In addition, cigarette smokers seem to be deficient in zinc, a trace metal positively related to birth weight. Cadmium from cigarettes may be responsible in part for this zinc deficiency, because there is a zinc-cadmium interaction in the maternal-fetal placental unit of the smoking mother.[409] Other dietary deficiencies, such as carotene and cholesterol, may also contribute to the smoking–birth weight relationship.[410] Finally, there is a smoking-caffeine interaction that may inhibit fetal growth in utero for women who are heavy smokers and heavy coffee drinkers. Such women have significant increases in placental size and decreases in birth weight.[411] Although deficits in birth weight are reversed by 6 months of age, the long-term effects of these nutritional deficiencies are unknown but potentially important in view of hypotheses relating fetal nutrition to long-term risks for chronic disease.[412]

More recent data have suggested that the magnitude of risk for having an infant with low birth weight is also modified by maternal genotype. For example, one case-control study of 741 cigarette-smoking mothers found that certain polymorphisms in maternal aryl hydrocarbon hydroxylase and glutathione-S-transferase genes were associated with low infant birth weights, presumably because they affected the metabolism of toxic substances in cigarette smoke.[413]

Lactation and Breast-Feeding

Nicotine is found in breast milk of smoking mothers, and the concentration of nicotine parallels the number of cigarettes smoked.[414] Although there are case reports of "nicotine poisoning" in newborns of heavy smokers, in which individual children have irritability, restlessness, diarrhea, and tachycardia, clinical illnesses such as these are relatively uncommon. The major issue is that the volume of breast milk from cigarette-smoking women is smaller than the volume of breast milk from nonsmoking women, and, therefore, breast milk output is insufficient to support the energy requirements of the fetus.[415] In addition, perhaps because of this problem, smoking mothers are likely to terminate breast-feeding earlier than nonsmoking mothers.

Childhood Disease

Perhaps the major area of new information is the growing recognition that fetal exposure to maternal cigarette smoke in utero is associated with a wide variety of potentially lethal disorders in later childhood and adult life. With maternal smoking, it is now clear that fetal nicotine concentrations are, on average, 90% of maternal values throughout gestation.[416] Of greatest concern is that fetal exposure in utero is associated with an increased cancer risk in offspring. There is approximately a twofold increased risk of non-Hodgkin's lymphoma, acute lymphoblastic leukemia, and Wilms' tumor in children of smoking mothers in comparison with those of nonsmoking mothers, and a dose-response relationship is also evident.[417] This increase in cancer risk is further substantiated by the finding that there are smoking-related DNA adduct changes that are present in the placentas of smoking mothers.[418,419]

There is also evidence that maternal cigarette smoking may be associated with the development of childhood asthma.[420] It is likely that the maternal smoking effect on asthma is related to in utero exposure.[421] Infants born to smoking mothers have a lower flow at FRC than do those born to nonsmoking mothers. In addition to these decreased flow rates, there are also changes in lung volume, specifically FRC.[422]

Acute respiratory illnesses such as pneumonia and bronchitis are also more common in infants exposed to in utero and environmental tobacco smoke than in nonexposed infants, particularly during the first year of life. Harlap and Davies studied 10,072 births in Israel between 1965 and 1968 and found that infants of mothers reporting smoking during pregnancy experienced approximately a 25% increase in hospitalization rates for pneumonia and bronchitis in relation to children of nonsmoking mothers.[423] These findings have been confirmed by Taylor and Wadsworth, who suggested that the bulk of this effect is due to in utero exposure.[424] In addition, a study by Tager and associates suggests that the abnormalities in early infant lung function are associated with the development of lower respiratory illness during the first year of life.[425]

Epidemiologic studies have also documented that what was previously thought to be a postnatal effect of maternal cigarette smoking on long-term growth in lung function is actually caused by in utero exposure. Cunningham and coworkers studied 8863 nonsmoking white children aged 8 to 12 years from 22 North American cities. Forced expiratory flow between 25% and 75% of VC and forced expiratory volume in 0.75 second were 4.9% and 1.7% lower, respectively, in children of women who smoked during pregnancy than in unexposed children. No effect of postnatal exposure was seen.[426] These investigators confirmed their findings in an inner-city population of 493 white and 383 African-American school children aged 9 to 11 years and found that the effects were stronger on African-American children than on white children and stronger for boys than for girls.[427]

These studies were cross sectional, and exposure assessment was therefore retrospective; however, prospective data are now available. Tager and coworkers defined a cohort of 159 infants who were prospectively observed over the first 2 years of life, with lung function measurements at 2 to 6 weeks of age and then at 4 to 6, 9 to 12, and 15 to 18 months. The maximal flow at FRC was used as the measure of lung function. At 1 year of age, infant girls exposed to maternal smoke in utero were predicted to have a 16% reduction in maximal flow at FRC, whereas boys had a 5% reduction in comparison with unexposed infants. Postnatal exposure had no effect.[428] This finding

was confirmed in a second, larger birth cohort from Australia with a different measure of lung function (peak tidal expiratory flow/total expiratory time).[429]

In summary, these studies demonstrate long-lasting deficits in lung function caused by in utero exposure to cigarette smoke that persist into early adolescence.

In addition to cancer, acute and chronic respiratory conditions, and reduced lung function, both strabismus and attention deficit disorder may be linked with maternal smoking during pregnancy.[430,431]

Smoking Cessation during Pregnancy

Marks and coworkers completed a cost-benefit/cost-effectiveness analysis of smoking cessation for pregnant women.[432] Simply on the basis of reduction of neonatal intensive care unit use and not even considering the long-term health consequences of in utero exposure, these investigators found that smoking cessation programs would save $77 million, or approximately $3 per $1 spent. A randomized controlled trial of smoking cessation in an academic clinic documented a statistically significant 20% quit rate in intervention subjects, which was twice the rate observed in controls.[433] Metaanalyses of multiple controlled trials have documented an approximately 50% increase in smoking cessation associated with prenatal smoking cessation interventions.[434,435]

All physicians should advise pregnant smokers of the aforementioned risks and provide assistance in smoking cessation.[436] Smoking cessation strategies should focus on behavioral interventions such as counseling, educational materials, and frequent reinforcement, because the safety and efficacy of pharmacologic interventions such as nicotine replacement, bupropion, and nortriptyline have not been established during pregnancy.[437]

References

1. ACOG technical bulletin. Pulmonary disease in pregnancy. Number 224—June 1996. American College of Obstetricians and Gynecologists. Int J Gynaecol Obstet 1996;54:187.
2. Thomson KJ, Cohen ME: Studies on the circulation in pregnancy. II. Vital capacity observations in normal pregnant women. Surg Gynecol Obstet 1938;66:591.
3. Gilroy RJ, Mangura BT, Lavietes MH: Rib cage and abdominal volume displacements during breathing in pregnancy. Am Rev Respir Dis 1988;137:668.
4. McGinty AP: Comparative effects of pregnancy and phrenic nerve interruption on the diaphragm and their relation to pulmonary tuberculosis. Am J Obstet Gynecol 1938;35:237.
5. Mobius W: Atmung und Schwangerschaft. Med Wochenschr 1961;103:1389.
6. Little AB, Biliar RB: Progestogens. In Fuchs F, Klopper A (eds): Endocrinology of Pregnancy. New York, Harper & Row, 1983, p 92.
7. Yannone ME, McCurdy JR, Goldfien A: Plasma progesterone levels in normal pregnancy, labor, and the puerperium. II. Clinical data. Am J Obstet Gynecol 1968;101:1058.
8. Lyons HA, Antonio R: The sensitivity of the respiratory center in pregnancy and after the administration of progesterone. Trans Assoc Am Physicians 1959;72:173.
9. Prowse CM, Gaensler EA: Respiratory and acid-base changes during pregnancy. Anesthesiology 1965;26:381.
10. Bayliss DA, Millhorn DE: Central neural mechanisms of progesterone action: Application to the respiratory system. J Appl Physiol 1992;73:393.

11. Skatrud JB, Dempsey JA, Kaiser DG: Ventilatory response to medroxyprogesterone acetate in normal subjects: Time course and mechanism. J Appl Physiol 1978;44:939.

12. Gaensler EA: Lung displacement: Abdominal enlargement, pleural space disorders, deformities of the thoracic cage. In Fenn WO, Rahn H (eds): Handbook of Physiology: Respiration, vol. 2. Washington, D.C., American Physiological Society, 1965, p 1623.

13. Bayliss DA, Cidlowski JA, Millhorn, DE: The stimulation of respiration by progesterone in ovariectomized cat is mediated by an estrogen-dependent hypothalamic mechanism requiring gene expression. Endocrinology 1990;126:519.

14. Brien TC, Dalrymple IJ: Longitudinal study of the free cortisol index in pregnancy. Br J Obstet Gynaecol 1976;83:361.

15. O'Connell M, Welsh GW: Unbound plasma cortisol in pregnant and Enovid-E treated women as determined by ultrafiltration. J Clin Endocrinol Metab 1969;29:563.

16. Peterson RE: Corticosteroids and corticotropins. In Fuchs F, Klopper A (eds): Endocrinology of Pregnancy. New York, Harper & Row, 1983, p 112.

17. Dörr HG, Heller A, Versmold HT, et al: Longitudinal study of progestins, mineralocorticoids, and glucocorticoids throughout human pregnancy. J Clin Endocrinol Metab 1989;68:863.

18. Chrousos GP, Torpy DJ, Gold, PW: Interactions between the hypothalamic-pituitary-adrenal axis and the female reproductive system: Clinical implications. Ann Intern Med 1998;129:229.

19. Crapo RO: Normal cardiopulmonary physiology during pregnancy. Clin Obstet Gynecol 1996;39:3.

20. Kendrick AH: Comparison of methods of measuring static lung volumes. Monaldi Arch Chest Dis 1996;51:431.

21. Cugell DW, Frank NR, Gaensler EA, Badger TL: Pulmonary function in pregnancy. I. Serial observations in normal women. Am Rev Tuberc 1953;67:568.

22. Alaily AB, Carrol KB: Pulmonary ventilation in pregnancy. Br J Obstet Gynaecol 1978;85:518.

23. Bevan DR, Holdcroft A, Loh L, et al: Closing volume and pregnancy. BMJ 1974;1:13.

24. Russell IF, Chambers WA: Closing volume in normal pregnancy. Br J Anaesth 1981;53:1043.

25. Garcia-Rio F, Pino-Garcia, JM, Serrano S, et al: Comparison of helium dilution and plethysmographic lung volumes in pregnant women. Eur Respir J 1997;10:2371.

26. Baldwin GR, Moorthi DS, Whelton JA, MacDonnell KF: New lung functions and pregnancy. Am J Obstet Gynecol 1977;127:235.

27. Cameron SJ, Bain HH, Grant IW: Ventilatory function in pregnancy. Scott Med J 1970;15:243.

28. Brancazio LR, Laifer SA, Schwartz T: Peak expiratory flow rate in normal pregnancy. Obstet Gynecol 1997;89:383.

29. Garrard GS, Littler WA, Redman CW: Closing volume during normal pregnancy. Thorax 1978;33:488.

30. Gee JB, Packer BS, Millen JE, Robin ED: Pulmonary mechanics during pregnancy. J Clin Invest 1967;46:945.

31. Milne JA, Mills RJ, Howie AD, Pack AI: Large airways function during normal pregnancy. Br J Obstet Gynaecol 1977;84:448.

32. Rubin A, Russo N, Goucher D: The effect of pregnancy upon pulmonary function in normal women. Am J Obstet Gynecol 1956;72:963.

33. Contreras G, Gutieárrez M, Beroiáza T, et al: Ventilatory drive and respiratory muscle function in pregnancy. Am Rev Respir Dis 1991;144:837.

34. Nava S, Zanotti E, Ambrosino N, et al: Evidence of acute diaphragmatic fatigue in a "natural" condition. The diaphragm during labor. Am Rev Respir Dis 1992;146:1226.

35. Bedell GN, Adams RW: Pulmonary diffusing capacity during rest and exercise: A study of normal persons and persons with atrial septal defect, pregnancy, and pulmonary disease. J Clin Invest 1962;41:1908.

36. Krumholz RA, Echt CR, Ross JC: Pulmonary diffusing capacity, capillary blood volume, lung volumes, and mechanics of ventilation in early and late pregnancy. J Lab Clin Med 1964;63:648.

37. Gazioglu K, Kaltreider NL, Rosen M, Yu PN: Pulmonary function during pregnancy in normal women and in patients with cardiopulmonary disease. Thorax 1970;25:445.

38. Krous HF, Campbell GA, Fowler MW, et al: Maternal nicotine administration and fetal brain stem damage: A rat model with implications for sudden infant death syndrome. Am J Obstet Gynecol 1981;140:743.

39. Milne JA, Mills RJ, Coutts JR, et al: The effect of human pregnancy on the pulmonary transfer factor for carbon monoxide as measured by the single-breath method. Clin Sci Mol Med 1977;53:271.

40. Rees GB, Pipkin FB, Symonds EM, Patrick JM: A longitudinal study of respiratory changes in normal human pregnancy with cross-sectional data on subjects with pregnancy-induced hypertension. Am J Obstet Gynecol 1990;162:826.

41. Knuttgen HG, Emerson K Jr: Physiological response to pregnancy at rest and during exercise. J Appl Physiol 1974;36:549.

42. Pernoll ML, Metcalfe J, Kovach PA, et al: Ventilation during rest and exercise in pregnancy and postpartum. Respir Physiol 1975;25:295.

43. Pernoll ML, Metcalfe J, Schlenker TL, et al: Oxygen consumption at rest and during exercise in pregnancy. Respir Physiol 1975;25:285.

44. Spätling L, Fallenstein F, Huch A, et al: The variability of cardiopulmonary adaptation to pregnancy at rest and during exercise. Br J Obstet Gynaecol 1992;99(Suppl 8):1.

45. Wolfe LA, Kemp JG, Heenan AP, et al: Acid-base regulation and control of ventilation in human pregnancy. Can J Physiol Pharmacol 1998;76:815.

46. Lotgering FK, Gilbert RD, Longo LD: Maternal and fetal responses to exercise during pregnancy. Physiol Rev 1985;65:1.

47. Edwards MJ, Metcalfe J, Dunham MJ, Paul MS: Accelerated respiratory response to moderate exercise in late pregnancy. Respir Physiol 1981;45:229.

48. McMurray RG, Mottola MF, Wolfe LA, et al: Recent advances in understanding maternal and fetal responses to exercise. Med Sci Sports Exerc 1993;25:1305.

49. Andersen GJ, James GB, Mathers NP, et al: The maternal oxygen tension and acid-base status during pregnancy. J Obstet Gynaecol Br Commonw 1969;76:16.

50. Blechner JN, Cotter JR, Stenger VG, et al: Oxygen, carbon dioxide, and hydrogen ion concentrations in arterial blood during pregnancy. Am J Obstet Gynecol 1968;100:1.

51. Dayal P, Murata Y, Takamura H: Antepartum and postpartum acid-base changes in maternal blood in normal and complicated pregnancies. J Obstet Gynaecol Br Commonw 1972;79:612.

52. Fadel HE, Northrop G, Misenhimer HR, Harp RJ: Normal pregnancy: A model of sustained respiratory alkalosis. J Perinat Med 1979;3:195.

53. Lucius H, Gahlenbeck H, Kleine HO, et al: Respiratory functions, buffer system, and electrolyte concentrations of blood during human pregnancy. Respir Physiol 1970;9:311.

54. MacRae DJ, Palavradji D: Maternal acid-base changes in pregnancy. J Obstet Gynaecol Br Commonw 1967;74:11.

55. Boutourline-Young H, Boutourline-Young E: Alveolar carbon dioxide levels in pregnant, parturient, and lactating subjects. J Obstet Gynecol Br Emp 1956;63:509.

56. Templeton A, Kelman GR: Maternal blood-gases (PA_{O_2}-Pa_{O_2}), physiological shunt and VD/VT in normal pregnancy. Br J Anaesth 1976;48:1001.

57. Andersen GJ, Walker J: The effect of labour on the maternal blood-gas and acid-base status. J Obstet Gynaecol Br Commonw 1970;77:289.

58. Lim VS, Katz AI, Lindheimer MD: Acid-base regulation in pregnancy. Am J Physiol 1976;231:1764.

59. Awe RJ, Nicotra MB, Newsom TD, Viles R: Arterial oxygenation and alveolar-arterial gradients in term pregnancy. Obstet Gynecol 1979;53:182.

60. Ang CK, Tan TH, Walters WA, Wood C: Postural influence on maternal capillary oxygen and carbon dioxide tension. BMJ 1969;4:201.

61. Longo LD: Respiratory gas exchange in the placenta. In Fishman AP, Farhi LE, Tenney SM, Geiger SR (eds): Handbook of Physiology: The Respiratory System. Bethesda, Md., American Physiological Society, 1987, p 351.

62. Polvi HJ, Pirhonen JP, Erkkola RU: The hemodynamic effects of maternal hypo- and hyperoxygenation in healthy term pregnancies. Obstet Gynecol 1995;86:795.

63. Yancey MK, Moore J, Brady K, et al: The effect of altitude on umbilical cord blood gases. Obstet Gynecol 1992;79:571.

64. Kitanaka T, Alonso JG, Gilbert RD, et al: Fetal responses to long-term hypoxemia in sheep. Am J Physiol 1989;256:R1348.

65. Moore LG, Rounds SS, Jahnigen D, et al: Infant birth weight is related to maternal arterial oxygenation at high altitude. J Appl Physiol 1982;52:695.

66. Hanka R, Lawn L, Mills IH, et al: The effects of maternal hypercapnia on foetal oxygenation and uterine blood flow in the pig. J Physiol (Lond) 1975;247:447.

67. Levinson G, Shnider SM, DeLorimier AA, Steffenson JL: Effects of maternal hyperventilation on uterine blood flow and fetal oxygenation and acid-base status. Anesthesiology 1974;40:340.

68. Motoyama EK, Rivard G, Acheson F, Cook CD: The effect of changes in maternal pH and PCO_2 on the PO_2 of fetal lambs. Anesthesiology 1967;28:891.

69. Wulf KH, Kunzel W, Lehmann V: Clinical aspects of placental gas exchange. In Longo LD, Bartels H (eds): Respiratory Gas Exchange and Blood Flow in the Placenta. Bethesda, Md., U.S. Department of Health, Education, and Welfare, 1972, p 505.

70. Zeldis SM: Dyspnea during pregnancy. Clin Chest Med 1992;13:567.

71. Gilbert R, Auchincloss JH Jr: Dyspnea of pregnancy. Clinical and physiological observations. Am J Med Sci 1966;252:270.

72. Gilbert R, Epifano K, Auchincloss JH Jr: Dyspnea of pregnancy: A syndrome of altered respiratory control. JAMA 1962;182:1073.

73. Milne JA, Howie AD, Pack AI: Dyspnea during normal pregnancy. Br J Obstet Gynaecol 1978;85:260.

74. Lehmann V: Dyspnea in pregnancy. J Perinat Med 1975;3:154.

75. Field SK, Bell SG, Cenaiko DF, Whitelaw WA: Relationship between inspiratory effort and breathlessness in pregnancy. J Appl Physiol 1991;71:1897.

76. Garciá-Rio F, Pino JM, Goámez L, et al: Regulation of breathing and perception of dyspnea in healthy pregnant women. Chest 1996;110:446.

77. Moore LG, McCullough RE, Weil JV: Increased HVR in pregnancy: Relationship to hormonal and metabolic changes. J Appl Physiol 1987;62:158.

78. Hytten FE, Leitch I: Respiration. In: The Physiology of Human Pregnancy. Oxford, U.K., Blackwell Scientific Publications, 1971, p 111.

79. Corrao WM, Braman SS, Irwin RS: Chronic cough as the sole presenting manifestation of bronchial asthma. N Engl J Med 1979;300:633.

80. Greenberger PA: Asthma in pregnancy. Clin Chest Med 1992;13:597.

81. Greenberger PA: Pregnancy and asthma. Chest 1985;87:85S.

82. Greenberger PA, Patterson R: Current concepts. Management of asthma during pregnancy. N Engl J Med 1985;312:897.

83. National Asthma Education Program: Report of the Working Group on Asthma and Pregnancy. Management of Asthma during Pregnancy [NIH publication no. 93-3279]. Bethesda, Md., National Institutes of Health, 1993.

84. Turner ES, Greenberger PA, Patterson R: Management of the pregnant asthmatic patient. Ann Intern Med 1980;93:905.

85. Schatz M, Harden K, Forsythe A, et al: The course of asthma during pregnancy, post partum, and with successive pregnancies: A prospective analysis. J Allergy Clin Immunol 1988;81:509.

86. Juniper EF, Daniel EE, Roberts RS, et al: Improvement in airway responsiveness and asthma severity during pregnancy. A prospective study. Am Rev Respir Dis 1989;140:924.

87. Gluck JC, Gluck P: The effects of pregnancy on asthma: A prospective study. Ann Allergy 1976;37:164.

88. Williams DA: Asthma and pregnancy. Acta Allergol 1967;22:311.

89. Schatz M, Hoffman C: Interrelationships between asthma and pregnancy: Clinical and mechanistic considerations. Clin Rev Allergy 1987;5:301.

90. Stenius-Aarniala RSM, Hedman J, Teramo KA: Acute asthma during pregnancy. Thorax 1996;51:411.

91. Schaefer G, Silverman F: Pregnancy complicated by asthma. Am J Obstet Gynecol 1961;82:182.

92. Gordon M, Niswander KR, Berendes H, Kantor AG: Fetal morbidity following potentially anoxigenic obstetric conditions. VII. Bronchial asthma. Am J Obstet Gynecol 1970;106:421.

93. Demissie K, Breckenridge MB, Rhoads CG: Infant and maternal outcomes in the pregnancies of asthmatic women. Am J Respir Crit Care Med 1998;158:1095.

94. Kallen B, Rydhstroem H, Aberg A: Asthma during pregnancy—a population based study. Eur J Epidemiol 2000;16:167.

95. Liu S, Wen SW, Demissie K, et al: Maternal asthma and pregnancy outcomes: A retrospective cohort study. Am J Obstet Gynecol 2001;184:90.

96. Wen SW, Demissie K, Liu S: Adverse outcomes in pregnancies of asthmatic women: Results from a Canadian population. Ann Epidemiol 2001;11:7.

97. Nelson-Piercy C: Asthma in pregnancy. Thorax 2001;56:325.

98. Perlow JH, Montgomery D, Morgan MA, et al: Severity of asthma and perinatal outcome. Am J Obstet Gynecol 1992;167:963.

99. Schatz M, Zeiger RS, Hoffman CP: Intrauterine growth is related to gestational pulmonary function in pregnant asthmatic women. Kaiser-Permanente Asthma and Pregnancy Study Group. Chest 1990;98:389.

100. Fitzsimons R, Greenberger PA, Patterson R: Outcome of pregnancy in women requiring corticosteroids for severe asthma. J Allergy Clin Immunol 1986;78:349.

101. Schatz M, Patterson R, Zeitz S, et al: Corticosteroid therapy for the pregnant asthmatic patient. JAMA 1975;233:804.

102. McFadden ER Jr, Gilbert IA: Asthma. N Engl J Med 1992;327:1928.

103. National Asthma Education and Prevention Program: Expert Panel Report 2. Guidelines for the Diagnosis and Management of Asthma [NIH publication no. 97-4051]. Bethesda, MD, National Institutes of Health, 1997.

104. Smith LJ: Leukotrienes in asthma: The potential therapeutic role of antileukotriene agents. Arch Intern Med 1996;156:2181.

105. Malmstrom K, Rodriguez-Gomez G, Guerra J, et al: Oral montelukast, inhaled beclomethasone, and placebo for chronic asthma. A randomized, controlled trial. Montelukast/Beclomethasone Study Group. Ann Intern Med 1999;130:487.

106. Schatz M: Asthma during pregnancy: Interrelationships and management. Ann Allergy 1992;68:123. [Published erratum appears in Ann Allergy 1992;68:305.]

107. Boulet LP, Becker A, Berube D, et al: Canadian asthma consensus report. Canadian Asthma Consensus Group. CMAJ 1999;161 (11, Suppl):S1.

108. Schatz M: The efficacy and safety of asthma medications during pregnancy. Semin Perinatol 1997;25:145.

109. Schatz M, Zeiger RS, Harden K, et al: The safety of asthma and allergy medications during pregnancy. J Allergy Clin Immunol 1997;100:301.

110. Misenhimer HR, Margulies SI, Panigel M, et al: Effects of vasoconstrictive drugs on the placental circulation of the rhesus monkey. A preliminary report. Invest Radiol 1972;7:496.

111. Akerlund M, Andersson KE: Effects of terbutaline on human myometrial activity and endometrial blood flow. Obstet Gynecol 1976;47:529.

112. Caritis SN, Mueller-Heubach E, Morishima HO, Edelstone DI: Effect of terbutaline on cardiovascular state and uterine blood flow in pregnant ewes. Obstet Gynecol 1977;50:603.

113. Lunell NO, Joelsson I, Lewander R, et al: Utero-placental blood flow and the effect of beta 2–adrenoceptor stimulating drugs. Acta Obstet Gynecol Scand 1982;108(Suppl):25.

114. Brennan SC, McLaughlin MK, Chez RA: Effects of prolonged infusion of beta-adrenergic agonists on uterine and umbilical blood flow in pregnant sheep. Am J Obstet Gynecol 1977;128:709.

115. Rayburn, WF, Atkinson BD, Gilbert K, Turnbull G: Short-term effects of inhaled albuterol on maternal and fetal circulations. Am J Obstet Gynecol 1994;171:770.

116. Banerjee BN, Woodard G: Teratologic evaluation of metaproterenol in the rhesus monkey (*Macaca mulatta*). Toxicol Appl Pharmacol 1971;20:562.

117. Heinonen OP, Slone D, Shapiro S: Birth Defects and Drugs in Pregnancy. Littleton, Mass., Publishing Sciences Group, 1977.

118. Schatz M, Zeiger RS, Harden KM, et al: The safety of inhaled beta-agonist bronchodilators during pregnancy. J Allergy Clin Immunol 1988;82:686.

119. Tepperman HM, Beydoun SN, Abdul-Karim RW: Drugs affecting myometrial contractility in pregnancy. Clin Obstet Gynecol 1977;20:423.

120. Andersson KE, Bengtsson LP, Ingemarsson I: Terbutaline inhibition of midtrimester uterine activity induced by prostaglandin F2alpha and hypertonic saline. Br J Obstet Gynecol 1975;82:745.

121. Liggins GC, Vaughan GS: Intravenous infusion of salbutamol in the management of premature labour. J Obstet Gynaecol Br Commonw 1973;80:29.

122. Zilianti M, Aller J: Action of orciprenaline on uterine contractility during labor, maternal cardiovascular system, fetal heart rate, and acid-base balance. Am J Obstet Gynecol 1971;109:1073.

123. Ingemarsson I: Effect of terbutaline on premature labor: A double-blind placebo-controlled study. Am J Obstet Gynecol 1976; 125:520.

124. Benedetti TJ, Hargrove JC, Rosene KA: Maternal pulmonary edema during premature labor inhibition. Obstet Gynecol 1982;59:33S.

125. Elliott HR, Abdulla U, Hayes PJ: Pulmonary oedema associated with ritodrine infusion and betamethasone administration in premature labour. BMJ 1978;2:799.

126. Mabie WC, Pernoll ML, Witty JB, Biswas MK: Pulmonary edema induced by betamimetic drugs. South Med J 1983;76:1354.

127. Wilson J: Utilisation du cromoglycate de sodium au cours de la grossesse. Acta Ther 1982;8(suppl):45.

128. Stenius-Aarniala B, Riikonen S, Teramo K: Slow-release theophylline in pregnant asthmatics. Chest 1995;107:642.

129. Mintz S: Pregnancy and asthma. In Weiss EB, Segal MS (eds): Bronchial Asthma: Mechanisms and Therapeutics. Boston, Little, Brown, 1976, p 971.

130. Neff RK, Leviton A: Maternal theophylline consumption and the risk of stillbirth. Chest 1990;97:1266.

131. Coutinho EM, Vieira Lopes AC: Inhibition of uterine motility by aminophylline. Am J Obstet Gynecol 1971;110:726.

132. Carter BL, Driscoll CE, Smith GD: Theophylline clearance during pregnancy. Obstet Gynecol 1986;68:555.

133. Frederiksen MC, Ruo TI, Chow MJ, Atkinson AJ Jr: Theophylline pharmacokinetics in pregnancy. Clin Pharmacol Ther 1986;40:321.

134. Arwood LL, Dasta JF, Friedman C: Placental transfer of theophylline: Two case reports. Pediatrics 1979;63:844.

135. Labovitz E, Spector S: Placental theophylline transfer in pregnant asthmatics. JAMA 1982;247:786.

136. Position statement. The use of newer asthma and allergy medications during pregnancy. Ann Allergy Asthma Immunol 2000;84:475.

137. Sidhu RK, Hawkins DF: Prescribing in pregnancy. Corticosteroids. Clin Obstet Gynaecol 1981;8:383.

138. Fainstat T: Cortisone-induced congenital cleft palate in rabbits. Endocrinology 1954;55:502.

139. Bongiovanni, AM, McPadden AJ: Steroids during pregnancy and possible fetal consequences. Fertil Steril 1960;2:181.

140. Snyder RD, Snyder D: Corticosteroids for asthma during pregnancy. Ann Allergy 1978;41:340.

141. Warrell DW, Taylor R: Outcome for the foetus of mothers receiving prednisolone during pregnancy. Lancet 1968;1:117.

142. Popert AJ: Pregnancy and adrenocortical hormones: Some aspects of their interaction in rheumatic diseases. BMJ 1962;1:967.

143. Walsh SD, Clark FR: Pregnancy in patients on long-term corticosteroid therapy. Scott Med J 1967;12:302.

144. Oppenheimer EH: Lesions in the adrenals of an infant following maternal corticosteroid therapy. Bull Johns Hopkins Hosp 1964;114:146.

145. Reinisch JM, Simon NG, Karow WG, Gandelman R: Prenatal exposure to prednisone in humans and animals retards intrauterine growth. Science 1978;202:436.

146. Arad I, Landau H: Adrenocortical reserve of neonates born of long-term, steroid-treated mothers. Eur J Pediatr 1984;142:279.

147. Kallen B, Rydhstroem H, Aberg A: Congenital malformations after the use of inhaled budesonide in early pregnancy. Obstet Gynecol 1999;93:392.

148. Greenberger PA, Patterson R: Beclomethasone diproprionate for severe asthma during pregnancy. Ann Intern Med 1983;98:478.

149. Dombrowski MP, Brown CL, Berry SM: Preliminary experience with triamcinolone acetonide during pregnancy. J Matern Fetal Med 1996;5:310.

150. American College of Obstetricians and Gynecologists (ACOG) and American College of Allergy, Asthma and Immunology (ACAAI). The use of newer asthma and allergy medications during pregnancy. Ann Allergy Asthma Immunol 2000;84:475.

151. Gelber M, Sidi Y, Gassner S, et al: Uncontrollable life-threatening status asthmaticus—an indicator for termination of pregnancy by cesarean section. Respiration 1984;46:320.

152. Atkinson AR: Pregnancy and alpha-1-antitrypsin deficiency. Postgrad Med J 1987;63:817.

153. Dempsey OJ, Godden DJ, Martin PD, Danielian PJ: Severe α1-antitrypsin deficiency and pregnancy. Eur Respir J 1999;13:1492.

154. Giesler CF, Buehler JH, Depp R: Alpha-1-antitrypsin deficiency. Severe obstructive lung disease and pregnancy. Obstet Gynecol 1977;49:31.

155. Kennedy SH, Barlow DH, Redman CWG: Pre-eclampsia in a woman with homozygous PiZZ alpha-1-antitrypsin deficiency. Case report. Br J Obstet Gynaecol 1987;94:1103.

156. Kuller JA, Katz VL, McCoy MC, Bristow CL: Alpha₁-antitrypsin deficiency and pregnancy. Am J Perinatol 1995;12:303.

157. Lalli CM, Raju L: Pregnancy and chronic obstructive pulmonary disease. Chest 1981;80:759.

158. Weiss ST, Weinberger SE, Weiss JW, Johnson TS: Normal pregnancy and delivery in a woman with severe underlying lung disease. Thorax 1981;36:878.

159. Barker AF: Bronchiectasis. N Engl J Med 2002;346:1383.

160. Teirstein AS: Bronchiectasis. In Rovinsky JJ, Guttmacher AF (eds): Medical, Surgical, and Gynecologic Complications of Pregnancy. Baltimore, Williams & Wilkins, 1965, p 144.

161. Howie AD, Milne JA: Pregnancy in patients with bronchiectasis. Br J Obstet Gynaecol 1978;85:197.

162. Templeton A: Intrauterine growth retardation associated with hypoxia due to bronchiectasis. Br J Obstet Gynaecol 1977;84:389.

163. Thaler I, Bronstein M, Rubin AE: The course and outcome of pregnancy associated with bronchiectasis. Case report. Br J Obstet Gynaecol 1986;93:1006.

164. Rosenstein BJ, Cutting GR: The diagnosis of cystic fibrosis: A consensus statement. J Pediatr 1998;132:589.

165. Siegel B, Siegel S: Pregnancy and delivery in a patient with cystic fibrosis of the pancreas: Report of a case. Obstet Gynecol 1960;16:438.

166. Hilman BC, Aitken ML, Constantinescu M: Pregnancy in patients with cystic fibrosis. Clin Obstet Gynecol 1996;39:70.

167. Johnson SR, Varner MW, Yates SJ, Hanson R: Diagnosis of maternal cystic fibrosis during pregnancy. Obstet Gynecol 1983;61:2S.

168. Kotloff RM, FitzSimmons SC, Fiel SB: Fertility and pregnancy in patients with cystic fibrosis. Clin Chest Med 1992;13:623.

169. Rodgers HC, Knox AJ, Toplis PJ, Thornton SJ: Successful pregnancy and birth after IVF in a woman with cystic fibrosis. Hum Reprod 2000;15:2152.

170. Cohen LF, di Sant'Agnese PA, Friedlander J: Cystic fibrosis and pregnancy. A national survey. Lancet 1980;2:842.

171. Edenborough FP: Women with cystic fibrosis and their potential for reproduction. Thorax 2001;56:649.

172. Kent NE, Farquharson DF: Cystic fibrosis and pregnancy. CMAJ 1993;149:809.

173. Corkey CW, Newth CJ, Corey M, Levison H: Pregnancy in cystic fibrosis: A better prognosis in patients with pancreatic function? Am J Obstet Gynecol 1981;140:737.

174. Edenborough FP, Stableforth DE, Webb AK, et al: Outcome of pregnancy in women with cystic fibrosis. Thorax 1995;50:170.

175. Palmer J, Dillon-Baker C, Tecklin JS, et al: Pregnancy in patients with cystic fibrosis. Ann Intern Med 1983;99:596.

176. Ahmed R, Wielinski CL, Warwick WJ: Effect of pregnancy on CF. Pediatr Pulmonol Suppl 1995;12:289.

177. Edenborough FP, Mackenzie WE, Stableforth DE: The outcome of 72 pregnancies in 55 women with cystic fibrosis in the United Kingdom 1977-1996. Br J Obstet Gynaecol 2000;107:254.

178. Fiel SB, Fitzsimmons S: Pregnancy in patients with cystic fibrosis. Pediatr Pulmonol Suppl 1997;16:111.

179. Frangolias DD, Nakielna EM, Wilcox PG: Pregnancy and cystic fibrosis: A case-controlled study. Chest 1997;111:963.

180. Gilljam M, Antoniou M, Shin J, et al: Pregnancy in cystic fibrosis. Fetal and maternal outcome. Chest 2000;118:85.

181. Fiel SB: Pulmonary function during pregnancy in cystic fibrosis: Implications for counseling. Curr Opin Pulm Med 1996;2:462.

182. Elias S, Annas GJ, Simpson JL: Carrier screening for cystic fibrosis: Implications for obstetric and gynecologic practice. Am J Obstet Gynecol 1991;164:1077.

183. Boggess KA, Easterling TR, Raghu G: Management and outcome of pregnant women with interstitial and restrictive lung disease. Am J Obstet Gynecol 1995;173:1007.

184. King TE Jr: Restrictive lung disease in pregnancy. Clin Chest Med 1992;13:607.

185. American Thoracic Society: Statement on sarcoidosis. Am J Respir Crit Care Med 1999;160:736.

186. Newman LS, Rose CS, Maier LA: Sarcoidosis. N Engl J Med 1997;336:1224.

187. Mayock RL, Sullivan RD, Greening RR, Jones R Jr: Sarcoidosis and pregnancy. JAMA 1957;164:158.

188. Reisfield DR: Boeck's sarcoid and pregnancy. Am J Obstet Gynecol 1958;75:795.

189. Reisfield DR, Yahia C, Laurenzi GA: Pregnancy and cardiorespiratory failure in Boeck's sarcoid. Surg Gynecol Obstet 1959;109:412.

190. Agha FP, Vade A, Amendola MA, Cooper RF: Effects of pregnancy on sarcoidosis. Surg Gynecol Obstet 1982;155:817.

191. Dines DE, Banner EA: Sarcoidosis during pregnancy. Improvement in pulmonary function. JAMA 1967;200:726.

192. Fried KH: Sarcoidosis and pregnancy. Acta Med Scand 1964; 425(Suppl):218.

193. O'Leary JA: Ten-year study of sarcoidosis and pregnancy. Am J Obstet Gynecol 1962;84:462.

194. Selroos O: Sarcoidosis and pregnancy: A review with results of a retrospective study. J Intern Med 1990;227:221.

195. Haynes de Regt R: Sarcoidosis and pregnancy. Obstet Gynecol 1987;70:369.

196. Scadding JG: Sarcoidosis. London, Eyre & Spottiswoode, 1967.

197. Given FT Jr, DiBenedetto RL: Sarcoidosis and pregnancy: Report of 5 cases and 1 maternal death. Obstet Gynecol 1963;22:355.

198. Johnson S: Lymphangioleiomyomatosis: Clinical features, management, and basic mechanisms. Thorax 1999;54:254.

199. Crausman RS, King TE Jr: Pulmonary lymphangioleiomyomatosis. UpToDate [online] 2002;10.1.

200. Eliasson AH, Phillips YY, Tenholder MF: Treatment of lymphangioleiomyomatosis. A meta-analysis. Chest 1989;96:1352.

201. Matsui K, Takeda K, Yu ZX, et al: Downregulation of estrogen and progesterone receptors in the abnormal smooth muscle cells in pulmonary lymphangioleiomyomatosis following therapy. Am J Respir Crit Care Med 2000;161:1002.

202. Johnson S, Tattersfield AE: Clinical experience of lymphangioleiomyomatosis in the UK. Thorax 2000;55:1052.

203. Weinberger SE: Recent advances in pulmonary medicine (2). N Engl J Med 1993;328:1462.

204. Shafer RW, Kim DS, Weiss JP, Quale JM: Extrapulmonary tuberculosis in patients with human immunodeficiency virus infection. Medicine (Baltimore) 1991;70:384.

205. Freeth A: Routine x-ray examination of the chest at an antenatal clinic. Lancet 1953;1:287.

206. Selikoff IJ, Dorfmann HL: Management of tuberculosis. In Rovinsky JJ, Guttmacher AF (eds): Medical, Surgical, and Gynecologic Complications of Pregnancy. Baltimore, Williams & Wilkins, 1965, p 111.

207. Stanton SL: Routine radiology of the chest in antenatal care. J Obstet Gynaecol Br Commonw 1968;75:1161.

208. Bonebrake CR, Noller KL, Loehnen CP, et al: Routine chest roentgenography in pregnancy. JAMA 1978;240:2747.

209. Mattox JH: The value of a routine prenatal chest x-ray. Obstet Gynecol 1973;41:243.

210. Swartz HM, Reichling BA: Hazards of radiation exposure for pregnant women. JAMA 1978;239:1907.

211. Turner AF: The chest radiograph in pregnancy. Clin Obstet Gynecol 1975;18:65.

212. Mole RH: Radiation effects on pre-natal development and their radiological significance. Br J Radiol 1979;52:89.

213. American Thoracic Society: Treatment of tuberculosis and tuberculosis infection in adults and children. Am J Respir Crit Care Med 1994;149:1359.

214. Hamadeh MA, Glassroth J: Tuberculosis and pregnancy. Chest 1992;101:1114.

215. Ormerod P: Tuberculosis in pregnancy and the puerperium. Thorax 2001;56:494.

216. Snider D: Pregnancy and tuberculosis. Chest 1984;86:10S.

217. Vallejo JG, Starke JR: Tuberculosis and pregnancy. Clin Chest Med 1992;13:693.

218. Hedvall E: Pregnancy and tuberculosis. Acta Med Scand 1953;147(Suppl):1.

219. Flanagan P, Hensler NM: The course of active tuberculosis complicated by pregnancy. JAMA 1959;170:783.

220. Giercke HW: Tuberkuloseablaufe kurz nach Schwangerschaftsbeendigung. Ztschr Tuberk 1956;108:1.

221. de March A: Tuberculosis and pregnancy. Five- to ten-year review of 215 patients in their fertile age. Chest 1975;68:800.

222. Schaefer G, Zervoudakis IA, Fuchs FF, David S: Pregnancy and pulmonary tuberculosis. Obstet Gynecol 1975;46:706.

223. Bjerkedal T, Bahna SL, Lehmann EH: Course and outcome of pregnancy in women with pulmonary tuberculosis. Scand J Respir Dis 1975;56:245.

224. Golditch IM: Tuberculosis meningitis and pregnancy. Am J Obstet Gynecol 1971;110:1144.

225. Stands JW, Jowers RG, Bryan CS: Miliary-meningeal tuberculosis during pregnancy: Case report, and brief survey of the problem of extra-pulmonary tuberculosis. J S C Med Assoc 1977;73:282.

226. Coden J: Tuberculous peritonitis in pregnancy. BMJ 1972;3:153.

227. Myers JP, Perlstein PH, Light IJ, et al: Tuberculosis in pregnancy with fatal congenital infection. Pediatrics 1981;67:89.

228. Niles RA: Puerperal tuberculosis with death of infant. Am J Obstet Gynecol 1982;144:131.

229. Good JT Jr, Iseman MD, Davidson PT, et al: Tuberculosis in association with pregnancy. Am J Obstet Gynecol 1981;140:492.

230. Small PM, Fujiwara PI: Management of tuberculosis in the United States. N Engl J Med 2001;345:189.

231. Joint Tuberculosis Committee of the British Thoracic Society: Chemotherapy and management of tuberculosis in the United Kingdom: Recommendations 1998. Thorax 1998;53:536.

232. Bothamley G: Drug treatment for tuberculosis during pregnancy. Safety considerations. Drug Saf 2001;24:553.

233. Davidson PT: Managing tuberculosis during pregnancy. Lancet 1995;346:199.

234. Atkins JN: Maternal plasma concentration of pyridoxal phosphate during pregnancy: Adequacy of vitamin B_6 supplementation during isoniazid therapy. Am Rev Respir Dis 1982;126:714.

235. Murray J, Sonnenberg P, Shearer SC, Godfrey-Faussett P: Human immunodeficiency virus and the outcome of treatment for new and recurrent pulmonary tuberculosis in African patients. Am J Respir Crit Care Med 1999;159:733.

236. Byrd RB, Horn BR, Solomon DA, Griggs GA: Toxic effects of isoniazid in tuberculosis chemoprophylaxis. Role of biochemical monitoring in 1,000 patients. JAMA 1979;241:1239.

237. Moulding TS, Redeker AG, Kanel GC: Twenty isoniazid-associated deaths in one state. Am Rev Respir Dis 1989;140:700.

238. Snider DE Jr, Caras GJ: Isoniazid-associated hepatitis deaths: A review of available information. Am Rev Respir Dis 1992; 145:494.

239. Franks AL, Binkin NJ, Snider DE Jr, et al: Isoniazid hepatitis among pregnant and postpartum Hispanic patients. Public Health Rep 1989;104:151.

240. American Thoracic Society: Targeted tuberculin testing and treatment of latent tuberculosis infection. Am J Respir Crit Care Med 2000;161:S221.

241. Warkany J: Antituberculous drugs. Teratology 1979;20:133.

242. Snider DE Jr, Layde PM, Johnson MW, Lyle MA: Treatment of tuberculosis during pregnancy. Am Rev Respir Dis 1980;122:65.

243. Lowe CR: Congenital defects among children born to women under supervision or treatment for pulmonary tuberculosis. Br J Prev Soc Med 1964;18:14.

244. Scheinhorn DJ, Angelillo VA: Antituberculous therapy in pregnancy. Risks to the fetus. West J Med 1977;127:195.

245. Bobrowitz ID: Ethambutol in pregnancy. Chest 1974;66:20.

246. Lewit T, Nebel L, Terracina S, Karman S: Ethambutol in pregnancy: Observations on embryogenesis. Chest 1974;66:25.

247. Rizk NW, Kalassian KG, Gilligan T, et al: Obstetric complications in pulmonary and critical care medicine. Chest 1996;110:791.

248. Conway N, Birt BD: Streptomycin in pregnancy: Effect on the foetal ear. BMJ 1965;2:260.

249. Robinson GC, Cambon KG: Hearing loss in infants of tuberculous mothers treated with streptomycin during pregnancy. N Engl J Med 1964;271:949.

250. Potworowska M, Sianozecka E, Szufladowicz R: Ethionamide treatment and pregnancy. Pol Med J 1966;5:1152.

251. Goble M, Iseman MD, Madsen LA, et al: Treatment of 171 patients with pulmonary tuberculosis resistant to isoniazid and rifampin. N Engl J Med 1993;328:527.

252. Iseman MD: Treatment of multidrug-resistant tuberculosis. N Engl J Med 1993;329:784.

253. Blackall PB: Tuberculosis: Maternal infection of the newborn. Med J Aust 1969;2:1055.

254. Cantwell MF, Shehab ZM, Costello AM: Congenital tuberculosis. N Engl J Med 1994;330:1051.

255. Ramos AD, Hibbard LT, Craig JR: Congenital tuberculosis. Obstet Gynecol 1974;43:61.

256. Voyce MA, Hunt AC: Congenital tuberculosis. Arch Dis Child 1966;41:299.

257. Starke JR: Tuberculosis: An old disease but a new threat to the mother, fetus, and neonate. Clin Perinatol 1997;24:107.

258. Finn R, St Hill CA, Govan AJ, et al: Immunological responses in pregnancy and survival of fetal homograft. BMJ 1972;3:150.

259. Montgomery WP, Young RC Jr, Allen MP, Harden KA: The tuberculin test in pregnancy. Am J Obstet Gynecol 1968;100:829.

260. Present PA, Comstock GW: Tuberculin sensitivity in pregnancy. Am Rev Respir Dis 1975;112:413.

261. Weinstein L, Murphy T: The management of tuberculosis during pregnancy. Clin Perinatol 1974;1:395.

262. Centers for Disease Control and Prevention: Update: Fatal and severe liver injuries associated with rifampin and pyrazinamide for latent tuberculosis infection, and revisions in American Thoracic Society/CDC recommendations—United States, 2001. JAMA 2001;286:1445.

263. Espinal MA, Reingold AL, Lavanera M: Effect of pregnancy on the risk of developing active tuberculosis. J Infect Dis 1996;173:488.

264. Boggess KA, Myers ER, Hamilton CD: Antepartum or postpartum isoniazid treatment of latent tuberculosis infection. Obstet Gynecol 2000;96:757.

265. Richey SD, Roberts SW, Ramin KD, et al: Pneumonia complicating pregnancy. Obstet Gynecol 1994;84:525.

266. Ramsey PS, Ramin KD: Pneumonia in pregnancy. Obstet Gynecol Clinic North Am 2001;28:553.

267. Berkowitz K, LaSala A: Risk factors associated with the increasing prevalence of pneumonia during pregnancy. Am J Obstet Gynecol 1990;163:981.

268. Madinger NE, Greenspoon JS, Ellrodt AG: Pneumonia during pregnancy: Has modern technology improved maternal and fetal outcome? Am J Obstet Gynecol 1989;161:657.

269. Hopwood HG Jr: Pneumonia in pregnancy. Obstet Gynecol 1965;25:875.

270. Rodrigues J, Niederman MS: Pneumonia complicating pregnancy. Clin Chest Med 1992;13:679.

271. Benedetti TJ, Valle R, Ledger WJ: Antepartum pneumonia in pregnancy. Am J Obstet Gynecol 1982;144:413.

272. Eisenberg VH, Eidelman LA, Arbel R, Ezra Y: Legionnaire's disease during pregnancy: A case presentation and review of the literature. Eur J Obstet Gynecol 1997;72:15.

273. American Thoracic Society: Guidelines for the initial management of adults with community-acquired pneumonia: Diagnosis, assessment of severity, and initial antimicrobial therapy. Am J Respir Crit Care Med 2001;163:1730.

274. Bartlett, JG, Mundy, LM: Community-acquired pneumonia. N Engl J Med 1995;333:1618.

275. Irving WL, James DK, Stephenson T, et al: Influenza virus infection in the second and third trimesters of pregnancy: A clinical and seroepidemiological study. Br J Obstet Gynaecol 2000;107:1282.

276. Bridges CB, Fukuda K, Cox NJ, et al: Prevention and control of influenza: Recommendations of the Advisory Committee on Immunization Practices. MMWR Recomm Rep 2001;50 (RR-4):1.

277. Pandit PB, Chitayat D, Jefferies AL, et al: Tibial hemimelia and tetralogy of Fallot associated with first trimester exposure to amantadine. Reprod Toxicol 1994;8:89.

278. Broussard RC, Payne DK, George RB: Treatment with acyclovir of varicella pneumonia in pregnancy. Chest 1991;99:1045.

279. Chapman SJ: Varicella in pregnancy. Semin Perinatol 1998;22:339.

280. Cox SM, Cunningham FG, Luby J: Management of varicella pneumonia complicating pregnancy. Am J Perinatol 1990;7:300.

281. Harris RE, Rhoades ER: Varicella pneumonia complicating pregnancy. Obstet Gynecol 1965;25:734.

282. Mendelow DA, Lewis GC Jr: Varicella pneumonia during pregnancy. Obstet Gynecol 1969;33:98.

283. Nathwani D, Maclean A, Conway S, Carrington D: Varicella infections in pregnancy and the newborn. A review prepared for the UK Advisory Group on Chickenpox on behalf of the British Society for the Study of Infection. J Infect 1998;36(Suppl 1):59.

284. Pickard RE: Varicella pneumonia in pregnancy. Am J Obstet Gynecol 1968;101:504.

285. Smego RA Jr, Asperilla MO: Use of acyclovir for varicella pneumonia during pregnancy. Obstet Gynecol 1991;78:1112.

286. Chapman SW, Bradsher RE Jr, Campbell GD, et al: Practice guidelines for the management of patients with blastomycosis. Clin Infect Dis 2000;30:679.

287. Davies SF: An overview of pulmonary fungal infections. Clin Chest Med 1987;8:495.

288. Ely EW, Peacock JE Jr, Haponik EF, Washburn RG: Cryptococcal pneumonia complicating pregnancy. Medicine 1998;77:436.

289. Stevens DA: Coccidioidomycosis. N Engl J Med 1995;332:1077.

290. Wheat J, Sarosi G, McKinsey D, et al: Practice guidelines for the management of patients with histoplasmosis. Clin Infect Dis 2000;30:688.

291. Peterson CM, Schuppert K, Kelly PC, Pappagianis D: Coccidioidomycosis and pregnancy. Obstet Gynecol Surv 1993;48:149.

292. Harris RE: Coccidioidomycosis complicating pregnancy. Report of 3 cases and review of the literature. Obstet Gynecol 1966;28:401.

293. Walker MP, Brody CZ, Resnik R: Reactivation of coccidioidomycosis in pregnancy. Obstet Gynecol 1992;79:815.

293a. Drutz DJ, Huppert M, Sun SH, McGuire WL: Human sex hormones stimulate the growth and maturation of Coccidioides immitis. Infect Immunol 1981;32:897.

294. Powell BL, Drutz DJ, Huppert M, Sun SH: Relationship of progesterone- and estradiol-binding proteins in Coccidioides immitis to coccidioidal dissemination in pregnancy. Infect Immun 1983;40:478.

295. Barbee RA, Hicks MJ, Grosso D, Sandel C: The maternal immune response in coccidioidomycosis. Is pregnancy a risk factor for serious infection? Chest 1991;100:709.

296. Catanzaro A: Pulmonary mycosis in pregnant women. Chest 1984;86:14S.

297. Wack EE, Ampel NM, Galgiani JN, Bronnimann DA: Coccidioidomycosis during pregnancy. An analysis of ten cases among 47,120 pregnancies. Chest 1988;94:376.

298. Smale LE, Waechter KG: Dissemination of coccidioidomycosis in pregnancy. Am J Obstet Gynecol 1970;107:356.

299. Purtilo DT: Opportunistic mycotic infections in pregnant women. Am J Obstet Gynecol 1975;122:607.

300. King CT, Rogers PD, Cleary JD, Chapman SW: Antifungal therapy during pregnancy. Clin Infect Dis 1998;27:1151.

301. Sobel JD: Use of antifungal drugs in pregnancy. A focus on safety. Drug Saf 2000;23:77.

302. Ellinoy BR: Amphotericin B usage in pregnancy complicated by cryptococcosis. Am J Obstet Gynecol 1973;115:285.

303. Ismail MA, Lerner SA: Disseminated blastomycosis in a pregnant woman: Review of amphotericin B usage during pregnancy. Am Rev Respir Dis 1982;126:350.

304. Silberfarb PM, Sarosi GA, Tosh FE: Cryptococcosis and pregnancy. Am J Obstet Gynecol 1972;112:714.

305. Jick SS: Pregnancy outcomes after maternal exposure to fluconazole. Pharmacotherapy 1999;19:221.

306. Mastroiacovo P, Mazzone T, Botto LD, et al: Prospective assessment of pregnancy outcomes after first trimester exposure to fluconazole. Am J Obstet Gynecol 1996;175:1645.

307. Sorensen, HT, Nielsen GL, Olesen C, et al: Risk of malformations and other outcomes in children exposed to fluconazole in utero. Br J Clin Pharmacol 1999;48:234.

308. Aleck KA, Bartley DL: Multiple malformation syndrome following fluconazole use in pregnancy: Report of an additional patient. Am J Med Genet 1997;72:253.

309. Bar-Oz B, Moretti ME, Bishai R, et al: Pregnancy outcome after in utero exposure to itraconazole: A prospective cohort study. Am J Obstet Gynecol 2000;183:1994.

310. Executive summary from the World Symposium on Primary Pulmonary Hypertension 1998, Evian, France, September 6-10, 1998, cosponsored by the World Health Organization, www.who.int/cardiovascular_diseases/resources/publications/en/.

311. Weiss BM, Hess OM: Pulmonary vascular disease and pregnancy: Current controversies, management strategies, and perspectives. Eur Heart J 1999;21:104.

312. Dawkins KD, Burke CM, Billingham ME, Jamieson SW: Primary pulmonary hypertension and pregnancy. Chest 1986;89:383.

313. McCaffrey RM, Dunn LJ: Primary pulmonary hypertension in pregnancy. Obstet Gynecol Surv 1964;19:567.

314. Abboud TK, Raya J, Noueihed R, Daniel J: Intrathecal morphine for relief of labor pain in a parturient with severe pulmonary hypertension. Anesthesiology 1983;59:477.

315. Demas NW: Maternal death due to primary pulmonary hypertension. Trans Pac Coast Obstet Gynecol Soc 1973;40:64.

316. Weiss BM, Zemp L, Seifert B, Hess OM: Outcome of pulmonary vascular disease in pregnancy: A systematic overview from 1978 through 1996. J Am Coll Cardiol 1998;31:1650.

317. Nelson DM, Main E, Crafford W, Ahumada GG: Peripartum heart failure due to primary pulmonary hypertension. Obstet Gynecol 1983;62:58S.

318. Kempf H, Linares C, Corvol P, Gasc JM: Pharmacological inactivation of the endothelin type A receptor in the early chick embryo: A model of mispatterning of the branchial arch derivatives. Development 1998;125:4931.

319. Badalian SS, Silverman RK, Aubry RH, Longo J: Twin pregnancy in a woman on long-term epoprostenol therapy for primary pulmonary hypertension. J Reprod Med 2000;45:149.

320. Easterling TR, Ralph DD, Schmucker BC: Pulmonary hypertension in pregnancy: Treatment with pulmonary vasodilators. Obstet Gynecol 1999;93:494.

321. Goodwin TM, Gherman RB, Hameed A, Elkayam U: Favorable response of Eisenmenger syndrome to inhaled nitric oxide during pregnancy. Am J Obstet Gynecol 1999;180:64.

322. Lam GK, Stafford RE, Thorp J, et al: Inhaled nitric oxide for primary pulmonary hypertension in pregnancy. Obstet Gynecol 2001;98:895.

323. Stewart R, Tuazon D, Olson G, Duarte AG: Pregnancy and primary pulmonary hypertension: Successful outcome with epoprostenol therapy. Chest 2001;119:973.

324. Barnard GR, Artigas A, Brigham KL, et al: The American-European consensus conference on ARDS: Definitions, mechanisms, relevant outcomes, and clinical trial coordination. Am J Respir Crit Care Med 1994;149:818.

325. Brower RG, Ware LB, Berthiaume Y, Matthay MA: Treatment of ARDS. Chest 2001;120:1347.

326. Ware LB, Matthay MA: The acute respiratory distress syndrome. N Engl J Med 2000;342:1334.

327. Catanzarite V, Willms D, Wong D, et al: Acute respiratory distress syndrome in pregnancy and the puerperium: Causes, courses, and outcomes. Obstet Gynecol 2001;97:760.

328. Mabie WC, Barton JR, Sibai BM: Adult respiratory distress syndrome in pregnancy. Am J Obstet Gynecol 1992;167:950.

329. Van Hook JW: Acute respiratory distress syndrome in pregnancy. Semin Perinatol 1997;21:320.

330. Acute Respiratory Distress Syndrome Network: Ventilation with lower tidal volumes as compared with traditional tidal volumes for acute lung injury and acute respiratory distress syndrome. N Engl J Med 2000;342:1301.

331. Campbell LA, Klocke RA: Implications for the pregnant patient. Am J Respir Crit Care Med 2001;163:1051.

332. Masson RG: Amniotic fluid embolism. Clin Chest Med 1992;13:657.

333. Clark SL, Hankins GDV, Dudley DA, et al: Amniotic fluid embolism: Analysis of the national registry. Am J Obstet Gynecol 1995;172:1158.

334. Resnik R, Swartz WH, Plumer MH, et al: Amniotic fluid embolism with survival. Obstet Gynecol 1976;47:295.

335. Davies S: Amniotic fluid embolus: a review of the literature. Can J Anesth 2001;48:88.

336. Courtney LD: Amniotic fluid embolism. Obstet Gynecol Surv 1974;29:169.

337. Dudney TM, Elliott CG: Pulmonary embolism from amniotic fluid, fat, and air. Progr Cardiovasc Dis 1994;36:447.

338. Adamsons K, Mueller-Heubach E, Myers RE: The innocuousness of amniotic fluid infusion in the pregnant rhesus monkey. Am J Obstet Gynecol 1971;109:977.

339. Spence M, Mason KG: Experimental amniotic fluid embolism in rabbits. Am J Obstet Gynecol 1974;119:1073.

340. Clark SL, Cotton DB, Gonik B, et al: Central hemodynamic alterations in amniotic fluid embolism. Am J Obstet Gynecol 1988;158:1124.

341. Anderson DG: Amniotic fluid embolism: A reevaluation. Am J Obstet Gynecol 1967;98:336.

342. Peterson EP, Taylor HB: Amniotic fluid embolism. An analysis of 40 cases. Obstet Gynecol 1970;35:787.

343. Courtney LD, Boxall RR, Child P: Permeability of membranes of dead fetus. BMJ 1971;1:492.

344. Sperry K: Landmark perspective: Amniotic fluid embolism. To understand an enigma. JAMA 1986;255:2183.

345. Masson RG, Ruggieri J, Siddiqui MM: Amniotic fluid embolism: Definitive diagnosis in a survivor. Am Rev Respir Dis 1979;120:187.

346. Dolyniuk M, Orfei E, Vania H, et al: Rapid diagnosis of amniotic fluid embolism. Obstet Gynecol 1983;61:28S.

347. Rodgers GP, Heymach GJ: Cryoprecipitate therapy in amniotic fluid embolization. Am J Med 1984;76:916.

348. Locksmith GJ: Amniotic fluid embolism. Obstet Gynecol Clin North Am 1999;26:435.

349. Hsieh YY, Chang CC, Li PC, et al: Successful application of extracorporeal membrane oxygenation and intra-aortic balloon counterpulsation as lifesaving therapy for a patient with amniotic fluid embolism. Am J Obstet Gynecol 2000;183:496.

350. Katz M, Robertson PA, Creasy RK: Cardiovascular complications associated with terbutaline treatment for preterm labor. Am J Obstet Gynecol 1981;139:605.

351. Pisani RJ, Rosenow EC: Pulmonary edema associated with tocolytic therapy. Ann Intern Med 1989;110:714.

352. Perry KG Jr, Morrison JC, Rust OA, et al: Incidence of adverse cardiopulmonary effects with low-dose continuous terbutaline infusion. Am J Obstet Gynecol 1995;173:1273.

353. Hatjis CG, Swain M: Systemic tocolysis for premature labor is associated with an increased incidence of pulmonary edema in the presence of maternal infection. Am J Obstet Gynecol 1988;159:723.

354. Lamont RF: The pathophysiology of pulmonary oedema with the use of beta-agonists. Br J Obstet Gynaecol 2000;107:439.

355. Nimrod CA, Beresford P, Frais M, et al: Hemodynamic observations on pulmonary edema associated with a beta-mimetic agent. A report of two cases. J Reprod Med 1984;29:341.

356. MacLennan FM, Thomson MA, Rankin R, et al: Fatal pulmonary oedema associated with the use of ritodrine in pregnancy. Case report. Br J Obstet Gynaecol 1985;92:703.

357. Engelhardt T, Webster NR: Pulmonary aspiration of gastric contents in anaesthesia. Br J Anaesth 2000;84:420.

358. Baggish MS, Hooper S: Aspiration as a cause of maternal death. Obstet Gynecol 1974;43:327.

359. Rowe TF: Acute gastric aspiration: Prevention and treatment. Semin Perinatol 1997;21:313.

360. Mucklow RG, Larard DG: The effect of the inhalation of vomitus on the lungs. Br J Anaesth 1963;35:153.

361. Mendelson CL: The aspiration of stomach contents into the lungs during obstetric anesthesia. Am J Obstet Gynecol 1946;52:191.

362. Wolfe JE, Bone RC, Ruth WE: Effects of corticosteroids in the treatment of patients with gastric aspiration. Am J Med 1977;63:719.

363. Heffner JE, Sahn SA: Pleural disease in pregnancy. Clin Chest Med 1992;13:667.

364. Light RW: Pleural Diseases, 3rd ed. Philadelphia, Lea & Febiger, 1995.

365. Sahn SA: State of the art. The pleura. Am Rev Respir Dis 1988;138:184.

366. Gourgoulianis KI, Karantanas AH, Diminikou G, Molyvdas PA: Benign postpartum pleural effusion. Eur Respir J 1995;8:1748.

367. Hughson WG, Friedman PJ, Feigin DS, et al: Postpartum pleural effusion: A common radiologic finding. Ann Intern Med 1982;97:856.

368. Udeshi UL, McHugo JM, Crawford JS: Postpartum pleural effusion. Br J Obstet Gynaecol 1988;95:894.

369. Munsell WP: Pneumomediastinum: A report of 28 cases and review of the literature. JAMA 1967;202:689.

370. Gemer O, Popescu M, Lebowits O, Segal S: Pneumomediastinum in labor. Arch Gynecol Obstet 1995;255:47.

371. Bard R, Hassini N: Pneumomediastinum complicating pregnancy. Respiration 1975;32:185.

372. Brandfass RT, Martinez DM: Mediastinal and subcutaneous emphysema in labor. South Med J 1976;69:1554.

373. Crean PA, Stronge JM, FitzGerald MX: Spontaneous pneumomediastinum in pregnancy. Br J Obstet Gynaecol 1981;88:952.

374. Karson EM, Saltzman D, Davis MR: Pneumomediastinum in pregnancy: Two case reports and a review of the literature, pathophysiology, and management. Obstet Gynecol 1984;64:39S.

375. Gorbach JS, Counselman FL, Mendelson MH: Spontaneous pneumomediastinum secondary to hyperemesis gravidarum. J Emerg Med 1997;15:639.

376. Schwartz M, Rossoff L: Pneumomediastinum and bilateral pneumothoraces in a patient with hyperemesis gravidarum. Chest 1994;106:1904.

377. VanWinter JT, Nichols FC III, Pairolero PC, et al: Management of spontaneous pneumothorax during pregnancy: Case report and review of the literature. Mayo Clin Proc 1996;71:249.

378. Dhalla SS, Teskey JM: Surgical management of recurrent spontaneous pneumothorax during pregnancy. Chest 1985;88:301.

379. Reid CJ, Biurgin GA: Video-assisted thoracoscopic pleurodesis for persistent spontaneous pneumothorax in late pregnancy. Anaesth Intensive Care 2000;28:208.

380. Gaensler EA, Patton WE, Verstraeten JM, Badger TL: Pulmonary function in pregnancy. III. Serial observations in patients with pulmonary insufficiency. Am Rev Tuberc 1953;67:779.

381. Novy MJ, Edwards MJ: Respiratory problems in pregnancy. Am J Obstet Gynecol 1967;99:1024.

382. Hung CT, Pelosi M, Langer A, Harrigan JT: Blood gas measurements in the kyphoscoliotic gravida and her fetus: Report of a case. Am J Obstet Gynecol 1975;121:287.

383. Smythe AR, Gallery GP Jr, Kraynack B: Assessment of severe pulmonary disease in pregnancy with Swan-Ganz monitoring. A report of two cases. J Reprod Med 1985;30:133.

384. Kleinman JC, Kopstein A: Smoking during pregnancy, 1967-80. Am J Public Health 1987;77:823.

385. Ventura SJ, Martin JA, Curtin SC, Mathews TJ: Report of final natality statistics, 1996 [Monthly Vital Statistics Report, vol 46, no. 11, supplement]. Hyattsville, Maryland: National Center for Health Statistics, June 30, 1998.

386. Camilli AE, McElroy LF, Reed KL: Smoking and pregnancy: A comparison of Mexican-American and non-Hispanic white women. Obstet Gynecol 1994;84:1033.

387. Andres RL, Day MC: Perinatal complications associated with maternal tobacco use. Semin Neonatol 2000;5:231.

388. Kleinman JC, Pierre MB Jr, Madans JH, et al: The effects of maternal smoking on fetal and infant mortality. Am J Epidemiol 1988;127:274.

389. Meyer MB, Tonascia JA: Maternal smoking, pregnancy complications, and perinatal mortality. Am J Obstet Gynecol 1977;128:494.

390. Heffner LJ, Sherman CB, Speizer FE, Weiss ST: Clinical and environmental predictors of preterm labor. Obstet Gynecol 1993;81:750.

391. Wisborg K, Henriksen TB, Hedeguard M, Secher NJ: Smoking during pregnancy and preterm birth. Br J Obstet Gynecol 1996;103:800.

392. Zabriskie JR: Effect of cigarette smoking during pregnancy: Study of 2000 cases. Obstet Gynecol 1963;21:405.

393. Kline J, Stein ZA, Susser M, Warburton D: Smoking: A risk factor for spontaneous abortion. N Engl J Med 1977;297:793.

394. Morrow RJ, Ritchie JW, Bull SB: Maternal cigarette smoking: The effects on umbilical and uterine blood flow velocity. Am J Obstet Gynecol 1988;159:1069.

395. Garn SM, Johnston M, Ridella SA, Petzold AS: Effect of maternal cigarette smoking on Apgar scores. Am J Dis Child 1981;135:503.

396. Bureau MA, Monette J, Shapcott D, et al: Carboxyhemoglobin concentration in fetal cord blood and in blood of mothers who smoked during labor. Pediatrics 1982;69:371.

397. Longo LD: The biological effects of carbon monoxide on the pregnant woman, fetus, and newborn infant. Am J Obstet Gynecol 1977;129:69.

398. Asmussen I: Ultrastructure of the human placenta at term. Observations on placentas from newborn children of smoking and non-smoking mothers. Acta Obstet Gynecol Scand 1977;56:119.

399. Golding J: Sudden infant death syndrome and parental smoking—a literature review. Paediatr Perinat Epidemiol 1997;11:67.

400. Malloy MH, Hoffman HJ, Peterson DR: Sudden infant death syndrome and maternal smoking. Am J Public Health 1992;82:1380.

401. Alm B, Milerad J, Wennergren G, et al: A case-control study of smoking and sudden infant death syndrome in the Scandinavian countries, 1992 to 1995. The Nordic Epidemiological SIDS Study. Arch Dis Child 1998;78:329.

402. Lieberman E, Torday J, Barbieri R, et al: Association of intrauterine cigarette smoke exposure with indices of fetal lung maturation. Obstet Gynecol 1992;79:564.

403. Czeizel AE, Kodaj I, Lenz W: Smoking during pregnancy and congenital limb deficiency. BMJ 1994;308:1473.

404. Wyszynski DF, Duffy DL, Beaty TH: Maternal cigarette smoking and oral clefts: A meta-analysis. Cleft Palate Craniofac J 1997;34:206.

405. Li DK, Mueller BA, Hickok DE, et al: Maternal smoking during pregnancy and the risk of congenital urinary tract anomalies. Am J Public Health 1996;86:249.

406. Weiss ST, Tager IB, Schenker M, Speizer FE: The health effects of involuntary smoking. Am Rev Respir Dis 1983;128:933.

407. Ellard GA, Johnstone FD, Prescott RJ, et al: Smoking during pregnancy: The dose dependence of birth weight deficits. Br J Obstet Gynecol 1996;103:806.

408. Haste FM, Brooke OG, Anderson HR, et al: Nutrient intakes during pregnancy: Observations on the influence of smoking and social class. Am J Clin Nutr 1990;51:29.

409. Kuhnert BR, Kuhnert PM, Debanne S, Williams TG: The relationship between cadmium, zinc, and birth weight in pregnant women who smoke. Am J Obstet Gynecol 1987;157:1247.

410. Metcoff J, Costiloe P, Crosby WM, et al: Smoking in pregnancy: Relation of birth weight to maternal plasma carotene and cholesterol levels. Obstet Gynecol 1989;74:302.

411. Beaulac-Baillargeon L, Desrosiers C: Caffeine-cigarette interaction on fetal growth. Am J Obstet Gynecol 1987;157:1236.

412. Conter V, Cortinovis I, Rogari P, Riva L: Weight growth in infants born to mothers who smoked during pregnancy. BMJ 1995;310:768.

413. Wang X, Zuckerman B, Pearson C, et al: Maternal cigarette smoking, metabolic gene polymorphism, and infant birth weight. JAMA 2002;287:195.

414. Perlman HH, Dannenberg AM, Sokoloff N: Excretion of nicotine in breast and urine from cigarette smoking. JAMA 1942;120:1003.

415. Vio F, Salazar G, Infante C: Smoking during pregnancy and lactation and its effects on breast-milk volume. Am J Clin Nutr 1991;54:1011.

416. Donnenfeld AE, Pulkkinen A, Palomaki GE, et al: Simultaneous fetal and maternal cotinine levels in pregnant women smokers. Am J Obstet Gynecol 1993;168:781.

417. Stjernfeldt M, Berglund K, Lindsten J, Ludvigsson J: Maternal smoking during pregnancy and risk of childhood cancer. Lancet 1986;1:1350.

418. Everson RB, Randerath E, Santella RM, et al: Detection of smoking-related covalent DNA adducts in human placenta. Science 1986;231:54.

419. Everson RB, Randerath E, Santella RM, et al: Quantitative associations between DNA damage in human placenta and maternal smoking and birth weight. J Natl Cancer Inst 1988;80:567.

420. Weitzman M, Gortmaker S, Walker DK, Sobol A: Maternal smoking and childhood asthma. Pediatrics 1990;85:505.

421. Gilliand FD, Li YF, Peters JM: Effects of maternal smoking during pregnancy and environmental tobacco smoke on asthma and wheezing in children. Am J Respir Crit Care Med 2001;163:429.

422. Hanrahan JP, Tager IB, Segal MR, et al: The effect of maternal smoking during pregnancy on early infant lung function. Am Rev Respir Dis 1992;145:1129.

423. Harlap S, Davies AM: Infant admissions to hospital and maternal smoking. Lancet 1974;1:529.

424. Taylor B, Wadsworth J: Maternal smoking during pregnancy and lower respiratory tract illness in early life. Arch Dis Child 1987;62:786.

425. Tager IB, Hanrahan JP, Tosteson TD, et al: Lung function, pre- and post-natal smoke exposure, and wheezing in the first year of life. Am Rev Respir Dis 1993;147:811.

426. Cunningham J, Dockery DW, Speizer FE: Maternal smoking during pregnancy as a predictor of lung function in children. Am J Epidemiol 1994;139:1139.

427. Cunningham J, Dockery DW, Gold DR, Speizer FE: Racial differences in the association between maternal smoking during pregnancy and lung function in children. Am J Respir Crit Care Med 1995;152:565.

428. Tager IB, Ngo L, Hanrahan JP: Maternal smoking during pregnancy: Effects of lung function during the first 18 months of life. Am J Respir Crit Care Med 1995;152:977.

429. Stick SM, Burton PR, Gurrin L, et al: Effects of maternal smoking during pregnancy and a family history of asthma on respiratory function in newborn infants. Lancet 1996;348:1060.

430. Hakim RB, Tielsch JM: Maternal cigarette smoking during pregnancy. A risk factor for childhood strabismus. Arch Ophthalmol 1992;110:1459.

431. Milberger S, Biederman J, Faraone SV, et al: Is maternal smoking during pregnancy a risk factor for attention deficit hyperactivity disorder in children? Am J Psychiatry 1996;153:1138.

432. Marks JS, Koplan JP, Hogue CJ, Dalmat ME: A cost-benefit/cost-effectiveness analysis of smoking cessation for pregnant women. Am J Prev Med 1990;6:282.

433. Hartmann KE, Thorp JM, Pahel-Short L, Koch MA: A randomized controlled trial of smoking cessation intervention in pregnancy in an academic clinic. Obstet Gynecol 1996;87:621.

434. Dolan-Mullen P, Ramirez G, Groff JY: A meta-analysis of randomized trials of prenatal smoking cessation interventions. Am J Obstet Gynecol 1994;171:1328.

435. Lumley J, Oliver S, Waters E: Interventions for promoting smoking cessation during pregnancy. Cochrane Database Syst Rev 2000;(2):CD001055.

436. ACOG educational bulletin. Smoking cessation during pregnancy [Number 260, September 2000]. American College of Obstetricians and Gynecologists. Int J Gynaecol Obstet 2001;75:345.

437. Benowitz NL, Dempsey DA, Goldenberg RL, et al: The use of pharmacotherapies for smoking cessation during pregnancy. Tob Control 2000;9(Suppl 3):III91.

NEUROLOGIC COMPLICATIONS

James O. Donaldson and Thomas P. Duffy

Underlying neurologic conditions can complicate and be complicated by pregnancy or arise as secondary complications of pregnancy. The spectrum of disorders ranges from commonplace backache to life-threatening seizures with eclamptic encephalopathy; previous effective drug management of epilepsy may become erratic as pregnancy evolves, and the teratogenic threat of necessary medications becomes an appropriate source of anxiety. Because of the complexity of many of these disorders and their potential for worsening during pregnancy, a close collaboration between the neurologist and obstetrician is necessary to ensure optimal fetal and maternal outcomes.

LEG CRAMPS

Painful muscle cramps are experienced to varying degrees by more than 25% of women during the second half of pregnancy, usually at night or immediately when movement is initiated upon awakening. The gastrocnemius muscle commonly cramps, but the thigh and gluteal muscles may also be involved. Leg cramps of pregnant women cannot be distinguished clinically and electromyographically from a "charley horse," the cramp of a poorly trained muscle. However, excellent conditioning does not protect pregnant women from muscle cramps. The cause of the cramps remains unknown.

The traditional treatment has been supplementation of dietary calcium intake, although the evidence for calcium reduction of muscle cramps is weak.[1] The best evidence of a positive intervention for these troublesome symptoms is administration of magnesium lactate or citrate. Salt depletion, dehydration, uremia, hypothyroidism, and hypomagnesemia may cause or worsen muscle cramps.

RESTLESS LEGS SYNDROME

The restless legs syndrome, which afflicts about 10% of pregnant women, is often mistaken for muscle cramps.[2] The two are quite distinct, however: Patients with restless legs syndrome complain that 10 to 20 minutes after getting into bed, a creeping, wormy, burning ache develops within

their legs. The more the urge to allow the legs to fidget is resisted, the greater the urge becomes until it can no longer be withstood. Walking about may help. Sometimes similar but milder symptoms may develop while the individual is seated, as in a theater or restaurant.

During pregnancy, restless leg syndrome is idiopathic, although women with iron deficiency may experience symptom improvement with correction of this deficiency. Pregnant women who supplement their diet with folic acid, 0.5 mg orally daily, appear to be less likely to develop restless legs syndrome. This condition can be mimicked by caffeinism and may be associated with polyneuropathy, vascular insufficiency, and uremia. Severe symptoms may warrant low doses of levodopa or pergolide.[3]

MYOTONIC MUSCULAR DYSTROPHY

Myotonic muscular dystrophy is an inherited systemic disease characterized by myopathic weakness of the neck, face, and distal limbs and by myotonia, which is clinically demonstrated most easily in the thenar muscles and tongue. Smooth muscle and myometrium may be involved by the dystrophic process, resulting in delayed gut motility and prolonged labor, but only skeletal muscle has a T-tubular system and can generate myotonic discharges. Weakness may worsen during pregnancy. Myotonia, whether part of myotonic muscular dystrophy or a feature of myotonia congenita (Thomsen's disease), may worsen during the second half of pregnancy.[4] If the condition is symptomatic, phenytoin may be warranted.

Ovarian function has been poorly investigated in myotonic muscular dystrophy, although 80% of men develop testicular atrophy at some stage of the disease. In women, spontaneous and habitual abortion and premature labor are not uncommon.[4] Postpartum hemorrhage can result from uterine inertia. In contrast, uterine contractions are strong in myotonia congenita.

Whether hypoventilation and chronic respiratory acidosis are present should be determined before labor. Pulmonary function should be evaluated before labor to identify the potential threat of respiratory decompensation during delivery. Regional anesthesia should be used whenever possible.[5] Depolarizing muscle relaxants (e.g., succinylcholine chloride) may cause severe spasms and hyperthermia. Curariform drugs may be used.

Severe fetal and neonatal myotonic muscular dystrophy may coexist with subclinical and mild, unrecognized disease in the mother. In utero manifestations include polyhydramnios from fetal swallowing dysfunction and arthrogryposis multiplex congenita from myopathic inactivity. Both may be detected in the second trimester by ultrasonography. Infants present as "floppy babies" with facial diplegia. Myotonia is not present. Almost half have talipes. Neonatal deaths are caused by respiratory distress and feeding problems.

The autosomal dominant gene responsible for myotonic muscular dystrophy is on chromosome 19; a disease-specific DNA probe is available for diagnosis.[6] Reproductive counseling is appropriate for women with myotonic muscular dystrophy.[7]

POLYMYOSITIS

Polymyositis is a subacute, symmetric inflammatory disease affecting primarily proximal limb and trunk muscles. The presence of dermatomyositis indicates that the skin is also involved. Among women of reproductive age, polymyositis is commonly associated with collagen-vascular diseases. The response to aggressive corticosteroid therapy is monitored by serial tests of muscle strength and measurements of serum creatine phosphokinase and erythrocyte sedimentation rate. The use of azathioprine and cyclophosphamide is reserved for refractory cases and should be avoided during pregnancy and among women with reproductive potential. Fetal wastage is correlated with the presence of an underlying disease and the activity of the polymyositis; the degree of fetal wastage reflects the level of maternal disease.[8,9] Mothers should be reassured that no effects of polymyositis/dermatomyositis have been demonstrated in surviving newborns.

MYASTHENIA GRAVIS

Myasthenia gravis is an autoimmune disease with immunoglobulin G antibody directed against nicotinic acetylcholine receptors of striated muscle. It is clinically characterized by fluctuating fatigability of ocular, facial, oropharyngeal, and, to a lesser extent, limb muscles. Smooth muscle and myometrium are spared. Thus, myasthenia gravis does not prolong labor and uterine involution. Uterine inertia responds normally to oxytocin. Hypermagnesemia inhibits the release of acetylcholine. Thus, if a myasthenic woman is administered magnesium sulfate for toxemia, she may develop apnea and marked weakness.[10]

The effect of pregnancy on myasthenia gravis cannot be predicted from its effect during a previous pregnancy or from any feature of the maternal disease, including severity.[11,12] Approximately equal numbers of patients experience improvement, worsening, and no change during pregnancy. Infections are a common cause of myasthenia exacerbations.[13] Abortion does not induce a remission if the disease has been exacerbated. Postpartum deterioration of myasthenia gravis is common enough that follow-up visits are recommended every 2 weeks for the first 6 weeks after childbirth.

Regional anesthesia is preferred.[11,14] If the patient is being treated with pyridostigmine and neostigmine, which block acetylcholinesterase, large amounts of procaine and congeners should be avoided, because the hydrolysis of these drugs by plasma cholinesterase has been inhibited and convulsions may result. Instead, lidocaine is recommended. If an inhalation anesthetic is to be used, ether should be avoided and narcotics administered judiciously. Curare and scopolamine are contraindicated.

The risk of a pregnancy-associated exacerbation of myasthenia gravis is lessened by a transsternal thymectomy early in the course of the disease.[15] It is appropriate for patients to wait approximately 1 year after surgery for the myasthenia to stabilize before becoming pregnant. Azathioprine should be avoided, if possible, in young myasthenic women with the potential for childbearing, because of its possible teratogenic effect. Prednisone and courses of plasmapheresis can be used during pregnancy.[16] Pyridostigmine and neostigmine are quaternary ammonium compounds that do not cross the placenta or the blood-brain barrier. Negligible amounts are secreted in breast milk.

Of the offspring of mothers with generalized myasthenia gravis, 12% to 30% develop transient neonatal myasthenia gravis.[17] Manifestations vary from a slack jaw, for which a finger is needed to support the infant's jaw to suckle normally, to a "floppy baby," in which the infant is unable to feed and displays a feeble cry and weak Moro reflex. Ptosis and ophthalmoplegia are not characteristics of transient neonatal myasthenia gravis but are seen with congenital myasthenia gravis.

Curiously, few manifestations of fetal myasthenia gravis occur. Mothers of affected infants report strong in utero movement, and polyhydramnios has not been reported. Arthrogryposis has been reported in congenital myasthenia but only rarely in neonatal myasthenia. Clearly, the immunoglobulin G passes the placenta; titers of antibody to acetylcholine receptors are approximately equal in maternal blood and cord blood. α-Fetoprotein may block the antibody and protect the fetus.

Neonatal myasthenia gravis abates spontaneously in 2 to 4 weeks. Eighty percent of patients require anticholinesterase therapy; some need assisted respiration. Exchange transfusion has been successfully used in the treatment of this condition.[17a]

GUILLAIN-BARRÉ SYNDROME

Guillain-Barré syndrome is an inflammatory demyelinating polyneuropathy characterized by areflexia and symmetric weakness of limb and facial muscles, loss of sensory perception, and autonomic symptoms. Respiration and swallowing may be paralyzed. Usually, bladder function remains intact. Symptoms commonly worsen for 1 to 4 weeks before spontaneously improving. Plasmapheresis within the first 10 days after the onset of weakness improves the speed of recovery. Most young patients regain full function.

The coexistence of Guillain-Barré syndrome and pregnancy is coincidental.[18] *Campylobacter jejuni* infection is the antecedent event in approximately 30% of cases of Guillain-Barré syndrome; pregnant women should take special care in handling and preparing food to prevent such infection.[19] The natural history of the disease is unaltered by pregnancy except that the gravid uterus may affect bladder control and diminish respiratory reserve. Premature labor may occur in severe cases in the third trimester, but severe disease earlier in pregnancy is not associated with spontaneous abortion. Uterine contractions are not affected.

Treatment consists of plasmapheresis or high-dose intravenous human immune globulin early in the course of the disease.[20] Prevention of complications requires the consistent, constant care of nurses, physical therapists, and physicians. Corticosteroid therapy is usually reserved for patients in whom symptoms have failed to improve by 4 to 6 weeks after the onset of weakness.

There are no fetal or neonatal manifestations of maternal Guillain-Barré syndrome. Breast-feeding is allowed.

GESTATIONAL POLYNEUROPATHY

Gestational polyneuropathy is a dying-back axonal neuropathy similar to the neuropathy of thiamine deficiency among alcoholic persons. It may be associated with hyperemesis gravidarum and Wernicke's encephalopathy.[21] Treatment consists of an adequate diet supplemented with vitamins. Thiamine should be administered parenterally for at least 1 week if Wernicke's encephalopathy is present.

BELL'S PALSY

Bell's palsy is a sudden, unilateral neuropathy of the seventh cranial nerve that causes weakness of the forehead and lower face and may cause ipsilateral ageusia, if the lesion is proximal to the branching off of the chorda tympani. The incidence of Bell's palsy in pregnant women is approximately three times higher than in nonpregnant women of the same age. A clustering of cases in the third trimester implies a sevenfold increased risk for that period. Onset of the condition during pregnancy appears associated with the development of the hypertensive disorders of pregnancy. Pregnant women who develop Bell's palsy should be closely monitored for hypertension or preeclampsia.[22-24] The prognosis is particularly good, for full recovery, if the onset is within the last 2 weeks of pregnancy. A short course of high-dose corticosteroids is indicated for complete unilateral facial weakness occurring earlier in pregnancy.[24a]

CARPAL TUNNEL SYNDROME

Twenty to 40 percent of pregnant women experience nocturnal hand pain.[25] Probably fewer than 5% have electromyographic evidence of a carpal tunnel syndrome.[26] The symptoms of median nerve entrapment at the wrist are easily confused with acroparesthesias caused by postural kinking of blood vessels at the thoracic outlet. In both cases, women awaken at night with a tingling hand. In carpal tunnel syndrome, paresthesias are usually limited to the index, middle, and ring fingers. A Tinel sign may be elicited by tapping the median nerve at the wrist, and the sensation of pinpricks may be blunted in the cutaneous distribution of the median nerve. Symptomatic treatment with nocturnal splinting of the wrist held in midposition is the recommended treatment, because in most cases, symptoms abate in the puerperium. If the abductor pollicis brevis and opponens pollicis are weak, permanent relief of symptoms by division of the transcarpal ligaments is indicated.

MERALGIA PARESTHETICA

Meralgia paresthetica is a painful dysesthesia along the lateral thigh caused by entrapment of the purely sensory lateral femoral cutaneous nerve as it passes beneath the inguinal ligament. Obesity and the rapid weight gain of pregnancy are predisposing factors. This nuisance develops in the third trimester and slowly, spontaneously resolves in the puerperium.[27] No treatment is indicated.

MATERNAL OBSTETRIC PALSY

The fetal head and forceps may compress segments of the lumbosacral plexus and individual peripheral nerves against the pelvic wall.[28,29] The typical patient is a short, overweight primipara whose labor is lengthy because of cephalopelvic disproportion. Patients may not be aware of their weakness as long as they remain in bed. Sometimes patients recall a stab of pain into a thigh, knee, or ankle during labor. Modern obstetric care and greater use of cesarean section have reduced the frequency of this complication of childbirth, whereas around 1900, fully 3.2% of 2480 deliveries in three series were complicated by femoral neuropathy alone.

The most common maternal obstetric palsy is postpartum footdrop. The lumbosacral trunk constituted from L4 and L5 roots can be compressed by the fetal brow against the sacral ala. This syndrome is characteristically unilateral and occurs on the side opposite the presentation of the vertex (right occiput anterior presentation is equivalent to left brow posterior presentation). If the site of compression is lower, nerves derived from the S1 root can be involved, in addition to L4 and L5 nerves, to produce an intrapelvic sciatic neuropathy.[28] Footdrop may also be caused by compression of the common peroneal nerve between leg holders and the fibular head.

In most instances, the prognosis is excellent because only the myelin sheath is distorted, and marked improvement is expected within 8 weeks. If axons are crushed and wallerian degeneration occurs, recovery is slow and usually incomplete. Electromyography helps to distinguish the two situations.

The risk of permanent weakness with recurrent intrapartum injury is unknown. Cephalopelvic disproportion is a predisposing factor to recurrence. Unless the fetus of a subsequent pregnancy is much smaller, women who have had axonal degeneration should undergo cesarean section. Women who recovered promptly and fully from this lesion may have a trial of labor but should expect a cesarean section if dystocia develops.

BACKACHE

Postural backache induced by exaggeration of the lumbar lordotic curve is a universal complaint during pregnancy, usually beginning in the fifth to eighth months.[30] Fifteen percent of affected women rate their pain as severe, with peak intensity in the evening and at night. Sometimes a pattern develops: periods of rest alternating with household chores. Pain is localized to the low back or to the sacroiliac region. If pain travels into a leg, it lacks the radicular quality of discogenic pain and does not go beyond the knee.

Anything that increases lumbar lordosis, such as wearing high-heeled shoes, or any preexisting condition that limits adaptability of the back muscles increases backache. Swimming is highly recommended. Women who experience distressing back pain during one pregnancy are strongly advised to start a conditioning program before becoming pregnant again.

LUMBAR DISK DISEASE

Prolapse of an intervertebral disk is unusual during pregnancy. Unless impaired sphincter function dictates a neuroimaging study on an urgent basis, conservative therapy with strict bed rest for 10 days is recommended. Magnetic resonance imaging (MRI), if available, is preferred to computed tomographic (CT) myelography, which causes significant fetal x-ray exposure. Bulging intervertebral disks are common in both pregnant and nonpregnant women of childbearing age.[31] Lumbar laminectomy and discectomy have been performed without incident during pregnancy. If a disk is herniated near term, cesarean section prevents the excruciating radicular pain that results from bearing down during labor.

SPINAL CORD TRANSECTIONS

Paraplegic and even quadriplegic women can successfully deliver vaginally. The obstetrician must anticipate and avoid complications.[32,33] Because more urinary incontinence and urinary tract infections can be expected, meticulous catheter care is a requirement, and acidification of urine with vitamin C, 500 mg four times daily, may be recommended. A high-bulk diet, stool softeners, and adequate fluid intake may help prevent constipation. Pressure sores and poor wound healing are always a concern, especially among anemic patients. Blood transfusions may be warranted.

Premature labor is an expected hazard. Weekly antenatal visits should begin in the 28th week of pregnancy and the patient should be hospitalized by the 32nd week. Cesarean section is performed only for obstetric indications.

Breast-feeding can be successful. The milk "let-down" phenomenon is normal.

The level of the spinal cord lesion can affect childbirth. All patients have sacral anesthesia. Patients with cauda equina lesions have relaxed perineal muscles, although they perceive labor pain because uterine sensory nerves enter the spinal cord at T11 and T12. If the lesion is above T11, labor is painless, although local somatic reflex arcs may be activated, resulting in sustained clonus and extensor and flexor muscle spasms. If the lesion is above T5 to T6 (i.e., above the outflow of the splanchnic autonomic nerves), labor can trigger release of large amounts of catecholamines. This autonomic stress syndrome, or autonomic hyperreflexia, is clinically characterized by brief paroxysms of severe hypertension, throbbing headaches, sweating, and flushed skin.[32] Patients may time their contractions by these symptoms. Intracranial hemorrhage and cardiac arrhythmias may cause death. Regional anesthesia is necessary to control autonomic hyperreflexia. β-Blocking agents may be helpful.

MYELOPATHY

The development of nontraumatic myelopathy during pregnancy is an indication for a neuroimaging study and often for examination of cerebrospinal fluid (CSF). In order to limit fetal exposure to radiation, MRI is preferred to CT myelography, especially with lumbar and thoracic lesions. However, time may be of the essence, and whatever technique is readily available should be used.

A common cause of acute transverse myelopathy during pregnancy is a vascular malformation.[34] Exacerbations during previous pregnancies, and sometimes during menstruation, may lead to an initial misdiagnosis of multiple sclerosis, although the CSF is normal and there are no signs or symptoms of a lesion above the foramen magnum. Several mechanisms may explain worsening during pregnancy. The gravid uterus can mechanically shift venous return from the inferior vena cava to vertebral and epidural veins. Also, estrogens directly dilate these arteriovenous shunts in a manner analogous to the production of spider "nevi" and palmar erythema during pregnancy.

Meningiomas, ependymomas, and other tumors of the spinal cord can cause rapid deterioration in the second half of pregnancy.[35] Spontaneous epidural hematomas can occur.

CHOREA GRAVIDARUM

Chorea gravidarum is any chorea, or hemichorea, acquired during pregnancy; the clinical picture is of extrapyramidal symptoms such as involuntary movements, lack of coordination and slurred speech.[36] Before penicillin curtailed rheumatic heart disease, many cases of chorea gravidarum were documented. Sixty percent of affected patients had experienced Sydenham's chorea. Some had acute rheumatic fever. The prognosis was poor, principally because of associated heart disease. Now it is a rarity just as likely to be linked with systemic lupus erythematosus and/or the antiphospholipid antibody syndrome. Oral contraceptives may also induce chorea, usually hemichorea.

Chorea gravidarum usually begins in the first half of pregnancy and persists until the early puerperium. Almost one third of affected patients become asymptomatic in the third trimester. The reasons are unclear. Estrogen can stimulate postsynaptic dopamine receptor activity. However, that does not help explain why a patient who has chorea gravidarum with one pregnancy may not experience it with subsequent pregnancies.

Haloperidol at doses up to 20 mg or more daily may be required in violent chorea to prevent hyperthermia and rhabdomyolysis.

WILSON'S DISEASE

Wilson's disease (hepatolenticular degeneration) is an inborn error of copper metabolism that usually manifests in the second decade of life. Until the introduction of chelation therapy with D-penicillamine, only rarely did women with Wilson's disease become pregnant and reach term. Once treated successfully, women with Wilson's disease can become pregnant and deliver normal infants.

All patients should be maintained on chelation therapy to prevent rebound of the disease; most affected women take D-penicillamine, 0.5 to 1 g/day, plus vitamin B_6, 50 to 100 mg/day, to counter the antipyridoxine effect of D-penicillamine.[37] Trientine with zinc sulfate is an effective alternative to penicillamine.[38,38a] An improvement in symptoms may be noted, although there is no consistent change, if any, in any parameter of copper metabolism during the pregnancies of women with Wilson's disease. If a cesarean section is planned, a reduction of the D-penicillamine dosage to 0.25 g/day has been recommended because the drug can impair wound healing. Breast-feeding is permitted. Breast milk contains normal amounts of copper.

Myasthenia gravis can result from antibodies to acetylcholine receptors that have been structurally altered by chronic D-penicillamine therapy. The son of one woman with Wilson's disease and myasthenia gravis induced by D-penicillamine developed neonatal myasthenia gravis.[39]

MULTIPLE SCLEROSIS

Multiple sclerosis is a multifocal demyelinating disease of the central nervous system clinically characterized by exacerbations and remissions occurring over decades. The cause is unknown. There is no specific cure. Short-term, high-dose corticosteroid therapy may be used for relapses during pregnancy but should be used with caution.

Multiple sclerosis rarely affects fertility, but it does alter family patterns. Women who develop multiple sclerosis choose to have fewer children and have more elective abortions than do normal women. Age and disability are often major factors in their decisions. The use of oral contraceptives does not alter the course of multiple sclerosis.[40] Breast-feeding is also not a determinant. The relapse rate for the entire pregnancy year approximates that for a nonpregnant year. This pattern also occurs in other autoimmune diseases, perhaps because α-fetoprotein acts as an immunosuppressive substance.

Uncomplicated multiple sclerosis has almost no effect on pregnancy.[41] The incidence of premature labor, complicated deliveries, toxemia, and stillbirths, and the duration of labor, are all as expected in the general population. Spinal anesthesia is usually not recommended for use in patients with multiple sclerosis; instead, epidural anesthesia is used.[42,42a] Breast-feeding is permitted. It is important for the new mother with multiple sclerosis to get enough rest.

Treatment with interferon-β is not recommended during pregnancy but may be resumed post partum, unless the woman is breast-feeding. Intravenous immunoglobulin in the postpartum period may potentially reduce the incidence of postpartum relapse.[43]

BRAIN TUMORS

The incidence of brain tumors in pregnant women is low and significantly decreased in comparison with nonpregnant women; this has been attributed to the altered hormonal milieu of pregnancy. When tumors do develop, the histologic types are very similar to those in nonpregnant women. The presenting symptoms of brain tumors may be masked in pregnancy, inasmuch as nausea and vomiting may be attributed to hyperemesis; headache may occur in pregnancy, but new-onset, persistent headache with nausea, vomiting, or neurologic signs mandates neuroimaging with CT scanning or MRI.[44] Some brain tumors enlarge during pregnancy and shrink post partum, at least temporarily.[45,46] Presumably, estrogen receptors in meningiomas, neurofibromas, and other tumors activate tumor growth.[47] Most tumors become symptomatic in the second half of pregnancy. Approximately one third of affected patients die during pregnancy, especially those with malignant gliomas, choroid plexus papillomas, and most infratentorial tumors except acoustic neuromas.[46] Tentorial herniation may occur during labor. Brain tumors account for almost 10% of maternal deaths. Pituitary tumors rarely cause maternal death.

Dangerous tumors necessitate intervention and treatment regardless of gestational age during pregnancy. More benign tumors, most meningiomas, and acoustic neuromas are tackled several weeks post partum, with steroids and anticonvulsants administered until fetal viability is achieved.[48] Accepted indications for therapeutic abortion include intracranial hypertension, uncontrolled seizures, and vision failure. Many women with malignant gliomas choose to have abortions. For them, another pregnancy is inadvisable and should be terminated early if it occurs.

PITUITARY ADENOMAS

Both a normal pituitary gland and prolactin-secreting adenomas swell during pregnancy. An expanding pituitary lesion, usually manifesting during the third trimester or early postpartum period, may be caused by lymphocytic hypophysitis.[49] Whether this enlargement becomes symptomatic depends on the initial size of the tumor; only 5% of microadenomas measuring less than 10 mm in diameter become symptomatic, whereas an estimated 35% of macroadenomas do. Some clinicians recommend pregestational resection of macroadenomas. In affected patients, headache usually develops in the first half of pregnancy and precedes vision disturbances by at least 1 month. Macroadenomas can cause deficits in other pituitary hormones.

The difference in the natural history of these two categories of prolactinomas directs the management of these tumors before and during pregnancy.[50] Larger prolactinomas are more likely to occur in women who have had surgery or radiation therapy before ovulation is induced with bromocriptine[51] or cabergoline. Transsphenoidal hypophysectomy is usually preferred to radiation because the latter often produces chronic hypopituitarism. Neither modality is necessarily curative. During pregnancy, women with microadenomas are observed with bedside determination of visual fields; women with macroadenomas usually have formal perimetry each month. Repeat CT scanning or MRI is warranted if the patient becomes symptomatic.[52] Periodic measurements of prolactin levels are of no benefit.

Early vision disturbances may be monitored carefully or treated with bromocriptine[51] or cabergoline according to the judgment of the clinician and the circumstances of each case, such as stage of gestation. If visual acuity becomes less than 20/50 or if the visual field defects encroach on nasal sectors, treatment becomes mandatory. If the fetus is viable, delivery is an option. Patients who fail to experience improvement with drug treatment are automatically candidates for surgery, as are patients with sudden blindness or pituitary apoplexy.

Most women with pituitary adenomas can deliver vaginally. Although suckling releases prolactin, there is no objective evidence that either microadenomas or macroadenomas enlarge during breast-feeding. Postpartum CT scanning or MRI should be done to detect enlargement of the adenoma.

CHORIOCARCINOMA

Choriocarcinoma is a highly invasive trophoblastic tumor that usually manifests as irregular uterine bleeding months after a molar pregnancy or miscarriage. About 15% accompany or follow a normal pregnancy.[35] Cerebral metastases may cause the presenting complaints during pregnancy or as much as 4 years later.[53] Metastatic tumor penetrates vascular walls and proliferates. The artery may be occluded, producing a large stroke or multiple small strokes. Alternatively, the weakened artery may rupture, causing intracerebral hemorrhage, subarachnoid hemorrhage, or a subdural hematoma. Large solitary masses may cause focal seizures and hemiplegia. The tumor may also invade the spinal column and pelvic structures, including the lumbosacral plexus. Aggressive chemotherapy and radiation therapy have successfully treated some intracranial metastases.[54]

PSEUDOTUMOR CEREBRI

Pseudotumor cerebri (idiopathic intracranial hypertension) is the syndrome of increased intracranial pressure in the absence of an intracranial mass lesion. Headache may be the only complaint, and the cause may be overlooked unless a funduscopic examination is performed and papilledema is observed. Other signs and symptoms include diminished visual acuity, loss of color vision, defects in visual fields, and horizontal diplopia caused by abducens nerve palsy. CT scans rule out a mass lesion. In the pseudotumor cerebri syndromes of obese young women and pregnant women, the CSF protein concentration is commonly less than 20 mg/dL.

Pseudotumor cerebri associated with pregnancy usually begins in obese women who are 3 to 5 months pregnant and lasts 1 to 3 months before spontaneously abating. For some women, abatement does not begin until the puerperium. Pseudotumor cerebri infrequently recurs with subsequent pregnancies. Pseudotumor cerebri has occurred in thin women who are taking oral contraceptives. Obese women with active pseudotumor cerebri who become pregnant usually experience worsening of symptoms. Why some obese women develop pseudotumor cerebri is unknown, but the extraovarian production of estrogen by adipocytes may be involved.

The treatment of pseudotumor cerebri during pregnancy consists of repeated lumbar punctures, restriction of gross excesses in caloric intake, and, in more serious instances, corticosteroid therapy. If all fails and vision is being lost, fenestration of the optic nerve sheath or lumboperitoneal shunting must be considered in order to prevent blindness.[55]

HEADACHE

The most common headache during pregnancy is the muscle contraction/tension variety characterized by persistent band-like squeezing pain or an exploding sensation often localized to the vertex. Typically, symptoms worsen late in the day and may start immediately upon eye opening each morning, if not before. Palpation of hard posterior cervical muscles evokes pain. The neurologic examination, including funduscopy, yields normal findings. Most patients have a history of headache of varying intensity but similar quality dating back years. Symptoms of depression and anxiety are frequently present. During pregnancy, these headaches are worsened by postural changes and by new situational problems.

The basic treatment for occasional muscle contraction headaches is muscle massage, application of heat or ice packs to the neck, and simple analgesics. Acetaminophen is usually preferred to aspirin for frequent use during pregnancy.[56,57] If these headaches become a regular feature of life, a tricyclic antidepressant, such as amitriptyline, 50-75 mg at bedtime, is good prophylaxis. Diazepam is not effective over the long term and should not be used regularly during pregnancy because sedating metabolites are trapped in the fetus and slowly eliminated by newborns.

Classic Migraine

Classic migraine is a distinct clinical syndrome. Typically, a 20- to 30-minute prodrome of scintillating visual hallucinations and scotomata precedes severe unilateral headache and nausea. Oral contraceptives worsen these headaches, as may perimenstrual estrogen withdrawal.[58] Pregnancy, on the other hand, is a protected time for many women, particularly those with a history of menstrual migraine.[59,60] Complicated migraine with hemiplegia and basilar artery migraine are prone to worsen during pregnancy.[61,62] Many agents are available for prescription for migraines.[63]

Ergot alkaloids taken early enough in the prodromal phase can ameliorate the headache phase. During pregnancy, however, ergot is best avoided, because it is feared, whether true or not for all ergot compounds, that its oxytocic property could prematurely stimulate uterine contractions. Instead, analgesics and phenothiazine antiemetic suppositories give good symptomatic relief for occasional migraines. Propranolol HCl, 10 to 40 mg orally 4 times daily, is effective prophylactic treatment for frequent classic migraine. Experience has shown this to be acceptably safe during pregnancy despite earlier concerns about fetal bradycardia and other effects.[64] Newer agents such as the triptans should be prescribed with caution during pregnancy.[65]

CEREBROVASCULAR DISEASE

Cerebrovascular disease in young adults, particularly pregnant women, is seldom simple. Because a wide variety of relatively rare types of cerebrovascular disease are collectively commonplace during pregnancy, an aggressive approach is needed to properly diagnose each case, enabling sound counsel concerning prognosis, treatment, and management of pregnancy and childbirth. Angiography is often needed. High-quality cerebral angiography may still be needed if magnetic resonance angiography does not define the situation. An underlying systemic disease should always be suspected.

Cerebral Ischemia

Ancient literature ascribed most strokes during pregnancy to thrombosis of cerebral veins, but cerebral angiography has documented arterial occlusion as the most likely cause during pregnancy and the first postpartum week.[66,67] Old literature that indicated the incidence of cerebral infarction and transient ischemic attacks increased fivefold to tenfold during pregnancy has been disputed, although an increased incidence post partum has been confirmed.[66,68] Approximately 30% of ischemic strokes occur in each of the second and third trimesters. Twenty-five percent occur in the first postpartum week alone. Death is uncommon unless caused by other manifestations of a primary condition of which the stroke was symptomatic.

In pregnant women, the site of occlusion is more likely to be the middle cerebral artery (35%) than the carotid artery (20%); the opposite ranking occurs in nonpregnant women with strokes.[66] No occlusion is found in 25% of patients.

Vertebrobasilar stroke is rare in young adults and during pregnancy; however, an unusually high proportion (25% to 40%) of strokes associated with oral contraceptives are vertebrobasilar. Middle cerebral artery occlusions, even bilateral occlusions, have also occurred with use of oral contraceptives. The prevalence of middle cerebral artery occlusions in pregnancy and with use of oral contraceptives raises suspicion of emboli from or through the heart as a major cause of stroke in these circumstances.[66]

Atherosclerosis

Atherosclerosis is the principal cause of stroke in older patients, but few strokes during pregnancy can be attributed to premature atherosclerosis.[67] Most affected patients can be identified by the presence of diabetes mellitus, chronic hypertension, and hyperhomocystinemia. A history of cigarette smoking is commonplace.

Mitral Valve Prolapse

The prevalence of mitral valve prolapse among women with pregnancy-associated cerebral ischemia is unknown. Use of new diagnostic criteria (three-dimensional analysis of the shape of the valve) reduces markedly the frequency of the occurrence of mitral valve prolapse.[69] The click-murmur of mitral valve prolapse, however, usually becomes inaudible as cardiac output increases during pregnancy. Prophylactic anticoagulation is not indicated. Intrapartum antibiotics lessen the risk of bacterial endocarditis.

Atrial Fibrillation

Atrial fibrillation may be associated with oral terbutaline therapy during pregnancy; discontinuation of this agent should be considered when the complication occurs.[70] Atrial fibrillation can be a dangerous condition during pregnancy. The risk of embolism is estimated at 10% to 23%, with a 2% to 10% risk of cerebral embolism. In addition, pregnancy aggravates underlying heart disease. Anticoagulation with a heparinoid is recommended throughout pregnancy for chronic fibrillation.

Paradoxical Embolism

The risk of phlebitis in the legs and pelvis increases during pregnancy and is greatest after uterine manipulation and cesarean section. Pulmonary emboli from this source may increase right atrial pressure enough to open an anatomically patent but previously physiologically closed foramen ovale. Thereafter, clots may cross to the left side of the heart and be pumped to cerebral, renal, and peripheral arteries. Sometimes bits of a clot trapped in the foramen ovale break off one at a time to cause recurrent embolic episodes. Until the advent of transesophageal echocardiography with a microbubble test, the diagnosis was usually made by a pathologist.

Subacute Bacterial Endocarditis

Approximately 20% of patients with subacute bacterial endocarditis present with stroke and subarachnoid hemorrhage.

Streptococcus viridans is the most common bacterial agent during pregnancy, especially among patients with rheumatic heart disease. Enterococcal endocarditis is often associated with abortion, uterine curettage, and insertion of an intrauterine device. Acute staphylococcal endocarditis occurs among drug addicts.

Peripartum Cardiomyopathy

In peripartum cardiomyopathy, all chambers of the heart are enlarged. Mural thrombi are expected. The combination of stroke and congestive heart failure is often fatal. Anticoagulation is recommended, especially if mural thrombus can be demonstrated by ultrasonography.

Hypotension

Pregnant women with hypotension can suffer infarction of the anterior pituitary gland (Sheehan's syndrome),[71] the optic chiasm, and border zones between major cerebral arterial distributions. Usually hypotension results from acute intrapartum blood loss, amniotic fluid embolism, and spinal anesthesia. Also at risk are patients with rheumatic heart disease and peripartum cardiomyopathy who have no cardiac output in reserve. Patients with chronic hypertension are at greater risk because of an increased lower limit of the autoregulation of cerebral perfusion by blood pressure.

Arteritis

Systemic lupus erythematosus is associated with encephalopathy and seizures, to a lesser degree with ischemic stroke, and rarely with subarachnoid hemorrhage. Women with neurologic symptoms caused by active systemic lupus erythematosus usually have decreasing levels of C3 complement and increasing titers of anti-DNA antibody. High-dose corticosteroid therapy is recommended during pregnancy and for at least 2 months post partum to prevent puerperal exacerbations.

Takayasu's Disease

Takayasu's disease is a progressive obliterative arteritis of the aorta and its major branches that occurs predominantly in women of childbearing age. Stroke is often a late manifestation that is uncommon during pregnancy. Headache, syncope, and jaw claudication are more common symptoms. The course during pregnancy is variable. Regional anesthesia should be used with caution because of the risk of hypotension.

Thrombotic Thrombocytopenic Purpura

Thrombotic thrombocytopenic purpura (TTP) shares many features with eclampsia, which creates challenging diagnostic and therapeutic dilemmas. Both disorders are characterized by traumatic hemolysis, thrombocytopenia, renal dysfunction, and neurologic abnormalities that may include seizures, stupor, and coma. The molecular pathophysiologic processes of acquired TTP—an antibody-induced deficiency of a metalloproteinase, ADAMTS—enables

a serologic diagnosis of TTP. In the absence of such information, the recommendation is to manage the constellation as eclampsia with delivery of the infant if a viable stage of maturity has been reached. In the absence of this option, specific treatment for TTP with plasmapheresis and plasma infusions is indicated.[72] The neurologic manifestations of TTP may precede the florid onset of the full syndrome by several months. A low platelet count may point to the diagnosis. Weakness and aphasia may be transient or persistent. Headache, confusion, and seizures are common. TTP does not cause subarachnoid hemorrhage.

Anticoagulation Therapy

Prophylaxis with low-dose aspirin (65 mg/day), which the Collaborative Low-dose Aspirin Study in Pregnancy (CLASP) proved to be safe during the second and third trimesters,[73] is reasonable for any pregnant woman who has had a cerebral ischemic event.

The indications for anticoagulation during pregnancy include deep venous thrombosis, atrial fibrillation, peripartum cardiomyopathy, and hypercoagulable states. Heparin is used during pregnancy because it is a large molecule that does not cross the placenta. Low-molecular-weight heparin does not cause maternal calcium wasting and is easy to administer.[74,75] Warfarin, which does cross the placenta, is a teratogen and can cause fetal hemorrhage, especially during birth.

Cerebral Phlebothrombosis

Aseptic cerebral phlebothrombosis can be caused by polycythemia, hyperviscosity syndromes, sickle cell disease, homocystinuria, paroxysmal nocturnal hemoglobinuria, hereditary coagulopathies, antiphospholipid antibody, and leukemia. Among healthy young women, the principal associations are with the puerperium, the use of oral contraceptives, and the factor V Leiden deletion.[67,76-78]

The majority of cases occur 3 days to 4 weeks post partum; 80% of cases begin in the second and third weeks after childbirth. Age and parity are indeterminate factors. Labor and delivery are usually normal. The incidence is estimated at 1 case per 10,000 deliveries in Europe and North America. In India the incidence is 40 to 50 times higher, and most cases occur soon after delivery.[79] Dehydration is probably a major factor in these cases.

The disease begins with a progressively intense headache. A seizure, either focal or generalized, heralds weakness and other cortical symptoms. Papilledema may be caused by the mass effect of an intracerebral hematoma or by obstruction of the superior sagittal sinus by clot. Progressive weakness, recurrent seizures, and deepening stupor imply propagation of the clot and are thus poor prognostic signs. Rapid progression of thrombosis increases the likelihood of hemorrhagic venous cerebral infarction because it allows less time for anastomotic veins to enlarge and provide an alternative drainage route. Coexistent phlebitis in the legs and pelvis is another poor prognostic sign.

The diagnosis of cerebral venous thrombosis can be established by both angiography and MRI. Both techniques have pitfalls and limitations; thus, both may be needed in some cases. CT scanning is less likely to establish the diagnosis but is the best way to detect acute intracerebral bleeding.

Treatment with heparin can stop thrombus formation and improves the prognosis for most patients.[76,77,80] The risk is intracerebral bleeding, especially if hemorrhagic infarction already exists. Direct thrombolysis has also achieved a good outcome in early pregnancy.[81-83]

The traditional mortality rate of approximately 25% has been significantly diminished to 10% or less by the aggressive use of anticoagulation.[80] Patients who survive usually do very well. Recurrences have been reported but are unlikely.[84] Prophylactic anticoagulation during a subsequent pregnancy is not indicated, because this is almost exclusively a condition occurring in the puerperium.

Subarachnoid Hemorrhage

Spontaneous subarachnoid hemorrhage occurs once or twice per 10,000 deliveries and accounts for 10% of maternal deaths, a percentage that increases as the maternal death rate from other causes decrease. The most common cause of spontaneous subarachnoid hemorrhage for women younger than 25 years is an arteriovenous malformation; most of these women are primiparas. For women 25 years and older, congenital berry aneurysms are the most common cause; most of these women are multiparas.[34,85,86] Arteriovenous malformations commonly bleed for the first time during the second trimester and during labor.[87] Aneurysms initially bleed in the third trimester, with the rate increasing as term is approached. Cocaine abuse can cause previously asymptomatic lesions to bleed, in addition to intracerebral bleeding de novo.[88]

Approximately one third of all spontaneous subarachnoid hemorrhages at any age are caused by bleeding disorders; sickle cell disease; bacterial endocarditis; metastatic tumor, including choriocarcinoma; and a long list of increasingly rare conditions, including ectopic endometriosis and moyamoya disease.[89] Usually, a circumspect documentation of history, a physical examination, and simple blood tests rule out the "other causes." Hereditary hemorrhagic telangiectasia may involve the brain; a family history and peripheral telangiectasias may suggest this disorder.

The presumptive clinical diagnosis must be confirmed by the demonstration of subarachnoid blood by CT scanning or by examination of CSF. The CT scan also shows intracerebral bleeding and secondary hydrocephalus and, in the case of multiple aneurysms, may suggest which one bled; a noncontrast CT scan identifies a subarachnoid hemorrhage in 95% of cases. Four-vessel cerebral angiography is needed to fully define an arteriovenous malformation and to detect multiple berry aneurysms.

The recommendation that patients be evaluated and surgically treated as if they were not pregnant, unless they are in active labor, is based on the natural history of this potentially lethal condition during pregnancy. Intrapartum rebleeding induced by Valsalva's maneuver, which almost irresistibly accompanies hard labor pain, should be avoided. If possible, the responsible aneurysm

should be obliterated or the arteriovenous malformation excised before childbirth, which can then be accomplished vaginally without special fears. Hypothermia and controlled hypotension during intracranial surgery can be used safely during pregnancy with monitoring of fetal heart rate.[90] Nimodipine has been safely used during pregnancy for vasospasm.[34] Experienced, practiced surgeons are recommended for this type of management.[91]

If curative surgery cannot be accomplished, many obstetricians plan to deliver these women by elective cesarean section at 38 weeks.[27,85,91a] Some allow labor for a multiparous woman with an aneurysm that bled in the first trimester if bearing down can be controlled by panting and regional anesthesia. In some cases, a cesarean section is immediately followed by aneurysm surgery.[92] Women with large arteriovenous malformations should deliver by cesarean section, although women with an adequate pelvis may be considered for vaginal delivery with regional anesthesia.[87]

If multiple aneurysms exist, only the one that bled need be tackled during pregnancy. The exception is probably an aneurysm measuring more than 10 mm in diameter, which is more likely to bleed at any time. The rate of death from subarachnoid hemorrhage in pregnancy is 30% to 35%.

ECLAMPTIC HYPERTENSIVE ENCEPHALOPATHY

The occurrence of convulsions distinguishes eclampsia from less severe forms of toxemia. The eclamptic convulsions may be described as focal, multifocal, generalized, or generalized with focal features. The accepted definition does not include cortical blindness as a differential point, although the pathologic process and neuroradiologic findings are identical to those of cortical blindness.[93-95] The gross neuropathologic findings of eclamptic brains include patches of petechial hemorrhages in the cortical ribbon of gray matter, which are sometimes found compacted into a subcortical "hematoma"; streak hemorrhages in the corona radiata; and single or multiple hemorrhages in the deep gray matter, the caudate nucleus, and the pons.[46] The cortical petechiae are common in the occipital lobes and in watersheds between the territories of major cerebral arteries. The classic microscopic lesion is a ring hemorrhage around a capillary or precapillary occluded by fibrinoid material. In 40% of cases, large, deep cerebral hematomas coexist with a hepatic hematoma of approximately the same age. Overall, cerebral lesions account for 40% of eclamptic deaths. Nevertheless, survivors infrequently develop epilepsy and other neurologic sequelae.[96]

Neurologic studies are not usually the first step for the obstetrician facing this emergency. A grossly bloody CSF probably indicates a poor prognosis, although CSF with a red blood cell count less than 3000/mm³ does not. CSF protein may be normal or increased to 150 mg/dL. The electroencephalogram may show variation from posterior slow waves with occasional epileptiform discharges to electrical status epilepticus. Posterior slowing may persist for 6 to 12 months.

The active management of eclamptic women with either generalized cerebral edema or major hematomas is best performed after delivery in an intensive care unit accustomed to neurologic cases.[86,97,98] Maintaining blood pressure within the zone of autoregulation is critical and is made more complicated by increased intracranial pressure. The ventilation of obtunded patients is especially important because the upper limit of autoregulation is inversely proportional to partial pressure of carbon dioxide. Thus, hyperventilation may both decrease cerebral edema and increase the upper limit of autoregulation. Diffuse cerebral edema in eclampsia is caused by generalized disruption of the blood-brain barrier. Thus, an osmotic agent such as mannitol could be predicted to be ineffective, if not dangerous, by increasing cerebral water content and by inducing pulmonary edema. High-dose corticosteroid therapy may be effective, as it is in vasogenic cerebral edema with metastatic tumors.

Neuroradiologic investigations of eclampsia are identical to those of hypertensive encephalopathy of different origins.[99] MRI is a more sensitive technique than CT scanning in the detection of small cortical lesions and edema.[93,99,100] CT scanning has the advantages of being quicker and detecting acute larger hemorrhages better. Both techniques may show an almost unique pattern of arcuate zones of edema in the internal and external capsules. In contrast to hypodense wedge of cytotoxic edema that appears on CT scans about 2 days after a standard ischemic stroke, CT and MRI evidence of cerebral edema in toxemia is apparent soon after the eclamptic crisis and disappears in a few days. This is compatible with vasogenic cerebral edema. Furthermore, MRI signal changes after gadolinium demonstrate the porosity of the blood-brain barrier in areas adjacent to previously demonstrated lesions.[99] Single photon emission computed tomography can be used with increased blood flow in affected areas.[99]

Arteriography shows angiospasm, such as that which can occur 3 days after rupture of a berry aneurysm and sometimes with sympathomimetic stimulation.[101] Arteriography is rarely done in standard cases of eclampsia but is often needed in late postpartum eclampsia, which has a broader differential diagnosis, including cerebral venous thrombosis.

The conventional wisdom holds that the cerebral manifestations of eclampsia are caused by severe vasoconstriction.[85] This may explain microinfarctions that can be intermixed in the patches of petechial hemorrhage, but it does not explain the hemorrhages. These can be explained as the failure of the constriction to limit perfusion and pressure through thinly walled cerebral capillaries, which rupture because of that force, thereby causing vasogenic cerebral edema and ring hemorrhages. In physiologic terms, the upper limit of the autoregulation of cerebral perfusion of blood pressure, which is proportional to mean arterial blood pressure, has been exceeded. Cerebral eclampsia is hypertensive encephalopathy in previously normotensive women.[102]

This scheme explains why a teenager who customarily has a blood pressure of 90/50 can be eclamptic at 140/90, a blood pressure that will not cause eclamptic convulsions in a woman who customarily has a blood pressure of 110/70.

The highest systolic blood pressure in a series of 52 pathologically proven cases of eclampsia was less than 160 in 25%, between 160 and 195 in 50%, and over 200 in 25%.[95] The standard blood pressure criteria for eclampsia are thus too rigid.

The best prophylaxis for eclamptic convulsions is antihypertensive therapy.[103] The agent chosen should decrease systemic vascular resistance but not directly affect cerebral arteries. Hydralazine, nitroprusside, nifedipine, nimodipine, and diazoxide are effective choices. An active convulsion can be stopped with diazepam, 5 to 10 mg intravenously, without affecting fetal partial pressure of oxygen, partial pressure of carbon dioxide, or pH.[104]

Magnesium sulfate is a mainstay of the treatment of eclampsia in North America, although it is neither an effective antihypertensive agent nor an effective anticonvulsant drug. Its "therapeutic" blood level has been a matter of debate since it was originally introduced.[105,106] Most regimens also include an antihypertensive drug such as hydralazine.

Two studies, which ostensibly support the use of magnesium sulfate for the prevention of both convulsions in women with severe preeclampsia and recurrent eclamptic convulsions, unfortunately did not evaluate the blood pressure at the time of any subsequent convulsions.[107,108] Critically elevated blood pressure could well have continued to cause fresh cerebral lesions of hypertensive encephalopathy and more eclamptic seizures. Prophylactic anticonvulsant therapy may not be indicated.[103]

EPILEPSY

The objective is to keep the pregnant patient with epilepsy seizure free while minimizing adverse effects on the pregnancy and fetus, including possible teratogenic effects. This is not a simple task. More information has become available to help physicians understand the complex interactions of maternal epilepsy, anticonvulsant metabolism, teratogenicity, and genetics, in addition to the fetal effects and neonatal metabolism of anticonvulsants.[109]

The effect of pregnancy on epilepsy can be predicted best from the prepregnancy seizure frequency.[109a] Women who suffer convulsions at least monthly in spite of an optimal anticonvulsant regimen can almost uniformly expect more seizures during pregnancy.[110] Women who have been seizure free for the 9 months before pregnancy have a 25% chance of experiencing worsening. Longer periods of control imply an even better prognosis.[111]

Hormones directly affect seizure threshold. Estrogens activate seizure foci; progestins dampen activity. Presumably this explains true gestational epilepsy: that is, the occurrence of convulsions, often focal seizures, only during pregnancy. Hormonal fluctuations also explain the perimenstrual exacerbations experienced by up to 70% of women with severe epilepsy. However, a history of menstrual epilepsy is not a clue to the course of epilepsy during pregnancy. Oral contraceptives do not worsen epilepsy for most women. Anticonvulsants increase hepatic estrogen metabolism and thus cause a higher rate of both breakthrough bleeding and contraceptive failure.[112]

Other factors affecting the course of epilepsy during pregnancy include noncompliance with the prescribed drug regimen, insomnia, salt and water retention, mild compensated respiratory alkalosis, and the random variation of seizure frequency.[110,111,113,114] The most important factor is the increased apparent plasma clearance of anticonvulsants during pregnancy. Of women who maintain blood levels determined to be therapeutic before pregnancy, only 10% experience worsening during pregnancy.

The course of pregnancy is affected more by maternal age and parity, socioeconomic status, the degree of prenatal care, and other maternal diseases than by epilepsy. Among the complications of pregnancy, bleeding is the only consistent association with maternal epilepsy.[115] The rate of spontaneous abortion is not increased. Stillbirths, however, are more likely. The offspring of epileptic women have a fourfold higher incidence of developing epilepsy and febrile convulsions. Anecdotal evidence indicates the risk to be still higher if both parents are epileptic.

Although fetal bradycardia occurs during and for 20 minutes after a maternal grand mal episode, a fetus appears to be resilient in the event of an isolated maternal convulsion. Only rarely have fetal death and intraventricular hemorrhages been attributed to a maternal convulsion. On the other hand, status epilepticus is an immediate threat to both mother and fetus; the risk of maternal death doubles, and the chance of fetal death is 50%. There may be a long-term effect of maternal convulsions on intellectual performance in childhood.[116]

Anticonvulsant metabolism is altered during pregnancy in a different manner for each drug.[117,118] The volume of distribution increases for all drugs. Each drug crosses the placenta. At term, maternal blood and cord blood levels are approximately equal. The gastrointestinal absorption of phenytoin can be markedly reduced. The hepatic metabolism of primidone, carbamazepine, and phenytoin increases. The renal excretion of phenobarbital increases. The sum effect is that the apparent plasma clearance (i.e., total daily dose divided by blood level) decreases. Most of this change is reversed in the first 6 weeks post partum.

To maintain blood levels previously established to be therapeutic, blood levels should be measured monthly, or more frequently if seizures occur, and then the dosage should be adjusted accordingly.[119] Free, protein-unbound anticonvulsant levels are preferred if available.[118] Some physicians recommend adjustment only if convulsions occur. If the dosage has been increased during pregnancy, blood levels rise during the puerperium and can reach toxic levels unless blood levels are monitored and appropriate changes made in the treatment regimen.

The literature concerning the teratogenicity of anticonvulsants is full of contradictions. Statistical methods are often queried. If the malformation in question is common and has been associated with other factors, a large investigational series is necessary to prove that a small increase in risk is statistically significant. A basic problem is separating the risk attributable to anticonvulsants from the risk attributable to the presence of maternal epilepsy of varying severity. But whatever the contributions of either maternal epilepsy and/or anticonvulsant ingestion to the problem, the infants of epileptic mothers do have a higher incidence of birth defects.[120] Prospective and retrospective studies differ on the relative risk. In the largest controlled series, a Norwegian study with 3879 infants in each group, the absolute risk increased from 3.5% to 4.4% if the mothers were epileptic.

Some drugs are clearly teratogenic. Trimethadione is considered to be a teratogen for humans because a cluster of malformations, including heart defects, was high. Cardiac malformations are not usually associated with other anticonvulsants, although lithium has been implicated in cases of Ebstein's anomaly.[121] In utero exposure to valproic acid is associated with a 1% to 2% risk of a neural tube defect.[122] A smaller risk has been associated with carbamazepine. Serious neural tube defects can usually be detected with high-resolution ultrasonography and determination of α-fetoprotein levels early enough to consider abortion. In addition, treatment with the combination of valproic acid, carbamazepine, and phenobarbital may be particularly risky.[123]

Orofacial clefting is the most common major malformation that has been attributed to anticonvulsants, particularly phenytoin in rodents.[124] Many factors contribute to this common malformation. There may be a genetic link between epilepsy and orofacial clefts, because epileptic patients have twice the expected incidence of orofacial clefts, and the incidence of epilepsy is more common than expected in the extended families of patients with orofacial clefts.

The cluster of malformations known as the fetal hydantoin syndrome is not specific for any anticonvulsant or any combination of anticonvulsants, although distal digital hypoplasia and hypertelorism are most strongly linked to phenytoin. Once again, genetics plays a major role. Many of the dysmorphic features ascribed to the fetal anticonvulsant syndrome (e.g., epicanthus), in addition to stature and head circumference, are more strongly linked to parental characteristics than to maternal epilepsy.[125] The role of genetics is well illustrated by a case of heteroparental dizygotic twins. Both had been exposed to hydantoin, but only one had the fetal anticonvulsant syndrome.[126]

One mechanism by which genetics could affect the infants of epileptic women is epoxide hydrolase deficiency, which could shift anticonvulsant metabolism to potentially teratogenic pathways. Monotherapy is preferred; drug-drug interactions produce metabolites that could also inhibit this enzyme.[123] A second potential mechanism for the teratogenicity of anticonvulsants is the malabsorption of folic acid.[120] This is a feature of all commonly used anticonvulsants; phenytoin and phenobarbital cause the greatest effect. Supplementation of dietary folate is advisable, with checking erythrocyte folate levels, before conception occurs. The optimal dose of folic acid has not been determined and probably varies. A dosage of 0.4 to 1 mg/day is reasonable for most women with a dose of 5 mg reserved for women with a family history of spina bifida.

A coagulopathy resulting from a deficiency of vitamin K–dependent clotting factors is present at birth in half of neonates whose mothers took phenytoin, phenobarbital, primidone, or carbamazepine during pregnancy.[127]

Far fewer are symptomatic; in rare cases, death has been reported. This complication has not been reported with carbamazepine monotherapy. Maternal blood levels of clotting factors are normal. An injection of phytonadione, 1 mg, should be given to the neonate after birth. If evidence of bleeding exists, fresh-frozen plasma is required until the vitamin K works. Maternal ingestion of vitamin K_1, 20 mg orally each day for 2 weeks before delivery, resulted in normal cord blood clotting function.[127]

Infants whose mothers took phenobarbital and primidone during pregnancy may have transiently retarded growth and develop a phenobarbital withdrawal syndrome characterized by hyperactivity and feeding problems just after being taken home.[128] Insecure mothers often mistake this syndrome for their own inability to care for their new babies.

Breast-feeding is usually successful.[113] The concentration of anticonvulsants in human breast milk is much lower than that in blood for phenytoin, carbamazepine, and phenobarbital and slightly lower for primidone and ethosuximide. Thus, neonatal blood levels are low unless the infant's metabolism is very slow and milk levels are relatively high. Phenobarbital and primidone may sedate some infants and result in poor suckling, but this is not commonplace. A blood level measurement resolves the issue if there is a question.

DIAGNOSTIC PROCEDURES

The most cost-effective diagnostic procedure is a thoughtful consultation with a neurologist. Depending on the clinical situation, pregnancy is not an absolute contraindication to any neurodiagnostic procedure. Electroencephalography and electromyography can be performed without risk. Abdominal lead shields reduce fetal radiation exposure to right-angle scatter except during filming of lumbar spines and myelography, which should be avoided if possible, particularly during the first trimester.[129] Transfemoral cerebral angiography is favored over brachial and direct carotid studies because the images are of high quality and the complication rate is lower, although the fetus does receive brief exposure during abdominal fluoroscopy.[114] CT scanning of the head and neck exposes the fetus to approximately the same minimal dose of radiation as do plain radiographs of the skull and cervical spine. The fetal dose of radiation from CT scanning of the lumbar spine is approximately half that from lumbar myelography. No fetal effect has been found after MRI of the gravid human uterus. MRI is the preferred method of imaging the thoracic and lumbar regions during pregnancy.

References

1. Young GL, Jewell D: Interventions for leg cramps in pregnancy. Cochrane Database Syst Rev 2002;(1):CD000121.
2. Goodman JDS, Brodie C, Ayida GA: Restless leg syndrome in pregnancy. BMJ 1988;297:1101.
3. Earley CJ: Clinical practice. Restless legs syndrome. N Engl J Med 2003;348:2103.
4. Jaffe R, Mock M, Abramowic J, et al: Myotonic dystrophy and pregnancy: A review. Obstet Gynecol Surv 1986;41:272.
5. Camann WR, Johnson MD: Anesthetic management of a parturient with myotonia dystrophica: A case report. Reg Anesth 1990;15:41.
6. Shelbourne P, Davies J, Buxton J, et al: Direct diagnosis of myotonic dystrophy with a disease-specific DNA marker. N Engl J Med 1993;328:471.
7. Magee AC, Hughes AE, Kidd A, et al: Reproductive counseling for women with myotonic dystrophy. J Med Genet 2002;39:E15.
8. Rosenzweig BA, Rotmensch S, Binette SP, et al: Primary idiopathic polymyositis and dermatomyositis complicating pregnancy: Diagnosis and management. Obstet Gynecol Surv 1989;44:162.
9. Silva CA, Sultan SM, Isenberg DA: Pregnancy outcome in adult-onset idiopathic inflammatory myopathy. Rheumatology 2003;42:1168.
10. Bashuk RG, Krendel DA: Myasthenia gravis presenting as weakness after magnesium administration. Muscle Nerve 1990;13:708.
11. Fennell DF, Ringel SP: Myasthenia gravis and pregnancy. Obstet Gynecol Surv 1987;41:414.
12. Plauche WC: Myasthenia gravis in mothers and their newborns. Clin Obstet Gynecol 1991;34:82.
13. Djelmis J, Sostarko M, Mayer D, Ivanisevic M: Myasthenia gravis in pregnancy: Report on 69 cases. Eur J Obstet Gynecol Reprod Biol 2002;104:21.
14. Warren TM, Fletcher M: Anaesthetic management of the obstetric patient with neurological disease. Clin Anaesthesiol 1986;4:291.
15. Eden RD, Gall SA: Myasthenia gravis and pregnancy: A reappraisal of thymectomy. Obstet Gynecol 1983;62:328.
16. Watson WJ, Katz VL, Bowes WA: Plasmapheresis during pregnancy. Obstet Gynecol 1990;76:451.
17. Morel E, Eymard B, Vernet–der Garabedian N, et al: Neonatal myasthenia gravis: A new clinical and immunological appraisal of 30 cases. Neurology 1988;38:138.
17a. Pasternak JF, Hageman J, Adams MA, et al: Exchange transfusion in neonatal myasthenia. J Pediatr 1981;99:644-6.
18. Ahlberg G, Ahlmark G: The Landry-Guillain-Barré syndrome and pregnancy. Acta Obstet Gynecol Scand 1978;57:377.
19. Smith JL: *Campylobacter jejuni* infection during pregnancy: Long-term consequences of associated bacteremia, Guillain-Barré syndrome, and reactive arthritis. J Food Prot 2002;65:696.
20. Hurley TJ, Brunson AD, Archer RL, et al: Landry Guillain-Barré Strohl syndrome in pregnancy: Report of three cases treated with plasmapheresis. Obstet Gynecol 1991;78:482.
21. Berkwitz NJ, Lufkin NH: Toxic neuronitis of pregnancy. Surg Gynecol Obstet 1932;54:743.
22. Cohen Y, Lavie O, Granovsky-Grisaru S, et al: Bell palsy complicating pregnancy: A review. Obstet Gynecol Surv 2000;55:184.
23. Gillman GS, Schaitkin BM, May M, Klein SR: Bell's palsy in pregnancy: A study of recovery outcomes. Otolaryngol Head Neck Surg 2002;126:26.
24. Shmorgun D, Chan WS, Ray JG: Association between Bell's palsy in pregnancy and pre-eclampsia. Q J Med 2002;95:359.
24a. Hilsinger RL, Adour KK, Doty HE: Idiopathic facial paralysis, pregnancy, and the menstrual cycle. Ann Otol Rhinol Laryngol 1975;84:433.
25. McLeannan HG, Oats JN, Walstab JE: Survey of hand symptoms in pregnancy. Med J Aust 1987;147:542.
26. Ekman-Ordeberg G, Salgeback S, Ordebert G: Carpal tunnel syndrome in pregnancy. Acta Obstet Gynecol Scand 1987;66:233.
27. Pearson MF: Meralgia paresthetica: With reference to its occurrence in pregnancy. J Obstet Gynaecol Br Commonw 1957;64:427.
28. Feasby TE, Burton SR, Hahn AF: Obstetrical lumbosacral plexus injury. Muscle Nerve 1992;15:937.
29. Rosenbaum RB, Donaldson JO: Peripheral nerve and neuromuscular disorders. Neurol Clin 1994;12:461.
30. Ostgaard HC, Andersson GBJ: Previous back pain and risk of developing back pain in a future pregnancy. Spine 1991;16:32.
31. Weinreb JC, Wolbarsht LB, Cohen JM, et al: Prevalence of lumbosacral intervertebral disk abnormalities on MR images in pregnant and asymptomatic nonpregnant women. Radiology 1989;170:125.
32. Hughes SJ, Short DJ, Usherwood MMcD, et al: Management of the pregnant woman with spinal cord injuries. Br J Obstet Gynaecol 1991;98:513.
33. Nygaard I, Bartscht KD, Cole S: Sexuality and reproduction in spinal cord injured women. Obstet Gynecol Surv 1990;45:727.

34. Dias MS, Selchar LN: Intracranial hemorrhage from aneurysms and arteriovenous malformations during pregnancy and the puerperium. Neurosurgery 1990;27:855.

35. Pihl K, Malstrom H, Simonsen E: Choriocarcinoma presenting with cerebral metastases after full-term pregnancy. Acta Obstet Gynecol Scand 1990;69:433.

36. Karageyim AY, Kars B, Dansuk R, et al: Chorea gravidarum: A case report. J Matern Fetal Neonatal Med 2002;12:353.

37. Scheinberg IH, Sternlieb I: Pregnancy in penicillamine-treated patients with Wilson's disease. N Engl J Med 1975;293:1300.

38. Schilsky ML: Treatment of Wilson's disease: What are the relative roles of penicillamine, trientine, and zinc supplementation? Curr Gastroenterol Rep 2001;3:54.

38a. Walsche JM: The management of pregnancy in Wilson's disease treated with trientine. Q J Med 1986;58:81.

39. Masters CL, Dawkins RL, Zilko PJ, et al: Penicillamine-associated myasthenia gravis, antiacetylcholine receptor, and antistriational antibodies. Am J Med 1977;63:689.

40. Dwosh E, Guimond C, Duquette P, Sadovnick AD: The interaction of MS and pregnancy: A critical review. Int MS J 2003;10:38.

41. Davis RK, Maslow AS: Multiple sclerosis in pregnancy: A review. Obstet Gynecol Surv 1992;47:290.

42. Dalmas AF, Texier C, Ducloy-Bouthors AS, Krivosic-Horber R: Obstetrical analgesia and anaesthesia in multiple sclerosis. Ann Fr Anesth Reanim 2003;22:861.

42a. Bader AM, Hunt CO, Datta S, et al: Anesthesia for the obstetric patient with multiple sclerosis. J Clin Anesth 1988;1:21.

43. Lorenzi AR, Ford HL: Multiple sclerosis and pregnancy. Postgrad Med J 2002;78:460.

44. Swensen R, Kirsch W: Brain neoplasms in women: A review. Clin Obstet Gynecol 2002;45:904.

45. Haas JF, Janish W, Staneczek W: Newly diagnosed primary intracranial neoplasms in pregnant women: A population-based assessment. J Neurol Neurosurg Psychiatry 1986;49:874.

46. Roelvink NCA, Kamphorst W, Van Alphen HSM, et al: Pregnancy-related primary brain and spinal tumors. Arch Neurol 1987; 44:209.

47. Saitoh Y, Oku Y, Izumoto S, et al: Rapid growth of a meningioma during pregnancy: Relationship with estrogen and progesterone receptors. Neurol Med Chir (Toyko) 1989;29:440.

48. Allen J, Eldridge R, Koerber T: Acoustic neuroma in the last months of pregnancy. Am J Obstet Gynecol 1974;119:516.

49. Vizner B, Talan-Hranilovic J, Gnjidic Z, et al: Lymphocytic adeno-hypophysitis simulating a pituitary adenoma in a pregnant woman. Coll Antropol 2002;26:641.

50. Molitch ME: Pregnancy and the hyperprolactinemic woman. N Engl J Med 1985;312:1364.

51. Konopka P, Raymond JP, Merceron RE, et al: Continuous administration of bromocriptine in the prevention of neurological complications in pregnant women with prolactinomas. Am J Obstet Gynecol 1983;146:935.

52. Steinn AL, Levenick MN, Kletsky OA: Computed tomography versus magnetic resonance imaging for the evaluation of suspected pituitary adenomas. Obstet Gynecol 1989;73:996.

53. Picone O, Castaigne V, Ede C, Fernandez H: Cerebral metastases of a choriocarcinoma during pregnancy. Obstet Gynecol 2003; 102:1380.

54. Kanazawa K, Takeuchi S: Clinical analysis of intracranial metastases in gestational choriocarcinoma: A series of 15 cases. Aust N Z J Obstet Gynaecol 1985;25:16.

55. Huna-Baron R, Kupersmith MJ: Idiopathic intracranial hypertension in pregnancy. J Neurol 2002;249:1078.

56. Bremer HA, Wallenburg HCS: Aspirin in pregnancy. Fetal Matern Med Rev 1992;4:37.

57. Rudolph AM: Effects of aspirin and acetaminophen in pregnancy and the newborn. Arch Intern Med 1981;141:358.

58. Silberstein SD, Merriam GR: Estrogens, progestins, and headache. Neurology 1991;41:786.

59. Mattsson P: Hormonal factors in migraine: A population-based study of women aged 40 to 74 years. Headache 2003;43:27.

60. Silberstein SD: Headaches and women: Treatment of the pregnant and lactating migraineur. Headache 1993;33:533.

61. Jacobson SL, Redman CWG: Basilar migraine with loss of consciousness in pregnancy: Case report. Br J Obstet Gynaecol 1989; 96:495.

62. Mandel S: Hemiplegic migraine in pregnancy. Headache 1988;28:414.

63. Diener HC, Limmroth V: Advances in pharmacological treatment of migraine. Expert Opin Investig Drugs 2001;10:1831.

64. Frishman WH, Chesner M: Beta-adrenergic blockers in pregnancy. Am Heart J 1988;115:147.

65. Loder E: Safety of sumatriptan in pregnancy: A review of the data so far. CNS Drugs 2003;17:1.

66. Cross JN, Castro PO, Jennett WB: Cerebral strokes associated with pregnancy and the puerperium. BMJ 1968;3:214.

67. Donaldson JO, Lee NS: Arterial and venous stroke associated with pregnancy. Neurol Clin 1994;12:583.

68. Kittner SJ, Stern BJ, Feeser BR, et al: Pregnancy and the risk of stroke. N Engl J Med 1996;335:768.

69. Gilon D, Buonanno FS, Joffe MM, et al: Lack of evidence of an association between mitral-valve prolapse and stroke in young patients. New Engl J Med 1999;341:8.

70. Lashgari S, Kueck AS, Oyelese Y: Atrial fibrillation in pregnancy associated with oral terbutaline therapy. Obstet Gynecol 2003;101:814.

71. Sheehan HL, Stanfield JB: The pathogenesis of postpartum necrosis of the pituitary gland. Acta Endocrinol 1961;37:479.

72. Allford SL, Hunt BJ, Rose P, et al: Guidelines on the diagnosis and management of the thrombotic microangiopathic haemolytic anaemias. Br J Haematol 2003;120:556.

73. CLASP: A randomised trial of low-dose aspirin for the prevention and treatment of pre-eclampsia among 9364 pregnant women. CLASP (Collaborative Low-dose Aspirin Study in Pregnancy) Collaborative Group: Lancet 1994;343:619.

74. Fejgin MD, Lourwood DL: Low molecular weight heparins and their use in obstetrics and gynecology. Obstet Gynecol Surv 1994; 49:424.

75. Sturridge F, DeSwiet M, Letsky E: The use of low molecular weight heparin for thromboprophylaxis in pregnancy. Br J Obstet Gynaecol 1994;101:69.

76. Ameri A, Bousser MG: Cerebral venous thrombosis. Neurol Clin 1992;10:87.

77. Cantuá C, Barinagarrementeria F: Cerebral venous thrombosis associated with pregnancy and puerperium: Review of 67 cases. Stroke 1993;24:1880.

78. Zuber M, Toulon P, Marnet L, Mas JL: Factor V Leiden mutation in cerebral venous thrombosis. Stroke 1996;27:1724.

79. Srinivasan K: Puerperal cerebral venous and arterial thrombosis. Semin Neurol 1988;8:222.

80. Einhäupl KM, Villringer A, Meister W, et al: Heparin treatment in sinus venous thrombosis. Lancet 1991;338:597.

81. Chow K, Gobin YP, Saver J, et al: Endovascular treatment of dural sinus thrombosis with rheolytic thrombectomy and intra-arterial thrombolysis. Stroke 2000;31:1420.

82. Philips MF, Bagley LJ, Sinson GP, et al: Endovascular thrombolysis for symptomatic cerebral venous thrombosis. J Neurosurg 1999;90:65.

83. Weatherby SJ, Edwards NC, West R, Heafield MT: Good outcome in early pregnancy following direct thrombolysis for cerebral venous sinus thrombosis. J Neurol 2003;250:1372.

84. Mehraein S, Ortwein H, Busch M, et al: Risk of recurrence of cerebral venous and sinus thrombosis during subsequent pregnancy and puerperium. J Neurol Neurosurg Psychiatry 2003;74:814.

85. Dias MS: Neurovascular emergencies in pregnancy. Clin Obstet Gynecol 1994;37:337.

86. Raps EC, Galetta SL, Flamm ES: Neurointensive care of the pregnant woman. Neurol Clin 1994;12:601.

87. Sadasivan B, Malik GM, Lee C, et al: Vascular malformations and pregnancy. Surg Neurol 1990;33:305.

88. Mercado A, Johnson G, Calver D, et al: Cocaine, pregnancy, and postpartum intracerebral hemorrhage. Obstet Gynecol 1989; 73:467.

89. Williams DL, Martin IL, Gully RM: Intracerebral hemorrhage and moyamoya disease in pregnancy. Can J Anaesth 2000;47:996.

90. Minielly R, Yuzde AA, Drake CG: Subarachnoid hemorrhage secondary to ruptured cerebral aneurysm in pregnancy. Obstet Gynecol 1979;53:64.

91. Trivedi RA, Kirkpatrick PJ: Arteriovenous malformations of the cerebral circulation that rupture in pregnancy. J Obstet Gynaecol 2003;23:484.

91a. Laidler JA, Jackson IJ, Redfern N: The management of caesarean sections in a patient with an intracranial arteriovenous malformation. Anaesthesia 1989;44:490.

92. Whitburn RH, Laishley RS, Jewkes DA: Anaesthesia for simultaneous caesarean section and clipping of intracerebral aneurysm. Br J Anaesthesiol 1990;64:642.

93. Digre KB, Varner MW, Osborn AG, et al: Cranial magnetic resonance imaging in severe preeclampsia vs. eclampsia. Arch Neurol 1993; 50:399.

94. Donaldson JO: The brain in eclampsia. Hypertens Pregnancy 1994;13:15.

95. Sheehan HL, Lynch JB: Pathology of Toxaemia of Pregnancy. Edinburgh, Churchill Livingstone, 1973.

96. Sibai BM, Spinnato JA, Watson DL, et al: Eclampsia. IV: Neurological findings and future outcome. Am J Obstet Gynecol 1985;152:184.

97. Richards AM, Moodley J, Graham DI, et al: Active management of the unconscious eclamptic patient. Br J Obstet Gynaecol 1986; 93:554.

98. Royburt M, Seidman DS, Serr DM, et al: Neurologic involvement in hypertensive disease of pregnancy. Obstet Gynecol Surv 1991;46:656.

99. Schwartz RB, Jones KM, Kalina P, et al: Hypertensive encephalopathy: Findings on CT, MR imaging, and SPECT imaging in 14 cases. AJR Am J Roentgenol 1992;159:379.

100. Richards A, Graham D, Bullock R: Clinicopathological study of neurological complications due to hypertensive disorders of pregnancy. J Neurol Neurosurg Psychiatry 1988;51:416.

101. Raps EC, Galetta SL, Braderick M, et al: Delayed peripartum vasculopathy: Cerebral eclampsia revisited. Ann Neurol 1993;33:222.

102. Belfort MA, Varner MW, Dizon-Townson DS, et al: Cerebral perfusion pressure, and not cerebral blood flow, may be the critical determinant of intracranial injury in preeclampsia: A new hypothesis. Am J Obstet Gynecol 2002;187:626.

103. Brown MA, Buddle ML: Is it safe to withhold convulsion prophylaxis in preeclamptic women without neurological features? Hypertens Pregnancy 1998;17:13.

104. Yeh SY, Paul RH, Cordeno L, et al: A study of diazepam during labor. Obstet Gynecol 1974;43:363.

105. Dayicioglu V, Sahinoglu Z, Kol E, Kucukbas M: The use of standard dose magnesium sulphate in prophylaxis of eclamptic seizures: Do body mass index alterations have any effect on success? Hypertens Pregnancy 2003;22:257.

106. Sibai BM, Ramanathan J: The case for magnesium sulfate in preeclampsia-eclampsia. Int J Obstet Anesth 1992;1:167.

107. Which anticonvulsant for women with eclampsia? Evidence from the Collaborative Eclampsia Trial. Lancet 1995;345:1455.

108. Lucas M, Leveno K, Cunningham G: The comparison of magnesium sulfate with phenytoin for the prevention of eclampsia. N Engl J Med 1995;333:201.

109. Yerby MS: Clinical care of pregnant women with epilepsy: Neural tube defects and folic acid supplementation. Epilepsia 2003;44:33.

109a. Devinsky O, Yerby MS: Women with epilepsy: Reproduction and effects of pregnancy on epilepsy. Neurol Clin 1994;12:479.

110. Knight AH, Rhind EG: Epilepsy and pregnancy: A study of 153 pregnancies in 59 patients. Epilepsia 1975;16:99.

111. Schmidt D, Canger R, Ayanzini G, et al: Change of seizure frequency in pregnant epileptic women. J Neurol Neurosurg Psychiatry 1983;46:751.

112. Mattson RH, Cramer JA, Darney PD, et al: Use of oral contraceptives by women with epilepsy. JAMA 1986;256:238.

113. Delgado-Escueta AV, Janz D: Consensus guidelines: Preconception counseling, management, and care of the pregnant woman with epilepsy. Neurology 1992;42(Suppl 5):149.

114. Pennell PB: The importance of monotherapy in pregnancy. Neurology 2003;60(11, Suppl 4):S31.

115. Hiilesmaa VK, Bardy A, Terano R: Obstetric outcome in women with epilepsy. Am J Obstet Gynecol 1985;152:499.

116. Gaily EK, Kantola-Sorsa E, Granström M-L: Specific cognitive dysfunction in children with epileptic mothers. Dev Med Child Neurol 1990;32:403.

117. Lander CM, Eadie MJ: Plasma antiepileptic drug concentrations during pregnancy. Epilepsia 1991;32:257.

118. Yerby MS, Friel PN, McCormick K, et al: Pharmacokinetics of anticonvulsants in pregnancy: Alterations in plasma protein binding. Epilepsy Res 1990;5:223.

119. Katz JM, Devinsky O: Primary generalized epilepsy: A risk factor for seizures in labor and delivery? Seizure 2003;12:217.

120. Dansky LV, Rosenblatt DS, Andermann E: Mechanisms of teratogenesis: Folic acid and antiepileptic therapy. Neurology 1992; 42(Suppl 5):32.

121. Friis ML, Hauge M: Congenital heart defects in liveborn children of epileptic parents. Arch Neurol 1985;42:374.

122. Oakeshott P, Hunt GM: Valproate and spina bifida. BMJ 1989; 298:1300.

123. Lindhout D: Pharmacogenetics and drug interactions: Role in antiepileptic-drug–induced teratogenesis. Neurology 1992; 42(Suppl 5):43.

124. Friis ML, Holm NV, Sindrup EH, et al: Facial clefts in sibs and children of epileptic patients. Neurology 1986;36:346.

125. Gaily E, Granström M-L, Hiilesmaa V, et al: Minor abnormalities in offspring of epileptic mothers. J Pediatr 1988; 112:520.

126. Phelan MC, Pellock MM, Nance WE: Discordant expression of fetal hydantoin syndrome in heteropaternal twins. N Engl J Med 1982; 397:397.

127. Deblay MF, Vert P, Andre M, et al: Transplacental vitamin K prevents haemorrhagic disease of infant of epileptic mother. Lancet 1982;1:1247.

128. Gaily E, Granström M-L: A transient retardation of early postnatal growth in drug-exposed children of epileptic mothers. Epilepsy Res 1989;4:147.

129. Swartz HM, Reichling BA: Hazards of radiation exposure for pregnant women. JAMA 1978;239:1908.

20

PREGNANCY AND THE RHEUMATIC DISEASES

Carl A. Laskin

In dealing with any disease in pregnancy, physicians must consider the effect of the pregnancy on the disease and the effect of the disease on the pregnancy. The multisystemic nature of rheumatic diseases creates some very difficult problems for general internists, rheumatology specialists, and obstetricians. In some cases, the underlying disease is a nuisance, whereas in other situations, the disease is life-threatening for both mother and fetus. An added complication is the effect of antirheumatic drugs on pregnancy. Although many of these agents can be used during pregnancy, some must be avoided for up to 3 months before conception and throughout the pregnancy. The ideal scenario is to assess and advise the patient before a pregnancy so that the pregnancy can be begun electively and safely. Unfortunately, many patients arrive at their physicians' office already pregnant, at which point the assessment is directed toward keeping both mother and fetus alive and well until delivery.

Although there are many rheumatic diseases, this chapter focuses on the entities more commonly encountered by the practitioner.

IMMUNOREGULATION IN CONNECTIVE TISSUE DISEASES AND PREGNANCY

The pathogenesis of most rheumatic diseases is immunologic. In addition, the majority of these diseases predominantly affect women. It therefore follows that the hormonal changes occurring in pregnancy often have a significant effect on the manifestations of the underlying disease. In some cases, pregnancy adversely affects the disease, whereas in other circumstances, the disease manifestations are ameliorated during pregnancy.

The hallmark of a number of connective tissue diseases is the presence in the serum of circulating autoantibodies. The mechanism whereby tissue injury is induced in connective tissue diseases can, in some cases, be correlated with the presence of these autoantibodies.

Autoantibodies may induce immune injury in connective tissue disease in two ways. First, they may react with antigens directly; for example, the Coombs antibody reacts with antigens on the surface of red blood cells, which results in cell damage (cytotoxic mechanism). Alternatively, the autoantibodies can combine with the antigen to form immune complexes. When these complexes are fixed in tissues, they trigger an inflammatory response (immune complex mechanism).

The cause of excessive autoantibody production—the basis of both mechanisms of tissue injury—is still not clear. However, current research tends to implicate abnormal regulating mechanisms of the immune response. Antibody production is modulated in part by the cell-mediated immune system through helper and suppressor T lymphocytes. A deficiency of T lymphocyte suppressor cells in patients who have a connective tissue disease is believed to result in unchecked autoantibody production and eventually in immune injury.

Inflammation is the end result of the immune response in most cases of immunologically mediated tissue damage. The clinical manifestations vary according to the site of inflammatory involvement, and the specific organs involved tend to vary from one disease to another (e.g., the joints in rheumatoid arthritis [RA] and many extraarticular sites in systemic lupus erythematosus [SLE]).

Normally during pregnancy, a number of alterations occur in lymphocyte function, humoral immunity, and the inflammatory response, which must be appreciated in an investigation of a suspected connective tissue disease. Human pregnancy appears to be associated with an altered immune response mediated both by cellular mechanisms (increased suppressor T cell function and decreased B cell function), and by a humoral mechanism, which in turn is mediated by pregnancy zone proteins.[1] In contrast to the immunoregulatory changes seen in normal pregnancy, in many autoimmune diseases there is an impairment of suppressor T cell activity, which leads to polyclonal B cell activation and the subsequent production of autoantibodies. The superimposition of pregnancy on the "immune background" of a connective tissue disease may therefore "correct" the immunologic abnormalities seen in that connective tissue disorder.

MANAGEMENT OF REPRODUCTION IN THE RHEUMATIC DISEASES

Pregnancies in women with rheumatic diseases should be planned in order to avoid disease complications to both mother and fetus and to prevent birth defects from medication. During a prepregnancy consultation, the internist must categorize the patient on the basis of the current condition and the past history of the disease in order to follow the patient's progress throughout the pregnancy and postpartum. The internist is thus in a position to counsel the patient about a future pregnancy and is prepared to manage the pregnancy medically. A pragmatic approach to this consultation involves determining (1) the clinical profile, (2) the laboratory profile, (3) the timing and pattern of the most recent disease flare, and (4) the medications being used.

Clinical Profile

This profile is derived from the current history and physical examination findings. In addition, the physician must obtain the previous history to appreciate how the disease manifested and what usually characterizes a flare.

Laboratory Profile

Current laboratory tests are used to document the routine and serologic laboratory parameters of the disease. The test results that best reflect the patient's disease state are used as indicators of disease activity during pregnancy.

Most Recent Disease Flare

Determining when the most recent exacerbation of the disease occurred provides information with which to counsel the patient appropriately about the timing of pregnancy. It is the internist's responsibility to advise the patient when it is safest to attempt a pregnancy. This information becomes part of the clinical profile.

Medications

Although a number of medications are used in the treatment of various rheumatic diseases, many of the diseases are treated with the same medications, which thereby simplifies the necessary knowledge base of the consultant. Before a pregnancy, the safety of the patient's medications in pregnancy should be determined. It is important to bear in mind that many of the drugs used in the treatment of rheumatic diseases are long-acting. In these cases, unsafe medication must be discontinued months before conception.

RHEUMATOID ARTHRITIS

RA is a chronic systemic inflammatory disease of unknown origin, manifested primarily in the joints. The disease occurs worldwide and has no racial predilection. It is common, occurring in 1% to 2% of the population, and affects two to three times more women than men. RA occurs at any age, but in most patients, the onset occurs between the ages of 20 and 60. Various infective agents, including bacteria, mycoplasma, and a number of viruses, have been implicated as the source of persistent antigenic stimulation, which is thought to initiate the inflammatory manifestations.[2]

The clinical picture of RA is one of a symmetric, inflammatory polyarthritis predominantly affecting small and medium-sized joints, accompanied by morning stiffness and constitutional symptoms of fatigue and malaise. The disease course is characterized by exacerbations and remissions of synovitis.[3] Extraarticular manifestations underscore the systemic nature of RA.

Laboratory findings in RA include normochromic, normocytic anemia; elevations in platelet count and erythrocyte sedimentation rate (ESR); and hypergammaglobulinemia. Leukopenia is seen in patients with RA and hypersplenism (Felty's syndrome). Rheumatoid factor is an antiimmunoglobulin and is detected in the serum of 75% to 80% of patients with RA, usually by means of the latex fixation test. Other antibodies, such as antinuclear factor, occur in 20% of patients and even more often in those with Felty's syndrome. Synovial fluid analysis reveals an inflammatory exudate with polymorphonuclear cells and lymphocytes. Radiographs may reveal soft tissue swelling; osteoporosis, often in a juxtaarticular distribution; marginal erosions; joint space narrowing; and, in severe cases, subluxation or ankylosis. The cervical spine may be involved, showing atlantoaxial subluxation, which in turn can lead to cord compression. Pathologic findings in the joints reveal synovial lining cell hyperplasia and a mononuclear cell infiltrate. In more advanced disease, the synovial membrane has villous projections with lymphoid nodules and pannus formation.[3]

The diagnosis of RA is based on the clinical and laboratory features outlined previously. The American College of Rheumatology has revised the classification criteria for RA.[2,3] Objective evidence for synovitis for a minimum of 6 weeks must be demonstrated, and other conditions must be ruled out.

Effect of Pregnancy on Rheumatoid Arthritis

Few diseases other than RA can be so dramatically affected by pregnancy. Almost 80% of women with RA experience remission, the majority in the first few weeks of pregnancy.[4] Hench first noted the marked improvement in rheumatoid disease in 33 of 34 pregnancies occurring in 20 patients with RA.[5] The tendency of RA to improve during pregnancy has been noted in several retrospective reports.[6] Persellin reported his own experience, reviewed the literature, and concluded that 203 (74%) of 274 pregnancies in patients with RA were associated with some degree of improvement.[7]

In most patients, improvement occurred in the first trimester, and an additional smaller group experienced improvement in the second and third trimesters. Often, medication taken before pregnancy can be discontinued because of the significant clinical improvement. In addition, remission in one pregnancy often indicates that a similar remission may be expected in subsequent pregnancies. Indeed, a protective effect of pregnancy against the development of RA has been shown.[8,9]

It is important to note that although most patients experience improvement during pregnancy, many experience a relapse between 6 weeks and 6 months post partum.[10] Spector and Da Silva reviewed studies of pregnancy and RA and confirmed this finding.[11] They also observed that although RA rarely develops during pregnancy, there is an increased risk of developing RA during the postpartum period. Some studies have suggested that both a postpartum flare and onset of RA may be associated with breast-feeding. Barrett and colleagues found that women breast-feeding for the first time had increased disease activity 6 months post partum.[12] A high level of the proinflammatory hormone prolactin is thought to underlie both the increased incidence of postpartum flares and onset of the disease.

In a prospective study, Barrett and colleagues found that greater than 25% of women still had significant disability during pregnancy.[13] Although other measures of disease activity showed a trend toward improvement, only 16% of this large prospective study of 140 women with RA were in complete remission during pregnancy.

Despite a number of attempts, there has been little success in predicting with any certainly which women with RA will experience remission during pregnancy. It is known that disease duration, functional class, and rheumatoid factor positivity have no predictive value with regard to remission. This improvement should occur by the end of the first trimester. However, a smaller but still significant percentage of women show no improvement, and they may require continued intervention to control the disease manifestations. Studies suggest that the effects of pregnancy on the clinical disease may be more variable than has been generally accepted.

Amelioration of Rheumatoid Arthritis during Pregnancy

The mechanism for the remission-inducing effect of pregnancy on RA is still unknown. It was initially thought to be mediated by the increase in blood cortisone levels during pregnancy.[5,14] However, several studies have shown that steroids alone could not fully explain the improvement during pregnancy.[10] There has been no correlation between the change in RA disease activity and plasma concentrations of corticosteroids. Plasma cortisol levels return to normal within 5 days of delivery, but the RA does not flare for 4 to 6 weeks post partum. More recent studies have questioned the effect of oral contraceptives in RA, suggesting that at best they may be weak modulators of the disease.[15]

The effect of plasma focuses attention on the role of nonhormonal plasma constituents in pregnancy. As outlined earlier, pregnancy zone protein has a suppressive effect on the inflammatory activity of polymorphonuclear cells. The timing of improvement in RA parallels the rise in concentration of pregnancy zone protein during pregnancy. The lack of improvement noted in approximately 25% of patients may be related to these women's inability to synthesize sufficient amounts of pregnancy zone protein.[7,16] In addition, increased suppressor cell function and decreased B cell response in pregnancy may counteract the depressed T suppressor cell function noted in RA. This is supported by the lower incidence of rheumatoid factor in pregnant women with RA in comparison with nonpregnant controls with RA.[6] Furthermore, cytokine production is dramatically altered during pregnancy. The immune response shifts from predominantly T helper 1 to T helper 2 lymphocytes, illustrated by a change in balance of cytokine production of the respective T helper cell subsets.[4,17-20] Supporting evidence indicates that a shift to T helper 2 cytokines during pregnancy may underlie the amelioration of RA, whereas the shift back to T helper 1 cytokine predominance is responsible for the postpartum flare.[4,17-20]

It has been suggested that fetal-maternal disparity in class II human leukocyte antigen (HLA) may be related to remission or improvement of RA during pregnancy.[21] Further studies in this area are needed, because the concept remains controversial.[10,21-24]

Effect of Rheumatoid Arthritis on Pregnancy

This aspect of the relationship between RA and pregnancy has not been thoroughly investigated. Kaplan and Diamond suggested that RA has no significant effect on the patient's ability to have a normal pregnancy, delivery, and infant.[25] Nelson and associates found no evidence of infertility in patients with RA, but there was diminished fecundity (the probability of achieving a pregnancy within one menstrual cycle).[26] The same group reported a prospective case-control study that showed no adverse pregnancy outcome in women who later developed RA.[27]

Studies suggest that oral contraceptives may protect against RA and perhaps against more severe disease, although the mechanism for this phenomenon is not clear.[15] Although this finding remains controversial, evidence from a report about a prospective inception cohort of 132 women with recent onset of RA indicates that oral contraceptive use and pregnancy do not influence long-term disease outcome.[28] Multiparous patients with a history of long-term oral contraceptive use showed a trend toward having less radiographic joint damage and a better functional level, but these data were not statistically significant. Regardless of these reported findings, there still is no evidence to promote the use of estrogenic agents in the prevention or treatment of RA in women.[29]

Management of Rheumatoid Arthritis during Pregnancy

Because the cause of RA remains unknown, a cure is not currently possible. It is, however, possible to control inflammation and thus relieve pain, restore function, and prevent deformities and damage resulting from persistent inflammation through a combination of drug therapy, patient education, physiotherapy, and occupational therapy.

Ideally, the patient becomes pregnant electively after a prepregnancy assessment and with an effective treatment regimen that includes only drugs known to be safe and efficacious during pregnancy. Although most antiinflammatory agents can be continued before conception, the regimen should be reevaluated once the woman is pregnant. Naproxen and ibuprofen are nonsteroidal antiinflammatory drugs (NSAIDs) with a good safety profile in pregnancy. With only minor safety issues to be considered, corticosteroids such as prednisone can be continued throughout the pregnancy. Antimalarial agents such as hydroxychloroquine are somewhat controversial, but several cohort studies have supported their safety in pregnancy.[30-35] Sulfasalazine in most cases can be continued with little risk to mother and fetus.[31,36,37] Immunosuppressive agents are more of an issue. Azathioprine (AZA) can be continued throughout pregnancy, but methotrexate (MTX) should be discontinued about 3 months before conception.[31] Interestingly, it is also advisable for men to discontinue MTX at least 3 months before attempting to conceive.[37] A woman might conceive while taking an anti–tumor necrosis factor α (TNF-α) inhibitor (infliximab and etanercept), but there are too few data regarding their safety during pregnancy to make any recommendations.

Because most women with RA experience an improvement during pregnancy, many of their medications can be discontinued for the duration of the pregnancy. In contrast, for those with disease that either remains active or flares during pregnancy, treatment should be directed at controlling the inflammatory process. The physician must balance the risk of a medication to the fetus with the benefits to the health of the mother. Often the physician and patient must resort to prednisone to control a moderate to severe flare of disease.

The postpartum flare is equally challenging to treat. One of the problems encountered is the reluctance of the breast-feeding mother to take any medication whatsoever. Under these circumstances, the usual drugs of choice are naproxen, ibuprofen, and prednisone. All of these agents are considered safe for breast-feeding in the dosages usually used to treat active RA.[37,38]

Nonpharmacologic therapy such as appropriate bed rest, physiotherapy, occupational therapy, and nutrition remain as important mainstays of therapy for active RA.

Labor and Delivery in Rheumatoid Arthritis

There have been no published reports of particular obstetric problems in pregnant women with RA, although these may occur if there is significant hip involvement. Disease involving the cervical spine with atlantoaxial subluxation may be a potential problem because of excessive flexion of the neck during anesthesia.

Family Planning

There is no evidence that RA adversely affects conception, and therapeutic abortion is not indicated. Pregnancy is not harmful to the mother with RA or to the baby, but consideration should be given, before a pregnancy is contemplated, to the emotional stress involved and the additional work required in caring for the newborn.

SYSTEMIC LUPUS ERYTHEMATOSUS

SLE is a chronic systemic disease with diverse clinical and laboratory manifestations and a course characterized by variability. The clinical manifestations result from inflammation of multiple organ systems, especially the joints, skin, kidneys, nervous system, and serous membranes. The disease tends to affect young women in the second, third, and fourth decades of life but may occur in any age group. The prevalence of SLE is 100 per 100,000, which is about 10% as common as RA.[39] The clinical and laboratory heterogeneity of this disease frequently makes the diagnosis and management difficult. In 1982, the American College of Rheumatology proposed classification criteria whereby the presence of any four render a high probability of a diagnosis of SLE (Table 20–1).[40]

Current concepts of the pathogenesis of SLE are that it is an autoimmune disease in which autoantibodies cause specific cytotoxic damage in some cases (e.g., hemolytic anemia, thrombocytopenia) and immune complexes lead to inflammation in other cases (e.g., nephritis, dermatitis, central nervous system [CNS] involvement).

TABLE 20–1   American College of Rheumatology 1982 Revised Criteria for Classification of Systemic Lupus Erythematosus

1. Butterfly rash
2. Discoid lupus
3. Photosensitivity
4. Oral ulcers
5. Arthritis
6. Serositis
   a. Pleuritis
   b. Pericarditis
7. Renal disorder
   a. Persistent proteinuria (>0.5 g/day)
   b. Cellular casts
8. Neurologic disorder
   a. Seizures
   b. Psychosis
9. Hematologic disorder
   a. Hemolytic anemia with reticulocytosis
   b. Leukopenia (<4000/mm^3)
   c. Lymphopenia (<1500/mm^3) or thrombocytopenia (<100,000/mm^3)
10. Immunologic disorder
    a. Positive lupus erythematosus cell preparation
    b. Anti–dsDNA antibody
    c. Anti–Sm antigen
    d. False-positive result of test for syphilis
11. Antinuclear antibody

The mechanism of excess autoantibody production and immune complex formation is not well understood, although current investigation is focused on abnormal regulator functions and the possibility of a slow-acting viral infection.[41] In addition, certain genetic factors may be important, as indicated by a number of family and twin studies for SLE and the finding of an increased frequency of HLA-DRB1*02 and HLA-DRB1*03 and null alleles of the fourth component of complement in patients with SLE.[42]

In addition to the common findings of arthritis and rash, clinical evidence of glomerulonephritis is found in more than 50% of cases. Histologically, six classes of SLE-associated glomerulonephritis have been recognized by the World Health Organization.[43] The prognosis seems to be somewhat better with mesangial and membranous glomerulonephritis and somewhat graver in the proliferative forms.[43] CNS inflammation in SLE may manifest with neurologic or psychiatric manifestations, or a combination.

Laboratory Findings

Patients with SLE have hypergammaglobulinemia, a wide array of autoantibodies, and circulating immune complexes in their serum. Perhaps the most important autoantibody that manifests in this disease, from a pathogenetic point of view, is anti–dsDNA antibody, which is frequently correlated with disease activity and, specifically, with SLE-associated nephritis.

A depressed complement level tends to be correlated with disease activity, especially SLE-associated nephritis. In most patients, the presence of anti–dsDNA antibody and a low complement level may be predictive of either the presence of disease activity or an impending flare.[44]

Systemic Lupus Erythematosus and Fertility

Although SLE may influence pregnancy outcome, studies indicate that it does not affect the chances of conception. One large study from Mexico reported that the fertility rate in patients with SLE was the same as that in the general population.[45] Although the evidence to date indicates that fertility rates are normal in patients with SLE, these findings must be interpreted with some degree of caution. In women with SLE in whom disease is under good control, the fertility rates are probably normal. However, as with any active inflammatory disease, patients with active SLE may be expected to have ovulatory abnormalities, including anovulation. In addition, the role of medications must be considered. In patients with a history of major organ disease, such as diffuse proliferative glomerulonephritis, the use of cyclophosphamide at some point in the disease course would have adverse effects on ovarian function. In this situation, fertility would definitely be affected.

Prepregnancy Assessment

Few diseases mandate as accurate an assessment before pregnancy as SLE. The clinician should adhere to characterizing the patient with regard to clinical profile, laboratory profile, date of most recent disease flare, and medications currently used. The heterogeneity of this disease, with its associated myriad of clinical manifestations, is responsible for some of the most challenging clinical problems for an internist. The superimposition of pregnancy with its dynamically changing physiology only increases the challenge. Using a methodical approach allows the physician to grasp the more subtle nuances of the patient's disease and therefore be better able to distinguish between disease activity and physiologic or pathophysiologic changes caused by pregnancy.

Effect of Pregnancy on Systemic Lupus Erythematosus

The predictable physiologic and immunologic changes seen in all pregnancies also affect women with SLE, but not in predictable ways. Although there may be some consistency in the disease response to pregnancy among many women with SLE, there are still a significant number in whom the disease simply does not behave as expected. In contrast to RA, disease exacerbation appears to be more common than amelioration during pregnancy in SLE. Indeed, the exacerbation of SLE during pregnancy was reported as long ago as 1952.[46] In 1962, Garenstein and associates reported the increased incidence of flares in SLE during the first 20 weeks of pregnancy and again in the first 8 weeks post partum.[47] This could not be confirmed by Mund and coworkers in 1963.[48] However, in 1975, Zurier concluded that patients with SLE frequently had exacerbations of disease activity either during pregnancy or in the early postpartum period.[49] In 1977, Grigor and colleagues reported an increased incidence of exacerbations, mainly in the puerperium.[50] However, in more recent reports on patients both with mild disease and with disease under control before and during pregnancy, the incidence of flares during and after the pregnancy has been significantly lower. Thus, in the series reported by Tozman and associates[51] and by Zulman and colleagues,[52] postpartum flares were not frequently seen. In a case-control prospective study comparing pregnant and nonpregnant patients with SLE with similar disease manifestations, Lockshin and coworkers found no increased frequency of flares in patients with SLE during pregnancy.[53,54] On the other hand, Petri concluded that pregnancy does induce flares in patients with SLE.[55] Petri's pregnant patients had a frequency of 1.63 flares per person years, in comparison with a rate of 0.64 to 0.65 flares in the pregnant population after delivery or in nonpregnant control subjects. Ruiz-Irastorza and colleagues who used similar methods to monitor their patients during pregnancy, also found that 65% of their pregnant patients had flares during the pregnancy, in comparison with 42% of the control group.[56] In a study of 60 patients with 103 pregnancies, Cortes-Hernandez and coworkers discovered that 33% of patients experienced flares during the pregnancy; 26% of those experienced flares in the second trimester and 51% in the postpartum period.[57] These authors showed that significant predictors of a flare included discontinuation of antimalarial treatment, a history of more than three flares before pregnancy, and a score of 5 during these flares. This score indicates active disease on the SLE Disease Activity Index, a validated measure of disease activity in SLE.

It might be argued that patients who had flares of disease during the pregnancy would have been treated and would therefore be less likely to have flares after delivery. The discrepancy between the studies might be explained by a number of reasons, including dissimilar entry criteria, different definitions of a flare, distinct patient populations, and different controls.[55,56] In a study of 61 pregnancies in 46 patients with SLE, Urowitz and coworkers used the SLE Disease Activity Index to assess flares.[58] In comparison with both control groups, there was no increased frequency of SLE flares during pregnancy. Indeed, there was a reduced chance of flare during pregnancy in a patient with inactive disease.

In a large retrospective analysis, 555 women with a diagnosis of SLE were found to have a significant increase in adverse pregnancy outcomes in comparison with a control population of 600,000.[59] These adverse pregnancy outcomes were not limited to manifestations of underlying SLE; they included hypertension, renal disease, preterm delivery, nonelective cesarean section, postpartum hemorrhage, and delivery-related deep venous thrombosis.

In the experience of many clinicians, pregnancy sometimes leads to recrudescence of severe nephritis in patients with SLE who are not sufficiently treated with steroids.[56] However, Tozman and associates[51] noted that renal disease did not recur during pregnancy in 11 of 18 patients who had had some evidence of SLE-associated nephritis during the course of their illness. The prognosis was best in patients who had a remission of the disease at the onset of pregnancy. Similarly, Jungers and colleagues[60] found that a recurrence of SLE-associated nephritis was unusual if pregnancy occurred after a complete, sustained remission of at least several months. Huong and associates obtained similar results, in which maternal and fetal outcomes were good in women with a history of SLE-associated nephritis who had normal renal function or mild renal impairment at the onset of pregnancy.[61] These investigators rarely observed deterioration of renal function as a result of the pregnancy, but they did find a higher risk of preeclampsia and premature birth. Moroni and coauthors noted the initial development of nephritis in 23% of 13 patients with SLE during a pregnancy.[62] They also reported 27% occurrence of a renal flare in 51 patients with SLE and known renal involvement. These authors conclude that the only predictor of a favorable maternal outcome in a pregnancy is quiescence of renal disease.

CNS involvement in SLE can be as difficult to diagnose as it is to treat. Unfortunately, there is little reported in the literature regarding pregnancy and CNS involvement in SLE. Of the few studies reported, this manifestation is associated with significant maternal and fetal risks. El-Sayed and associates reported that in three of five pregnancies, there was a flare of CNS involvement in SLE in women with a history of this manifestation.[63] Severe adverse fetal outcomes occurred in two of the pregnancies. Suffice to say that moderate to severe active SLE represents a high-risk situation for both mother and fetus.

Toxemia of Pregnancy versus Flare of Systemic Lupus Erythematosus

One of the more common clinical dilemmas facing the internist and obstetrician in the management of pregnancy in women with SLE is to distinguish preeclampsia from a flare of the underlying disease. The onset of edema and hypertension in pregnancy in such patients is characteristic of both preeclampsia and active SLE-associated nephritis. Treatment of these two conditions is very different, which emphasizes the importance of an accurate diagnosis. In the absence of other signs of SLE or any serologic abnormalities, the occurrence of edema and hypertension and a recent increase in serum uric acid levels favor a diagnosis of preeclampsia. However, the presence of serologic abnormalities, such as a decrease in serum complement and elevation of anti–dsDNA antibody titers or the presence of other systemic features of SLE, suggests the onset of an SLE flare. Knowledge of the specific clinical and laboratory manifestations of previous flares in the individual patient assists in differentiating these two conditions. This important clinical differentiation was discussed by Zulman and colleagues.[52]

Therapeutic Abortion

In the presteroid era, it was common practice to terminate pregnancy in patients with active SLE. However, with successful treatment of active disease with corticosteroids, this practice has become less frequent. Patients are more likely to have inactive SLE at the onset of pregnancy because of earlier diagnosis and more effective prepregnancy therapy, as well as appropriate prepregnancy counseling. In addition, careful monitoring and early treatment of active disease during pregnancy have allowed the successful completion of pregnancy without significant detriment to the mother or child in many cases. Another indication for therapeutic abortion in the past was a history of serious renal disease. However, as discussed previously, more recent studies have shown that a history of serious renal disease need not be a contraindication to continuation of a pregnancy.

Several older reports indicated a high incidence of disease exacerbation after a therapeutic abortion, occasionally leading to a fatal outcome.[64] However, a study by Zulman and colleagues revealed no detrimental short- or long-term physical effects of therapeutic abortions in 10 pregnant women with SLE.[52]

Effect of Systemic Lupus Erythematosus on Pregnancy

Adverse pregnancy outcome is more common in SLE than in any other rheumatic disease. Appropriate prepregnancy counseling is essential for maximizing the probability of a successful result for both the mother and neonate. Maintaining the viability of the pregnancy and the health of the mother requires close collaboration between the obstetrician/perinatologist and internist/rheumatologist.

Spontaneous Abortion, Prematurity, and Stillbirth

Whereas a patient with SLE may conceive normally, her chances of maintaining the pregnancy are reduced. In the past, the incidence of adverse outcomes in SLE pregnancies, including prematurity, spontaneous abortion, and intrauterine death, approached 50%.[47,50,55,56,59,65-67] A review of the literature determined that the rate of spontaneous abortion in SLE has steadily declined from 50% to less than 20% since 1960 ($r^2 = 0.711$) (Fig. 20-1).[68] The pregnancy outcomes in my own clinic from the period 2000 to 2003 were compared to those reported in the literature since the early 1960s. Predicting an adverse outcome in the pregnant woman with SLE remains a difficult task. Several risk factors, including antiphospholipid antibodies, hypocomplementemia, and hypertension during pregnancy, have been proposed.[57] Although some authorities have found the birth weight of infants born to mothers with SLE is lower than normal, others have shown that birth weight was not reduced, despite the fact that placental size was reduced in comparison with that in controls.[69]

Several factors have been proposed to explain the increased frequency of fetal loss in SLE: (1) active SLE resulting in decidual vasculitis, compromising placental blood supply and consequent deprivation of the fetus; (2) trophoblast-reactive lymphocytotoxic antibodies; (3) anti-Ro/SSA and anti-La/SSB antibodies associated with destruction of the fetal cardiac conduction system leading to intrauterine death; and (4) the lupus anticoagulant (LAC) and antiphospholipid antibodies, with resulting ischemic pregnancy loss often associated with placental insufficiency caused by thrombosis.

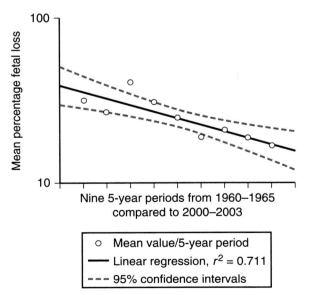

Figure 20–1. Change in fetal loss rates in pregnancies among women with systemic lupus erythematosus (SLE), 1960 to 2003. The rate of fetal loss in SLE pregnancies since the early 1960s has decreased from a mean of 43% in the period 1960 to 1965 to 17% in the period 2000 to 2003. (From Clark CA, Spitzer KA, Laskin CA: Decrease in pregnancy loss rates in SLE over a 40-year period [abstract]. Arthritis Rheum 2003;48 Suppl:S180.)

Although decidual vasculopathy has been documented in the placentas of some patients with SLE, this has not been uniformly seen.[69,70] Hanly and associates concluded that the observed reduction in placental size in patients with SLE may impair the capacity of the placenta to tolerate additional insults.[69] Studies suggest that uterine-umbilical artery Doppler velocimetry in pregnant patients with SLE may identify the fetus at risk for adverse perinatal outcome.[71] Patients with normal flow in both arteries had normal outcomes; patients with reduced velocity in one uterine artery delivered newborns with reduced birth weight; and reduced flow velocity in both arteries was associated with perinatal losses.

The relationship between active SLE in the mother and fetal outcome has been controversial, primarily because of a lack of uniform assessment of disease activity.[55,72,73] In two studies, investigators using validated measures of disease activity found no correlation between disease activity at onset of pregnancy and fetal outcome.[57,73] However, more recently, active renal disease, proteinuria, the presence of LAC, or anticardiolipin antibody in the mother were found to be predictive for fetal loss (including spontaneous abortion and stillbirth) in patients with SLE. Hypertension and active SLE were found to be correlated with poor fetal outcome, defined as prematurity or intrauterine growth restriction.[66,72-75]

The presence of trophoblast-reactive lymphocytotoxic antibodies has been proposed as the reason for loss of pregnancy in patients with SLE, because their incidence in pregnancies in the case of patients with SLE ending in live births was lower than in those resulting in spontaneous abortions.[76] Similarly, the presence of antilymphocyte antibodies was found to correlate with pregnancy losses in patients with recurrent fetal loss but without clinical evidence of SLE.[77]

Anti-Ro/SSA and anti-La/SSB antibodies are thought to be involved in the pathogenesis of congenital heart block in the neonatal SLE syndrome (see "The Newborn" section). These antibodies have been shown to bind to neonatal rabbit heart tissue and to inhibit membrane repolarization.[78,79] These changes may lead to the destruction of the fetal cardiac conductive system and may lead to intrauterine death.

Lupus Anticoagulant, Antiphospholipid Antibodies, and Pregnancy

LAC is an acquired inhibitor of coagulation in vitro present in 5% to 18% of patients with SLE.[80,81] The inhibitor is an immunoglobulin G or M antibody to specific phospholipids that interfere with the conversion of prothrombin to thrombin by the prothrombin-converting complex of factor Va, factor Xa, and calcium that assembles on the surface of a phospholipid micelle during the in vitro activated partial thromboplastin time (aPTT) assay. Plasma samples found to have a prolonged aPTT, indicating anticoagulant activity, are then tested with a 50/50 mix with platelet-poor and normal plasma. Repeated prolongation of the aPTT confirms the presence of a global inhibitor to coagulation, the LAC. The phospholipid dependence of the LAC can be further confirmed by reversing the prolongation of the aPTT through the addition of excess phospholipid. Several tests assess the LAC; no one test has greater significance.[82] Indeed, it has been proposed that a panel of at least four tests for the LAC be undertaken to definitely detect its presence.[83-86]

"Lupus anticoagulant" is a misnomer in that patients who have the abnormality do not have a bleeding tendency but rather tend to be hypercoagulable with a risk of venous and/or arterial thrombosis. The term *anticoagulant* is merely a reflection of the in vitro artifact of the prolonged aPTT.[87,88] In addition, an association among the presence of LAC, recurrent pregnancy loss, preeclampsia, and placental abruption has been noted.[81,89-91] Anticardiolipin antibody is one of a family of antibodies directed against specific phospholipids and has been thought to cross react with LAC. Although the terms *anticardiolipin antibody* and *lupus anticoagulant* have been used interchangeably to indicate antiphospholipid antibodies among patients with SLE, it has been shown that the correlation between the two antibodies was not as strong as expected. Lockshin and coworkers showed that although LAC or anticardiolipin antibody was associated with fetal loss, a high level of anticardiolipin antibody may be a better predictor of fetal distress or fetal death among pregnant patients with SLE.[89] Two studies suggest that the presence of the anticardiolipin antibody or features of the antiphospholipid syndrome are associated with increased risk for fetal loss among patients with SLE.[67,73] However, this has not been universally found, and the correlation remains controversial.[69,72] Among the issues in contention are the association of antiphospholipid antibodies with early or only late pregnancy losses, the significance of immunoglobulins M and A isotypes of anticardiolipin antibodies, and the predictive value of the presence of LAC or anticardiolipin antibody and the need for intervention in women with no thromboembolic or adverse obstetric history.[92,93] All these findings have renewed interest in the possible association of LAC activity and recurrent pregnancy loss, both in patients with SLE and in those without features of SLE.[87,88,90,94,95] Some authors have attempted to treat women with the laboratory abnormality with moderately high doses of corticosteroids to suppress the anticoagulant and have claimed that this has resulted in live births.[96] However, one study of the use of prednisone and aspirin in patients with autoantibodies and recurrent fetal loss showed no benefit over placebo.[97] Some studies have provided evidence supporting the use of heparin and aspirin in the treatment of recurrent pregnancy loss in women with antiphospholipid antibodies.[98-100] Other studies, however, have challenged these findings and reported a high success rate with the use of aspirin alone in such patients.[101] Further randomized, controlled trials of therapy of this condition are clearly necessary.[102,103] Successful pregnancy outcomes with low-molecular-weight heparin and aspirin in patients with recurrent fetal loss who have autoantibodies, including antiphospholipid antibodies, have been reported,[104] but results from additional randomized controlled studies with this form of therapy that are currently under way are needed to confirm earlier findings.

The Newborn

In general, but with notable exceptions, the neonate born at term to a woman with SLE is at no greater risk for congenital abnormalities than are those of the general population. A number of children of mothers with SLE have been found to have transient serologic abnormalities, skin lesions, and congenital heart block.[78,79,105,106] These abnormalities are usually associated with a very specific autoimmune disorder, which in turn results from the presence of specific autoantibodies, anti-Ro/SSA and anti-La/SSB, in the serum of the mother. The association of these antibodies with the neonatal syndrome, especially congenital heart block, is so striking that it is wise to evaluate all children born to mothers with SLE for congenital cardiac rhythm anomalies and, conversely, to investigate mothers of babies born with complete heart block for signs of SLE.

The neonatal SLE syndrome is characterized by SLE-associated dermatitis, a variety of systemic and hematologic abnormalities, and isolated congenital heart block.[79] This syndrome is thought to result from placental transfer of a maternal immunoglobulin G antibody. The syndrome usually resolves spontaneously by 8 to 9 months of age. It has been suggested that the anti-Ro/SSA antibody may be a marker for the development of neonatal SLE syndrome.[79] Anti-Ro/SSA and anti-La/SSB antibodies are antibodies to nonhistone nuclear antigens detected by immunodiffusion. They have been found in the sera of 70% of patients with Sjögren's syndrome and in 25% to 30% of patients with SLE. Initially, seven of eight mothers of infants with neonatal SLE syndrome were found to have the anti-Ro/SSA antibody.[107] It now appears that antibodies to Ro/SSA or La/SSB, or both, are almost universally found in the sera of parturient mothers and newborns with SLE.[79] Moreover, a very high correlation was found between isolated congenital heart block and anti-Ro/SSA antibody in maternal serum, regardless of whether the mother had a connective tissue disease or not.[108] The presence of these antibodies in the mother is associated with a 3% to 5% risk of giving birth to a baby with neonatal SLE syndrome. After one pregnancy results in neonatal SLE syndrome, the risk doubles in a subsequent pregnancy. Brucato and colleagues failed to find any case of congenital heart block among the offspring of 53 women with SLE and anti-Ro/SSA antibodies and noted the occurrence of congenital heart block in 2% of pregnancies from mothers with other connective tissue diseases and anti-Ro/SSA antibodies.[109] It appears, however, that anti-Ro/SSA antibodies do not affect other pregnancy outcomes.[110]

The finding of immunoglobulin deposits in the cardiac tissue of an infant who died of congenital heart block has been proposed as evidence to support the hypothesis that the antibody is transmitted transplacentally and may act on cardiac tissue to produce the heart block.[79] The presence of Ro/SSA antigen in fetal tissues as well as in adult skin, areas where tissue injury occurs with anti-Ro/SSA–associated disease, lends further credibility to this hypothesis.[111]

Management of Systemic Lupus Erythematosus and Pregnancy

Prepregnancy Assessment

Ideally, both an internist-rheumatologist and an obstetrician should manage a patient with SLE about to embark on a pregnancy. As previously stated, documentation of the clinical and laboratory profiles of the patient are most helpful for ensuring appropriate medical management of the pregnancy. The patient should be counseled before the pregnancy about the impact of pregnancy on SLE and of SLE on both pregnancy and the infant.

Ideally, SLE should be inactive at the time that pregnancy is contemplated. Inactive or well-controlled disease necessitates fewer drugs; this in turn has less risk of an adverse impact on the pregnancy. Should the disease flare during the pregnancy, treatment must be implemented as quickly as possible. The physician must determine the manifestations and extent of disease exacerbation and then select the safest, most effective therapy. The mother's health must be deemed the first priority and treatment directed accordingly. Because prednisone has few adverse effects on the fetus, it should be used without hesitation as is necessary. NSAIDs, antimalarial agents, and AZA have good safety profiles in pregnancy and can be used in most circumstances. A detailed discussion of medication use in pregnancy appears later in this chapter.

Monitoring During Pregnancy

The internist and obstetrician should assess the pregnant patient with SLE with almost equal frequency. At these visits, signs and symptoms of an impending flare should be sought on history and physical examination, and blood samples should be drawn for serologic evaluation. A rise in anti–dsDNA antibody titer and a decrease in complement may be predictive of an exacerbation of SLE. It must be remembered that serum complement is an acute-phase reactant that rises somewhat in a normal pregnancy. Therefore, in a patient with SLE, a decrease in complement may still be within normal range but has the same significance as a low complement in a nonpregnant patient. This change in complement value must be monitored, and therapy should be adjusted accordingly. There are now a number of validated measures of disease activity, and these may be used to identify a flare both in the clinical setting and for research purposes.[112]

Delivery

The decision with regard to the type of delivery should be obstetric. Most patients with SLE can successfully deliver vaginally. Corticosteroid supplementation should be given to cover the labor or cesarean delivery in patients currently receiving steroids or those recently treated with these drugs. There is currently no rationale for automatically increasing steroids in the postpartum period as prophylaxis against a postpartum flare.

Breast-Feeding

The potential problems raised by breast-feeding involve its possible effect on the disease process and the possible transmission of medications through the breast milk to the infant. There is suggestive but conflicting evidence linking hyperprolactinemia seen in the nursing mother with disease exacerbation.[113-116] Breast-feeding also demands time and energy of the mother, and this might lead to undue fatigue in some patients. In general, if the physician is considering only the effect on disease activity, the decision regarding breast-feeding should be left up to the mother, encouragement given for the decision made. If significant amounts of corticosteroids (>40 mg of prednisone) or cytotoxic or other disease-suppressive medications are necessary to control disease activity, it would probably be wise not to breast-feed.

Contraception

There is still significant controversy regarding the role of oral contraceptives in inducing SLE. The controversy was sparked in 1968, when Schleicher reported the development of a positive LE preparation in addition to some vague symptoms compatible with a systemic disease in 19 healthy women taking oral contraceptives.[117] After discontinuation of the oral contraceptives, the test results became negative. In the same year, a study of 3014 women taking oral contraceptives revealed the incidence of rheumatic disease to be no higher than that found in the general population.[118] Also in the same year, Dubois and coworkers could not find these autoantibodies in 39 patients taking the contraceptive medication.[119]

In 1971, Chapel and Burns reported the development of mild SLE in two patients taking oral contraceptives. Their symptoms improved after the drug was discontinued.[120] In a prospective cohort study of 121,645 women, Sanchez-Guerrero and associates found that past use of oral contraceptives was associated with a slightly increased risk of developing SLE (relative ratio, 1.9 for past users vs. those who never used them).[121]

There is evidence of increased incidence of thrombosis, vasculitis, and hypertension in women using estrogen-containing oral contraceptives, especially in those with antiphospholipid antibodies.[122] In women with SLE, appropriate counseling should be undertaken before they start taking oral contraceptives, to ensure that the potential risks of these agents are understood. However, in women with antiphospholipid antibodies, it would be prudent to avoid estrogen-containing oral contraceptives and encourage them to use other methods of contraception.

Some patients using the intrauterine device (IUD) complain of dysmenorrhea and recurrent infections, especially if taking prednisone and cytotoxic drugs. In those cases, patients should discontinue this method of contraception and consider other types of birth control, such as the diaphragm, condom, and spermicidal preparation, preferably in combination.

Ovulation Induction

Although, as a group, patients with SLE do not have an increased risk of infertility, there are women with SLE who may require ovulation induction therapy for fertility problems. The administration of high doses of exogenous follicle-stimulating hormone with its consequent hyper-estrogenicity raises concerns regarding this form of therapy. Five cases that suggest that such therapy may be deleterious for these patients have been reported. In four women, there was exacerbation of disease activity, and one woman died.[123] In 19 women who underwent 68 cycles of ovulation induction therapy, an acceptable pregnancy rate occurred, although the rates of both fetal and maternal complications were high.[124] Although ovulation induction therapy is not contraindicated in patients with SLE, physicians who plan to advise the use of this therapy in these patients should do so with caution.

Genetic Counseling

Although it was initially believed that the incidence of SLE in families is no higher than in the general population, this is no longer thought to be true. The frequency of SLE among first- or second-degree relatives is estimated to be between 5% and 12%.[125] However, this estimate not only is based on clinical evidence of disease but also includes family members with positive serologic profiles but no clinical disease. Therefore, although the risk is present, it is probably less than 5%, which is not sufficient to advise against pregnancy.

SERONEGATIVE SPONDYLOARTHROPATHIES

The diseases included in the group of seronegative spondyloarthropathies have been distinguished from RA by the absence of the rheumatoid factor; hence the term *seronegative*. The group includes ankylosing spondylitis (AS) as the prototype, as well as reactive arthritis, psoriatic arthritis, and the arthritis of ulcerative colitis and Crohn's disease (enterocolitic arthropathies).[126] Since 1980, it has become clear that these diseases are distinct clinical entities with closely linked clinical manifestations. As a group, these diseases share several articular and nonarticular manifestations, although the distinction of a particular disease is possible in most cases. The common articular features of the seronegative arthropathies include sacroiliitis, spondylitis, seronegative polyarthritis, and dactylitis.

Sacroiliitis manifests as low back pain of inflammatory character. Inflammatory back pain is aggravated by rest and improves with activity and is accompanied by significant stiffness and, often, pain early in the morning. Radiographs show evidence of sacroiliitis in the form of erosions, sclerosis, and in advanced cases, total ankylosis with loss of joint contour. The involvement tends to be symmetric in classic AS and often unilateral in reactive and psoriatic arthritides.

Spondylitis, which is inflammation of the apophyseal joints of the spine, is common in this group of diseases.

It is most severe in AS, manifesting with inflammatory low back pain and progressing to marked muscle spasm and often deformities with ankylosis later in the course of the disease. In AS, the whole spine is affected, starting at the thoracolumbar junction and spreading up into the neck and down throughout the lumbar spine. In reactive arthritis, psoriatic arthritis, and the enterocolitic arthropathies, the spondylitis is not widespread, and skip lesions are common. Radiographs show the classic syndesmophytes arising from the vertebral margins in AS with nonmarginal syndesmophytes in other entities.

Seronegative polyarthritis is classically an asymmetric form of inflammatory arthritis, often involving large joints as well as the distal interphalangeal joints, which are commonly spared in RA. There is often a periosteal reaction, and ankylosis may occur.

Dactylitis is inflammation extending from the joint to involve part or all of the digits and is a common feature among the diseases of this group.

The following extraarticular features of seronegative spondyloarthropathies may appear; a psoriasiform rash and nail changes are seen more frequently in patients with psoriatic arthritis and reactive arthritis than in those with classic AS. Ocular inflammation is one of the most common manifestations in all seronegative diseases. The inflammation usually involves the uveal tract. Genitourinary inflammation is seen, particularly in reactive arthritis and AS. Buccal and genitourinary ulcerations are common in all entities of this group. Aortic insufficiency is seen most frequently in classic AS.

Another feature of this group of diseases is strong familial aggregation, which occurs not only within each entity but also among the entities of the group. Further evidence that these clinical entities are an interrelated group of disorders comes from the strong association between HLA antigen B27 and several of these diseases. The discovery of the association with HLA-B27 may be relevant to the study of the origin of these conditions.[127,128]

The diagnosis of seronegative arthropathy is based on the clinical features, both articular and extraarticular, and the radiologic evidence of sacroiliitis and spondylitis. Laboratory investigations are not particularly helpful except for a negative rheumatoid factor. The ESR is usually normal, although it may be quite high in the presence of severe disease. HLA typing may sometimes be useful in a case difficult to diagnose.

With the exception of psoriatic arthritis, seronegative diseases are traditionally thought to be much more common in men than in women. The diagnosis of AS in women is often missed, perhaps because it is usually milder in women than in men.[129]

Seronegative Disease in Pregnancy

There are very few reports on the association of seronegative diseases and pregnancy. Hart reported on 14 pregnancies in patients with AS.[130] He concluded that there was no apparent change in the progress of the disease and that childbirth had little effect on its course. Ostensen and Husby reviewed the literature on AS and pregnancy and reported that although pregnancy does not improve the course of the spondylitis, there appears to be no adverse effects on the pregnancy.[131]

Although McHugh and Laurent reported improvement in the arthritis in only 4 of 12 pregnancies,[132] a prospective study of 20 pregnancies in 15 patients with psoriatic arthritis revealed improvement in 16 cases in both skin and joint disease.[133] As with RA, remission during pregnancy is common in psoriatic arthritis, and there is frequently a flare of the disease post partum.

In general, the course of AS is independent of the pregnancy. A flare of AS is not uncommon during pregnancy, but this may be because of the natural history of the disease or the mechanical strain on the back and weight-bearing joints in pregnancy.

Treatment of Seronegative Disease

The treatment of early seronegative disease is similar to that of RA: namely, control of inflammation. NSAIDs, usually in high doses, represent the treatment of choice. This may present a particular concern in pregnancy, in which the use of such agents after the 28th week may be problematic. In severe inflammatory disease, corticosteroids in moderately high doses may be necessary. These agents do not raise the same concerns as NSAIDs in late pregnancy. Psoriatic arthritis has been shown to be a more severe disease[134] and may necessitate more aggressive therapy, including the use of gold, antimalarial agents, penicillamine, or sulfasalazine therapy. MTX has been used in the treatment of psoriatic arthritis, with encouraging results, particularly when severe skin involvement occurs simultaneously.

An important aspect of treatment in seronegative diseases, particularly sacroiliitis and spondylitis, is physical therapy with the appropriate exercise program. Postural and breathing exercises are especially important for the pregnant woman with this condition.

PROGRESSIVE SYSTEMIC SCLEROSIS (SCLERODERMA)

Progressive systemic sclerosis (PSS) is an uncommon connective tissue disease of unknown cause, manifested by fibrosis and degenerative vascular changes in the skin, joints, and many internal organs.[135] The disease has a global distribution, with a reported incidence of 2 to 12 cases per million people per year, and affects three to four times as many women as men. PSS may occur at any age, but in most patients, the onset occurs between the ages of 30 and 50 years.

Early lesions of PSS often show a mononuclear cell infiltrate. Serologic abnormalities are common in this disease, and there is occasionally an association with other autoimmune diseases. The main pathologic lesion found in established PSS is vascular, consisting of concentric proliferation of the intima and fibrosis of the adventitia of small arteries and arterioles.[136] This had led to the hypothesis that an unknown agent initiates the mononuclear inflammatory response around small arteries, leading to marked fibroblastic proliferation, which in turn results

in the severe sclerosis of the small arteries and interstitium. This process leads to tissue induration and vascular insufficiency, which underlie the clinical features of this disease.

The most common feature of PSS is Raynaud's phenomenon, which often precedes the other clinical features by many years. Skin involvement often manifests with edema, followed by induration. The skin later becomes tight and bound down (sclerodactyly), with resultant contractures. This may be associated with hyperpigmentation and ulcerations, particularly over bone prominences. Telangiectasia (dilated blood vessels) commonly occurs on fingertips, lips, tongue, and face. Calcification in the soft tissues (calcinosis) may develop in patients with long-standing disease. Many patients present with polyarthralgia, and small effusions are occasionally detected. Muscle involvement, ranging from noninflammatory myopathy to a frank myositis, may develop. Dysphagia is a frequent manifestation of the esophageal dysmotility that occurs in a large number of patients with PSS. Esophageal involvement may lead to esophagitis that may result in strictures. Intestinal motility disorders associated with diarrhea and malabsorption may occur. Myocardial fibrosis may lead to significant myocardial insufficiency, arrhythmias, cardiomyopathy, and sudden death. The pericardium may also be involved. Dyspnea often signifies pulmonary fibrosis or the onset of pulmonary hypertension.

Renal involvement is a major cause of death in PSS. It is typically manifested by the abrupt onset of malignant hypertension, leading to rapidly progressive renal insufficiency. Renal disease and pulmonary hypertension in PSS are the most ominous prognostic signs of this disease.[137]

Laboratory manifestations of PSS include anemia, which is usually normochromic and normocytic, but in cases of rapidly progressive renal failure, a microangiopathic hemolytic anemia occurs with a high frequency. Many patients have an elevated ESR, and hypergammaglobulinemia is common. Antinuclear antibodies occur in 30% to 90% of patients with PSS. These commonly give a speckled pattern on human laryngeal tumor cell substrates. Elevated peripheral renin activity levels have been found in patients with PSS, even without clinically apparent renal disease.

The course of the disease is quite variable. Patients with the CREST (calcinosis, Raynaud's phenomenon, esophageal involvement, sclerodactyly, and telangiectasia) variant are thought to have a more benign disease with a better prognosis. Pulmonary hypertension and renal disease are indicators of more severe disease and carry a grave prognosis.[137] The diagnosis of PSS is based on the clinical manifestations. The American College of Rheumatology has devised preliminary criteria for the diagnosis of systemic sclerosis, determining proximal scleroderma as a major criterion and sclerodactyly, digital pitting scars, and bibasilar pulmonary fibrosis as minor criteria; one major or two minor criteria are necessary for the diagnosis.[138]

Effect of Scleroderma on Pregnancy

The association of PSS and pregnancy is unusual, first because PSS is a rare disease, and second because it often begins in the fourth or fifth decade, after the major child-bearing years. Although some studies have found an increase in the prevalence of infertility in women with PSS,[139-141] Steen and Medsger showed that there was no significant difference in infertility rates in comparison with a group with RA and neighborhood controls after adjusting for other contributing factors.[142] Similarly, Sampaio-Barros and associates found that 79% of 150 women with PSS had a total of 406 pregnancies, an average of 3.4 per patient.[143] However, it is important to note that 364 of these pregnancies occurred before the onset of disease and, therefore, only 42 occurred after the diagnosis.

An increased incidence of spontaneous abortions in women with systemic sclerosis was found in a case-controlled study including healthy controls.[144] These results were supported by a study from Great Britain, which showed both an increased rate of infertility and an increased incidence of spontaneous abortions in women destined to develop PSS.[139,140] Other investigators have found fetal deaths occurring in 14% of pregnancies, the majority in the first trimester and before the onset of disease.[143] Patients with PSS had higher rates of pregnancies ending with perinatal deaths and more infants with low birth weights than did the control populations. In a case-controlled study, Steen and colleagues found no differences in the frequencies of miscarriage or perinatal death between the patients with PSS and either those with RA or a neighborhood control group.[142] They did note, however, a slightly increased rate of preterm births and small full-term infants among their patients with PSS. In their prospective study of pregnancy in PSS, Steen and colleagues documented miscarriages in 18% and prematurity in 26% of all patients.[141] Of note, more adverse outcomes occurred in patients with diffuse PSS. However, Steen suggested that "these risks of miscarriage or prematurity should not discourage women from becoming pregnant."[145] Two reports highlighted the fact that even patients with severe PSS may have successful pregnancies if their complications are adequately treated.[146,147]

Effect of Pregnancy on Scleroderma

The early literature on PSS and pregnancy included case reports describing patients with diffuse disease and unfavorable outcomes, with worsening of disease during pregnancy and maternal deaths.[145,148] A review of case series totaling 103 patients revealed that the disease began during pregnancy in 9 patients, worsened during pregnancy in 32 patients, was stable in 35 patients, and remitted in 11 patients.[149] The one case-controlled study that addressed the question of maternal morbidity was conducted by questionnaire.[144] Overall, maternal complications reported on the questionnaires were neither more frequent nor more severe in the patients with PSS than in the patients with RA or in the neighborhood control group. A prospective study of pregnancy in PSS was reported in 1996.[141] In this study of 67 pregnancies in 50 women with PSS, symptoms remained stable in 61% of the pregnancies; 20% experienced improvement, usually in Raynaud's symptoms; and the remainder noted worsening. Two women had an end-stage renal crisis. In a more recent study,

58 (14%) of 406 pregnancies in a group of women with PSS resulted in fetal death.[143] Of interest, the majority (50) of the 58 fetal deaths occurred before disease onset, whereas only 8 occurred after diagnosis. Of course, this may be a direct result of the lower number of pregnancies in this population after disease onset.

Most authors agree that if PSS progresses rapidly, with cardiac or renal disease, the effect of pregnancy may be serious and may lead to sudden worsening of renal function and death.[150-152] In addition, esophagitis is often aggravated by pregnancy, and therapy, including elevation of the head of the bed and ingestion of antacids or use of H_2 blockers, is indicated. Raynaud's phenomenon usually improves during pregnancy, probably because of the peripheral vasodilatation characteristic of pregnancy.[153]

It is clear from the case-control studies that pregnancy in PSS is not as rare as was initially thought. Many patients do well during pregnancy, whereas in some, disease exacerbation may be precipitated by the pregnancy. Therefore, patients with PSS should be monitored closely, both by the internist/rheumatologist and by the obstetrician, and blood pressure and renal function should be evaluated frequently.

Treatment

There is no effective treatment for PSS. Current modes of therapy are aimed at suppression of the microvascular abnormalities and inhibition of the processes that give rise to overgrowth of collagen.[135] Supportive measures include patient education, avoidance of exposure to cold, and use of physical therapy designed to preserve hand function and minimize contractures.

Various pharmacologic agents are used in the treatment of PSS. Antihypertensive agents, such as reserpine and methyldopa, and a variety of vasodilators, especially the calcium channel antagonists, have been used to control Raynaud's phenomenon. Corticosteroids have only a transient effect on the skin but may be useful in the treatment of the myositis. Treatment of acid reflux with antacids, H_2 blockers, proton pump inhibitors, and metoclopramide for esophageal dysmotility is recommended and may be continued during pregnancy. Patients with severe renal disease may require dialysis.

Most of the pharmacologic agents used for PSS have not been tried in pregnancy and should be avoided. In the presence of rapidly progressive cardiac or renal disease, immediate termination of pregnancy is recommended.

An anesthesia consultation before delivery may be very beneficial because the pregnant patient with PSS represents a particularly difficult challenge during delivery. Physical limitations caused by contractures of the skin, hips, and extremities can complicate the delivery. The delivery room should be kept warm, as should the intravenous fluids; in addition, thermal socks and warm compresses should be used to minimize problems caused by Raynaud's phenomenon, which can occur during labor and delivery.[153] Post partum, the patient's blood pressure should be carefully monitored to alert the physician to the onset of a renal crisis.

In general, PSS has no impact on maternal and fetal outcomes. The adverse outcomes described in earlier literature do not seem to be as frequent as once thought. However, these patients should be attended by a perinatologist because of the higher risk of prematurity and smallness for gestational age in infants. Appropriate prepregnancy planning, coupled with close monitoring and aggressive therapeutic intervention by both the obstetrician and internist/rheumatologist, carries a higher probability of a successful pregnancy outcome for both mother and neonate.

POLYMYOSITIS/DERMATOMYOSITIS

Polymyositis (PM) is a diffuse inflammatory disease of striated muscle with an estimated incidence of 1 per 280,000. It affects twice as many women as men, with a peak incidence in the fifth and sixth decades. The origin of polymyositis/dermatomyositis (PM/DM) remains unknown, but there is evidence to support the role of immunologic factors in pathogenesis.[150]

Clinically, PM/DM manifests with symmetric proximal muscle weakness of variable intensity of either acute or gradual onset, with or without the typical dermatomyositis rash. The latter is a dusky erythematous eruption on the face, neck, and arms in association with a violaceous rash over the eyelids. Other skin manifestations include mucous membrane lesions, scaly lesions over the knuckles, bullous lesions, and exfoliative dermatitis. Raynaud's phenomenon is common. A mild arthritis occurs in about one third of cases. Transient pneumonitis and pulmonary fibrosis may occur. Cardiac manifestations include rhythm and conduction disturbances. Myocardial inflammation has also been described. Dysphagia, abdominal pain, and, in rare cases, gastrointestinal hemorrhage may occur. Renal involvement, however, is uncommon in PM/DM.

Laboratory manifestations include an elevated ESR, leukocytosis, and elevated muscle enzyme levels (creatine phosphokinase, serum glutamic-oxaloacetic transaminase, and aldolase). Urinary creatine concentration is also elevated. Serologic abnormalities include positive rheumatoid factor and antinuclear factor in some patients. Antibodies to *Toxoplasma* organisms have been detected in patients with PM. An antinuclear antibody specific for Jo-1 has been described in PM. Both electromyographic studies and muscle pathologic specimens show characteristic features.

The diagnosis of PM is based on the clinical features of muscle weakness with or without the rash, the enzyme elevation, and the typical electromyographic and biopsy findings.

Pregnancy in Polymyositis/Dermatomyositis

The rarity of PM/DM explains the paucity of literature on the disease in pregnancy. The few reports that exist deal mainly with a description of the clinical scenario and the outcome. There are now 22 case reports of 32 pregnancies associated with PM/DM.[154-160] In one group of 17 cases,

the disease developed during pregnancy or in the immediate postpartum period. In 12 of these cases, the mother's disease was active throughout pregnancy, and in the remainder, the disease went into remission. There was one maternal death. There were 10 healthy newborns, 1 premature birth, 2 spontaneous abortions, 2 neonatal deaths and 2 stillbirths. In another group of 15 cases, the disease antedated the pregnancy. Only one patient developed a minor flare during the pregnancy. There were 12 healthy newborns, 1 neonatal death, 1 stillborn, and 1 spontaneous abortion. There are no prospective studies of PM/DM during pregnancy. Overall, of the 32 pregnancies reported, there were 9 pregnancy losses (28%), which is similar to the rates reported in SLE and PSS. Thus, despite the limited experience managing the disease in pregnancy, it appears that the disease may have an adverse affect on the pregnancy.

Treatment of Polymyositis/Dermatomyositis

In addition to supportive measures, including rest, physiotherapy, and analgesics, corticosteroids remain the drug of choice in this disease. The dosage required is often high, up to 1 mg/kg/day of prednisone. This therapy results in improvement in both the clinical and the biochemical changes in this disease, but the response tends to be slow. The use of MTX and AZA has been reported and is usually reserved for refractory cases.[161] Both AZA and corticosteroids have been used successfully during pregnancy.

VASCULITIC SYNDROMES

The group of vasculitic syndromes comprises a broad spectrum of uncommon diseases resulting from inflammation and necrosis of blood vessels. This process may involve vessels of different types, sizes, and locations, characterized by various clinical manifestations with or without identifiable precipitating factors. Recognition and understanding of specific entities in this group have been difficult because of the confusion surrounding the classification of these disorders. The prevailing classification is complex but necessary not only for academic reasons but also to provide a rational basis for therapy. These diseases are so rare that most internists/rheumatologists and obstetricians never encounter a patient with one of these conditions during a pregnancy. Only polyarteritis nodosa (PAN) and Wegener's granulomatosus are discussed in detail, because there have been no reports of pregnancy occurring in combination with any of the other disorders.[162]

Polyarteritis Nodosa

The characteristic clinical manifestations of PAN are those of systemic disease with multiple organ involvement, resulting from necrotizing angiitis of small and medium-sized muscular arteries, often in a segmental manner. Patients present with fever, malaise, fatigue, myalgias, and arthralgias. Hypertension is common.

Abdominal pain (resulting from intestinal infarction), mononeuritis multiplex, and evidence of coronary arteritis may be present. Hematuria and casts, signifying renal involvement with either vasculitis or glomerulitis, are frequent. Skin manifestations include subcutaneous nodules and purpuric rashes. Hepatitis may occur as a result of liver involvement with vasculitis or may be related to hepatitis B antigenemia. Other manifestations include epididymitis or involvement of the ovaries or other parts of the genitourinary tract.

Pathologically, the lesions consist of leukocytic infiltrate, initially with polymorphonuclear cells and later with mononuclear cells, in the vessel wall. Intimal proliferation is followed by evidence of degeneration and necrosis of the vessel wall. Thrombosis, ischemia, and infarction give rise to the various clinical manifestations. Lesions at all stages of development are found simultaneously, and aneurysmal dilatation is common. Anemia, eosinophilia, an elevated ESR, and hypergammaglobulinemia are commonly found, as are rheumatoid factor, antinuclear factor, and hepatitis B antigen and antibody. Immune complexes are thought to play a role in the pathogenesis of PAN. One complex currently under investigation is the hepatitis B antigen-antibody complex. Hepatitis C has also been associated with PAN.

The association of PAN with pregnancy is rare; only 13 cases of PAN and pregnancy have been reported.[163-168] Seven of the cases resulted in maternal death, each in the postpartum period. In all these patients, the onset of disease occurred during pregnancy or the early puerperium. Another patient, in whom Churg-Strauss vasculitis was diagnosed during her first pregnancy, had two subsequent spontaneous abortions and presented during her fourth pregnancy with an exacerbation of the disease, which proved fatal.[167] The five patients who survived received diagnoses and were treated before pregnancy. The fetal outcomes were good, and 10 infants survived. However, vasculitis in an infant of a woman who had a long history of cutaneous polyarteritis nodosa was reported.[169] The development of PAN in pregnancy may be confused with toxemia, but a fulminating diastolic hypertension in the presence of multisystem involvement should alert the clinician to the possibility of PAN.

The treatment of choice for PAN is high-dosage prednisone therapy. There are reports suggesting that cytotoxic medications may be helpful, particularly in aggressive renal disease and hypertension.[170,171] In the rare cases of the association of pregnancy with PAN, prompt diagnosis and treatment with control of the underlying disease is important. Therapeutic termination of pregnancy is indicated only for prevention of teratogenic side effects from cytotoxic drugs, but it does not appear to be necessary to ameliorate disease activity.[163]

Wegener's Granulomatosis

This entity has a distinctive clinicopathologic complex of necrotizing granulomatous vasculitis of the upper and lower respiratory tracts, necrotizing glomerulonephritis, and a variable disseminated small-vessel vasculitis. The clinical features include severe paranasal sinusitis, nasopharyngeal ulceration with nasal septal perforations and saddlenose deformity, and pulmonary infiltrates, occasionally with cavitation. Proteinuria, hematuria, and red blood cell casts with ensuing renal failure are the hallmark of generalized Wegener's granulomatosis. Skin involvement, with papules and ulcerations, is common. Coronary vasculitis and pancarditis, various ocular manifestations, and both cranial and peripheral nerve involvement occur in a large number of patients. Anemia, leukocytosis, hypergammaglobulinemia, and elevated ESR are characteristic laboratory features of Wegener's granulomatosis.[172] The presence of the antineutrophil cytoplasmic antibody directed against proteinase 3 is both sensitive and specific for Wegener's granulomatosis.[172,173]

Eighteen cases of Wegener's granulomatosis have been reported in relation to pregnancy.[174,175] In five patients, Wegener's granulomatosis was diagnosed before pregnancy, and all had healthy babies; only one pregnancy was complicated by preeclampsia. In five other patients, the diagnosis was made during pregnancy. Of these, one resulted in a therapeutic abortion at 13 weeks, and one neonate died at 1 month. One mother died 1 month after delivery, one required hemodialysis, and the other mothers experienced improvement. All were treated with oral corticosteroids, four also had oral cyclophosphamide, and one was given AZA therapy. Three patients in whom the disease was diagnosed after delivery did well. It appears that, as in PAN, if the underlying disease is under control at the time of conception, pregnancy has no deleterious effect on the disease and the disease has no adverse effect on the mother or infant.

The treatment of Wegener's granulomatosis is currently based on a combination of adequate steroid dose and oral cyclophosphamide.[172,176] Because of the paucity of cases, it is impossible to develop guidelines for treatment during pregnancy. However, because the disease may otherwise be fatal, the use of cytotoxic medications even during pregnancy may be indicated.

ANTIRHEUMATIC DRUG THERAPY AND REPRODUCTION

Any assessment of the patient with rheumatic disease who is contemplating a pregnancy requires careful consideration of past medication exposure and current pharmacologic therapy. Most drugs can be used while the patient is attempting to conceive, but some must be discontinued months before conception, and yet others merely require discontinuation once conception is confirmed. The use of specific agents varies, depending on the disease and its manifestations. This section reviews current medications used in treating most rheumatic disorders with some reference to their use in specific diseases. The safety profile of the various drugs is indicated with reference to the U.S. Food and Drug Administration safety ratings of drugs in pregnancy (Table 20–2). In addition, in certain instances, the internist must be aware of the implications of administering these medications to a patient trying to conceive. Specific reference is made to these issues as necessary.

TABLE 20–2   U.S. Food and Drug Administration Classification of Drugs in Pregnancy

A	Controlled studies show no risk
B	No evidence of risk in humans
C	Risk cannot be ruled out
D	Positive evidence of risk
X	Contraindicated in pregnancy

Nonsteroidal Antiinflammatory Drugs

The drugs most commonly used in the treatment of most rheumatic diseases are NSAIDs, which inhibit cyclooxygenase, thereby blunting the inflammatory response. They are the mainstay in the day-to-day treatment of RA and are used frequently for any disease characterized by arthritis. With the over-the-counter availability of some of these agents, it is especially important that both the internist and obstetrician be aware of all medications that the patient might be taking, prescribed or self-administered.

Many NSAIDs can actually contribute to difficulties conceiving, by inhibiting the prostaglandin-dependent event of follicular rupture and thereby preventing the release of the oocyte from the follicle.[177] In these cases, luteinization and oocyte maturation remain unaffected. Prostaglandins are also important in the motility of the fallopian tubes. Theoretically, NSAIDs could alter this function by inhibiting motility and the passage of the oocyte down the fallopian tube.[178,179] These effects might occur in a woman with RA who is dependent on the use of a nonsteroidal agent. Although any NSAID is capable of inhibition of the ovulatory event, indomethacin has been the agent most often studied.[177]

The use of aspirin in pregnancy, particularly the low-dose formulation of 80 mg, has become fairly common. The 80-mg dose has been used to prevent pregnancy loss, preeclampsia, and other adverse pregnancy outcomes.[103,180] Evidence supporting such use is still far from conclusive, but there appears to be little risk in using this dose during pregnancy. A metaanalysis found an increase in the incidence of gastroschisis (from 1 per 100,000 to 1 per 1000) in neonates exposed to aspirin during the first trimester.[184] This side effect, however, is nonetheless very uncommon, which further attests to the safety profile of aspirin at this dosage. Aspirin is capable of prolonging labor and can complicate delivery with an increase in antepartum and postpartum bleeding. For this reason, aspirin has a Food and Drug Administration rating of C/D when used in the third trimester. These problems can be avoided by discontinuing the aspirin at least 4 weeks before the expected delivery date.

Approximately 0.1% to 21% of the dose of aspirin reaches the infant through breast milk. This appears to be of concern only in high doses. The American Academy of Pediatrics (AAP) recommends both that aspirin be used cautiously and that breast-feeding mothers avoid high dosages.[185]

Most other NSAIDs have been used infrequently in pregnancy; therefore, there is little in the literature regarding their safety. Among those most studied are naproxen, ibuprofen, and indomethacin. Naproxen and ibuprofen appear to have the best safety record. The fetal risk is classified as category B, but when these drugs are used in high doses, the risk is classified as category C. During parturition, these drugs are classified as category D because of increased risks to the baby, such as intracranial hemorrhage at delivery, premature closure of the ductus arteriosus, and impaired renal function, as evidenced by a decrease in amniotic fluid volume. It is recommended that NSAIDs be discontinued 6 to 8 weeks before the expected delivery. It is best to plan with the patient to start to decrease the dose of the drug at approximately the 25th week and to discontinue these agents between the 28th and 32nd weeks.

The AAP considers naproxen and ibuprofen to be compatible with breast-feeding. Again, the lowest effective dose should be used.

The side effects regarding reproduction and pregnancy of the traditional NSAIDs, naproxen and ibuprofen, are shared by the newer cyclooxygenase 2 specific inhibitors, celecoxib and rofecoxib. These include potential inhibitory effects on ovulation, fallopian tube motility, and inhibition of blastocyst implantation during the time of conception.[186-189] With regard to pregnancy, the cyclooxygenase 2 inhibitors share the tocolytic effects of naproxen, ibuprofen, and indomethacin, as well as the adverse effects on renal blood flow.[190] The latter occurring in the fetus therefore affect amniotic fluid volume, as do the less specific cyclooxygenase inhibitors. These findings, however, have all been demonstrated in animal studies, inasmuch as there is little experience in humans. Although there appears to be little risk should conception occur while the patient is taking cyclooxygenase 2 inhibitors, too little experience exists to support the use of these agents in pregnancy.

Antimalarial Agents

The antimalarial class of drugs is used extensively in both RA and SLE. In RA, they are considered convenient and safe second-line agents. In SLE, they are used for the manifestations of arthritis and dermatitis. The major side effect is retinal toxicity, necessitating 6- to 12-month assessments by an ophthalmologist. Although chloroquine has been used extensively in the treatment of either condition, the more common agent is hydroxychloroquine, which presumably has less retinal toxicity. The antimalarial agents are long-acting drugs requiring about 6 to 12 weeks before any effect can be clinically detected.

The literature supports the use of antimalarial agents during pregnancy in patients with RA or SLE.[30] Khamashta and coauthors described a case-control study of 36 pregnancies in patients with SLE who took hydroxychloroquine.[191] Of the 36 pregnancies exposed to hydroxychloroquine, 31 resulted in live births, a frequency similar to that of the control group. Both Parke and Levy and associates described their experience and that of others supporting the use of hydroxychloroquine in pregnancy.[33,35] In a survey study of 78 SLE experts in North America and the United Kingdom, Al-Herz and associates found that 69% of respondents continue antimalarial therapy during pregnancy.[30] None of these physicians ever noted any fetal toxicity, nor was a pregnancy ever terminated unless requested by the patient. Of the respondents, 63% advised continuation of the drugs post partum in breast-feeding mothers. In a follow-up study of 21 children born to mothers who had taken an antimalarial drug during pregnancy, Klinger and colleagues found no evidence of ocular toxicity.[192] These authors concluded that antimalarial drugs taken during pregnancy do not appear to pose a significant risk of ocular toxicity to the offspring. With regard to breast-feeding, hydroxychloroquine has been deemed compatible by the AAP. In conclusion, antimalarial drugs can be used in pregnancy because the risk of disease exacerbation on withdrawal of the drugs exceeds any risk of fetal toxicity by continuing treatment.

Corticosteroids

Corticosteroids, most notably prednisone, are commonly used in the treatment of many rheumatic diseases. In many cases, their use is essential for gaining rapid control of a life-threatening disease process. Patients with RA respond to low dosages of prednisone, because the synovitis of this disease is very sensitive in most cases to corticosteroids; it is unusual to require more than 20 mg of prednisone daily to control the arthritis. Dosages in the range of 5 to 10 mg per day are typical.

In SLE, the prednisone dose tends to be higher, because disease manifestations are less sensitive. In patients with minor organ disease such as arthritis, dermatitis, or serositis, dosages in the range of 20 to 40 mg of prednisone per day usually suffice. Major organ disease, including renal and CNS involvement, are more commonly treated with 40 to 80 mg of prednisone per day. There is no indication to increase the dosage of prednisone routinely post partum in women with SLE unless there is a flare of the underlying disease. The appropriate dosage of prednisone for the patient is the minimally effective dosage.

The use of prednisone in pregnancy is associated with few side effects on the fetus. The drug must be used if the maternal clinical condition warrants its use regardless of the pregnant state. Maternal side effects of prednisone are usually proportional to the dosage used. In pregnancy, hypertension and diabetes mellitus are the more common side effects. In a double-blind, randomized, controlled trial, Laskin and coauthors found the incidence of hypertension to be 13% and that of diabetes mellitus to be 15% in the prednisone-treated group, in comparison with 5% for both of these disorders in the placebo-treated group.[97] The other side effects of corticosteroid use, including cushingoid features and loss of bone mass, occur in pregnancy, as they would in the nonpregnant woman.

Fetal side effects are few and are not of major concern. Case-control studies have shown a small but significant increase in orofacial clefting in the children of mothers treated with corticosteroids in the first trimester.[193,194] A metaanalysis showed the prevalence of orofacial cleft at 1 per 400, in comparison with the 1 per 800 expected in any pregnancy.[195] The risk of this congenital anomaly is still very low, but when prednisone is prescribed to the mother, she must be informed of this risk. Counseling such a patient must also include an explanation of the risk involved in *not* taking corticosteroids. In addition to the small risk of orofacial clefting, there was an increase in premature births in mothers treated with steroids.[195] Laskin and coauthors found premature births, at 37 weeks and earlier, in 62% of the prednisone-treated group, in comparison with 11% of the placebo-treated group.[97] All the neonates, however, were appropriate size for gestational age. Although prednisone is class D when used in the first trimester, the physician must weigh the risks to the mother of avoiding the drug against the low risk of fetal toxicity.

The AAP classifies prednisone as compatible with breast-feeding. There is minimal neonatal exposure with maternal dosages up to 40 mg of prednisone daily.

Sulfasalazine

Sulfasalazine is the only drug originally developed for the treatment of RA.[196] Although initial studies were not successful, it has been used effectively since the early 1980s in the treatment of RA. Its use in pregnancy is reported most extensively in patients with inflammatory bowel disease, for whom it appears to be safe.[197-199] There are no reported problems with fertility in women treated with sulfasalazine. In contrast, men treated with sulfasalazine often are found to have low sperm counts with low motility. At least 2 months are necessary to correct this condition after drug withdrawal.[200-201]

In spite of levels in breast milk of 40% to 60% of the maternal concentration, most neonates exhibit no adverse effects breast-feeding from mothers treated with sulfasalazine.[202] There is a report of bloody diarrhea in one infant exposed to sulfasalazine in breast milk.[203] Because of this latter report, the AAP classifies sulfasalazine as a drug to be administered to breast-feeding mothers with caution.

Azathioprine

AZA is an immunosuppressive agent often used in the treatment of more severe manifestations of certain rheumatic disorders. It is used extensively for its corticosteroid-sparing properties, which allow lower doses of corticosteroids to be used in a patient treated with AZA. Of all of the immunosuppressive agents, AZA appears to be the safest one to be used in pregnancy. Although AZA almost freely crosses the placental barrier, the fetal liver lacks the enzyme to convert AZA to 6-mercaptopurine, the active metabolite of the drugs[204]; therefore, the fetus is not exposed to 6-mercaptopurine, and this is to be protective for the fetus. There have been no reports of congenital anomalies in the offspring of women with SLE treated throughout their pregnancies with AZA.[205] Although some sporadic anomalies have been reported, including spontaneous abortions, intrauterine growth restriction, and prematurity, the abnormalities might just as easily be attributed to concurrent medication or the underlying disease in the mother.[197,204,206] The benefit of AZA in improving pregnancy outcome in women with SLE supports the use of this agent in pregnancy when coupled with the low probability of congenital anomalies.[38]

There are few data regarding the safety of breast-feeding in women treated with AZA. It is known that AZA is secreted in breast milk, but because of the lack of data, the AAP recommends that mothers not breast-feed when taking AZA.

Methotrexate

MTX is a folic acid antagonist that has been used with great success in treating RA. It has been used to a lesser extent in the treatment of SLE. MTX use in pregnancy has been implicated in causing spontaneous abortions as a result of its embryotoxicity. Indeed, MTX is used almost routinely as an abortifacient, particularly in the treatment of an ectopic pregnancy. The drug is well known to cause numerous fetal anomalies and has been associated with intrauterine growth restriction.[38,204] For these reasons, MTX is not to be used in pregnancy. Many authorities recommend that, if a woman taking MTX becomes pregnant, the pregnancy be electively terminated.

Because MTX binds to maternal tissues, it is recommended that it be discontinued 3 months before the woman conceives. A similar recommendation is given to men taking MTX who are planning a pregnancy. Although there are currently no reports of adverse pregnancy outcomes despite paternal exposure to MTX before conception, until better evidence exists, both men and women should avoid MTX for three months before attempting to conceive.[207]

Although MTX is excreted in breast milk to only a small degree, there is concern that it may bind to neonatal tissues with subsequent accumulation and toxicity.[208] Because of this potential toxicity, the AAP regards MTX as contraindicated in breast-feeding mothers.

Cyclophosphamide

Cyclophosphamide is a cytotoxic, alkylating agent used in the treatment of severe major organ disease in SLE and vasculitis. It is known to be embryotoxic and is associated with many fetal anomalies after exposure in the first trimester. It is teratogenic in early pregnancy but does not appear to be associated with anomalies if used in the second or third trimester. The drug should be avoided during pregnancy unless it is necessary for a life-threatening problem in the second or third trimester. Even under those circumstances, the mother must be counseled about the potential risks to both herself and her unborn child. Similarly, cyclophosphamide is contraindicated during breast-feeding because of the risk of neutropenia, immunosuppression, growth disturbances, and potential carcinogenesis in the newborn.[38,208]

Leflunomide

Leflunomide is a pyrimidine synthesis inhibitor used in the treatment of active RA. The active metabolite has a half-life of 2 weeks. The drug is in class X and is contraindicated in pregnancy because of dose-related teratogenicity and embryotoxicity when administered to animals in equivalent human dosages.[38] The drug should not be given to a woman until pregnancy has been ruled out. Furthermore, she should be taking an effective contraceptive. Leflunomide is of sufficiently low molecular weight that it is probably crosses the placental barrier, but this has not been confirmed, and the consequences of the drug in the fetal circulation are unknown at this time. The concern about this drug in both men and women contemplating a pregnancy is sufficient that the manufacturer has devised an elimination protocol in the case of inadvertent pregnancy or if pregnancy is contemplated, because it may take up to 2 years to eliminate the drug and for levels to become undetectable. Unfortunately, the elimination protocol probably is clinically ineffective if the woman is already pregnant; most physicians therefore advocate termination of the pregnancy in this circumstance.

There is no information regarding breast-feeding during leflunomide therapy. However, in view of the great concern regarding possible side effects, breast-feeding should probably not be undertaken. There is no recommendation from the AAP regarding leflunomide at this time.

Etanercept

Etanercept is a TNF-α inhibitor used in the treatment of RA. There are very few data on use of the drug in pregnancy other than a few case reports in the product insert and some animal studies.[209] In the animal studies, in which 60 to 100 times the dosage in humans was used, no fetal anomalies resulted. The human case reports also indicate that the agent does not appear to be teratogenic. Until further experience is reported, etanercept should be avoided during pregnancy. Similarly, there is insufficient information available to recommend the use of this drug in the breast-feeding mother.

Infliximab

Infliximab is another TNF-α inhibitor used in the treatment of active RA. Only a few abstracts have been published; they indicated that no anomalies occurred in women who became pregnant while taking infliximab.[209,210] Animal studies using up to 10 times the human dosage failed to show any adverse fetal effects. However, because so few data are available, this drug should not be used during pregnancy at this time. It therefore follows that that there are also few data available about the use of infliximab in breast-feeding. Hence, women taking infliximab should not breast-feed.

References

1. Bulla R, Bossi F, Radillo O, et al: Placental trophoblast and endothelial cells as target of maternal immune response. Autoimmunity 2003;36:11.
2. Firestein G: Etiology and pathogenesis of rheumatoid arthritis. In Kelley WN, Harris ED, Ruddy S, Sledge CB (eds): Textbook

of Rheumatology, vol 1, 5th ed. Philadelphia, WB Saunders, 1997, p 851.

3. Harris ED Jr: Clinical features of rheumatoid arthritis. In Kelley WN, Harris ED, Ruddy S, Sledge CB (eds): Textbook of Rheumatology, vol 1, 5th ed. Philadelphia, WB Saunders, 1997, p 896.

4. Ostensen M, Villiger PM: Immunology of pregnancy—pregnancy as a remission inducing agent in rheumatoid arthritis. Transpl Immunol 2002;9:155.

5. Hench PS: The amelioration effect of pregnancy on chronic atrophic (infectious) rheumatoid arthritis, fibrositis and intermittent hydrarthrosis. Proc Mayo Clin 1938;13:161.

6. Bulmash JM: Rheumatoid arthritis and pregnancy. Obstet Gynecol Ann 1978;8:276.

7. Persellin RH: The effect of pregnancy on rheumatoid arthritis. Bull Rheum Dis 1977;27:922.

8. Hazes JMW, Dukmans BAC, Vandenbroucke JP, et al: Pregnancy and the risk of developing rheumatoid arthritis. Arthritis Rheum 1990;33:1770.

9. Silman A, Kay A, Brennan P: Timing of pregnancy in relation to the onset of rheumatoid arthritis. Arthritis Rheum 1992;35:152.

10. Nelson JL, Ostensen M: Pregnancy and rheumatoid arthritis. Rheum Dis Clin North Am 1997;23:195.

11. Spector TD, Da Silva JAP: Pregnancy and rheumatoid arthritis: An overview. Am J Reprod Immunol 1992;28:222.

12. Barrett JH, Brennan P, Fiddler M, Silman A: Breast-feeding and postpartum relapse in women with rheumatoid and inflammatory arthritis. Arthritis Rheum 2000;43:1010.

13. Barrett JH, Brennan P, Fiddler M, Silman AJ: Does rheumatoid arthritis remit during pregnancy and relapse post partum? Results from a nationwide study in the United Kingdom performed prospectively from late pregnancy. Arthritis Rheum 2000;42:1219.

14. Plotz CM, Goldenberg A: Rheumatoid arthritis. In Ravinsky JJ, Gutman AF (eds): Medical, Surgical and Gynecological Complications of Pregnancy, 2nd ed. Baltimore, Williams & Wilkins, 1965, p 720.

15. Bijlsma JWJ, Van Den Brink HR: Estrogens and rheumatoid arthritis. Am J Reprod Immunol 1992;28:231.

16. Neely NT, Persellin RH: Activity of rheumatoid arthritis during pregnancy. Texas Med 1977;73:59.

17. Shimoaka Y, Hidaka Y, Tada H, et al: Changes in cytokine production during and after normal pregnancy. Am J Reprod Immunol 2000;44:143.

18. Elenkov IJ, Wilder RL, Bakalov VK, et al: IL-12, TNF-alpha, and hormonal changes during late pregnancy and early postpartum: Implications for autoimmune disease activity during these times. J Clin Endocrinol Metab 2001;86:4933.

19. Weetman AP: The immunology of pregnancy. Thyroid 1999;9:643.

20. Van Roon JA, Bijlsma JW, Lafeber FP: Suppression of inflammation and joint destruction in rheumatoid arthritis may require a concerted action of Th2 cytokines. Curr Opin Investig Drugs 2002;3:1011.

21. Nelson JL, Hughes KA, Smith AG, et al: Maternal-fetal disparity in HLA class II alloantigens and the pregnancy-induced amelioration of rheumatoid arthritis. N Engl J Med 1993;329:466.

22. Nelson JL, Hughes KA, Smith AG, et al: Remission of rheumatoid arthritis during pregnancy and maternal-fetal class II alloantigen disparity. Am J Reprod Immunol 1992;28:226.

23. Van der Horst-Bruinsma IE, de Vries RR, de Buck PD, et al: Influence of HLA–class II incompatibility between mother and fetus on the development and course of rheumatoid arthritis of the mother. Ann Rheum Dis 1998;57:286.

24. Brennan P, Barrett J, Fiddler M, et al: Maternal-fetal HLA incompatibility and the course of inflammatory arthritis during pregnancy. J Rheumatol 2000;27:2843.

25. Kaplan D, Diamond H: Rheumatoid arthritis and pregnancy. Clin Obstet Gynecol 1965;8:286.

26. Nelson JL, Koepsell RD, Dugowson CE, et al: Fecundity before disease onset in women with rheumatoid arthritis. Arthritis Rheum 1993;36:7.

27. Nelson JL, Voigt LF, Koepsell TD, et al: Pregnancy outcome in women with rheumatoid arthritis before disease onset. J Rheumatol 1992;19:18.

28. Drossaers-Bakker KW, Zwinderman AH, van Zeben D, et al: Pregnancy and oral contraceptive use do not significantly influence

outcome in long term rheumatoid arthritis. Ann Rheum Dis 2002;61:405.

29. Cutolo M, Villaggio B, Craviotto C, et al: Sex hormones and rheumatoid arthritis. Autoimmun Rev 2002;1:284.

30. Al-Herz A, Schulzer M, Esdaile JM: Survey of antimalarial use in lupus pregnancy and lactation. J Rheumatol 2002;29:700.

31. Ostebsen M, Ramsey-Goodman R: Treatment of inflammatory rheumatic disorders in pregnancy: What are the safest treatment options? Drug Saf 1998;19:389.

32. Costedoat-Chalumeau N, Amoura Z, Duhaut P, et al: Safety of hydroxychloroquine in pregnant patients wih connective tissue diseases: A study of 133 cases compared with a control group. Arthritis Rheum 2003;48:3207.

33. Levy RA, Vilela VS, Cataldo MJ, et al: Hydroxychloroquine (HCQ) in lupus pregnancy: Double-blind and placebo-controlled study. Lupus 2001;10:401.

34. Borden MB, Parke AL: Antimalarial drugs in systemic lupus erythematosus: Use in pregnancy. Drug Saf 2001;24:1055.

35. Parke A, West B: Hydroxychloroquine in pregnant patients with systemic lupus erythematosus. J Rheumatol 1996;23:1715.

36. Rains CP, Noble S, Faulds D: Sulfasalazine. A review of its pharmacological properties and therapeutic efficacy in the treatment of rheumatoid arthritis. Drugs 1995;50:137.

37. Janseen NM, Genta MS: The effects of immunosuppressive and anti-inflammatory medications on fertility, pregnancy and lactation. Arch Intern Med 2000;160:610.

38. Ramsey-Goldman R, Schilling E: Immunosuppressive drug use during pregnancy. Rheum Dis Clin North Am 1997;23:149.

39. Gladman DD, Urowitz, MB: Systemic lupus erythematosus—clinical features. In Klippel JH, Dieppe PA (eds): Rheumatology. St. Louis, Mosby, 1997, p 7.1.

40. Tan EM, Cohen AS, Fries J, et al: Criteria for the classification of systemic lupus erythematosus. Arthritis Rheum 1982;25:53.

41. Hahn BH: Pathogenesis of systemic lupus erythematosus. In Kelley WN, Harris ED, Ruddy S, Sledge CB (eds): Textbook of Rheumatology, vol 2, 5th ed. Philadelphia, WB Saunders, 1997, p 1015.

42. Arnett FC: The genetics of human lupus. In Wallace DJ, Hahn BH (eds): Dubois' Lupus Erythematosus, 5th ed. Baltimore, Williams & Wilkins, 1997, p 77.

43. Gladman DD, Urowitz MB, Cole E, et al: Kidney biopsy in SLE. 1. A clinical-morphologic correlations. Q J Med 1989;73:1125.

44. Urowitz MB, Gladman DD: Clinical monitoring. In Schur P (ed): The Clinical Management of Systemic Lupus Erythematosus, 2nd ed. New York, Lippincott Williams & Wilkins, 1996, p 225.

45. Fraga A, Mintz G, Orozco J, et al: Sterility and fertility rates, fetal wastage and maternal morbidity in systemic lupus erythematosus. J Rheumatol 1974;1:293.

46. Ellis FA, Bereston ES: Lupus erythematosus associated with pregnancy and menopause. AMA Arch Dermatol Syphilol 1952; 69:170.

47. Garenstein M, Poliak VE, Kark RM: Systemic lupus erythematosus and pregnancy. N Engl J Med 1962;267:165.

48. Mund A, Simson J, Rothfield N: Effect of pregnancy on the course of systemic lupus erythematosus. JAMA 1963;183:917.

49. Zurier RB: Systemic lupus erythematosus and pregnancy. Clin Rheum Dis 1975;1:613.

50. Grigor RR, Shervington PC, Hughes GRV, et al: Outcome of pregnancy in systemic lupus erythematosus. Proc R Soc Med 1977;70:99.

51. Tozman ECS, Urowitz MB, Gladman DD: Systemic lupus erythematosus and pregnancy. J Rheumatol 1980;7:624.

52. Zulman MI, Talal N, Hoffman GS, et al: Problems associated with the management of pregnancies in patients with systemic lupus erythematosus. J Rheumatol 1980;7:37.

53. Lockshin MD, Reinitz E, Druzin ML, et al: Lupus pregnancy: Case control study demonstrating absence of lupus exacerbations during and after pregnancy. Am J Med 1984;77:893.

54. Lockshin MD: Pregnancy does not cause systemic lupus erythematosus to worsen. Arthritis Rheum 1989;32:665.

55. Petri M: Hopkins lupus pregnancy center: 1987-1996. Rheum Dis Clin North Am 1997;23:1.

56. Ruiz-Irastorza G, Lima F, Alves J, et al: Increased rate of lupus flare during pregnancy and the puerperium: A prospective study of 78 pregnancies. Br J Rheumatol 1996;35:133.

57. Cortes-Hernandez J, Ordi-Ros J, Paredes F, et al: Clinical predictors of fetal and maternal outcome in systemic lupus erythematosus: A prospective study of 103 pregnancies. Rheumatology (Oxford) 2002;41:643.

58. Urowitz MB, Gladman DD, Farewell VT, et al: Lupus and pregnancy studies. Arthritis Rheum 1993;36:1392.

59. Yasmeen S, Wilkins EE, Field NT, et al: Pregnancy outcomes in women with systemic lupus erythematosus. J Matern Fetal Med 2001;10:91.

60. Jungers P, Dougados M, Pelissier C, et al: Lupus nephropathy and pregnancy. Arch Intern Med 1982;142:771.

61. Huong DL, Wechsler B, Vauthier-Brouzes D, et al: Pregnancy in past or present lupus nephritis: A study of 32 pregnancies from a single centre. Ann Rheum Dis 2001;60:599.

62. Moroni G, Quaglini S, Banfi G, et al: Pregnancy in lupus nephritis. Am J Kidney Dis 2002;40:713.

63. El-Sayed YY, Lu EJ, Genovese MC, et al: Central nervous system lupus and pregnancy: 11-year experience at a single center. J Matern Fetal Neonatal Med 2002;12:99.

64. Morris EK: Pregnancy in rheumatoid arthritis and systemic lupus erythematosus. N Z J Obstet Gynecol 1969;9:136.

65. Friedman EA, Rutherford JW: Pregnancy and lupus erythematosus. Obstet Gynecol 1956;8:601.

66. Lima F, Buchanan NMM, Kamashta MA, et al: Obstetric outcome in systemic lupus erythematosus. Semin Arthritis Rheum 1995;25:184.

67. Martinez-Rueda JO, Arce-Salinas CA, Kraus A, et al: Factors associated with fetal loss in severe systemic lupus erythematosus. Lupus 1996;5:113.

68. Clark CA, Spitzer KA, Laskin CA: Decrease in pregnancy loss rates in SLE over a 40-year period [abstract]. Arthritis Rheum 2003;48 Suppl:S180.

69. Hanly JG, Gladman DD, Rose TH, et al: Lupus pregnancy: A prospective study of placental changes. Arthritis Rheum 1988;31:358.

70. Abramowsky CR, Vegas ME, Swinehart G, et al: Decidual vasculopathy of the placenta in lupus erythematosus. N Engl J Med 1980;303:668.

71. Guzman E, Schulman H, Bracero L, et al: Uterine-umbilical artery Doppler velocimetry in pregnant women with systemic lupus erythematosus. J Ultrasound Med 1992;11:275.

72. Rahman P, Gladman DD, Urowitz MB: Clinical predictors of fetal outcome in systemic lupus erythematosus. J Rheumatol 1998;25:760.

73. Petri M, Allbritton J: Fetal outcome of lupus pregnancy: A retrospective case-control study of the Hopkins Lupus Cohort. J Rheumatol 1993;20:650.

74. Le Thi Huong DR, Wechsler B, Piette J-C, et al: Pregnancy and its outcomes in SLE. Q J Med 1994;87:721.

75. Julkunen H, Jouhikainen T, Kaaja R, et al: Fetal outcomes in lupus pregnancy: A retrospective case control study of 242 pregnancies in 112 patients. Lupus 1993;2:125.

76. Bresnihan B, Grigor RR, Oliver M, et al: Immunological mechanism for spontaneous abortion in systemic lupus erythematosus. Lancet 1977;2:1205.

77. Soloninka CA, Laskin CA, Wither J, et al: Clinical utility and specificity of anticardiolipin antibodies. J Rheumatol 1991;18:2849.

78. Alexander E, Buyon JP, Provost TT, et al: Anti-Ro/SSA antibodies in the pathophysiology of congenital heart block in neonatal lupus syndrome: An experimental model. Arthritis Rheum 1992;35:176.

79. Tseng CE, Buyon JP: Neonatal lupus syndrome. Rheum Dis Clin North Am 1997;23:31.

80. Gladman DD, Urowitz MB, Tozman ECS, et al: Haemostatic abnormalities in systemic lupus erythematosus. Q J Med 1983;52:424.

81. Parke AL: Antiphospholipid antibody syndromes. Rheum Dis Clin North Am 1989;15:275.

82. Petri M, Nelson L, Weiner E, et al: The automated modified Russell viper venom time test.

83. Laboratory heterogeneity of the lupus anticoagulant: A multicentre study using different clotting assays on a panel of 78 samples. Hemostasis Committee of the "Société Française de Biologie Clinique." Thromb Res 1992;15:349.

84. Legnani C, Palareti G, Boggian O, et al: An evaluation of several laboratory tests and test combinations in the detection of lupus anticoagulant. Int J Clin Lab Res 1992;22:106.

85. Jain A, Dash S, Marwaha N, et al: Assays for lupus anticoagulant: The sensitivity of different assays. Med Lab Sci 1991;48:31.

86. Clark-Soloninka CA, Spitzer KA, Nadler JN, Laskin CA: Evaluation of screening 590 plasma samples for the lupus anticoagulant using a panel of four tests. Arthritis Rheum 1998;41:S168.

87. Elias M, Eldor A: Thromboembolism in patients with the "lupus" type circulating anticoagulant. Arch Intern Med 1984;144:510.

88. Mueh JK, Herbst KD, Rapaport SI: Thrombosis in patients with lupus anticoagulant. Ann Intern Med 1980;92:156.

89. Lockshin MD, Druzin ML, Goei S, et al: Antibody to cardiolipin as a predictor of fetal distress or death in pregnant patients with systemic lupus erythematosus. N Engl J Med 1985;313:152.

90. Carreras LO, Machin SJ, Deman R, et al: Arterial thrombosis, intrauterine death and "lupus" anticoagulant: Detection of immunoglobulin interfering with prostacyclin formation. Lancet 1981;1:244.

91. Geis W, Branch DW: Obstetric implications of antiphospholipid antibodies: Pregnancy loss and other complications. Clin Obstet Gynecol 2001;44:2.

92. Oshiro BT, Silver RM, Scott JR, et al: Antiphospholipid antibodies and fetal death. Obstet Gynecol 1996;87:489.

93. Clark CA, Spitzer KA, Laskin CA: The spectrum of the antiphospholipid syndrome: A matter of perspective. J Rheumatol 2001;28:1939.

94. Out HJ, Bruinse HW, Chrustuaebs GCML, et al: A prospective, controlled multicenter study on the obstetric risks of pregnant women with antiphospholipid antibodies. Am J Obstet Gynecol 1992;167:26.

95. Vinatier D, Dufour P, Cosson M, Houpeau JL: Antiphospholipid syndrome and recurrent miscarriages. Eur J Obstet Gynecol Reprod Biol 2001;96:37.

96. Lubbe WFF, Pamer SJ, Butler WS, et al: Fetal survival after prednisone suppression of maternal lupus anticoagulant. Lancet 1983;2:1361.

97. Laskin CA, Bombardier C, Hannah M, et al: Prednisone and aspirin in women with autoantibodies and unexplained recurrent fetal loss. N Engl J Med 1997;337:148.

98. Rai R, Cohen H, Dave M, Regan L: Randomised controlled trial of aspirin and aspirin plus heparin in pregnant women with recurrent miscarriage associated with phospholipid antibodies (or antiphospholipid antibodies). BMJ 1997;314:253.

99. Kutteh WH: Antiphospholipid antibody–associated recurrent pregnancy loss: Treatment with heparin and low-dose aspirin is superior to low-dose aspirin alone. Am J Obstet Gynecol 1996;174:1584.

100. Huong DL, Wechsler B, Bletry O, et al: A study of 75 pregnancies in patients with antiphospholipid syndrome. J Rheumatol 2001;28:1939.

101. Farquharson RG, Quenby S, Greaves M: Antiphospholipid syndrome in pregnancy: A randomized, controlled trial of treatment. Obstet Gynecol 2002;100:408.

102. Shehata HA, Nelson-Piercy C, Khamashta MA: Management of pregnancy in antiphospholipid syndrome. Rheum Dis Clin North Am 2001;27:643.

103. Empson M, Lassere M, Craig JC, Scott JR: Recurrent pregnancy loss with antiphospholipid antibody: A systematic review of therapeutic trials. Obstet Gynecol 2002;100:135.

104. Laskin CA, Ginsberg J, Farine D, et al: Low molecular weight heparin and ASA therapy in women with autoantibodies and unexplained recurrent fetal loss (U-RFL). Society of Perinatal Obstetricians abstracts. Am J Obstet Gynecol 1997;176:S125.

105. Bridge RG, Folley FE: Placental transmission of the lupus erythematosus factor. Am J Med Sci 1954;227:1.

106. Jackson R: Discoid lupus erythematosus in a newborn infant of a mother with lupus erythematosus. Pediatrics 1964;33:425.

107. Weston WL, Harmon C, Peebles C, et al: A serologic marker for neonatal lupus erythematosus. Br J Dermatol 1982;107:377.

108. Scott JS, Maddison PJ, Taylor PV, et al: Connective tissue disease antibodies to ribonucleoproteins and congenital heart block. N Engl J Med 1983;309:209.

109. Brucato A. Frassi M, Franceschini F, et al: Risk of congenital complete heart block in newborns of mothers with anti-Ro/SSA

antibodies detected by counterimmunoelectrophoresis. Arthritis Rheum 2001;44:1832.

110. Brucato A, Doria A, Frassi M, et al: Pregnancy outcome in 100 women with autoimmune diseases and anti-Ro/SSA antibodies: A prospective controlled study. Lupus 2002;11:716.

111. Lee LA, Harmon CE, Huff C, et al: The demonstration of SSA/Ro antigen in human fetal tissues and in neonatal and adult skin. J Invest Dermatol 1985;85:143.

112. Urowitz MB, Gladman DD: Measures of disease activity and damage in SLE. Baillieres Clin Rheumatol 1998;12:406.

113. Mok CC, Wong RW, Lau CS: Exacerbation of systemic lupus erythematosus by breast feeding. Lupus 1998;7:569.

114. Ostensen M: Sex hormones and pregnancy in rheumatoid arthritis and systemic lupus erythematosus. Ann N Y Acad Sci 1999;876:131.

115. Cooper GS, Dooley MA, Treadwell EL, et al: Hormonal and reproductive risk factors for development of systemic lupus erythematosus: Results of a population-based, case-control study. Arthritis Rheum 2002;7:1809.

116. Jara LJ, Vera-Lastra O, Miranda JM, et al: Prolactin in human systemic lupus erythematosus. Lupus 2001;10:748.

117. Schleicher EM: LE cells after oral contraceptives. Lancet 1968;1:821.

118. Gill D: Rheumatic complaints of women using antiovulatory drugs. J Chron Dis 1968;21:435.

119. Dubois EL, Strain L, Ehn M, et al: LE cells after oral contraceptives. Lancet 1968;2:679.

120. Chapel RA, Burns RE: Oral contraceptives and exacerbation of lupus erythematosus. Am J Obstet Gynecol 1971;110:366.

121. Sanchez-Guerrero J, Karlson EW, Liang MH, et al: Past use of oral contraceptives and the risk of developing systemic lupus erythematosus. Arthritis Rheum 1997;40:804.

122. Lakasing L, Khamashta M: Contraceptive practices in women with systemic lupus erythematosus and/or antiphospholipid syndrome: What advice should we be giving? J Fam Plan Reprod Health Care 2001;27:7.

123. Le Thi Huong D, Wechsler B, Piette J-C, et al: Risks of ovulation induction therapy in systemic lupus erythematosus. Br J Rheumatol 1996;35:1184.

124. Guballa N, Sammaritano L, Schwartzman S, et al: Ovulation induction and in vitro fertilization in systemic lupus erythematosus and antiphospholipid syndrome. Arthritis Rheum 2000;43:550.

125. Winchester R: Genetic susceptibility to systemic lupus erythematosus. In Lahita RG (ed): Systemic Lupus Erythematosus, 2nd ed. New York, Churchill Livingstone, 1992, p 65.

126. Wright V, Moll JMH: Seronegative Polyarthritis. New York, North Holland, 1976.

127. Benjamin R, Parham P: HLA-B27 and disease: A consequence of inadvertent antigen presentation. Rheum Dis Clin North Am 1992;18:11.

128. Moll JMH: The place of psoriatic arthritis in the spondarthritides. Baillieres Clin Rheumatol 1994;8:395.

129. Gladman DD, Brubacher B, Langevitz P, et al: The spondyloarthropathies of psoriatic arthritis and ankylosing spondylitis: Genetic and gender effects. Clin Invest Med 1993;16:1.

130. Hart FD: Medical diseases in pregnancy. Proc R Soc Med 1959;52:771.

131. Ostensen M, Husby G: Ankylosing spondylitis and pregnancy. Rheum Dis Clin North Am 1989;15:241.

132. McHugh NJ, Laurent MR: The effect of pregnancy on the onset of psoriatic arthritis. Br J Rheumatol 1989;28:50.

133. Ostensen M: The effect of pregnancy on ankylosing spondylitis, psoriatic arthritis, and juvenile rheumatoid arthritis. Am J Reprod Immunol 1992;28:235.

134. Gladman DD: Natural history of psoriatic arthritis. Baillieres Clin Rheumatol 1994;8:379.

135. Seibold JR: Scleroderma. In Kelley WN, Harris ED, Ruddy S, Sledge CB (eds): Textbook of Rheumatology, vol 1, 5th ed. Philadelphia, WB Saunders, 1997, p 1133.

136. Mariq HR, LeRoy EC: Progressive systemic sclerosis: Disorders of the microcirculation. Clin Rheum Dis 1979;5:81.

137. Lee P, Langevitz P, Alderdice CA, et al: Mortality in systemic sclerosis (scleroderma). Q J Med 1992;82:139.

138. Masi A, for Subcommittee for Scleroderma Criteria of the American Rheumatism Association Diagnostic and Therapeutic Criteria Committee: Preliminary criteria for the classification of systemic sclerosis (scleroderma). Arthritis Rheum 1980;23:581.

139. Silman AJ, Black C: Increased incidence of spontaneous abortion and infertility in women with scleroderma before disease onset: A controlled study. Ann Rheum Dis 1988;47:441.

140. Englert H, Brennan P, McNeil D, et al: Reproductive function prior to disease onset in women with scleroderma. J Rheumatol 1992;19:1575.

141. Steen VD, Brodeur M, Conte C: Prospective pregnancy (PG) study in women with systemic sclerosis (Ssc). Arthritis Rheum 1996; 39(Suppl 9):S151.

142. Steen VD, Medsger TA Jr: Fertility and pregnancy outcome in women with systemic sclerosis. Arthritis Rheum 1999;42:763.

143. Sampaio-Barros PD, Samara AM, Marques Neto JF: Gynaecologic history in systemic sclerosis. Clin Rheumatol 2000;19:184.

144. Giordano M, Valentini G, Lupoli S, et al: Pregnancy and systemic sclerosis. Arthritis Rheum 1985;28:237.

145. Steen VD: Scleroderma and pregnancy. Rheum Dis Clin North Am 1997;23:133.

146. Spiera H, Krakoff L, Fishbane-Mayer J: Successful pregnancy after scleroderma hypertensive renal crisis. J Rheumatol 1989;16:1587.

147. Wilson AG, Kirby JD: Successful pregnancy in a woman with systemic sclerosis while taking nifedipine. Ann Rheum Dis 1990;49:51.

148. Avrech OM, Golan A, Pansky M, et al: Raynaud's phenomenon and peripheral gangrene complicating scleroderma in pregnancy—diagnosis and management. Br J Obstet Gynaecol 1992;99:850.

149. Black CM: Systemic sclerosis and pregnancy. Baillieres Clin Rheumatol 1990;4:105.

150. Maymon R, Fejgin M: Scleroderma in pregnancy. Obstet Gynecol Surv 1989;44:530.

151. Brown AN, Bolster MB: Scleroderma renal crisis in pregnancy associated with massive proteinuria. Clin Exp Rheumatol 2003;21:114.

152. Mok CC, Kwan TH, Chow L: Scleroderma renal crisis sine scleroderma during pregnancy. Scand J Rheumatol 2003;32:55.

153. Steen VD: Session 6: Connective tissue disease and pregnancy: Pregnancy in systemic sclerosis. Scand J Rheumatol 1998;27:72.

154. Rosenzweig BA, Rotmensch S, Binette SP, et al: Primary idiopathic polymyositis and dermatomyositis complicating pregnancy: Diagnosis and management. Obstet Gynecol 1989;44:162.

155. Satoh M, Ajmani AK, Hirakata M, et al: Onset of polymyositis with autoantibodies to threonyl-tRNA synthetase during pregnancy. J Rheumatol 1994;21:1564.

156. Harris A, Webley M, Usherwood M, Burge S: Dermatomyositis presenting in pregnancy. Br J Dermatol 1995;133:783.

157. Wortman RL: Inflammatory diseases of muscle and other myopathies. In Kelley WN, Harris ED, Ruddy S, Sledge CB (eds): Textbook of Rheumatology, vol 2, 5th ed. Philadelphia, WB Saunders, 1997, p 1177.

158. Tsai A, Lindheimer MD, Lamberg SI: Dermatomyositis complicating pregnancy. Obstet Gynecol 1973;41:570.

159. Baines AB, Link DA: Childhood dermatomyositis and pregnancy. Am J Obstet Gynecol 1983;145:335.

160. Houck W, Melnick C, Gast MJ: Polymyositis in pregnancy. A case report and a review of the literature. J Reprod Med 1987;32:208.

161. Silman AJ: Pregnancy and scleroderma. Am J Reprod Immunol 1992;28:238.

162. Valente RM, Hall S, O'Duffy JD, Conn DL: Vasculitis and related disorders. In Kelley WN, Harris ED, Ruddy S, Sledge CB (eds): Textbook of Rheumatology, vol 2, 5th ed. Philadelphia, WB Saunders, 1997, p 1079.

163. Nagey PA, Fatier KJ, Cinder J: Pregnancy complicated by periarteritis nodosa: Induced abortion as an alternative. J Obstet Gynecol 1983;147:103.

164. Pitkin RM: Polyarteritis nodosa. Clin Obstet Gynecol 1983;26:579.

165. Aya AG, Hoffet M, Mangin R, et al: Severe preeclampsia superimposed on polyarteritis nodosa. Am J Obstet Gynecol 1996;174:1659.

166. Fernandes SR, Cury CP, Samara AM: Pregnancy with a history of treated polyarteritis nodosa. J Rheumatol 1996;23:1119.

167. Connolly JO, Lanham JG, Partridge MR: Fulminant pregnancy-related Churg-Strauss syndrome. Br J Rheumatol 1994;33:776.

168. Ramsey-Goldman R: The effect of pregnancy on the vasculitides. Scand J Rheumatol Suppl 1998;107:116.

169. Stone MS, Olson RR, Weismann DN, et al: Cutaneous vasculitis in the newborn of a mother with cutaneous polyarteritis nodosa. J Am Acad Dermatol 1993;28:101.

170. Fauci AS, Katz P, Haynes BF, Wolff SM: Cyclophosphamide therapy of severe systemic necrotizing vasculitis. N Engl J Med 1979;301:235.
171. Leib ES, Restive C, Paulus HE: Immunosuppressive and corticosteroid therapy of polyarteritis nodosa. Am J Med 1979;67:941.
172. Duna GF, Galperin C, Hoffman GS: Wegener's granulomatosus. Rheum Dis Clin North Am 1995;20:949.
173. Gross WL: Antineutrophil cytoplasmic autoantibody testing in vasculitides. Rheum Dis Clin North Am 1995;20:987.
174. Luisiri P, Lance NJ, Curran JJ: Wegener's granulomatosus in pregnancy. Arthritis Rheum 1997;40:1354.
175. Auzary C, Huong DT, Wechsler B, et al: Pregnancy in patients with Wegener's granulomatosus: Report of five cases in three women. Ann Rheum Dis 2000;59:800.
176. Hoffman G: Treatment of Wegener's granulomatosus: Time to change the standard of care. Arthritis Rheum 1997;40:2099.
177. Killick S, Elstein M: Pharmacologic production of luteinized unruptured follicles by prostaglandin synthetase inhibitors. Fertil Steril 1987;47:773.
178. Elder MG, Myatt L, Chaudhuri G: The role of prostaglandins in the spontaneous motility of the fallopian tube. Fertil Steril 1977;28:86.
179. Laszlo A, Nadasy GL, Monos E, Zsolnai B: Effect of pharmacological agents on the activity of the circular and longitudinal smooth muscle layers of human fallopian tube ampullar segments. Acta Physiol Hung 1988;72:123.
180. Lee RM, Silver RM: Recurrent pregnancy loss: Summary and clinical recommendations. Semin Reprod Med 2000;18:433.
181. Franklin RD, Kutteh WH: Antiphospholipid antibodies (APA) and recurrent pregnancy loss: Treating a unique APA positive population. Hum Reprod 2002;17:2981.
182. Ahmed AS: Pre-eclampsia: Prevention. J R Soc Health 2003;123:9.
183. Grandone E, Brancaccio V, Colaizzo D, et al: Preventing adverse obstetric outcomes in women with genetic thrombophilia. Fertil Steril 2002;78:371.
184. Kozer E, Nikfar S, Costei A, et al: Aspirin consumption during the first trimester of pregnancy and congenital anomalies: a meta-analysis. Am J Obstet Gynecol 2002;187:1623.
185. American Academy of Pediatrics Committee on Drugs: The transfer of drugs and other chemicals into human milk. Pediatrics 1994;93:137.
186. Mertz HL, Liu J, Valego NK, et al: Inhibition of cyclooxygenase-2: Effects on renin secretion and expression in fetal lambs. Am J Physiol Regul Integr Comp Physiol 2003;284:R1012.
187. Sakai M, Tanebe K, Sasaki Y, et al: Evaluation of the tocolytic effect of a selective cyclooxygenase-2 inhibitor in a mouse model of lipopolysaccharide-induced preterm delivery. Mol Hum Reprod 2001;7:595.
188. Sookvanichsilp N, Pulbutr P: Anti-implantation effects of indomethacin and celecoxib in rats. Contraception 2002;65:373.
189. Lim H, Paria BC, Das SK, et al: Multiple female reproductive failures in cyclooxygenase 2–deficient mice. Cell 1997;91:197.
190. Stika CS, Gross GA, Leguizamon G, et al: A prospective randomized safety trial of celecoxib for treatment of preterm labor. Am J Obstet Gynecol 2002;187:653.
191. Khamashta MA, Buchanan NM, Hughes GR: The use of hydroxychloroquine in lupus pregnancy: The British experience. Lupus 1996;5(Suppl 1):S65.
192. Klinger G, Morad Y, Westall CA, et al: Ocular toxicity and antenatal exposure to chloroquine or hydroxychloroquine for rheumatic diseases. Lancet 2001;358:813.
193. Carmichael SL, Shaw GM: Maternal corticosteroid use and risk of selected congenital anomalies. Am J Med Genet 1999;86:242.
194. Rodriguez-Pinilla E, Martinez-Frias ML: Corticosteroids during pregnancy and oral clefts: A case-control study. Teratology 1998;58:2.
195. Park-Wyllie L, Mazzotta P, Pastuszak A, et al: Birth defects following maternal exposure to corticosteroids: A prospective cohort study and meta-analysis of epidemiological studies. Teratology 2000;62:385.
196. Day RO: Sulphasalazine. In Kelley WN, Harris ED, Ruddy S, Sledge CB (eds): Textbook of Rheumatology, vol 1, 5th ed. Philadelphia, WB Saunders, 1997, p 741.
197. Ostensen MA: Treatment with immunosuppressive and disease modifying drugs during pregnancy and lactation. Am J Reprod Immunol 1992;28:148.
198. Ferrero S, Ragni N: Inflammatory bowel disease: Management issues during pregnancy. Arch Gynecol Obstet [epub 2003; April 30].
199. Rajapakse R, Korelitz BI: Inflammatory bowel disease during pregnancy. Curr Treat Options Gastroenterol 2001;4:245.
200. Toovey S, Hudson E, Hendry WF, Levi AJ: Sulphasalazine and male infertility: Reversibility and possible mechanism. Gut 1981;22:445.
201. Freeman JC, Reece VAC, Venables CW: Sulphasalazine and spermatogenesis. Digestion 1982;23:68.
202. Jarnerot G, Into-Malmberg MB: Sulphasalazine treatment during breast feeding. Scand J Gastroenterol 1979;14:869.
203. Branski D, Kerem E, Gross-Kieselstein E, et al: Bloody diarrhea—a possible complication of sulfasalazine transferred through human breast milk. J Pediatr Gastroenterol Nutr 1986;5:316.
204. Janssen NM, Genta MS: The effects of immunosuppressive and anti-inflammatory medications on fertility, pregnancy, and lactation. Arch Intern Med 2000;160:610.
205. Bermas BL, Hill JA: Effects of immunosuppressive drugs during pregnancy. Arthritis Rheum 1995;38:1722.
206. Davison JM, Lindheimer MD: Pregnancy in renal transplant patients. J Reprod Med 1982;27:613.
207. French AE, Koren G, Motherisk Team: Effect of methotrexate on male fertility. Can Fam Physician 2003;49:577.
208. Committee on Drugs, American Academy of Pediatrics: The transfer of drugs and other chemicals into human milk. Pediatrics 1994;93:137.
209. Chakravarty EF, Sanchez-Yamamoto D, Bush TM: The use of disease modifying antirheumatic drugs in women with rheumatoid arthritis of childbearing age: A survey of practice patterns and pregnancy outcomes. J Rheumatol 2003;30:241.
210. Antoni CE, Furst D, Manger B, et al: Outcome of pregnancy in disease receiving Remicade (infliximab) for the treatment of Crohn's disease or rheumatoid arthritis [Abstract]. Arthritis Rheum 2001;44(Suppl):S53.

21

IMMUNOLOGY OF PREGNANCY

David A. Clark

The importance of the immune system is evident from acquired immunodeficiency syndrome, the disease that destroys it. If an organism's immune system cannot distinguish nonself from self, and, thus, reject nonself that is dangerous (e.g., pathogens), the organism dies. However, the reproduction of mammals requires a certain degree of "tolerance" for nonself. The gametes of the male are foreign to the female, and conceptus resulting from sperm fertilizing the oocyte is 50% foreign DNA. The survival of the embryo during gestation has been viewed as a paradoxically successful allograft (because the male is foreign by virtue of individual specific alloantigens expressed on the surface of male cells),[1] as a successful tumor,[2] and as a typical symbiotic host-parasite relationship in which the fetus is the parasite that can be terminated if the life of the mother is threatened.[3]

The success of reproduction is currently believed to depend on (1) special properties of fetal trophoblast cells that are "foreign" to, but are species compatible with, the mother[3,4] and (2) a degree of compromise of the mother's defense mechanisms, minimizing the chance of rejection of the intrauterine fetoplacental unit as an "innocent bystander."[5,6] Alterations in the defense system occur as local phenomena in the uterus and as systemic changes that may be beneficial (e.g., rheumatoid arthritis remits) or harmful (e.g., certain severe infections, including those that lead to infertility, miscarriage, or premature parturition, occur).[3,6-13] Conversely, lack of local or systemic compromise can lead to problems such as infertility, clinical miscarriages, pregnancy gestosis (preeclampsia), and premature labor in the absence of a specifically identified agonist.[3,7-12]

The objective of this chapter is to describe the current understanding of local and systemic alterations linked to the success of pregnancy and what may go wrong to cause disease.

BRIEF SUMMARY OF THE IMMUNE SYSTEM

Host defense mechanisms that preserve the integrity of the organism consist of sets of cells and molecules with special functions. Preserving the organism's integrity requires an ability to recognize a threat (i.e., danger).[14] Such threats usually come from outside the organism and manifest at a cutaneous or mucosal surface. Not surprisingly, the skin is a particularly effective site for inducing an immune response to a foreign protein (i.e., antigen), and lymphomyeloid cells that mediate host defenses are present in significant numbers at the interface between inside and outside.[15] This is particularly evident in mucosal tissues, in which some of the lymphocytes and precursors of antigen-presenting cells (APCs) may reside within the epithelium (intraepithelial lymphocytes).[16-19] At mucosal sites, such as the intestine, a particularly high concentration of "antigen" in the form of food, yeast, and bacteria exists. If the host's immune system were to respond to such antigens, the host would quickly turn into a large ball composed mainly of immune system cells. Thus, a distinction must be made so that responses develop against only what is dangerous, and there must be control mechanisms to allow the host to tolerate the presence of innocuous but foreign material.[14]

The term *immune system* usually refers to antigen-specific thymus-derived (T) lymphocytes responsible for cell-mediated immunity and bone marrow–derived (B) lymphocytes that make antibodies.[19] The function of these cells depends on antigen processing and presentation. Various cell types can present antigen, but macrophages and, in particular, a subset of phagocytic cells that mature into dendritic cells are particularly important. It is now clear that the antigen-specific immune system is merely a more specific targeting system developed by vertebrates, and its function is controlled and regulated to a major extent by lymphomyeloid cells, which constitute the innate or natural immune system.[19] When inflammation ensues, the vascular and blood coagulation systems are also involved. A schematic diagram illustrating this division of labor is shown in Figure 21–1.

The most primitive defensive cells are phagocytic and participate in the inflammatory response; they include macrophages and polymorphonuclear leukocytes. Related molecules include those of the coagulation system and complement series of enzymes that attract inflammatory cells and that provide binders, such as C3b, which attach to invaders and secure them to C3b receptors on

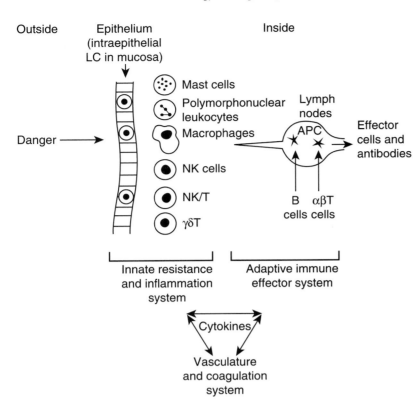

Figure 21–1. Potential responders to external "danger" presenting at an epithelial surface, such as the female genital tract. Other mucosal surfaces, such as gut and lung, have phagocytic macrophage cells within the epithelium to sample luminal contents. APC, antigen-presenting cell; B cell, bone marrow–derived immunocompetent lymphocyte; LC, lymphocyte; NK, natural killer; T cell, thymus-derived lymphocyte in the classical sense, but term is currently used for any cell expressing T cell receptor (TCR) for antigen on its surface, including NK/T, TCR αβ, and TCR γδ (a proportion of which develop without the need for a thymus).

phagocytic cells.[19] At a slightly more advanced level of evolution of innate defenses, natural killer (NK) cells provide a rapid initial response to infection and have surface receptors, known as killer inhibitory receptors, for major histocompatibility complex (MHC) self molecules, which inhibit killing of the organism's own cells.[20] The vertebrate classical immune system adds T lymphocytes that have the additional property of "memory," resulting in a more rapid response on second exposure to the same foreign antigen and a distinct change in circulation pattern after education by antigen.

Of the T cells, some have classical αβ receptors that recognize eight- or nine–amino acid peptides presented in the groove of MHC self molecules. Triggering requires coreceptor interactions between CD8 and class I MHC and between CD4 and class II MHC; several other types of adhesion receptor–ligand interaction may also act to strengthen the binding so that a sufficient T cell receptor occupancy is achieved to activate the cell.[19] A second signal is then required, or the T cell dies; the second signal can be provided by two pathways. A subset of macrophage-like phagocytic cells processes antigen at the initial site of encounter and then migrates via blood or lymphatic vessels to the spleen and lymph nodes, where they mature into very powerful APCs, called *dendritic cells.*[21] These cells express antigen on the surface of their dendrite-like processes, which is an efficient way to optimize delivery of the first signal. Dendritic cells (see APC in Fig. 21-1) also express surface molecules, such as B7, which interacts with CD28 on the T cell, and CD40 ligand, which interacts with CD40, and a variety of other adhesion ligand-receptor pairs; these interactions deliver the second signal.

Once the second signal is received, T cell growth and differentiation into effector cells can occur in response to small peptides in the milieu called *cytokines.* There are second signals that either turn off the system, as in B7 interaction with CTLA4 (present on certain T cells)[22] or deliver signals that lead to "tolerance." An example of this latter signaling is provided by the OX-2, now designated as CD200, a molecule that is expressed on subpopulations of "dendritic" APCs, as well as on fetal trophoblast cells and on as yet-unidentified cells in uterine decidua[23,24]. CD200 + antigen stimulates certain types of T cells to act as "suppressor T cells" by release of the cytokines interleukin (IL)-10 and transforming growth factor (TGF)-β.[23,24] CD200 can also bind to small activated antigen-presenting macrophages and stimulates production of indole amine 2,3-dioxygenase (IDO) which degrades the essential amino acid tryptophan[25]; αβ T cells reacting to antigen on such macrophages are thought to die.

A second type of T cell has γδ receptors, and cells of this type are rendered immunosuppressive by CD200 + antigen.[22,24,25] A significant portion of such cells develop in the absence of a thymus gland, need not express CD4 or CD8, have receptor specificity dictated by germline genes (and thus are said to be canonical), and clearly belong to the innate resistance system because they respond rapidly to antigen, show little evidence of "memory," and developed before the evolution of vertebrates[26,27]. Most γδ T cells reside at mucosal and epithelial surfaces and do not recirculate. Some γδ T cells recognize antigen in the absence of an APC and can bind to complex carbohydrate antigens as well as low-molecular-weight phosphoantigens and heat shock proteins; heat shock proteins are expressed by damaged cells. This type of recognition is similar to but more specific than that exhibited by NK cells and macrophages. γδ T cells can also recognize non-polymorphic MHC antigens, such as human leukocyte antigen (HLA)-G and HLA-E and CD1 in the mouse.[26,27] Although peptides associated with the antigen-binding groove on MHC molecules can modify recognition by γδ T cells, the γδ receptor does not directly recognize or bind to peptides in the groove. The recognition repertoire of γδ T cells differs among various subsets defined by which of the nine γ chains is used; importantly, the $γ_1$ chain defines a unique T cell subset that can recognize and react to trophoblast cells.[28]

Activated T cells of the αβ and γδ type may exhibit antigen-specific killing, may produce cytokines that enhance or suppress inflammation, and may "help" B cells become mature plasma cells that secrete the B cell receptor in the form of antibody molecules.[19] Antibody molecules increase the probability of an interaction with antigen, can be secreted at mucosal surfaces to prevent passage of antigen across and into the organism (e.g., immunoglob-ulin A [IgA]), and can interact with receptors of phago-cytic cells and with complement components. Antibody usually does not bind the small peptides seen by αβ T cell receptors but instead reacts with large proteins, peptides, and carbohydrates. The γδ T cell receptor for antigen is similar in many respects to antibody.[26] However, antigen recognition by γδ T cells may be restricted by CD1, as mentioned earlier. γδ T cells at mucosal surfaces commonly express NK cell markers, which has led to the suggestion that γδ T cells may represent an intermediary step in development between NK cells and αβ T cells (which are present only in vertebrates).[26,27]

The αβ T cell system is destroyed by human immuno-deficiency virus infection, and the consequences underline the importance of αβ T cells, particularly type 1 helper T (Th1) cells for inflammation/cell-mediated immunity and type 2 helper T (Th2) cells for antibody responses (Table 21–1).[19] However, resistance during the initial stages of infection is mediated by the innate resistance system, which includes macrophages, NK cells, and natu-ral T cells. Natural T cells may be αβ or γδ, bear activation receptors of NK cells, and act immediately, without the need for a preliminary proliferation step, as part of the normal immune response.[27,29-32] Recognition of these cell types is preprogrammed and may include production of proinflammatory cytokines of the Th1 variety (e.g., IL-1, IL-12, interferon-γ [INF-γ], tumor necrosis factor [TNF]) in response to particular archetypal motifs on pathogens or Th2 reactions (e.g., IL-4, IL-10) in response to other patterns and motifs.[30]

As explained earlier, activation of conventional αβ T cells involves recognition of antigen (short eight- to nine–amino acid peptides) bound to a groove of the organism's own MHC antigens, but the nature and vigor of the response seem to be determined by the innate sys-tem. Activated αβ helper T cells exposed to IFN-γ and IL-12 develop into Th1-type cells, and those exposed to IL-4 develop into Th2-type cells.[19,32] The role proposed for the innate system is to recognize and respond immediately to what is "dangerous" and to direct the subsequent response to the αβ T cells of the adaptive immune system.[30]

TABLE 21–1   Th1, Th2, and Th3 Cytokines

Effector Classification	Distinctive Cytokines	Common/Shared Cytokines
Th0	Any Th1 + any Th2 + shared cytokines	—
Th1	IL-2, IFN-γ, TNF-β, IL-12, IL-15, IL-17, IL-18	IL-3, IL-6, GM-CSF, TNF-α
Th2	IL-4, IL-5, IL-6, IL-9, IL-10, IL-13	IL-3, GM-CSF, ± TNF-α
Th3	TGF-βs	Unknown

Data from Janeway CA Jr, Travers P: Immunobiology, 3rd ed. New York, Garland Publishing, 1997, and from Mosmann TR, Sad S: The expanding universe of T-cell subsets: Th1, Th2, and more. Immunol Today 1996;17:138-146, and updated from the literature to 2003.
GM-CSF, granulocyte-macrophage colony–stimulating factor; IFN, interferon; IL, interleukin; TGF, transforming growth factor; Th1, Th2, and Th3, helper T cell types 1, 2, and 3; TNF, tumor necrosis factor.

The requirement for such direction may explain, in part, why the organism may have circulating αβ T cells to its own self antigens and yet not mount a self-destructive immune response.[14] A good example of "danger" is bacterial lipopolysaccharide (LPS) (or endotoxin). Chronic injection of strains of mice that do not ordinarily develop autoanti-bodies can lead to production of these strains in sufficient quantities to be pathogenic.[33] Antibody responses are usually linked to production of Th2 cytokines. LPS also stimulates production of proinflammatory Th1-type cytokines, such as TNF-α, and IFN-γ, and increases expression of B7 on APCs. The lipid A of LPS associates with a plasma LPS-binding protein, binds to the CD14 molecule on APCs, and is then "presented" to Toll-like receptor.[34] Toll-like receptor then delivers the activating signal to the APC. At least nine Toll-like receptor recep-tors have been identified, and each has a different speci-ficity that determines its ability to react with particular pathogen-associated molecular patterns. Lipid A binds in mice to Toll-like receptor 4, bacterial flagellin to Toll-like receptor 5, double-stranded RNA to Toll-like receptor 3, and bacterial DNA to Toll-like receptor 9. It is not known whether all Toll-like receptor ligands are presented via CD14. Expression of CD14 depends on coexpression on the cell of the MD-1 molecule, and inhibiting MD-1 expression diminishes both αβ T cell responses to antigen and responses to LPS.[35] Although production of cytokines such as TNF-α result from this signaling,[36] it appears that the ability of cytokines such as TNF-α to act optimally on a target cell bearing a TNF-α receptor requires the presence of a Toll-like receptor signal; TNF-α cannot produce shock without LPS, and blocking CD14 via inhibition of MD-1 prevents responses to TNF-α.[35,37] The importance of these interactions in pregnancy are explained later.

Danger signals, when present, do not invariably lead to harmful responses. This has two explanations: (1) The individual may not have αβ T cells specific for epitopes on self antigens to which effector cells (cytotoxic T lympho-cyte or helper T cell) must be generated to inflict actual damage on an organ, or (2) there may be mechanisms that promote "tolerance" via active suppression through IL-4 and IL-10. Some Toll-like receptor ligands stimulate Th2 rather than Th1 cytokine production.[38] Mucosa-associated T cells may also produce TGF-βs, which are potent immunosuppressants; these T cells have been called Th3[39] and may be responsible for nonreactivity in the intestine (i.e., oral tolerance) to the many antigens that are normally associated with intestinal contents (i.e., food antigens). CD200 may also exert a direct inhibitory effect on the response of cells to Toll-like receptor ligands.

One of the best experiments demonstrating the physiologic importance of suppression by T cells in preventing autoimmune disease promotion by normal levels of endogenous danger signals were those involving neonatal thymectomy in mice.[40] Thymectomy on day 1 of life (but not later) leads to autoimmune oophoritis by removing the suppressor T cells specific for autoantigen in this tissue before they emigrate from the thymus to the periphery. Antibody to antigen can also inhibit T cell responses,[19] but because antibody does not normally bind to the peptide in the groove of the MHC on the APC, a direct competition for the same epitope that is seen (i.e., recognized) by T cells is unlikely to occur. Anti-MHC antibody may sterically interfere with T cell recognition (i.e., blocking antibody) but usually only in the artificial setting of transplantation of allogeneic tissue.

There are several pathways by which a pathogen can take advantage of the phenomenon of tolerance. A foreigner can be invisible (i.e., express no recognizable antigens or signal 1 or fail to induce, through Toll-like receptor, the upregulation of signal 2 molecules on APCs), can be invulnerable (i.e., resist mechanisms that normally kill foreigners; such resistance is similar to evasion mechanisms exhibited by successful bacterial pathogens), or can inhibit (i.e., actively suppress of any attack).[41] Both antibody and T cells can "turn off" (i.e., suppress) inflammation and antigen-specific rejection responses, and this provides an opportunity for a parasite to inhibit rejection indirectly. The mammalian embryo is a type of parasite that appears to peacefully coexist with the immunocompetent mother, notwithstanding direct contact with maternal uterine tissues, and it is this type of parasitic relationship that is the focus for the remainder of this chapter.

STAGES IN THE PARASITE'S LIFE CYCLE

Figure 21-2 illustrates early events in mammalian reproduction. Gametes bear antigens to which the female can respond.[42] In a female with autoimmunity to the zona pellucida that envelopes the oocytes, infertility may develop as a result of autoimmune oophoritis.[43] This can lead to premature menopause. Removal of the thymus of mice on day 1 of life (but not on day 2) can lead to spontaneous oophoritis, and grafting day 1 thymocytes to thymectomized neonates restores protection of the oocytes.[40] This suggests that suppressor T cells specific for ovarian autoantigens mature and leave the thymus between days 1 and 2 after birth, and thymectomy therefore prevents them from doing so; these are probably αβ T cells. A similar autoimmune infertility can be created by thymectomizing male mice.[39] Gamete antigens are also thought to be sequestered; that is, they are not normally presented by an APC to the T and B cells of the host. Trauma can achieve exposure, however, and in vasectomized males, antisperm antibodies can be induced and may block restoration of fertility by vasectomy reversal surgery.[44] The antibodies of primary importance are those within

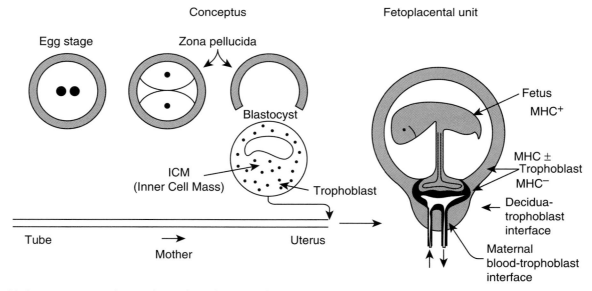

PREGNANCY AS PARASITISM: LIFE CYCLE OF A FETAL ALLOGRAFT

Figure 21–2. Host-parasite relations during the early stages of mammalian reproduction. MHC, major histocompatibility complex. (Reprinted from Clark DA, Arck PC, Chaouat G: Why did your mother reject you? Immunogenetic determinants of the response to environmental selective pressure expressed at the uterine level. Am J Reprod Immunol 1999;41:5-22.)

the genital tract, usually IgA or immunoglobulin G (IgG), which impair sperm function. Production of the latter can occur by agglutination, immobilization in cervical mucus, and masking of surface molecules on sperm required for binding to the zona pellucida. Although the female genital tract is immunocompetent to deal with infectious organisms, and although the female genital mucosa may be repeatedly assaulted by millions of spermatozoa, seldom does the female make antisperm antibodies. The lack of a response may result from low levels of surface antigen and the presence of immunosuppressive substances in semen. The major immunosuppressive factors include prostaglandin E and TGF-β.[45] Immunosuppression does not always prevent an immune response in the female. Some women make antisperm antibodies; the most important antisperm antibodies from the standpoint of fertility are those that are present in the genital tract, primarily IgA and IgG. A woman can also be sensitized to antigen in seminal plasma, and this has been responsible for the clinical phenomenon of postintercourse anaphylaxis. Fortunately, desensitization is possible.[46,47]

Certain nonspecific factors in human seminal plasma may promote implantation of blastocysts[48]; the possible mechanism of this effect is discussed later. It is also suggested that an active immune response to certain antigens specific for the male may elicit an immune response that reduces the chance of pregnancy-induced hypertension by enabling the fetal trophoblast to better invade the walls of maternal spiral arteries and convert them into low-resistance conduits through which large volumes of blood may be pumped to provide the nutrition required by the parasite during its final growth phase (the third trimester in humans).[9] Otherwise, the parasite needs to activate mechanisms to boost maternal blood pressure to obtain the necessary flow. The regulation of trophoblast growth and invasion is thought to depend on expression of particular adhesion receptors (integrins) on the trophoblast[49,50]; a differential sensitivity to inhibition by TGF-β_1 and TGF-β_3 (but not TGF-β_2) that is caused by binding of the former to the TGF-β_1 and TGF-β_3 receptor, endoglin[51]; and effects of other cytokines on growth, motility, and differentiation, as are discussed later. Finally, when the parasite is mature, it sends signals to the mother that restore contractile vigor to uterine musculature; thus, labor ensues and the parasite is expelled into the outside world to become an independent being.[52] Cytokines similar to those that cause abortion (IL-1, TNF-α, INF-γ) have been implicated in triggering parturition and may be produced by fetal membranes or by lymphomyeloid cells responding to infection.[13]

IMMUNOLOGIC ASPECTS OF PREGNANCY

It is clear from Figures 21–1 and 21–2 that the interaction between an intrauterine parasite at the mucosal surface of the uterus and the maternal defense system can be conveniently considered in several ways:

1. Local effects of pregnancy on the uterus
2. Effects of the local uterine immune system on the pregnancy (i.e., parasite)

3. Systemic effects of pregnancy on maternal immunity
   a. Effects due to the hormonal alterations of pregnancy
   b. Nonhormonal mechanisms used by the parasite
4. Effects of maternal systemic immunity on the pregnancy (i.e., parasite)

Local Effects of Pregnancy on the Uterus

The epithelium and stroma that line the mammalian uterus undergo cyclic growth, differentiation, and regression in response to estradiol and progesterone secreted by the ovary. In primates, actual necrosis, sloughing, and external expulsion of blood and tissue (menstruation) occur. However, in other species, such as rodents, the cells appear to die by apoptosis and are reabsorbed. In association with the cycle, there are distinct patterns of accumulation of different lymphomyeloid cell subsets in the uterine lining.[53] In humans, granulated NK-like cells accumulate in the luteal phase. These cells carry the CD56 surface marker but (unlike classical NK cells in blood) lack CD16, the receptor for the crystallized fragment end of IgG. With necrosis, polymorphonuclear leukocytes appear. Initial necrosis is caused by spasm of spiral arteries when progesterone levels fall. There is then relaxation and bleeding that facilitate sloughing of the outer two thirds of the uterine lining. Then bleeding stops and the epithelium regenerates from remnants of glands in the remaining stroma, and lymphocytes reenter the epithelium to repopulate the intraepithelial lymphocyte compartment. Hemostasis at the time of menstruation is a complex process in which cytokines play an important role.[53] Excessive bleeding at the time of menses is associated with certain types of intrauterine devices that attract maternal macrophages and stimulate Th1 cytokine production; excessive bleeding as also seen with progestogen-only contraceptive agents that lead to endometrial atrophy. Interestingly, the tendency to bleed in this situation has been linked to increased numbers of T cells, macrophages, and decreased numbers of granulated NK-lineage (CD56+ type) cells in the endometrium[54] (Table 21–2). Interestingly, some women untroubled by unscheduled bleeding (see Table 21–2) can have an acellular/atrophic endometrium.[55]

When conception occurs in a normal cycle in the human, there is a 6-day period of development to the blastocyst stage, and as the time of implantation approaches, the frequency of the uterine intraepithelial lymphocyte decreases and the cytotoxic activity of the intraepithelial lymphocyte diminishes.[18,56] The blastocysts adhere to the epithelium; trophoblast cells penetrate it and establish an invasive front of syncytiotrophoblast.[57] Lacunar spaces develop and fill with maternal blood from the ends of digested vessels, but, to keep the pressure low, there is a significant degree of occlusion by trophoblasts in the form of a plug (endovascular trophoblasts). Human chorionic gonadotropin produced by syncytiotrophoblasts appears in the bloodstream at the time of implantation and is thought to maintain hormone secretion by the corpus luteum. Estradiol and progesterone lead to transformation

TABLE 21–2   Endometrial Granulated Lymphocytes in Women Receiving Levonorgestrel (Norplant) Progestogen Contraception

Group	Number	Unevaluable*	Evaluable	No. Cells per Square Millimeter (mean ± 1 SEM)†
No bleeding	12	6	6	$P < .025$ { 391 ± 93
Bleeding	19	0	19	160 ± 23
		$P < .01$		

Data represent combined result of study reported in Human Reproduction,[54] confirmed and updated for endometrial granulated cells stained by phloxine tartrazine.
*Unevaluable means endometrial biopsy tissue was fibrotic and acellular; these were found in women who did not suffer from unscheduled bleeding while taking levonorgestrel contraceptive, which is in agreement with the findings of Hadisaputra et al.[55]
†Cell counts were done only on samples with identifiable endometrium.
SEM, standard error of the mean.

of stromal cells into decidual cells. Within the early decidua, there is an infiltrate of lymphomyeloid cells.[57] Because early human implantation site material is difficult to obtain for study through modern cell identification technology, knowledge about the infiltrate is limited. It is known from pregnancy termination tissue, however, that by 6 to 8 weeks of human gestation, the maternal lymphomyeloid cells dominant in the decidua are the CD56+ CD16− NK-related cells (decidual granulated lymphocytes [dGLs]).[57-60] There are also macrophages, which are T lymphocytes of predominantly the CD8+ phenotype. T cells include those with $\alpha\beta$ and $\gamma\delta$ T cell receptor for antigen; some of the latter also express CD56 (i.e., they are NK T cells).[53,58-60] Extravillous cytotrophoblasts from columns anchoring the developing placenta to the uterine wall invade the decidua and maternal spiral arteries, and, in close association, dGLs and macrophages are present.[58] After the first trimester, the frequency of dGL cells diminishes.[58]

Rodent pregnancy has provided important models for understanding cellular and molecular events important in humans, but, in addition to similarities, there are some differences that should be noted. In the mouse, for example, the male ejaculate passes directly into the uterus without any filtering via the cervical mucus that is present in humans.[61] Bacteria are present in the mouse uterus, and there is a proinflammatory response with an exudate of polymorphonuclear leukocytes and production of Th1-type cytokines, notably TNF-α and IL-1.[62] Shortly thereafter, the inflammation ceases, and large nonspecific CD8+ cells with immunosuppressive activity appear.[63] These are hormonally recruited and correspond to large nonspecific suppressor cells found in the endometrium during the human luteal phase.[53,64] It is unknown whether CD8 is present on these human cells. In the circulating blood in early pregnancy, there are CD8+ $\gamma\delta$ T cells of the γ_1 subtype, and these cells bear progesterone receptors; in response to the gestational hormone progesterone, these cells release IL-10 and a progesterone-induced blocking factor.[65] In rodent pregnancy, as exemplified by the mouse, the blastocyst lodges in a narrow crypt, dissolves the epithelium on both sides, and induces a primary decidual reaction at the embryonic end, opposite the end from which the trophoblast grows to cross the uterine lumen and establish a placenta.[66] There is a primary decidual transformation at the nonplacental end, and lymphomyeloid cells are

excluded from this zone. In decidua that develop at the site of attachment of α placenta-forming trophoblast, in contrast, an infiltrate of NK-like cells and macrophages may be seen.[67]

Mouse blastocyst implantation occurs approximately 4.5 days after mating (as in humans, implantation tends to occur at night), and a distinct placenta and fetus develop 8.5 to 9.5 days after mating, corresponding to 5 to 6 weeks of human gestation (or 21 days after fertilization).[68] In mice and rats, implantation requires formation of prostaglandins that alter vascular permeability.[69] At the time of formation of a placenta, the large immunosuppressor cells disappear in both the mouse and human decidua, and small lymphocytic suppressor cells appear.[64,70] In the human, these cells are CD56+ CD16− and appear to release a suppressor factor related to TGF-β_2.[71] In the mouse, the cells are predominantly $\gamma\delta$ T cells, a proportion of which also express NK surface markers.[72,73] Interestingly, it is only a proportion of the CD56+ cells in the human that make TGF-β_2, and a similar proportion of CD56+ cells express T cell receptor $\gamma\delta$.[60,71,74] The generation or activation of these cells, both in the mouse and human, seems to represent a response to trophoblasts, probably a $\gamma\delta$ T cell response.[65,70,75,76] Both in humans and in mice, there is downregulation of T cell receptor expression by a trophoblast-derived factor that is yet to be fully characterized.[77,78] Therefore, it is evident that changes in uterine cell populations during pregnancy may be induced by hormones or products of the parasite itself, which is its fetal trophoblast. This process is similar to events that occur with other types of parasite-host interactions.[79]

There are some differences between pregnancy in rodents and humans in addition to those already mentioned. In the mouse, a subset of NK-lineage cells enlarges to 20 μm or more in diameter and contains large numbers of PAS+ granules.[80] These cells accumulate in decidua, muscle, and the mesentery that contains the uterus. This area has become known as the metrial gland (MG), and the large granulated cells are known as MG cells.[80] MG cells produce a variety of cytokines, as do human CD56+ CD16− dGLs.[80,81] The possible role of these cytokines on the embryo qua parasite is described in the next section. However, in the mouse, nitric oxide produced by MG cells causes arterial relaxation, and lack of MG cells leads to retention of thick-walled vessels, hypoperfusion (or the parasite with attendant growth restriction), and fetal deaths (abortions). These problems can be prevented with IFN-γ in the absence of MG cells, which indicates that this cytokine, rather than nitric oxide, is of pivotal importance in maternal vascular remodeling during placentation, and the role of MG cells is to produce IFN-γ.[82,83] MG cells are not particularly effective in lysing NK cell–susceptible target cells but may kill trophoblasts[83]; however, in humans, dGL (CD56+ CD16−) cells do not kill freshly isolated trophoblasts that have not been cultured in vitro but do have NK cell activity.[84]

During pregnancy in humans or rodents, there is also a suppression of contractility of the uterine musculature. This sedative state disappears at the time of parturition. Progesterone has been proposed as the major sedative agent, and TNF-α and IL-1 (probably of placental trophoblast origin), as well as prostaglandin $F_{2\alpha}$, have been proposed as major stimulants of contractility.[13] When there are multiple implanted embryos (typical of rodents and occasionally occurring in humans), the demise of one of the embryos usually (but not always) leads to resorption without external expulsion of uterine contents, because expulsion would terminate the remaining viable intrauterine embryo or embryos.[68] Resorption is achieved by a dissociation of the processes that lead to the demise of the embryo from those that result in uterine muscle contraction. Indeed, even in humans, in whom typically there is a single fetus and placenta, embryonic demise may be accompanied by nonexpulsion if muscle sedation is maintained; this is clinically called a "missed" abortion.

Local Effects of the Uterine Immune System on the Pregnancy

The effect of antisperm antibodies on male gametes has been mentioned earlier. Reduced fertility and, in rare cases, abortions may occur in which antisperm IgG antibody binds two sperm together, resulting in dispermic fertilization. Once fertilization occurs (and pregnancy begins), however, there are no further effects. The dividing cells within the zona pellucida are shielded from cytotoxic effects of antibody and cytolytic cells, such as cytotoxic T cells that would otherwise recognize paternal MHC on the dividing zygote and kill it.[85] In contrast, cytokines may have significant effects. Cytokines arise in the mouse by bacterial stimulation of lymphomyeloid cells in the uterine wall, and bacterial endotoxins (LPSs) entering with the ejaculate, via bowel absorption or via injection systemically by an investigator, boost Th1/proinflammatory mediators.[13,61,62,69,86,87]

In humans, it appears that retrograde menstruation in some women elicits an inflammatory response in the pelvic peritoneum; the endometrium implants and grows and can be identified as endometriosis.[88,89] In other women, there is no visible pathologic process. The high levels of cytokines (IL-1, TNF-α, IFN-γ) in pelvic fluid can increase cytokine levels in the fallopian tube fluid, where there can be inhibition of fertilization and inhibition of cell division within the zona pellucida.[89,90]

When the blastocyst hatches from the zona, expression of cell surface MHC antigens is shut off, at least in the mouse, where such determinations are possible. It is not entirely clear what happens with expression of minor histocompatibility antigens, because immunity to minor antigens can cause rejection of blastocysts transplanted to a nonuterine site but not if the blastocysts are placed in the uterus of the preimmunized female.[91] Minor histocompatibility antigens are now thought to be self peptides bound to the organism's own MHC; thus, both major and minor antigens would be expected to disappear together. It seems most likely that this shutting off may be incomplete at the time of hatching (and transference to a nonuterine site) but may be complete at the time when contact occurs with the uterine epithelium to begin implantation. Production of IDO by the trophoblast, or induction of IDO production in macrophage-type cells that infiltrate the implantation site appears to be important at the time of implantation, and this suggests that complete shutting off of production of paternal antigens does not occur. Soluble class I MHC and minor paternal transplantation antigens may be taken up by maternal APCs and presented to maternal T cells; this is the process of indirect antigen presentation, in contrast to recognition of antigen attached to cells of the donor blastocyst. IDO+ APCs inactivate T cells that recognize antigens presented indirectly. The ability of the trophoblast to attach to, invade, and grow out into uterine tissues is inhibited by Th1 cytokines.[89] Therefore, implantation may be arrested. Such a mechanism may also account for so-called chemical pregnancies that occur in women in whom the initial stages of implantation are successful; losses of chemical pregnancies appear to be twice as common as the loss of a clinically evident pregnancy (i.e., a spontaneous miscarriage/abortion).[92] Similar "occult" losses can be produced in mice by inhibiting IDO in vivo, and this allows maternal T cells to recognize paternal minor antigens and precipitate deposition of the C3 component of complement so as to cause pregnancy failure.[91,93]

Deleterious cytokines in women with unexplained infertility who have an increased number of lymphocytes and macrophages in their pelvic peritoneal fluid[89] may explain, in part, why transfer of in vitro fertilized (IVF) embryos at the blastocyst stage may have a higher success rate than transfer at the four- to eight-cell stage.[94] The latter may be growth inhibited and may never reach the blastocyst stage.

Certain cytokines may enhance implantation. In the mouse, macrophage colony–stimulating factor (M-CSF/CSF-1), produced largely by uterine glandular epithelium in response to gestational hormones, is important[95]; mice deficient in this cytokine (genotype op/op) suffer from implantation failure, which appears to relate to the loss of macrophages rather than to M-CSF/CSF-1 itself.[95] Affected males are also hypospermic.[96] The defect in spermatogenesis and implantation can, to some extent, be corrected by G-CSF treatment, and restoration of tissue macrophage levels may be responsible.[95,97] Macrophages produce various cytokines that can benefit trophoblast growth. Granulocyte-macrophage colony–stimulating factor (GM-CSF), which is produced by activated T cells, was once thought to be such a mediator but is produced by non-T cells such as epithelium, and its growth-stimulating effects on trophoblasts may be due to a "contaminant."[98,99]

However, TGF-β in seminal plasma may act to stimulate epithelial production of GM-CSF, which may enhance implantation.[99] Furthermore, GM-CSF can suppress the cytotoxic activity of natural effector cells against trophoblasts, if CD8+ T cells are present,[100] and CD8+ cells play an important role in the peri-implantation phase, illustrated in Figure 21–2. A more detailed summary of key stages in the human implantation process is provided in Figure 21–3. An attachment and initial trophoblast invasion through uterine epithelium (A) is distinguished from the peri-implantation phase (B).[101] One analysis strongly suggested that a large proportion of "occult" chemical pregnancies (which fail) represent otherwise normal embryos, particularly in infertile couples.[102] In humans, CD56+ CD16− dGL cells appear to produce GM-CSF in significant quantities,[81,103] and, as in the mouse, CD8+ T cells are present in the decidua. An abnormality in uterine lymphocytic cells compatible with a shift toward Th1-type cells and a decrease in Th2-type cells has been associated with infertility, and similar changes in peripheral blood cells have been linked to failure of transfers of in vitro–fertilized embryos.[104,105] In any analysis of "implantation failure," it is important to distinguish failure at the attachment phase from failure during the peri-implantation phase. The latter can represent a maternal T cell–mediated "rejection" of the embryo as an allograft (the concept of the "fetal allograft" is discussed later). Occult failures do occur in mice, in which it is possible to analyze mechanisms.[87,91]

Once implantation has been completed and a distinct fetus and placenta form (see Fig. 21–2), a different set of positive and negative influences on the parasite are described.[70,81] Failure at this point occurs as spontaneous abortion or resorption, which occurs after the time of occult losses described previously. A variety of pathogenic mechanisms have been suggested as causes of such failures. In humans, loss is often a solitary reproductive event (sporadic miscarriage) occurring with an incidence of 5% to 15%, but in a subset of couples (2% to 4%), this loss may be recurrent.[106-111] In humans, most explanations for recurrent loss do not appear to be supported by good evidence.[106-108] In sporadic abortion, chromosomal abnormalities may account for 60% to 70% of the losses and have been thought of as random accidents.[109] Of the people with recurrent abortions, 55% of those with three abortions or more and no live births have a trophoblast karyotype abnormality, as do 35% of those with multiple abortions and one live birth.[111] Finding an explanation for loss of chromosomally normal embryos has been the focus of intense interest of immunologists, and a variety of mechanisms and treatments have been advocated.

Four main paradigms have been explored as a basis for abortions (Table 21–3). The *fetal allograft model* enunciated by Medawar in 1953[1] suggested that embryos were rejected like organ allografts (e.g., kidney, heart, skin) because embryos inherited and should express paternal MHC antigens that are foreign to the mother (unless the mother and father have identical HLA). Mediators of allograft rejection are primarily cytotoxic T lymphocytes, Th1 cytokine–producing T cells, and antibodies that facilitate killing by phagocytic cells and NK cells (antibody-dependent cell-mediated cytotoxicity).[19] Th1 cytokine production by T cells and macrophage activation are considered relevant to certain aspects of rejection, because in normal pregnancy, there is a Th1-to-Th2 shift, and a Th1 response may cause abortions (at least in mice).[5,6,81,112] Blood transfusion should inhibit rejection (and abortion) through allogeneic leukocytes that cause transfusion-related immunomodulation (a Th1-to-Th2 shift in cytokine

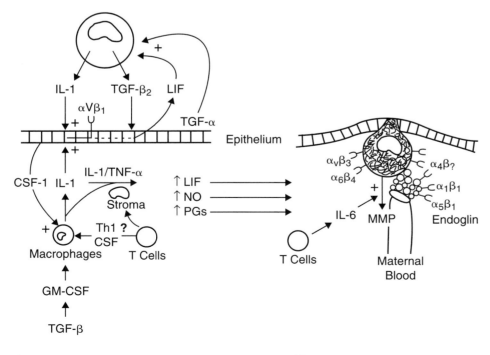

Figure 21–3. Key events in implantation. **A,** Phase of initial attachment and trophoblast invasion in the human. **B,** Peri-implantation phase in humans. $\alpha_V\beta_1$ is a type of integrin receptor with a V-type α chain and type 1 β chain (note related integrin receptors are illustrated); endoglin is a type of receptor for TGF-β_1 and TGF-β_3. CSF, colony-stimulating factor; GM-CSF, granulocyte-macrophage colony–stimulating factor; IL, interleukin; LIF, leukemia inhibitory factor; MMP, matrix metalloproteinases; NO, nitric oxide; PGs, prostaglandins; TGF, transforming growth factor; Th1, type 1 helper T cell; TNF-α, tumor necrosis factor α. (From Ghazeeri GS, Clark DA, Kutteh WH: Immunological factors in implantation. Infertil Reprod Med Clin North Am 2001;12:315.)

TABLE 21–3   Paradigms of the Fetomaternal Relationship

Model	Basis for Concepts
1. Fetal allograft	Transplantation immunology: rejection/tolerance
2. Immunotrophism	Trophic role postulated for immune system plus evidence that lymphokines can act as growth factors
3. Tumor	Tumor immunology
4. Th1/Th2	Empirical correlation of T helper cytokine phenotypes with outcome of pregnancy and effects on maternal infections
5. Parasite	Immunoparasitology

Th1 and Th2, helper T cell types 1 and 2.

pattern)[113], and this appears to depend on the presence of adequate amounts of CD200+ alloantigenic dendritic cells in the blood.[114] Experiments with inbred strains of rats and mice have enabled investigators to show that the mother could react against and reject tissues of the fetus during pregnancy, but only if the fetus was removed from its cocoon of trophoblast cells.[3,4,81,115] Trophoblasts proved resistant to all forms of antigen-specific transplantation immunity, even when MHC alloantigens were expressed.[4,116,117] The only exception was anti-MHC antibody plus a xenogeneic source of complement that could kill mouse trophoblasts in vitro and abort mice in vivo.[118] Trophoblast cells (in humans) express complement inhibitor proteins, but abortions are not associated with any deficiency of such inhibitors such as CD46.[119] In humans and possibly rats, truncated MHC lacking alloantigenic determinants was identified on a subset of trophoblasts (HLA-G and HLA-E in humans; Qa, TL, and CD1 in mice),[120] and this observation bolstered the prevailing prejudice that trophoblasts were nonantigenic except in the example of occult pregnancy failure. Transplantation immunology mediated by αβ T cells did not seem to be relevant to trophoblasts. How then might the Th1/Th2 effect be explained in the later occurring clinical miscarriages?

The next paradigm was based on the observation that trophoblasts formed a barrier to lymphocyte traffic into the fetus by interposing themselves between the fetal and maternal circulations so as to effect a complete separation.[1,121] Trophoblasts were resistant to classical forms of allograft rejection, and trophoblasts were stimulated to grow by T cell–derived cytokines.[122] The *immunotrophism* model, as advocated by Wegmann,[122] suggested that T cells recognized antigens on trophoblasts and produced cytokines that stimulated trophoblast growth and differentiation, thus leading to a better barrier so that maternal lymphocytes could not enter into the fetus and destroy the real fetal allograft. Indeed, trophoblasts may express molecules that discriminate against passage of sensitized maternal lymphocytes into the fetus,[123] but substantial numbers of putatively maternal immunocompetent cells appear to pass without causing harm,[124-126] just as there is traffic of fetal cells into the mother that does not cause graft-versus-host disease.[126] Furthermore, alloimmunization against paternal MHC appeared to prevent abortions

and to promote fetal and placental growth in certain mouse mating combinations,[127,128] even where no FAS/FAS ligand interaction was possible[129]; similar effects were seen in humans with primary recurrent miscarriages,[106,107,110,130,131] but evidence that conventional T cells (i.e., bearing T cell receptor αβ) could recognize antigens on trophoblasts could not be demonstrated.[132] However, trophoblast recognition by γδ T cells (isolated from the uterine decidua of pregnant mice by fusing the decidual lymphocytes with a tumor cell to generate immortal hybridoma cell lines in tissue culture) was shown by Heyborne and colleagues, but only IL-2, a Th1 cytokine that stimulates abortions, was reported.[28] The demonstration that most of the cytokines affecting trophoblast growth came from non-T cells in the uterus provided a further blow to the model, as did demonstration of successful pregnancies in mice with severe combined immunodeficiency disease.[133] Furthermore, αβ T cell depletion in vivo did not prevent abortions in mice.[134] Finally, Kinsky and colleagues[135] showed that an injection of activated NK cells caused abortion in mice, and Baines and associates prevented spontaneous abortions in the CBA × DBA/2 mouse model by anti–NK cell antibodies and antimacrophage antibodies.[136,137] Thus, pregnancy failure did not result from lack of immunotrophism.

NK cells could not kill trophoblasts, but when the NK cells were activated by culturing with IL-2, the NK cells transformed into lymphokine-activated killer cells (LAKs), which were able to kill a variety of nonantigenic tumor cells resistant to cytotoxic T lymphocyte and NK. LAKs could also kill NK-resistant trophoblast cells that had been cultured in vitro, both in the mouse system and in humans.[138-140] Conventional NK cells (found in blood) that accumulate at implantation sites destined to abort in mice[136] also accumulate as CD56+-CD16+ cells in the endometrium of women who have recurrent miscarriages, and higher levels than normal have been found in peripheral blood.[141-144] These findings led to the *embryo as a tumor model,* in which the natural effector system was paramount in causing rejection by a direct cell contact killing mechanism.[2,145] However, it was not possible to demonstrate LAKs or trophoblast killing in situ in abortion sites; freshly isolated human trophoblast cells that had not been cultured in vitro overnight were not sensitive to killing by LAKs.[84] Furthermore, macrophages seemed just as important, at least in the CBA × DBA/2 mouse mating combination, the most widely used laboratory system for the study of abortion mechanisms.[68,70,80,127,128,136,137] Macrophages, activated by IFN-γ from NK cells of Th1 cells, were proposed to secrete toxic levels of nitric oxide, which mediates immunity to bacteria, viruses, parasites, and prostaglandins.[79,137,145,146] Study of *Leishmania* infection in mouse pregnancy showed the Th1-to-Th2 shift systemically prevented effective rejection of the infection; however, in animals that mounted the necessary Th1 response, the intrauterine embryos were aborted.[147] Th1 responses were also seen in the CBA × DBA/2 abortion model and in women with recurrent abortions.[81,112,148,149] These data supported the idea of Th1/Th2 balance as a determinant of pregnancy outcome; hence the *Th1/Th2 paradigm.*[6]

The technology used by Heyborne and colleagues to clone γδ T cells from the mouse uterine lining by fusion to an "immortal hybridoma cell line" appeared to have biased cytokine response toward Th1[28], the default pattern dictated by the hybridoma cell line. We have reported that freshly isolated decidual γδ T cells express Th2/Th3 cytokines without the need for an artificial activation stimulus in vitro.[72,150,151] In abortion-prone CBA × DBA/2 matings, there was an abnormal increase in Th1-type γδ cells immediately after implantation, which predisposed to abortion if there was a second signal, and these appear now to be primarily NK γδ T cells able to produce the Th1 cytokines TNF-α and IFN-γ.[32,150,151] Potential second signals included production of Th1 cytokines by circulating systemic T cells, bacterial endotoxin (which triggers TNF-α production by macrophages), and psychic stress which, through release of the neuropeptide substance P, activates macrophages to produce TNF-α (and probably IL-12), and mast cells to produce TNF-α and IFN-γ.[69,152,153] The potential cellular interactions generating TNF-α + IFN-γ are illustrated in Figure 21–4. Because mast cells play an important role in antiparasite immunity, and because the fetus is, de facto, a parasite that depends on the mother during gestation but whose development can be terminated when the mother's life or health is threatened (so as to best preserve those already born who will continue the species), my colleagues and I propose a new paradigm, the embryo as a parasite model,[81] and this analogy has been used as a basis for the previous discussion.

The parasite model did not resolve the question as to how the embryo was rejected, but the NK-macrophage interaction illustrated in Figure 21–4 did provide a testable framework. In vivo elimination of either NK cells or macrophages in the CBA × DBA/2 system prevented abortions, and the ability of either an injection of TNF-α or an injection of IFN-γ to boost the abortion rate was eliminated.[154] If both cytokines were injected in these animals, however, more than 80% of embryos were aborted.[154] Suppression of ovarian hormone secretion was ruled out as a cause of abortions, and that left vascular endothelial cells as the next most likely cause. In response to these cytokines, endothelial cells increase expression of the procoagulant fibrinogen-like peptide 2 (FGL2) prothrombinase molecule that directly converts prothrombin to thrombin. Antibody to FGL2 effectively blocked abortions.[154]

When prothrombin is converted to thrombin, in addition to generation of fibrin clot that chokes off blood supply to the placenta, endothelial cells are stimulated to release IL-8 (human) or macrophage inflammatory protein 2 (mouse), which attracts polymorphonuclear leukocytes. Polymorphonuclear leukocytes are cytotoxic to cytokine-activated endothelial cells.[155] Antigranulocyte antibody also dramatically reduced abortions but not as effectively as did anti-FGL2.[155] Anticoagulation with heparin (which activates antithrombin III) or with hirudin (a direct antithrombin) also reduced the abortion rate.[156] Together with findings of microthrombi, hemorrhage at the trophoblast-decidual junction, and polymorphonuclear leukocyte infiltration in mouse resorption sites, these data have indicated that abortions in CBA × DBA/2 mice are caused by a vascular autoamputation mechanism triggered by the Th1 cytokines produced by NK cells, macrophages, T cells, and mast cells.[114,154,155]

Cytokines such as IL-10 and TGF-β₂ that derive from trophoblast-activated γδ Th2/Th3-type cells antagonize these processes.[147,150,151,157] IL-4 and IL-3 may act similarly. In the mouse, this process is dependent on expression of CD200, as mentioned previously.[24,81] Indeed, injections of TNF-α plus IFN-γ only slightly increase FGL2 expression but dramatically reduce expression of CD200.[24] Soluble CD200 can act as a rescue molecule and blocks abortion of implantation sites expressing high levels of FGL2.[24] In mice and in humans, subnormal levels of TGF-β₂⁺ cells in decidua have been associated with recurrent abortions.[70,158-160] Inhibition of expression of CD200 appears to be as important as upregulation of FGL2 as a basis for abortion.

There is evidence for vascular events as a basis for human abortions,[161] as summarized in Table 21–4, and my colleagues and I have found increased expression of FGL2 messenger RNA associated with miscarriage of chromosomally normal embryos, as distinct from loss of abnormal embryos, in which FGL2 levels were usually normal.[24,50] CD200 is expressed on the trophoblast cells of successful human pregnancies.[162] The similarities between the mouse and human are striking. A vascular mechanism leading to abortion is also seen in other situations leading

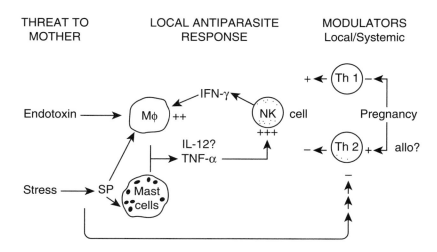

THREAT TO MOTHER

LOCAL ANTIPARASITE RESPONSE

MODULATORS Local/Systemic

Figure 21–4. Effector mechanisms that act to eliminate (reject) the implanted fetoplacental unit. Note that stress can exert a direct inhibitory effect on systemic Th2-type CD8⁺ suppressor cells, which are thought to express progesterone receptors in early pregnancy.[65,81] allo, alloimmune stimulation; IFN, interferon; IL, interleukin; M, macrophage; NK, natural killer lineage cell (which may include NKγδT cells); SP, substance P; Th1 and Th2, types 1 and 2 helper T cells; TNF, tumor necrosis factor.

TABLE 21–4 Association of Abortion of Embryos of Normal Karyotype with Vascular Events

Histologic Finding	Normal Karyotype (N = 51)* (%)†	Abnormal Karyotype (N = 133)* (%)
Decidual vasculitis	43	32
Decidual thrombi	37	28
Chronic intervillositis	14	7
Villous infarcts	16	5

*By logistic regression, if a fetus was viable (as indicated by presence of nucleated red cells), positive predictive value for a normal karyotype was 97%.
†P < 0.05.
Data from Salafia C, Maier D, Vogel C, et al: Placental and decidual histology in spontaneous abortion: Detailed description and correlations with chromosome number. Obstet Gynecol 1993;82:295-303. Adapted from Clark D, Arck PC, Chaouat G: Why did your mother reject you? Immunogenetic determinants of the response to environmental selective pressure expressed at the uterine level. Am J Reprod Immunol 1999;41:5-22.

to recurrent human abortions. Antiphospholipid antibodies that have been associated with recurrent abortions, particularly antiphosphatidyl serine and antiphosphatidyl ethanolamine, bind to annexin V on endothelial cells[163]; annexin V is an antithrombotic molecule on endothelium, and its neutralization leads to the same procoagulant state as does upregulation of FGL2.

It is possible that similar events underlie development of preeclampsia, intrauterine fetal distress, and premature labor. Preeclampsia in humans has been related to inadequate extravillous trophoblast growth into decidual arterial walls, perhaps caused by cytokines antagonistic to this process, although increased expression of FGL2 prothrombinase has been implicated.[50] As already mentioned, Th1-type cytokines may precipitate emptying of the uterus. Nitric oxide is a potent sedative for uterine muscle and a vasodilator that has been used to treat preeclampsia and premature labor clinically.[164] Some dissociation might be predicted between embryo rejection through macrophages and NK cells (which should upregulate nitric oxide production) and levels of nitric oxide that promote successful pregnancy in humans and

in mice.[82,83,137] Stress and infection have also been strongly linked to prematurity in humans.[8,52,165-167] Little is known about the underlying mechanisms. There is a mouse model of endotoxin-triggered prematurity[7] and a similar model in rabbits[168]; indeed, in endotoxin-treated pregnant rabbits, an intravenous injection of TGF-β_2 prevented prematurity.[168] Thus, Th2/Th3 cytokines that prevent abortions may also prevent other complications in pregnancy. These data suggest that CD200 + antigen will prove to be an important mechanism preventing such pathologic processes. At present, the only technique for administering CD200 to women is by transfusion of freshly isolated allogeneic blood mononuclear leukocytes.[110,114,133,169] Perhaps that is the mechanism accounting for the association of prior blood transfusion with a lowered risk of preeclampsia.[9]

Figure 21–4 illustrates some mechanisms for generating sufficient TNF-α plus IFN-γ to trigger abortion/resorption, but it has also been mentioned that for these cytokines to act, a Toll-like receptor signal must also be present.[114] This provides a fail-safe situation in which a pregnancy will be terminated (to save the health or life of the mother) only if there is real danger. In mice with low levels of spontaneous loss attributable to housing in clean cage conditions, it is difficult to abort with cytokines or stress, and anti–MD-1 antibody, which reduces levels of CD14 that present Toll-like receptor ligands to Toll-like receptors, abrogates abortions after injection of TNF-α plus IFN-γ.[25,114] This finding has led to the insight that an important effect of the cytokines may be to increase absorption of LPS and related Toll-like receptor ligands through mucosal surfaces such as the intestine.[114] This concept is illustrated in Figure 21–5, for which supportive data are given elsewhere.[114,170]

Systemic Effects of Pregnancy on Maternal Immunity

The systemic shift from Th1 to Th2 (cell-mediated immunity to antibody production/humoral immunity), associated with successful pregnancy, has been implicated in

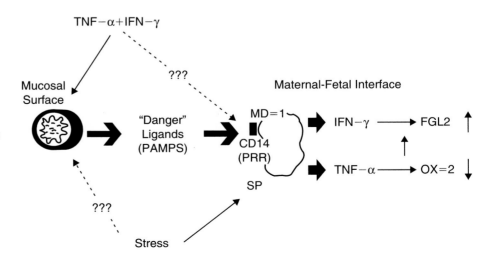

Figure 21–5. Danger signals and cytokine-triggered abortions. Effect of cytokines generated in Figure 20–3 as well as direct SP-mediated effects of stress are illustrated. OX-2 is now known as CD200. FGL2, fibrinogen-like peptide 2; IFN-γ, interferon γ; PAMPS, pathogen-associated molecular patterns; PRR, pattern recognition receptors; SP, substance P; TNF-α, tumor necrosis factor α. (Adapted from Clark DA, Chaouat G, Gorczynski RM: Thinking outside the box: Mechanisms of environmental selective pressures on the outcome of the materno-fetal relationship. Am J Reprod Immunol 2002;47:275.)

causing a slight but sometimes significant increase in susceptibility to certain infectious diseases.[5,6,147] The gestational hormone progesterone can promote a Th1-to-Th2 shift in vitro, as may expression of nonclassical MHC such as HLA-G,[171] but whether either mechanism explains what occurs in vivo is uncertain. Alloactivated T cells express progesterone receptors, and progesterone has been reported to stimulate a CD8 γ_1 subset to release a 34-kD molecule that suppresses NK cell activity and IL-12 release.[65,172] NK cell cytolytic activity is usually normal during the first trimester and is decreased in the late second and in the third trimesters.[173] Progesterone-stimulated CD8+ "suppressor T cells" might act to reduce abnormally elevated levels of blood NK activity that have been linked with subsequent abortion,[174] as well as to suppress Th1 cytokine production and promote Th2.[112,172]

Pregnancy can also induce remission in certain autoimmune/inflammatory diseases, most notably rheumatoid arthritis, in which the evidence is quite solid.[175] Remission occurs in 75% of affected women, is more likely to occur if there is an HLA-D–incompatible fetus, and usually begins in the first trimester.[175] A few weeks after parturition, the arthritis relapses. Indeed, autoimmune disease may be precipitated by parturition, and thyroid autoimmunity is probably the most common example of this in humans.[176] Remission of arthritis in pregnancy led to the discovery of cortisone, but it is not cortisol or gestational hormones that cause remission.[177] The association with an HLA-D–incompatible fetus suggests that transplacental passage of fetal leukocytes (which can begin in the first trimester) is producing a transfusion-related immunomodulation; transfusions promote a Th1-to-Th2 shift, and injection of paternal leukocytes has been reported to improve rheumatoid arthritis in some patients.[113,178]

Important clues to the mechanism of arthritis remission have been obtained by studying collagen-induced arthritis in DBA/1 mice. Pregnancy resulting from a mating with a histocompatible DBA/1 male induces remission, which corresponds in timing with the development of TGF-β_2/IL-10–producing, trophoblast-dependent $\gamma\delta$ T cells in decidua.[179,180] There is some evidence that these types of cells may be present in bone marrow and in inflamed synovia.[180] If histoincompatible DBA/2 males are used to generate pregnancy, the arthritis remits 2 days earlier and before the development of TGF-β_2 $\gamma\delta$ cells,[180] as illustrated in Figure 21-6. At this time, CD8+ suppressor cells with progesterone receptors that produce IL-10 and a progesterone-induced blocking factor that inhibits NK-type cells are present. TGF-β_2–related suppression is much weaker in human decidua than in the mouse, so a CD8+ T cell–mediated component might be more important.[71] CD8+ $\alpha\beta$ T cells recognize class I MHC antigens (HLA-A, HLA-B, HLA-C, and possibly HLA-G) but usually not class II MHC antigens (HLA-D). The CD8+ T cells that produce progesterone-induced blocking factor are $\gamma\delta$ T cells and are γ_1, which renders them able to recognize trophoblast cells (as well as certain heat shock proteins on stressed cells).[24,65] The induction of these CD8+ γ_1 cells in vivo can be triggered by paternal alloantigen if CD200 is also present.[114] Soluble CD200 can arrest development of collagen-induced arthritis, as can soluble CTLA4 that binds B7, but these cause arthritis only to stabilize, not to improve.[181,182] Further work is necessary to determine the exact mechanism

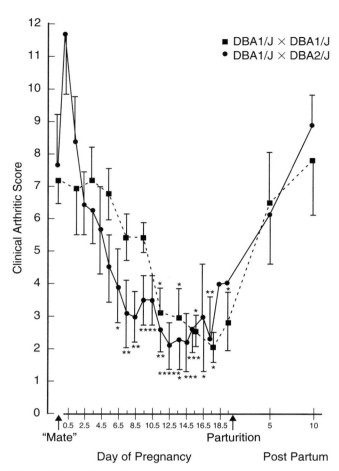

Figure 21–6. Effect of pregnancy on severity of collagen-induced arthritis in DBA/1 mice. The mice were immunized against collagen and then became pregnant; a high rate of severe arthritis developed after parturition. The maximum joint score for severity was 4 × 4 paws, or 16. The effect of a second pregnancy is shown for syngeneic (DBA/1) matings[176] and allogeneic (DBA/2) matings.[177] Data points represent mean +/– SEM. * represents P < 0.05 compared to control, **P < 0.025, and ***P < 0.0125. From Hidaka Y, Tamaki H, Iwatani Y, et al: Prediction of post-partum Graves' thyrotoxicosis by measurement of thyroid stimulating antibody in early pregnancy. Clin Endocrinol 1994; 41:7. From Persellin RH: The effect of pregnancy on rheumatoid arthritis. Bull Rheum Dis 1976–1977;27:922.

by which pregnancy causes remission of rheumatoid arthritis in mice and humans.

On occasion, local immune responses to antigens on the conceptus have systemic effects. One example is herpes gestationis, a rash that is related to an immune infiltrate in the placenta and increased expression of class II HLA-D antigens in the placenta.[183] Parturition is curative, but a high rate of spontaneous abortion may end the problem much earlier in pregnancy.

Systemic Immune Effects on the Pregnancy

In general, systemic immune responses have little effect on an intrauterine pregnancy unless they are autoimmune responses. It is notoriously difficult to immunize against allogeneic pregnancy,[115] and patients who have allografted kidneys usually reject neither the graft nor the intrauterine parasite. Injection/infusion of allogeneic blood mononuclear leukocytes may promote fetal and placental growth, sometimes to a striking degree, if given 10 to 14 days after the missed menses.[130] There has been considerable controversy surrounding the therapeutic use of leukocytes to prevent recurrent miscarriages in humans; this controversy is largely attributable to lack of understanding of the mechanism and to defects in the design, execution, and analysis of clinical trials. A review with updated metaanalysis of clinical trials provides convincing evidence of efficacy of freshly isolated paternal blood mononuclear leukocytes given to patients who do not have autoimmunity.[131] In contrast, cells stored overnight before injection lose efficacy in mice and humans, and in both species, this is linked to loss of cell surface CD200.[131] Stored cells are still sufficiently alloantigenic to induce anti-HLA antibodies in some women, but such antibodies are not protective. Originally described as "blocking antibodies" because of one of the in vitro methods used to detect them, their action in vivo has nothing to do with blocking recognition of antigens on trophoblasts by hypothesized aggressive maternal T cells, because trophoblasts lacks the HLA determinants against which these antibodies are directed. The most likely target for the antibodies generated by infusing freshly isolated allogeneic mononuclear leukocytes is the leukocytes themselves. In the absence of antibody, protection against abortion wanes after 80 to 90 days (but can be restored by injecting a small number of freshly isolated paternal cells as a booster immunization), whereas with antibody, protection is prolonged for more than 5 months.[115,131] The most likely mechanism is immunologic enhancement of survival of CD200+ paternal dendritic cells. The immunotherapeutic effect that prevents abortion does not seem to be caused by inducing an immune response in the woman; instead, it is the consequences of providing a sufficient number of CD200+ cells bearing paternal antigen(s) similar to epitopes that are present at the fetal-maternal interface. A large dose of soluble CD200 would be as effective, as has been shown in a mouse model of cytokine-triggered recurrent abortions.[24]

Autoantibodies can cross placental trophoblast tissues and affect the fetus; antibody-mediated immunity to infectious agents may also do so. Antigen or primed memory cells may also cross the placenta and induce a state of priming.[184] The most successful approach to immunization against pregnancy in humans has involved a human chorionic gonadotropin vaccine.[185] Antisperm antigen vaccines have also been developed in animal systems as an alternative,[186,187] but this immunity has, in some cases, been linked to an increased loss through abortions.[68] As illustrated by *Leishmania* infection, a more dramatic demonstration of the effects of systemic immunity has been obtained in mice than in humans.[127] It is nonetheless important to recall the lesson taught by Charles Darwin: Species may differ in special ways, and this makes each unique, but there are important significant homologies and commonalities. Without animal studies, we would not have known what to look for in humans. Animal studies are important in their own right, because domestic animal production may be affected by reduced fertility and early pregnancy loss, thus reducing the supply of food and driving up its cost. The causes of such wastage are known in some[10-12] but not all situations, as in humans. Physicians, however, gain clues from animal studies that allow them to understand mechanisms of human disease and, from this understanding, to treat them more effectively. Immunology is playing an increasing practical role in this quest.

Acknowledgments

The author's work has been supported by grants from the Medical Research Council of Canada (now the Canadian Institutes for Health Research), the Arthritis Society of Canada, and the World Health Organization, Geneva, Switzerland.

References

1. Medawar PB: Some immunological and endocrinological problems raised by evolution of viviparity in vertebrates. In Society for Experimental Biology, Evolution Symposium, No. 11. New York, Academic Press, 1953, pp 320-328.
2. Loke YW: Experimenting with human extravillous trophoblast: A personal view. Am J Reprod Immunol 1990;24:22.
3. Clark DA, Arck PC, Jalali R, et al: Psycho-neuro-cytokine/ endocrine pathways in immunoregulation during pregnancy. Am J Reprod Immunol 1996;35:352.
4. Simmons RL, Russell PS: The immunologic problem of pregnancy. Adv Obstet Gynecol 1963;85:583.
5. Krishnan L, Guilbert LJ, Russell AS, et al: Pregnancy impairs resistance of C57Bl/6 mice to *Leishmania* major infection and causes decreased antigen-specific IFN-γ response and increased production of T helper 2 cytokines. J Immunol 1996;156:644.
6. Wegmann TG, Lin H, Guilbert L, Mossman TR: Bidirectional cytokine interactions in the maternal-fetal relationship: Is successful pregnancy a TH2 phenomenon? Immunol Today 1993;14:353.
7. Chaouat G: Synergy of lipopolysaccharide and inflammatory cytokines in murine pregnancy: Alloimmunization prevents abortion but does not affect the induction of preterm delivery. Cell Immunol 1994;157:328.
8. McGregor JA, French JI, Witkin S: Infection and prematurity: Evidence based approaches. Curr Opin Obstet Gynecol 1996;8:628.
9. Clark DA: Does immunological intercourse prevent pre-eclampsia? Lancet 1984;344:73.
10. Foley GL, Schlafer DH: Bacterial endotoxemia and reproductive effects in ruminants. Vet Clin North Am 1994;10:491.
11. Doucet F, Bernard S: In vitro cellular responses from sheep draining lymph node cells after subcutaneous inoculation with *Salmonella abortus ovis*. Vet Res 1997;28:165.
12. Jones GI, Low JC, Machell J, Armstrong K: Comparison of five tests for the detection of antibodies against chlamydial (epizootic) abortion of ewes. Vet Res 1997;141:164.
13. Laham N, Brennecke SP, Rice GE: Interleukin-8 release from human gestational tissue explants: The effects of lipopolysaccharide and cytokines. Biol Reprod 1997;57:616.
14. Matzinger P: Tolerance, danger, and the extended family. Annu Rev Immunol 1994;12:991.
15. Dunn DA, Gadenne AS, Simha S, et al: T-cell receptor V beta expression in normal human skin. Proc Natl Acad Sci U S A 1993;90:1267.
16. Klein JR: T cell development in the intestinal mucosa: Clues to a novel immune-endocrine network? Adv Neuroimmunol 1996;6:397.
17. Maric I, Holt PG, Perdue MH, et al: Class II MHC antigen (Ia)–bearing dendritic cells in the epithelium of the intestine. J Immunol 1996;156:1408.
18. Givan AL, White HD, Stern JE, et al: Flow cytometric analysis of leukocytes in the female reproductive tract: Comparison of fallopian tube, uterus, cervix, and vagina. Am J Reprod Immunol 1997;38:350.
19. Janeway CA Jr, Travers P: Immunobiology, 3rd ed. New York, Garland Publishing, 1997.
20. King A, Hiby SE, Verma S, et al: Uterine NK cells and trophoblast HLA class I molecules. Am J Reprod Immunol 1997;37:459.
21. Henderson RA, Watkins SC, Flynn JL: Activation of human dendritic cells following infection with *Mycobacterium tuberculosis*. J Immunol 1997;159:635.

22. Bluestone JA: Is CTLA-4 a master switch for peripheral T cell tolerance? J Immunol 1997;158:1989.

23. Gorczynski RM, Chen Z, Fu XM, Zeng H: Increased expression of the novel molecules OX-2 is involved in prolongation of renal allograft survival. Transplantation 1998;65:1106.

24. Clark DA, Ding JW, Yu G, et al: Fgl2 prothrombinase expression in mouse trophoblast and decidua triggers abortion but may be countered by OX-2. Mol Hum Reprod 2001;7:185.

25. Gorczynski RM, Johnston N, Yu G, Clark DA: Does successful allopregnancy mimic transplantation tolerance? Graft 2001;4:345.

26. Chien YH, Jores R, Crowley MP: Recognition by γ/δ T cells. Annu Rev Immunol 1996;14:511.

27. Boismenu R, Havran WL: An innate view of γδ T cells. Curr Opin Immunol 1997;9:57.

28. Heyborne K, Fu Y-X, Nelson A, et al: Recognition of trophoblasts by γδ T cells. J Immunol 1994;153:2918.

29. Bendelac A, Lantz O, Quimby ME, et al: CD1 recognition by mouse NK1+ T lymphocytes. Science 1995;268:863.

30. Medzhitov R, Janeway CA Jr: Innate immunity: Impact on the adaptive immune response. Curr Opin Immunol 1997;9:4.

31. Mosmann TR, Sad S: The expanding universe of T-cell subsets: Th1, Th2, and more. Immunol Today 1996;17:138.

32. Clark DA, Croitoru K: TH1/TH2,3 imbalance due to cytokine-producing NK, γδ T and NK-γδ T cells in murine pregnancy decidua in success or failure of pregnancy. Am J Reprod Immunol 2002;45:257.

33. Hang L, Slack JH, Amundson C, et al: Induction of murine autoimmune disease by polyclonal B cell activation. J Exp Med 1983;157:874.

34. Schnare M, Barton GM, Holt AC, et al: Toll-like receptors control activation of adaptive immune responses. Nature Immunol 2001;2:947.

35. Gorczynski RM, Chen Z, Clark DA, et al: Regulation of gene expression of MD-1 regulates subsequent T cell activation and cytokine production. J Immunol 2000;164:1925.

36. Held TK, Weihua X, Kavarolanu DV, et al: γ Interferon augments macrophage activation by lipopolysaccharide by two different mechanisms, at the signal transduction level and via an autocrine mechanism involving tumor necrosis factor α and interleukin 1. Infect Immun 1999;67:206.

37. Neilson IR, Neilson KA, Yunis EJ, et al: Failure of tumor necrosis factor to produce hypotensive shock in the absence of endotoxin. Surgery 1989;106:439.

38. Pulendran B, Kumar P, Cutler CW, et al: Lipopolysaccharides from distinct pathogens induce different classes of immune responses in vivo. J Immunol 2001;167:5067.

39. Chen Y, Kuchroo VK, Inobe J, et al: Regulatory T cell clones induced by oral tolerance: Suppression of autoimmune encephalomyelitis. Science 1994;265:1237.

40. Sakaguchi S, Sakaguchi S: Organ-specific autoimmune disease induced in mice by elimination of T cell subsets. J Immunol 1989;142:471.

41. Clark DA: Decidua-placenta immunologic interactions. In Chaouat G (ed): Immunology of the Fetus. Boca Raton, Fla, CRC Press, 1990, pp 161-170.

42. Tsuji Y: Carbohydrate antigens recognized by antisperm antibodies. In Kurpisz M, Fernandez N (eds): Immunology of Human Reproduction. Oxford, U.K., Bios Scientific Publishers, 1995, pp 23-32.

43. Bagavant H, Fusi FM, Baisch J, et al: Immunogenicity and contraceptive potential of a human zona pellucida 3 peptide vaccine. Biol Reprod 1997;56:764. [Published erratum appears in Biol Reprod 1997;56:1361.]

44. Fox M: Failed vasectomy reversal: Is a further attempt worthwhile using microsurgery? Eur Urol 1997;31:436.

45. Imade GE, Baker HW, de Kretser DM, et al: Immunosuppressive activities in the seminal plasma of infertile men: Relationship to sperm antibodies and autoimmunity. Human Reprod 1997;12:256.

46. Bernstein JA, Sugaran R, Bernstein DI, et al: Prevalence of human seminal plasma hypersensitivity among symptomatic women. Ann Allergy Asthma Immunol 1997;78:54.

47. Drout M, Sabbah A, Hassoun S: Thirteen cases of allergy to human seminal plasma. Allergy 1997;52:112.

48. Coulam CB: Immunotherapy for spontaneous abortion. In Hunt JS (ed): Immunobiology of Reproduction, Serono Symposia USA. New York, Springer-Verlag, 1994, pp 303-315.

49. Burrows TD, King A, Loke YW: Trophoblast migration during human placental implantation. Hum Reprod Update 1996;2:307.

50. Knackstedt M, Ding JW, Arck PC, et al: Activation of the novel prothrombinase, fgl2, as a basis for the pregnancy complications spontaneous abortion and pre-eclampsia. Am J Reprod Immunol 2001;46:196.

51. Caniggia I, Taylor CV, Ritchie JW, et al: Endoglin regulates trophoblast differentiation along the invasive pathway in human placental villous explants. Placenta 1997;138:4977.

52. Steinborn A, Kuhnert M, Halberstadt F: Immunomodulatory cytokines induce term and premature parturition. J Perinat Med 1996;24:381.

53. Clark DA, Daya S: Macrophages and other migratory cells in the endometrium: Relevance to uterine bleeding. In d'Arcangues C, Fraser IS, Newton JR, Olind V (eds): Contraception and Mechanisms of Uterine Bleeding. Cambridge, U.K., Cambridge University Press, 1990, pp 363-382.

54. Clark DA, Wang S, Rogers P, et al: Endometrial lymphomyeloid cells in abnormal bleeding due to levonorgestrel (Norplant). Human Reprod 1996;11:1438.

55. Hadisaputra W, Affandi B, Witjaksono J, et al: Endometrial biopsy collection from women receiving Norplant. Human Reprod 1996;11(Suppl 2):31.

56. White HD, Crassi KM, Givan AL, et al: CTL activation within the female reproductive tract. J Immunol 1997;158:3017.

57. Hamilton WJ, Boyd JD, Mossman HW: Human Embryology. Cambridge, U.K., Heffer, 1962.

58. Bulmer JN: Immune cells in decidua. In Kurpisz M, Fernandez N (eds): Immunology of Human Reproduction. Oxford, U.K., Bios Scientific Publishers, 1995, pp 313-334.

59. Vassiliadou N, Bulmer JN: Quantitative analysis of T lymphocyte subsets in pregnant and nonpregnant human endometrium. Hum Reprod 1996;55:1017.

60. Mincherva-Nilsson L, Kling M, Hammarstrom S, et al: γδT cells of human early pregnancy decidua. Evidence for local proliferation, phenotypic heterogeneity, and extrathymic differentiation. J Immunol 1997;159:3266.

61. Parr EL, Parr MB: Deposition of C3 on bacteria in the mouse uterus after mating. J Reprod Immunol 1988;12:315.

62. Choudhri R, Wood GW: Production of interleukin-1, interleukin-6, and tumor necrosis factor alpha in the uterus of pseudopregnant mice. Biol Reprod 1993;49:596. [Published erratum appears in Biol Reprod 1993;49:1385.]

63. Clark DA, Brierly J, Banwatt D, Chaouat G: Hormone-induced pre-implantation Ly-2+ murine uterine suppressor cells persist after implantation and may reduce the spontaneous abortion rate. Cell Immunol 1989;123:334.

64. Daya S, Clark DA, Devlin C, et al: Preliminary characterization of two types of suppressor cells in the human uterus. Fertil Steril 1985;44:778.

65. Clark DA: T cells in pregnancy: Illusion and reality. Am J Reprod Immunol 1999;41:233.

66. Enders AC, Welsh AO: Structural interactions of trophoblast and uterus during hemochorial placenta formation. J Exp Zool 1993;266:578.

67. Gendron RL, Baines MG: Infiltrating decidual natural killer cells are associated with spontaneous abortion in mice. Cell Immunol 1988;113:261.

68. Clark DA: Animal models of recurrent pregnancy loss. In Coulam CB, Faulk WP, McIntyre JA (eds): Immunological Obstetrics. New York, Norton, 1992, pp 428-436.

69. Clark DA, Banwatt D, Chaouat G: Effect of prostaglandin synthesis inhibitors on spontaneous and endotoxin-induced abortion in mice. J Reprod Immunol 1993;24:29.

70. Clark DA, Lea RG, Podor T, et al: Cytokines determining the success or failure of pregnancy. Ann N Y Acad Sci 1991;626:524.

71. Clark DA, Vince G, Flanders KC, et al: CD56+ lymphoid cells in human first trimester decidua as a source of novel TGF-β2–related immunosuppressive factors. Hum Reprod 1994;9:2270.

72. Clark DA, Merali F, Hoskin D, et al: Decidua-associated suppressor cells in abortion-prone DBA/2-mated CBA/J mice that release bioactive transforming growth factor β2–related immunosuppressive molecules express a bone marrow–derived natural suppressor cell marker and γδ T cell receptor. Biol Reprod 1997;56:1351.

73. Clark DA, Arck PC, Steele-Norwood D, et al: Th1/Th2 balance determines outcome of pregnancy via fgl2 prothrombinase-triggered inflammation. FASEB J 1998;12:A880.

74. Hayakawa S, Shiraishi H, Saitoh S, Satoh K: Decidua as a site of extrathymic Vγ1 T-cell differentiation. Am J Reprod Immunol 1996;35:233.

75. Slapsys RM, Younglai E, Clark DA: A novel suppressor cell develops in uterine decidua in response to fetal trophoblast-type cells. Regional Immunol 1988;1:182.

76. Daya S, Johnson PM, Clark DA: Trophoblast induction of suppressor type cell activity in human endometrial tissue. Am J Reprod Immunol 1989;19:65.

77. Volumene JL, Mognetti B, de Smedt D, et al: Induction of transient murine T cell anergy by a low molecular weight compound obtained from supernatants of human placental cultures is linked to defective phosphorylation of TCR CD3 chain. Am J Reprod Immunol 1997;38:168.

78. Morri T, Nishikawa K, Saito S, et al: T cell receptors are expressed but down-regulated on intradecidual T lymphocytes. Am J Reprod Immunol 1993;29:1.

79. Scott PA, Sher A: Immunoparasitology. In Paul WE (ed): Fundamental Immunology, 3rd ed. New York, Raven Press, 1993, pp 1179-1210.

80. Croy BA, Guimond MJ, Luross J, et al: Uterine natural killer cells do not require interleukin-2 for their maturation or differentiation. Am J Reprod Immunol 1997;37:463.

81. Clark DA, Arck PC, Chaouat G: Why did your mother reject you? Immunogenetic determinants of the response to environmental selective pressure expressed at the uterine level. Am J Reprod Immunol 1999;41:5.

82. Ashkar AA, Di Santo JP, Croy BA: Interferon γ contributes to initiation of uterine vascular modification, decidual integrity, and uterine natural killer cell maturation during normal murine pregnancy. J Exp Med 2000;192:259.

83. Hunt JS, Miller L, Vassmer D, Croy BA: Expression of the inducible nitric oxide synthetase gene in mouse uterine leukocytes and potential relationships with uterine function during pregnancy. Biol Reprod 1997;57:827.

84. Ferry BL, Sargent IL, Starkey PM, Redman CWG: Cytotoxic activity against trophoblast and choriocarcinoma cells of large granular lymphocytes from human early pregnancy decidua. Cell Immunol 1991;132:140.

85. Ewoldsen MA, Ostlie NS, Warner CM: Killing of mouse blastocyst stage embryos by cytotoxic T lymphocytes directed to major histocompatibility complex antigens. J Immunol 1987;138:2764.

86. Pajkrt D, Comoglio L, Tiel-van Buul MCM, et al: Attenuation of the proinflammatory response by recombinant human IL-10 in human endotoxemia. J Immunol 1997;158:3971.

87. Muzikova E, Clark DA: Is spontaneous resorption in the DBA/2-mated CBA/J mouse due to a defect in "seed" or "soil"? Am J Reprod Immunol 1995;33:81.

88. Ho HN, Wu MY, Yang YS: Peritoneal cellular immunity and endometriosis. Am J Reprod Immunol 1997;38:400.

89. Hill JA: Endometriosis: Immune cells and their products. In Hunt JS (ed): Immunobiology of Reproduction, Serono Symposia USA. New York, Springer-Verlag, 1994, pp 23-33.

90. Haimovici F, Anderson DJ: Cytokines and growth factors in implantation. Microsc Res Tech 1993;25:201.

91. Clark DA, Yu G, Levy GA, et al: Procoagulants in fetus rejection: The role of the OX-2 (CD200) tolerance signal. Semin Immunol 2001;13:255.

92. Lea RG, Clark DA: Macrophages and other migratory cells in endometrium relevant to implantation. Baillieres Clin Obstet Gynecol 1991;5:25.

93. Mellor AL, Sivakumar J, Chandler P, et al: Prevention of T cell–driven complement activation and inflammation by tryptophan catabolism during pregnancy. Nature Immunol 2001;2:64.

94. Janny L, Menezo YJ: Maternal age effect on early human embryonic development and blastocyst formation. Mol Reprod Dev 1996;45:31.

95. Pollard JW: Role of colony-stimulating factor-1 in reproduction and development. Mol Reprod Dev 1997;46:54.

96. Pollard JW, Dominguez MG, Mocci S, et al: Effect of the colony-stimulating factor-1 null mutation, osteopetrotic (csfm(op)), in the distribution of macrophages in the male mouse reproductive tract. Biol Reprod 1997;56:1290.

97. Watanabe H, Tatsumi K, Yokoi H, et al: Ovulation defect and its restoration by bone marrow transplantation in osteopetrotic mutant mice of Mitf^fmi/Mitf^fmi genotype. Biol Reprod 1997;57:1394.

98. Lea RG, Clark DA: Effects of decidual supernatants and lymphokines on murine trophoblast growth in vitro. Biol Reprod 1992;148:778.

99. Robertson SA, Sharkey DJ: The role of semen in induction of maternal immune tolerance to pregnancy. Semin Immunol 2001;13:243.

100. Clark DA, Chaouat G, Mogil R, Wegmann TG: Prevention of spontaneous abortion in DBA/2-mated CBA/J mice by GM-CSF involves CD8+ T cell–dependent suppression of natural effector cells. Cell Immunol 1994;154:143.

101. Ghazeeri GS, Clark DA, Kutteh WH: Immunological factors in implantation. Infertil Reprod Med Clin North Am 2001;12:315.

102. Clark DA: Is there any evidence for immunologically mediated or immunologically modifiable early pregnancy failure? J Assisted Reprod Genetics 2003;20:73.

103. King A, Jokhi PP, Burrows TD, et al: Functions of human decidual NK cells. Am J Reprod Immunol 1996;35:258.

104. Stewart-Akers AM, Krasnow JS, Brekosky J, DeLoria JA: Endometrial leukocytes are altered numerically and functionally in women with implantation defects. Am J Reprod Immunol 1998;39:1.

105. Kwak-Kim JYH, Chung-Bang HS, Ng SC, et al: Increased T helper 1 cytokine responses by circulating T cells are present in women with recurrent pregnancy losses and in infertile women with multiple implantation failures after IVF. Human Reprod 2003;18;767.

106. Clark DA, Coulam CB: Is there an immunological cause of repeated pregnancy wastage? Adv Obstet Gynecol 1995;3:321.

107. Clark DA, Daya S, Coulam CB, et al: Implications of human trophoblast karyotype for the evidence-based approach to the understanding, investigation, and treatment of recurrent spontaneous abortion. The Recurrent Miscarriage Immunotherapy Trialists Group. Am J Reprod Immunol 1996;35:495.

108. Rai R, Clifford K, Regan L: The modern preventative treatment of recurrent miscarriage. Br J Obstet Gynaecol 1996;103:106.

109. Boue J, Boue A, Lazar P: Retrospective and prospective epidemiologic studies of 1500 karyotyped spontaneous human abortions. Teratology 1975;12:11.

110. Recurrent Miscarriage Immunotherapy Trialists Group: Worldwide collaborative observational study and meta-analysis on allogeneic leukocyte immunotherapy for recurrent spontaneous abortion. Am J Reprod Immunol 1994;32:55.

111. Coulam CB, Stephenson M, Stern JJ, Clark DA: Immunotherapy for recurrent pregnancy loss: Analysis of results from clinical trials. Am J Reprod Immunol 1996;35:352.

112. Makhseed M, Raghupathy R, Azizieh F, et al: Th1 and Th2 cytokine profiles in recurrent aborters with successful pregnancy and with subsequent abortions. Human Reprod 2001;16:2219.

113. Blumberg N, Heal JM: The transfusion immunomodulation theory: The Th1/Th2 paradigm and an analogy with pregnancy as a unifying mechanism. Semin Hematol 1996;33:329.

114. Clark DA, Chaouat G, Gorczynski RM: Thinking outside the box: Mechanisms of environmental selective pressures on the outcome of the materno-fetal relationship. Am J Reprod Immunol 2002;47:275.

115. Wegmann TG, Waters CA, Drell DW, Carlson GA: Pregnant mice are not primed but can be primed to fetal alloantigens. Proc Natl Acad Sci U S A 1979;76:2410.

116. Zuckerman FA, Head J: Murine trophoblast resists cell mediated lysis. I. Resistance to allospecific cytotoxic T lymphocytes. J Immunol 1987;139:2856.

117. Zuckerman FA, Head J: Murine trophoblast resists cell-mediated lysis. II. Resistance to natural killer cell mediated cytotoxicity. Cell Immunol 1988;116:274.

118. Zuckerman FA, Head JR: Possible mechanism of non-rejection of the feto-placental allograft: Trophoblast resistance to lysis by cellular immune effectors. Transplant Proc 1987;19(1, Pt 1):554.

119. Hill JA, Melling GC, Johnson PM: Immunohistochemical studies of human uteroplacental tissues from first-trimester spontaneous abortions. Am J Obstet Gynecol 1995;173:90.

120. Bainbridge D, Ellis S, Le Bouteiller P, et al: HLA-G remains a mystery. Trends Immunol 2001;22:548.

121. Hunziker R, Gambel P, Wegmann TG: Placenta as a selective barrier to cellular traffic. J Immunol 1984;133:667.

122. Wegmann TG: Maternal T cells promote placental growth and prevent spontaneous abortion. Immunol Lett 1988;17:297.

123. Hunt JS, Vassamer D, Ferguson TA, Miller L: Fas ligand is positioned in mouse uterus and placenta to prevent trafficking of activated leukocytes between mother and conceptus. J Immunol 1997;158:4122.

124. Zhang L, Miller RG: The correlation of prolonged survival of maternal skin grafts with the presence of naturally transferred maternal T cells. Transplantation 1993;56:918.

125. Piotrowski P, Croy BA: Maternal cells are widely distributed in murine fetuses in utero. Biol Reprod 1996;54:1103.

126. Papadogiannakis N: Traffic of leukocytes through the maternofetal placental interface and its possible consequences. Curr Topics Microbiol Immunol 1997;222:141.

127. Chaouat G, Clark DA, Wegmann TG: Genetic aspects of the CBA × DBA/2 and B10 × B10.A models of murine pregnancy failure and its prevention by lymphocyte immunization. In Beard RW, Sharp F (eds): Early Pregnancy Failure: Mechanisms and Treatment. Ashton-under-Lyne, U.K., Peacock Press, 1988, pp 89-102.

128. Kiger N, Chaouat G, Kolb JP, et al: Immunogenetic studies of spontaneous abortions in mice: Preimmunization of the mother with allogeneic spleen cells. J Immunol 1985;134:2966.

129. Chaouat G, Clark DA: FAS/FAS ligand interaction at the placental interface is not required for the success of pregnancy in anti-paternal MHC preimmunized mice. Am J Reprod Immunol 2001;45:108.

130. Mowbray JF, Underwood JL: Effect of paternal lymphocyte immunisation on birthweight and pregnancy outcome. In Chaouat G, Mowbray JF (eds): Cellular and Molecular Biology of the Materno-Fetal Relationship, vol 212. Paris, Colloque INSERM/John Libbey Eurotext, 1991, pp 295-302.

131. Clark DA, Coulam CB, Daya S, et al: Unexplained sporadic and recurrent miscarriage in the new millennium: A critical analysis of immune mechanisms and treatments. Hum Reprod Update 2001;7:501.

132. King A, Gardner L, Loke YW: Human decidual leukocytes do not proliferate in response to either extravillous trophoblast or allogeneic peripheral blood lymphocytes. J Reprod Immunol 1996;30:67.

133. Croy BA, Chapeau C: Evaluation of the pregnancy immunotrophism hypothesis by assessment of the reproductive performance of young adult mice of genotype scid/scid.bg/bg. J Reprod Fertil 1990;88:231.

134. Clark DA, Lea RG, Denburg J, et al: Transforming growth factor-β related suppressor factor in mammalian pregnancy decidua: Homologies between the mouse and human successful pregnancy and in recurrent unexplained abortion. In Chaouat G, Mowbray JF (eds): Molecular and Cellular Biology of the Materno-Fetal Relationship, vol 212. Paris, INSERM Colloque/John Libbey Eurotext, 1991, pp 171-179.

135. Kinsky R, Delage G, Rosin M, et al: A murine model of NK cell mediated resorption. Am J Reprod Immunol 1990;23:73.

136. deFogerolles R, Baines MG: Modulation of natural killer activity influences resorption rates in CBA × DBA/2 matings. J Reprod Immunol 1987;11:147.

137. Baines MG, Duclos AJ, Antecka E, et al: Decidual infiltration and activation of macrophages leads to early embryo loss. Am J Reprod Immunol 1997;37:471.

138. Grimm EA: Human lymphokine-activated killer cells (LAK cells) as a potential therapeutic modality. Biochim Biophys Acta 1986;865:267.

139. Drake BL, Head J: Murine trophoblast can be killed by lymphokine-activated killer cells. J Immunol 1989;143:9.

140. King A, Loke YW: Human trophoblast cells and JEG choriocarcinoma cells are sensitive to lysis by IL-2–stimulated decidual NK cells. Cell Immunol 1990;129:435.

141. Lachapelle MH, Miron P, Hemmings R, et al: Endometrial T, B, and NK cells in patients with recurrent spontaneous abortion. J Immunol 1996;156:4027.

142. Vassiliadou N, Bulmer JN: Immunohistochemical evidence for increased numbers of "classic" CD56+ natural killer cells in the endometrium of women suffering spontaneous early pregnancy loss. Hum Reprod 1996;11:1559.

143. Maruyama T, Makino T, Sugi T, et al: Flow-cytometric analysis of immune cell populations in human decidua from various types of first-trimester pregnancy. Hum Immunol 1992;34:212.

144. Coulam CB, Beaman KD: Reciprocal alteration in circulating TJ6+ CD19+ and TJ6+ CD56− leukocytes in early pregnancy predicts success or miscarriage. Am J Reprod Immunol 1995;34:219.

145. Clark DA: Host immunoregulatory mechanisms and the success of the conceptus fertilized in vivo and in vitro. In Beard RW, Sharp F (eds): Early Pregnancy Loss: Mechanisms and Treatment. Ashton-under-Lyne, U.K., Peacock Press, 1988, pp 215-227.

146. Silver RM, Edwin SS, Trautman MS, et al: Bacterial lipopolysaccharide-mediated fetal death. Production of a newly recognized form of inducible cyclooxygenase (COX-2) in murine decidua in response to lipopolysaccharide. J Clin Invest 1995;95:725.

147. Krishnan L, Guilbert LJ, Wegmann TG, et al: T helper 1 response against Leishmania major in pregnant C57Bl/6 mice increases implantation failure and fetal resorptions. Correlation with increased IFN-γ and TNF and reduced IL-10 production by placental cells. J Immunol 1996;156:653.

148. Hill JA, Anderson DJ, Polgar K: T helper 1–type cellular immunity to trophoblast in women with recurrent spontaneous abortions. JAMA 1995;273:1933.

149. Marzi M, Vigano A, Trabettoni D, et al: Characterization of type 1 and type 2 cytokine production in physiologic and pathologic human pregnancy. Clin Exp Immunol 1996;106:127.

150. Arck PC, Ferrick DA, Steele-Norwood D, et al: Regulation of abortion by γδ T cells. Am J Reprod Immunol 1997;37:87.

151. Arck PC, Ferrick DA, Steele-Norwood D, et al: Murine T cell determination of pregnancy outcome. I. Effects of strain, αβ T cell receptor, γδ T cell receptor, and γδ T cell subsets. Am J Reprod Immunol 1997;37:492.

152. Arck P, Merali F, Stanisz A, et al: Stress-induced murine abortion associated with substance P–dependent alteration in cytokines in maternal uterine decidua. Biol Reprod 1995;53:814.

153. Markert U, Arck PC, McBey BA, et al: Stress-triggered abortions are associated with alterations of granulated cells in the decidua. Am J Reprod Immunol 1997;37:94.

154. Clark DA, Chaouat G, Arck PC, et al: Cytokine-dependent abortion in CBA × DBA/2 mice is mediated by the procoagulant fgl2 prothrombinase. J Immunol 1998;160:545.

155. Bratt J, Palmblad J: Cytokine-induced neutrophil-mediated injury of human endothelial cells. J Immunol 1997;159:912.

156. Clark DA, Ding JW, Chaouat G, et al: The emerging role of immunoregulation of fibrinogen-related procoagulant fgl2 in the success or spontaneous abortion of early pregnancy in mice and humans. Am J Reprod Immunol 1999;42:37.

157. Chaouat G, Menu E, Clark DA, et al: Control of fetal survival in CBA × DBA/2 mice by lymphokine therapy. J Reprod Fertil 1990;89:447.

158. Clark DA, Drake B, Head JR, et al: Decidua associated suppressor activity and viability of implantation sites in allopregnant C3H mice. J Reprod Immunol 1990;17:253.

159. Lea RG, Flanders KC, Harley CB, et al: Release of TGF-β2–related suppressor factor from postimplantation murine decidual tissue can be correlated with the detection of a subpopulation of cells containing RNA for TGF-β2. J Immunol 1992;148:778.

160. Lea RG, Underwood J, Flanders KC, et al: A subset of patients with recurrent spontaneous abortion is deficient in transforming growth factor β2–producing "suppressor cells" in uterine tissue near the implantation site. Am J Reprod Immunol 1995;34:52.

161. Salafia C, Maier D, Vogel C, et al: Placental and decidual histology in spontaneous abortion: Detailed description and correlations with chromosome number. Obstet Gynecol 1993;82:295.

162. Keil A, Yu K, Manuel J, et al: The "tolerance-promoting" molecule OX-2 is expressed in fetal trophoblast cells that cocoon the "fetal allograft" and may prevent pregnancy loss caused by cytokine-activation of fgl2 prothrombinase. Am J Reprod Immunol 2001;46:31.

163. Rand JH, Wu XX, Andree HAM, et al: Pregnancy loss in the antiphospholipid antibody syndrome: A possible thrombogenic mechanism. N Engl J Med 1997;227:154.

164. Lees C, Langford E, Brown AS, et al: The effects of S-nitrosoglutathione on platelet activation, hypertension, and uterine and fetal Doppler in severe preeclampsia. Obstet Gynecol 1996;88:14.

165. Bhagwanani SG, Seagraves K, Dieker LJ, et al: Relationship between prenatal anxiety and perinatal outcome in nulliparous women: A prospective study. J Natl Med Assoc 1997;89:93.

166. Sandman CA, Wadhwa PD, Chicz-Demet A, et al: Maternal stress, HPA activity, and fetal/infant outcome. Ann N Y Acad Sci 1997;814:266.

167. Goepfert AR, Goldenberg RL: Prediction of prematurity. Curr Opin Obstet Gynecol 1996;8:417.

168. Bry K, Hallman M: Transforming growth factor–β_2 prevents preterm delivery induced by interleukin 1α and tumor necrosis factor–α in the rabbit. Am J Obstet Gynecol 1993;168:1318.

169. Tranchot-Diallo J, Gras G, Parnet-Mathieu F, et al: Modulation of cytokine expression in pregnant women. Am J Reprod Immunol 1997;37:215.

170. Gorczynski RM, Hadidi S, Yu G, Clark DA: The same immunoregulatory molecules contribute to successful pregnancy and transplantation. Am J Reprod Immunol 2002;48:18.

171. Clark DA: HLA-G finally does something! Am J Reprod Immunol 1997;38:75.

172. Szekeres-Bartho J, Wegmann TG: A progesterone-dependent immunomodulatory protein alters the Th1/Th2 balance. J Reprod Immunol 1996;31:81.

173. Baines MG, Pross HF, Millar KG: Spontaneous human lymphocyte-mediated cytotoxicity against tumor target cells. VI. The suppressive effect of normal pregnancy. Am J Obstet Gynecol 1978;130:741.

174. Aoki K, Kajiura S, Matsumoto Y, et al: Preconceptional natural-killer-cell activity as a predictor of miscarriage. Lancet 1995;345:1340.

175. Nelson JL, Hughes KA, Smith AG, et al: Maternal-fetal disparity in HLA class II alloantigens and the pregnancy-induced amelioration of rheumatoid arthritis. N Engl J Med 1993;329:466.

176. Hidaka Y, Tamaki H, Iwatani Y, et al: Prediction of post-partum Graves' thyrotoxicosis by measurement of thyroid stimulating antibody in early pregnancy. Clin Endocrinol 1994;41:7.

177. Persellin RH: The effect of pregnancy on rheumatoid arthritis. Bull Rheum Dis 1976-1977;27:922.

178. Smith JB, Fort JG: Treatment of rheumatoid arthritis by immunization with mononuclear white cells. J Rheumatol 1996;23:220.

179. Waites GT, Whyte A: Effect of pregnancy on collagen-induced arthritis. Clin Exp Immunol 1987;67:467.

180. Clark DA, Manuel J, Arck PC, et al: Is remission of collagen-induced arthritis in pregnant DBA/1 mice relevant to remission of rheumatoid arthritis in human pregnancy? Am J Reprod Immunol 1996;35:464.

181. Gorczynski RM, Chen Z, Yu K, et al: CD200 immunoadhesin suppresses collagen-induced arthritis in mice. Clin Immunol 2001;101:328.

182. Ijima K, Murakami M, Okamoto H, et al: Successful gene therapy via intraarticular injection of adenovirus vector containing CTLA4IgG in a murine model of type II collagen–induced arthritis. Hum Gene Ther 2001;12:1063.

183. Black MM: New observations on pemphigoid "herpes gestationis." Dermatol 1994;189(Suppl 1):50.

184. Gill TJ III, Karasic RB, Antoncic J, et al: Long-term follow-up of children born to women immunized to tetanus toxoid during pregnancy. Am J Reprod Immunol 1991;25:69.

185. Talwar GP, Singh O, Gupta SK, et al: The HSD-hCG vaccine prevents pregnancy in women: feasibility study of a reversible safe contraceptive vaccine. Am J Reprod Immunol 1997;37:153.

186. Diekman AB, Goldberg E: Sperm antigens: Where are the private specificities? In Kurpisz M, Fernandez N (eds): Immunology of Human Reproduction. Oxford, U.K., Bios Scientific Publishers, 1995, pp 1-21.

187. Lea IA, Adoyo P, O'Rand MG: Autoimmunogenicity of the human sperm protein Sp17 in vasectomized men and identification of linear B epitopes. Fertil Steril 1997;67:355.

22

THE SKIN IN PREGNANCY

Cheryl F. Rosen

In this chapter, the physiologic changes that occur in the skin during pregnancy are reviewed, along with the specific dermatoses of pregnancy and intrahepatic cholestasis of pregnancy (ICP).

PIGMENTATION

An early sign of pregnancy is an increase in pigmentation of the skin, affecting primarily the areolae, the genitalia, and the abdominal midline. The pigmentation may continue to increase throughout pregnancy and may not completely regress post partum. Although increased levels of estrogen, progesterone,[1] and proopiomelanocortin-derived peptides, such as adrenocorticotropic hormone (ACTH), α-melanocyte-stimulating hormone (MSH), β-MSH, and β-endorphin,[2,3] may be involved, this has not been established. The darkening of the skin along the vertical midline of the abdominal wall is termed *linea nigra*. There is a tendency for new scars to be more pigmented than usual. Vertical demarcation lines between areas of different normal degrees of pigmentation, notably on the lower extremities, have been described.[4] Linear melanonychia, which are pigmented vertical lines on one or more nails, may be present during pregnancy.[5]

MELASMA

Melasma is a common disorder of facial hyperpigmentation (Fig. 22–1). It was previously termed *chloasma* or the *mask of pregnancy*. Macular areas of uniform brown pigmentation develop, mainly on the malar eminences, the forehead, the angles of the jaw, and the perioral area. Melasma occurs in 50% to 70% of pregnant women[6] and is more common in women with darker skin. Melasma usually diminishes after delivery, but it may persist. Sunlight exposure is involved in the origin of melasma in both pregnant and nonpregnant women. There are two types of melasma, epidermal and dermal, according to the location of the increased melanin in the skin.[7] Wood's lamp, which emits narrow-band ultraviolet A radiation, can be used to determine the site of melanin deposition.

Epidermal hyperpigmentation appears enhanced by the light of the lamp, whereas increased melanin in the dermis is not enhanced.

Melasma can be treated with topical preparations containing varying concentrations of tretinoin, hydroquinone (a tyrosinase inhibitor), and a corticosteroid.[8] One possible mixture is 4% hydroquinone powder in equal parts of tretinoin 0.025% cream and desonide cream, to be applied nightly. Protection from sunlight, including the use of a broad-spectrum sunscreen and a hat with a wide brim, is an important aspect of treatment of melasma. In a randomized double-blind study, a combination of 5% glycolic acid and 2% kojic acid (another tyrosinase inhibitor) appeared to be as effective as a combination of 5% glycolic acid and 2% hydroquinone.[9] In that study, 39 women treated half the face with each cream. None of the women had complete

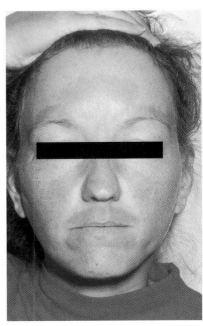

Figure 22–1. Melasma. Hypermelanosis on both cheeks, above eyebrows, on midforehead, above upper lip, and on chin.

resolution of the pigmentation, but all were judged to have improvement, between 10% to 90%. The average reduction in pigmentation was 58%.

Other treatments include tretinoin cream, 15% to 20% azalaic acid cream, and chemical peels using a number of agents including trichloroacetic acid.[10,11] The topical treatments for melasma may cause irritation with daily use. If this develops, the products can be used every other day. Treatments are thought to be more successful in women with epidermal melasma. The benefit of laser treatment for melasma has not been established.[10] Chemical peels and laser treatment should be used with caution in women of color.

HAIR

Telogen Effluvium

The normal human hair cycle consists of three phases: anagen, the growing phase; catagen, the brief transitional phase; and telogen, the resting phase. Telogen hairs remain in place until pushed out by new anagen hairs. It is normal to lose 100 to 150 hairs a day. During pregnancy, the anagen phase is prolonged until the postpartum period, when synchronous conversion to telogen occurs.[12] This results in telogen effluvium, a marked increase in telogen hair loss in the postpartum period. In a cohort of 98 postpartum women, 90% began to lose hair between 8 and 16 weeks post partum; in two thirds of these women, hair volume returned to normal in 4 to 6 months.[13] Hair loss was diffuse in 20%, frontal in 11%, and more noticeable over the anterior third of the scalp in 60%.

There is no active treatment for telogen effluvium. Women can be reassured that most of the shed hair will grow back. Cosmetically significant hair loss may not occur in subsequent pregnancies.

Androgenic Alopecia

Women may first become aware of diffuse or frontal thinning after a pregnancy. This is more likely to happen if the pregnancy occurs in the middle 20s to early 30s, the same age when early signs of androgenic alopecia begin to appear in nonpregnant women.

Hirsutism

Mild degrees of hirsutism may appear around the 20th week of pregnancy but almost always completely disappear after delivery. This phenomenon remains unexplained.

The most common cause of hirsutism in pregnancy is polycystic ovary disease.[14] Hirsutism developing for the first time or increasing rapidly during pregnancy should prompt an examination for signs of virilization. If these signs are present, further evaluation is required.

If the increase in hair growth does not resolve after delivery, and if investigation does not uncover an endocrine abnormality that necessitates systemic therapy, the unwanted hair can be removed by several methods, including shaving, plucking, waxing, electrolysis, and laser treatment.

BLOOD VESSELS

The mother's vascular system undergoes profound changes to accommodate the growing fetus. There is a substantial increase in blood volume, vascular distention, capillary permeability, and angiogenesis.[15] Placental angiogenesis factor and vascular endothelial growth factor are involved in the proper development of the placenta.[16,17]

Spider Telangiectasia and Palmar Erythema

There is an increased incidence of spider telangiectasia and palmar erythema during pregnancy. The telangiectasia are much more common in white women. According to a review of several papers, 67% of white women and 11% of black women developed spider telangiectasia between the second and fifth months of pregnancy.[18] Palmar erythema is seen almost as frequently as spider telangiectasia in white women but is three times more common than vascular spiders in black women.[18] Palmar erythema and telangiectasia resolve in the postpartum period in the majority of women.

Angiomatous Growths

Cherry angiomas are benign, erythematous, nonblanching papules, ranging in size from pinpoint to several millimeters. They usually occur on the trunk and may first appear during pregnancy. Although some may regress post partum, larger angiomas are likely to persist.

Unilateral nevoid telangiectatic syndrome is a collection of vascular "spiders" in a dermatomal distribution. One woman developed this syndrome while taking oral contraceptives. The telangiectasia increased in number and size during pregnancy and faded dramatically 2 weeks post partum.[19,20] Involved skin showed markedly increased numbers of estrogen and progesterone receptors, which were absent to negligible in uninvolved skin; these findings are suggestive of an etiologic role for estrogen.

Because telangiectasia and angiomas often resolve spontaneously, treatment of these lesions, if desired, should be postponed until the postpartum period. Low-voltage, fine-needle electrodesiccation and pulsed dye laser therapy can be used.

Varicosities

Varicose veins are common in pregnancy. They often appear for the first time during pregnancy. Existing varicosities may worsen. Varicose veins occur most commonly on the legs, the vulva, and the perianal area. Familial predisposition and parity are factors in the development of varicosities. During pregnancy, the gravid uterus is thought to compress the pelvic plexus. Blood vessel walls are thought to be more distensible as a result of the softening of connective tissue that accompanies pregnancy. Women may experience discomfort or pain from the varicosities in the legs and vulva. Hemorrhoids may be problematic. Deep venous thrombosis is a rare complication. Varicosities usually do not resolve completely after delivery.

Conservative treatment includes leg elevation, sleeping in a Trendelenburg or lateral decubitus position, and avoidance of prolonged standing. It is important to provide support for the varicose veins of the legs. Support stockings can be very helpful in easing discomfort.

Persistent large varicosities may ultimately necessitate surgery. If the patient is interested in cosmetic improvement, smaller varicosities may be amenable to treatment with sclerotherapy, in which hypertonic saline or other sclerosing agents are injected into the vessels. Persistent hemorrhoids necessitate evaluation for possible surgical treatment.

EDEMA

Nonpitting edema of the face, hands, ankles, and feet occurs in 50% to 70% of women in the last trimester of pregnancy.[21] Edema normally subsides soon after delivery.

Treatment is similar to conservative management of leg varicosities. Women can be advised to remove rings from their fingers when they first notice the edema appearing.

CUTIS MARMORATA

A transitory, erythematous reticulate mottling of the skin can occur in pregnant women when exposed to cold temperatures.[21] The erythematous skin blanches on pressure, and the condition is thought to be caused by vascular instability. Cutis marmorata is a benign phenomenon and is frequently seen in children. However, when a reticulate pattern is persistent and does not blanche, livedo reticularis enters the differential diagnosis. Livedo reticularis may also be a benign idiopathic disorder, but collagen vascular diseases must be ruled out by the appropriate investigations.

CONNECTIVE TISSUE

Skin Tags

Skin tags are also called *acrochordons*. Large lesions are known as *fibroepithelial polyps*. In the past, skin tags were called *molluscum fibrosum gravidarum*. They are small, skin-colored to hyperpigmented, polypoid lesions with a predilection for certain areas: the neck, axillae, groin, and inframammary folds. Clinically and histologically, there is no difference between lesions that develop during pregnancy and those developing at other times (Fig. 22–2). Skin tags tend to appear during the second half of pregnancy and increase in size and number. They are benign. Small skin tags may resolve during the postpartum period. If they persist, they can be removed for cosmetic reasons by cryotherapy, or they can be snipped off with

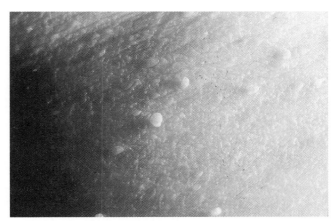

Figure 22–2. Skin tags (acrochordons). Seen on the neck and in areas with creases, such as eyelids, axillae, and inframammary folds; smaller skin tags may involute after delivery.

a pair of scissors, either with or without local anesthesia. Larger lesions may removed by scissors or electrodesiccation, after local anesthesia.

Striae Gravidarum

Stretch marks (striae gravidarum or striae distensae) begin as pink to violaceous linear bands showing dermal and epidermal atrophy. Striae usually occur on the abdomen, breasts, buttocks, and thighs. They are said to occur in 90% of pregnant white women and are less common in Asian and black women.[21] Continuous stretching of the skin over the abdomen and the increased levels of glucocorticoids associated with pregnancy are thought to lead to the development of striae.[22] In in vitro models, glucocorticoids led to a decrease in the number of fibroblasts in the dermis and a decrease in collagen synthesis.[23]

Dermal glycosaminoglycan content is increased in striae.[24] The amount of vertical fibrillin fibers beneath the dermal-epidermal junction and elastin fibers in the papillary dermis was found to be significantly reduced in striae in comparison with normal skin of pregnant women. The elastin and fibrillin fibers in the deep dermis were realigned, with fibers oriented parallel to the dermal epidermal junction. No alterations were observed in the other extracellular matrix components.[24]

Many topical preparations have been tried to prevent the formation of striae. A Cochrane Collaboration review found one preparation to be helpful.[25] In a placebo-controlled trial, a cream containing *Centella asiatica* extract, α-tocopherol, and collagen-elastin hydrolysates was associated with development of striae in fewer women (odds ratio, 0.41; 95% confidence interval, 0.17 to 0.99). However, this was found only in women who had developed striae during an earlier pregnancy.

There is no uniformly successful treatment for striae. Topical tretinoin has been used with varying success.[26-28] The pulsed dye laser has been used to treat striae, having a greater effect on erythema.[29] With time, the violaceous or erythematous color fades, and the striae become less obvious.

Gingivitis of Pregnancy

Edema and hyperemia of the gingivae are very common during pregnancy. Gingivitis develops in 35% to 50% of pregnant women.[21] Gingivitis may begin in the first trimester and is progressive. The papillae become congested and edematous, may bleed easily, and may be painful. Women should be encouraged to seek care from a dentist.

Pyogenic Granuloma

A pyogenic granuloma is a benign vascular growth, a lobular capillary hemangioma. This lesion is not unique to pregnancy, but it may occur in 5% of pregnant women.[21] It may appear on the oral mucosa or on the skin. When these lesions occur on the mucosa, they have also been termed *granuloma gravidarum* or *epulis*. The lesions are typically erythematous moist papules with a collarette of skin at the base. The surface may be crusted. The lesions bleed easily. They grow rapidly initially and then remain stable and may resolve completely after delivery. Histologic examination shows a proliferation of new blood vessels and endothelial cells within a loose granulation tissue.[30] Surgical removal or treatment with a pulsed dye laser may be required because the lesions often persist, and their tendency to bleed makes them a nuisance.

DERMATOSES OF PREGNANCY

Over the years, many pruritic eruptions have been described in pregnant women. This led to a confusing situation in which there seemed to be more names for diseases than there were actual disorders. There seems to be a reluctance to abandon the historical names for conditions. To clarify the situation, Holmes and Black proposed a simplified classification for the specific dermatoses of pregnancy.[31,32] This classification includes pemphigoid gestationis, pruritic urticarial papules and plaques of pregnancy (PUPPP) (known as *polymorphic eruption of pregnancy* in the United Kingdom), prurigo of pregnancy, and pruritic folliculitis of pregnancy. To this classification another category must be added: intrahepatic cholestasis of pregnancy (ICP). It is not considered a specific dermatosis, inasmuch as there are no primary skin lesions; however, it is specific to pregnancy.

Pemphigoid gestationis and ICP are associated with an increased risk to the fetus, whereas PUPPP, prurigo of pregnancy, and pruritic folliculitis are not.[33]

It is important to remember that pregnant women may also develop itchy skin eruptions that are not specific to pregnancy. Flares of eczema may be particularly common.[34] Impetigo herpetiformis, a rare generalized pustular eruption, is now generally considered to be pustular psoriasis occurring during pregnancy.[35,36]

Intrahepatic Cholestasis of Pregnancy

Women with ICP note the onset of generalized pruritus, generally after the 30th week of gestation. ICP results from an abnormality of biliary transport from the liver to the small intestine.[37] There are no primary skin lesions, but secondary skin changes, often excoriations, are seen. When jaundice is not present but the biochemical abnormalities to be discussed are detected, the term *pruritus gravidarum* is sometimes used.[35] ICP resolves in the postpartum period.

The incidence of ICP varies considerably around the world. In Scandinavia, Bolivia, and Chile, prevalence rates of 3%, 9%, and 16% have been reported. In Europe (0.1% to 1.5%), Canada (0.5%), and Australia and the United States (0.07% to 0.6%), the incidence is lower.[35]

Estrogens and progestins have been implicated in causing ICP. Estrogen interferes with bile acid secretion across the hepatocyte membrane.[38] Progestins inhibit hepatic glucuronyl transferase, which reduces the hepatic clearance of estrogens, allowing their effect on bile secretion to be enhanced. The use of micronized progesterone to prevent premature labor was seen to trigger ICP.[39] The serum concentrations of various progesterone metabolites are altered in the blood of women with ICP, in comparison with unaffected pregnant women. Monosulfated and disulfated progesterone metabolites are increased,[38] and the ratio of 3α-hydroxylated steroids to 3β-hydroxylated steroids is increased. It is unclear whether these alterations are primary or secondary. Mutations in genes encoding bile transport proteins are being identified.[37]

A positive family history is found in approximately 50% of women with ICP.[40] There is a high recurrence rate (40% to 50%) with subsequent pregnancies.

Laboratory Findings

Serum bile acid levels are elevated in women with ICP; the degree of elevation is correlated with severity of pruritus.[38] They may be elevated 10 to 100 times the normal value. Liver function test values, including those of alkaline phosphatase, transaminases (alanine and aspartate aminotransferase), 5′-nucleotidase, cholesterol, and triglycerides, are mildly elevated. Jaundiced patients have a mild to moderate increase in bilirubin. Malabsorption of fat may occur and can result in vitamin K deficiency.[38]

Cholestatic changes are noted on liver biopsy. Dilated biliary canaliculi, staining of hepatocytes with bile pigment, and minimal inflammation are seen.[38] Because there are no primary skin lesions, skin biopsies are not helpful.

The role of hepatitis C in ICP has been investigated. Of pregnant women with hepatitis C, 20% developed ICP, in contrast to only 0.78% of women who were hepatitis C seronegative.[41]

Differential Diagnosis

Other causes of jaundice, such as viral or drug-induced hepatitis and biliary tract obstruction, must be ruled out by laboratory tests.

Fetal Prognosis

With ICP, there is an increased incidence of fetal distress, stillbirths, and premature births. Meconium staining of the amniotic fluid has been noted.[42] However, babies born to women who have had ICP do not have evidence of abnormal development.[42] Close fetal surveillance with induction of labor at the first sign of fetal distress is recommended.[43] At 38 weeks' gestation, induction of labor is suggested.[43] Delivery by 38 weeks has reduced the perinatal mortality rate to 2.0% to 3.5%.[37]

Treatment

Delivery of the baby leads to resolution of the pruritus. Mild pruritus may be treated with soothing lotions and cool compresses. Antihistamines are usually not helpful.

Cholestyramine, an anion exchange resin that binds bile acids, has been used to treat the pruritus of ICP.[44] In an uncontrolled trial, 80 pregnant women with ICP were treated with cholestyramine; 70% improved. However, most of the women in this study may have had mild pruritus that was more easily controlled. The cholestatic biochemical abnormalities are not improved by taking cholestyramine. Guar gum can increase the fecal elimination of bile acids and has been suggested as an adjunct to ursodeoxycholic acid (UDCA) therapy.[45]

UDCA is a naturally occurring hydrophilic bile acid. It stimulates the excretion of hydrophobic bile acids and sulfated progesterone metabolites. Theoretically, UDCA should decrease total bile acids in the mother and in the fetus. Interventions for treating ICP have been analyzed in a review in which the authors found insufficient evidence to support the use of any treatment for ICP.[46] In a second review, the investigators stated that although further study with larger randomized controlled trials are needed, the available data support a role for UDCA, with improvement in maternal and fetal morbidity.[43] A regimen of 1 g/day in divided doses was recommended in that review.[43] UDCA is safe for the pregnant woman and the fetus.

Pemphigoid (Herpes) Gestationis

Definition

Clinical and immunopathologic similarities to bullous pemphigoid (BP) have led to an attempt to replace the term *herpes gestationis* with *pemphigoid gestationis*.[31,47] Adoption of this terminology prevents confusion of this disease with an eruption caused by a herpesvirus.

Clinical Features

Pemphigoid gestationis is an intensely itchy eruption that usually begins around the second or third trimester of pregnancy. This condition is rare, occurring in 1 per 50,000 pregnancies in North America and in 1 per 40,000 pregnancies in the United Kingdom.[35,48] In 50% to 85% of cases, the eruption first appears as urticarial erythematous papules and plaques in or around the umbilicus (Fig. 22–3). The lesions enlarge to become polycyclic, annular, or targetoid urticarial plaques with tense vesicles or bullae (Fig. 22–4).[49] Lesions spread to the arms and legs; the face, mucosal surfaces, palms, and soles are spared. Ultimately, the eruption is a generalized vesicobullous disease. In rare cases, no vesicles or bullae develop. This nonbullous form can be diagnosed by immunohistologic techniques.[47]

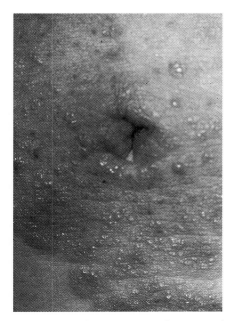

Figure 22–3. Pemphigoid gestationis. Erythematous plaque surmounted by tense vesicles spreading from within the umbilicus to surrounding abdominal skin.

Pemphigoid gestationis persists after delivery, with an average postpartum duration of 12 to 60 weeks.[35] It is very common to have a postpartum flare. Pemphigoid gestationis often recurs in subsequent pregnancies, but recurrences may be less severe.[47] Recurrences may occur after the use of oral contraceptives.

Histopathology

The histologic examination of a typical bulla of pemphigoid gestationis reveals a subepidermal vesicle with a mixed, perivascular infiltrate consisting of lymphocytes, histiocytes, and eosinophils. Eosinophilic spongiosis, in which numerous eosinophils are visible within the epidermis of the urticarial plaques, is seen.[50]

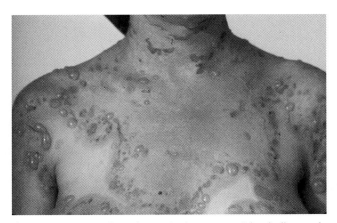

Figure 22–4. Pemphigoid gestationis. Tense vesicles, bullae, and erosions along an urticarial border in an annular and polycyclic pattern on the anterior chest.

Immunopathology

To confirm the diagnosis of pemphigoid gestationis, a perilesional skin biopsy specimen should be obtained for direct immunofluorescence examination. Pemphigoid gestationis is defined by the presence of linear deposits of the third component of complement (C3) along the dermal-epidermal junction. Thus, 100% of positive biopsy specimens in pemphigoid gestationis show the C3 deposits. Deposition of immunoglobulin G (IgG) is seen in 30% of cases. Immunoelectron microscopy demonstrates that IgG and C3 are deposited in the lamina lucida of the dermal-epidermal junction. The antibody belongs to the IgG_1 major subclass and recognizes a 180-kD protein, the BP antigen 2 (BP180 or BPAg2). BPAg2 is a transmembrane glycoprotein found in hemidesmosomes, the cellular structures that bind the basal keratinocytes to the dermal-epidermal junction.[51] BPAg2 is type XVII collagen. The antibody binds to epitopes within the extracellular noncollagenous domain of BPAg2 called NC16A.[52] Linear C3 and IgG deposits are found in the skin of babies of affected mothers; the infants rarely demonstrate clinical disease.[36]

A genetic predisposition to pemphigoid gestationis is strongly suggested by an increased frequency of the human leukocyte antigen class II antigens DR3 and DR4.[53] These haplotypes are also observed in patients with other autoimmune diseases.

Differential Diagnosis

The differential diagnoses include other bullous diseases such as BP, pemphigus vulgaris, erythema multiforme, and PUPPP. Despite some overlap in the morphologic appearance of lesions and in immunohistologic features, pemphigoid gestationis differs from BP in that the latter is more common in people older than 60 years. According to histologic examination, destruction of basal keratinocytes is not a feature of BP, but can be seen in pemphigoid gestationis.

The vesicles in pemphigus vulgaris are usually flaccid and rupture easily, whereas those of pemphigoid gestationis and BP are tense. Pemphigus vulgaris often manifests with mucous membrane involvement. Histologic examination reveals an intraepidermal bulla with acantholysis of epidermal cells. Direct immunofluorescence examination reveals intercellular deposition of IgG between keratinocytes, and the sera of patients with pemphigus have IgG antibodies that react with a protein called desmoglein 1.

Although both pemphigoid gestationis and erythema multiforme can present with targetoid lesions that histologically show vacuolar destruction of basal keratinocytes, immune deposits at the basement membrane zone and circulating IgG antibody are not features of erythema multiforme.

Early and nonbullous stages of pemphigoid gestationis can be differentiated from PUPPP by the absence of immune deposits and circulating antibodies in PUPPP.

Treatment

The goal of treatment is to prevent the formation of new lesions and to control pruritus. Mild cases may respond to topical steroids and antihistamines. However, most patients need systemic therapy. The mainstay of treatment is systemic steroids in the form of prednisone, usually in the range of 40 to 80 mg/day initially.[49] The maintenance steroid dosage may need to be adjusted upward for postpartum flares and for exacerbations associated with menses.[47] Minocycline and nicotinamide were used to treat one woman with severe recurrent pemphigoid gestationis.[54] For persistent postpartum flares, immunosuppressive therapy has been used in one patient.[55]

Fetal Risk

The outcomes of 254 pregnancies in 74 women with immunofluorescence-confirmed pemphigoid gestationis were studied.[56] No evidence for an increased rate of spontaneous abortion or significant fetal mortality was found. The study did confirm an increased incidence of prematurity and a slight increase in the number of infants small for gestational age. Treatment with systemic corticosteroids did not increase or decrease these risks. According to a review of articles published between 1966 and 1999, pregnancies affected by pemphigoid gestationis should be considered high risk until more definitive information becomes available.[33]

Only 5% to 10% of babies born to mothers with pemphigoid gestationis develop skin lesions. The lesions resolve spontaneously.

Pruritic Urticarial Papules and Plaques of Pregnancy

Clinical Features

PUPPP is a pruritic eruption that appears during the last few weeks of pregnancy. It is the most common dermatosis of pregnancy. The typical lesions are erythematous papules that coalesce into large urticarial plaques.[57,58] The papules first appear on the abdomen (Fig. 22–5), particularly within striae, and spread to the thighs (Fig. 22–6).

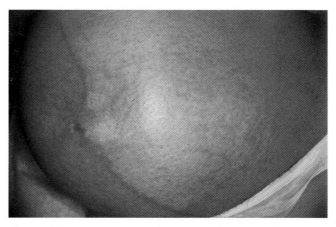

Figure 22–5. Pruritic urticarial papules and plaques of pregnancy (PUPPP). Also known as polymorphic eruption of pregnancy. Erythematous, urticarial papules first appear on the abdomen; note pigmented line running vertically along the midabdomen (linea nigra).

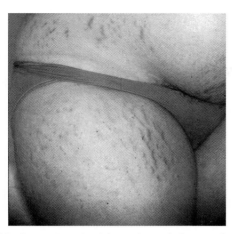

Figure 22–6. Pruritic urticarial papules and plaques of pregnancy (PUPPP). Erythematous papules have spread to sides of abdomen and thighs, particularly within striae distensae (stretch marks).

Papules are very edematous and may become vesicular. The lesions can involve the extremities, chest, and back, but the face is spared. Despite the pruritus, excoriations are rare. There is an increased incidence of PUPPP in twin and other higher order pregnancies.[59]

The pruritus and the eruption persist until delivery. Resolution may occur in the early postpartum period, but the eruption may persist for 3 to 4 weeks post partum. Recurrence is rare, as is onset in the postpartum period. No related maternal deaths have been reported, and there is no increase in fetal morbidity or mortality.

Diagnosis

The histologic features of PUPPP are nonspecific. There is a perivascular lymphohistiocytic infiltrate in the superficial to middle dermis. Occasional eosinophils are noted. Edema of the epidermis (spongiosis) and papillary dermis may be seen. No antibodies to any component of the skin are found in PUPPP. Direct immunofluorescence examination of both lesional and perilesional skin yields negative findings.

The major differential diagnosis is pemphigoid gestationis (Table 22–1), particularly in the early urticarial phase.[47] PUPPP and pemphigoid gestationis differ in the usual time of onset during pregnancy, and the immunofluorescent findings are negative in PUPPP and diagnostically positive in pemphigoid gestationis. Idiopathic urticaria and drug eruptions should be considered in the differential diagnosis.

Treatment

Treatment is aimed at relieving pruritus. Potent topical steroids can be beneficial. Antihistamines and colloidal oatmeal baths and lubrication may offer symptomatic relief.

Prurigo of Pregnancy

Prurigo of pregnancy remains poorly defined. The clinical features include grouped excoriated or crusted papules over the abdomen and extensor surfaces of the arms and legs.[34,59] The appearance has been described as eczematous.

TABLE 22–1   Pruritic Eruptions Unique to Pregnancy

Characteristics	Cholestasis of Pregnancy	Pemphigoid Gestationis*	Pruritic Urticarial Papules and Plaques of Pregnancy†
Prevalence	<1% of pregnancies (United States)	1:50,000 pregnancies	1:160 pregnancies
Onset	Third trimester	Second trimester or earlier	Last few weeks of pregnancy
Course	Clears within a few days of delivery	Persists after delivery for as long as 12-60 weeks	Generally clears after delivery but may persist for 3-4 weeks
Recurrence with subsequent pregnancies	Yes	Yes	No
Skin lesions	Excoriations; rarely, jaundice	Erythematous papules, plaques, polycyclic and annular wheals; vesicles and large, tense bullae are typical	Papules, plaques, polycyclic wheals, microvesicles
Location of eruption	Areas accessible to scratching	Starts and is most prominent around the umbilicus	Starts within striae on the abdomen and may spare the periumbilical area
Direct immunofluorescence findings	Negative	Linear deposits of C3 in DEJ of uninvolved skin	Negative
Indirect immunofluorescence findings	Negative	IgG antibody that binds complement to epidermal aspect of saline split normal skin	Negative
Treatment	Soothing antipruritic lotions, antihistamines, cholestyramine, ursodeoxycholic acid	Systemic steroids: >40-80 mg prednisone per day initially	Topical steroids, antihistamines; rarely, systemic steroids
Fetal risk	Increased incidence of fetal distress and prematurity	Increased incidence of prematurity and small for gestational age babies	None

*Also known as herpes gestationis.
†Also known polymorphic eruption of pregnancy.
DEJ, dermal epidermal junction; IgG, immunoglobulin G.

Histologic features are nonspecific, with a perivascular lymphocytic infiltrate in the dermis. Immunofluorescence test results are negative.

There is no risk to the mother or the fetus.

Treatment is directed toward controlling the pruritus.[36]

Pruritic Folliculitis of Pregnancy

The first report of pruritic folliculitis described six pregnant women who developed a generalized, pruritic, papular eruption that was clinically and histologically consistent with noninfectious folliculitis.[60] All lesions were excoriated. The eruption occurred between the fourth and ninth months of pregnancy and cleared spontaneously after delivery; the infants were normal. Direct immunofluorescence was negative for immune deposits. Investigations of more patients have been documented in other studies.[34,61] There is no evidence of any maternal or fetal risk. It is not clear whether pruritic folliculitis is a distinct entity.

Impetigo Herpetiformis

Impetigo herpetiformis has come to be regarded as the occurrence of pustular psoriasis during pregnancy. It usually begins in the third trimester. There may not be a personal or family history of psoriasis. Recurrence in subsequent pregnancies is often seen.

Clinical Features

Pustules develop on erythematous patches that enlarge centrifugally, resulting in annular to polycyclic lesions (Figs. 22–7 and 22–8). New pustules arise in waves, often at the edges of the patches. The extremities, primarily flexures, and the trunk and the oral mucosa may be involved. Systemic symptoms, fever, malaise, diarrhea, and vomiting may occur.[36]

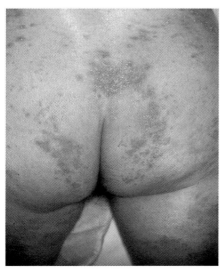

Figure 22–7. Impetigo herpetiformis. Erythematous papules and plaques surmounted by superficial pustules on buttocks and thighs.

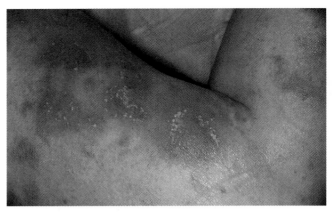

Figure 22–8. Impetigo herpetiformis. Note the tendency of the pustules to form arcs and circles.

Diagnosis

As in pustular psoriasis, the histologic appearance is characterized by collections of neutrophils beneath the stratum corneum of the epidermis (subcorneal pustules) and within the epidermis (spongiform pustules). Affected women may have leukocytosis and hypocalcemia.

Treatment

The mainstay of therapy is systemic corticosteroids.[35] The eruption usually clears in the postpartum period, but there are reports of prolonged persistence. Impetigo herpetiformis is associated with an increased risk of placental insufficiency, stillbirth, and neonatal death.[36]

References

1. Snell RS, Turner R: Skin pigmentation in relation to the menstrual cycle. J Invest Dermatol 1966;47:147.
2. Margioris AN, Grino M, Protos P, et al: Corticotropin-releasing hormone and oxytocin stimulate the release of placental proopiomelanocortin peptides. J Clin Endocrinol Metab 1988;66:922.
3. Margioris AN, Grino M, Rabin D, et al: Human placenta and the hypothalamic-pituitary-adrenal axis. Adv Exp Med Biol 1988;245:389.
4. Vazquez M, Ibanez MI, Sanchez JL: Pigmentary demarcation lines during pregnancy. Cutis 1986;38:263.
5. Fryer JM, Werth VP: Pregnancy-associated hyperpigmentation: Longitudinal melanonychia. J Am Acad Dermatol 1992;26:493.
6. Wade TR, Wade SL, Jones HE: Skin changes and diseases associated with pregnancy. Obstet Gynecol 1978;52:233.
7. Sanchez NP, Pathak MA, Sato S, et al: Melasma: A clinical, light microscopic, ultrastructural, and immunofluorescence study. J Am Acad Dermatol 1981;4:698.
8. Kligman AM, Willis I: A new formula for depigmenting human skin. Arch Dermatol 1975;111:40.
9. Garcia A, Fulton JE Jr: The combination of glycolic acid and hydroquinone or kojic acid for the treatment of melasma and related conditions. Dermatol Surg 1996;22:443.
10. Grimes PE: Melasma. Etiologic and therapeutic considerations. Arch Dermatol 1995;131:1453.
11. Perez-Bernal A, Munoz-Perez MA, Camacho F: Management of facial hyperpigmentation. Am J Clin Dermatol 2000;1:261.
12. Lynfield YL: Effect of pregnancy on the human hair cycle. J Invest Dermatol 1960;35:323.
13. Schiff BL, Kern AB: Study of postpartum alopecia. Arch Dermatol 1963;87:609.

14. Fayez JA, Bunch TR, Miller GL: Virilization in pregnancy associated with polycystic ovary disease. Obstet Gynecol 1974;44:511.
15. Parmley T, O'Brien TJ: Skin changes during pregnancy. Clin Obstet Gynecol 1990;33:713.
16. Geva E, Ginzinger DG, Zaloudek CJ, et al: Human placental vascular development: Vasculogenic and angiogenic (branching and non-branching) transformation is regulated by vascular endothelial growth factor-A, angiopoietin-1, and angiopoietin-2. J Clin Endocrinol Metab 2002;87:4213.
17. Cross JC, Hemberger M, Lu Y, et al: Trophoblast functions, angiogenesis and remodeling of the maternal vasculature in the placenta. Mol Cell Endocrinol 2002;187:207.
18. Barankin B, Silver SG, Carruthers A: The skin in pregnancy. J Cutan Med Surg 2002;6:236.
19. Uhlin SR, McCarty KS Jr: Unilateral nevoid telangiectatic syndrome. The role of estrogen and progesterone receptors. Arch Dermatol 1983;119:226.
20. Wilkin JK, Smith JG Jr, Cullison DA, et al: Unilateral dermatomal superficial telangiectasia. Nine new cases and a review of unilateral dermatomal superficial telangiectasia. J Am Acad Dermatol 1983;8:468.
21. Wong RC, Ellis CN: Physiologic skin changes in pregnancy. J Am Acad Dermatol 1984;10:929.
22. Davey CM: Factors associated with the occurrence of striae gravidarum. J Obstet Gynaecol Br Commonw 1972;79:1113.
23. Booth BA, Tan EM, Oikarinen A, Uitto J: Steroid-induced dermal atrophy: Effects of glucocorticosteroids on collagen metabolism in human skin fibroblast cultures. Int J Dermatol 1982;21:333.
24. Watson RE, Parry EJ, Humphries JD, et al: Fibrillin microfibrils are reduced in skin exhibiting striae distensae. Br J Dermatol 1998;138:931.
25. Young GL, Jewell D: Creams for preventing stretch marks in pregnancy. Cochrane Database Syst Rev 2000;(2):CD000066.
26. Elson ML: Treatment of striae distensae with topical tretinoin. J Dermatol Surg Oncol 1990;16:267.
27. Rangel O, Arias I, Garcia E, et al: Topical tretinoin 0.1% for pregnancy-related abdominal striae: An open-label, multicenter, prospective study. Adv Ther 2001;18:181.
28. Pribanich S, Simpson FG, Held B, et al: Low-dose tretinoin does not improve striae distensae: A double-blind, placebo-controlled study. Cutis 1994;54:121.
29. Jimenez GP, Flores F, Berman B, et al: Treatment of striae rubra and striae alba with the 585-nm pulsed-dye laser. Dermatol Surg 2003;29:362.
30. Sills ES, Zegarelli DJ, Hoschander MM, et al: Clinical diagnosis and management of hormonally responsive oral pregnancy tumor (pyogenic granuloma). J Reprod Med 1996;41:467.
31. Holmes RC, Black MM: The specific dermatoses of pregnancy: A reappraisal with special emphasis on a proposed simplified clinical classification. Clin Exp Dermatol 1982;7:65.
32. Holmes RC, Black MM: The specific dermatoses of pregnancy. J Am Acad Dermatol 1983;8:405.
33. Sherard GB 3rd, Atkinson SM Jr: Focus on primary care: Pruritic dermatological conditions in pregnancy. Obstet Gynecol Surv 2001;56:427.
34. Vaughan Jones SA, Hern S, Nelson-Piercy C, et al: A prospective study of 200 women with dermatoses of pregnancy correlating clinical findings with hormonal and immunopathological profiles. Br J Dermatol 1999;141:71.
35. Kroumpouzos G, Cohen LM: Dermatoses of pregnancy. J Am Acad Dermatol 2001;45:1.
36. Al-Fares SI, Jones SV, Black MM: The specific dermatoses of pregnancy: A re-appraisal. J Eur Acad Dermatol Venereol 2001;15:197.
37. Dixon PH, Weerasekera N, Linton KJ, et al: Heterozygous MDR3 missense mutation associated with intrahepatic cholestasis of

pregnancy: Evidence for a defect in protein trafficking. Hum Mol Genet 2000;9:1209.
38. Kroumpouzos G: Intrahepatic cholestasis of pregnancy: What's new. J Eur Acad Dermatol Venereol 2002;16:316.
39. Bacq Y, Sapey T, Brechot MC, et al: Intrahepatic cholestasis of pregnancy: A French prospective study. Hepatology 1997;26:358.
40. Shornick JK: Dermatoses of pregnancy. Semin Cutan Med Surg 1998;17:172.
41. Paternoster DM, Fabris F, Palu G, et al: Intra-hepatic cholestasis of pregnancy in hepatitis C virus infection. Acta Obstet Gynecol Scand 2002;81:99.
42. Reyes H: The spectrum of liver and gastrointestinal disease seen in cholestasis of pregnancy. Gastroenterol Clin North Am 1992;21:905.
43. Jenkins JK, Boothby LA: Treatment of itching associated with intrahepatic cholestasis of pregnancy. Ann Pharmacother 2002;36:1462.
44. Rampone A, Rampone B, Tirabasso S, et al: Prurigo gestationis. J Eur Acad Dermatol Venereol 2002;16:425.
45. Riikonen S, Savonius H, Gylling H, et al: Oral guar gum, a gel-forming dietary fiber, relieves pruritus in intrahepatic cholestasis of pregnancy. Acta Obstet Gynecol Scand 2000;79:260.
46. Burrows RF, Clavisi O, Burrows E: Interventions for treating cholestasis in pregnancy. Cochrane Database Syst Rev 2001;(4):CD000493.
47. Shornick JK, Bangert JL, Freeman RG, et al: Herpes gestationis: Clinical and histologic features of twenty-eight cases. J Am Acad Dermatol 1983;8:214.
48. Yancey KB: Herpes gestationis. Dermatol Clin 1990;8:727.
49. Jenkins RE, Hern S, Black MM: Clinical features and management of 87 patients with pemphigoid gestationis. Clin Exp Dermatol 1999;24:255.
50. Morrison LH, Anhalt GJ: Herpes gestationis. J Autoimmun 1991;4:37.
51. Diaz LA, Ratrie H 3rd, Saunders WS, et al: Isolation of a human epidermal cDNA corresponding to the 180-kD autoantigen recognized by bullous pemphigoid and herpes gestationis sera. Immunolocalization of this protein to the hemidesmosome. J Clin Invest 1990;86:1088.
52. Lin MS, Gharia M, Fu CL, et al: Molecular mapping of the major epitopes of BP180 recognized by herpes gestationis autoantibodies. Clin Immunol 1999;92:285.
53. Engineer L, Bhol K, Ahmed AR: Pemphigoid gestationis: A review. Am J Obstet Gynecol 2000;183:483.
54. Loo WJ, Dean D, Wojnarowska F: A severe persistent case of recurrent pemphigoid gestationis successfully treated with minocycline and nicotinamide. Clin Exp Dermatol 2001;26:726.
55. Jolles S: A review of high-dose intravenous immunoglobulin (hdIVIg) in the treatment of the autoimmune blistering disorders. Clin Exp Dermatol 2001;26:127.
56. Shornick JK, Black MM: Fetal risks in herpes gestationis. J Am Acad Dermatol 1992;26:63.
57. Lawley TJ, Hertz KC, Wade TR, et al: Pruritic urticarial papules and plaques of pregnancy. JAMA 1979;241:1696.
58. Yancey KB, Hall RP, Lawley TJ: Pruritic urticarial papules and plaques of pregnancy. Clinical experience in twenty-five patients. J Am Acad Dermatol 1984;10:473.
59. Kroumpouzos G, Cohen LM: Specific dermatoses of pregnancy: An evidence-based systematic review. Am J Obstet Gynecol 2003;188:1083.
60. Zoberman E, Farmer ER: Pruritic folliculitis of pregnancy. Arch Dermatol 1981;117:20.
61. Roger D, Vaillant L, Fignon A, et al: Specific pruritic diseases of pregnancy. A prospective study of 3192 pregnant women. Arch Dermatol 1994;130:734.

23

Neoplastic Diseases

Barbara Burtness

Cancer has a bimodal age distribution. It is a hereditary disease, in which case it may manifest in childhood, and it is a disease of acquired genetic abnormalities, in which case it most often manifests in middle and old age. Cancer manifests much less frequently in the childbearing years. The incidence of cancer in pregnant women is similar to that of other women of childbearing age; cancer complicates 1 per 1000 pregnancies and accounts for only 5% of maternal deaths.[1] Because more women today choose to delay childbearing, the co-occurrence of pregnancy and cancer may increase.

REPRODUCTIVE RISK FACTORS AND CANCER

Reproductive characteristics are important risk factors for many cancers, which is suggestive of a role for endogenous hormones in cancer suppression or promotion in different malignancies. Age at menarche has an effect on the incidence of several solid tumors. Menarche at 14 years of age or older is associated with a lower risk of colorectal cancer.[2] An older age at menarche is also protective against breast cancer in the United States.[3] Among pairs of twins with the concordant development of breast cancer, earlier puberty is associated with an earlier age at breast cancer diagnosis, whereas other reproductive characteristics such as parity have no such association.[4]

The use of oral contraceptives for 96 months or longer reduces the risk of colorectal cancer by 40%.[2] Use of oral contraceptives for a longer duration probably increases the relative risk of breast cancer modestly. This effect is greatest for the contraceptive agents that deliver the highest dose of estrogen and it is higher in younger women.[5] The use of infertility treatments, with the exception of the use of human menopausal gonadotropin for longer than 6 months, does not increase the risk of breast cancer in relation to women who have been evaluated for infertility but have not undergone medical therapy for infertility.[6]

Whether use of oral contraceptives for longer than 5 years increases the incidence of superficial spreading melanoma, as suggested by the small study of Holly and coworkers, is controversial.[7] The association was not confirmed by a case-control study of 276 women with melanoma, which found no effect of any reproductive characteristic on the risk of any subtype of melanoma.[8] Prospective studies of women with familial dysplastic nevus syndrome—a hereditary disorder in which patients have variable numbers of dysplastic nevi and are at increased risk for malignant melanoma—have documented a doubling of the rate of change of nevi during pregnancy.[9]

Unopposed estrogen replacement therapy leads to an increase in the risk of endometrial cancer. However, small case-control and prospective studies suggest that this increase in risk is abolished by the use of estrogen/progestin combinations.[10,11] The Women's Health Initiative randomly assigned 16,608 women either to combination hormone replacement therapy with conjugated equine estrogen and progestin or to placebo treatment. The study was halted after 5.2 years of follow-up because the estimated hazard ratio for invasive breast cancer in the hormone replacement recipients was 1.26. The risks of several other chronic diseases were increased as well; all-cause mortality is not yet affected.[12] These randomized prospective data confirmed the findings of a metaanalysis reported by the Collaborative Group on Hormonal Risk Factors in Breast Cancer involving 52,705 women with breast cancer and 108,411 control subjects, in which the relative risk of breast cancer increased by 1.023 for each year of exposure to hormone replacement therapy; the relative risk after 5 years of exposure was 1.35.[13] According to the New Mexico Women's Health Study, a case-control study, this effect was greater for Hispanic women than for non-Hispanic white women.[14]

Initial reports that induced abortion predisposes to breast cancer have not been confirmed by large case-control studies.[15] Because most subjects in such studies underwent one or few abortions, the question of an increased risk of breast cancer is not answered for women who have had 10 or more abortions. Late age at first pregnancy is a powerful risk factor for breast cancer in the United States. First delivery of a full-term newborn after 35 years of age confers a risk of breast cancer triple that of first delivery by age 18.[16] There is an increase in the incidence of breast cancer in the years after a first delivery, which is most marked among women who first gave birth after age 30.[17] A protective effect of pregnancy is manifest by 15 years after delivery. A prospective study monitoring more than 800,000 parous Norwegian women for a median of 16 years showed an increase in risk of breast cancer for an interval of 4 years after delivery; this was followed by a decades-long decrease in risk.[18] Increased parity is also thought to be protective, although this variable has been difficult to separate from age at first birth and the transient increase in risk in the postpartum period.

Increasing parity up to three births reduces the risk of ovarian cancer, with association weakening with increasing age at last birth.[19] Parity is also protective against endometrial cancer, which appears to be a cancer strongly linked to total lifetime exposure to unopposed estrogen.[20]

Use of diethylstilbestrol in pregnancy conferred a relative risk of breast cancer of 1.34 (i.e., the risk of breast cancer was 34% higher if the woman had taken diethylstilbestrol) in a prospective study of more than 500,000 gravid women; this finding withstood multivariate analysis.[21] Changes in breast cancer incidence have been reported in patients with infertility and those who have undergone follicular stimulation, but the relative importance of the cause of infertility remains unclear.[22,23] Increased rates of spontaneous abortion result from cytogenetic translocations, some of which may coincidentally also result in the loss of tumor suppressor gene function, and thus raise the risk of breast or other cancer.

Prolonged lactation was studied in a case-control study of 136 women with endometrial cancer and 933 control subjects, which included patients from developing countries. An apparent protective effect of increasing duration of lactation and months of lactation per pregnancy was noted, but this declined with time elapsed since the cessation of breast-feeding, and there was no protective effect among women older than 55.[24] A history of prolonged lactation and younger age at lactation, after adjustment for parity, age at first delivery, family history, and age at menopause, have also been shown to have a protective effect on the risk of premenopausal breast cancer.[25] Last, age at menopause influences the likelihood that breast cancer will develop. A late menopause raises the risk, and surgical menopause reduces the risk. The effect of surgical menopause is greatest if it occurs before 35 years of age.[26]

Birth weight is a risk factor for breast cancer. According to a nested case-control study within cohorts of the Nurses' Health Studies, in which self-administered questionnaires were given to mothers of 582 nurses, higher birth weight carried a higher risk of breast cancer.[27]

Maternal age of 45 or older confers a relative risk of 1.3 for breast cancer in the daughters.[28]

The implications of these reproductive risks for subsequent pregnancies in the cancer survivor are discussed later in this chapter, but it is clear from these data that a large number of risk factors that reflect very dramatic changes in the hormonal milieu are associated with relative risks that are, on the whole, not dramatic, usually less than twofold. These risk factors have been strongest for breast, ovarian, and endometrial cancer but have been little studied for other cancers.

Women who carry mutations in the breast cancer susceptibility genes BRCA1 (located at chromosome 17q21) or BRCA2 (chromosome 13q12-13) have lifetime breast cancer risks ranging from 65% to 90%. BRCA1 is a tumor suppressor gene; both the gene and its promoter have estrogen-binding elements, and BRCA1 expression is increased during puberty and pregnancy.[29] BRCA1 messenger RNA levels remain higher in postlactational animals than in age-matched virgins.[30] Small reports suggest an increased rate of pregnancy-associated and oral contraceptive–induced breast cancers among BRCA1 and BRCA2 carriers.[31] Until larger studies are available, BRCA1 and BRCA2 carriers should not be counseled that increased parity is protective against breast cancer; they should consider reducing exposure to exogenous hormones, with the possible exception of hormone replacement therapy in the setting of prophylactic oophorectomy.

PROBLEMS IN STAGING CANCER IN THE PREGNANT PATIENT

The appropriate procedures for determining the stage of a cancer are determined by the cancer and its site. In most cancers, imaging studies are used to establish both the local extent of the tumor and to search for secondary deposits of cancer. Imaging with plain radiographs, mammograms, computed tomographic (CT) scans, and nuclear medicine studies expose the fetus and mother to variable amounts of radiation, the risks of which are discussed later. Positron emission tomography is an important adjunct to CT scanning in the staging of many cancers but should not be used in pregnancy. Ultrasonography and magnetic resonance (MR) studies are preferred in most situations of cancer in pregnancy, to avoid radiation exposure. The safety of MR imaging in the first trimester is not established, and there are no data on the safety of MR contrast agents. Breast-feeding should be interrupted for 36 to 48 hours after the administration of MR contrast agents. Liver function tests have poor sensitivity for predicting the presence of liver metastases in nonpregnant patients; in pregnancy, this is compounded by low specificity because of physiologic elevation of the alkaline phosphatase level.

Assessment of early-stage Hodgkin's disease may necessitate a laparotomy to exclude tumor outside the planned radiation field, and staging of ovarian cancer necessitates laparotomy and a defined series of node samples. The risks of abdominal surgery in pregnancy are reviewed later.

TUMOR MARKERS IN PREGNANCY

Many of the antigens that can be measured in the serum in cancer patients to follow the burden of cancer are oncofetal proteins, expressed normally in the developing fetus and abnormally in the presence of cancer. An example is α-fetoprotein, which is useful in monitoring a pregnancy to detect fetal neural tube defects but which, when its levels are elevated in the nonpregnant adult, is strongly associated with the presence of a germ cell tumor, hepatocellular cancer, or, more rarely, adenocarcinoma. If such tumor markers are to be used to monitor a pregnant patient with cancer, it is necessary to distinguish between the fetal and malignant expression of the antigen. Immunoblotting characteristics of some of these markers are distinct for the forms measured during normal pregnancy and in the presence of malignancy.[32] For α-fetoprotein, although there are several possible immunoreactive species, the pattern seen with pregnancy resembles that seen with hepatocellular carcinoma.[33] The β subunit of human chorionic gonadotropin (β-hCG) is measured to detect pregnancy. β-hCG is also used to monitor most forms of trophoblastic disease. When the β-hCG level is elevated, the distinction between recurrent disease and a new conceptus must be made on other grounds. Thyroglobulin is used in the follow-up of well-differentiated thyroid cancer. This marker is not elevated among healthy pregnant women in iodine-replete areas, but it may be altered in the setting of iodine deficiency or benign thyroid disease of pregnancy.[34,35] A newer generation of serum markers, the tyrosine kinase growth factor receptors, does not yet have defined roles, but these markers may also be elevated in pregnancy.[36]

THERAPEUTIC INTERVENTIONS DURING PREGNANCY

Anticancer therapies may be teratogenic and mutagenic, and in the management of cancer in the pregnant patient, the effects of therapy on the developing fetus are an important consideration. Interactions between environmental exposures and hereditary mutations are important in cancer causation in all age groups. The increase in the incidence of childhood cancers to the current level of approximately 12 per 100,000 may relate to maternal and in utero exposures to carcinogens. Cancer incidence trends, which show steady increases over time in the occurrence of cancer even in children younger than 1 year, suggest that the effects of such exposures can be transmitted from one generation to the next.[37] Some childhood cancers are likely to be caused by in utero exposures; for example, chromosomal analyses of infant leukemia occurring in twins demonstrate that the genetic abnormality of infant leukemia is acquired in utero.[38]

The prognosis, the risks of the cancer and the therapy to the mother, and the risks of pregnancy must also be taken into account in helping the patient to make a decision about continuing the pregnancy and in managing both the pregnancy and the malignancy should she choose to continue the pregnancy.

Surgical Intervention

Anesthetic considerations are of prime importance in deciding on surgery during pregnancy. General anesthesia is a more complex issue in pregnancy because blood volume and cardiac output increase. The anesthetic drugs themselves are relatively safe for the fetus. Neither nitrous oxide nor halothane has been demonstrated to be teratogenic or to cause fetal death. Both agents may relax the uterus and thus diminish the risk of premature labor. Of 5405 operations, predominantly laparoscopies and laparotomies, performed for nonobstetric reasons in a population of 720,000 pregnant women, surgery increased rates of pregnancy complications, including prematurity, intrauterine growth retardation, and neonatal death. The incidence of congenital anomalies when surgery had been performed during gestation was slightly higher than expected. The relative contributions of surgery and anesthesia in comparison with the underlying conditions that mandated surgery during pregnancy are not known.[39] Premature labor and fetal loss after surgery during pregnancy are most tightly related to the surgical procedure itself; rates are highest for abdominal and pelvic surgery. Percutaneous drainage of adnexal cysts for symptoms of impending torsion has been performed during pregnancy without complication.[40]

Extraabdominal surgery is less likely to be complicated by abortion, and reports of successful surgical management of malignancy in gravid women include resection of a supraglottic larynx cancer,[41] resection of vulvar cancer with bilateral groin lymph node dissection,[42] and mastectomies and local excisions of breast cancers.

Radiotherapy

The potential adverse consequences of fetal radiation exposure include fetal loss, fetal anomalies, low birth weight, cancer in later life, and, at least theoretically, transmission of genetic abnormalities to future generations.[43] Pregnant survivors of the atom bomb explosions had children among whom rates of microcephaly and mental retardation were increased. The incidence of mental retardation was linked to radiation dose, ranging from 2.4% when the exposure was 10 to 50 rad to 18-40% when the exposure was 50 to 100 rad. No forebrain injury occurred with exposure during the first 8 weeks after conception. The risk of injury was greatest for fetuses between 8 and 15 weeks of gestational age. In addition to mental retardation, growth delay and stunting were seen.[44]

New DNA fragments are sevenfold more common among children of workers who participated in cleanup of the Chernobyl reactor accident than among siblings conceived before the accident.[45] Swedish health registries have been monitored for evidence that excess fetal anomalies and childhood cancers may have been seen in the regions of Sweden where radioactive fallout in the wake of the Chernobyl disaster was highest.[46] As of 1994, three Swedish children who were in utero at the time of the accident have developed leukemia. Because of the small numbers, it is possible that this increase was attributable to random variation; however, the association between low-level radiation in utero and childhood cancer has been described frequently.[47] This effect is enhanced in the presence of maternal smoking. There is no threshold dose of radiation to which the fetus may be exposed, especially in the third trimester, without raising the risk of childhood cancer. Childhood cancer can result from exposure even to single plain radiographs. The case-control and population studies and the experimental evidence from animal models have been reviewed.[48]

In addition to concerns about the effects of radiation on the fetus, there is a question of whether the risks of radiation to the pregnant woman herself may be increased in relation to the risks in a nonpregnant adult. Increased susceptibility to chromosomal damage after radiation has been demonstrated toward the end of gestation in pregnant mice. Ricoul and associates established short-term cultures with the lymphocytes and serum of pregnant women, radiated the cultures, and compared them with similarly cultured and radiated lymphocytes from non-pregnant women; they demonstrated increased chromosomal breakage in metaphases in the lymphocytes of pregnant women. This increased radiosensitivity reverted immediately after delivery.[49]

Pregnant women are exposed to radiation during the course of diagnostic procedures, such as mammography, CT scanning, and plain radiography, and in the workplace and environment. A single plain radiographic study involves an exposure of less than 10 rad and can be undertaken if necessary; however, ultrasonography or MR imaging are preferred, because both appear to be without harmful effects for the fetus, and should be substituted if possible.[50] Fluoroscopic procedures result in much higher doses of radiation and should be avoided. Diagnostic studies that utilize radionuclides are contraindicated.

Women may also be exposed therapeutically, as when radiotherapy is used to treat early-stage Hodgkin's disease. About 4000 women per year receive radiotherapy, predominantly to the neck and thorax, during pregnancy. With appropriate shielding, the dose to the fetus can be reduced by approximately 50%.[51] Radiation to the breast or chest wall in the treatment of breast cancer results in an absorbed fetal dose of 0.05 Gy early in pregnancy. Once the fetus is close to the diaphragm late in pregnancy, the dose is higher than 1 Gy. According to the assumptions of Stovall and coworkers,[51] 0.05 Gy is the threshold for risk of malformation, and at 1 Gy, this risk is 40%. Although systemic radioiodine therapy is strictly contraindicated in pregnancy, a case has been reported in which radioiodine was administered for the treatment of thyroid cancer to a woman believed not to be pregnant, but in whom a 24-week-old fetus was discovered after 3700 MBq had been administered in the 2nd and 22nd weeks of pregnancy. The pregnancy was terminated because of concerns about fetal damage, and the fetus was examined. Significant radiation effect was noted in the thyroid, but there were no other malformations and karyotypic analysis showed no gross chromosomal aberrations.[52]

Among British medical radiographers, a study performed by mailed questionnaire revealed no significant increase in major congenital anomalies, but slight increases in chromosomal anomalies and childhood

cancer were seen.[53] The International Commission on Radiological Protection recommends a dose limit of 0.2 mSv per month to the abdominal surface of a pregnant health care worker who works with patients who have received technetium 99m or iodine 133. With a distributed source of these radioisotopes to radiate an anthropomorphic phantom, the fetal dose when a nurse or radiology technologist cares for an adult treated with technetium 99m is estimated to be up to 86 µSv. The fetal dose to a radiology technologist after iodine 133 administration is up to 9 µSv. Thus, current recommendations are that a pregnant imaging technologist not perform more than six technetium scans or one iodine scan per day.[54]

Chemotherapy

The U.S. Food and Drug Administration assigns drugs into specific pregnancy risk categories. Category C refers to drugs for which animal data demonstrate adverse fetal effects; category D drugs are those for which human evidence of adverse effects exists; and category X drugs are those for which evidence of an adverse effect exists and the risk is seen as clearly outweighing the possible benefits. Although chemotherapeutics are rarely assigned to category X because of the life-threatening nature of many cancers, detailed information about the risks to mother and fetus allows optimization of the systemic therapy and influences decisions about continuation and management of the pregnancy. A comprehensive review of this subject has been published.[55] Long-term follow-up of 84 children whose mothers received chemotherapy for hematologic malignancies during pregnancy revealed no cancers, leukemias, or developmental abnormalities.[56]

Conventional Cytotoxic Chemotherapy

Pregnant patients are almost always specifically excluded from initial safety trials of new drugs, and large prospective series of the use of chemotherapy during pregnancy have not been performed. Physicians treating cancer during pregnancy are left to rely on animal models of teratogenesis, retrospective studies, and case reports in choosing chemotherapy. A registry of pregnancy outcomes after use of chemotherapy during gestation is kept at the University of Oklahoma. The registry currently contains more than 280 cases. It can be contacted by phone during business hours, 9:00 AM to 5:00 PM Central Standard Time, at 405-271-8685 or through electronic mail at john-mulvihill@ouhsc.edu. Practitioners are urged to report all use of chemotherapy during pregnancy to the registry and also to receive current information from the registry on any chemotherapy agent or regimen intended for use in a pregnant patient, before therapy is begun.

Certain predictions can be made on the basis of the known physiology of pregnancy. Renal clearance is increased in pregnancy; the volume of third-space fluid is increased; and the plasma volume is increased. Thus, renally excreted drugs clear more rapidly in pregnancy, with the exception of methotrexate, which accumulates in the third space; the delay in its elimination increases toxicity.

Almost all cytotoxic agents cross the placenta, and most are teratogenic during the first trimester. The use of chemotherapy in the first trimester increases the rate of fetal loss. Among fetuses that survive to term, the incidence of malformations is increased up to 20%.[57] Use of certain chemotherapy agents in the second and third trimesters, when organogenesis is complete, does not detectably increase the rate of fetal malformations. Use of chemotherapy at any time in pregnancy results in lower birth weight.[58,59] The long-term consequences of in utero exposure to chemotherapy are not known. They potentially include delayed growth and learning delays; delayed carcinogenesis in the child or subsequent generations; and delayed cardiotoxicity from anthracycline exposure.

Alkylating agents act by binding covalently to DNA. This results in tumor cell death by apoptosis or by failure of the damaged DNA to serve as an effective template at the time of cell replication. This group includes the commonly used agents cyclophosphamide, ifosfamide, busulfan, melphalan, and chlorambucil, as well as the organoplatinum agents. Use of chlorambucil in the first trimester has resulted in a syndrome of renal aplasia, cleft palate, and skeletal anomalies, echoing abnormalities seen in the rat model.[60] Animal models of teratogenesis after exposure to cyclophosphamide have demonstrated that the percentage of cells undergoing apoptosis is radically increased after cyclophosphamide damage to DNA.[61] Ectrodactylia has been seen in humans after in utero exposure to cyclophosphamide.

The organoplatinum agent cisplatin causes renal and ototoxicity. In the mouse model, cisplatin crosses the placenta in substantial amounts only after day 13. Fetal levels are higher than maternal levels after day 17, which is evidence of active transport of cisplatin across the placenta.[62] The mother's renal function should be monitored carefully, and she should undergo serial audiographic evaluations. Fetal ototoxicity can be detected by monitoring changes in fetal heart rate in response to stimulation by an artificial larynx held 10 inches from the maternal abdomen.[63] The sensitivity and specificity of this test for cisplatin-induced fetal ototoxicity are unknown. Gestational diabetes and preeclampsia have been reported in a pregnant woman receiving carboplatin chemotherapy, but no causative relationship was established.

The alkylating agents are metabolized predominantly in the liver. The fetus and newborn may lack hepatic enzymes involved in alkylating agent metabolism. The placenta allows excretion of these drugs into the maternal circulation, which results in metabolism by the maternal liver, but if substantial levels remain in the neonatal circulation after delivery, when the placental route is no longer available, the neonate may require support through a period of cytopenia.

The antifolate agents such as methotrexate are abortifacients. Of 36 pregnant patients who received a folate antagonist in the first trimester, 26 had spontaneous abortions within weeks. The majority of fetuses in six pregnancies subsequently aborted, and four delivered at term had multiple malformations. Two aborted fetuses appeared normal, and two infants born with multiple anomalies survived. Methotrexate should be strictly avoided in any circumstance in which the mother is considering continuing the pregnancy.[64] Multiple anomalies have been reported in a child who was conceived at a time when the mother was receiving cytosine arabinoside, and a trisomy was reported in a fetus aborted 4 weeks after exposure to the same agent early in the second trimester.[65]

The anthracyclines and anthracenediones act as topoisomerase II inhibitors. The most commonly used member of this class in the United States is doxorubicin. This agent has been used extensively in the second and third trimesters of pregnancy in the adjuvant therapy of breast cancer and in the treatment of advanced breast cancer, lymphomas, and Hodgkin's disease. It is not known to increase the incidence of fetal anomalies, but it is associated with treatment-related leukemias.[66] Whether its use during pregnancy increases the likelihood of childhood leukemia is not known. Epirubicin has a similar spectrum of activity as doxorubicin, and a case has been reported of a healthy infant delivered after four cycles of epirubicin-containing chemotherapy given in the second and third trimesters of pregnancy.[67] Idarubicin is preferred to doxorubicin for the induction of remission in acute myeloid leukemia. Its use during the second trimester of pregnancy has been associated with fetal death.[68]

Little is known about the safety in late pregnancy of the taxanes, a novel class of antineoplastic agents that act by promoting microtubule assembly. Animal models have demonstrated fetal death and ossification delay when taxanes are given during the period of organogenesis. Docetaxel at higher cumulative doses can be complicated by a syndrome of fluid retention, which may be difficult to manage in pregnancy. Both docetaxel and paclitaxel are important in the management of a broad spectrum of solid tumors. No reports of malformations occurring after the use of vincristine alone in any trimester are known. Vincristine is useful in the management of lymphoma and lymphoblastic leukemias.

Chemotherapeutic agents are commonly excreted in breast milk. Those that have been found in breast milk include hydroxyurea, cyclophosphamide, cisplatin, doxorubicin, and methotrexate.[69] Breast-feeding is contraindicated when there is a possibility that chemotherapeutic agents would be fed to the infant.

Cytotoxic Therapy in Human Immunodeficiency Virus Infection

Women who are pregnant and infected with human immunodeficiency virus (HIV) receive a recommendation to take antiretroviral therapy to reduce the transmission of HIV to the child, as well as for its benefits in improving quality of life and prolonging survival in the mother.[70,71] HIV infection is a recognized risk factor for cervical cancer and lymphoma, which are among the cancers most commonly diagnosed during pregnancy. The best method of combining chemotherapy with therapy directed against HIV infection is determined by the patient's stage of HIV infection and history of antiretroviral therapy. An important goal in treating HIV infection is to avoid the induction of resistance to antiretroviral agents. Because such resistance may be fostered by starting and stopping therapy, continuation of the regimen the patient has been following, if at all feasible, is preferred. When overlapping toxic effects of chemotherapy and antiretroviral therapy develop, dose reductions should in most cases be made in the chemotherapeutic agents rather than the antiretroviral agents. It is difficult to combine zidovudine with myelosuppressive chemotherapy because zidovudine is myelosuppressive in its own right. It is not advisable to administer didanosine (ddL, Videx) and zalcitabine (ddC, Hivid) simultaneously with neurotoxic chemotherapy such as the vinca alkaloids or paclitaxel, because they cause neuropathy. Neither the nonnucleoside reverse transcriptase inhibitors nevirapine and delavirdine nor the protease inhibitors saquinavir mesylate, ritonavir, indinavir sulfate, and nelfinavir mesylate have been tested for safety or efficacy in pregnancy. Because of their contributions to the well-being of the mother and because reduced viral load in the mother is likely to further decrease the risk of viral transmission to the fetus, protease inhibitors are increasingly prescribed during pregnancy. To date, evidence of fetal harm has not been reported.

Enfuvirtide is an HIV fusion inhibitor that is active in drug-resistant HIV infection. Animal data contain no evidence for harmful effects in pregnancy, but human data are not available. As with all antiretroviral use in pregnancy, practitioners are urged to report their cases to the Antiretroviral Pregnancy Registry at 800-258-4263 or *www.apregistry.com.*

Biologic and Targeted Therapies

The differentiating agent all-*trans*-retinoic acid (ATRA) is used in the treatment of acute promyelocytic leukemia. This agent, in common with all retinoids, has known teratogenicity.[72] If its use is indicated in the first trimester, termination of pregnancy should be recommended. ATRA may induce the retinoic acid syndrome, which can develop as early as the second day after initiation of therapy.[73] This syndrome is characterized by fever, weight gain, respiratory distress, interstitial pulmonary infiltrates, and pleural and pericardial effusions and is often associated with leukocytosis. The consequences of this syndrome for fetal viability are unknown. When the retinoic acid syndrome develops, retinoic acid is withheld; dexamethasone is administered, and the retinoic acid can be reintroduced at a lower dosage once the symptoms have resolved.

The interferons are a group of naturally occurring proteins with immunomodulating, antiproliferative, and differentiating activity. Interferon-alfa is used in the therapy of chronic myelogenous leukemia and myeloma and in the adjuvant therapy of melanoma. Its teratogenetic potential is unknown, but a case has been reported of interferon use in the therapy of myeloma in the first 7 weeks of pregnancy, without apparent adverse effect.[74] Corticosteroids are important lympholytic agents and are utilized in many antiemetic regimens. Animal models and retrospective reviews of use of steroids in pregnant women demonstrate a high incidence of cleft palate after in utero exposure to steroids. Other adverse effects include stillbirth, prematurity, masculinization of infant girls, and hypoadrenalism necessitating corticosteroid supplementation. Corticosteroids may also worsen maternal glucose intolerance and the attendant risks of hyperglycemia to the mother and fetus.

Imatinib, a highly active inhibitor of the bcr-abl fusion protein, as well as of c-kit and the platelet-derived growth factor receptor, is teratogenic in rats at dosages equivalent to the maximal human dosage and increases postimplantation embryonic loss. It appears in rat milk. At present, it is contraindicated during pregnancy and lactation. Common side effects anticipated in the mother are myelosuppression, nausea, edema, fatigue, headaches, myalgias, arthralgias, diarrhea, and rash.

Trastuzumab, a humanized antibody that targets the growth factor receptor Her-2/*neu*, has not been studied in pregnant humans. No fetal harm has been demonstrated in a monkey model, but placental transfer to the fetal monkey has been demonstrated.

Gefitinib is an anilinoquinazolone that inhibits the kinase activity of the epidermal growth factor receptor (EGFR) in vitro in nanomolar concentrations. It is associated with a modest rate of objective responses in non–small cell lung cancer and squamous cell cancer of the head and neck. It was approved by the U.S. Food and Drug Administration for use in advanced non–small cell lung cancer in 2003; its use in other settings remains under study. Animal studies yielded no evidence for genotoxicity or teratogenicity, but at maternally toxic dosages, fetal weight was reduced and neonatal mortality increased in rabbit and rat models. EGFR is expected to be important in fetal development, and gefitinib should not be used during pregnancy until further data become available.

Thalidomide has now returned to the therapeutic armamentarium as an inhibitor of vascular neogenesis for the treatment of cancers dependent on a tumor-specific microvasculature, exploiting the very activity that caused so much suffering during the years thalidomide was prescribed for use by pregnant women. Thalidomide causes severe birth defects in 20% to 30% of exposed fetuses.[75] The effects of thalidomide are most apparent after exposure at days 27 through 40 of gestation and may arise after even a single dose of thalidomide. The commonly seen abnormalities include phocomelia, short stature, and osseous defects. Facial hemangiomata and atresia of the esophagus and duodenum are also seen. The use of thalidomide in pregnancy is absolutely contraindicated; patients receiving thalidomide are extensively counseled about the teratogenicity of the agent and about contraception.

The mixed estrogen-antiestrogen agent tamoxifen is the most commonly used hormonal agent in the treatment of primary and advanced breast cancer. The drug was designed initially for use as an oral contraceptive, for which purpose it was completely inefficacious, actually enhancing fertility.[76] Tamoxifen has caused reversible developmental changes in fetal rats and monkeys exposed during all stages of gestation.

Supportive Care in the Pregnant Cancer Patient

The symptoms of cancer and the morbid nature of many anticancer therapies can cause fatigue, appetite disturbance, and emotional distress; the most debilitating symptom is pain, which may be severe. Opioids are widely used for the palliation of cancer pain in patients with curable and incurable disease, although adjuvant pharmacologic agents, neurosurgical approaches, and therapy for the underlying malignancy are also important. Long-term exposure to opioids in utero may lead to opioid dependence in the fetus, with resultant drug withdrawal syndrome and growth retardation after delivery. Systemic levels of opioid can be minimized by intrathecal delivery of morphine if appropriate.[77]

Chemotherapy for cancer is commonly emetogenic. Premedication with an antiemetic is used for all emetogenic chemotherapy agents, and patients are also supplied with some combination of the oral antiemetics prochlorperazine, lorazepam, dexamethasone, or 5-hydroxytryptamine type 3 antagonists for outpatient management of delayed emesis. Consistent data about the use of any of these agents in pregnancy are not available. Administration of the 5-hydroxytryptamine type 3 antagonist ondansetron is not associated with teratogenic effects in animals at any stage of gestation. Despite early reports of an association with oral clefts, large retrospective studies of benzodiazepine use in pregnancy have not supported this association.[78] Retrospective series document that normal infants have been delivered after use of phenothiazines, such as prochlorperazine, during pregnancy. Use of antinausea drugs during pregnancy was associated with a nonsignificant increase in incidence of childhood leukemia in a small series.[79] Potential fetal complications of steroid use have been discussed previously.

The oxazaphosphorine alkylating agents cyclophosphamide and ifosfamide undergo hepatic metabolism; this results in the generation of an active metabolite, acrolein, which is renally excreted and causes hemorrhagic cystitis. For this reason, when used in a high dose, these agents are given with hyperhydration or the acrolein-binding agent mesna (sodium 2-mercaptoethane sulfonate), greatly reducing but not eliminating the risk of hemorrhagic cystitis. BK viruria is associated with a higher incidence of hemorrhagic cystitis after oxazaphosphorine chemotherapy.[80] Hemorrhagic cystitis should be managed with further doses of mesna if it manifests during the first several half-lives after drug administration. Continuous bladder irrigation with normal saline, antispasmodic agents, and pain medication are indicated. Refractory bleeding should be evaluated with cystoscopy to exclude tumor, polyp, trauma, and other causes of persistent hematuria. Severe hemorrhagic cystitis during pregnancy can result in preterm labor.[81]

Total parenteral nutrition is indicated for cancer patients with some frequency. It may be required because of (1) mechanical interference of a tumor with the alimentary tract, (2) postsurgical complications, (3) chemotherapy-induced mucositis or emesis, or (4) cachexia induced by the cancer itself. There is also increasing use of total parenteral nutrition in pregnancy for other causes of malnutrition. Parenteral lipid emulsion can lead to fat deposits in the chorionic villi, and this has been reported in association with fetal death at 22 weeks' gestation.[82]

Malignant hypercalcemia resulting from paraneoplastic secretion of parathyroid hormone–related protein or from widespread bone metastases may be seen in the advanced stages of breast and lung cancer and with some lymphomas. Intravenous bisphosphonate therapy, usually with pamidronate, is the therapy of choice for malignant hypercalcemia.[83] Bisphosphonates foster recalcification of bone metastases and reduce skeletal complications of breast cancer.[84] Limited data support the use of bisphosphonates in pregnancy; they should be used only if the indication for therapy is compelling, as with symptomatic hypercalcemia.[85]

Tobacco Cessation

Approximately 30% of women in the United States who conceive are smokers. The physician's role in personalizing the risks of continued tobacco use is central to the decision to quit for many smokers. In the case of cancer during pregnancy, the risks of continued tobacco exposure to the fetus and the mother should be emphasized. Patients may be unaware that radiation is more effective if tobacco is discontinued and that this may be the case for chemotherapy as well. Survivors of many tobacco-induced cancers remain at high risk for second cancers. Chemoprevention with retinoids should not be given during pregnancy; these agents are highly teratogenic.

FERTILITY AND PREGNANCY IN CANCER SURVIVORS

No difference in survival after radical or conservative surgery for unilateral ovarian cancer was demonstrated among 72 Mexican women. Resumption of menses occurred within 6 months in 89% of those who underwent conservative surgery, and there was a cumulative pregnancy rate of 59% in the 22 women who remained premenopausal.[86] Conservative treatment of endometrial cancer by curettage and progestin therapy without hysterectomy can preserve fertility with the subsequent use of gamete intrafallopian transfer. Such a patient was successfully delivered of a triplet pregnancy by cesarean section at 30 weeks and underwent hysterectomy as definitive therapy for cancer after delivery.[87]

Among 405 former childhood cancer patients surveyed by questionnaire, 148 reported 280 pregnancies. These resulted in 230 live full-term births and 17 live premature births. Records of 81% of the liveborn infants were reviewed. Of these, 3.3% had congenital anomalies; this incidence is similar to that in the general population.[88] The risk of cancer among children of survivors of childhood cancer has been measured in 5847 children of more than 14,000 survivors of cancer diagnosed in childhood or adolescence in the Nordic countries during the 1940s and 1950s. The follow-up period totaled 86,780 person-years. Excess retinoblastomas and nervous system tumors were observed, but there was no evidence for an excess of nonhereditary cancer.[89]

Chemotherapy, such as that used for the therapy of advanced stages of Hodgkin's disease or for the adjuvant therapy of breast cancer, can cause menopause, and the risk of temporary or permanent cessation of menses is related to the age at treatment, the drugs used, and the cumulative dose. Recurrence of ovarian function is usually heralded by resumption of menses and, in rare cases, by pregnancy. When patients are treated with high-dose chemotherapy necessitating marrow support for the treatment of hematologic, breast, or ovarian malignancies, cessation of menses is highly likely whether the patient receives total-body irradiation or chemotherapy. Of 708 postpubertal women treated with high-dose cyclophosphamide, with or without high-dose busulfan and total-body irradiation, 110 recovered normal gonadal function, and 32 of those women became pregnant.[90] The chance of recovering gonadal function for patients who received such therapy as adults varied with the therapy. Of 73 patients who received conditioning with high-dose busulfan and cyclophosphamide, only 1 retained gonadal function, whereas of 103 who received high-dose cyclophosphamide alone, 56 did so. Among patients who underwent total-body irradiation as part of the treatment, preservation of fertility was related to the total radiation dose. Of those who received conditioning when prepubertal, 28% retained fertility, and 9 of 196 ultimately became pregnant. Pregnancies were more likely to result in babies with low or very low birth weight and were more likely to be complicated by preterm labor; also, among patients who received total-body irradiation, the risk of spontaneous abortion appeared increased. All pregnancies in survivors of high-dose chemotherapy should be managed as high-risk pregnancies.[90] Among women who are older than 18 years of age when they undergo high-dose chemotherapy or total-body irradiation with allogeneic bone marrow transplantation, preservation of fertility is unlikely.[91] A few cases have been reported of such patients who have successfully become pregnant after implantation of in vitro fertilized ova. In three cases the ova were donated, and in three cases the ova were harvested from the patient before the administration of high-dose chemotherapy.[92]

Pregnancy after treatment for breast cancer has not been demonstrated to raise the risk of breast cancer recurrence, and multiple pregnancies may in fact be protective.[93] In one series from Finland, breast cancer survivors who became pregnant and delivered were found to have a fivefold or 80% lower risk of breast cancer recurrence than stage- and age-matched breast cancer survivors who acted as control subjects. The authors argued that this represented a "healthy mother effect": namely, that breast cancer survivors who became pregnant received mild enough adjuvant therapy that they retained fertility and were asymptomatic at the time of conception, although no differences in management of survivors who became pregnant and those who did not were actually identified.[94]

Women who deliver after treatment for breast cancer may choose to breast-feed their children. If the involved breast was conserved by use of limited surgery followed by radiotherapy to the breast, lactation from that breast is rarely possible. Higgins and Haffty reviewed 11 patients who became pregnant after breast conservation. Three patients chose to suppress lactation with bromocriptine. Of the remaining seven, four had some evidence of milk production, but lactation was normal in only one.[95]

Women who have received iodine 133 therapy for thyroid cancer do not appear to have an increased risk of complications of pregnancy or of having fetuses with anomalies if they receive adequate thyroid replacement and if pregnancy is deferred until the radionuclide is completely eliminated.[96]

CANCER SITES

Cervical Cancer in Pregnancy

Cervical cancer is the most commonly diagnosed malignancy during pregnancy and the postpartum period. The incidence of cervical intraepithelial neoplasia is 1.3 per 1000 pregnancies, and the incidence of invasive disease is 1 per 2200 pregnancies.[97] Worldwide, it is the most commonly diagnosed cancer in women, and in many parts of the world, it is still the leading cause of cancer death among women. Pregnancy has been reported to be associated with an increased prevalence of human papillomavirus (HPV), the causative agent of cervical cancer. Clinical progression of HPV infection may be seen in pregnancy; this has been attributed to the integration of the HPV genome 3′ downstream to the glucocorticoid response element. The 70 types of HPV are divided into low- and high-risk types. The highest cancer risk is associated with types 16, 18, 31, and 45.[98] The prevalence of high-risk HPV is reported to be increased during pregnancy.[99] A HPV-16 L1 virus-like particle vaccine reduced the incidence of HPV-16 infection and of HPV-16-related cervical intraepithelial neoplasia in a randomized trial.[100]

Diagnosis

Speculum examination and Papanicolaou (Pap) smear should be performed in all pregnant women at the first antenatal visit. The Pap smear should be reported in the terminology of the Bethesda System of reporting,[101] which includes an assessment of the adequacy of the specimen for interpretation. If the specimen is not adequate for interpretation, the Pap smear should be repeated, because half of false-negative Pap smears result from inadequate sampling. The appropriate further management for a Pap smear finding of atypical squamous cells of undetermined significance (accounting for up to 9% of all Pap smear results) or low-grade squamous intraepithelial lesion is not agreed upon. A clinical trial is currently ongoing to determine whether testing for HPV can discern cases of early abnormality in which more invasive testing is indicated. Gross lesions must always be sampled for biopsy, because hemorrhage or necrosis may obscure Pap results.

In cases in which there is evidence of higher grade dysplasia, colposcopy with cytologic examination and directed biopsy is the procedure of choice for establishing whether invasive disease is present. The transformation zone is physiologically everted in pregnancy, rendering colposcopic assessment easier. Bleeding from biopsy sites is increased because of hyperemia. If multiple biopsies are required, several colposcopies may be performed, or minimal conization with a free-hand–guided laser may be used. Miniconization is also indicated if the initial biopsies disclosed microinvasion. In a series of miniconizations that included 85 pregnant women, no significant complications were observed.[102] Full conization, even with exclusion of the cervical canal to avoid rupture of the membranes, leads to more blood loss in the pregnant patient and raises the risks of abortion and preterm delivery. These risks are highest in the first trimester, which is when early series have reported the risk of abortion to be as high as 33%. Fetal death may follow chorioamnionitis.[103-105] Excess blood loss may be noted if conization is performed in the third trimester.[103] Endocervical curettage should be avoided because of the risk of hemorrhage or of rupture of the membranes. When cervical intraepithelial neoplasia or microinvasive disease less than 3 mm in depth is diagnosed, the patient may be observed and conization performed after delivery. Fewer than 10% of patients with cervical intraepithelial neoplasia in a small series had progression to microinvasive disease during this planned delay.[106]

Staging of invasive cervical cancer typically involves a CT scan of the pelvis, but MR studies are preferred in pregnancy to avoid exposing the fetus to ionizing radiation. Lymphangiography and intravenous pyelography are contraindicated if the pregnancy is to be continued. MR and physical examination can be used to determine lymph node involvement. Laparoscopic lymph node staging is considered experimental. Advanced-stage cervical cancer often invades bladder or ureters, and this should be assessed with ultrasonography and cystoscopy. Stage Ia cervical cancer can be stratified into Ia_1 and Ia_2 on the basis of the depth of invasion. The depth of invasion of a Ia_1 cancer is no more than 3 mm, and that of a Ia_2 cancer is no more than 5 mm. In addition to depth of invasion, the presence or absence of lymphovascular invasion should be considered.

Management

All patients with stage Ia cancers can consider continuing the pregnancy. For stage Ia_1 cancers without invasion of the lymphovascular space, the pregnancy can be continued to term, and the definitive cancer procedure is then chosen according to the patient's wishes with regard to further childbearing. If the patient desires more children, therapeutic conization to negative margins can be used as definitive therapy. In a series of 93 nonpregnant patients with minimally invasive disease managed by this approach, 1 patient suffered a fatal recurrence, and 92 patients had no evidence of recurrence.[104] If a patient with stage Ia_1 disease does not intend further childbearing, a vaginal hysterectomy can be performed 6 weeks post partum. Among patients with stage Ia_2 disease or lymphatic or vascular invasion, there is at least a 5% risk of metastases to regional nodes.[107] In such patients, the delay in definitive therapy should be minimized by a cesarean section once fetal maturity has been attained. Definitive therapy of the cervical cancer, consisting of an immediate modified radical hysterectomy with pelvic lymph node dissection, can then be undertaken.

Patients with stage Ib or IIa cervical cancer also require hysterectomy with pelvic lymphadenectomy. In the pregnant patient, this results in a delay in definitive therapy until delivery. Sood and coworkers reported on 11 patients who underwent hysterectomy after a mean treatment delay of 16 weeks (range, 3 to 40 weeks) because of pregnancy. All had early-stage disease, and this subgroup of 11 patients was selected from a population of 85 patients in whom cervical cancer was diagnosed during pregnancy. None of these 11 patients suffered a recurrence at a median follow-up time of 33 months.[108] Other series have reported on median treatment delays of 109 and 144 days.[109,110] A small cohort study did not demonstrate any alteration in the outcome of early-stage cervical cancer in the setting of pregnancy in comparison with control subjects who were not pregnant.[111] Thus, in early-stage cervical cancer, the previous practice of hysterectomy with the fetus in utero for cancers diagnosed in the first two trimesters may not be necessary; however, data on which to base a decision to delay definitive therapy are scarce. Cesarean section at the earliest time of fetal maturity with immediate modified radical hysterectomy and pelvic lymph node dissection is also appropriate for stage Ib and IIa cervical cancers.

For locally advanced cancers, radiotherapy is the treatment of choice. If the cancer is discovered during the first trimester and external beam radiation is given, spontaneous abortion often results. If spontaneous abortion does not occur, curettage should be performed. If cancer is discovered during the second trimester, abortion followed by radiotherapy is recommended; however, cervical cancer is generally slowly progressive, and the exact consequences of delay in this setting are not known. If cancer is discovered during the third trimester, it is common to delay therapy until maturation of the fetal lungs.

The use of neoadjuvant (primary or preoperative) chemotherapy in cervical cancer is being studied. Response rates of up to 100% have been reported for cisplatin-based polychemotherapy in previously untreated patients.[112] A small randomized study of neoadjuvant chemotherapy showed an advantage for neoadjuvant therapy over surgery at interim analysis. In subset analysis, the benefit of the neoadjuvant approach appeared to be confined to bulky tumors. The question of whether controlling disease progression of a locally advanced cervical cancer with chemotherapy can allow continuation of a pregnancy has not been studied.[113] Chemotherapy also has activity in cervical cancer metastatic to distant organs, but such stage IVb cancers are not curable. Chemotherapy may be given to a pregnant patient, but her decision whether to continue the pregnancy should be informed by this evidence about her prognosis.

If the antepartum diagnosis of cervical cancer is not made and the patient delivers vaginally, seeding of the episiotomy site with cancer cells may occur and manifest as an episiotomy site recurrence within 12 weeks to 2 years after delivery. If cervical cancer is diagnosed at or after vaginal delivery, consideration should be given to regular colposcopy of the episiotomy site, with or without random biopsies, for the first 2 years after delivery.[114]

Trophoblastic Diseases

Trophoblastic disease complicates fewer than 2 per 1000 pregnancies in the United States but as many as 1 per 120 in some areas of Asia and South America. These diseases manifest across a spectrum from molar pregnancies to metastatic choriocarcinoma. The rarest manifestations are invasive mole, also known as choriocarcinoma destruens, and the placental-site trophoblastic tumors. Invasive trophoblastic disease is most common after a molar pregnancy but may also develop in the wake of a normal pregnancy or abortion. The most powerful predisposing factor is higher maternal age. Maternal age over 50 increases the risk over 400-fold. There is also a modest increase in risk for maternal age younger than 15 years. A previous history of hydatidiform mole is also a risk factor. The risk of a second mole is 1 per 76, but the risk of a third mole is 1 per 6.5.[115] There is a great geographic variation in the incidence and some evidence for an effect of low-dose background radiation in increasing risk.[116]

Molar Pregnancies

Hydatidiform moles may manifest with first-trimester bleeding, passage of clots or grape-like villi, an abnormally enlarging uterus, absence of fetal development in a patient with an elevated β-hCG level, hyperemesis, early onset of toxemia, or, in cases of invasive trophoblastic disease, uterine rupture. A normal fetus develops synchronously with fewer than 1% of molar pregnancies. If the diagnosis of coexisting normal pregnancy and hydatidiform mole is made late in the pregnancy, it is possible to attempt to allow the pregnancy to continue and treat the trophoblastic disease definitively after delivery, although the risk of metastasis from treatment delay is not known. Preeclampsia and maternal bleeding usually preclude carrying the pregnancy to term and, indeed, only in their absence should the diagnosis be delayed until near term.[117] Ultrasonography with color-flow Doppler imaging is the mainstay of diagnosis; this modality usually visualizes the mass, which is highly vascular and sometimes has a necrotic center, and can determine whether a normal fetus is present. MR imaging can also show focal tumor masses, pathologic vasculature, and loss of uterine zonal anatomy.[118] Partial moles are biparental and usually triploid, whereas complete moles are derived from diploid paternal genetic material and maternal cytoplasmic material and are usually diploid.[119] Flow cytometry can distinguish between diploid and triploid moles; however, the prognostic distinction between partial moles and complete moles is based on histologic criteria. None of 43 triploid or tetraploid moles described by Sunde and coworkers were complicated by persistent trophoblastic disease. The confidence intervals for risk of persistent disease after a triploid mole were 0% to 2.7% in that series.[120] Complete moles are more likely to be complicated by persistent trophoblastic disease; nonmetastatic trophoblastic disease develops after 15% of complete molar pregnancies, in comparison with 5.5% after partial molar pregnancies.[121]

Molar pregnancies are treated by evacuation. Passage of clots may represent spontaneous abortion of the mole but do not lead to complete evacuation. The β-hCG level should become undetectable within 10 weeks; delayed decline or persistent detectable β-hCG levels are indicative of residual local or metastatic disease. For this reason, β-hCG determinations are performed weekly until the level is 0 mIU/mL and are continued monthly for the next 6 months. Patients should be counseled to avoid pregnancy during this period of follow-up because the normal rise in β-hCG during pregnancy will confound follow-up. The impact of immediate pregnancy on the risk of recurrence is not understood, and the patient's prognosis is much more certain once the β-hCG level has normalized. Oral hormonal contraception can be recommended without concern that it will increase the risk of recurrence.[122] If there is a concern that a rise in β-hCG level is caused by conception, the distinction between a persistent mole and a normal pregnancy is aided by ultrasonography with color-flow Doppler imaging. Serum progesterone levels are useful in making this distinction when the β-hCG level is below 1000 mIU/mL, when ultrasonography is least likely to be helpful. A progesterone level below 2.5 ng/mL is predictive of trophoblastic disease with a sensitivity of 83% and a specificity of 95%; a level higher than 10 ng/mL is correlated with the presence of a viable pregnancy.[123] Management of subsequent pregnancies in the patient with a history of molar pregnancy should include ultrasonography in the first trimester to confirm the presence of a normal pregnancy, careful histopathologic review of the products of conception or the placenta, and measurement of the β-hCG level 6 weeks after delivery.[121]

Follow-up should also include regular examinations and chest radiographs to search for lung metastases (Table 23–1). Risk factors for persistent disease include a β-hCG level higher than 100,000 mIU/mL, an abnormally enlarged uterus, and a theca lutein cyst larger than 6 cm. Weekly color-flow Doppler imaging is under investigation as a means of monitoring regression of disease in the postevacuation period.[124] Persistent gestational trophoblastic disease may be classified in the World Health Organization or Charing Cross scoring systems as low or high risk.[125] Among patients with low-risk disease treated with adjuvant low-dosage methotrexate and folinic acid or single-agent dactinomycin, the relapse rate at 5 years is 3%.[126] The advisability of adjuvant chemotherapy for women at highest risk has not been established. Methotrexate/actinomycin D combination chemotherapy is likely to be successful in 80% of patients with persistent disease.[127]

If the β-hCG level rises after an initial fall that follows evacuation of the hydatidiform mole, or if there is a

TABLE 23–1	Follow-up of Molar Pregnancy
After evacuation	β-hCG measurements weekly until values = 0 mIU/mL, then monthly for 6 months
	Counseling of patient to avoid pregnancy during this initial follow-up period
	Regular pelvic examination and chest radiographs
Subsequent pregnancy	Ultrasonography with Doppler imaging to confirm normal pregnancy
	Serum progesterone if β-hCG value <1000 mIU/mL
	Careful histopathologic review of the products of conception
	β-hCG measurement 6 weeks after delivery

β-hCG, β-human chorionic gonadotropin.

plateau in the β-hCG level, additional evaluation with pelvic examination and transvaginal ultrasonography and color Doppler imaging are indicated for identifying persistent disease and, if necessary, ruling out normal pregnancy. A search for evidence of metastatic disease should also be made with CT scanning of the chest, abdomen, and pelvis and with MR imaging of the brain. Once the absence of metastases has been established, chemotherapy can be initiated without dilatation and curettage or other attempt at biopsy. These latter procedures place the patient at risk for uterine perforation without aiding in management. The β-hCG level should be measured immediately before the first dose of chemotherapy, to provide a baseline against which to assess the response.[128] The β-hCG level should fall by at least one log in the first 18 days. This marker is followed closely until it normalizes, and then tumor marker measurements and chest radiographs are performed every month for 1 year. If methotrexate therapy fails, dactinomycin or other salvage chemotherapy is attempted. Hysterectomy is reserved for chemotherapy-refractory localized disease; chemotherapy is preferable to hysterectomy, not only because it preserves fertility but also because the cure rate in the prechemotherapy era was only 60% for locally confined disease.

Chorioadenoma destruens is a form of molar pregnancy that is locally invasive. It manifests in the first 6 months after treatment of a molar pregnancy with uterine enlargement caused by myometrial invasion without endometrial invasion. Transvaginal ultrasonograms show a well-defined spheric and echogenic mass in the myometrium.[129] Pelvic masses and peritoneal extension may also be present. Pulmonary emboli with infarction can occur as a result of embolization of chorionic villi. The clinical presentation and the findings on ventilation perfusion scans and pulmonary angiography are indistinguishable from those of thromboemboli to the lungs.[130] The disease is staged with CT scanning of the chest, abdomen, pelvis, and brain to distinguish this syndrome from metastatic choriocarcinoma. Radioimmunoscintigraphy with antibodies to β-hCG can identify metastases in some cases, but its role in the management of invasive trophoblastic disease has not yet been established.[131]

Placental-site trophoblastic disease is the rarest of the trophoblastic conditions. It manifests most commonly with vaginal bleeding but may also be detected because of preeclampsia, virilization, amenorrhea, or the nephrotic syndrome. Uterine nodules are palpable. Ultrasonography or MR studies may disclose the presence of vascular lakes or sinusoids.[132] Placental-site trophoblastic disease is usually cured with wide excision, consisting of complete hysterectomy, with or without salpingo-oophorectomy.[133] In patients with no extrapelvic disease and an antecedent pregnancy interval of less than 4 years, the disease is entirely curable with surgery and combination chemotherapy; lung metastases and longer interval of antecedent pregnancy are grave prognostic indicators.[134]

Choriocarcinoma

Choriocarcinoma, the malignant and usually metastatic form of trophoblastic disease, is a rapidly growing tumor with the potential for brain metastases and hemorrhage. It has rarely been known to manifest first through the symptoms of brain metastases.[135] Choriocarcinoma is preceded by a molar pregnancy in many cases and may also develop in the period after delivery of a normal fetus or after spontaneous or therapeutic abortion. The ultrasound appearance of malignant choriocarcinoma may be similar to that seen with chorioadenoma destruens, except with the rare occurrence of cervical choriocarcinoma.[136] The disease is staged with CT scans of the chest, abdomen, and pelvis and with MR imaging of the brain.

Treatment with chemotherapy, to which choriocarcinoma is highly sensitive, should be initiated promptly. Hysterectomy is deferred because the uterus is highly vascular before treatment, bleeding complications can be minimized by a response to primary chemotherapy, and control of systemic disease is the most important goal of therapy. Treatment is chosen by the patient's score in the combined International Federation of Gynecology and Obstetrics/World Health Organization system.[125] Patients with low-risk disease are treated with methotrexate, with or without actinomycin D. Patients with high-risk disease receive combination chemotherapy consisting of cycles of etoposide, dactinomycin, high-dose methotrexate, and leucovorin rescue alternating with cycles of vincristine and cyclophosphamide.[115,137] Those with brain metastases should also receive steroids and whole brain radiotherapy. Brain metastases do not preclude the possibility of a cure, especially if they are not associated with neurologic symptoms, if they did not develop while the patient was receiving chemotherapy, and if the largest metastasis is less than 3 cm.[138,139] Choriocarcinoma is, as mentioned, highly sensitive to radiotherapy, and patients with this cancer were excluded from the landmark randomized trial that established the curative potential of resection of a solitary brain metastasis, on the basis of the expectation that their disease could be cured by radiotherapy alone.[140] Fewer than 20% of patients do not achieve cure. The presence of hepatic metastases and the coexistence of hepatic and cerebral metastases are risk factors for treatment-refractory disease.[141] Among patients with resistant or recurrent disease, a minority responds nonetheless to second-line chemotherapy with platinum-based chemotherapy or paclitaxel.[142] Case and single-arm studies have shown a role in treatment-refractory disease for high-dose chemotherapy with stem cell or autologous marrow rescue.[143,144] There may be a limited role for salvage surgery to resect metastatic disease that is chemotherapy refractory, if the number of metastatic sites is small.[145] Several cases are reported to have been cured by chemoembolization of hepatic metastases.[146]

Endometrial Cancer

The mean age at diagnosis of endometrial cancer is 60 years; the disease is rare during pregnancy. Women with a history of prolonged exposure to unopposed estrogen are at higher risk of developing endometrial cancer, and pregnancy is protective. Tamoxifen, an agent that binds to the estrogen receptor variously as an agonist or antagonist, increases the risk of endometrial cancer by twofold to sixfold.[147] This drug is increasingly prescribed for the adjuvant therapy of breast cancer or as a breast cancer chemopreventive agent in premenopausal women.

Ovarian Cancer in Pregnancy

Diagnosis

Ovarian carcinoma is not the most likely cause of a pelvic mass diagnosed during pregnancy. The majority of adnexal masses that manifest during pregnancy are benign and resolve during the first trimester. As with endometrial cancer, ovarian cancer is rare in women of childbearing age, although among women who carry certain mutations of the BRCA1 gene, the risk of ovarian cancer development before menopause is increased.[148] Ueda and Ueki reported on 106 cases in which ovarian masses were resected from pregnant women. Of these, 29% were caused by physiologic enlargement; 66% were benign neoplasms; and 5% contained ovarian cancer. The incidence of benign tumors was 1 per 112 deliveries, and that of malignant tumors was 1 per 1684 deliveries.[149] The possibility of ovarian cancer is strong enough that histologic evaluation of all adnexal masses that persist after 16 weeks of pregnancy must be considered.

Color-flow Doppler imaging may be helpful in detecting hypervascularity, and ultrasonography is useful for distinguishing simple from complex cysts. Laparotomy for diagnostic purposes and to resect the mass may be complicated by postoperative spontaneous abortion. Surgical diagnosis and management are safer during the second trimester, and masses persisting into the second trimester should be surgically evaluated if they are not simple cysts.[150] A case has been reported of successful outcome of a 9-week pregnancy despite bilateral salpingo-oophorectomy for ovarian cancer.[151]

A retrospective series of 10 serous neoplasms of low malignant potential of ovarian or peritoneal origin manifesting during pregnancy was reported from the pathology department of the M. D. Anderson Cancer Center. Multiple areas of microinvasion were seen in most cases, all cases had marked epithelial proliferation, and two had abdominal or distant metastases. Histologic or clinical downgrading of the tumors was noted after delivery or termination of the pregnancy in some cases. Despite the poor clinical and histologic features, all patients were alive without evidence of disease at the time of the report, after follow-up periods of 2 months to 20 years.[152]

Ovarian masses may contain teratoma. Simultaneous teratoma in the mother and fetus has been described. Histologic features suggested a clonal origin for the intracranial mass of the fetus and the ovarian mass in the mother, but polymorphisms of DNA microsatellites in the two tumors were more consistent with independent origins for the two tumors.[153]

Management

Low-grade ovarian cancer that is confined to the ovaries, without ascites or tumor on the external ovarian surfaces, has an excellent 5-year prognosis, and resection with appropriate surgical staging is adequate management. If the patient wishes to preserve fertility and only one ovary is grossly involved, the contralateral ovary can yield a biopsy sample but can be preserved.[154] Patients with early-stage tumors who have a worse prognosis on the basis of high-grade histologic findings, ascites, or pelvic tumor extension are offered adjuvant chemotherapy, usually with the combination of cisplatin and paclitaxel, although the optimal adjuvant therapy for these patients is not yet established. Patients with advanced disease undergo debulking surgery, followed by combination chemotherapy. Trials are ongoing to determine whether intraperitoneal therapy offers an advantage over cisplatin/paclitaxel combination therapy for patients with minimal residual intraabdominal disease.[155,156]

Breast Cancer

Breast cancer, in industrialized societies, is predominantly a disease of aging and is not common during pregnancy. In the United States, fewer than 4% of breast cancers manifest during pregnancy or the first postpartum year, but among patients who are younger than 35 years of age at the time of breast cancer diagnosis, more than 25% are pregnant or in the first postpartum year.[157] In Zaria, Nigeria, where most breast cancers develop before menopause, 26% of all cases seen in women younger than 50 years of age develop while the patient is pregnant or lactating.[158]

For women with a first pregnancy at the age of 30 years or older, pregnancy increases the risk of breast cancer over the first 3 to 4 postpartum years but decreases the lifetime risk of breast cancer.[18] Because the latency period before manifestation of such pregnancy-associated breast cancers is short, it seems likely that the hormonal changes of pregnancy act to promote growth or transformation of abnormal clones that are already present at the time of conception. Murine models demonstrate accelerated growth of mammary cancers in pregnancy on the basis of 130-fold higher levels of messenger RNA for the mitogenic growth factor insulin-like growth factor II.[159]

Diagnosis

Early detection is crucial if breast cancer is to be cured (Table 23–2), and mammography has been demonstrated to help reduce cause-specific and overall mortality among women older than 50 years.[160,161] Mammography is not routinely recommended for women younger than 50 years of age, but it also helps reduce cause-specific mortality rates among women aged 40 to 49.[162] Mammography is not routinely recommended during pregnancy, because its sensitivity is reduced during pregnancy; the general population of pregnant women is not at high risk for the disease; and radiation exposure to the fetus should always be minimized. Women who are at increased risk for early-onset breast cancer because of mantle radiotherapy, an identified genetic mutation, family history, late age during first-term pregnancy, use of alcohol, prolonged use of hormonal contraception, prior personal history of

TABLE 23–2   Early Detection of Cancer during Pregnancy

First antenatal visit	Family history of cancer
	Personal risk factors for cancer
	Pap smear; repeat if results are inadequate
	Hemoccult test of stool
	Examination of nevi
	Breast examination
Subsequent visits	Follow-up examination of all nevi; biopsy of lesions that change in size, color, variegation, or outline
	Ultrasonography and biopsy of suspect or enlarging breast lesions or inflammatory changes of the breast
	Doppler flow study of all adnexal masses persisting into the second trimester; laparoscopic biopsy of hypervascular or complex masses

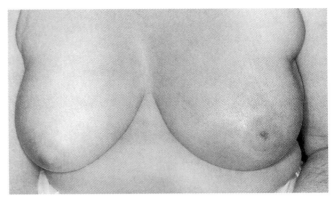

Figure 23–1. The erythema and swelling of the left breast are characteristic of inflammatory breast cancer. (From Skarin AT [ed]: Slide Atlas of Diagnostic Oncology, Breast Cancer, vol 6, 2nd ed. New York, Gower Medical Publishers, 1992.)

breast cancer, or abnormal histologic findings on breast biopsy, and who are planning pregnancy, especially a first pregnancy after age 35, may consider screening mammography before becoming pregnant.[4]

Referral centers report the unfortunate fact that the diagnosis of breast cancer during and after pregnancy is frequently delayed. Women with postpartum breast cancer (within 5 years of delivery) had slightly larger tumors than a control group of women with breast cancer that developed before the age of 50.[157] It has been hypothesized that the more advanced stage of breast cancers diagnosed during pregnancy or during the postpartum period is attributable to faster growth and more invasive properties of breast cancer in the hormonal milieu of pregnancy.[163] Although this is probable, it is not the only factor: at Memorial Sloan-Kettering Cancer Center, more than 50% of patients who are seen for a postpartum breast cancer have a palpable mass that developed and was detected during pregnancy but that was monitored clinically without imaging or biopsy. The mean size of these cancers was a relatively large 3.5 cm, in comparison with 2 cm for cancers diagnosed before delivery.[164] As expected, larger tumor size is correlated with a higher likelihood of the prognostically adverse finding of metastases to the axillary lymph nodes. Nugent and O'Connell found axillary lymph node involvement in 74% of pregnancy-associated breast cancers, in comparison with 37% of nonpregnant premenopausal women.[165] Clinicians may be uncertain about a new mass in the breast because the physiologic changes of pregnancy include increased density and hypertrophy of the breast. These changes are least marked early in pregnancy, and a thorough breast examination should be performed at the first antenatal visit. It is common for a pregnant patient to have each antenatal visit with a different provider in an obstetric group practice, so that she is familiar with everyone who might be present at her delivery. This makes evaluation of changes in the breast more difficult. Thus, for patients at highest risk for breast cancer during pregnancy—those with a personal history of breast cancer, a strong family history, a known genetic predisposition to breast cancer, or a history of thoracic radiotherapy—consideration should be given to having a single provider monitor the breast examination or to having the patient monitored by her breast surgeon during the pregnancy.

Inflammatory breast cancer is a syndrome of erythema, warmth, and induration of the breast, with or without peau d'orange; it typically evolves over a period of 3 months or less (Fig. 23–1). The abnormalities may be diffuse in the breast; on occasion, they extend beyond the breast onto the chest wall. The appearance of inflammation is secondary to emboli of breast cancer to the dermal lymphatic vessels, which obstruct lymphatic drainage in the breast. Without prompt therapy, the prognosis of this uncommon syndrome (which represents fewer than 3% of all newly diagnosed breast cancers in the United States) is for rapid progression and death, and even with prompt and aggressive therapy, the risk of recurrence remains high.[166] The diagnosis of inflammatory breast cancer in association with pregnancy is also commonly delayed. This distinction is somewhat more difficult on clinical grounds in lactating women, because lactation is one of the few clinical settings in which mastitis occurs with any frequency. Lack of a response to antibiotics and lack of an abscess cavity suggest the possibility of inflammatory breast cancer. The sensitivity of mammography during lactation may be improved if the patient breast-feeds or expresses milk immediately before mammography is performed.

New breast masses should not be attributed to the changes of pregnancy without investigation. Breast ultrasonography is the modality of choice, but mammography can be considered because the fetal dose from a single mammogram is low. In a retrospective series of 85 women who received a diagnosis of breast cancer while pregnant or during the first postpartum year, 21 underwent mammography before biopsy. In these women, 23 cancers were diagnosed, and 18 of these cancers were visualized mammographically. Breast sonography demonstrated a focal solid mass in all six cases in which it was performed. This retrospective study is limited because it is not known why mammography was performed in those 21 women or how many pregnant women were evaluated by mammography and ultimately found to have only benign disease. Also, findings were not correlated to the timing of mammography in relation to delivery. Nonetheless, this experience demonstrates that the breast of a pregnant woman can be evaluated by mammography.[167] A normal mammogram never rules out breast cancer in a palpable mass, and this is the case during pregnancy as well. Multiple core biopsies or local excision should be performed to rule out cancer in any dominant mass, except a simple cyst. If inflammatory changes are present, the biopsy should always include overlying skin so that the dermal lymphatic vessels may be assessed.

Prognostic Features

The most important prognostic feature of a primary breast cancer is whether it has metastasized to the axillary lymph nodes (Fig. 23–2). When four axillary nodes are involved, the risk of recurrence by 10 years in the absence of adjuvant chemotherapy is 75%. Involvement of 10 nodes or more carries a 100% risk of recurrence by 10 years. Adjuvant chemotherapy delays the median time to recurrence in this group but is not curative.[168] Cancers that have not spread to an axillary node have an approximately 30% risk of recurrence at 10 years.[169] Among node-negative tumors, recognizing those with a substantial risk of recurrence is more difficult. Size is helpful, especially if the tumor size is 1 cm or smaller.[170] Overexpression of hormone receptors is predictive of a longer time to recurrence, but with long follow-up, the ultimate risks of recurrence are similar in untreated hormone receptor–negative and –positive cases.[171] Markers of growth rate have been reproducibly prognostic in large series with long follow-up.[172,173] Detection of micrometastases in the bone marrow is an adverse prognostic indicator in node-positive or node-negative breast cancer.[174]

Gene amplification of the ligandless growth factor receptor Her-2/neu is associated with a more aggressive phenotype, relatively resistant to some forms of chemotherapy, and often with absence of nuclear hormone receptors.[175,176] Trastuzumab is a humanized antibody to the Her-2/neu protein that is active in Her-2/neu amplified

advanced breast cancers and under study in stage II and III breast cancer.[177]

The prognosis, if the most recent birth was less than 2 years before the diagnosis of breast cancers, is worse than that if the most recent birth was more than 5 years before diagnosis; the hazard ratio for death is 2.7.[178]

Management

The sequence of local excision of tumor to tumor-free margins followed by radiation to the remainder of the breast is established as a good alternative to mastectomy in women who are not pregnant if the tumor is less than 4 cm in size, unifocal, and without inflammatory features.[179,180] Among nonpregnant women, the risks of local recurrence, distant metastases, and death are the same after mastectomy or lumpectomy and after radiation. The same has not been demonstrated for breast conservation in pregnancy. Pregnant patients are explicitly excluded from randomized trials of breast conservation. Because of the increased density of the breast on a mammogram during pregnancy, the sensitivity of mammography for multifocal cancer may be reduced. Last, therapeutic radiation must not be given to the breast during pregnancy because of unacceptable radiation exposure to the fetus. If breast conservation is chosen, radiation would be delayed until after delivery. A randomized study has demonstrated that radiation after lumpectomy can be safely delayed for the duration of adjuvant chemotherapy, but this study excluded pregnant women.[181] The hormonal milieu of pregnancy might lead to a greater risk of progression during this delay. Anecdotal reports of breast conservation during pregnancy exist; however, no prospective series have defined the local and distant recurrence rates after breast conservation in pregnancy. In the absence of such data, a pregnant woman in whom breast cancer is diagnosed during the first or second trimester and who intends to continue the pregnancy should receive a strong recommendation for mastectomy. The mastectomy

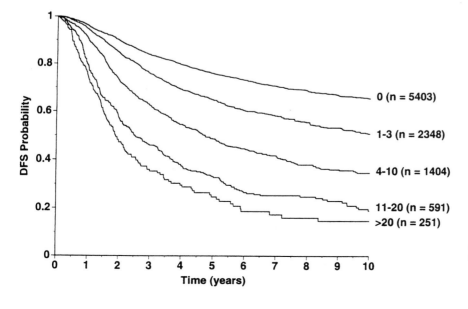

Figure 23–2. Disease-free survival (DFS) by number of positive axillary lymph nodes. Data from the San Antonio Data Base; median length of follow-up, 51 months. (From Clark G: Prognostic and predictive factors. In Harris JR, Lippman ME, Morrow M, Hellman S [eds]: Diseases of the Breast. Philadelphia, Lippincott-Raven, 2000, p 491.)

should include dissection of the ipsilateral axilla. The procedure of sentinel node biopsy should be substituted for a conventional lymph node biopsy only at centers that have established the sensitivity and specificity of this approach in their own series. If it is to be performed in a pregnant woman, it should be done with a dye rather than a radioactive tracer, but this may reduce the utility of the procedure. A positive sentinel node is an indication for completion of the axillary node dissection to ascertain the extent of axillary node involvement, whereas a negative sentinel node is only rarely found if other axillary nodes are involved.[182]

Recommendations about adjuvant therapy depend on the size of the tumor, its biologic characteristics, and the extent of axillary lymph node involvement. If the breast cancer is diagnosed during the third trimester, adjuvant therapy can usually be delayed until after delivery. For a tumor with a poor prognosis, delivery by cesarean section at the time of fetal maturity should be undertaken to minimize the delay in beginning adjuvant therapy. The adjuvant therapy can then be chosen without regard to its risks to the fetus, although the infant cannot be breast-fed. If the cancer is diagnosed early in the pregnancy and the pregnancy is to be continued, adjuvant therapy cannot be initiated until the second trimester. The commonly used regimen of cyclophosphamide, methotrexate, and 5-fluorouracil is not an option for the pregnant patient, because the toxic effects of methotrexate in the mother may be unacceptably increased and because methotrexate, as reviewed earlier, is an abortifacient and causes fetal malformations with a high frequency.

The alternative regimen of doxorubicin and cyclophosphamide has been demonstrated to have similar adjuvant efficacy and is preferred in this setting.[183] Adjuvant regimens in which dose intensity is increased and a taxane is added are preferred for patients with node-positive disease.[184,185] The use of myeloablative doses necessitating stem cell support remains experimental at present.[186] The toxic effects of such approaches to the pregnant patient and the fetus are not known, but because toxicity in non-pregnant patients is high, and because infectious and bleeding complications are common, it seems likely that these approaches will not be well tolerated during pregnancy. Use of such therapies should be delayed until after delivery. Because these regimens are most often considered in women with the highest risk of dying of breast cancer and the shortest expected survival times, termination of the pregnancy followed by experimental adjuvant therapy merits consideration. Tamoxifen is indicated as a component of adjuvant therapy in premenopausal women with hormone-receptor positive cancers. The risk reduction from use of tamoxifen in these patients is greater than that from chemotherapy.

The sequence of mastectomy followed by adjuvant chemotherapy is no longer the preferred approach for patients with locally advanced or inflammatory breast cancers. The risk of local recurrence is high when locally advanced or inflammatory cancers are treated with initial mastectomy. Hormonal therapy of receptor-positive tumors can lead to excellent responses, but these responses may take months and in premenopausal women are most likely if tamoxifen is given together with ovarian ablation.[187] Response rates to initial chemotherapy are 60% to 90%, and complete responses are confirmed by pathologic findings in about 20% of patients.[188] The tumor can be monitored well clinically while it is large, but imaging studies are helpful in response assessment. Mammograms may show increased calcifications with response; MR imaging is used increasingly in pregnant and nonpregnant patients to monitor the size of a primary breast tumor while the patient is receiving chemotherapy.[189] The finding of involved axillary nodes at the time of resection after a response to primary chemotherapy is an adverse prognostic indicator.[190] All patients who have been treated for locally advanced disease should receive further adjuvant chemotherapy after resection, and if the prognosis is known to be poor on the basis of the extent of axillary involvement, consideration should be given to dose-intensive therapy, possibly with hematopoietic support. All patients with locally advanced disease require chest wall radiotherapy after completion of all systemic therapy, to reduce the risk of local recurrence.

The median length of survival of patients with metastatic breast cancer that responds to hormones is less than 3 years; that of those with disease that is refractory to hormone treatment is less than 2 years. The conventional approach is to give palliative therapy with hormonal treatment, followed by combination chemotherapy with agents to which the patient has not previously been exposed. In the setting of pregnancy, it was traditional to encourage the patient to make decisions with the well-being of the fetus foremost in her mind, because her expectation of survival was low. However, optimal hormonal therapy of metastatic breast cancer in a premenopausal woman requires ovarian ablation, which would preclude continuance of the pregnancy. In addition, experimental approaches that intensify therapy and that are neither tested in pregnancy nor likely to be safe in pregnancy may offer a hope of cure to some women with metastatic disease that responds to chemotherapy and is confined to a few metastases.

Continuation of pregnancy by any subset of pregnant women with breast cancer is not absolutely contraindicated by current information. As discussed earlier, there is some evidence that pregnancy may foster growth or transformation of breast cancers, but the small series that have compared breast cancer outcomes after therapeutic abortion or with continuation of pregnancy have failed to demonstrate a difference.[165,191] In the discussion about therapeutic abortion with a pregnant patient who has breast cancer, the clinician should review these data but should also emphasize that these small, retrospective studies, although likely to be the only information that will ever be available, are not definitive. They are subject to bias if therapeutic abortion is chosen more often by patients with the most advanced disease, thus reducing the ability to detect an advantage for termination of pregnancy. The discussion of therapeutic abortion should also cover the patient's individual risk for recurrence and death, which is based on tumor size, the extent of nodal involvement, the histologic characteristics and growth fraction of the cancer, the presence or absence of hormone receptors, and whether there is evidence for distant metastasis. Recommendations of therapies should be placed in the context of trimester of pregnancy, how much of a delay in therapy will be caused by continuation of the pregnancy, and the probable risks of this delay. The decision to continue or terminate the pregnancy should take into account not only the impact of the pregnancy on the breast cancer and the impact of therapy on the fetus but also long-term issues, such as who will take responsibility for the child if the mother is disabled by or dies of metastatic breast cancer. This question is especially complicated if the child has long-term sequelae of in utero exposure to chemotherapy. In summary, many patients have undergone mastectomy and received adjuvant chemotherapy during the latter trimesters of pregnancy without complication, but the risks of this approach are not fully known.

Stage for stage, pregnant women with breast cancer have the same recurrence-free and overall survival expectations as age-matched patients who had breast cancers that were not associated with pregnancy.[165,192] The risk that a subsequent pregnancy might stimulate growth of micrometastatic disease and lead to a relapse of the breast cancer has long been debated. No series has demonstrated an adverse effect of subsequent pregnancy on the course of breast cancer, and multiple pregnancies after therapy for breast cancer may be somewhat protective against recurrence.[93,191,193] Most of these series are subject to the bias that only healthy women choose to or are able to become pregnant.[194] An age- and stage-matched case-control study of women who became pregnant within 6 months of mastectomy, diminishing the opportunity for bias by difference in breast cancer outcome, found a survival advantage with subsequent pregnancy.[192]

An often-quoted recommendation is that women delay further childbearing by 2 years after the diagnosis of breast cancer. This recommendation is derived from a report published in 1977 and is based on 21 years of experience (thus reflecting practice patterns beginning in 1956), which demonstrated that the peak time of breast cancer recurrence is at 2 years.[165] The author of that study argued that women who had not had a relapse by 2 years were less likely to have a relapse or to have aggressive disease when they did so, and thus they could most safely consider becoming pregnant. The risk of recurrence of breast cancer is lower today than it was in 1956 or 1977. Mammography and enhanced awareness of the advantages of prompt treatment of breast cancer have led to detection at lower stages and smaller tumor sizes in the earliest stage, and the use of adjuvant chemotherapy decreases the overall risk of recurrence and delays recurrence for patients destined to have relapses. The median length of time until recurrence for nonpregnant patients treated with adjuvant chemotherapy with the popular regimen of cyclophosphamide, methotrexate, and 5-fluorouracil is 83 months.[168] A large metaanalysis of various forms of polychemotherapy without subsequent hormonal manipulation demonstrated a median length of time until relapse of more than 5 years for node-positive patients. The median survival of the node-negative patients, with 10 years of follow-up, had not yet been reached.[195] Thus, although a short time from diagnosis to development of metastatic disease remains an adverse

prognostic indicator, the 2-year mark should not be considered a watershed for any group of breast cancer survivors.

The decision by a survivor of breast cancer to become pregnant is a personal one. The physician can assist the patient by providing individual information about the risk of recurrence and by informing her that the possibility that the pregnancy will accelerate a relapse of the cancer is not high. The single case-control study reported in 1968 cannot be taken as definitive proof that pregnancy will actually be beneficial, because of the concern about selection bias.[190]

Thyroid Cancer in Pregnancy

Differentiated thyroid cancer is an indolent disease in nonpregnant adults, but in pregnant women, this cancer may take a more aggressive clinical course. Thyroid nodules that develop during pregnancy should be evaluated with ultrasonography and cytologic sampling obtained by fine-needle aspiration, if indicated. Further evaluation is clearly needed for rapidly enlarging nodules, those enlarging despite suppressive therapy, solid lesions larger than 2 cm, cystic nodules larger than 4 cm, and those associated with cervical nodes.[196] Of 40 cases of thyroid nodules in pregnant patients, 25 (62.5%) were found to be benign on cytologic examination.[197] If the biopsy sample contains any evidence of a papillary carcinoma, even if the histologic appearance is mixed, if the size is small and the patient is younger than 40 years, the disease is likely to be indolent, and the long-term prognosis is among the best reported for any cancer. In such patients, definitive therapy may be deferred until after delivery. If the patient is older than 40 years, if the tumor is large, if there is concern that the histologic findings may be of a higher grade, or if the patient cannot tolerate a treatment delay for psychologic reasons, resection can be performed after the first trimester.

The current surgical recommendation is for near-total thyroidectomy. This allows preservation of the recurrent laryngeal nerve in almost all cases, so that quality of life is better than with total thyroidectomy, and the amount of residual thyroid tissue is small enough to permit good radioablation. The most effective modality in the management of well-differentiated thyroid cancer is suppression with exogenous thyroid hormone. This should be initiated in the postoperative period in the pregnant patient as anticancer therapy, as well as for prevention of congenital hypothyroidism in the fetus. There is no indication to hasten delivery in such cases.

Hormone replacement can be stopped after delivery, and the patient can be monitored until she is profoundly hypothyroid. At this point, uptake of radioactive iodine is maximized, and thyroid scanning is most sensitive. If there is evidence of uptake of radioactive iodine, demonstrating residual or metastatic thyroid tissue, the patient should undergo radioablation. This should then be followed by reinstitution of thyroid hormone supplementation with the goal to suppress thyroid-stimulating hormone levels. The patient should never breast-feed her child after either a thyroid scan or therapeutic iodine ablation. It is conventional to withdraw thyroid hormone supplementation temporarily after 1 year and again after 3 years to permit follow-up radioiodine scanning. This practice has no demonstrated impact on survival, and many patients become severely symptomatic during the period when they are not taking thyroid supplementation. Among the patients at the lowest risk, this practice may not be necessary. Conception after radioiodine ablation is associated with a slightly higher risk of miscarriage, which is most pronounced in the first year after therapy with iodine 133.[198]

Melanoma

Cutaneous melanoma among white persons is increasing in incidence more rapidly than any other malignancy. Although increased awareness has led to earlier detection, the fatality rate is also increasing. Thickness is the principal determinant of the risk of recurrence and death after diagnosis of melanoma; thus, failure to promptly recognize a melanoma can have a significant and negative impact on the patient's chances for a cure.

Pregnancy can be associated with generalized hyperpigmentation. This has led to an expectation that hyperpigmented lesions will darken and change during pregnancy, so that physicians have not been disposed to recommend biopsy of nevi that change in size or configuration during pregnancy. However, a melanoma should be suspected in any case of a change in a pigmented lesion (Fig. 23–3). Attention should be paid to changes in color, outline, size, symmetry, and the degree of variegation of pigmentation. Lesions larger than 6 mm in diameter are worrisome, and bleeding and ulceration are late and ominous findings. Because of the importance of early diagnosis, people with many nevi are best monitored by a dermatologist with experience in managing pigmented lesions; however, examination of the skin with attention to pigmented lesions should be part of routine health care, and nevi should be assessed at antenatal visits (see Table 23–2). Consultation of an atlas of pigmented lesions may be helpful in assessing nevi that appear atypical.[199] In the United States, the overwhelming majority of melanomas occur in white persons, but it is important to remember that, worldwide, 40% of melanomas arise in nonwhite persons.

Although pregnancy has not been found to influence whether a melanoma will develop, the diagnosis of melanoma in pregnancy, like the diagnosis of breast cancer, appears to be delayed. The mean thickness of a melanoma diagnosed during pregnancy is larger than that of lesions diagnosed in nonpregnant women.[200] A case-control study of 100 pregnant women with diagnoses of melanoma was published at a median follow-up of over 6 years; it revealed an increased incidence of lymph node metastases and of recurrent and metastatic disease among the patients who had been pregnant at the time of diagnosis. At this length of follow-up, in a series this size, the difference in survival was not statistically significant; however, multivariate analysis showed that pregnancy had a significant association with the development of metastases, which suggests that longer follow-up may show a survival difference.[201]

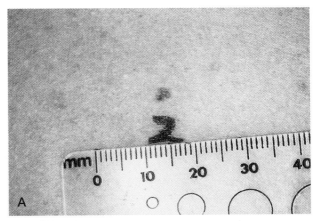

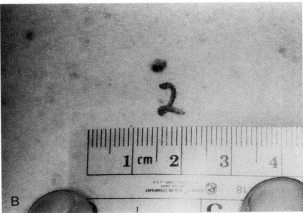

Figure 23–3. Dysplastic nevus (**A**) in a nonpregnant woman. The same nevus (**B**) during a subsequent pregnancy. It has increased in size and darkened. These changes indicate the need for biopsy. (From Ellis DL: Pregnancy and sex steroid hormone effects on nevi of patients with the dysplastic nevus syndrome. J Am Acad Dermatol 1991;25:467.)

Prognosis

Melanomas are categorized by growth pattern. About 70% of melanomas are of the superficial spreading type. These are generally flat lesions with irregular areas of deep pigmentation, arising from preexisting nevi. Nodular melanomas are the next most common type. These are larger, more rapidly growing lesions that are most likely to arise in previously uninvolved areas of skin. Lentigo maligna melanomas are indolent lesions with a low metastatic potential. They occur most often in postmenopausal women and are rare in women of childbearing age. Acral lentiginous melanomas are also rare in women of childbearing age, and most are seen in patients of African, Asian, or Native American ancestry.

Prognosis in melanoma is determined by microstaging. The Breslow system determines the height of the lesion from the granular layer to the deepest point of penetration.[202] Tumor depth appears to be a continuous variable, but depth of 0.76 mm or greater is the criterion for categorizing a node-negative cancer as stage II, which worsens the prognosis for 15-year survival rates from 85% to 50%. Involvement of regional nodes is the criterion for categorizing a tumor as stage III, which is associated with a 10-year survival rate of 25%, and the number of involved nodes has greater predictive power than the size of the nodal mass.[203] The median length of survival of patients with limited nodal metastases is less than 3 years. Median length of survival in the presence of distant metastases is 7 months if the metastases are in skin and less if viscera are involved.

Management

The initial diagnostic procedure for a lesion smaller than 1.5 cm is an excisional biopsy to the depth of the subcutaneous fat and with a 2-mm margin. This narrow margin avoids unnecessarily disfiguring scars for lesions found to be benign, but reexcision is mandated if the lesion is found to be malignant. For large lesions, or in areas of the body where scarring will be most noticeable, an incisional biopsy should be performed. Reexcision is necessary if malignant melanoma is diagnosed. The margins at reexcision are determined by the thickness of the lesion on microstaging.[204] No difference in survival was demonstrated among patients randomly assigned to resection margins of 1 or 3 cm.[205]

Sentinel lymph node biopsy allows the surgeon to limit the morbidity of a full lymph node dissection to patients with demonstrable lymph node metastases.[206,207] If this approach is to be taken during pregnancy, it should be performed as originally described, with a vital blue dye rather than with the more sensitive technetium technique, because the safety of this procedure in pregnancy is not established.[208]

Five-year disease-free and overall survival rates can be improved by the use of adjuvant systemic interferon in patients at high risk for recurrence on the basis of a depth greater than 4 mm or the presence of limited lymph node metastases. This was demonstrated initially with an intensive interferon-alfa regimen consisting of 1 month of 20 million U/m^2/day intravenously for 5 days of every week, followed by 11 months of thrice-weekly subcutaneous therapy with 10 million U/m^2.[209] Subsequent and ongoing studies that have assessed the role of lower dosage interferon regimens, which cause fewer constitutional symptoms and less hematologic and hepatic toxicity, have not yet defined another active regimen. The safety of interferon in pregnancy is not well known, nor is there information about the use of this adjuvant therapy during pregnancy. There exists an isolated case report of interferon use during the first trimester.[74] The role of radiotherapy to a therapeutically dissected regional lymph node basin is still to be determined. A single pilot study suggests an effect on the risk of local recurrence.[210] A randomized trial is currently testing this approach.

The goal of therapy for metastatic melanoma is purely palliative. This may involve resection or radiation of individual metastases to relieve local symptoms or systemic therapy. Combination chemotherapy regimens, with or without biologic or hormonal therapy, have not yet been demonstrated to be superior to single-agent chemotherapy in overall survival. The palliative intent of such therapy should be borne in mind, and an attempt should be made to minimize the symptoms of therapy. Some patients, especially those who are asymptomatic, may

elect not to receive systemic therapy of uncertain benefit. If metastatic melanoma arises during pregnancy, therapeutic abortion may be considered in the first or second trimester because of the exceedingly short expected duration of survival. Chemotherapy with dacarbazine or other alkylating agents may be given after the first trimester in cases in which the pregnancy is continued. Although cases of melanoma metastatic to the placenta or the fetus have been reported, these are rare outcomes and should not influence the decision about therapy or continuation of the pregnancy.

Colorectal Cancer

Colorectal cancer is rare during pregnancy, because it manifests uncommonly during the childbearing years, except in patients with ulcerative colitis or an inherited predisposition. When it is diagnosed in the unscreened population, it usually manifests with bleeding but may manifest with obstruction, and this has been described in pregnancy.[211] The curability of colon cancer is greatest for the earliest lesions, and screening has a dramatic impact on cause-specific survival in the middle-aged population. In families with a known hereditary predisposition to colon cancer because of a mutation in the FAP/APC or hMSH2 genes, regular full colonoscopy for screening should be initiated when the family members are approximately 10 years younger than the youngest age at which a family member was afflicted or at age 30, whichever is younger.[212] Colon cancer deaths in the early 30s are not uncommon in such families. If a family history of young-onset colorectal cancer is obtained, and the patient's age justifies screening, this should be arranged during the early postpartum period while the patient is still in regular contact with the health care system. If on routine antenatal evaluation the patient is found to have occult blood in the stool, colonoscopy should not be delayed.

Advances in the management of metastatic disease led to an improvement in median survival from 9 to 20 months during the 1990s. Studies are currently under way to determine the role of irinotecan, oxaliplatin, EGFR-directed therapies, and angiogenesis inhibitors in stages II and III disease.

Hepatocellular Cancer in Pregnancy

Hormonal promotion of hepatocellular carcinoma has long been recognized. In geographic areas endemic for hepatitis B, neonatal infection with hepatitis B is associated in boys with a peak in incidence of hepatocellular cancer at the time of puberty. Oral contraceptives are known to cause hepatic adenomas and hepatocellular carcinoma at a low frequency. Peripartum manifestation of hepatocellular carcinoma is also recognized in chronic hepatitis B carriers, although hepatocellular carcinoma in pregnancy is rare; this may be partially explained by reduced fertility of women with advanced cirrhosis.[213] The only curative approach to hepatocellular carcinoma is removal of the tumor. This can be accomplished by hepatic lobectomy for a small cancer if the function of the remaining liver permits or by orthotopic liver transplantation if cirrhosis precludes hepatic resection. For patients with inoperable tumors, palliative local therapies such as cryotherapy, chemoembolization, or ethanol ablation are promising.

Gastric Cancer

Gastric cancer is rare in pregnancy, even in parts of the world where gastric cancer is still a leading form of cancer. There were only 14 pregnancy-associated cases of gastric cancer in a series of 2325 consecutive cases reported from Japan. The pregnancy-associated cases tended to be of higher grade, but the rate of survival after curative surgery was similar to that found in nonpregnant patients.[214] Metastatic gastric cancer may manifest with ovarian metastases. These ovarian metastases are known as Krukenberg's tumor (Fig. 23-4).

HEMATOLOGIC MALIGNANCIES IN PREGNANCY

Acute Leukemia

The incidence of leukemia in pregnant women is not known to differ from that in nonpregnant women, and the manifestation of leukemia is usually the same in the pregnant patient. Acute leukemias are generally accompanied by problems caused by a paucity of normal cells: anemia and its symptom of easy fatigability, infection, or bleeding. A routine complete blood cell count determination at an antenatal visit may also lead to the diagnosis. The complete blood cell count demonstrates a variable

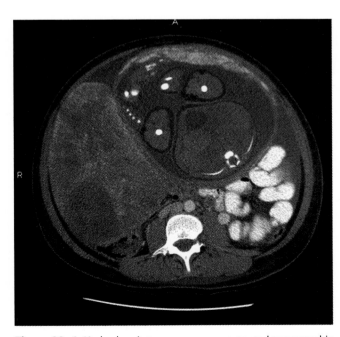

Figure 23-4. Krukenberg's tumor, seen on computed tomographic image.

degree of anemia and thrombocytopenia and usually shows a leukocytosis with the presence of blasts, although, in rare cases, the white blood cell count may be depressed. Acute leukemias may also present because of symptoms of leukostasis, which arises in the setting of leukocytosis. This most commonly manifests with ocular or central nervous system symptoms but may manifest with fetal loss, which in rare cases has been the presenting symptom of acute leukemia in the pregnant woman.

The diagnosis of leukemia is confirmed by an examination of the bone marrow with histochemical stains and by cytogenetics. Leukemias are described by the French-American-British (FAB) classification on the basis of histologic features, but in some cases, immunophenotyping, specific cytogenetic abnormalities, or molecular probes for recognized DNA sequence abnormalities give more specific prognostic information and are better guides to therapy than the FAB class. In addition, the distinction between myeloid and lymphoid leukemias in the most undifferentiated leukemias may be made on the basis of immunophenotyping.

If left untreated, all acute leukemias have a rapidly fatal course; however, with appropriate chemotherapy, complete remissions are expected in more than 70% of patients. Pregnancy does not decrease the likelihood of a complete remission. Placental involvement by acute leukemia has been reported several times. In a case of acute monocytic leukemia diagnosed at 29 weeks of pregnancy and managed conservatively until fetal maturity at 33 weeks, a leukemic infiltrate was detected in the basal plate of the placenta. The infant was normal.[215]

The clinical consequences of cytopenia can be exaggerated in pregnancy because of preexisting anemia and because of the risks of bleeding and infection associated with pregnancy and labor. Rapid reduction in white blood cell count can be achieved with cytotoxic agents, such as hydroxyurea, at the risk of a tumor lysis syndrome in which rapid release of intracellular contents can lead to hyperkalemia, hyperphosphatemia, ectopic apatite crystal formation with resultant hypocalcemia and renal tubular dysfunction, hyperuricemia, and urate nephropathy. It is preferable to use leukapheresis to remove white blood cells from the circulation, allowing a reduction in white blood cell count and blood viscosity at less risk. This approach is practical during pregnancy. The therapy for acute leukemias results in prolonged periods of marrow suppression, and all patients undergoing induction chemotherapy for acute leukemia require extensive supportive care, including transfusions and treatment of infection. Pregnancies complicated by leukemia must be managed as high-risk pregnancies. The incidences of spontaneous abortion, stillbirth, growth retardation, and prematurity are all increased in the presence of maternal leukemia.[59,216] The risks of delivery in the mother if she is thrombocytopenic or neutropenic are increased. Thus, to maximize the chance for complete remission and cure and to decrease the risks of delivery, induction therapy should be initiated promptly. If the pregnancy is in the first trimester, the risk of congenital anomalies is high, and termination of the pregnancy should be considered. If fetal maturity has been attained at the time of diagnosis, elective delivery by cesarean section can be accomplished before induction therapy. For pregnancies in the second and third trimesters, a good pregnancy outcome is likely, and there is no contraindication to continuation of the pregnancy and initiation of induction therapy. Intensive postremission therapy is safest for the mother and fetus after delivery or for the mother after termination of the pregnancy.

Acute Myeloid Leukemia

Initial therapy of acute myeloid leukemia consists of continuous infusion cytarabine and an anthracycline (either idarubicin or doxorubicin) to induce complete remission. Complete remissions can be expected in 70% of adult patients, and inclusion of additional agents in the induction regimen has not been proved to enhance the complete remission rate. Postremission therapy is important for achieving disease-free survival of long duration. Among younger patients, the use of intensive postremission therapy with high-dose cytarabine or, if an allogeneic bone marrow donor is available, with allogeneic bone marrow transplantation improves the 3-year survival rate and should be considered. With intensive postremission therapy, approximately one third of patients of childbearing age achieve prolonged disease-free survival.

Acute promyelocytic leukemia, M3 in the FAB classification, is caused by a balanced translocation between chromosomes 15 and 17, in which portions of the promyelocytic leukemia gene are juxtaposed with the retinoic acid receptor α gene, which results in a fusion protein.[217,218] This disease is distinct from the other subtypes of acute myeloid leukemia. It can be complicated by bleeding caused by disseminated intravascular coagulation, fibrinolysis, and proteolysis, either at the time of presentation or during induction chemotherapy, and induction therapy carries a higher mortality rate than in the other subtypes. Nevertheless, the complete response rate and long-term survival rate are favorable. The morbidity from this syndrome is reduced if complete remission is induced with the differentiating agent ATRA, which binds to the abnormal retinoic acid receptor. Remissions induced by ATRA are not durable, and patients are given both conventional induction chemotherapy after complete remission is achieved and maintenance therapy with ATRA for 1 year. Induction with sequential differentiating and cytotoxic therapy and maintenance differentiation therapy confers a significant survival advantage over cytotoxic chemotherapy alone.[219] There is almost no experience with the use of this approach in pregnancy. Twenty-three cases of acute promyelocytic leukemia in pregnancy have been reviewed. Of these, 19 resulted in live births, including 8 in which chemotherapy had been administered late in pregnancy and 3 in which ATRA had been administered late in pregnancy. Complete remission was induced in 72%. In cases complicated by disseminated intravascular coagulation at presentation, fetal loss did not result.[220]

Acute Lymphoblastic Leukemia

The initial treatment for acute lymphoblastic leukemia is combination therapy with vincristine and prednisone. The inclusion of an anthracycline, cyclophosphamide, and asparaginase increases the complete response rate and extends the time to relapse. Intensive postremission therapy has been accepted as integral to the achievement of long-term survival rates of about 33%. In some high-dosage consolidation regimens, chemotherapy penetrates the central nervous system, perhaps obviating the need for central nervous system prophylaxis with radiotherapy or intrathecal chemotherapy. Patients who are at high risk for relapse by virtue of an initial white blood cell count exceeding 35×10^6/mL, older age, adverse karyotype, or slow remission are considered for allogeneic bone marrow transplantation in first remission.

Chronic Leukemias

Chronic Myelogenous Leukemia

The cause of almost all chronic myelogenous leukemia (CML) is the formation of a novel protein tyrosine kinase by a translocation that results in juxtaposition of the BCR and ABL genes.[221] After a chronic phase of generally 1 to 5 years, acceleration and transformation to acute leukemia are expected. The International Randomized Study of Interferon and STI571 established imatinib, a novel, oral, small molecular inhibitor of the bcr-abl fusion kinase, as the standard initial therapy in newly diagnosed CML on the basis of hematologic and cytogenetic response rate, rapidity of response, tolerability, and proportion of patients who are progression free at 1 year.[222] Imatinib is also active in previously treated CML, in the accelerated phase, and in blast crisis. Allogeneic stem cell transplantation during the chronic phase is potentially curative in the minority of patients who are suitable candidates for this therapy, but the rate of mortality from this approach is high.[223] The optimal integration of allogeneic transplantation in the management of CML in the imatinib era remains to be defined.

For CML in the chronic phase, conservative management during pregnancy may be appropriate. Complications from an exceedingly high white blood cell count causing altered blood viscosity may lead to retinal vein occlusion, cerebrovascular accidents, and placental dysfunction. Leukapheresis can be used to control the white blood cell count during the first trimester. Once organogenesis is complete and the use of alkylating agents is safer, hydroxyurea therapy can be instituted for control of the white blood cell count.[224] Imatinib and high-dosage chemotherapy should not be given during pregnancy but, rather, should be delayed.

Chronic Lymphocytic Leukemia

This disease, most common in elderly persons, has been reported in a pregnant woman only once. The patient was managed conservatively during the pregnancy and required antibiotic and transfusion support. A normal infant was delivered.[225] Because the course of this disease is often indolent and the timing of therapy is not known to affect outcome, a conservative approach to management during pregnancy is appropriate.

Lymphoma

Non-Hodgkin's Lymphomas

The average age at presentation for non-Hodgkin's lymphomas is 42; thus, many patients present with these diseases during the childbearing years.[226] The incidence of lymphoma is rapidly increasing, predominantly among HIV-infected people.[227] This may lead to an increase in the coincidence of lymphoma with pregnancy. A case was reported in which histologic evidence of B cell lymphoma in the placenta, discovered on routine examination, preceded by 9 months the diagnosis of immunoblastic lymphoma in the HIV-infected mother.[228] The non-Hodgkin's lymphomas are categorized by the World Health Organization/Revised European-American Lymphoma classification as indolent, aggressive, highly aggressive, and localized indolent.[229] They are further divided histologically, and by cell of origin. Indolent lymphomas are uncommon during pregnancy, and in most cases, because of their slow growth, management can be deferred until after delivery at the time of fetal maturity. The localized indolent lymphomas—extranodal marginal zone B cell lymphoma of the mucosa-associated lymphoid tissue type and primary cutaneous anaplastic large cell lymphoma—generally remain localized. Regressions may be seen after treatment for *Helicobacter pylori* or *Borrelia,* respectively.

Chemotherapy is curative for a proportion of patients who have aggressive lymphomas, and the likelihood of cure is predicted by the patient's performance status, β_2-microglobulin level, lactate dehydrogenase level, and the extent of the disease, including whether there is extranodal involvement, adjusted for age.[230] The cytogenetic profile of the cancer and biologic markers of growth rate also have prognostic significance. The standard combination of cyclophosphamide, doxorubicin, vincristine, and prednisone can feasibly be given after the first trimester, and pregnancy does not adversely affect the prognosis.[231] Combination chemotherapy given at standard dosages achieves cure in approximately 40% of patients with intermediate or high-grade advanced-stage non-Hodgkin's lymphoma. Rituximab is a therapeutic monoclonal antibody directed against the CD20 moiety with activity in B cell lymphomas; there are no data on the use of rituximab in pregnancy. Patients who suffer relapse after cyclophosphamide, doxorubicin, vincristine, and prednisone combination chemotherapy can be expected to respond to salvage chemotherapy, but salvage chemotherapy is not likely to be curative. A multicenter trial conducted in Europe compared salvage chemotherapy with a shorter course of the same salvage chemotherapy followed by high-dosage chemotherapy with autologous bone marrow transplantation. This study demonstrated an improvement in overall survival at 5 years from 32% to 51% among patients who received consolidation with high-dosage chemotherapy.[232] This approach is also offered to patients with an extremely poor prognosis, on the basis of a retrospective subset analysis of a randomized study of standard therapy followed by conventional-dosage maintenance therapy versus high-dosage therapy, which showed an advantage to high-dosage chemotherapy among patients with high-risk disease according to the age-adjusted index.[233] Therapy should be initiated at conventional dosages for patients in whom poor-prognosis lymphoma is diagnosed, according to the age-adjusted index, or for those who develop recurrent lymphoma during pregnancy. High-dosage chemotherapy is most appropriate for the patient with a poor prognosis who responds to conventional dosages of chemotherapy and thus does not need to initiate treatment during the pregnancy. On the other hand, chemotherapy for lymphoma is myelosuppressive, and the long-term prognosis for patients with poor risk and relapsed disease is not excellent. Under these circumstances, some patients prefer to terminate the pregnancy. Non-Hodgkin's lymphoma arising during pregnancy can metastasize to the placenta; this can lead to neonatal death.[234] Histopathologic samples of the products of conception or placenta should be studied carefully for evidence of lymphoma at every birth or abortion in a mother with lymphoma.

Bilateral primary breast lymphoma is an unusual manifestation of lymphoma, is most common with high-grade lymphomas and lymphoblastic leukemia, and has an association with pregnancy.[235] In a small series from Nigeria, two thirds of patients with bilateral breast masses were found to have bilateral Burkitt's lymphoma of the breast, which invariably manifested during pregnancy or lactation. The mean age at manifestation of Burkitt's lymphoma was 22 years, in comparison with 37 years for bilateral mammary carcinoma.[236] The reason for breast involvement when these cancers are found in pregnancy is not clear. The breast mass resulting from lymphoma characteristically is more rounded, smoother, and less hard than the mass of mammary adenocarcinoma. Breast lymphoma may also manifest as enlargement of one or both breasts. This has been confused with the physiologic changes of pregnancy.[237] Breast lymphoma does not have pathognomonic mammographic characteristics. The mammogram may show multiple bilateral masses, and the masses are unlikely to contain calcifications, but these findings do not exclude mammary carcinoma, and, as with mammary carcinoma, the mammogram may be normal.[238] When mammary carcinoma is present in both breasts, it may be present as synchronous primary tumors or as metastasis to the contralateral breast, by which time other manifestations of metastatic disease would commonly be present. Whatever the clinical findings, the diagnosis of lymphoma requires a sufficient sample of tissue for assessment of tissue architecture and for special staining tests to be performed. A large-core biopsy or open biopsy is preferable to fine-needle aspiration for the diagnosis of lymphoma, as for the diagnosis of adenocarcinoma.

Hodgkin's Disease

Hodgkin's disease usually arises in lymph nodes and occurs most commonly in the neck. Because of the prominence of the inflammatory response in Hodgkin's disease, it is important for accurate diagnosis to obtain a generous specimen for histologic evaluation. This is obtained generally through an excisional lymph node biopsy. Nodular sclerosis is the most common subtype of

Hodgkin's disease. This subtype is most common in adolescents and young adults and frequently affects women.

The standard management of early-stage Hodgkin's disease has been local radiotherapy, without any systemic treatment. This approach demands a high degree of certainty that there is no undetected disease outside the radiation field, and it has been traditional for staging to include lymphangiography and exploratory laparotomy with splenectomy. Long-term results with chemotherapy followed by limited-field radiotherapy appear to be similar, with a lower risk of second malignancies, and can be considered for patients who do not undergo laparotomy. This approach has the advantages for the pregnant patient of avoiding abdominal surgery during pregnancy and of delaying radiotherapy. Thoracic irradiation for Hodgkin's disease can be accomplished during pregnancy with the use of abdominal shielding, but some radiation exposure of the fetus is inevitable.

Advanced-stage Hodgkin's disease is treated with combination chemotherapy. The first-line regimen consists of doxorubicin, bleomycin, vinblastine, and dacarbazine.[239] This regimen is preferable to the first reported curative chemotherapy in this disease—nitrogen mustard, vincristine, procarbazine, and prednisone—because of its lesser effect on fertility and because it is less leukemogenic.[240] Patients who have a relapse after radiotherapy may achieve cure by chemotherapy with a first-line regimen. Reintroduction of the same chemotherapy is often effective if the relapse after chemotherapy occurs after a long disease-free interval, but patients with short disease-free periods have a lower likelihood of cure with a second trial of chemotherapy. Dose-intensive approaches with autologous hematopoietic support have also been used in such patients.

References

1. Sachs BP, Penzias AS, Brown DAJ, et al: Cancer-related maternal mortality in Massachusetts, 1954-1985. Gynecol Oncol 1990;36:395.
2. Martinez ME, Grodstein F, Giovanucci E, et al: A prospective study of reproductive factors, oral contraceptive use, and risk of colorectal cancer. Cancer Epidemiol Biomarkers Prev 1997;6:1.
3. Brinton LA, Schairer CS, Hoover RN, Fraumeni JF Jr: Menstrual factors and risk of breast cancer. Cancer Invest 1988;6:245.
4. Hamilton AS, Mack TM: Puberty and genetic susceptibility to breast cancer in a case-control study in twins. N Engl J Med 2003;348:2313.
5. Malone K, Daling J, Weiss N: Oral contraceptives in relation to breast cancer. Epidemiol Rev 1993;15:80.
6. Burkman RT, Tang MT, Malone KE, et al: Infertility drugs and the risk of breast cancer: Findings from the National Institute of Child Health and Human Development Womens Contraceptive and Reproductive Experiences Study. Fertil Steril 2003;79:844.
7. Holly EA, Weiss NS, Liff JM: Cutaneous melanoma in relation to exogenous hormones and reproductive factors. J Natl Cancer Inst 1983;70:827.
8. Holman CD, Armstrong BD, Heenan PJ: Cutaneous malignant melanoma in women: Exogenous sex hormones and reproductive factors. Br J Cancer 1984;50:673.
9. Ellis DL: Pregnancy and sex steroid hormone effects on nevi of patients with the dysplastic nevus syndrome. J Am Acad Dermatol 1991;25:467.
10. Smith DC, Prentice R, Thompson DJ, Herrmann WL: Association of exogenous estrogen and endometrial carcinoma. N Engl J Med 1975;293:1164.
11. Voigt LF, Weiss NS, Chu J, et al: Progestagen supplementation of exogenous oestrogens and risk of endometrial cancer. Lancet 1991;338:274.
12. Writing Group for the Women's Health Initiative Investigators: Risks and benefits of estrogen plus progestin in healthy postmenopausal women: Principal results from the Women's Health Initiative randomized controlled trial. JAMA 2002;288:321.
13. Breast cancer and hormone replacement therapy: Collaborative reanalysis of data from 51 epidemiological studies of 52,705 women with breast cancer and 108,411 women without breast cancer. Lancet 1997;350:1047.
14. Li R, Gilliland FD, Baumgartner K, Samet J: Hormone replacement therapy and breast cancer risk in Hispanic and non-Hispanic women. Cancer 2002;95:960.
15. Melbye M, Wohlfahrt J, Olsen JH, et al: Induced abortion and the risk of breast cancer. N Engl J Med 1997;336:81.
16. MacMahon B, Cole P, Lin TM, et al: Age at first birth and breast cancer risk. Bull WHO 1970;43:209.
17. Lambe M, Hsieh C-C, Trichopoulos D, et al: Transient increase in risk of breast cancer after giving birth. N Engl J Med 1994;331:5.
18. Albrektsen G, Heuch I, Kvale G: The short-term and long-term effect of a pregnancy on breast cancer risk: A prospective study of 802,457 parous Norwegian women. Br J Cancer 1995;72:480.
19. Albrektsen G, Heuch I, Kvale G: Reproductive factors and incidence of epithelial ovarian cancer: A Norwegian prospective study. Cancer Causes Control 1996;7:421.
20. Parazzina F, La Vecchia C, Bocciolone L, Franceschi S: The epidemiology of endometrial cancer. Gynecol Oncol 1991;41:1.
21. Calle EE, Mervis CA, Thun MJ, et al: Diethylstilbestrol and risk of fatal breast cancer in a prospective cohort of US women. Am J Epidemiol 1996;144:645.
22. Brzezinski A, Peretz T, Mor-Yosef S, Schenker JG: Ovarian stimulation and breast cancer: Is there a link? Gynecol Oncol 1994;52:292.
23. Cowan LD, Gordis L, Tonasicia JA, Jones GS: Breast cancer incidence in women with a history of progesterone deficiency. Am J Epidemiol 1981;114:209.
24. Rosenblatt KA, Thomas DB: Prolonged lactation and endometrial cancer. WHO Collaborative Study of Neoplasia and Steroid Contraceptives. Int J Epidemiol 1995;24:499.
25. Newcomb PA, Storer BE, Longnecker MP, et al: Lactation and a reduced risk of premenopausal breast cancer. N Engl J Med 1994;330:81.
26. Trichopoulos D, MacMahon B, Cole P: Menopause and breast cancer risk. J Natl Cancer Inst 1972;48:605.
27. Michels KB, Trichopoulos D, Robins JM, et al: Birthweight as a risk factor for breast cancer. Lancet 1996;348:1542.
28. Holmberg L, Ekbom A, Calle E, et al: Parental age and breast cancer mortality. Epidemiology 1995;6:425.
29. Marquis ST, Rajan JV, Wynshaw-Boris A, et al: The developmental pattern of Brca 1 expression implies a role in differentiation of the breast and other tissues. Nat Genet 1995;11:17.
30. Rajan JV, Wang M, Marquis ST, Chodosh LA: Brca2 is coordinately regulated with Brca1 during proliferation and differentiation in mammary epithelial cells. Proc Natl Acad Sci 1996;93:13078.
31. Grabrick DM, Hartman LC, Cerhan JR, et al: Risk of breast cancer with oral contraceptive use in women with a family history of breast cancer. JAMA 2000;284:1791.
32. Barbati A, Lauro V, Orlacchio A, Cosmi EV: Immunoblotting characterization of CA125 in biological fluids: Difference between pregnancy and cancer CA 125 origin. Anticancer Res 1996;16:3621.
33. Chen RJ, Chen CK, Chang DY, et al: Immunoelectrophoretic differentiation of alpha-fetoprotein in disorders with elevated alpha-fetoprotein levels or during pregnancy. Acta Oncol 1995;34:931.
34. Berghout A, Endert E, Ross A, et al: Thyroid function and thyroid size in normal pregnant women living in an iodine replete area. Clin Endocrinol 1994;41:375.
35. Pedersen KM, Laurberg P, Iversen E, et al: Amelioration of some pregnancy-associated variations in thyroid function by iodine supplementation. J Clin Endocrinol Metab 1993;77:1078.
36. Meden H, Marx D, Fattahi A, et al: Elevated serum levels of a c-erbB-2 oncogene product in ovarian cancer patients and in pregnancy. J Cancer Res Clin Oncol 1994;120:378.
37. Gurney JG, Davis S, Severson RK, et al: Trends in cancer incidence among children in the U.S. Cancer 1996;78:532.

38. Ford AM, Ridge SA, Cabrera ME, et al: In utero rearrangements in the trithorax-related oncogene in infant leukaemias. Nature 1993; 363:358.

39. Mazze RI, Kallen B: Reproductive outcome after anesthesia and operation during pregnancy: A registry study of 5405 cases. Am J Obstet Gynecol 1989;161:1178.

40. Platek DN, Henderson CE, Goldberg GL: The management of a persistent adnexal mass in pregnancy. Am J Obstet Gynecol 1995;173:1236.

41. Pytel J, Gerlinger I, Arany A: Twin pregnancy following in vitro fertilisation coinciding with laryngeal cancer. ORL J Otorhinolaryngol Relat Spec 1995;57:232.

42. Gitsch G, van Eijkeren M, Hacker NF: Surgical therapy of vulvar cancer in pregnancy. Gynecol Oncol 1995;56:312.

43. Hall EJ: Scientific view of low-level radiation risks. Radiographics 1991;11:509.

44. Otake M, Schull WJ: In utero exposure to A-bomb radiation and mental retardation: A reassessment. Br J Radiol 1984;57:409.

45. Weinberg HS, Korol AB, Krizhner VM, et al: Very high mutation rate in offspring of Chernobyl accident liquidators. Proc R Soc Lond B Biol Sci 2001;268:1001.

46. Ericson A, Kallen B: Pregnancy outcome in Sweden after the Chernobyl accident. Environ Res 1994;67:149.

47. Harvey EB, Bioce JD Jr, Honeyman M, Flannery JT: Prenatal x-ray exposure and childhood cancer in twins. N Engl J Med 1985;312:541.

48. Doll R, Wakeford R: Risk of childhood cancer from fetal irradiation. Br J Radiol 1997;70:130.

49. Ricoul M, Sabatier L, Dutrillaux B: Increased chromosome radiosensitivity during pregnancy. Mutat Res 1997;374:73.

50. Mattison DR, Angtuaco T: Magnetic resonance imaging in prenatal diagnosis. Clin Obstet Gynecol 1988;31:353.

51. Stovall M, Blackwell CR, Cundiff J, et al: Fetal dose from radiotherapy with photon beams: Report of AAPM Radiation Therapy Committee Task Group No. 36. Med Phys 1995;22:63.

52. Arndt D, Mehnert WH, Franke WG, et al: Radioiodine therapy during an unknown remained pregnancy and radiation exposure of the fetus: A case report. Strahlenther Onkol 1994;170:408.

53. Roman E, Doyle P, Ansell P, et al: Health of children born to medical radiographers. Occup Environ Med 1996;53:73.

54. Mountford PJ, Steele HR: Fetal dose estimates and the ICRP abdominal dose limit for occupational exposure of pregnant staff to technetium-99m and iodine-131 patients. Eur J Nucl Med 1995;22:1173.

55. Leslie KK: Chemotherapy and pregnancy. Clin Obstet Gynecol 2002;45:153.

56. Aviles A, Neri N: Hematological malignancies and pregnancy: A final report of 84 children who received chemotherapy in utero. Clin Lymphoma 2001;2:173.

57. Gililland J, Weinstein L: The effects of cancer chemotherapeutics agents on the developing fetus. Obstet Gynecol Surv 1983;38:6.

58. Sweet DL, Kinzie J: Consequences of radiotherapy and antineoplastic therapy for the fetus. J Reprod Med 1976;17:241.

59. Zuazu J, Julia A, Sierra J, et al: Pregnancy outcomes in hematologic malignancies. Cancer 1991;67:3.

60. Glantz JC: Reproductive toxicology of alkylating agents. Obstet Gynecol Surv 1994;49:709.

61. Torchinsky A, Savion S, Gorivodsky M, et al: Cyclophosphamide-induced teratogenesis in ICR mice: The role of apoptosis. Teratog Carcinog Mutagen 1995;15:179.

62. Koph-Maier P: Stage of pregnancy-dependent transplacental passage of 195m-Pt after cisplatin therapy. Eur J Cancer Clin Oncol 1983;19:533.

63. Henderson CE, Elia G, Garfinkel D, et al: Platinum chemotherapy during pregnancy for serous cystadenocarcinoma of the ovary. Gynecol Oncol 1993;49:92.

64. Capizzi R: Hematologic neoplasms during pregnancy. In Brodsky I, Kahn SB, Hoyer JH (eds): Cancer Chemotherapy II, the 22nd Hahnemann Symposium. New York, Grune & Stratton, 1972, p 131.

65. Maurer LH, Jackson-Forcier R, McIntyre OR, Benirschke K: Fetal group C trisomy after cytosine arabinoside and thioguanine. Ann Intern Med 1971;75:809.

66. DeCillis A, Anderson S, Bryant J, et al: Acute myeloid leukemia (AML) and myelodysplastic syndrome (MDS) on NSABP B-25: An update. Proc Am Soc Clin Oncol 1997;16:130a.

67. Goldwasser F, Pico JL, Cerrina J, et al: Successful chemotherapy including epirubicin in a pregnant non-Hodgkin's lymphoma patient. Leuk Lymphoma 1995;20:173.

68. Reynoso EE, Huerta F: Acute leukemia and pregnancy: Fatal fetal outcome after exposure to idarubicin during the second trimester. Acta Oncol 1994;33:709.

69. Egan PC, Costanza ME, Dodion P, et al: Doxorubicin and cisplatin excretion into human breast milk. Cancer Treat Rep 1985;69:1387.

70. Connor EM, Sperling RS, Gelber R, et al: Reduction of maternal-infant transmission of human immunodeficiency virus type I with zidovudine treatment. N Engl J Med 1994;331:1173.

71. Sperling RS, Shapiro BE, Coombs RW, et al: Maternal vial load, zidovudine treatment and the risk of transmission of human immunodeficiency virus type 1 from mother to infant. Pediatrics AIDS Clinical Trial Group Protocol 076 Study Group. N Engl J Med 1996;335:1621.

72. Means AL, Gudas LJ: The roles of retinoids in vertebrate development. Annu Rev Biochem 1995;64:201.

73. Frankel SR, Eardley A, Lauwers G, et al: The "retinoic acid syndrome" in acute promyelocytic leukemia. Ann Intern Med 1992; 117:292.

74. Sakata H, Karamitsos J, Kundaria B, DiSaia PJ: Case report of interferon alfa therapy for multiple myeloma during pregnancy. Am J Obstet Gynecol 1995;172:217.

75. Lenz W, Knapp K: Die Thalidomid-Embryopathie [Thalidomide embryopathy]. Dtsch Med Wochenschr 1962;87:1232.

76. Harper MJK, Walpole AL: A new derivative of triphenylethylene: Effect on implantation and mode of action in rats. J Reprod Fertil 1967;13:101.

77. Wen YR, Hou WY, Chen YA, et al: Intrathecal morphine for neuropathic pain in a pregnant cancer patient. J Formos Med Assoc 1996;95:252.

78. Rosenberg L, Mitchell AA, Parsells JL, et al: Lack of relation of oral clefts to diazepam use during pregnancy. N Engl J Med 1983; 309:1282.

79. Cocco P, Rapallo M, Targhetta R, et al: Analysis of risk factors in a cluster of childhood acute lymphoblastic leukemia. Arch Environ Health 1996;51:242.

80. Bedi A, Miller CB, Hanson JL, et al: Association of BK virus with failure of prophylaxis against hemorrhagic cystitis following bone marrow transplantation. J Clin Oncol 1995;13:1103.

81. Fakhoury GF, Daikoku NH, Parikh AR: Management of severe hemorrhagic cystitis in pregnancy. A report of two cases. J Reprod Med 1994;39:485.

82. Jasnosz KM, Pickeral JJ, Graner S: Fat deposits in the placenta following maternal total parenteral nutrition with intravenous lipid emulsion. Arch Pathol Lab Med 1995;119:555.

83. Body JJ, Dumon JC: Treatment of tumor-induced hypercalcemia with the bisphosphonate pamidronate: Dose-response relationship and influence of tumor type. Ann Oncol 1994;5:359.

84. Hortobagyi GN, Theriault RL, Porter L, et al: Efficacy of pamidronate in reducing skeletal complications in patients with breast cancer and lytic bone metastases. Protocol 19 Aredia Breast Cancer Study Group. N Engl J Med 1996;335:1785.

85. Illidge TM, Hussey M, Godden CW: Malignant hypercalcemia in pregnancy and antenatal administration of intravenous pamidronate. Clin Oncol (R Coll Radiol) 1996;8:257.

86. Gonzalez-Lira G, Escudero-De Los Rios P, Salazar-Martinez E: Conservative surgery for ovarian cancer and effect on fertility. Int J Gynaecol Obstet 1997;56:155.

87. Kimming R, Strowitzki T, Muller-Hocker J, et al: Conservative treatment of endometrial cancer permitting subsequent triplet pregnancy. Gynecol Oncol 1995;58:255.

88. Green DM, Fiorella A, Zevon MA, et al: Birth defects and childhood cancer in offspring of survivors of childhood cancer. Arch Pediatr Adolesc Med 1997;151:379.

89. Sankila R, Olsen JH, Anderson H, et al: Risk of cancer among offspring of childhood cancer survivors. N Eng J Med 1998;338:1339.

90. Sanders JE, Hawley J, Levy W, et al: Pregnancies following high-dose cyclophosphamide with or without high-dose busulfan or total-body irradiation and bone marrow transplantation. Blood 1996;87:3045.

91. Spinelli S, Chiodi S, Baciglaupo A, et al: Ovarian recovery after total body irradiation and allogeneic bone marrow transplantation: Long-term follow up of 79 females. Bone Marrow Transplant 1994;14:373.

92. Lipton JH, Virro M, Solow H: Successful pregnancy after allogeneic bone marrow transplant with embryos isolated before transplant. J Clin Oncol 1997;15:3347.

93. Clark RM, Reid J: Carcinoma of the breast in pregnancy and lactation. Int J Radiat Oncol Biol Phys 1978;4:693.

94. Sankila R, Heinavaara S, Hakulinen T: Survival of breast cancer patients after subsequent term pregnancy: "Healthy mother effect." Am J Obstet Gynecol 1994;170:818.

95. Higgins S, Haffty BG: Pregnancy and lactation after breast-conserving therapy for early stage breast cancer. Cancer 1994;73:2175.

96. Casara D, Rubello D, Saldadini G, et al: Pregnancy after high therapeutic doses of iodine-131 in differentiated thyroid cancer: Potential risks and recommendations. Eur J Nucl Med 1993;20:192.

97. Hacker NF, Berek JS, Lagasse LD, et al: Carcinoma of the cervix associated with pregnancy. Obstet Gynecol 1982;59:735.

98. Crum CP, Nuovo GJ: Genital Papillomaviruses and Related Neoplasms. New York, Raven Press, 1991.

99. Fife KH, Katx BP, Roush J, et al: Cancer-associated human papillomavirus types are selectively increased in the cervix of women in the first trimester of pregnancy. Am J Obstet Gynecol 1996;174:1487.

100. Koutsky LA, Ault KA, Wheeler CM, et al: A controlled trial of human papilloma virus type 16 vaccine. N Engl J Med 2002; 347:1645.

101. Cervical cancer. NIH Consens Statement 1996;14:1.

102. Bekassy Z: Laser miniconization procedure. Int J Gynaecol Obstet 1996;55:237.

103. Averette HE, Nasser N, Yakow SL, Little WA: Cervical conization in pregnancy: Analysis of 180 operations. Am J Obstet Gynecol 1970;106:543.

104. Burghardt E, Girardi F, Lahousen M, et al: Microinvasive carcinoma of the uterine cervix (International Federation of Gynecology and Obstetrics Stage IA). Cancer 1991;67:1037.

105. Hannigan EV, Whitehouse HH, Atkinson WD, Becker SN: Cone biopsy during pregnancy. Obstet Gynecol 1982;60:450.

106. Madej JG Jr: Colposcopy monitoring in pregnancy complicated by CIN and early cervical cancer. Eur J Gynaecol Oncol 1996;17:59.

107. Delgado G, Bundy BN, Fowler WC, et al: A prospective surgical pathological study of stage I squamous carcinoma of the cervix: A Gynecologic Oncology Group study. Gynecol Oncol 1989;36:314.

108. Sood AK, Sorosky JI, Krogman S, et al: Surgical management of cervical cancer complicating pregnancy: A case-control study. Gynecol Oncol 1996;63:294.

109. Duggan B, Muderspach LI, Roman LD, et al: Cervical cancer in pregnancy: Reporting on planned delay in therapy. Obstet Gynecol 1993;82:598.

110. Sorosky JI, Squatrito R, Ndubisi BU, et al: Stage I squamous cell cervical carcinoma in pregnancy: Planned delay in therapy awaiting fetal maturity. Gynecol Oncol 1995;59:207.

111. van der Vange N, Weverling GJ, Ketting BW, et al: The prognosis of cervical cancer associated with pregnancy: A matched cohort study. Obstet Gynecol 1995;85:1022.

112. Dottino PR, Plaxe S, Beddoe A, et al: Induction chemotherapy followed by radical surgery in cervical cancer. Gynecol Oncol 1991;40:7.

113. Sardi J, Sananes C, Giaroli A, et al: Results of a prospective randomized trial with neoadjuvant chemotherapy in stage IB, bulky squamous carcinoma of the cervix. Gynecol Oncol 1993;49:153.

114. Cliby WA, Dodson MK, Podratz KC: Cervical cancer complicated by pregnancy: Episiotomy site recurrences following vaginal delivery. Obstet Gynecol 1994;84:179.

115. Bagshawe KD, Dent J, Webb J: Hydatidiform mole in England and Wales 1973-1983. Lancet 1986;2:673.

116. Ujeno Y: Epidemiological studies of human fetal development in areas with various doses of natural background radiation. II: Relationship between incidences of hydatidiform mole, malignant hydatidiform mole, and chorioepithelioma and gonad dose equivalent rate of natural background radiation. Arch Environ Health 1985;40:181.

117. Chen FP: Molar pregnancy and living normal fetus coexisting until term: Prenatal biochemical and sonographic diagnosis. Hum Reprod 1997;12:853.

118. Preidler KW, Luschin G, Tamussino K, et al: Magnetic resonance imaging in patients with gestational trophoblastic disease. Invest Radiol 1996;31:492.

119. Roberts DJ, Mutter GL: Advances in the molecular biology of gestational trophoblastic disease. J Reprod Med 1994;39:201.

120. Sunde L, Mogensen B, Olsen S, et al: Flow cytometric DNA analyses of 105 fresh hydatidiform moles, with correlations to prognosis. Anal Cell Pathol 1996;12:99.

121. Berkowitz RS, Bernstein MR, Laborde O, Goldstein DP: Subsequent pregnancy experience with gestational trophoblastic disease. New England Trophoblastic Disease Center, 1965-1992. J Reprod Med 1994;39:228.

122. Curry SL, Schlaerth JB, Kohorn EI, et al: Hormonal contraception and trophoblastic sequelae after hydatidiform mole (a Gynecologic Oncology Group study). Am J Obstet Gynecol 1989;160:805.

123. Rodriguez GC, Hughes CL, Soper JT, et al: Serum progesterone for the exclusion of early pregnancy in women at risk for recurrent gestational trophoblastic neoplasia. Obstet Gynecol 1994;84:794.

124. Maymon R, Schneider D, Shulman A, et al: Serial color Doppler flow of uterine vasculature combined with serum beta-hCG measurements for improved monitoring of patients with gestational trophoblastic disease. A preliminary report. Gynecol Obstet Invest 1996;42:201.

125. Kohorn EI, Goldstein DP, Hancock BW, et al: Combining the staging system of the International Federation of Gynecology and Obstetrics with the scoring system of the World Health Organization for Trophoblastic Neoplasia: Report of the Working Committee of the International Society for the Study of Trophoblastic Disease and International Gynecologic Cancer Society. Int J Gynecol Cancer 2001;10:84.

126. McNeish IA, Strickland S, Holden L, et al: Low-risk persistent gestational trophoblastic disease: outcome after initial treatment with low-dose methotrexate and folinic acid from 1992 to 2000. J Clin Oncol 2002;20:1838.

127. Berkowitz RS, Goldstein DP, Bernstein MR: Ten years' experience with methotrexate and folinic acid as primary therapy for gestational trophoblastic disease. Gynecol Oncol 1986;23:111.

128. Kennedy AW: Persistent nonmetastatic gestational trophoblastic disease. Semin Oncol 1995;22:161.

129. Schneider DF, Bukovsky I, Weinraub Z, et al: Transvaginal ultrasound diagnosis and treatment follow-up of invasive gestational trophoblastic disease. J Clin Ultrasound 1990;18:110.

130. Seckl MJ, Rustin GJS, Newlands ES, et al: Pulmonary embolism, pulmonary hypertension and choriocarcinoma. Lancet 1991;338:1313.

131. Begent RH, Bagshawe KD, Green AJ, Searle F: The clinical value of imaging with antibody to human chorionic gonadotrophin in the detection of residual choriocarcinoma. Br J Cancer 1987; 55:657.

132. Munyer TP, Callen PW, Filly RA, et al: Further observations on the sonographic spectrum of gestational trophoblastic disease. J Clin Ultrasound 1981;9:349.

133. Finkler NJ: Placental site trophoblastic tumor. Diagnosis, clinical behavior and treatment. J Reprod Med 1991;36:27.

134. Papadopoulos AJ, Foskett M, Seckl MJ, et al: Twenty-five years' clinical experience with placental site trophoblastic tumors. J Reprod Med 2002;47:460.

135. Flam F, Holtz A: Case report: Choriocarcinoma presenting with brain metastases. Neurol Res 1994;16:403.

136. Hertz BH, Yee JM, Porges RF: Primary cervical choriocarcinoma: Case report and review of the literature. J Ultrasound Med 1993;12:59.

137. Bower M, Newlands ES, Holden L, et al: EMA/CO for high-risk gestational trophoblastic tumors: Results from a cohort of 272 patients. J Clin Oncol 1997;15:2636.

138. Evans AC Jr, Soper JT, Clarke-Pearson DL, et al: Gestational trophoblastic disease metastatic to the central nervous system. Gynecol Oncol 1995;59:226.

139. Small W Jr, Lurain JR, Shetty RM, et al: Gestational trophoblastic disease metastatic to the brain. Radiology 1996;200:277.

140. Patchell RA, Tibbs PA, Walsh JW, et al: A randomized trial of surgery in the treatment of single metastases to the brain. N Engl J Med 1990;322:494.

141. Crawford RA, Newlands E, Rustin GJ, et al: Gestational trophoblastic disease with liver metastases: The Charing Cross experience. Br J Obstet Gynaecol 1997;104:105.

142. Gerson R, Serano A, Del Carmen Bello M, et al: Response of choriocarcinoma to paclitaxel. Case report and review of resistance. Eur J Gynaecol Oncol 1997;18:108.

143. Lotz JP, Andre T, Donsimoni R, et al: High dose chemotherapy with ifosfamide, carboplatin, and etoposide combine with autologous bone marrow transplantation for the treatment of poor-prognosis

germ cell tumors and metastatic trophoblastic disease in adults. Cancer 1995;75:874.

144. van Biesen K, Verschraegen C, Mehra R, et al: Complete remission of refractory gestational trophoblastic disease with brain metastases treated with multicycle ifosfamide, carboplatin, and etoposide and stem cell rescue. Gynecol Oncol 1997;65:366.

145. Lehman E, Gershenson DM, Burke TW, et al: Salvage surgery for chemorefractory gestational trophoblastic disease. J Clin Oncol 1994;12:2737.

146. Lang EK: Reduced systemic toxicity from superselective chemoembolization compared with systemic chemotherapy in patients with high-risk metastatic gestational trophoblastic disease. Cardiovasc Intervent Radiol 1997;20:280.

147. Fisher B, Constantino JP, Redmond CK, et al: Endometrial cancer in tamoxifen-treated breast cancer patients: Findings from the National Surgical Adjuvant Breast and Bowel Project (NSABP) B-14. J Natl Cancer Inst 1994;86:527.

148. Struewing JP, Hartge P, Nacholder S, et al: The risk of cancer associated with specific mutations of BRCA1 and BRCA2 among Ashkenazi Jews. N Engl J Med 1997;336:1401.

149. Ueda M, Ueki M: Ovarian tumors associated with pregnancy. Int J Gynaecol Obstet 1996;55:59.

150. Grendys EC Jr, Barnes WA: Ovarian cancer in pregnancy. Surg Clin North Am 1995;75:1.

151. Colavita M, Gerzetti G, Baiocchi G, et al: Successful outcome of a 9-week pregnancy managed by bilateral salpingo-oophorectomy for ovarian cancer: case report. Eur J Gynaecol Oncol 1996;17:522.

152. Mooney J, Silva E, Tornos C, Gershenson D: Unusual features of serous neoplasms of low malignant potential during pregnancy. Gynecol Oncol 1997;65:30.

153. Poremba C, Dockhorn-Dworniczak B, Merritt V, et al: Immature teratomas of different origin carried by a pregnant mother and her fetus. Diagn Mol Pathol 1993;2:131.

154. Schwartz PE: Surgical management of ovarian cancer. Arch Surg 1981;116:99.

155. Alberts DS, Liu PY, Hannigan EV, et al: Phase III study of intraperitoneal (IP), cisplatin (CDDP)/intravenous (IV), cyclophosphamide (CPA) versus IV CDDP/IV CPA in patients with optimal disease stage III ovarian cancer: A SWOG-GOG-ECOG Intergroup study (INT 0051) (Abstract 760). Proc Am Soc Clin Oncol 1995; 14:273.

156. McGuire WP, Hoskins WJ, Brady MF, et al: Cyclophosphamide and cisplatin compared with paclitaxel and cisplatin in patients with stage III and stage IV ovarian cancer. N Engl J Med 1996;334:1.

157. von Schoultz E, Johansson H, Wilking N, Rutqvist LE: Influence of prior and subsequent pregnancy on breast cancer prognosis. J Clin Oncol 1995;13:430.

158. Hassan I, Muhammed I, Attah MM, Mabogunje O: Breast cancer during pregnancy and lactation in Zaria, Nigeria. East Afr Med J 1995;72:280.

159. Huynh H, Alpert L, Pollak M: Pregnancy-dependent growth of mammary tumors is associated with overexpression of insulin-like growth factor II. Cancer Res 1996;56:3651.

160. Roberts MM, Alexander FE, Anderson TJ, et al: Edinburgh trial of screening for breast cancer: Mortality at seven years. Lancet 1990;335:241.

161. Shapiro S, Venet W, Strax P, et al: Current results of the breast cancer screening trial: The Health Insurance Plan (HIP) of Greater New York study. In Day NE, Miller AB (eds): Screening for Breast Cancer. Toronto, Ontario, Canada, Sam Huber Publishing, 1988.

162. Tabar L, Duffy S, Burhenne L: New Swedish breast cancer detection results for women aged 40-49. Cancer 1993;72:1437.

163. DiFronzo LA, O'Connell TX: Breast cancer in pregnancy and lactation. Surg Clin North Am 1996;76:267.

164. Petrek JA, Dukoff R, Rogatko A: Prognosis of pregnancy-associated breast cancer. Cancer 1991;67:869.

165. Nugent P, O'Connell TX: Breast cancer in pregnancy. Arch Surg 1985;120:1221.

166. Jaiyesemi IA, Buzdar AU, Hortobagyi G: Inflammatory breast cancer: A review. J Clin Oncol 1992;10:1014.

167. Liberman L, Giess CS, Dershaw DD, et al: Imaging of pregnancy-associated breast cancer. Radiology 1994;191:245.

168. Bonadonna G, Valagussa P, Moliterni A, et al: Adjuvant cyclophosphamide, methotrexate, and fluorouracil in node-positive breast cancer. N Engl J Med 1995;332:901.

169. Carter CL, Allen C, Henson DE: Relation of tumor size, lymph node status, and survival in 24,740 breast cancer cases. Cancer 1989; 63:181.

170. Rosen PP, Groshen S, Kinne DW, Norton L: Factors influencing prognosis in node-negative breast carcinoma: Analysis of 767 T1N0M0/T2N0M0 patients with long-term follow-up. J Clin Oncol 1993;11:2090.

171. Quiet CA, Ferguson DJ, Weichselbaum RR, et al: The natural history of node-negative breast cancer: A study of 826 patients with long follow-up. J Clin Oncol 1995;13:1144.

172. Burtness BA: Histologic markers and long-term prognosis in breast cancer. Cancer J Sci Am 1997;3:211.

173. Silvestrini R, Daidone MG, Luisi A, et al: Cell proliferation in 3,800 node-negative breast cancers: Consistency over time of biological and clinical information provided by TLI. Int J Cancer 1997;74:122.

174. Diel IJ, Kaufmann M, Costa SD, et al: Micrometastatic breast cancer cells in bone marrow at primary surgery: Prognostic value in comparison with nodal status. J Natl Cancer Inst 1996;88:1652.

175. Slamon DJ, Clark GM, Wong SG, et al: Human breast cancer: Correlation of relapse and survival with amplification of the HER-2/neu oncogene. Science 1987;235:177.

176. Muss HB, Thor A, Berry DA, et al: c-erb B-2 expression and S-phase activity predict response to adjuvant therapy in women with node-positive early breast cancer. N Engl J Med 1994;330:1260.

177. Slamon DJ, Leyland-Jones B, Shak S, et al: Use of chemotherapy plus a monoclonal antibody against HER2 for metastatic breast cancer that overexpresses HER2. N Engl J Med 2001;344:783.

178. Daling JR, Malone KE, Doody DR, et al: The relation of reproductive factors to mortality in breast cancer. Cancer Epidemiol Biomarkers Prev 2002;11:235.

179. Fisher B, Redmond C, Poisson R, et al: Eight-year results of a randomized clinical trial comparing total mastectomy and lumpectomy with or without irradiation in the treatment of breast cancer. N Engl J Med 1989;320:822.

180. Veronesi U, Salvadori B, Luini A, et al: Conservative treatment of early breast cancer: Long-term results of 1232 cases treated with quadrantectomy, axillary dissection, and radiotherapy. Ann Surg 1990;211:250.

181. Recht A, Come SE: Sequencing of irradiation and chemotherapy for early-stage breast cancer. Oncology 1994;8:19.

182. Veronesi U, Paganelli G, Galimberti V, et al: Sentinel-node biopsy to avoid axillary dissection in breast cancer with clinically negative lymph-nodes. Lancet 1997;349:1864.

183. Fisher B, Brown AM, Dimitrov NV, et al: Two months of doxorubicin-cyclophosphamide with and without interval reinduction therapy compared with 6 months of cyclophosphamide, methotrexate, and fluorouracil in positive-node breast cancer patients with tamoxifen-nonresponsive tumors: Results from the National Surgical Adjuvant Breast and Bowel Project B-15. J Clin Oncol 1990;8:1483.

184. Citron ML, Berry DA, Cirrincione C, et al: Randomized trial of dose-dense versus conventionally scheduled and sequential versus concurrent combination chemotherapy as postoperative adjuvant treatment of node-positive primary breast cancer: First report of Intergroup Trial C9741/Cancer and Leukemia Group B Trial 9741. J Clin Oncol 2003;21:1431.

185. Burtness BA, Windsor S, Holston B, et al: Adjuvant sequential dose-dense doxorubicin, paclitaxel and cyclophosphamide (ATC) for high-risk breast cancer is safe in the community setting. Cancer J Sci Am 1999;5:224.

186. Rodenhuis S, Bontenbal M, Beex LVAM, et al. High dose chemotherapy with hematopoietic stem-cell rescue for high-risk breast cancer. N Eng J Med 2003;349:7.

187. Buzzoni R, Biganzoli L, Bajetta E, et al: Combination goserelin and tamoxifen therapy in premenopausal advanced breast cancer: A multicentre study by the ITMO group. Br J Cancer 1995;71:1111.

188. Bonadonna G, Veronesi U, Brambilla C, et al: Primary chemotherapy to avoid mastectomy in tumors with diameters of three centimeters or more. J Natl Cancer Inst 1990;82:1539.

189. Abraham DC, Jones RC, Jones SE, et al: Evaluation of neoadjuvant chemotherapeutic response of locally advanced breast cancer by magnetic resonance imaging. Cancer 1996;78:91.

190. Botti C, Vici P, Lopez M, et al: Prognostic value of lymph node metastases after neoadjuvant chemotherapy for large-sized operable carcinoma of the breast. J Am Coll Surg 1995;181:202.

191. White TT, White WC: Breast cancer and pregnancy: A report of 49 cases followed 5 years. Ann Surg 1956;144:384.

192. Peters PV: The effect of pregnancy in breast cancer. In Forrest APM, Kunkler PB (eds): Prognostic Factors in Breast Cancer. Baltimore, Williams & Wilkins, 1968, pp 65–80.

193. Cooper DR, Butterfield J: Pregnancy subsequent to mastectomy for cancer of the breast. Ann Surg 1970;171:429.

194. Petrek JA: Pregnancy safety after breast cancer. Cancer 1994; 74:528.

195. Early Breast Cancer Trialists' Collaborative Group: Systemic treatment of early breast cancer by hormonal, cytotoxic, or immune therapy: 133 randomized trials involving 31,000 recurrences and 24,000 deaths among 75,000 women. Lancet 1992;339:1.

196. Doherty CM, Shindo ML, Rice DH, et al: Management of thyroid nodules during pregnancy. Laryngoscope 1995;105:251.

197. Tan GH, Gharib H, Goellner JR, et al: Management of thyroid nodules in pregnancy. Arch Intern Med 1996;156:2317.

198. Schlumberger M, De Vathaire F, Ceccarelli C, et al: Exposure to radioactive iodine-131 for scintigraphy or therapy does not preclude pregnancy in thyroid cancer patients. J Nucl Med 1996;37:606.

199. Mihm MC, Fitzpatrick TB, Brown MML, et al: Early detection of primary cutaneous malignant melanoma: A color atlas. N Engl J Med 1973;289:89.

200. MacKie RM, Bufalino R, Morabito A, et al: Lack of effect of pregnancy on outcome of melanoma. For The World Health Organisation Melanoma Programme. Lancet 1991;337:8742.

201. Slingluff C, Vollmer R, Reintgen D, Seigler HF: Malignant melanoma and pregnancy. An analysis of 100 consecutive cases. Ann Surg 1990;211:552.

202. Breslow A: Thickness, cross-sectional areas and depth of melanoma in the prognosis of cutaneous melanoma. Ann Surg 1970; 72:902.

203. Buzaid AC, Tinoco LA, Jendiroba D, et al: Prognostic value of size of lymph node metastases in patients with cutaneous melanoma. J Clin Oncol 1995;13:2361.

204. Cascinelli N, Marubini E, Morabito A, Bufalino R: Prognostic factors for stage I melanoma of the skin: A review. Stat Med 1985;4:265.

205. Veronesi U, Cascinelli N, Adamus J, et al: Thin stage I primary cutaneous melanoma: Comparison of excision with margins of 1 or 3 cm. N Engl J Med 1988;318:1159.

206. Albertini JJ, Cruse CW, Rapaport D, et al: Intraoperative radiolymphoscintigraphy improves sentinel node identification in melanoma patients. Ann Surg 1996;223:217.

207. Balch CM, Milton GW, Cascinelli N, et al: Elective node dissection: Pros and cons. In Balch CM, Houghton AN, Milton GW, et al (eds): Cutaneous Melanoma, 2nd ed. Philadelphia, JB Lippincott, 1992, p 345.

208. Morton DL, Wen DR, Wong JH, et al: Technical details of intraoperative lymphatic mapping for early stage melanoma. Arch Surg 1992;127:392.

209. Kirkwood JM, Strawderman MH, Ernstoff MS, et al: Adjuvant therapy of high-risk resected cutaneous melanoma: The Eastern Cooperative Oncology Group Trial EST 1684. J Clin Oncol 1996;14:7.

210. Balch CM, Reintgen DS, Kirkwood JM, et al: Cutaneous melanoma. In DeVita VT Jr, Hellman S, Rosenberg SA (eds): Cancer: Principles and Practice of Oncology, 5th ed. Philadelphia, Lippincott-Raven, 1997, p 1975.

211. Shioda Y, Koizumi S, Furuya S, et al: Intussusception caused by a carcinoma of the cecum during pregnancy: Report of a case and review of the literature. Surg Today 1993;23:556.

212. Eddy DM, Nugent FW, Eddy JF, et al: Screening for colorectal cancer in a high-risk population: Results of a mathematical model. Gastroenterology 1987;92:682.

213. Lau WY, Leung WT, Ho S, et al: Hepatocellular carcinoma during pregnancy and its comparison with other pregnancy-associated malignancies. Cancer 1995;75:2669.

214. Maeta M, Yamashiro H, Oka A, et al: Gastric cancer in the young, with special reference to 14 pregnancy-associated cases: Analysis based on 2,325 consecutive cases of gastric cancer. J Surg Oncol 1995;58:191.

215. Sjeikh SS, Khalifa MA, Marley EF, et al: Acute monocytic leukemia (FAB M5) involving the placenta associated with delivery of a healthy infant: Case report and discussion. Int J Gynecol Pathol 1996;15:363.

216. Baer MR: Management of unusual presentations of acute leukemia. Hematol Oncol Clin North Am 1993;7:275.

217. de The H, Chomienne C, Lanotte M, et al: The t(15;17) translocation of acute promyelocytic leukemia fuses the retinoic acid receptor α gene to a novel transcribed locus. Nature 1990;347:358.

218. Miller WH Jr, Warrell RP Jr, Frankel SR, et al: Novel retinoic acid receptor-alpha transcripts in acute promyelocytic leukemia responsive to all-*trans*-retinoic acid. J Natl Cancer Inst 1990;82:1932.

219. Tallman MS, Andersen JW, Schiffer CA, et al: All-*trans*-retinoic acid in acute promyelocytic leukemia. N Engl J Med 1997; 337:1021.

220. Hoffman MA, Wiernik PH, Kleiner GJ: Acute promyelocytic leukemia and pregnancy. A case report. Cancer 1995;76:2237.

221. Shtivelman E, Lifshitz B, Gale RP, Canaani E: Fused transcript of abl and bcr genes in chronic myelogenous leukaemia. Nature 1985;315:550.

222. O'Brien SG, Guilhot F, Larson RA: Imatinib compared with interferon and low-dose cytarabine for newly diagnosed chronic-phase chronic myelogenous leukemia. N Engl J Med 2003;348:994.

223. Goldman J, Szydlo R, Horowitz M, et al: Choice of pre-transplant treatment and timing of transplants for chronic myelogenous leukemia in chronic phase. Blood 1993;82:2235.

224. Fitzgerald JM, McCann SR: The combination of hydroxyurea and leucapheresis in the treatment of chronic myeloid leukaemia in pregnancy. Clin Lab Haematol 1993;15:63.

225. Chrisomalis L, Baxi LV, Heller D: Chronic lymphocytic leukemia in pregnancy. Am J Obstet Gynecol 1996;175:1381.

226. Cancer Facts and Figures—1994. Atlanta, American Cancer Society, 1994.

227. Rabkin C, Devesa SS, Zahm SH, Gail MH: Increasing incidence of non-Hodgkin's lymphoma. Semin Hematol 1993;30:286.

228. Pollack RN, Sklarin NT, Rao S, Divon MY: Metastatic placental lymphoma associated with maternal human immunodeficiency virus infection. Obstet Gynecol 1993;81:856.

229. Jaffe ES, Harris NL, Diebold J, et al: World Health Organization classification of neoplastic diseases of the hematopoietic and lymphoid tissues. A progress report. Am J Clin Pathol 1999; 111:S8.

230. Shipp MA: Prognostic factors in aggressive non-Hodgkin's lymphoma: Who has "high-risk" disease? Blood 1994;83:1165.

231. Fisher RI, Gaynor ER, Dahlberg S, et al: Comparison of a standard regimen (CHOP) with three intensive chemotherapy regimens for advanced non-Hodgkin's lymphoma. N Engl J Med 1993;328:1002.

232. Philip T, Guglielmi C, Hagenbeek A, et al: Autologous bone marrow transplantation (ABNT) versus conventional chemotherapy (DHAP) in relapsed non Hodgkin lymphoma (NHL): Final analysis of the Parma randomized study (216 patients). Proc ASCO 1995;14:390.

233. Haioun C, Lepage E, Gisselbracht C, et al: Comparison of autologous bone marrow transplantation with sequential chemotherapy for intermediate-grade and high-grade non-Hodgkin's lymphoma in first complete remission: A study of 464 patients. Groupe d'Eátude des Lymphomes de L'Adulte. J Clin Oncol 1994;12:2543.

234. Tsujimura T, Matusmoto K, Aozasa K: Placental involvement by maternal non-Hodgkin's lymphoma. Arch Pathol Lab Med 1993;117:325.

235. Selvais PL, Mazy G, Gosseye S, et al: Breast infiltration by acute lymphoblastic leukemia during pregnancy. Am J Obstet Gynecol 1993;169:1619.

236. Aghadiuno PU, Akang EE, Lapido JK: Simultaneous bilateral malignant breast neoplasms in Nigerian women. J Natl Med Assoc 1994;86:365.

237. Kirkpatrick AW, Bailey DJ, Weizel HA: Bilateral breast lymphoma in pregnancy: A case report and literature review. Can J Surg 1996;39:333.

238. Liberman L, Giess CS, Dershaw DD, et al: Non-Hodgkin lymphoma of the breast: Imaging characteristics and correlation with histopathologic features. Radiology 1994;192:157.

239. Santoro A, Bonadonna G: Prolonged disease-free survival in MOPP-resistant Hodgkin's disease with Adriamycin, bleomycin, vinblastine and dacarbazine (ABVD). Cancer Chemother Pharmacol 1979;2:101.

240. DeVita VT, Serpick AA, Carbone PP: Combination chemotherapy in the treatment of advanced Hodgkin's disease. Ann Intern Med 1970;73:891.

24

PSYCHIATRIC COMPLICATIONS

C. Neill Epperson and Kathryn Czarkowski

OVERVIEW

Psychiatric complications during pregnancy can represent an exacerbation of an ongoing psychiatric disorder, a resurgence of previously remitted symptoms, or the onset of a new illness. Millions of women suffer from mental illness during their childbearing years, and more than 50% of pregnancies are unplanned; these facts highlight the importance of prenatal counseling with regard to the natural history of various psychiatric disorders during pregnancy, as well as the potential risks associated with fetal exposure to psychotropic agents and/or maternal mental illness.

The most common psychiatric disorders, such as mood and anxiety disorders, are underreported by patients and underdiagnosed by primary care physicians. However, the majority of treatment for such disorders occurs in the primary care setting, not the psychiatrist's office. Thus, the overarching goal of this chapter is to summarize the clinical course and treatment of psychiatric disorders during pregnancy and the early puerperium, with a specific focus on disorders frequently encountered in the primary care setting. Methods of enhancing detection of ongoing or new mental illness in the pregnant patient, as well as basics of the consultation, are discussed. Finally, a brief overview of the natural history of mood, anxiety, psychotic, and eating disorders during pregnancy are included with specific recommendations for treatment.

Detection as the First Intervention

Although the myth of the "protective effects of pregnancy" has been dispelled in the medical field, the general lay population continues to perceive pregnancy as a time of relative well-being. Along with this myth, the ever-present stigma regarding mental disorders, which alter mood, cognition, and behavior, and the expectation that women with mental illness are compromised as mothers hinder women from revealing their psychiatric histories or their current symptoms to their obstetric providers.

Thus, the onus is on the clinician to create an overtly welcoming environment for disclosure. Pamphlets and posters educating women regarding mood and behavior changes during pregnancy and the postnatal period suggest to the client that the provider values her psychologic well-being. Personal and family psychiatric histories should be reviewed verbally with each new obstetric patient. An assessment of the client's current psychologic status can be facilitated by the use of self-rated questionnaires such as the 10-item Edinburgh Postnatal Depression Scale.[1] This user-friendly questionnaire is written for the layperson and can be scored by a clinician or clinic staff within several minutes. Studies from multiple countries with varied cultures and medical financing systems show that a score of 12.5 or higher indicates a case of clinical depression.[2] Because managed care does not yet cover psychologic assessments in the obstetric practice, it is important to use these techniques to create an environment that enhances the rapid detection of ongoing or new mental illness in the pregnant patient. Once a woman is found to require psychiatric intervention, valuable staff time can be saved by having previously developed a local referral network or collaboration with a specific mental health care provider who will readily evaluate new patients with varying means of payment.

Enhancing Detection: Summary

1. Place psychoeducational materials in office and in waiting rooms, examination rooms, and restrooms.
2. Medical history forms, including family and personal psychiatric history, should be reviewed at the first prenatal appointment.
3. Administer the Edinburgh Postnatal Depression Scale (or a similar measure). Review answers with the patient. Probe for other psychiatric symptoms and for use of psychotropic medications.
4. Review recent psychosocial stressors.
5. Assess patient's access to social and familial supports.
6. Develop a mental health provider referral list.

Consulting with the Pregnant Psychiatric Patient: The Basics

Consultations with pregnant women who suffer from a psychiatric disorder, regardless of the diagnosis, include discussion of the following facts: (1) Psychoactive medications readily cross the placenta; (2) there are potential risks associated with untreated maternal psychiatric illness as well as fetal exposure to psychotropic medications; and (3) many women experience relapse or worsening of symptoms if pharmacologic treatment is not continued or instituted when necessary.

The first issue is self-explanatory: The fetus is exposed to psychoactive substances ingested by the mother. However, it is not clear to what degree fetal exposure is influenced by factors such as maternal drug metabolism and medication pharmacokinetics. Moreover, the genetic make-up of the fetus could theoretically modulate the expression of in utero psychotropic exposure.

The second aspect of the consultation, assessment of risks of maternal illness versus psychotropic exposure on fetal well-being, poses several clinical conundrums. There is a relative dearth of data regarding the impact of in utero psychotropic exposure on long-term neurodevelopment (Table 24–1). Frequently, the patient's clinical course with regard to her symptoms and treatment is not completely clear. In contrast to the limited data regarding long-term sequelae of in utero exposure to psychotropic agents, it is well known that relapse of maternal mental illness is detrimental to the short- and long-term health of both the mother and her child or children. Symptoms affecting the unborn child can be as overt as deliberate maternal self-harm and can result in injury to or death of the fetus. Alternatively, they can be more insidious, revealing themselves in the form of poor attention to prenatal care or participation in unsafe behaviors such as cigarette smoking, heavy alcohol consumption, and/or use of other illicit substances.

Maternal anxiety and stress have been shown to have adverse effects on pregnancy outcome, infant/child neurodevelopment, and maternal postnatal mental health.[3-7] Anxiety and depression may be risk factors for preeclampsia,[4] preterm deliveries, and lower birth weights,[8-10] as well as for childhood behavioral and emotional disturbances.[5,11] Mediating mechanisms may include abnormal uterine blood flow[12] and increased cortisol transfer from mother to fetus.[13]

Together, these facts highlight the importance for clinicians working with pregnant women who are taking psychotropic medication to obtain a history with regard to the severity and chronicity of the patient's psychiatric illness. Only in collaboration with the prescribing physician should the obstetrician make recommendations about discontinuation of a psychotropic medication in a pregnant woman.

Discussing the Risks of Psychotropic Exposure

Discussion of the risks associated with specific medications should include review of their potential for (1) fetal teratogenicity, (2) neonatal withdrawal syndrome, and (3) behavioral teratogenicity. Medications are considered teratogenic when exposure to the drug during organogenesis (the first 12 weeks of gestation) results in an increased incidence of major birth defects in comparison with the baseline risk (2% to 4%) in the general population. *Neonatal withdrawal syndrome* refers to difficulties in physical and behavioral adjustment shortly after delivery; *behavioral teratogenicity* refers to long-term neurobehavioral disturbances related to antenatal drug exposure. The U.S. Food and Drug Administration classified medication into five categories (A, B, C, D, and X) to reflect the degree of risk to the fetus according to available animal and human data; however, this classification is outdated and unable to adequately elucidate the risks between categories or describe the risks associated with new medications as they become available.[14] In addition, data regarding the pregnancy safety profile of a particular medication cannot be generalized to its generic equivalent.

In summary, the task of the medical care provider for women of reproductive potential is clear. An environment welcoming full disclosure of psychiatric history and/or current symptoms is crucial. Moreover, a clinician caring for a woman with mental illness who wishes to become or who is already pregnant must be prepared to help her adequately weigh (1) the risk of relapse or deterioration of symptoms during pregnancy and its attendant risks of poor obstetric and perinatal outcome against (2) the risks associated with specific pharmacologic interventions.

PSYCHIATRIC DISORDERS DURING PREGNANCY AND THE PUERPERIUM

Affective Disorders

The Natural History

After puberty, girls and women are twice as likely as boys and men to experience a major depressive episode in the course of their lives.[15] The fact that peak onset is during the childbearing years could suggest that such reproductive events place a woman at increased risk of depression. Regardless of whether this association between depression and childbearing is causal or coincidental, this finding highlights the importance of symptom surveillance in this clinical population.

Although events in the media have drawn attention to postpartum depression, few realize that depression during pregnancy is common (10% to 13%).[16] Women at risk for antepartum and/or postpartum depression are those with a personal or family history of affective disorders (unipolar and bipolar), few social supports, marital conflict, or significant stressful life events.[2]

The risk of relapse of major depression during pregnancy is high in women with a history of major depression and in those who discontinue medication at the time of conception. Women must be cautioned about abrupt discontinuation of antidepressants, particularly of paroxetine (Paxil) and venlafaxine (Effexor), which can result in an unpleasant discontinuation syndrome. In addition, cessation of antidepressant treatment after achieving

TABLE 24-1   Profile of Psychotropic Medications during Pregnancy: At a Glance

Drug	Organ Teratogen	Neonatal Adaptation	Long-Term Neurodevelopment (LTD)
Antidepressants			
Fluoxetine (Prozac) Sertraline (Zoloft) Paroxetine (Paxil) Citalopram (Celexa) Bupropion (Wellbutrin) Venlafaxine (Effexor) Nefazodone (Serzone)	No increased risk of major birth defects reported Newer agents studied in small samples[18]	A few reports of NWS in infants exposed to fluoxetine or paroxetine at term[25,26]	Measures of cognitive function, temperament, attention all WNL in preschool age children exposed in utero to fluoxetine or a TCA[28] Bayley scale scores WNL in four sertraline-exposed children at 24 months[35]
Mood Stabilizers/Antiepileptic Drugs (AEDs)			
Lithium (Eskalith, Lithobid)	Ebstein's anomaly: 0.1%[36]	Old reports of "floppy baby" have not been confirmed in recent literature	No adequate data regarding neurodevelopment with lithium exposure
Carbamazepine (Tegretol) Valproic acid (Depakote)	Data from infants of women with epilepsy,[38,39,40] increased risk of neural tube defects	No systematic reports	Evidence of EEG abnormalities, minor neurologic dysfunction in offspring exposed to AEDs, particularly true for those exposed to multiple AEDs.[43] No difference between offspring exposed to carbamazepine and controls on neurobehavioral development.[45]
Gabapentin (Neurontin) Lamotrigine (Lamictal) Topiramate (Topamax) Ziprasidone (Geodon)	No increased risk of major birth defects reported in the Gabapentin Pregnancy Registry (N = 51)[79] or the Lamotrigine Registry (N = 168 monotherapy; N = 166 polytherapy).[46] Animal studies suggest topiramate may be more teratogenic than gabapentin or lamotrigine. Very little human data available[80] for it or ziprasidone	Not reported	No long-term studies
Anxiolytics/Sedatives			
Lorazepam (Ativan) Clonazepam (Klonopin) Alprazolam (Xanax) Diazepam (Valium) Secobarbital (Seconal Sodium, Novo-Secobarb)	Metaanalysis of risk of oral cleft indicates little to no risk[58]	Doses commonly used in clinical practice not commonly associated with NWS	No adequate studies addressing LTD with in utero exposure to benzodiazepines or barbiturates
Antipsychotics (Typical)			
Haloperidol (Haldol) Perphenazine (Trilafon)	No increased risk with high-potency antipsychotic agents	Rarely reported motoric symptoms; last case report for haloperidal in 2002 suggests risk for hypothermia[81]	No adequate studies addressing LTD with in utero exposure to antipsychotic agents
Antipsychotics (Atypical)			
Clozapine (Clozaril) Risperidone (Risperdal) Olanzapine (Zyprexa) Quetiapine (Seroquel)	Sample sizes reported are inadequate to rule out risks	None reported but not systematically studied	No studies to date

NWS, neonatal withdrawal syndrome; TCA, tricyclic antidepressant; WNL, within normal limits.

a partial clinical response, or before an adequate period of remission, has been demonstrated to increase the risk of relapse in nonpregnant women, and this finding may be applicable to pregnant women as well. Finally, antepartum depression is the strongest predictor of postpartum depression, and aggressive treatment should therefore be instituted before delivery.

The course of bipolar affective disorder (BPAD) is particularly unpredictable during pregnancy and the puerperium. Although there have been no prospective studies examining the relapse rate in women who discontinue treatment with mood stabilizers such as carbamazepine (Tegretol) and valproic acid (Depakote), Viguera and colleagues reported a heightened risk in women who rapidly discontinued their lithium treatment, in comparison with those who underwent a slow, controlled taper over 4 weeks.[17] Regardless of how rapidly lithium doses were tapered, the risk of relapse of bipolar illness in these women was 52% during pregnancy and 70% during the puerperium.

Treatment and Recommendations

Selective Serotonin Reuptake Inhibitors

Selective serotonin reuptake inhibitors (SSRIs) are considered first-line treatment for unipolar, nonpsychotic major depression. The safety profile with regard to the use of SSRIs (fluoxetine, sertraline, paroxetine, citalopram, fluvoxamine) during pregnancy is encouraging, because they have not been found to result in major fetal anomalies with first trimester use (see Table 24–1).[18,19] However, the drugs in this class have individual differences, which may render one more or less desirable in a given case. For example, the long half-life and active metabolite of fluoxetine (Prozac) may be less appropriate for a woman with antepartum depression whose past or current symptoms are consistent with hypomania and/or who have a first-degree relative with BPAD; these factors increase her chance of having SSRI-induced mania. Alternatively, a woman who desires to breast-feed may prefer to begin treatment with sertraline (Zoloft) or paroxetine (Paxil), both of which have been thoroughly investigated and found in nondetectable or very low quantities in plasma of infants exposed through maternal breast milk.[20]

The choice of which medication to institute in a pregnant woman with recurrent depression is typically dictated by her history of response to a particular agent. Women should be treated with dosages that result in remission of symptoms. Two reports suggested that, as with the tricyclic antidepressants (TCAs), pregnancy-related induction of the hepatic enzyme 2D6 may result in decreased maternal plasma SSRI levels. However, clinical stability may[21] or may not[22] be compromised.

With regard to neonatal adjustment, some concern has been raised, albeit inconsistently with peripartum use of fluoxetine[19,23,24] and paroxetine.[25,26] A comprehensive prospective investigation of neurodevelopment revealed no differences in measures of global intelligence quotient (IQ), temperament, mood, arousability, activity level, distractibility, or language or behavioral development in a group of toddlers and elementary school–aged children who had been exposed to fluoxetine during some part[27] or all[28] of the pregnancy.

Other investigators have found comparable results with regard to pregnancy and perinatal outcome with the SSRIs sertraline, paroxetine, and fluvoxamine; however, the children were exposed primarily in the first trimester, sample sizes have been smaller, and long-term neurodevelopment has not been adequately addressed.[29] Data demonstrating preferential safety of one SSRI over another are insufficient to warrant risking clinical stability by having a woman in remission switch from one SSRI to another during pregnancy.

Tricyclic Antidepressants

Although SSRIs are considered first-line treatment for major depression, TCAs, utilized primarily to augment SSRI treatment response, may also be used as a monotherapy. A review of 13 studies assessing the risk of congenital malformations after first trimester exposure to TCAs revealed no increased risk of congenital defects.[30] In rare instances, infants exposed to TCAs through delivery have developed a neonatal withdrawal syndrome, which included seizures in one case and gastrointestinal stasis in another. No differences were found in global IQ, language development, or behavioral development among a group of preschool-aged children exposed to TCAs in utero.[27]

Other Antidepressants

In a study of 125 infants, in utero exposure to venlafaxine (Effexor) was not associated with birth defects or perinatal complications.[31] Data about the effects of trazodone, nefazodone, or mirtazapine are scant. Limited animal data do not suggest teratogenicity; however, few or no human data are available.[32] Because of the limited and relatively worrisome data about monoamine oxidase inhibitor use during pregnancy, and because of the risk of hypertensive crises if the necessary dietary restrictions are not observed, monoamine oxidase inhibitors are relatively poor options for treatment of depression in pregnant women.

Nonpharmacologic Treatments

The lack of conclusive data regarding the safety of pharmacotherapy during pregnancy and women's hesitance to take medications while pregnant has led investigators to examine nonpharmacologic treatments for antepartum mood and anxiety disorders. Spinelli and colleagues recently reported efficacy of interpersonal psychotherapy in the treatment of depressed pregnant women.[33] This particular type of therapy is well suited for the pregnant population, inasmuch as most of these women are experiencing significant issues in their interpersonal relationships during this time. Morning bright light treatment is another form of somatic therapy that has been examined in antepartum depression with some success.[34,35] Light therapy has the advantages of being safe for the mother and fetus and of being less expensive and less subject to stigmatization than are medications.

Lithium

The treatment of BPAD can be complicated and often includes medications from several drug classes, including mood-stabilizing agents such as antiepileptic drugs (AEDs) and lithium. Lithium is effective in protecting women with BPAD from depressive or manic relapse and is used frequently as an augmentation strategy for women with recurrent unipolar depression who have had partial response to treatment with an SSRI.

Reevaluation of the relationship between lithium and congenital heart defects such as Ebstein's anomaly has greatly reduced the concern regarding the use of this medication during the first trimester.[30,36] Additional findings have suggested that women with BPAD should never be weaned rapidly from lithium and that most require continued treatment throughout pregnancy to maintain clinical stability. Relapse of BPAD or psychotic unipolar depression can be particularly grave, because the woman's judgment is impaired and she is likely to require multiple medications at higher dosages to regain stability. In the severest cases, electroconvulsive therapy (ECT) is a safe and relatively underutilized option.[37] Cases of self-limiting neonatal complications with second and third trimester lithium use were reported in the 1970s; however, more recent reports are lacking, and there have been no adequate evaluations of the neurodevelopment of infants exposed to lithium in utero.

Monthly monitoring of lithium levels is recommended during pregnancy until the last month, when weekly monitoring is preferable. Pregnancy-induced changes in body fluid and volume of distribution frequently result in reductions in lithium levels. However, increases in dosage should be based on resurgence of symptoms, not reductions in blood level. If the lithium dosage was increased during pregnancy, it should be reduced to the prepregnancy level after delivery, and the blood level should be monitored closely during the early puerperium. Rapid fluid shifts occurring within the first 48 hours after delivery can contribute to the emergence of lithium toxicity.

Antiepileptic Drugs

AEDs are also commonly used in the treatment of BPAD; however, data about the teratogenic effects of in utero exposure to AEDs have been obtained primarily from children born to women with epilepsy. Women with seizure disorders have children with an incidence of birth defects that is at least two to three times the population average of about 2%.[38] Prospective studies suggest that excess teratogenicity is attributable to AEDs rather than to epilepsy[39,40] and thus should be considered when AEDs are used to treat women with BPAD or other psychiatric disorders. Animal research has demonstrated that most anticonvulsant agents produce teratogenic effects.[30]

Both valproic acid and carbamazepine exposure (as monotherapy) in utero are associated with a higher incidence (approximately 1% to 5.4% and 0.5% to 1%, respectively) of neural tube defects than in the general population (0.038% to 0.096%).[40-42] A prospective study suggests a dosage-response relationship between valproic acid and neural tube defects, with an average daily dose being higher in exposed infants who develop neural tube defects (1640 ± 136 mg/day) compared to exposed infants without neural tube defects (941 ± 48 mg/day).[41] Another study found that offspring of women taking valproic acid ≥1000 mg/day were almost 4 times more likely to have a neural tube defect than offspring of women taking valproic acid ≤600 mg/day.[41a] Other major congenital defects suspected with valproic acid exposure are orofacial clefts, urogenital abnormalities, cardiac defects, and skeletal anomalies, although the exact risks are unclear.[32] A syndrome of facial dimorphism, nail dysplasia, digital hypoplasia, cleft lip and palate, cardiac defects, and cognitive abnormalities, initially identified as fetal hydantoin syndrome, is now recognized with other anticonvulsants, including carbamazepine and valproic acid. In addition to major congenital defects, infants exposed to AEDs in utero tend to have more minor malformations[42] that can occur independently or with syndromes associated with carbamazepine or valproic acid exposure.

Although the data are conflicting and the studies were conducted in nonpsychiatric populations, several reports have suggested that children of mothers with epilepsy and antenatal exposure to AEDs have developmental delays, lower intelligence, and neurologic dysfunction in comparison with controls.[43,44] A prospective, controlled study found no differences in global IQ in 36 infants exposed to carbamazepine monotherapy.[45] Thus, women with BPAD who require treatment with an AED should consider carbamazepine or one of the newer AEDs, such as lamotrigine, over valproic acid. Pregnant women who are treated with carbamazepine or valproic acid should also take high-dosage folic acid (4 mg/day) to decrease the risk of neural tube defects.

Newer Antiepileptic Drugs

Lamotrigine (Lamictal), gabapentin (Neurontin), and topiramate (Topamax) have been used in the treatment of neuropsychiatric disorders, particularly BPAD and schizoaffective disorder. A relatively large European database with lamotrigine suggests that it is not teratogenic with first trimester use.[46] Fewer but similar data are available for gabapentin and topiramate. There have been no controlled studies of the effect of these agents on neonatal adjustment or long-term neurodevelopment.

Antipsychotic Drugs

A metaanalysis evaluating the effect of antenatal exposure to the older high-potency antipsychotic drugs (APDs) such as haloperidol (Haldol), perphenazine (Trilafon), trifluoperazine (Stelazine), and fluphenazine (Prolixin) found no increased risk of fetal anomalies.[30] The relatively new atypical APDs are frequently included in the pharmacologic regimen of women with moderate to severe affective disorders, specifically both unipolar and bipolar disorders. Risperidone[47] (Risperdal), as well as other atypical APDs that block the neuronal postsynaptic 5-hydroxytryptamine (serotonin) 2A receptor,[48] have shown promise as an augmentation of SSRIs in the treatment of depression even when no psychotic features are present. Although there are few or no case reports of risperidone, clozapine (Clozaril), quetiapine (Seroquel), or ziprasidone (Geodon) use during pregnancy, olanzapine (Zyprexa), which is effective in the treatment of acute mania, has been prospectively assessed in a group of 37 pregnancies that resulted in 14 therapeutic abortions and 23 live births. There was no increase in overall birth defects or clustering of any particular defect in the infants born to the women taking olanzapine, 5 to 25 mg/day.[49] Olanzapine doses of 1.25 to 5 mg/day may be adequate when used as augmentation of SSRI treatment in major depression without psychotic features. Higher dosages are typically required for treatment of acute mania and/or psychotic depression. There have been no adequate investigations of the impact of typical or atypical APDs on neurodevelopment or neonatal adjustment. Case reports suggest that infants may experience transient anticholinergic effects, such as urine or bowel retention, if exposed to typical APDs late in gestation.[32]

Electroconvulsive Therapy

ECT remains one of the most effective treatments for severe major depression or mania. Because there have been no prospective, controlled trials of ECT administration during pregnancy, experience with this treatment modality is derived from more than 300 case reports and case series. Miller and colleagues found 28 reports of ECT-associated pregnancy complications—including transient, benign fetal arrhythmias, mild vaginal bleeding; abdominal pain; and self-limited uterine contractions—in a case series of 300 women who were treated with ECT during pregnancy.[37] There was no association between ECT and major congenital malformations. Guidelines for ECT use during pregnancy are available and should include a pre-ECT evaluation with pelvic examination, discontinuation of nonessential anticholinergic medication, uterine tocodynamometry, and intravenous hydration. During ECT, elevation of the right hip, intubation, reduction of excessive hyperventilation, and external fetal cardiac monitoring are recommended.

Anxiety Disorders

Natural History

Anxiety disorders such as panic disorder, generalized anxiety disorder (GAD), obsessive-compulsive disorder (OCD), and post-traumatic stress disorder (PTSD) are common during the childbearing years. Childbearing has been associated with the onset or worsening of panic disorder[50] and of OCD.[51,52] There are conflicting reports of whether subgroups of women with panic disorder have a newfound success in being able to wean themselves from their antianxiety medications during pregnancy.[53,54] One suggestion is that these women have fewer panic attacks during pregnancy as a result of progesterone-induced hyperventilation and relatively lower partial pressure of carbon dioxide.[55] However, many women cannot be successfully weaned from their antipanic medications.[54] Devastating sequelae of panic attacks, such as placental abruption[56] and preeclampsia,[4] as well as nonfatal consequences of heightened anxiety during pregnancy, such as earlier births, lower birth weight, neonatal irritability, and childhood behavioral problems, have all been reported.[5,9]

Partial or full PTSD occurs in up to 21% of pregnant women who have had a previous third trimester stillbirth,[57] and pregnant women experience some degree of PTSD symptoms, depression, and anxiety after other types of fetal loss. These women often complain of a lack of attachment to the fetus and a fear that they will not bond with the baby when and if the baby is successfully delivered. Women who suffer from PTSD secondary to rape or childhood sexual abuse may find the sexuality inherent in pregnancy and childbirth destabilizing and may need additional psychotherapeutic supports during this time of heightened reminders of their trauma. Women with OCD may neglect aspects of good prenatal care if their obsessions and/or compulsions interfere with rational ways of eating, sleeping, grooming, and/or cleaning. Women with OCD may also develop worrisome obsessions about the fetus, which increase their sense of shame and limit their ability to enjoy the pregnancy.

Treatment

Combination Pharmacotherapy and Cognitive-Behavioral Therapy

As with mood disorders, the treatment of anxiety disorders during pregnancy depends on the severity of current symptoms and on the likelihood of relapse if medications are discontinued. As mentioned previously, the sequelae of untreated maternal anxiety can have dire consequences and should be minimized through the use of appropriate psychopharmacology and/or psychotherapy. Cognitive-behavioral therapy, yoga, and relaxation training may limit the degree to which the patient relies on medications to resolve her symptoms. However, access to these interventions may be limited by time constraints, location, and/or financial resources and often require a significant degree of motivation in the patient, who may be very ill and may have few social supports.

Antidepressants, particularly the SSRIs and/or cognitive-behavioral therapy are the mainstay of treatment for panic disorder, as well as for GAD and OCD. TCAs are as effective as SSRIs in the treatment of panic disorder but are less effective for GAD and ineffective for OCD. Dosages of SSRIs necessary for the treatment of panic disorder and GAD are similar to those used in patients with depression. In women with OCD, SSRI dosages at the upper prescribing limit are usually necessary to obtain clinical efficacy. Individuals with OCD who have a partial response to treatment with SSRIs may benefit from addition of a low-dosage atypical neuroleptic such as risperidone or olanzapine to their ongoing SSRI regimen.

Benzodiazepines

Benzodiazepines are commonly prescribed in the psychiatric practice to treat anxiety, insomnia, and unpleasant side effects associated with other psychotropic agents. Although early case-control studies found that maternal benzodiazepine exposure increased the risk of cleft lip and cleft palate in infants, a more recent metaanalysis,[58] examining pooled data from cohort and case-control studies published between 1966 and 1998, found little association between antenatal benzodiazepine exposure and oral cleft or other major malformations.

There have been no reports linking lorazepam, clonazepam, or alprazolam to congenital defects in humans. Lorazepam is protein bound to a greater degree, lacks the multiple metabolites of clonazepam, and may therefore result in relatively less transfer of drug from the maternal to fetal circulation. Neonatal adjustment difficulties, including hypotonia and poor respiratory effort at birth, or symptoms of neonatal withdrawal within the first few days of delivery have been reported with heavy and prolonged use of benzodiazepines during pregnancy or high dosages given during parturition.[18] However, no such phenomena have been reported with dosages of benzodiazepines commonly prescribed today. It is not clear whether in utero exposure to benzodiazepines at any dosage and/or for any duration has adverse effects on neurodevelopment.[59]

Psychotic Disorders

Natural History

The mean age at onset of schizophrenia in women is during the late 20s, a time when many women contemplate becoming pregnant. In comparison with men, women have later disease onset, require lower dosages of APDs, and have a better overall prognosis.[60] However, the symptoms of schizophrenia are not ameliorated by pregnancy, and most affected women require continued pharmacotherapy, frequently from multiple drug classes. Whenever possible, efforts should be made to simplify the patient's medication regimen and thereby reduce polypharmacy that can increase the potential risks for the fetus. With their preferable side effect profile, the newer atypical APDs have become the mainstay of treatment for psychotic disorders, particularly schizophrenia. However, as with most newer medications, little is known about their safety for use during pregnancy. Women with schizophrenia are more likely to participate in behaviors known to increase the risk of intrauterine growth retardation, preterm birth, and perinatal death.[61] Smoking cigarettes, abusing cocaine or alcohol, and having low socioeconomic status place women with schizophrenia at particular risk of a poor pregnancy outcome. Notably, women with schizophrenia have a significant reduction in fertility in comparison with controls.[62] Women who have major depression with psychotic features should be treated for stability during pregnancy with a special focus on alleviating psychotic symptoms, because such symptoms in the postnatal period increase the risk of infanticide.

Treatment

Antipsychotic Drugs

As mentioned previously, studies evaluating the effect of antenatal exposure to high-potency APDs, primarily haloperidol, have often been conducted in nonpsychotic women treated for hyperemesis gravidarum and have not been associated with an increase in fetal birth defects. In addition, a small prospective study of the newer atypical APD olanzapine suggests that it is not associated with an increased risk for fetal anomalies.[49] Likewise, animal studies have also failed to demonstrate a teratogenic effect associated with olanzapine treatment.[63]

Clozapine, the first atypical APD to become available, has been invaluable to many individuals with schizophrenia who could either not tolerate the side effects of typical APDs or were unresponsive to these older agents. Approximately 30 cases of clozapine use during pregnancy have been documented. No major congenital anomalies were noted in 21 of the children.[18,32] Nine cases of adverse outcomes with clozapine use in pregnancy were reported to the U.S. Food and Drug Administration. Because information about all known exposures was lacking, it is possible that these abnormalities could have been caused by chance. These outcomes do not suggest that antenatal clozapine exposure increases fetal risk.[32] Although there are several case reports in the literature suggesting that peripartum use of typical APDs can result in neonatal complications, no difference in IQ was found between APD-exposed and nonexposed children tested at 4 years of age.[64]

When the older APDs are used at the dosages necessary to treat schizophrenia, coadministration of agents to control extrapyramidal symptoms is often required. Two studies suggested a possible association between benztropine exposure and major malformations, one linked first trimester trihexyphenidyl exposure to minor malformations, and conflicting reports exist about the teratogenic risk of diphenhydramine (Benadryl).[32]

As with mood and anxiety disorders, the goal of treatment should be remission of symptoms, and women with psychotic disorders are thus likely to require medications from several classes and at substantial dosages to attain and/or maintain clinical stability throughout pregnancy. Although it may be prudent to choose a typical APD such as haloperidol if a woman presents with new-onset psychosis during pregnancy, many women with schizophrenia have tried these agents and have already switched to one of the atypical APDs before conception. Emerging data indicate that these drugs, particularly olanzapine and clozapine, may not result in adverse fetal effects.

Eating Disorders

Natural History

The eating disorders anorexia nervosa and bulimia nervosa are distinguished by extreme eating patterns that may compromise maternal nutrition and fetal growth and development. A typical pattern of eating behavior of a person suffering from anorexia nervosa is an insistence on maintaining a below-normal body weight, whereas a person suffering from bulimia nervosa has periods of binge eating accompanied by self-induced vomiting; misuse of laxatives, diuretics, or other medications; fasting; or excessive exercise. More than 90% of all cases of eating disorders occur in girls and women who are of childbearing age.[65] Eating disorders are most common in individuals who were sexually abused as children or have a first-degree relative with a history of a psychiatric illness.[65,66]

Eating disorders in pregnant women have both physiologic and psychologic effects on the outcome of the pregnancy[67,68] and on subsequent infant development.[69] Specifically, women with anorexia nervosa have infants with higher rates of perinatal mortality,[70] obstetric complications,[67] and congenital abnormalities.[71] Bulimia nervosa sufferers experience extreme weight gain and specific pregnancy complications such as preeclampsia and hypertension.[72] In general, however, eating disorders in pregnancy have been associated with miscarriage, low birth weight, obstetric complications, and postpartum depression.[73] These outcomes necessitate the need for fastidious identification and evaluation of women with eating disorders who are contemplating pregnancy or who have already conceived.[65,73] Although studies from before 1990 suggested that eating disorders decrease during pregnancy, the disorders do not entirely disappear, and they reemerge after delivery.

Treatment and Recommendations

Nonpharmacologic Interventions

By proactively dealing with an eating disorder early in the pregnancy, the practitioner reduces the chances of pregnancy complications and establishes an open-method of communication with the patient. The patient's nutrition during pregnancy should also be an important part of the dialogue between the patient and physician, and the patient's daily caloric intake should be monitored. Referring the patient to a dietitian with experience in dealing with eating disorders may be helpful in promoting caloric intake. If a patient continues to restrict her diet severely during pregnancy, her physical state may deteriorate to the point of necessitating hospital admission for nutritional supplements.

Combination Therapy

The most practical approach to treating eating disorders during pregnancy would be the multidisciplinary approach. Cognitive-behavioral therapy and psychotherapy along with SSRIs and collaboration between all health care providers and supportive family members would be the ideal treatment strategy.[74] Studies have demonstrated that behavioral therapy is an essential component to the successful treatment of anorexia nervosa or bulimia nervosa. Although fewer studies have found successful results by using SSRIs solely to treat anorexia nervosa, data on bulimia nervosa are more promising and show fluoxetine specifically to be more effective than placebo but not as effective as cognitive-behavioral therapy alone.[75,76] More recent studies have examined the use of haloperidol and olanzapine in the treatment of anorexia nervosa.[77,78]

SUMMARY

Millions of childbearing women face the decision of whether to institute or continue taking psychotropic medication during pregnancy. Before recommending continuation, alteration, or induction of medications in preparation for or during pregnancy, the health care provider must determine the severity of illness, consider the mother's previous response to treatment and repercussions of untreated psychiatric illness, and review the potential adverse effects of the medication on the developing fetus. The provider and the patient must make a collaborative decision regarding treatment, and this decision must include a discussion and documentation of associated risks and benefits to both the mother and the unborn child.

Because the mother's decisions regarding the management of her illness may influence the course of her pregnancy and potentially the infant's outcome, input from the other medical professionals involved in the woman's pregnancy and the infant's care should be included whenever possible. A multidisciplinary approach to treatment of many of the most common psychiatric disorders is often preferable. A treatment plan that incorporates pharmacotherapy, psychotherapy, relaxation training, and case management and, if necessary, social service is likely to yield the best outcome for both the mother and her unborn child.

References

1. Cox JL, Holden JM, Sagovsky R: Detection of postnatal depression: Development of the 10-item Edinbugh Postnatal Depression Scale. Br J Psychol 1987;150:782-786.
2. O'Hara MW, Swain AM: Rates and risk of postpartum depression: A meta-analysis. Int Rev Psychiatry 1996;8:37.
3. Hughes P, Turton P, Hopper E, et al: Disorganised attachment behaviour among infants born subsequent to stillbirth. J Child Psychol Psychiatry 2001;42:791-801.
4. Kurki T, Vilho Hiilesmaa V, Raitasalo R, et al: Depression and anxiety in early pregnancy and risk for preeclampsia. Obstet Gynecol 2000; 95:487-490.
5. O'Conner TG, Herona J, Golding J, et al: Maternal antenatal anxiety and children's behavioral/emotional problems at 4 years. Br J Psychol 2002;180:502-508.
6. Groome LJ, Swiber MJ, Bentz LS, et al: Maternal anxiety during pregnancy: Effect on fetal behavior at 38-40 weeks of gestation. Dev Behav Pediatr 1995;16:391-396.
7. Hansen, D, Lou, HC, Olsen J: Serious life events and congenital malformations: A national study with complete follow-up. Lancet 2000;356:875-880.
8. Dole N, Savitz DA, Hertz-Picciotto I, et al: Maternal stress and preterm birth. Am J Epidemiol 2003;157:14-24.
9. Wadhwa, PD, Sandman CA, Porto M, et al: The association between prenatal stress and infant birth weight and gestational age at birth: A prospective investigation. Am J Obstet Gynecol 1993;169:858-865.
10. Copper RL, Goldenberg RL, Das A, et al: The preterm prediction study: Maternal stress is associated with spontaneous preterm birth at less than thirty-five weeks' gestation. National Institute of Child Health and Human Development Maternal-Fetal Medicine Units Network. Am J Obstet Gynecol 1996;175:1286-1292.
11. Susman EJ, Schmeelk KH, Ponirakis A, Gariepy JL: Maternal prenatal, postpartum and concurrent stressor and temperament in 3-year-olds: A person and variable analysis. Dev Psychopathol 2001;13:629-652.
12. Kent A, Hughes P, Omerod L, et al: Uterine artery resistance and anxiety in the second trimester of pregnancy. Ultrasound Obstet Gynecol 2002;19:177-179.
13. Gitau R, Cameron A, Fisk NM, Glover V: Fetal exposure to maternal cortisol. Lancet 1998;352:707-708.
14. Teratology Society, Public Affairs Committee: FDA classification of drugs for teratogenic risk. Teratology 1994;49:446-447.
15. Kessler RC, McGonagle KA, Swartz M, et al: Sex and depression in the National Comorbidity Survey I: Lifetime prevalence, chronicity, and recurrence. J Affect Disord 1993;29:85-96.
16. Evans J, Heron J, Francomb H, et al: Cohort study of depressed mood during pregnancy and after childbirth. BMJ 2001;323:257-260.
17. Viguera AC, Baldessarini RJ, Tondo L: Response to lithium maintenance treatment in bipolar disorders: Comparison of women and men. Bipolar Disord 2001;3:245-252.
18. Walter E, Epperson CN: Psychopharmacology during pregnancy. In Martin A, Leckman J, Lewis M, Cohen D (eds): Textbook of Child and Adolescent Psychopharmacology. New York, Oxford University Press, 2003, pp 642-653.
19. Chambers CD, Johnson KA, Dick LM, et al: Birth outcomes in pregnant women taking fluoxetine. N Engl J Med 1996;335:1010-1015.
20. Epperson CN, Ward-O'Brien D, Czarkowski KA, et al: Maternal sertraline treatment and platelet serotonin transport in breast-feeding mother/infant pairs. Am J Psychiatry 2001;158:1631-1637.
21. Hostetter A, Stowe ZN, Strader JR, et al: Dose of selective serotonin uptake inhibitors across pregnancy: Clinical implications. Depress Anxiety 2000;11:51-57.
22. Heikkinen T, Ekblad U, Palo P, Laine K: Pharmacokinetics of fluoxetine and norfluoxetine in pregnancy and lactation. Clin Pharmacol Ther 2003;73:330-337.
23. Cohen LS, Heller VL, Bailey JW, et al: Birth outcomes following prenatal exposure to fluoxetine. Biol Psychiatry 2000;48:996-1000.
24. Goldstein DJ: Effects of third trimester fluoxetine exposure on the newborn. J Clin Psychopharmacol 1995;15:417-420.
25. Costei AM, Kozer E, Ho T, et al: Perinatal outcome following third trimester exposure to paroxetine. Arch Pediatr Adolesc Med 2002;156:1129-1132.
26. Nordeng H, Lindemann R, Perminov KV, Reikvam A: Neonatal withdrawal syndrome after in utero exposure to selective serotonin reuptake inhibitors. Acta Pediatr 2001;90:288-291.
27. Nulman I, Rovet J, Stewart DE, et al: Neurodevelopment of children exposed in utero to antidepressant drugs. N Engl J Med 1997;336: 258-262.
28. Nulman I, Rovet J, Stewart DE, et al: Child development following exposure to tricyclic antidepressants or fluoxetine throughout fetal life: A prospective, controlled study. Am J Psychiatry 2002;159: 1889-1895.
29. Kulin NA, Pastuszak A, Sage SR, et al: Pregnancy outcome following maternal use of the new selective serotonin reuptake inhibitors: A prospective controlled multicenter study. JAMA 1998;279:609-610.

30. Altshuler LL, Cohen L, Szuba MP, et al: Pharmacologic management of psychiatric illness during pregnancy: Dilemmas and guidelines. Am J Psychiatry 1996;153:592-606.

31. Einarson A, Fatoye B, Sarkar M, et al: Pregnancy outcome following gestational exposure to venlafaxine: A multicenter prospective controlled study. Am J Psychiatry 2001;158:1728-1730.

32. Briggs GG, Freeman RK, Yaffe SJ: Drugs in Pregnancy and Lactation: A Reference Guide to Fetal and Neonatal Risk, 5th ed. Baltimore, Williams & Wilkins, 1998.

33. Spinelli MG, Endicott J: Controlled clinical trial of interpersonal psychotherapy versus parenting education program for depressed pregnant women. Am J Psychiatry 2003;160:555-562.

34. Oren DA, Wisner KL, Spinelli MG, et al: An open trial for morning light therapy for treatment of antepartum depression. Am J Psychiatry 2002;159:666-669.

35. Epperson CN, Jatlow PI, Czarkowski KA, Anderson GM: Maternal fluoxetine treatment in the postpartum period: Effects on platelet serotonin and plasma drug levels in breastfeeding mother-infant pairs. Pediatrics 2003;112:E425 [http://www.pediatrics.org].

36. Cohen LS, Friedman JM, Jefferson JW, et al: A reevaluation of risk of in utero exposure to lithium. JAMA 1994;271:146-150.

37. Miller LJ: Use of electroconvulsive therapy during pregnancy. Hosp Community Psychiatry 1994;45:444-450.

38. Kelly TE: Teratogenicity of anticonvulsant drugs. I: Review of the literature. Am J Med Genet 1984;19:413-434.

39. Jäger-Roman E, Deichl A, Jakob S, et al: Fetal growth, major malformations, and minor anomalies in infants born to women receiving valproic acid. J Pediatr 1986;108:997-1004.

40. Kaneko S, Otani K, Fukushima Y, et al: Teratogenicity of antiepileptic drugs: Analysis of possible risk factors. Epilepsia 1988;29:459-467.

41. Omtzigt JG, Nau H, Los FJ, et al: The disposition of valproate and its metabolites in the late first trimester and early second trimester of pregnancy in maternal serum, urine, and amniotic fluid: Effect of dose, co-medication, and the presence of spina bifida. Eur J Clin Pharmacol 1992;43:381-388.

41a. Samrén EB, vanDuijn CM, Christiaens GC, et al. Antiepileptic drug regimens and major congenital abnormalities in the offspring. Ann Neurol 1999;46:739-746.

42. Yerby MS, Leavitt A, Erickson DM, et al: Antiepileptics and the development of cognitive abnormalities. Neurology 1992;42:132-140.

43. Koch S, Titze K, Zimmermann RB, et al: Long-term neuropsychological consequences of maternal epilepsy and anticonvulsant treatment during pregnancy for school-age children and adolescents. Epilepsia 1999;40:1237-1246.

44. Gaily E, Kantola-Sorsa E, Granstrom M-J: Specific cognitive dysfunction in children with epileptic mothers. Dev Med Child Neurol 1990;32:403-414.

45. Scolnik D, Nulman I, Rovet J, et al: Neurodevelopment of children exposed in utero to phenytoin and carbamazepine monotherapy. JAMA 1994;271:767-770.

46. Tennis P, Eldridge RR: Preliminary results on pregnancy outcomes in women using lamotrigine. Epilepsia 2002;43:1161-1167.

47. Viner MW, Chen Y, Bakshi I, Kamper P: Low-dose risperidone augmentation of antidepressants in nonpsychotic depressive disorders with suicidal ideation [Letter]. J Clin Psychopharmacol 2003;23:104-106.

48. Marek GJ, Carpenter LL, McDougle CJ, Price LH: Synergistic action of 5-HT2A antagonists and selective serotonin reuptake inhibitors in neuropsychiatric disorders. Neuropsychopharmacology 2003;28:402-412.

49. Goldstein DJ, Cortin LA, Fung MC: Olanzapine-exposed pregnancies and lactation: Early experience. J Clin Psychopharmacol 2000;20:399-403.

50. Sholomskas DE, Wickamaratne PJ, Dogolo L, et al: Postpartum onset of panic disorder: A coincidental event? J Clin Psychiatry 1993;54:476-480.

51. Epperson CN, McDougle CJ, Brown RM, et al: Obsessive compulsive disorder during pregnancy and the puerperium. Presented at the New Research Poster Session, NR 12, Annual Meeting of the American Psychiatric Association, Miami Beach, Fla, May 22, 1995.

52. Williams KE, Koran LM: Obsessive-compulsive disorder in pregnancy, the puerperium, and the premenstruum. J Clin Psychiatry 1997;58:330-334.

53. Villeponteaux VA, Lydiard R, Laraia MT, et al: The effects of pregnancy on preexisting panic disorder. J Clin Psychiatry 1992;53:201-203.

54. Cohen LS, Sichel DA, Dimmock JA, Rosenbaum J: Impact of pregnancy on panic disorder: A case series. J Clin Psychiatry 1994;55:284-288.

55. Klein DF: False suffocation alarms, spontaneous panics and related conditions: An integrative hypothesis. Arch Gen Psychiatry 1993;50:306-317.

56. Cohen LS, Rosenbaum J, Heller VL: Panic attack–associated placental abruption: A case report. J Clin Psychiatry 1989;50:266-267.

57. Turton P, Hughes P, Evans CDH, Fainman D: Incidence, correlates and predictors of post-traumatic stress disorder in the pregnancy after stillbirth. Br J Psychol 2001;178:556-560.

58. Dolovich L, Addis A, Vaillancourt JMR, et al: Benzodiazepine use in pregnancy and malformations or oral clefts: Meta-analysis of cohort and case-control studies. BMJ 1998;317:839-843.

59. Viggedal G, Hagberg BS, Laegreid L, Aronsson M: Mental development in late infancy after prenatal exposure to benzodiazepines—a prospective study. J Child Psychol Psychiatry 1993;34:295-305.

60. Epperson CN, Yamamoto B, Wisner K: Gonadal steroids in the treatment of mood disorders. Psychosom Med 1999;61:676-697.

61. Bennedsen BE: Adverse pregnancy outcome in schizophrenic women: Occurrence and risk factors. Schizophr Res 1998;33:1-26.

62. Howard LM, Kumar C, Leese M, Thornicroft G: The general fertility rate in women with psychotic disorders. Am J Psychiatry 2002;159:991-997.

63. Hagopian GS, Meyers DB, Markham JK: Teratology studies of LY170053 in rats and rabbits. Teratology 1987;35:60a-61a.

64. Slone D, Siskind V, Heinonen OP, et al: Antenatal exposure to the phenothiazines in relation to congenital malformations, perinatal mortality rate, birth weight, and intelligence quotient score. Am J Obstet Gynecol 1977;128:486-488.

65. Little L, Lowkes E: Critical issues in the care of pregnant women with eating disorders and the impact on their children. J Midwifery Womens Health 2000;45:301-307.

66. Strober M, Freeman R, Lampert C, et al: Controlled family study of anorexia nervosa and bulimia nervosa: Evidence of shared liability and transmission of partial syndromes. Am J Psychiatry 2000;157:393-401.

67. Stewart DE, Raskin J, Garfinkel PE, et al: Anorexia nervosa, bulimia and pregnancy. Am J Obstet Gynecol 1987;157:1194-1198.

68. Lacey JH, Smith G: Bulimia nervosa: The impact of pregnancy on mother and baby. Br J Psychol 1987;150:777-781.

69. Stein A, Murray L, Cooper P, Fairburn CG: Infant growth in the context of maternal eating disorder and maternal depression: A comparative study. Psychol Med 1996;26:569-574.

70. Brinch M, Isager T, Tolstrup K: Anorexia and motherhood: Reproduction pattern and mothering behavior of fifty women. Acta Psychiatr Scand 1988;77:611-617.

71. Van der Spuy ZM, Steer PJ, McCusker M, et al: Outcome of pregnancy in underweight women after spontaneous and induced ovulation. BMJ 1988;296:962-965.

72. Fairburn CF, Welch SL: The impact of pregnancy on eating habits and attitudes to shape and weight. Int J Eat Disord 1990;9:153-160.

73. Erick M: Eating disorders: A few more thoughts. J Am Diet Assoc 2002;102:477.

74. James DC: Eating disorders, fertility, and pregnancy: Relationships and complications. J Perinat Neonatal Nurs 2001;15:36-48.

75. Mitchell JE, Fletcher L, Hanson K, et al: The relative efficacy of fluoxetine and manual-based self-help in the treatment of outpatients with bulimia nervosa. J Clin Psychopharmacol 2001;21:298-304.

76. Mitchell JE, Peterson CB, Myers T, Wonderlich S: Combining pharmacotherapy and psychotherapy in the treatment of patients with eating disorders. Psychiatr Clin North Am 2001;24:315-323.

77. Cassano GB, Miniati M, Pini S, et al: Six-month open trial of haloperidol as an adjunctive treatment for anorexia nervosa: A preliminary report. Int J Eat Disord 2003;33:172-177.

78. Malina A, Gaskill J, McConaha C, et al: Olanzapine treatment of anorexia nervosa: A retrospective study. Int J Eat Disord 2003;33:234-237.

79. Montouris G: Gabapentin exposure in human pregnancy: Results from the Gabapentin Pregnancy Registry. 2003;4:310-317.

80. Palmieri C, Canger R: Teratogenic potential of the newer antiepileptic drugs. CNS Drugs 2002;16:755-756.

81. Mohan MS, Patole SK, Whitehall JS: Severe hypothermia in a neonate following antenatal exposure to haloperidol. J Paediatr Child Health 2000;36:412-3.

25

SUBSTANCE ABUSE

Ellen D. Mason and Richard V. Lee

Drug and alcohol use during pregnancy is a common phenomenon and a significant public health issue. Since 1970, the lay public and the medical and the scientific communities have become increasingly aware that women's lifestyles and behaviors can adversely affect pregnancy outcomes, fetal growth, and long-term child development. The fetal alcohol syndrome (FAS) was first described in the 1970s, at a time when consumption of alcohol by women of reproductive age had became a social norm and was increasing in amount and frequency. A decade later, an epidemic of crack cocaine use during the 1980s, followed by a surge of inhaled opiate use in the 1990s, expanded the population of chemically dependent women and perinatally exposed children.

Studies of substance abuse during pregnancy document a high incidence of adverse and, sometimes, catastrophic perinatal outcomes associated with intrauterine drug and alcohol exposure. Adverse outcomes associated with perinatal substance exposures have an effect on many social systems, including the health care system, the criminal justice system, and the educational system, and on child protective agencies. Although exact data are not available, estimates of costs associated with treated perinatally exposed children are daunting. A single drug-exposed child with serious impairments may need up to $750,000 of health and special education services by age 18.[1] Bloss and colleagues estimated that it cost $1.9 billion dollars in 1992 to provide care for infants, children, and surviving adults in whom FAS and its sequelae were diagnosed.[2]

In the years after the peak of the crack cocaine epidemic, enormous national resources were mobilized to study the problem of perinatal alcohol and drug exposure through laboratory, epidemiologic, and clinical research. Expanded national research funding, together with greater allocation of philanthropic and local resources, has supported a "second wave" of increasingly rigorous investigation into the field of perinatal substance use. Results from many completed studies are now available, as are recent meta-analyses and reviews of the literature. This chapter is a discussion of the current state of knowledge regarding the effect of licit and illicit substances on maternal health, obstetric outcomes, fetal growth and development, and long-term child health status. The epidemiology of drug, alcohol, and tobacco use during pregnancy is reviewed, as are gender-specific issues of addiction in women. Approaches to screening pregnant women for substance use, management protocols for substance-exposed pregnancies, and recommendations for referral to substance abuse treatment are presented.

PREVALENCE AND DEMOGRAPHIC CORRELATES OF SUBSTANCE USE IN PREGNANCY

Substance use in pregnancy is a global phenomenon that affects all races, is present in all social classes, and is found in most regions. Accurate data on prevalence are difficult to obtain. Maternal self-report of drug or alcohol use in pregnancy generally provides underestimate of prevalence.[3-6] Denial, shame, and fears of sanction or even of criminal prosecution prevent women from providing true information when questioned during pregnancy. Studies of perinatal drug use done in single hospitals often report very high numbers of perinatally exposed infants, particularly when toxicology screening is selectively obtained on indigent minority women. Prevalence investigations that rely on single maternal urine toxicology tests to establish perinatal drug or alcohol use underestimate fetal exposure because they can detect only drugs used a few days before testing. Despite limitations, useful information about perinatal substance exposure is now available from around the world.

International reports from Europe, Asia, and Africa have documented increasing rates of perinatal drug and alcohol use, although screening methods in different countries vary considerably and the populations studied often do not represent the general population. Pregnancy-specific data are not available for the majority of countries; however, in 1999 the World Health Organization Global Illicit Drug Trends reported that 3% to 4% of the global population abuses one or more illicit drugs and that exposure, particularly intravenous drug use among women, has been increasing, especially in developing countries.[7,8] Increased use of alcohol, opiates, and amphetamines during pregnancy is reported worldwide in developed and developing countries.[9-12]

Of particular concern are reports that the prevalence of FAS is increasing in areas affected by political and economic challenges, such as South Africa.[13]

In the United States, estimates of alcohol and drug use by pregnant women have fluctuated somewhat since 1990 by region and in accordance with secular drug use trends. Reliable, generalizable data has been generated by statewide prevalence studies and well-designed national surveys. Between 1989 and 1992, four states—Rhode Island,[14] Ohio,[15] California,[16] and Utah[17]—carried out large-scale studies of perinatal substance use rates by performing anonymous tests on maternal or neonatal urine for metabolites of illicit drugs and for alcohol. From 1990 to 1991, South Carolina performed a statewide assessment of perinatal drug use that screened both maternal urine and neonatal meconium.[18] The California study revealed that 11.2% of pregnant women presenting to a hospital for delivery had used alcohol, cocaine, marijuana, benzodiazepines, amphetamines, barbiturates, opiates, methadone, or phencyclidine (PCP). Urine screens in Rhode Island yielded positive results for illicit drugs in 7.5% of pregnant women presenting for delivery. In South Carolina, screens yielded positive results for alcohol or at least one licit or illicit substance in 25.8% of pregnant women. The higher numbers of positive tests found in the South Carolina study may be attributed to the inclusion of neonatal meconium testing, inasmuch as this substance is a reservoir for drug metabolites and reflects fetal drug exposures occurring throughout the second and third trimesters.

A broader view of drug use during pregnancy is available from national survey data. From 1992 to 1993, the National Institute of Drug Abuse (NIDA) conducted a unique survey of perinatal drug use in pregnancy.[19] The survey gathered data from a large national sample of women who delivered in 52 urban and rural hospitals. Information on drug use was obtained by questionnaire as well as anonymous maternal urine toxicology testing. According to these data, 5.5% of the women who gave birth in 1992 used illicit drugs while they were pregnant. Marijuana and cocaine were the most frequently used illicit drugs; 2.9% of the women used marijuana, and 1.1% of the women used cocaine at some time during their pregnancy. The survey found a high incidence of cigarette and alcohol use among pregnant women. At some point during pregnancy, 20.4% of the women smoked cigarettes and 18.8% drank alcohol.

Recent information about maternal substance use is available from the 2001 and the 1999/2000 National Household Surveys on Drug Abuse (NHSDA).[20,21] These telephone surveys are designed to capture data on illicit drug use and nonmedical use of prescription drugs such as analgesics, tranquilizers, and stimulants in the general population of the United States. Women participating in these surveys are asked specifically whether they are pregnant and whether they have used illicit drugs in the month before the interview. Overall, in 2001, 3.7% of pregnant women questioned said that they had used drugs in the month before the survey. In the 1999/2000 survey, 3.0% said that they had used an illicit drug in the month before interview, and 12% said that they had drunk alcohol during that time period. Pregnant adolescents between the ages of 15 and 17 reported a higher use rate (15.1% in the 2001 survey) than did other women. Although rates of substance use by pregnant women in the general surveys may appear lower than those reported in the earlier, pregnancy-specific survey, it is important to remember that population-wide telephone surveys provide conservative estimates of alcohol and illicit drug use because they reflect use only in 1 month and not during the entire pregnancy. In addition, these surveys do not include corroborative measures such as urine toxicology testing, which yields additional positive results.

Specific findings from the NHSDA surveys reveal encouraging trends, as well as new areas of deep concern. Perhaps as a result of extensive public education campaigns directed toward prevention of birth defects, pregnant women contacted in the 1999/2000 survey reported significant decreases in alcohol use over the three trimesters and a trend toward decreasing drug use after the first trimester. Although exposure rates remain highest during the period of gestation in which the fetus is most vulnerable, when organogenesis is occurring, decreased use later may prevent adverse effects on fetal growth and the development of the central nervous system.

It is disturbing that the NHSDA survey reports rates of binge drinking by 8.8% of women during the first trimester and by 2.3% during the second trimester. Binge drinking, which is defined as drinking five or more drinks on the same occasion or at least once in 30 days, is associated with a high incidence of FAS.[22-24] Other disquieting information from the 2001 NHSDA survey, as well as from the Community Epidemiology Work Group (CEWG)[25] (the latter is a national working group that assesses drug abuse patterns and trends yearly by city and state), indicate that an increasing percentage of the United States population is using illicit drugs. These surveys report increases in the use of marijuana, cocaine, and hallucinogens, particularly the "club drug" 3,4-methylenedioxymethamphetamine (MDMA),[26] often referred to as "ecstasy."

Although popular opinion and the media tend to view perinatal substance use as essentially a problem of ethnic poor women, data from county, state, and national surveys refute this myth. The NIDA National Pregnancy and Health Survey found that 11.3% of African American women, 4.4% of non-Hispanic white women, and 4.5% of Hispanic women used illicit drugs during pregnancy. National prevalence date showed that white women had the highest rate of alcohol use of any group. In Utah, anonymous testing of prenatal patients' urine was performed in 10 clinics across the state. The patient population, which was 85% white and largely middle class, had a 5.5% rate of illicit drug use and a 5.2% rate of alcohol use. These rates were consistent with national data. A landmark study was done by Chasnoff and associates in Pinellas County, Florida, in 1989.[27] The investigators performed anonymous screens on all pregnant women registering for antenatal care in 5 public and 12 private clinics. Fifteen percent of the women had positive test results for alcohol, opiates, cocaine, or cannabinoids. Positive urine screens were not related to race or socioeconomic status as determined by insurance type. In this population, white women tended to have higher rates of cannabinoid use, whereas black women had higher rates of cocaine use.

Although race is not predictive of substance use per se during pregnancy, other factors appear to be strongly correlated. The 1992 NIDA Pregnancy and Health Survey found a strong link between cigarette smoking and the use of alcohol or illicit drugs. Socioeconomic status and age were correlated with specific drug use. Marijuana use was more common among younger women, and cocaine and alcohol, among older women. Rates of cocaine and marijuana use were higher in unmarried women, unemployed women, and women with less than 4 years of college. Of note, in the NIDA study, predictors for alcohol use during pregnancy were surprising. Women who drank during pregnancy tended to be college educated, to be working, and to have private health insurance.

PSYCHOSOCIAL CORRELATES OF SUBSTANCE ABUSING WOMEN

Pregnancy does not occur in a vacuum but is an event that is superimposed on the context and circumstances of women's lives. Substance-abusing women have a high incidence of social and psychologic comorbid conditions that affect their health status, their ability to engage in prenatal care, and their ability to succeed in drug abuse treatment. Comorbid conditions become more important considerations when the biologic and psychologic stress of pregnancy is added to an already fragile system.

Studies of women enrolled in substance abuse treatment programs indicate a high rate of coexisting psychiatric disorders, particularly affective and anxiety disorders. Depression is common in women who use opiates, cocaine, and alcohol.[28,29] The incidence of depression in substance-using pregnant women may be as high as 74%.[30,31] In a study of alcoholic women, one investigator found that suicide attempts were five times more frequent among the subjects than in a control population.[32] Substance-abusing women also have an unusually high incidence of post-traumatic stress disorder, ranging from 25% to 59%, as documented in multiple studies of either current or lifetime symptoms.[33-35]

In addition to grappling with the debilitating effects of mental illness, substance-using women are frequently affected by difficult issues stemming from childhood experiences. In studies of women seeking treatment for alcoholism or opiate dependency, investigators reported that up to 60% of enrollees had a parent or a close relative with a history of alcoholism or substance abuse.[36,37] Although intergenerational patterns of substance abuse are thought to have a genetic component, as demonstrated by twin and adoption studies,[38,39] environmental factors such as poor or neglectful parenting are implicated in adoption studies as well.[40,41] Tragically, a large number of alcoholic and drug-using women suffered abuse as children, particularly sexual abuse. Numerous studies, including large epidemiologic studies, have shown that the experience of abuse in childhood is a potent risk factor for drug abuse by women.[42,43] A study of adult twins by Kendler and colleagues[44] found that women who experienced any type of sexual abuse in childhood were approximately three times more likely than nonabused girls to become drug dependent as adults.

The difficult pasts of substance-abusing women are frequently followed by problematic, dangerous relationships in adult life. Substance-using women are often victims of domestic violence, which may increase in frequency and severity during pregnancy.[45] The combination of drug abuse and physical violence has been shown to result in adverse pregnancy outcomes, including abortions, miscarriages, and preterm labor.[46,47]

Studies of women in substance abuse treatment show that approximately two thirds have experienced violence from adult partners.[48,49] The abusive partner is often a substance user himself who has initiated his partner into drug abuse and who provides drugs and alcohol to the woman.

ADDICTION: BIOLOGY AND VOCABULARY

Psychoactive substance use began millennia before written records. During many epochs and in many societies, regular use of mood- and perception-altering drugs has been considered acceptable, normal behavior. The tradition of women using substances as part of their roles as shamans or curanderas is an ancient one.[50] In a very real sense, "drug abuse" is a culturally defined term. Most people in our society use at least one psychoactive substance, be it caffeine, nicotine, or alcohol, and many have experienced a transient or serious health consequence from such use. However, most substance users do not have a diagnosable disorder.

Because heroin, cocaine, and lysergic acid diethylamide (LSD) are illegal, society calls a single use of these substances "drug abuse." However, for the purposes of understanding the effects of regular alcohol or drug use on a pregnancy, it is important to distinguish between chronic or binge use of substances and a single or several exposures. Predictable biologic, psychologic, and physiologic consequences result from regular drug use. It is unclear whether a single or several uses of an illicit substance or prescription drug taken for recreational purposes during pregnancy (with the exception of binge alcohol use) can be unequivocally tied to a specific adverse pregnancy outcome. This observation is not to condone casual illicit drug use or to excuse the use of illicit drugs at any time during pregnancy. Rather, it is to establish the fact that substance abuse per se (i.e., excessive self-administration of chemicals that change the user's perceptions, mood, or consciousness) produces an intricate set of emotional, physical, and behavioral abnormalities that adversely affect maternal and fetal health.

Alcohol and all drugs of abuse act on the deep, central, and anterior regions of the brain: that is, the mesolimbic system, which flows from the locus ceruleus through the ventral tectum and nucleus accumbens to the amygdala and prefrontal cortex. These structures are associated with the sensation of pleasure and with development of rewarding, reinforcing behaviors. All substances of abuse affect mesolimbic dopaminergic pathways through a variety of mechanisms, facilitating dopamine release and preventing dopamine reuptake. Over time, repeated dopaminergic surges "rewire" neuronal circuitry. Other neurotransmitter systems and neuroreceptors are altered as well; ultimately, tolerance, as well as physical and psychologic dependence, is created. When a state of dependence is in effect, experience of withdrawal symptoms is inevitable when drug effects wear off.

Alcohol and all illicit drugs cross the placenta freely, entering the fetal circulation and the fetus's central nervous system, as they do in the adult. Substances of abuse taken during pregnancy therefore affect fetal neurotransmitter levels and fetal neuron development. It is hypothesized that perinatal exposure to substances of abuse has the potential to permanently change brain structure and function. Drug-seeking behaviors and withdrawal have been seen in perinatally exposed animal offspring. It remains unclear however, to what extent animal studies are predictive of human outcomes. This is especially true because human behaviors are shaped tremendously by the effects of postnatal environment and experiences.

The Vocabulary of Addiction

The official definition of *substance dependence*, according to the 4th edition of the *Diagnostic and Statistical Manual of Mental Disorders* (DSM-IV),[51] is a maladaptive pattern of substance use that leads to significant impairment or distress as manifested by three or more of the following occurring in a 12-month period:

1. tolerance, as defined by need for increasing amounts of the substance to achieve intoxication, or markedly diminished effect with continued use of the same amount of the substance
2. withdrawal, as manifested by withdrawal symptoms or prophylactic substance use to avoid withdrawal symptoms
3. increasing substance use over time
4. unsuccessful attempts to cut down or control substance use
5. inordinate time spent obtaining substances
6. abandonment of important social and occupational activities
7. continued substance use despite knowledge of a physical or psychologic problem that can be caused or worsened by use

The DSM-IV definition of *substance abuse* stipulates that one or more of the following occur in a 12-month period:

1. Substance use results in failure to fulfill major role obligations in work and personal life.
2. Substance use occurs in situations in which it is physically hazardous.
3. Substance use is associated with recurrent legal problems.
4. Substance use continues despite persistence of social or interpersonal problems.

From these definitions, it is clear that regular or binge use of substances during pregnancy nearly always meets criteria for abuse or dependence, because use at this time always has the potential to affect fetal development and pregnancy outcome.

DRUGS OF ABUSE: EFFECTS ON PREGNANCY AND OFFSPRING

Overview

Almost any substance taken by a pregnant woman has the potential to affect maternal health or fetal development. Most drugs of abuse (Tables 25–1 and 25–2) have been shown to have some deleterious effects during intrauterine life or on postnatal development. The clinician caring for pregnant women needs to distinguish between "casual" substance use, unassociated with dependence and addiction, and repeated or frequent use. The latter is much more clearly associated with specific drug effects and predictably results in disorganization of maternal life, poor hygiene, and poor nutritional status. The chaotic lifestyle associated with drug use during pregnancy increases the incidence of acute and chronic maternal infections, preterm labor, and premature birth and low birth weight.[52-54]

Numerous preclinical studies with animal models have tried to identify specific effects of specific drugs on fetal growth and development. Animal studies have unequivocally shown that fetal exposure to commonly abused drugs produces gross and microscopic structural abnormalities in offspring, particularly in the central nervous system. Intrauterine drug administration to pregnant animals results in developmental changes in brains of the exposed offspring, including alterations in neuronal numbers and density, in neuronal migration and differentiation, and in measurement of absolute amounts and ratios of neurotransmitters, such as dopamine and serotonin. What remains unclear is whether similar changes occur in exposed human brains and whether structural and functional alterations of the human central nervous system, if they occur, cause predictable, permanent impairments in global functions such as learning and behavior in children and adults. Current ongoing studies include structural and functional neuroimaging as part of the longitudinal evaluation of perinatally substance-exposed children.[55]

The difficulty of determining *drug-specific* effects of perinatal drug exposure arises in part from the immense problem of multiple confounding factors in human studies that measure child outcomes. Most studies of drug-exposed children have been done on urban populations of socially disadvantaged women and children who suffer from high

---

TABLE 25–1 Drugs of Abuse

Alcohol
Cocaine/amphetamines*
Opiates†
Marijuana
Sedatives/hypnotics‡
Hallucinogens
Phencyclidine
Volatile substances§
Nicotine

---

*Includes "designer drugs" such as 3,4-methylenedioxymethamphetamine (MDMA), methylenedioxyamphetamine (MDA), and methylphenidate (Ritalin).
†Includes synthetic opioids such as fentanyl and oxycodone (OxyContin).
‡Includes flunitrazepam (Rohypnol) and γ-hydroxybutyrate (GBH).
§Includes toluene, glue, aerosol propellants, gasoline, lighter fluid, correction fluid, etc.

TABLE 25–2 Effects of Substance Abuse on Pregnancy and Progeny

Mother	Fetus	Neonate
Withdrawal syndrome	Withdrawal syndrome	Withdrawal syndrome
Tolerance	Tolerance	Tolerance
Overdose	Intrauterine growth restriction	Congenital anomalies
Biochemical disarray	Teratogenesis	Developmental disorders
Death	Intrauterine fetal death	Sudden infant death syndrome
Coma	Congenital abnormalities	Congenital infection
Abruptio placentae	Premature labor	Child abuse/neglect
Addiction	Congenital infection	Trauma
Premature labor	Intrauterine infection	
Malnutrition	Premature delivery	
Infections		
Inadequate prenatal and medical care		
Physical and sexual abuse		
Chronic and acute illness		
Trauma		
Chaos, loss of social supports		

rates of poverty, violence, unemployment, poor nutrition, inadequate medical care, inadequate housing, and unstable family situations.[56] It is extremely difficult to control for the effects of these variables, particularly in smaller samples, when infant and child growth and development are evaluated longitudinally.

Apart from the issue of confounding variables, understanding the effects of drug and alcohol use in human pregnancy is hampered by difficulties in accurately ascertaining the quantity of drug exposure, the gestational timing of exposure, and the duration of exposure. In a study of outcomes in cocaine-using women in relation to frequency of use, "light" users were found to have obstetric outcomes that were the same as those in nonusers.[57] Additional uncertainty in outcomes is introduced by the incompletely characterized genetic heterogeneity of human drug metabolism and genetic variations in fetal susceptibility to drug induced harm.

Polysubstance use introduces additional complexity into the analysis of drug effects on pregnancy. It is well established that the majority of women who use drugs regularly during pregnancy use many substances concurrently. Combining drugs such as cocaine and alcohol can result in the formation of toxic intermediate compounds, such as cocaethylene, that may be more toxic than either drug alone.[58,59] Of more importance is that most drug-abusing women use alcohol and tobacco. Both of these are well known to cause fetal harm by themselves. Analyses of pregnancy outcomes in drug-using women are frequently uncorrected for the effects of these substances. In a database of 101 studies of effects of perinatal cocaine, 23% did not control for alcohol use, and 25% did not control for nicotine exposure.[60] Failure to control for nicotine exposure when drug effects on pregnancy are studied is particularly

problematic, because many adverse perinatal outcomes associated with drug and alcohol use are highly correlated with isolated nicotine exposure.[61-63] Tobacco by itself causes more low birth weight and infant mortality than any other substance.[64]

The literature on perinatal substance use continues to be affected by a bias against the publication of negative studies. The data available to clinicians are therefore not as robust as they might be. Koren and colleagues reviewed the rejection rate for manuscripts on cocaine use in pregnancy submitted for publication and found a higher rate of rejection of studies reporting negative effects than for studies reporting positive effects, even when the negative studies were more methodologically rigorous.[65] Reasons for this bias are not clear but may be related to maintenance of research funding and the editorial policies of journals, as well as the fact that research on illicit drugs has a moral dimension that is lacking in other areas of clinical investigation.

Because so much of what is currently known about the effects of illicit drugs on child health and development is drawn from studies that are methodologically flawed, it is encouraging that a multicenter, prospective cohort study of the effects of cocaine and opiate exposure during pregnancy that is more rigorous than previous studies is currently under way in the United States. The Maternal Lifestyles Study (MLS), which is being sponsored by the National Institute of Child Health and Human Development, is the largest clinical study that has ever been undertaken to date, to investigate the short- and long-term consequences of illicit drug exposure. The MLS, which consists of four peer review–selected research centers, has screened and enrolled 11,800 mother-infant dyads from 1993 to 1995. Drug exposure in this study was determined by a combination of maternal history, together with gas chromatography and mass spectroscopic analysis of cocaine or opiate metabolites in infant meconium. The study consists of three phases. Phase I addresses all outcomes up to hospital discharge of mother and infant. Phase II is a follow-up of a subsample of exposed infants and a matched comparison group assessed at 1 to 3 months of age, corrected for gestational age. Phase III of the MLS study extends follow-up into school age, through the seventh year of life.

The findings from phase I of the MLS up to and including the time of delivery have been published.[66] Important baseline characteristics of the study group include a 93% rate of alcohol/tobacco and marijuana use among the cocaine-/opiate-using women, in comparison with a 42% use rate among the control women. The investigators report a relatively low frequency of adverse acute obstetric effects in the cohort of drug-using women in comparison with previous studies. Common medical complications of pregnancy such as urinary tract infections and preeclampsia were low and equal in prevalence in both drug-using and control women. The authors did, however, note significantly elevated odds ratios for infectious complications such as syphilis, gonorrhea, hepatitis, and human immunodeficiency virus (HIV) infection in the substance-using mothers. Chlamydia and gonorrhea were commoner among cocaine-using women; hepatitis and HIV infection were commoner in the opiate-exposed cohort.

Hospitalization rates for both drug-using and control groups did not differ, although there was a 19-fold increase in hospitalization specifically related to violence among the substance-using mothers. Conditions that have traditionally been associated with cocaine use, such as antepartum hemorrhage (from placental abruption and placenta previa) were more prevalent in the exposed group but occurred overall in less than 3% of the substance-using mothers. Greater than expected use of prenatal care services by the substance-using group of women may explain, in part, the lower than expected incidence of medical and obstetric complications. Future publications from the MLS will focus on infant and child development measures, as well as measures of parenting and mother-child bonding.

Effects of Specific Substances of Abuse

Alcohol

Despite a decade-long public education campaign warning women about the dangers of drinking alcohol during pregnancy, alcohol use in pregnancy remains common and is a major cause of adverse pregnancy outcomes. Estimates of the prevalence of drinking during pregnancy vary. Approximately half of American women drink alcohol. Self-report data from the Behavioral Risk Factor Surveillance System,[67] a state-based survey sponsored by the Centers for Disease Control and Prevention, indicate that about 12% to 15% of women in the reproductive years drink frequently (defined as seven or more drinks per week or five or more drinks on any one occasion during the past month). Overall, the prevalence of heavy drinking in women 21 to 34 years of age increased from the 1960s through the early 1990s.[68] With the exception of increased heavy drinking among college-aged women, alcohol consumption in women has remained stable since the early 1990s. Drinking alcohol during pregnancy is correlated with maternal age of more than 35 years and with lack of prenatal care.[69]

Medical/Obstetric Complications of Alcohol Use

Well-established complications of chronic alcohol abuse and heavy alcohol use, such as hypertension, pancreatitis, alcoholic hepatitis, and alcohol withdrawal, occur in pregnant women as frequently as they do in nonpregnant women. Women who drink more than 2.0 to 2.9 drinks per day appear to have greater health risks than do men, including a higher relative risk for death from all causes.[70] Women also develop alcoholic liver disease sooner than men, after consuming lower levels of alcohol.[71] In a study of asymptomatic women undergoing outpatient treatment for alcoholism whose mean age was 39 ± 9.7 years, the risk of alcoholic cardiomyopathy and myopathy was higher among these women than in men.[72] It is thus disquieting that Witlin and colleagues noted an association between alcohol abuse and peripartum cardiomyopathy.[73] It is possible that as the age of first drinking decreases and heavier alcohol consumption by women of reproductive age becomes a social norm, the incidence of this serious pregnancy complication may rise.

Alcohol can affect reproductive function in a number of ways. Chronic heavy alcohol intake, defined as more than 10 drinks per week, is associated with significant decreases in fertility.[74] Advanced chronic liver disease has been associated with anovulatory cycles.[75] An increased risk of spontaneous abortion is reported among women who drink during pregnancy. It is unclear whether this is a direct affect of alcohol toxicity on the early conceptus or related to alcohol-induced maternal disorders. Pregnancy losses in general are commoner in women who drink heavily.[76,77] Oddly, although alcohol was once widely used as a tocolytic agent, drinking during the third trimester is associated with increased odds of preterm delivery.[78]

Alcohol abuse is associated with vitamin and mineral deficiencies that can lead to anemia or thrombocytopenia. Pregnant alcohol abusers have inadequate intake of essential nutrients at a time when nutritional requirements are increased. Alcohol-mediated malabsorption of food can result in deficiencies of thiamine, folic acid, pyridoxine, iron, zinc, and other micronutrients. Animal studies suggest that some nutritional deficiencies potentiate the teratogenicity of alcohol.[79-81] Additional studies suggest that enhanced nutrition during pregnancy can ameliorate alcohol's toxicity.[82,83] Differences in nutritional status may explain why FAS occurs disproportionately among the children of low-income women in comparison with those of women of higher socioeconomic status.[84]

Effects of Alcohol on the Fetus

Alcohol has been called the leading teratogen in the western world because a vast literature linking it with a wide spectrum of birth defects and fetal growth abnormalities has accumulated. It is, in fact, the only really predictable teratogen among the substances of abuse. Alcohol use during pregnancy is the commonest cause of mental retardation in the United States and is estimated to account for up to 5% of all congenital anomalies.[85,86] The teratogenicity of alcohol appears to be, in part, genetically determined, inasmuch as certain populations, such as the Apache and Ute tribes in the southwestern United States and aboriginal Canadians, have a much higher incidence of alcohol-related birth defects than does the general population.[87]

Fetal physiology is directly disrupted, throughout gestation, by the direct effects of alcohol and its primary metabolite acetaldehyde. Acetaldehyde is both cytotoxic and teratogenic. Very intriguing studies indicate that polymorphisms in the alleles of the alcohol dehydrogenase (ADH) 2 gene may result in differential ADH enzymatic activity in pregnant individuals, thereby producing higher acetaldehyde levels in some women than in others drinking equivalent amounts of alcohol. Low levels of acetaldehyde in women who metabolize acetaldehyde rapidly may explain the lower incidence and lack of alcohol-related birth defects seen in the children of some heavy drinkers and some members of high-risk populations.[88-90]

Although fetal toxicity is attributed to alcohol and its metabolites, there is a spectrum of mechanisms by which alcohol ingested during pregnancy interferes with normal maternal and fetal physiology. These metabolic abnormalities have been extensively studied and are still under investigation.[91-93] Administration of alcohol to pregnant animals results in decreased placental blood flow and alterations in critical placental functions such as amino acid transport. Alcohol-induced changes in maternal carbohydrate metabolism can cause maternal hypoglycemia. Alcohol has been shown to decrease fetal protein and DNA synthesis, inhibit cell migration, and increase the formation of free radicals. Abnormalities in insulin-like growth factors have also been demonstrated in alcohol-exposed fetuses, possibly accounting for some of the growth impairment frequently associated with fetal alcohol exposure.[94] Elevated erythropoietin levels found in the cord blood of human alcohol abusers are believed to be indirect evidence of chronic fetal hypoxemia.[95]

Fetal Alcohol Syndrome: Background and Definition

Warnings against drinking during pregnancy have been found in the writings of ancient Greek philosophers and in the Old Testament.[96] A publication in the late 19th century reported doubled infant mortality and stillborn rates among the children of drinking mothers in comparison with nondrinking mothers.[97] Remarkably, research on alcohol in multiple pregnant animal models done between 1900 and 1920 reported that alcoholic progeny produced smaller litters but "superior" offspring.[98] After a gap of 50 years, scientific observations regarding the deleterious effects of alcohol on human offspring appeared in 1968, when Lemoine and associates described a common pattern of birth defects born to alcoholic French mothers.[99] A landmark paper by Jones and colleagues that appeared 5 years later in the English literature described a constellation of malformations and growth abnormalities (FAS).[100] Since the early 1970s, the specific teratogenic effects of alcohol have been confirmed by a large body of animal research, as well as clinical and epidemiologic studies in humans.

The effects of alcohol on fetal development are partially dose dependent and partially genetically determined. Estimates of the prevalence of FAS in the United States range from 6.7 per 10,000 to 2 per 1000 live births.[101,102] Data from the Fetal Alcohol Syndrome Surveillance Network, which is sponsored by the Centers for Disease Control and Prevention, found rates of FAS ranging from 0.3 to 1.5 per 1000 live births.[103] There was considerable state-to-state variation. The highest prevalence was found in Alaska, a state with a large population of Native Americans and Alaska Natives. Quoted numbers vary, according to whether birth certificate data or aggregated data sources are used. Fetal alcohol effects are seen in approximately 30% to 40% of neonates whose mothers consumed two or more ounces of absolute alcohol daily throughout the first trimester.[104] Isolated alcohol-related birth defects and neurobehavioral abnormalities have been seen in children whose mothers consumed three to four drinks per week, or up to 0.3 ounces of absolute alcohol per day, while pregnant.[105,106] Lack of a clear safe lower threshold for consumption of alcohol in pregnancy has led to a recommendation of complete abstinence for women attempting pregnancy or who are known to be pregnant. However, two metaanalyses by Bishai and colleagues failed to show an increased risk for major malformations and perinatal complications in the fetuses of "social drinkers" (i.e., women consuming less than one drink per day).[107]

For women in whom pregnancy is newly diagnosed and whom alcohol consumption has been low, reassurance is reasonable.

The Fetal Alcohol Study Group of the Research Society on Alcoholism has developed specific diagnostic criteria for FAS (Table 25-3).[108] At least one characteristic from each of three categories must be present to make a diagnosis of FAS:

1. Growth restriction is present before or after birth, with a body length less than the 10th percentile for gestational or actual age. Unlike most other kinds of intrauterine malnutrition, the growth abnormalities of FAS do not respond to postnatal feeding. Affected individuals remain small and thin throughout life.
2. Facial dysmorphology is found and includes at least two of the following: microphthalmia; small palpebral fissures; absent or underdeveloped philtrum; shortened, upturned nose; thin upper lip; and hypoplastic, elongated, flattened midface. Facial abnormalities become less pronounced with time and may be undetectable by adolescence or young adulthood.
3. Central nervous system dysfunction is always present. In infancy, this may manifest as poor suckling, tremulousness, irritability, and abnormal motor development. In later life, varying degrees of mental retardation are noted, with significant intelligence quotient (IQ) deficits. The average IQ of a person with FAS is in the range of mild mental retardation (i.e., 60 to 75). Microcephaly is commonly observed. In addition to intellectual deficits, neurobehavioral abnormalities such as hyperactivity or attention deficit disorder are present.

The central nervous system is vulnerable to the toxic effects of alcohol throughout gestational life. Alcohol affects endogenous opiates and attenuates neurotransmitter levels in the brain, including γ-aminobutyric acid, glutamate, and dopamine.

Autopsy studies of individuals with FAS and of animals exposed to alcohol in utero show structural abnormalities in the hippocampus, as well as disruption of cortical cytoarchitecture.[109-111]

More recently, neuroimaging of FAS affected children with magnetic resonance imaging and computed tomography has demonstrated increased incidence of agenesis of the corpus callosum, abnormalities in the cerebellum, and decreased size of the basal ganglia.[112]

TABLE 25–3   Fetal Alcohol Syndrome

Category	Description
Growth restriction (prenatal or postnatal)	Weight
	Length
Central nervous system involvement	Developmental delay
	Intellectual impairment
	Neurologic/behavioral abnormalities
Facial dysmorphology	Microcephaly
	Microphthalmia
	Short palpebral fissures
	Poorly developed philtrum
	Thin upper lip
	Flat maxillary area

Behavioral problems, delayed language acquisition, and learning disabilities are commonly seen with FAS. Some of these problems can be attributed to primary central nervous system damage; however, abnormalities in the auditory system produced by facial maldevelopment also play a significant role. Delayed maturation of the auditory system, recurrent serous otitis media, and central hearing loss are common in affected children.[113] Early screening for hearing problems is essential for children with FAS.

Fetal Alcohol Effects

Perinatally exposed infants who do not meet all the criteria for FAS have been referred to as having fetal alcohol effects, alcohol-related birth defects, and alcohol-related neurodevelopmental disorder. Alcohol-related birth defects can occur in any structure, but cardiac or genitourinary structures are most commonly affected.[104] Oral clefts and ocular defects are frequently seen.[114,115] Alcohol-related behavioral anomalies occur in the absence of growth deficits and facial dysmorphology. Attention deficit disorder, poor memory and learning, poor impulse control, and impaired executive and social functioning have been described in early reports and more recent reviews.[116]

As children with FAS and fetal alcohol effects grow up, they face many challenges even when given special care and educational assistance from an early age. A disproportionate number of youths and adults with FAS come into conflict with the legal system. In a Canadian study, 23.3% of youths evaluated by the juvenile justice system were found to have a diagnosis of FAS or fetal alcohol effects.[117] A prospective study of a German cohort of children with FAS and fetal alcohol effects monitored to adulthood found that only 11.5% were able to live independently as adults.[118] An additional complication of FAS may be an increased susceptibility to alcoholism and substance abuse in later life.[119]

Cocaine

Epidemiology of Use

Despite the fact that indicators of cocaine/crack use have been stabilizing and decreasing for some time, cocaine continues to be a dominant drug of abuse in the United States. A national survey of illicit drug use in the United States, published in 2001, reports that 1.7 million Americans (0.7%) older than 12 years are current cocaine users and 406,000 (0.2%) are current crack users.[26] Data from the 2001 Community Epidemiology Work Group[25] show that crack use decreased as powder cocaine became more available in some parts of the country. Cocaine is the commonest drug mentioned in association with drug-related emergency department visits, as monitored by the Drug Abuse Warning Network. High percentages of arrested men and women continue to produce positive test results for cocaine and its metabolites, as documented by the Arrestee Drug Abuse Monitoring program of the National Institute of Justice.

Estimates of use by pregnant women vary widely. The NIDA National Pregnancy and Health Survey done in 1992 to 1993 found that 4.5% of African American women, 0.7% of Hispanic women, and 0.4% of white women used some form of cocaine. In a more recent case-control study in North Carolina involving a cohort of women enrolled in prenatal care,[5] the investigators ascertained cocaine use by three modalities. They identified cocaine use during pregnancy in 2% of the group on the basis of self-report, 5% to 6% on the basis of urine assays, and 13% to 15% on the basis of hair assays. In this study, African American ethnicity, low educational status, and low socioeconomic status were strongly predictive of positive hair assays.

General Effects

Cocaine is an ester of benzoic acid that is extracted from the leaves of the coca plant, *Erythroxylum coca*. Combining hydrochloric acid with raw coca paste produces cocaine hydrochloride, which can be snorted or injected. Further treatment of the hydrochloride salt with a base yields alkaloidal cocaine, also known as crack. Crack is heat stable and therefore suitable for inhalational use. All forms of cocaine produce rapid psychoactive effects characterized by a feeling of intense euphoria, increased energy, and alertness. Long-term use leads to tolerance, a blunted euphoric response, exhaustion, and depression.

Cocaine is a short-acting drug. Peak plasma levels are seen in 15 to 60 minutes, after which the drug is metabolized by hepatic and plasma cholinesterases to water-soluble metabolites such as norcaine, an active metabolite, and benzoylecgonine and ergonine, which are inactive metabolites. Plasma cholinesterase activity may be decreased in pregnant women, fetuses, and neonates; therefore, serum levels of the drug may be sustained in these groups.[120]

Cocaine is a powerful stimulant and vasoconstrictor. The drug works by inhibiting the reuptake and metabolism of norepinephrine and epinephrine at neural junctions, which results in activation of the central and peripheral autonomic nervous systems. In the brain, cocaine also impairs reuptake of dopamine. Increased concentrations of this neurotransmitter in the mesolimbic system and the mesocortex produce cocaine-induced euphoria.

Because of its low molecular weight, low ionization at physiologic pH, and high water and lipid solubility, cocaine crosses the placenta freely. Studies of isolated human placental cotyledons demonstrate rapid transfer of the drug and its metabolites.[121] Significant amounts of maternal cocaine are retained by the placenta, later leaching into the maternal and fetal circulations and presumably prolonging the toxicity of each bolus dose. Placental microsomal preparations have the ability to hydrolyze cocaine into inactive metabolites via placental cholinesterases.[122] In a study of primates who were given cocaine throughout pregnancy, total maternal dose was poorly correlated with neonatal exposure, as determined by quantitative analysis of the cocaine metabolite benzoylecgonine in neonatal hair.[123] These findings suggest a differential ability of individual placentas to degrade cocaine before it reaches the fetal compartment. A study of cocaine-exposed human dizygotic twins also showed large disparities in meconium cocaine concentrations of the twin dyads.[124] In animal models, fetal cocaine levels reach 14% to 17% of maternal levels five minutes after intravenous administration. Fetal drug levels remain consistently lower than maternal ones, in part because of cocaine-induced uterine artery vasoconstriction.

Maternal Effects of Cocaine
Cardiovascular Effects

Cocaine profoundly affects maternal hemodynamics. At moderate to high doses, it causes marked elevations in heart rate and blood pressure through stimulation of the adrenal glands and activation of the peripheral autonomic nervous system. In the pregnant woman, cocaine-mediated vasoconstriction decreases blood flow to the heart, brain, and uterus. Reduction in uterine blood flow has deleterious effects on the fetus and results in fetal tachycardia, hypertension, and hypoxemia.[125] The hormonal milieu of pregnancy appears to accentuate the cardiovascular effects of cocaine. When equal doses of cocaine are given to pregnant and nonpregnant sheep, a twofold greater hypertensive response is seen in the pregnant animals.[126] Cocaine administration was associated with exaggerated falls in cardiac output in pregnant rats, in comparison with nonpregnant rodents.[127]

The exaggerated cardiovascular responses to cocaine in pregnancy may be progesterone mediated,[128] and there is some evidence that they may be more pronounced in the third trimester.[129]

Uteroplacental Effects

Isolated strips of perfused uterine myometrium respond to cocaine with a dose-dependent increase in frequency, duration, and force of contractions.[130] Cocaine augments myometrial contractility through adrenergic and nonadrenergic mechanisms. Reports of the effect of cocaine on placental structures have been conflicting. Mooney and colleagues found evidence of chorionic villus hemorrhage and villus edema in placentas of cocaine users, in contrast to those of drug-free controls.[131] However, a subsequent study by Cejtin and associates, who controlled for use of other drugs by the parturients whose placentas were examined, revealed no increase in placental pathologic processes in comparison with controls.[132]

Medical Complications of Cocaine

Numerous adverse consequences of cocaine use have been described anecdotally and in retrospective case series with pregnant and nonpregnant populations. Complications of cocaine use result primarily from the sympathomimetic actions of the drug. Virtually every organ system can be affected. Cardiovascular complications of cocaine occurring in otherwise healthy subjects are reported. Arrhythmias, myocardial infarction, aortic dissection, and cardiomyopathy have been seen in pregnant women.[133-137] Hypertensive crisis caused by cocaine use during pregnancy can be mistaken for preeclampsia. If preexistent liver disease is also present, the patient's clinical picture mimics the HELLP (hemolysis, elevated liver enzymes, and low platelets) syndrome. In light of this, it is useful to know that a case-control study of pregnant chronic cocaine users did not find an increased prevalence of thrombocytopenia in comparison with nonusers.[138]

Catastrophic central nervous system complications associated with acute cocaine use in pregnant and postpartum women include cerebrovascular accidents and subarachnoid hemorrhage caused by aneurysmal rupture.[139,140]

Seizures may result from cocaine use, either as primary events[141] or in association with cardiac dysrhythmias. The hyperpyrexia produced by cocaine may lower seizure thresholds. Pulmonary complications of cocaine are associated mostly with smoking alkaloidal crack. Persistent cough and wheezing are common complaints.[142] Less frequently, pulmonary edema and bronchiolitis obliterans have been reported. "Crack lung" is the name for the triad of chest pain, hemoptysis, and diffuse alveolar infiltrates.[143]

The most common medical complication associated with cocaine use by pregnant women may be the increased incidence of infectious diseases. Numerous studies of cocaine-using women document a high prevalence of syphilis, hepatitis B and C, and HIV infections.[144,145] Although in vitro studies of cocaine showed that the drug is able to alter the function and numbers of CD4+ T cells and natural killer monocytes,[146] deficiencies of humeral and cellular immunity are probably not the major cause of excessive infection rates in cocaine-using pregnant women. Rather, the chaotic lifestyle associated with regular use of this drug is the primary culprit. Cocaine-using women enter prenatal care late or sometimes not at all. They exchange sex for drugs and, because of the disinhibiting effects of the drug on behavior and sexuality, engage in unsafe sexual practices. Studies of cocaine-using women engaged in prenatal care show marked decreases in infectious complications.[56]

Obstetric Complications of Cocaine

Epidemiologic studies consistently link cocaine use in pregnancy to a number of adverse obstetric outcomes. Associations between cocaine use and preterm labor and delivery, preterm rupture of membranes, placental abruption, and placenta previa are all well documented in studies that control for important confounders such as tobacco or other drug use.[147-149] Because cocaine predictably elevates systemic blood pressure, circulating catecholamine levels, and uterine contraction intensity, while decreasing uterine artery blood flow, these outcomes are biologically plausible. Premature infants born to cocaine-using mothers appear to fare better postnatally than unexposed infants of comparable weight[150] and have lower rates of sepsis and pneumonia. Intrauterine fetal stress with attendant chronic catecholamine excess has been shown to accelerate fetal lung maturity.[151]

Fetal, Neonatal, and Behavioral Effects of Cocaine

Episodic decreases in uterine blood flow and placental perfusion are probably responsible for the increased incidence of low birth weight and smallness for gestational age in infants born to cocaine-using women.[152,153] In vitro, cocaine has also been shown to decrease amino acid transport across the placental cotyledon.[154] Unlike the growth restriction associated with antenatal alcohol exposure, cocaine-mediated growth restriction may respond better to postnatal nutrition: Longitudinal follow-up of such children to 7 years of age has demonstrated better catch-up for children exposed to cocaine than for those exposed to alcohol.[155,156]

Although maternal cocaine use has been reported to cause congenital anomalies in many offspring, neither single cohort studies nor large epidemiologic studies, controlling for use of other substances, have confirmed that cocaine is a predictable teratogen.[157-160] The existence of a specific neonatal abstinence syndrome associated with perinatal cocaine exposure is also poorly substantiated by current literature[161-163] although neurobehavioral abnormalities such as tremulousness and increased startle responses have been detected with the Brazelton Neonatal Assessment Scale.[164]

Abundant evidence from animal studies has shown that cocaine affects the brain structurally and histochemically. In addition, cranial ultrasonograms of cocaine-exposed newborns demonstrate abnormalities such as subependymal hemorrhages and cysts.[165] The significance of these findings in terms of infant/child development and language acquisition is unclear. In a metaanalysis, Frank and colleagues reviewed the published literature on cocaine and child development.[166] Studies were included in the metaanalysis if they included a comparison group, recruited samples prospectively in the perinatal period, used anonymous assessors, and did not include a large proportion of subjects who were also exposed to multiple drugs or to HIV infection. Using these selection criteria, the reviewers found no convincing evidence that prenatal cocaine exposure is associated with specific "toxic" developmental effects different than those attributable to other factors, such as multiple drug exposure, impoverished environment, and poor parenting.

The analysis by Frank and colleagues does not imply that cocaine is without negative effects, nor does it minimize the risks of its use during pregnancy. Rather, it supports the theory that the effects of cocaine are much more subtle than initially reported. Better studies, such as the multicenter MLS referred to earlier in this chapter, are needed to help clinicians truly understand the specific actions of this substance in pregnancy and after birth.

In particular, while waiting for more definitive information, it is critical to avoid negative stereotyping of children known to be cocaine exposed. The findings from this metaanalysis also underscore the need to separate the broader social and legal ramifications of using cocaine from the study of its impact on perinatal health.

Amphetamines

Amphetamines have been popular drugs of abuse since the 1960s. Although the street availability of commercial amphetamines has declined significantly, clandestine laboratories produce a steady supply of the drugs. Methamphetamine is commonly referred to as "ice," "crank," "crystal," or "speed." Methamphetamine consumption remains high in the western and midwestern United States and in rural areas.[167] It can be inhaled, injected, or ingested orally. So-called designer amphetamine use, particularly MDMA, has virtually exploded since the early 1990s. By 2001, 8.1 million Americans had tried MDMA at least once, and 786,000 people (0.3% of the population) are classified as current users.[26]

Like cocaine, amphetamines are powerful sympathomimetic stimulants. Both substances act by blocking the reuptake of catecholamines through inhibition of monoamine transporters.[168] Unlike cocaine, high doses of amphetamines also release serotonin from central serotonin receptors or act directly on these receptors. Interaction with serotonin receptors causes the hallucinogenic effects of amphetamines commonly reported by users. The half-life of amphetamines is much longer than that of cocaine; thus, the effects of a single dose can last for up to 12 hours. Toxic effects of amphetamines, which may be dose dependent, include cardiac arrhythmias, retinal hemorrhage, seizures, strokes, and sudden death.[169]

Despite increasing use of methamphetamine, little information is available about its effects on pregnancy. As with cocaine, complications associated with amphetamine use arise primarily from vasospasm. Hence, maternal hypertension, premature labor, and placental hemorrhage have been reported.[170] Exposed infants have an increased incidence of low birth weight and neonatal seizures. Neonatal behavioral abnormalities similar to those associated with cocaine exposure have been described.[171] Isolated birth anomalies, particularly cardiac defects and oral clefts,[172] have been reported after antenatal amphetamine use. These studies are not controlled for other environmental effects and maternal health status; therefore, direct drug toxicity cannot be assumed.

MDMA is a relatively new drug; thus, information about it is very limited. The drug is frequently used at "rave" clubs and parties to provide increased energy for dancing and for mood enhancement. The drug is remarkable for masking thirst sensation. Users have developed cardiac and renal failure. Death, particularly from acute dehydration,[173] is not uncommon. Public teratology services in Canada and the Netherlands have collected data about MDMA exposures during pregnancy. They report that the drug is usually used in combination with alcohol binging, cigarettes, and other drugs.[174,175] In a single prospective study of 136 MDMA-exposed infants, 74 of whom were antenatally exposed to MDMA and not to other drugs, there was a 15.4% rate of anomalies.[176] Cardiac and musculoskeletal anomalies were frequent in this group.

Narcotics

Narcotic use continues to be common in the United States. Since the early 1990s, heroin usage has risen to a level not matched since the 1970s. In 2000 the number of new heroin users was 146,000, which was double the number seen 10 years earlier.[26] Rising heroin use has been attributed to increases in the purity of the drug and stable, low prices. Increasing heroin purity has led to a shift from parenteral use to nasal use. Currently, most heroin is snorted or sniffed, although pockets of intravenous use remain in certain regions. An important trend in narcotic use is the dramatic increase in recreational use of oxycodone (OxyContin). In 2001, approximately 957,000 persons older than 12 years had used this prescription medication nonmedically. Rising heroin use has been accompanied by a secondary rise in the use of methadone, primarily to treat heroin addiction. Enrollment in methadone treatment programs has increased steadily since 1994.[177]

Regardless of whether opiates are used illicitly or for the treatment of addiction or pain, physiologic dependence as a consequence of use is possible. When used regularly during pregnancy, opiate dependence and withdrawal occur in both the mother and the fetus. Additional maternal and obstetric complications of opiate use have been reported in the medical literature, but the majority of this information was collected when parenteral drug use among opiate-dependent pregnant women was the norm. Therefore, many of the frequently cited medical complications associated with heroin use, particularly infections such as HIV or bacterial endocarditis, are a consequence of unsterile injection of particulate matter and not direct effects of the drugs themselves.

Obstetric, Fetal, and Neonatal Complications of Narcotic Use

Diagnosis of pregnancy in heroin-addicted women may be delayed. Menstrual abnormalities are seen in 60% to 90% of heroin-dependent women.[178] Chronic heroin use reduces the release of luteinizing hormone from the hypothalamus and is therefore associated with anovulatory cycles.[179] Early symptoms of pregnancy such as nausea and fatigue and abdominal cramps may feel like withdrawal to the opiate-dependent woman, prompting her to increase drug use and delay medical evaluation.

Heroin is a short-acting drug with a half-life of minutes. Withdrawal begins approximately 6 to 8 hours after the last dose is taken. Because of these pharmacokinetics, alternating cycles of intoxication and withdrawal are the norm in heroin users. Narcotic withdrawal is uncomfortable but not injurious to the opiate-using mother. However, withdrawal at any stage of pregnancy potentially jeopardizes the conceptus. In early pregnancy, uterine contractions may result in spontaneous abortion. Later in pregnancy, withdrawal can initiate preterm labor. Fetal withdrawal can result in meconium passage and fetal distress.[180]

Whether a woman uses narcotics regularly or sporadically, the risk of unintended narcotic overdose exists. This is especially true when the heroin content of purchased bags varies or when a bag is adulterated with a more potent narcotic such as fentanyl or its congeners. The diagnosis of opiate overdose must be considered in pregnant women who present with coma, miotic pupils, and depressed respiration. Resuscitation with naloxone (Narcan), a narcotic antagonist, should be prompt. The dose, which is 0.1 mg/kg intramuscularly or intravenously, can be repeated within 10 to 30 minutes.

Use of narcotics in pregnancy is associated with late booking of prenatal care, preterm labor and delivery, low birth weight in infants of these women, anemia, poor nutrition, and a high prevalence of untreated disease.[181,182] Many of these complications undoubtedly result from the lifestyle associated with drug use and do not represent direct effects of narcotics on pregnancy. High rates of chronic infections, including HIV and hepatitis B and C, are seen in heroin-using women, although it is not known how high rates are for the noninjecting users.

Chronic narcotic use of any kind during pregnancy, whether for recreation or opiate addiction treatment, results in a neonatal abstinence syndrome in exposed infants. Abstinence symptoms are seen in 42% to 68% of heroin-exposed infants and in 63% to 85% of methadone-exposed infants.[183,184] Symptoms appear within 24 to 48 hours if the mother was using heroin. Infants born to methadone-maintained women experience withdrawal later, because the half-life of methadone is much longer than heroin. A methadone-exposed infant may be become ill as late as 2 weeks after birth. Neonatal withdrawal from methadone is often more severe and prolonged than heroin withdrawal. The neonatal abstinence syndrome resembles adult withdrawal in some ways and is characterized by sweating, excessive yawning, sneezing, fever, and gastrointestinal symptoms. In contrast to adult narcotic withdrawal, seizures are common in neonates experiencing severe withdrawal and may necessitate pharmacotherapy.

Long-term developmental and behavioral effects of perinatal heroin or methadone exposure are not well understood. No opiate has been found to be teratogenic. An increased rate of sudden infant death syndrome was reported in opiate-exposed infants; however, more recent studies have not found this to be true.[185] Newer data need to be collected, because current pediatric recommendations about supine infant positioning to prevent sudden infant death syndrome may have decreased this tragic outcome in opiate-exposed infants.

Marijuana

Although marijuana is unquestionably the most commonly used illicit drug among women of childbearing age, very little is known about its effects on human pregnancy. National survey data from 2001 indicate that 5.3% of the population currently use marijuana and that approximately 20 million persons are classified as frequent users.[186] Age at first use of marijuana has decreased steadily since the early 1990s. Use rates among high school students and young adults are climbing rapidly. The National Health and Pregnancy Survey of 1992 to 1993 found that 2.9% of women self-reported marijuana use during pregnancy. Regional studies report higher use rates in some populations. In a prospective multicenter study involving seven university-based prenatal clinics in the United States, Shiono and associates observed that 11% of 13,913 women entered into the study had either a positive history or a positive urine toxicology finding for marijuana use.[187] Self-report and urine toxicology results correlated poorly in this study, which may mean that use during pregnancy on a national basis may be seriously underestimated.

Marijuana is prepared from the plant *Cannabis sativa*. The principal active ingredient is Δ-9-tetrahydrocannabinol (THC). Inhalation of marijuana rapidly produces psychoactive effects that last for about 2 to 3 hours. Marijuana use results in physiologic changes: Blood pressure falls and pulse increases soon after inhaling. Few adverse health effects have been reported from marijuana use, although regular use causes many of the health problems associated with tobacco smoking. Habitual marijuana use is associated with chronic bronchitis and elevated blood carboxyhemoglobin levels.[188]

Effects in Pregnancy

Marijuana has been used by pregnant women for centuries.[189] Considering its long history, as well as its current popularity, it is astounding how little information is available about its effects on pregnancy outcomes, fetal growth, and long-term child development. In the first trimester, marijuana has been used as an antiemetic to reduce the nausea and vomiting of early pregnancy.[190] THC use has been shown to delay recognition of early pregnancy symptoms in women attempting conception.[191] Investigators have demonstrated two types of cannabinoid receptors in the human placenta.[192] These receptors affect serotonin transport across the placenta. In addition, they may regulate transfer of THC across the placenta, inasmuch as fetal THC levels have been shown to be lower than maternal ones.

Studies of the effects of marijuana when used after the first trimester are conflicting. Some studies have noted an association between marijuana exposure and shortened gestation, meconium staining, and lower birth weights. Two large, prospective studies, however, did not find any increases in preterm delivery and or decrements in birth weight when the data were controlled for parity and for alcohol and tobacco use.[187,193]

Marijuana has not been shown to be a teratogen in humans. Drug interactions are a critical factor, however, because substances such as marijuana may potentiate the effects of other drugs. In a study by Hingson and colleagues, there was a fivefold increase in the likelihood of finding characteristic fetal alcohol facies in infants born to women who used both marijuana and alcohol during pregnancy.[194] Fried and Makin prospectively recruited a cohort of pregnant regular marijuana users. Their neonates had increased tremors and startle responses.[195] Testing at 1 year of age did not show neurobehavioral abnormalities. Other investigators[196,197] have reported sleep abnormalities in marijuana-exposed infants that persist until age 3 years, although similar findings were absent in the cohort studied by Fried and Makin.

Two longitudinal cohort studies have been in progress since the early 1980s, monitoring cohorts of children who were perinatally exposed to marijuana. The first, headed by Fried and Makin, as mentioned, is the Ottawa Prenatal Prospective Study. This is a cohort of primarily white, predominantly middle class families with few risk factors. The other study is the Maternal Health Practices and Child Development Study (MHPCPD) in Pittsburgh, Pennsylvania. This cohort is an urban group of low socioeconomic status that is 50% African American. Serial developmental evaluation of exposed children in the Canadian cohort up to age 10 years has yielded essentially normal results. The Canadian group reported their findings on 9- to 12-year-olds and 13- to 16-year-olds from the cohort.[198] They did not find any physical abnormalities in comparison with control children; rather, they found subtle deficits in what they term "executive functions" in the exposed children: poorer self-regulatory abilities, mild attention deficits, and decreased ability to act on accumulated knowledge. Global intelligence (IQ) was unaffected by marijuana, as were language skills.

In contrast to the Canadian children, the MHPCPD group in Pittsburgh was significantly more impaired. At age 6, these children had deficits in height.[199] At age 10, the marijuana-exposed children were significantly hyperactive, inattentive, and delinquent.[200]

It is noteworthy that both the Canadian and the American cohorts display deficits consistent with perinatal damage to frontal lobe processes, albeit subtle ones. It underscores the fact that intrauterine drug exposure may cause complex abnormalities that can be determined only by specialized testing over a long time. These two studies also demonstrate that children growing up in disadvantaged circumstances appear to be far more affected by perinatal substance exposure than are children who have better environments. The ability of a good environment to modify the effects of exposures to drugs during intrauterine life underscores the enormous plasticity and resilience of the human brain, as well as the need for special evaluation and services for exposed children.

Miscellaneous Drugs of Abuse

Sedatives and Tranquilizers

Use of sedative agents remains a persistent problem in pregnancy. Many of these drugs, such as the benzodiazepines, are commonly prescribed by physicians. Others, such as γ-hydroxybutyrate and flunitrazepam (Rohypnol), are often manufactured illegally or smuggled into the United States. Self-medication with sedatives is common in women who use stimulants or alcohol in order to induce sleep and to treat symptoms of withdrawal and overstimulation. All sedatives and tranquilizers have the potential to induce tolerance and withdrawal symptoms in regular pregnant users and their offspring. The teratogenic potential of most of these agents remains unclear.

Maternal benzodiazepine use is problematic for the fetus. Early in pregnancy, these drugs may be associated with oral clefting and isolated anomalies.[201] In the third trimester, diazepam and related compounds diffuse readily across the placenta and accumulate in the fetal compartment.[202] Chronic use in pregnancy is associated with the "floppy baby" syndrome: that is, neonatal depression at the time of birth and, later, neonatal withdrawal symptoms.[203]

Short- and medium-acting barbiturates, once common drugs of abuse, are not frequently encountered now, because they are rarely prescribed and their distribution is tightly controlled. Nonetheless, it is wise to remember that these drugs have high addiction potential and that withdrawal from them is potentially fatal for adults and neonates. Long-acting barbiturates are often used to treat seizure disorders in pregnant women. Phenobarbital use during pregnancy can result in neonatal withdrawal symptoms,[204] which are usually managed expectantly by pediatricians.

Clinicians should be aware that depressant drugs are very commonly used as part of "rave" parties and the club culture that is a part of the lives of many young adults from all social strata. Rohypnol—also known, among other names, as "Rophy" or "roofies"—has gained notoriety as a "date rape drug." When mixed with alcohol, it produces somnolence, amnesia, and potential airway compromise. γ-Hydroxybutyrate, once available in health food stores, was withdrawn from the market after a series of fatalities in the 1990s. It is now a Schedule I drug that is manufactured by clandestine laboratories and distributed in powder or tablet form. Chronic use is associated with intense physical dependence and severe withdrawal symptoms. Information on the effects of these drugs in pregnancy is scant but expected to accumulate because of their frequency of use by young women.

Hallucinogens

Phencyclidine

PCP, also known as "angel dust," was originally developed as a dissociative anesthetic. It remains a common drug of abuse, although its popularity may be waning in some areas. Use and mortality in certain regions, however, remain high. Los Angeles reported 51 PCP-related deaths in 2000, down from 66 in 1997.[205] The drug is inexpensive to produce and may be taken in a variety of ways, such as swallowing, inhalation, and injection. Violent agitation and mood swings are common with this drug, making it particularly problematic for use by pregnant women. Intoxication is associated with combative behaviors that can result in maternal injuries and, potentially, fetal compromise. Fetal loss and fetal anomalies have been reported when PCP is used during pregnancy.[206] A case-control study of PCP use in pregnancy found an increase in maternal complications such as diabetes mellitus and syphilis infections among women who used PCP and significantly lower birth weights in their infants, in comparison with controls.[207]

Lysergic Acid Diethylamide

LSD remains popular in some areas of the United States.

Ingestion can result in an acute psychotic panic reaction, characterized by severe paranoia, confusion, and depression.[208] The drug has entered the club scene, where it is mixed with MDMA, a practice called "candy flipping." Contrary to popular belief, LSD does not produce chromosomal damage when used during pregnancy. It is difficult to evaluate the effects of this drug in pregnancy, because it is used intermittently and often with other substances.

Inhalants

Inhalation of volatile substances continues to be common in teenage patients and in rural areas. Approximately 17% of adolescents in the United States have used inhalants at least once.[209] Data from the National Pregnancy and Health survey indicate that approximately 12,000 pregnant women abuse inhalants each year.[19] A host of legally purchased substances can be abused, including aerosols, gasoline, paint thinner, correction fluid, and organic nitrites. Toluene use appears to be particularly problematic during pregnancy. Maternal complications include renal tubular acidosis, dysrhythmias, rhabdomyolysis, and preterm labor.[210] A significant percentage of toluene-exposed infants exhibit a pattern of embryopathy similar to that of FAS, including abnormal facies, central nervous system dysfunction, and growth deficiency.[211,212] The long-term effects of perinatal toluene exposure on development are not known.

Tobacco

The adverse effects of cigarette smoking on fetal growth and development are well documented. Tobacco is the most abused drug in pregnancy. Because its use is so common, it is the single largest preventable cause of low birth weight and infant mortality. Cigarette smoking rates are very high among substance-using women. Tobacco is a cofactor in generating the multiple morbid conditions associated with the use of drugs and alcohol in pregnancy.

IDENTIFYING AND MANAGING THE PREGNANT SUBSTANCE ABUSER

Most non-drug-using patients are motivated to seek medical care when they are ill, uncomfortable, or pregnant. Women who abuse drugs and alcohol, however, are engaged in activities that are considered shameful, dangerous, and, often, illegal. A substance-using pregnant woman may not consider herself as having a problem and may not want to stop using drugs. Unless she experiences an acute problem, she may not seek medical care or enroll in prenatal care. Even when enrolled in prenatal care, substance-using women may go to great lengths to conceal their habits.

Because drug, alcohol, and tobacco use is ubiquitous in prenatal populations, it is essential that clinicians screen all patients systematically and effectively. Substance abuse disorders are significantly underdiagnosed in women. Studies show that as many as 90% of cases are missed, particularly in women of upper socioeconomic status.[213,214] Despite good intentions, prenatal providers fail to screen for many reasons. Time constraints and poor reimbursement are some of the reasons why providers do not screen. Many physicians believe that substance abuse does not occur in their practices; the "not in my clinic/office" attitude is frequently encountered. Embarrassment, conflicted attitudes about their own use of substances, and unfamiliarity with documentation of substance use all contribute to missed opportunities for intervention and improved care in substance drug-exposed pregnancies.

Routine questioning about drug and alcohol use should be done at the first prenatal visit. Questions about substance use should be asked at the same time that other lifestyle information is being obtained, such as information about exercise, nutrition, caffeine intake, cigarette smoking, and use of nonprescription items such as supplements and "complementary" therapies. The questions should be asked in a direct, specific, and nonjudgmental way. Patients need to be assured of the confidentiality of the interview and to understand that their responses will not affect their ability to get medical care. Providers often unintentionally communicate to patients that positive responses to questions about drugs and alcohol use in pregnancy are unwelcome and unacceptable. Great care should be taken to ensure that a prenatal patient feels comfortable giving true answers to these sensitive questions. Patients need to understand why they are being questioned about their personal habits. The focus should be on the effect of alcohol and drug use on personal health and on pregnancy. Any patient who does give a history of drug use or alcohol use should be further questioned about frequency and quantity of use, routes of administration, and the social context of use. Patients who admit to isolated incidents of use or very occasional use should be questioned about use at follow-up visits.

Self-administered paper-and-pencil or computer questionnaires about drug and alcohol use have practical advantages but have not been found to be as effective as face-to-face interviews.[215] Many practitioners routinely use short, validated oral screening instruments such as the alcohol or drug CAGE questionnaire[216,217] when interviewing new patients. The American College of Obstetrics and Gynecology recommends use of the T-ACE questionnaire[218] (Table 25-4) for alcohol screening in pregnancy,[219] because it contains a question about alcohol tolerance, which is helpful in distinguishing the frequent drinker. Probably the shortest and highest yield approach for detecting high-risk drinking is to ask the two questions proposed by Cyr and Wartman[220]: "Have you ever had a drinking problem?" and "When was your last drink?" (A positive response to the second question is "within the past 24 hours.") This test has a specificity of 90% for persons meeting criteria for alcohol use or dependence.

Medical, Obstetric, and Social Clues to Substance Abuse

There are a number of items in a patient's medical, obstetric, or social history that should prompt a physician to take greater pains to obtain a thorough substance abuse history (Table 25-5). A family history of alcoholism has been found to be correlated very highly with the development of drug or alcohol dependency in female patients.[221] Social history and patient behavior are particularly important. A woman who has had multiple traumatic injuries, motor vehicle accidents, fights, assaults, recurrent financial or legal problems, or difficulty maintaining employment may be grappling with the disorganizing effects of an addiction. Failure to keep scheduled medical appointments, requests for mood-altering medications, and poor grooming together with poor weight gain may alert a clinician to the fact that a patient should be more carefully assessed or reassessed for chemical dependency.

Toxicology testing does not have a well-defined role in routine drug and alcohol screening during pregnancy. Illicit drug use can be detected in a myriad of biologic samples, including urine, saliva, and hair and nail clippings. However, unless medical necessity can be documented, testing for drugs without obtaining specific informed

TABLE 25-4   Alcohol Screening Questionnaire: T-ACE

"How many drinks can you hold?" (Tolerance: refers to number of drinks before passing out or falling asleep, with more than five being positive)
"Have close friends or relatives annoyed you by criticizing your drinking?"
"Have you ever felt you ought to cut down on your drinking?"
"Have you ever taken a drink first thing in the morning (eye opener) to steady your nerves or get rid of a hangover?"

From Sokol RJ, Martier SS, Ager JW: The T-ACE questions: Practical prenatal detection of risk-drinking. Am J Obstet Gynecol 1989;160:863.

TABLE 25-5   Clues to Substance Abuse

Medical Clues
Infections: human immunodeficiency virus (HIV), viral hepatitis B or C, endocarditis, skin infections, multiple sexually transmitted diseases, unusual infection sites
History of multiple traumatic injuries
Pancreatitis, abnormal liver functions, recurrent gastritis, or diarrhea
Chronic pain syndromes; repeated requests for analgesics, tranquilizers, and sedatives
Insomnia
Poor dental hygiene
Blackout spells
Loss of libido, sexual dysfunction
Depression, anxiety, suicide attempts
Tobacco use

Obstetric Clues

Past History
Multiple pregnancy loss
Premature labor
Preterm premature rupture of membranes
Placental abruption
Intrauterine growth restriction (IUGR)
Intrauterine fetal demise
Neonatal abstinence syndrome

Current History
Poor nutrition or weight loss
Unexplained fetal tachycardia
IUGR
Premature labor
Preterm premature rupture of membranes
Labile maternal blood pressure

Social/Behavioral Clues
Noncompliance, multiple missed/rescheduled appointments
History of substance abuse by spouse or family
Multiple emergency room visits
Abnormal affect: lethargy, agitation
Poor employment history
Criminal behavior/legal system involvement
Chaotic family situation, unstable housing, loss of custody of children
History of domestic, sexual, or childhood abuse
Relationship difficulties: family, social

consent from the patient is considered a violation of a woman's rights under the Fourth Amendment's protection against illegal search and seizure.[222,223] In cases of medical emergency, however, when maternal or fetal well-being is at stake, signature of a general consent to treatment is sufficient to justify ordering urine toxicology, as long as it is done in a nondiscriminatory manner consistent with institutional practices and policies.

Evaluation and Management of the Pregnant Substance User

If a woman is known to be abusing alcohol or drugs, meticulous maternal and fetal evaluation is essential (Table 25-6). Infections, including dental infections, should be assiduously sought and, if found, aggressively treated. Regardless of whether there is a history of parenteral drug use, HIV counseling and testing should be

TABLE 25–6 Evaluation of the Pregnant Substance Abuser

Physical Examination

General: nutritional status, height, weight
Dermatologic: infections, abscesses, bruises and scars from old injuries, icterus, needle tracks, palmar erythema
Dental: pyorrhea, abscessed caries
Ear/nose/throat: nasal mucosal erythema, atrophy, or damage
Pulmonary: rales, wheezes, evidence of chronic interstitial lung disease
Cardiovascular: murmurs (consistent with valvular heart disease, endocarditis, increased pulmonary artery pressure), dysrhythmias
Gastrointestinal: hepatomegaly, evidence of portal hypertension
Genitourinary: vaginal and rectal infections, stool guaiac
Lymphatic: lymphadenopathy in any location
Neurologic: mental status, tremor, hyperreflexia

Prenatal Panel

Hepatitis B and C antibody status
Baseline liver function tests
Purified protein derivative of tuberculin
Human immunodeficiency virus screens at baseline and 6 months later
Cervical cytologic assessments at baseline and 6 months later

offered at the first visit and repeated at 6-month intervals. Refusal to be tested should be documented by the clinician, and the HIV screen should be offered again at each subsequent prenatal visit. Immunization status should be investigated. If appropriate, tetanus toxoid and hepatitis B vaccine should be administered.

Particular attention should be paid to maternal nutritional status. Chemical dependency is highly correlated with poor nutrition. The anorectic effects of drugs of abuse, in combination with a drug- or alcohol-using lifestyle, mitigate against intake of adequate calories and micronutrients. In a prospective study of substance-abusing women in an urban area, serial blood samples were obtained during each trimester of pregnancy and analyzed for drugs of abuse, as well as for levels of folate, vitamin B_{12}, ferritin, and ascorbic acid. The investigators found an inverse relationship between illicit drug levels and micronutrients.[224]

Aggressive vitamin and mineral supplementation, as well as nutritional counseling, may help improve maternal status and pregnancy outcome.

Serial ultrasonography is very useful in managing a substance-exposed pregnancy. Early sonograms establish pregnancy dating. Morphologic survey in the second trimester detects anomalies. In the third trimester, sonograms document appropriate fetal growth.

In the latter part of pregnancy, beginning at 32 to 34 weeks, semiweekly nonstress tests or biophysical profiles should be ordered. This is especially important for the woman who continues to use drugs during pregnancy or who has delayed seeking prenatal care. Antepartum testing detects preterm contractions and evaluates fetal well-being. Clinicians should be aware that substances such as cocaine or methadone may diminish the reactivity of the nonstress test or reduce fetal activity in the biophysical profile.[225-227]

Substance-using women should be seen in prenatal care at intervals of no longer than 2 weeks. If the woman is unable to achieve abstinence or does not enter a drug rehabilitation program, it may be advisable to ask her to come to the office or clinic on a weekly basis. Many obstetric providers find caring for substance-using patients trying and frustrating. It is therefore important to remember that prenatal care itself has a tremendously positive effect on outcomes, even when women continue to use drugs. Numerous studies have demonstrated an independent effect of prenatal care in improving birth weight[228-230] and reducing perinatal mortality[231] in nonabstinent women.

In the postpartum period, substance-using women require a great deal of support and attention. If they are in early drug recovery, the potential for relapse is very high. If they are still using drugs, their ability to bond with and parent an infant is inadequate. Follow-up by social service agencies should be arranged before discharge, because postpartum substance abuse is associated with high rates of child abuse and neglect. A contraceptive method should be chosen. Follow-up visits with the prenatal provider should continue at 2-week intervals for the first 2 months, unless the patient is in residential or intensive outpatient drug rehabilitation treatment. Breast-feeding should certainly be discussed with the patient. It is important for women who use drugs and or abuse alcohol to know that these substances pass into breast milk and are dangerous to the breast-feeding infant. The American Academy of Pediatrics considers methadone compatible with breast-feeding, although caution and close observation of infants is necessary in such cases.[232] Breast-feeding while on methadone maintenance may ameliorate neonatal abstinence symptoms.[233]

Special Management Issues in Substance-Using Women

Pain

Physicians need to be skilled in the management of pain in patients with a history of alcohol or drug abuse. Addiction is not a reason to withhold analgesia. Brief courses of short-acting opiates are appropriate for acute problems, such as severe musculoskeletal derangement or trauma. It is important to make it absolutely clear to patients at the outset that the amount of medication prescribed in the outpatient setting will be limited in terms of number of pills, that return for prescription medication on a frequent basis may be necessary, and that any medication diversion will interfere with provision of further analgesic treatment.

Management of pain in labor should be proactive and nondiscriminatory. A common misconception is that chemically dependent women have a low pain threshold. The truth is that drug tolerance may necessitate the use of higher-than-usual doses of short-acting parenteral narcotics.[234] In the case of the opiate-dependent woman, the use of combined narcotic agonist-antagonists (e.g., nalbuphine [Nubain], butorphanol [Stadol]) must be avoided, because these agents may precipitate withdrawal in mother and fetus. If the patient is receiving methadone treatment, clinicians should be aware that maintenance doses of methadone do not provide analgesia in labor. Regional analgesia may be the best way to provide pain relief for a woman with a history of substance abuse.

The intoxicated gravida who presents in labor poses special problems. Stimulant intoxication, especially when accompanied by elevated blood pressure or seizures, may resemble preeclampsia. Treatment of hypertension with β blockers in the setting of recent cocaine ingestion may result in a paradoxical rise in blood pressure.[235] Combination α-β blockers are preferable.[236] Consultation with the anesthesiologist when there is evidence of recent drug use in a laboring woman is vital. Cocaine-intoxicated women requiring operative delivery have a higher risk of anesthetic complications, such as exaggerated hypotension from epidural anesthesia, diastolic hypertension after intubation, and higher rates of perioperative wheezing.[136,237]

Management of Alcohol Withdrawal/Detoxification

When a patient gives a history of chronic, heavy alcohol consumption, it is unwise to advise her to discontinue use "cold turkey." Abrupt cessation of alcohol use can result in physiologic withdrawal symptoms that may compromise maternal and fetal well-being. Isolated seizures, status epilepticus, or premature labor may occur during alcohol withdrawal. Delirium tremens can be fatal to the mother and the fetus. Alcohol-dependent pregnant women who are at high risk for withdrawal should undergo detoxification in a hospital setting, where mother and fetus can be closely monitored and medicated as needed.

Pregnant women who consume more than 8 oz (90 g) of absolute alcohol daily (eight 12-ounce beers, six 6-ounce glasses of wine, eight 1.2-ounce glasses of 80-proof liquor) are likely to have developed alcohol dependence. Inpatient withdrawal is necessary for these women, as well as for women who report lower alcohol consumption but who display signs of alcohol withdrawal in a social-setting detoxification unit or who give a history of withdrawal in the past.

Symptoms of withdrawal begin within 24 to 48 hours after cessation of drinking. The hallmark of alcohol withdrawal is pronounced autonomic hyperactivity. Sweating, tachycardia, and tremor are common. The presence of nausea; vomiting; transient tactile, visual, or auditory hallucinations; agitation; and grand mal seizures constitute full-blown alcohol withdrawal, also known as delirium tremens. The best validated tool for evaluating symptom severity and determining the level of intervention needed is the Clinical Institute Withdrawal Assessment Scale for Alcohol, revised (CIWA-Ar).[238] The CIWA-Ar score should be calculated frequently, hourly if necessary, when patients are symptomatic, to help guide medication dosing decisions. To avoid maternal or fetal compromise, it is recommended that pregnant patients with relatively low CIWA-Ar scores (i.e., 8-14; maximum score is 67) be considered candidates for pharmacotherapy.[239]

There are no controlled data to guide pharmacotherapy of alcohol withdrawal in pregnancy. In general, benzodiazepines are the drugs of choice for management of alcohol withdrawal (Table 25–7). However, avoidance of high-dose benzodiazepine therapy may be preferable in the first trimester and in the last weeks of pregnancy. Per consensus recommendations, phenobarbital is an acceptable alternative for management of alcohol withdrawal

TABLE 25–7   Management of Alcohol Withdrawal in Pregnancy

Admission to antepartum unit

Routine medications: thiamine, folic acid, prenatal vitamins

Monitoring for severity of withdrawal: agitation, anxiety, nausea and vomiting, headache, sweats, tremor, visual disturbances, tactile disturbances, auditory disturbances

Measurement of electrolytes and magnesium levels at baseline; repeat magnesium measurement if indicated by symptoms

Fetal assessments at regular intervals: fetal heart monitoring, nonstress tests as appropriate for gestational age

Nonpharmacologic interventions: reduction of stimuli, maintenance of hydration and body temperature, nutritional support, reality orientation, reassurance and support

Pharmacologic interventions (FDA pregnancy classification)

    Parenteral magnesium for patients developing signs and symptoms of hypomagnesemia

    Chlordiazepoxide (D), 25 to 50 mg q.i.d. for first 2 days, decreasing gradually to 10 mg four times a day for 8 to 10 days

    Phenobarbital (D), 15 to 60 mg q4-6h as needed for the first 2 days, gradually decreasing to 15 mg by the 4th day

    Diazepam (D), 10 mg q.i.d.: 10 mg every 2 hours as needed for withdrawal symptoms to a maximum of 100 mg/24 hours, decreasing gradually at a rate of 20% to 25% over approximately 5 days

From Mitchell JL (consensus panel chair): Treatment Improvement Protocol Series (TIPS): Pregnant Substance Abusing Women. Rockville, Md, U.S. Department of Health and Human Services, 1993.
FDA, U.S. Food and Drug Administration.

in pregnancy.[240,241] After stabilization in the hospital, an alcohol-detoxified gravida should be transferred to a treatment program for long-term care.

Naltrexone (ReVia), an opiate antagonist that reduces alcohol craving, may be started after detoxification. Information about the safety of this medication when used in pregnant women, however, is limited (FDA category C).

Management of Opiate Addiction: Methadone

Opiate-dependent pregnant women are candidates for methadone maintenance therapy. The rationale for substituting one narcotic for another during pregnancy is twofold. First, because of its long half-life, methadone maintenance prevents the alternating cycles of fetal narcotic depression and intrauterine withdrawal that are characteristic of heroin use. Second, methadone promotes better maternal rehabilitation, as measured by increased participation in prenatal care and in substance abuse treatment. If the patient is a parenteral drug user, methadone reduces needle use and thus reduces exposure to needleborne infections such as HIV.[242] Methadone maintenance in pregnancy should be used as part of a comprehensive drug rehabilitation treatment. It is not a stand-alone modality of care.

Despite its benefits, methadone maintenance treatment during pregnancy is not without drawbacks. Methadone causes a neonatal abstinence syndrome that is more severe and prolonged than the withdrawal seen in infants born to users of illicit narcotics such as heroin.[243,244] In addition, methadone-maintained gravidas often increase or continue their use of other illicit drugs, such as cocaine and marijuana.[245,246] Most authorities believe, however, that the benefits associated with methadone therapy, which include increased birth weight and reduced criminal activity and risk-taking behaviors, outweigh the risks of neonatal exposures and withdrawal, particularly because the neonate can be managed expectantly to reduce the severity of the abstinence syndrome.

Pregnancy alters the pharmacokinetics of methadone. For any given dose, plasma levels of the drug are lower in pregnant women. Increased intracellular fluid space and tissue reservoirs for storing methadone, as well as increased drug metabolism by the liver, placenta, and fetus,[247] account for this decline. As pregnancy progresses, the methadone dose may need to be increased or the dosing interval shortened from daily to twice daily, to maintain the same plasma level.[248]

Opiate-dependent women who conceive while taking methadone should continue to receive their prepregnancy dose initially. Opiate-dependent women who begin methadone maintenance during pregnancy may need to be hospitalized to determine an appropriate dose. Federal consensus guidelines advise individualizing methadone doses, with the goal of extinction of all subjective (cravings) and objective signs and symptoms of opiate withdrawal.[240] A reasonable approach to starting methadone therapy is to give 10 to 20 mg as an initial dose. Subsequent doses may be given in 5- to 10-mg increments every 4 to 6 hours over 24 hours, until all withdrawal symptoms are gone. On the second day, the total dose of the previous day can be given as a single dose (Table 25-8). A new idea for prescribing methadone is to use drug levels as a guide. In a prospective observational study, Drozdick and colleagues followed a cohort of methadone maintained pregnant women.[249] They found that methadone serum trough levels between 0.24 and 0.3 mg/L were needed to keep the women from experiencing symptoms of opiate withdrawal. The mean dose of methadone that was needed to render these women asymptomatic, however, was 100.0 ± 38.2 mg (range, 35 to 215 mg). At such doses, the incidence of severe neonatal withdrawal is greater than 90%.[250]

The practice of maintaining all opiate-dependent pregnant women on methadone has been called into question.[251] Legitimate alternatives to methadone maintenance, although not considered standard care, do exist. Opiate-dependent pregnant women can be safely detoxified

from methadone.[252] This should be done in an inpatient setting, slowly reducing the methadone dosage if the patient is already taking methadone . If the patient is not taking methadone, clonidine can be used to treat mild withdrawal symptoms and intermittent methadone doses to treat more severe ones. Detoxification from methadone requires the patient to be highly motivated, in a stable social situation, and willing to commit to close follow-up. It is safest to detoxify pregnant women between 14 and 32 weeks of pregnancy.[253] After detoxification, opiate-using pregnant women may be prescribed naltrexone, an opiate antagonist that blocks μ-opioid receptors,[254] and transferred to outpatient treatment.

As newer agents become available for treating opiate addiction, their safety and efficacy in pregnancy are being explored. l-Acetyl-α-methadol (LAAM), a long-acting methadone derivative, has been used successfully by pregnant women.[255] The advantage of LAAM over methadone is its prolonged duration of action, with suppression of symptoms for up to 72 hours. Usual doses are 30 to 100 mg every 2 to 3 days. The incidence of neonatal abstinence syndrome with LAAM is the same as with methadone.

In October of 2002, the Food and Drug Administration approved the use of buprenorphine for treatment of opiate dependence. Like methadone and LAAM, buprenorphine interacts with μ-opioid receptors. The dose is 8 to 12 mg sublingually every day. Buprenorphine has advantages over other receptor blockers: It has a higher safety margin, is less physically addicting, and has less potential for illicit diversion. Most important, buprenorphine can be dispensed from any physician's office without the cumbersome regulations that pertain to methadone or LAAM. A number of reports[256-259] have already appeared in the literature documenting use in pregnancy. Many of them suggest that there is less neonatal abstinence syndrome associated with maternal buprenorphine than with methadone. Buprenorphine may prove to be better than methadone for treating opiate dependency in pregnancy, but further studies of the drug are needed.

Substance Abuse Treatment

More pregnant women are referred into substance abuse treatment by the criminal justice system than by the health care community. Physicians are often unsure of how to access alcohol and drug rehabilitative services. They are frequently unfamiliar with the variety of treatment programs available to their patients and unable to help them select the type of care best suited for them. One of the most fundamental barriers to getting pregnant women who need treatment into care is their physicians' lack of belief that treatment works.

Not every pregnant woman who is using drugs or alcohol will accept a treatment referral. Denial, guilt, opposition from family and friends, and inadequate financial resources are all barriers to entering treatment. But pregnancy has been shown[260,261] to be a powerful motivation for many women to change, to discontinue substance use, to learn a new way of life, or to regain a lost one. When pregnant patients screen positively for at-risk alcohol use or illicit drug use, it is important for physicians to intervene

TABLE 25-8 Methadone Maintenance for the Opiate-Dependent Gravida

Evaluate for signs and symptoms of opiate withdrawal, if present
Obtain urine toxicologic profile, document nonmethadone opiate metabolites
Initiate methadone: give 10-20 mg PO
Evaluate patient every 4-6 hours
Repeat methadone dose, 5-10 mg PO every 4-6 hours, PRN for withdrawal symptoms
24 to 48 hours after admission, add total amount methadone given in 24 hours and give as a single oral dose; evaluate for overmedication (e.g., sedation)
Periodically reevaluate adequacy of methadone dose as pregnancy progresses

PO, per os (orally); PRN, pro re nata (as needed).

in a way that has been proved to increase patient motivation and willingness to make needed changes. A report from the Institute of Medicine recommended that obstetric providers conduct a specific and brief motivational interview with a woman at risk for an alcohol affected pregnancy,[262] using the FRAMES (Table 25–9) approach of Miller and Rollnick.[263] The same interview is appropriate for a pregnant woman who is using drugs. The physician begins by offering education about the effects of substance use on the pregnancy and on the fetus. Next, the physician makes recommendations for behavior change and lists options to achieve that change. The patient is invited to give feedback about the information and advice she has received. At all times during this process, the physician must remain sympathetic and supportive of the patient's self-efficacy. Avoidance of labels and confrontation in order to develop patient trust is crucial for ultimate success.

Patients who are in a state of "precontemplation"—that is, are not able to accept or understand that they have a problem—can benefit from repetition of the FRAMES intervention at future appointments. Even when this script is repeated, the physician should never lead the patient to believe that ongoing medical care is contingent on accepting the physician's beliefs about the patient's addiction.

Pregnant women who accept referral to substance abuse treatment should be evaluated by a specialist in addiction medicine. This may be a local psychiatrist, a specially trained social worker, or a licensed addiction counselor. Addiction medicine specialists establish severity of disease by using standardized criteria, screen for coexisting mental disorders such as depression, and determine the appropriate level of care needed for an individual patient. Although no single type of treatment is effective for everyone, pregnant women are usually best served by abstinence-based programs, which emphasize self-efficacy, family involvement, case management, and integration with primary care.[264] Studies have shown that residential treatment is often essential when pregnant women are homeless or trapped in chaotic, violent environments that include abusive people and other drug users.[265,266] Treatment programs that contain elements important for pregnant women, such as onsite child care, social services, and parenting classes, have superior client retention and lead to improved obstetric outcomes.[267-269]

Ultimately, it is essential to understand that substance use is a social problem as well as a biologic disease. As with other chronic diseases, such as hypertension, diabetes, or asthma, definitive cure is not a reasonable expectation. Stabilization during pregnancy and the postpartum period is an achievable goal. Treatment of the pregnant, substance-using woman engenders concern for two patients: the woman and the unborn child. The complex task of promoting the welfare of both is a balancing act that may be unequaled in clinical medicine.

References

1. U.S. General Accounting Office: Drug-Exposed Infants: A Generation at Risk. United States Report to the Chairman, Committee on Finance, U.S. Senate, Report No. GAO/HRD-90-138. Washington, D.C.: U.S. General Accounting Office, Human Resources Division, June 1990.
2. Bloss G, et al: NIDA Notes. Rockville, Md, U.S. Department of Health and Human Services, 1995. Available at www.nida.nih.gov.
3. Markovic N, Ness RB, Ceffilli D, et al: Substance use measures among women in early pregnancy. Am J Obstet Gynecol 2000;183:627.
4. Landsay MK, Carmichael S, Peterson H, et al: Correlation between self-reported cocaine use and urine toxicology in an inner city prenatal population. J Natl Med Assoc 1997;89:57.
5. Savitz DA, Henderson L, Dole N, et al: Indicators of cocaine exposure and preterm birth. Obstet Gynecol 2002;99:458.
6. Ostrea EM, Knapp DK, Tannenbaum L, et al: Estimates of illicit drug use during pregnancy by maternal interview, hair analysis, and meconium analysis. J Pediatr 2001;138:344.
7. Jamison DT, Creese T, Prentice T: The World Health Report 1999: Making a Difference (1-121). Geneva, Switzerland, World Health Organization, 1999.
8. United Nations Office for Drug Control and Crime Prevention: Global Illicit Drug Trends 2000. Available at *http://www.odccp.org/pdf/report_2000-12-21-1.pdf.*
9. Sherwood RA, Keating J, Kavvadia V, et al: Substance misuse in early pregnancy and relationship to fetal outcome. Eur J Paediatr 1999;158:488.
10. Kelly JJ, Davis PG, Henschke PN: The drug epidemic: Effects on newborn infants and health resource consumption at a tertiary perinatal centre. J Paediatr Child Health 2000;36:262.
11. May PA, Brooke L, Gossage JP, et al: Epidemiology of fetal alcohol syndrome in a South African community in the Western Cape Province. Am J Pub Health 2000;90:1905.
12. Addis A, Moretti ME, Ahmed Syed F, et al: Fetal effects of cocaine: An updated meta-analysis. Reprod Toxicol 2001;15:341.
13. Croxford J, Viljoen D: Alcohol consumption by pregnant women in the Western Cape. S Afr Med J 1999;89:962.
14. Hollinshead WH, Griffin JF, Scott HD, et al: Statewide prevalence of illicit drug use by pregnant women—Rhode Island. MMWR Morbid Mortal Wkly Rep 1990;39:225.
15. Buchi KF, Varner MW: Prenatal substance use in a western urban community. West J Med 1994;161:483.
16. Vega WA, Kolody B, Hwang J, et al: Prevalence and magnitude of perinatal substance exposures in California. N Engl J Med 1993;329:850.
17. Buchi KF, Varner MW, Chase RA: The prevalence of substance abuse among pregnant women in Utah. Obstet Gynecol 1993;81:239.
18. Nalty D: South Carolina Prevalence Study of Drug Use among Women Giving Birth. Columbia, S.C., South Carolina Commission on Alcohol and Drug Abuse, 1991.
19. National Institute of Drug and Alcohol Abuse: National pregnancy and health survey—drug use among women delivering livebirths (NCADI Publication No. 96-3819). Rockville, Md, 1996.
20. Illicit Drug Use. The NHSDA Report, July 23, 2001. Available at *http://www.samhsa.gov/oas/2k2/pregDU/pregDU.htm.*
21. Substance Use among Pregnant Women during 1999 and 2000. The NHSDA Report, May 17, 2002. Available at *www.samhsa.gov/oas/2k2/preg/preg.htm* (accessed February 11, 2004).
22. Gladstone J, Nulman I, Koren G: Reproductive risks of binge drinking during pregnancy. Reprod Toxicol 1996;10:1.
23. Pierce DR, West JR: Blood alcohol concentration: A critical factor for producing fetal alcohol effects. Alcohol 1986;3:269.
24. West JR, Goodlett CR, Bonthiuse DJ, et al: Manipulating peak blood alcohol concentrations in neonatal rats: A review of an animal

---

TABLE 25–9   FRAMES: Motivational Interviewing for Substance-Abusing Pregnant Women

F	Provide *feedback* on drinking/(drug use) behavior
R	Reinforce patient's *responsibility* for changing behavior
A	State your *advice* about changing behavior
M	Discuss a *menu* of options to change behavior
E	Express *empathy* for patient
S	Support patient's *self-efficacy*

From Miller WR, Rollnick S: Motivational Interviewing. New York, Guilford Press, 1991.

model for alcohol-related developmental effects. Neurotoxicology 1989;10:347.

25. Epidemiologic Trends in Drug Abuse: Proceedings of the Community Epidemiology Work Group—Highlights and Executive Summary, vol 1. Bethesda, Md, National Institute on Drug Abuse, Community Epidemiology Work Group, December 2001, pp 3-4.

26. Trends in Initiation of Substance Use. National Household Survey on Drug Abuse. Washington, D.C., Office of Applied Studies, Substance Abuse and Mental Health Services Administration, 2001. Available at *www.samhsa.gov/oas/NHSDA/2k1NHSDA/vol1/Chapter5.htm* (accessed February 11, 2004).

27. Chasnoff IJ, Landress HJ, Barrett ME: The prevalence of illicit-drug or alcohol use during pregnancy and discrepancies in mandatory reporting in Pinellas County, Florida. N Engl J Med 1990; 322:1202.

28. Rounsaville BJ, Weissman MM, Kleber H, et al: Heterogeneity of psychiatric diagnosis in treated opiate addicts. Arch Gen Psychiatry 1982;39:161.

29. Rounsaville BJ, Foley-Anton S, Carroll K, et al: Psychiatric diagnosis of treatment-seeking cocaine abusers. Arch Gen Psychiatry 1991; 48:43.

30. Burns K, Melamed J, Burns W, et al: Chemical dependence and clinical depression in pregnancy. J Clin Psychol 1985;41:851.

31. Hawley TL, Disney ER: Crack's children: The consequences of maternal cocaine abuse. Soc Policy Rep 1992;6(4):1.

32. Gomberg ES: Suicide risk among women with alcohol problems. Am J Pub Health 1989;79:1363.

33. Brown PJ, Rucupero PR, Stout R: PTSD substance abuse comorbidity and treatment utilization. Addict Behav 1995;20:251.

34. Dansky BS, Saladin ME, Brady KT, et al: Prevalence of victimization and posttraumatic stress disorder among women with substance use disorders: Comparison of telephone and in person assessment samples. Int J Addict 1995;30:1079.

35. Triffleman E, Marmar CR, Delucchi KL, Ronfeldt H: Childhood trauma and posttraumatic stress disorder in substance abuse inpatients. J Nerv Ment Dis 1995;183:172.

36. Gomberg ES: Women and alcoholism: Psychosocial issues. In: Women and Alcohol: Health Related Issues. National Institute on Alcohol Abuse and Alcoholism Research Monograph 16, Department of Health and Human Services Publication No. (ADM) 86-1139. Washington, D.C., U.S. Department of Health and Human Services, 1986, pp 78-120.

37. Binion VJ: A descriptive comparison of the families of origin of women heroin users and nonusers. In Colten ME, Tucker MB, Binion VJ, et al (eds): Addicted Women: Family Dynamics, Self Perceptions and Support Systems. Services Research Monograph Series. U.S. Department of Health, Education, and Welfare, Public Health Service Publication No. (ADM) 80-762. Washington, D.C., National Institute on Drug Abuse, 1979.

38. Cadoret RJ, Yates WR, Troughton E, et al: An adoption study of drug abuse/dependency in females. Compr Psychiatry 1996;37:38.

39. Kendler KS, Heath AC, Neale MC, et al: A population-based twin study of alcoholism in women. JAMA 1992;268:1877.

40. Cadoret RJ, Cain C, Grove WM: Development of alcoholism in adoptees raised apart from alcoholic biologic relatives. Arch Gen Psychiatry 1996;37:88.

41. Light JM: Estimating genetic and environmental effects of alcohol use and dependence from a national survey: A "quasi-adoption" study. J Stud Alcohol 1996;57:507.

42. Wilsnack SC, Vogeltanz ND, Klassen AD, Harris TR: Childhood sexual abuse and women's substance abuse: National survey findings. J Stud Alcohol 1997;58:264.

43. Miller BA, Downs WR, Gondoli DM, Keil A: The role of childhood sexual abuse in the development of alcoholism in women. Violence Vict 1987;2:157.

44. Kendler KS, Bulik CM, Silberg J, et al: Childhood sexual abuse and adult psychiatric and substance use disorders in women: An epidemiological and cotwin control analysis. Arch Gen Psychiatry 2000;57:953.

45. Amaro H, Fried LE, Cabral H, et al: Violence during pregnancy and substance use. Am J Pub Health 1990;80:575.

46. Hedin LW, Janson PO: Domestic violence during pregnancy. The prevalence of physical injuries, substance use, abortions and miscarriages. Acta Obstet Gynecol Scand 2000;79:623.

47. Thompson MP, Kingree JB: The frequency and impact of violent trauma among pregnant substance abusers. Addict Behav 1998; 23:257.

48. Miller B, Downs WR, Gondoli DM: Spousal violence among alcoholic women as compared to a random household sample of women. J Stud Alcohol 1989;50:553.

49. Miller BA, Downs WR, Testa M: Interrelationships between victimization experiences and women's alcohol use. J Stud Alcohol Suppl 1993;11:109.

50. Palmer C, Horowitz M: Shaman Woman, Mainline Lady: Women's Writings on the Drug Experience. New York, William Morrow, 1982.

51. American Psychiatric Association: Diagnostic and statistical manual of mental disorders, 4th ed. Washington, D.C., American Psychiatric Press, 1994.

52. Miller JM, Boudreaux MC: A study of antenatal cocaine use—chaos in action. Am J Obset Gynecol 1999;189:1427.

53. Burkett G, Gomez-Marin O, Yasin SY, et al: Prenatal care in cocaine-exposed pregnancies. Obstet Gynecol 1998;92:193.

54. Latt NC, Spencer JD, Beeby PJ, et al: Hepatitis C in injecting drug-using women during and after pregnancy. J Gastroenterol Hepatol 2000;15:175.

55. Tools for Pediatric Neuroimaging. Available at *http://neuro-www.mgh.harvard.edu/cma/tfpn*.

56. LaGasse LL, Seifer R, Lester BM: Interpreting research on prenatal substance exposure in the context of multiple confounding factors. Clin Perinatol 1999;26:39.

57. Richardson G, Day N: Maternal and neonatal effects of moderate cocaine use during pregnancy. Neurol Toxicol 1991;13:455.

58. Randall CL, Cook JL, Thomas SE, et al: Alcohol plus cocaine prenatally is more deleterious than either drug alone. Neurotoxicol Teratol 1999;21:673.

59. Snodgrass SR: Cocaine babies: A result of multiple teratogenic influences. J Child Neurol 1994;9:227.

60. Lester BM, LaGasse L, Brunner S: Data base of studies on prenatal cocaine exposure and child outcome. J Drug Issues 1997;27:487.

61. Kistin N, Handler A, Davis F, Ferre C: Cocaine and cigarettes: A comparison of risks. Paediatr Perinat Epidemiol 1996;10:269.

62. Lambers DS, Clark KE: The maternal and fetal physiologic effects of nicotine. Semin Perinatol 1996;20:115.

63. Habek D, Habek JC, Ivanisevic M, et al: Fetal tobacco syndrome and perinatal outcome. Fetal Diagn Ther 2002;17:367.

64. Shiono PH, Behrman RE: Low birth weight: Analysis and recommendations. Future Child 1995;5:4.

65. Koren GM, Graham K, Shear H, et al: Bias against the null hypothesis: The reproductive hazards of cocaine. Lancet 1989;2:1440.

66. Bauer CR, Shankaran S, Bada HS, et al: The Maternal Lifestyle Study: Drug exposure during pregnancy and short-term maternal outcomes. Am J Obstet Gynecol 2002;186:487.

67. Floyd RL, Ebrahim SH, Boyle CA, Gould DW: Observations from the CDC. Preventing alcohol-exposed pregnancies among women of childbearing age: The necessity of a preconceptional approach. J Womens Health Gend Based Med 1999;8:733.

68. Hilton ME: Trends in U.S. drinking pattern: Further evidence from the past twenty years. In Clark WB, Hilton ME (eds): Alcohol in America: Drinking Practices and Problems. Albany, N.Y., State University of New York Press, 1991, p 122.

69. Centers for Disease Control and Prevention: Sociodemographic and behavioral characteristics associated with alcohol consumption during pregnancy—United States, 1988. MMWR Morbid Mortal Wkly Rep 1995;44:261.

70. Bradley KA, Badrinath S, Bush K, et al: Medical risks for women who drink alcohol. J Gen Intern Med 1998;13:627.

71. Hall P: Factors influencing individual susceptibility to alcoholic liver disease. In: Alcoholic Liver Disease: Pathology and Pathogenesis, 2nd ed. London, Edward Arnold, 1995, pp 299-316.

72. Urbano-Marquez A, Estruch R, Fernandez-Sola J, et al: The greater risk of alcoholic cardiomyopathy in women compared with men. JAMA 1995;274:149.

73. Witlin AG, Mabie WC, Sibai BM: Peripartum cardiomyopathy: An ominous diagnosis. Am J Obstet Gynecol 1997;176:182.

74. Jenson TK, Hjollund NH, Henriksen TB, et al: Does moderate alcohol consumption affect fertility? Follow-up study among couples planning first pregnancy. BMJ 1998;317:505.

75. Lee W: Pregnancy in patients with chronic liver disease. Gasteroenterol Clin North Am 1992;21:889.

76. Abel EL: Maternal alcohol consumption and spontaneous abortion. Alcohol 1997;32:211.

77. Sokol RJ: Alcohol and spontaneous abortion [Letter]. Lancet 1980;2:1079.

78. Lundsberg LS, Bracken MB, Saftlas AF: Low to moderate gestational alcohol use and intrauterine growth retardation, low birthweight and preterm delivery. Ann Epidemiol 1997;7:498.

79. Keppen DL, Pysher T, Rennert M: Zinc deficiency acts as a coteratogen with alcohol in fetal alcohol syndrome. Pediatr Res 1985;19:944.

80. Flink FP: Mineral metabolism in alcoholism. In Kissen H, Beglieter H (eds): The Biology of Alcoholism. New York, Plenum Press, vol. 1 1971, pp 377-395.

81. Church MW, Jen KL, Pellizzon MA, et al: Prenatal cocaine, alcohol and undernutrition differentially alter mineral and protein content in fetal rats. Pharmacol Biochem Behav 1998;59:577.

82. Cano MJ, Ayala A, Murillo ML, Carreras O: Protective effect of folic acid against oxidative stress produced in 21-day postpartum rats by maternal ethanol chronic consumption during pregnancy and lactation period. Free Radic Res 2001;34:1.

83. Mitchell JJ, Paiva M, Heaton MB: Vitamin B and beta-carotene protect against ethanol combined with ischemia in an embryonic rat hippocampal culture model of fetal alcohol syndrome. Neurosci Lett 1999;263:189.

84. Bingol N, Schuster C, Fuchs M, et al: The influence of socioeconomic factors on the occurrence of fetal alcohol syndrome. Adv Alcohol Subst Abuse 1987;6:105.

85. Abel EL: Fetal alcohol syndrome: A comprehensive bibliography. Westport, Conn, Greenwood Press, 1988.

86. Abel EL, Sokol RJ: Incidence of fetal alcohol syndrome and economic impact of FAS-related anomalies. Drug Alcohol Depend 1987; 19:51.

87. Burd L, Moffatt MEK: Epidemiology of fetal alcohol syndrome in American Indians, Alaskan Natives and Canadian Aboriginal Peoples: A review of the literature. Public Health Rep 1994; 109:668.

88. Viljoen DL, Carr LG, Foroud TM, et al: Alcohol dehydrogenase-2*2 allele is associated with decreased prevalence of fetal alcohol syndrome in the mixed-ancestry population of the Western Cape Province, South Africa. Alcohol Clin Exp Res 2001;25:1719.

89. Stoler JM, Ryan Lm, Holmes LB: Alcohol dehydrogenase 2 genotypes, maternal alcohol use and infant outcome. J Pediatr 2002;141:780.

90. Eriksson CJ, Fukunaga T, Sarkola T, et al: Functional relevance of human ADH polymorphism. Alcohol Clin Exp Res 2001;25(5 Suppl ISBRA):157S.

91. Schenker S, Bay MK: Medical problems associated with alcoholism. Adv Intern Med 1998;43:27.

92. Shoemaker WJ, Baetge F, Azad R, et al: Effects of prenatal alcohol exposure on amine and peptide neurotransmitter systems. Monogr Neurol Sci 1983;9:130.

93. Rovinski B, Hosein EA, Lee H. Effect of maternal ethanol ingestion during pregnancy and lactation on the structure and function of the post-natal rat liver plasma membrane. Biochem Pharmacol 1984;33:311.

94. Singh SP, Ehmann S, Snyder AK: Ethanol induced changes in insulin-like growth factors and IGF gene expression in the fetal brain. Proc Soc Exp Biol Med 1996;212:349.

95. Halmesmake E, Teramo AK, Widness AJ, et al: Maternal alcohol abuse is associated with elevated fetal erythropoietin levels. Obstet Gynecol 1990;76:219.

96. Warner RH, Rosett HL: The effects of drinking on offspring: An historical survey of the American and British literature. J Stud Alcohol 1975;36:1395.

97. Sullivan WC: A note on the influence of maternal inebriety on the offspring. J Ment Sci 1899;45:489.

98. Randall CL: Alcohol and pregnancy: Highlights from three decades of research. J Stud Alcohol 2001;62:554.

99. Lemoine P, Haronesseau H, Borteyru JP, et al: Les enfants de parents alcoholique: Anomalies observees a propos de 127 cas [Children of alcoholic parents: Anomalies observed in 127 cases]. Ouest Med 1968;21:476.

100. Jones KL, Smith DW, Ullelan CN, et al: Patterns of malformation in the offspring of chronic alcoholic mothers. Lancet 1973; 1:1267.

101. Update: Trends in fetal alcohol syndrome—United States, 1979-1993. MMWR Morb Mortal Wkly Rep 1995;44:249.

102. Abel EL: An update on incidence of FAS: FAS is not an equal opportunity birth defect. Neurotoxicol Teratol 1995;17:437.

103. Fetal alcohol syndrome—Alaska, Arizona, Colorado and New York, 1995-1997. MMWR Morbid Mortal Wkly Rep 2002;51:4333.

104. Day NL, Richardson GA: Prenatal alcohol exposure: A continuum of effects. Semin Perinatal 1991;15:271.

105. Sood B, Delaney-Black V, Covington C, et al: Low-level prenatal alcohol exposure was associated with adverse behavioral outcomes in children at 6 to 7 years of age. Pediatrics 2001;108:E34.

106. Moore CA, Khoury MJ, Liu Y: Does light to moderate alcohol consumption during pregnancy increase the risk for renal anomalies among offspring? Pediatrics 1997;99:1.

107. Bishai R, Koren G: Maternal and obstetric effects of prenatal drug exposure. Clin Perinatol 1999;26:75.

108. Rosett HL: A clinical perspective of the fetal alcohol syndrome. Alcohol Clin Exp Res 1980;3:119.

109. Gressens P, Lammens M, Picard JJ, et al: Ethanol-induced disturbances of gliogenesis and neurogenesis in the developing murine brain: An in vitro and in vivo immunohistochemical and ultrastructural study. Alcohol 1992;27:219.

110. Miller MW, Robertson S: Prenatal exposure to ethanol alters the postnatal development and transformation of radial glia to astrocytes in the cortex. J Comp Neurol 1993;337:253.

111. West JR, Hodges CA, Balck AC: Prenatal exposure to ethanol alters the organization of hippocampal mossy fibers in rats. Science 1981;211:957.

112. Mattson SN, Riley EP: Brain anomalies in fetal alcohol syndrome. In Abel EL (ed): Fetal Alcohol Syndrome: From Mechanism to Prevention. Boca Raton, Fla, CRC Press, 1996, pp 51-58.

113. Church MW, Abel EL: Fetal alcohol syndrome: Hearing, speech, language and vestibular disorders. Obstet Gynecol Clin North Am 1998;25:85.

114. Shaw GM, Lammer EJ: Maternal periconceptual alcohol consumption and risk for orofacial clefts. J Pediatr 1999;134:298.

115. Stromland K: Ogonavdelningen for barn, Drotting Silvias barn—och ungdomssjukhus, Sahlgrenska univeritetssjukhuset/Ostra [Fetal alcohol syndrome—unnecessary suffering which has not become rarer. Eyes are affected in up to 90 per cent of the cases]. Lakartidningen 2000;97:5108.

116. National Institute on Alchol Abuse and Alcoholism: Tenth Special Report to the U.S. Congress on Alcohol and Health. Highlights from Current Research, NIH Publication No. 00-1583. Bethesda, Md, Department of Health and Human Services, 2000, pp 283-338.

117. Fast DK, Conry J, Loock CA: Identifying fetal alcohol syndrome among youth in the criminal justice system. J Dev Behav Pediatr 1999;20:370.

118. Loser H, Bierstedt T, Blum A: [Fetal alcohol syndrome in adulthood. A long-term study.] Dtsch Med Wocheschr 1999;124:412.

119. Spohr H, Willms J, Steinhauser H: Prenatal alcohol exposure and long-term developmental consequences. Lancet 1993;341:907.

120. Stewart DJ, Inahaba T, Lucasses M, et al: Cocaine metabolism: Cocaine and norcaine hydrolysis by liver and serum esterases. Clin Pharmacol Ther 1979;25:464.

121. Simone C, Derewlany LO, Oskamp M, et al: Transfer of cocaine and benzoylecgonine across the perfused human placental cotyledon. Am J Obstet Gynecol 1994;170:1404.

122. Little B, Roe K, Settle W, et al: A new placental enzyme in the metabolism of cocaine: An in vitro animal model. Am J Obstet Gynecol 1995;172:1441.

123. Bailey B, Morris P, McMartin KI, et al: Transplacental pharmacokinetics of cocaine and benzoylecgonine in plasma and hair of rhesus monkeys. Reprod Toxicol 1998;12:517.

124. Boskovic R, Klein J, Woodland C, et al: The role of the placenta in variability to fetal exposure to cocaine and cannabinoids: A twin study. Can J Physiol Pharmacol 2001;79:1044.

125. Chao CR: Cardiovascular effects of cocaine during pregnancy. Semin Perinatol 1996;20:107.

126. Woods JR, Plessinger MA: Pregnancy increase cardiovascular toxicity to cocaine. Am J Obstet Gynecol 1990;162:529.

127. Morishima HO, Cooper TB, Hara T, et al: Pregnancy alters the hemodynamic responses to cocaine in the rat. Dev Pharmacol Ther 1992;19:69.

128. Hurd WW, Betx AL, Dombrowski MP, et al: Cocaine augments contractility of the pregnant human uterus by both adrenergic and nonadrenergic mechanisms. Am J Obstet Gynecol 1998; 178:1077.

129. Church MW, Subramanian MG: Cocaine's lethality increases during late gestation in the rat: A study of "critical periods" of exposure. Am J Obstet Gyncol 1997;176:901.

130. Monga M, Weisbrodt NW, Andrs RL, et al: The acute effect of cocaine exposure on pregnant human myometrial contractile activity. Am J Obstet Gynecol 1993;169:782.

131. Mooney EE, Boggess KA, Herbert WN, et al: Placental pathology in patients using cocaine: An observational study. Obstet Gynecol 1998;91:925.

132. Cejtin HE, Young SA, Ungaretti J, et al: Effects of cocaine on the placenta. Pediatr Dev Pathol 1999;2:143.

133. Brody SL, Slovis CM, Wrenn KD: Cocaine-related medical problems: Consecutive series of 233 patients. Am J Med 1990;88:325.

134. Isner JM, Estes M, Thompson PD, et al: Acute cardiac events temporally related to cocaine abuse. N Engl J Med 1986;315:1438.

135. Madu EC, Shala B, Baugh D: Crack-cocaine–associated aortic dissection in early pregnancy—a case report. Angiology 1999;50:163.

136. Livingston JC, Mabie BC, Ramanathan J: Crack cocaine, myocardial infarction and troponin I levels at the time of cesarean delivery. Anesthesia Analgesia 2000;91:913.

137. Mendelson MA, Chandler J: Postpartum cardiomyopathy associated with maternal cocaine use. Am J Cardiol 1992;70:1092.

138. Miller JM, Nolan TE: Case-control study of antenatal cocaine use and platelet levels. Am J Obstet Gynecol 2001;184:434.

139. Mercado A, Johnson F, Calver K, et al: Cocaine, pregnancy and postpartum intracerebral hemorrhage. Obstet Gynecol 1989;73:467.

140. Iriye B, Asrat T, Adashek J: Intraventricular hemorrhage and maternal brain death associated with antepartum cocaine abuse. Br J Obstet Gynaecol 1995;102:68.

141. Myers JA, Earnest MP: Generalized seizures and cocaine abuse. Neurology 1984;34:675.

142. Tashkin DL, Khalsa ME, Gorelick D, et al: Pulmonary status of habitual cocaine smokers. Am Rev Respir Dis 1992;145:92.

143. Kissiner DG, Lawence WD, Selis JE, et al: Crack lung: pulmonary disease caused by cocaine abuse. Am Rev Respir Dis 1987; 136:1250.

144. Minkoff HL, McCalla S, Delke L, et al: The relationship of cocaine use to syphilis and human immunodeficiency virus among inner city parturient women. Am J Obstet Gynecol 1991;163:521.

145. Ward H, Pallecaros A, Green A: Health issues associated with increasing use of "crack" cocaine among female sex workers in London. Sex Transm Dis 2000;76:292.

146. Ruiz P, Cleary T, Nassiri M, et al: Human T lymphocyte subpopulation and NK cell alterations in persons exposed to cocaine. Clin Immunol Immunopathol 1994;70:245.

147. Macones GA, Sehdev HM, Harish M, et al: The association between maternal cocaine use and placenta previa. Am J Obstet Gynecol 1997;177:1097.

148. Sprauve ME, Lindsay MK, Herbert S, et al: Adverse perinatal outcome in parturients who use crack cocaine. Obstet Gynecol 1997; 89:674.

149. Dombrowski MP, Wolfe HM, Welch RA, et al: Cocaine abuse is associated with abruptio placentae and decreased birth weight but not shorter labor. Obstet Gynecol 1991;77:807.

150. Refuezo JS, Sokol RJ, Blackwell SC, et al: Cocaine use and preterm premature rupture of membranes: Improvement in neonatal outcome. Am J Obstet Gyecol 2002;186:1150.

151. Hanlon-Lundberg KM, Williams M, Rhim T, et al: Accelerated fetal lung maturity profiles and maternal cocaine exposure. Obstet Gynecol 1996;87:128.

152. Bandstra ES, Morrow CE, Nathony JC, et al: Intrauterine growth of full-term infants: Impact of prenatal cocaine exposure. Pediatrics 2001;108:1309.

153. Eyler FD, Behnke M, Conlon M, et al: Birth outcomes from a prospective, matched study of prenatal crack/cocaine use: Interactive and dose effects on health and growth. Pediatrics 1998;101:229.

154. Pastrakuljic A, Derewlany L, Koren G: The effects of cocaine and nicotine on amino acid transport across the human placental cotyledon perfused in vitro. J Pharmacol Exp Ther 2000;294:141.

155. Covington CY, Nordstrom-Klee B, Ager J, et al: Birth to age 7 growth of children prenatally exposed to drugs: A prospective cohort study. Neurotoxicol Teratol 2002;24:489.

156. Weathers WT, Crane MM, Sauvain KJ, et al: Cocaine use in women from a defined population: Prevalence at delivery and effects on growth in infants. Pediatrics 1993;91:350.

157. Benke M, Eyler FD, Garvan CW: The search for congenital malformations in newborns with fetal cocaine exposure. Pediatrics 2001; 107:E74.

158. Robbins LN, Mills JL, Krulewitch C, et al: Effects of in utero exposure to street drugs. Am J Pub Health 1993;83(Suppl):9.

159. Bauer CR: Perinatal effects of prenatal drug exposure: Neonatal aspects. Clin Perinatol 1999;26:87.

160. Holmes LB: Teratogen-induced limb defects. Am J Med Genet 2002;112:297.

161. Azuma SD, Chasnoff IJ: Outcome of children prenatally exposed to cocaine and other drugs: A path analysis of three year old data. Pediatrics 1993;92:396.

162. Coles CD: Saying "goodbye" to the crack baby. Neurotoxicol Teratol 1993;15:290.

163. Woods NS, Eyler FD, Conlon M, et al: Pygmalion in the cradle: Observer bias against cocaine exposed infants. J Dev Behav Pediatr 1998;19:283.

164. Chasnoff IJ, Burns W, Schnoll S, et al: Cocaine use in pregnancy. N Engl J Med 1985;313:666.

165. Smith LM, Qureshi N, Renslo R, et al: Prenatal cocaine exposure and cranial sonographic findings in preterm infants. J Clin Ultrasound 2001;29:72.

166. Frank DA, Augustyn M, Knight W, et al: Growth, development and behavior in early childhood following prenatal cocaine exposure: A systematic review. JAMA 2001;285:1613.

167. Methamphetamine: Abuse and Addiction. National Institute on Drug Abuse Research Report Series, Bethesda, Md, 1998. Available at *http://www.nida.nih.gov/ResearchReports/Methamph/Methamph.html* (accessed February 11, 2004).

168. Kandall SR: Perinatal effects of cocaine and amphetamine use during pregnancy. Bull N Y Acad Med 1991;67:240.

169. Bryson PD: Central nervous system stimulants. In: Comprehensive Review in Toxicology for Emergency Clinicians. Washington, D.C., Taylor and Francis, 1996, pp 482-495.

170. Oro AS, Dixon SD: Perinatal cocaine and methamphetamine exposure. Maternal and neonatal correlates. J Pediatr 1987;111:571.

171. Eriksson M, Larsson G, Winbladh B, Zetterstrom R: The influence of amphetamine addiction on pregnancy and the newborn infant. Acta Paediatr Scand 1978;67:95.

172. Thomas DB: Cleft palate, mortality and morbidity in infants of substance abusing mothers. J Paediatr Child Health 1995;31:457.

173. Leshner AI: A club drug alert. NIDA Notes 2000;14(6):1. Available at *http://www.nida.nih.gov/NIDA_Notes/NNVol14N6/DirRepVol14N6.html* (accessed February 11, 2004).

174. Ho E, Karimi-Tabesh L, Koren G: Characteristics of pregnant women who use ectasy (3,4-methylenedioxymethamphetamine). Neurol Teratol 2001;23:561.

175. Van Tonningen-van Driel MM, Garbis-Berkvens JM, Reuvers-Lodewijks WE: [Pregnancy outcome after ecstasy use; 43 cases followed by the Teratology Information Service of the National Institute for Public Health and Environment (RIVM).] Ned Tijdschrift Geneeskd 1999;143:27.

176. McElhatton PR, Bateman DN, Evans C, et al: Congenital anomalies after prenatal ecstasy exposure. Lancet 1999;354:1441.

177. Epidemiologic Trends in Drug Abuse: Proceedings of the Community Epidemiology Work Group—Highlights and Executive Summary, vol 1. Bethesda, Md, National Institute on Drug Abuse, Community Epidemiology Work Group, December 2001, pp 18-31.

178. Santen RJ, Sossky J, Bilic N, et al: Mechanism of action of narcotics in the production of menstrual dysfunction in women. Fertil Steril 1975;26:538.

179. Kreek MJ: Long-term pharmacotherapy for opiate (primarily heroin) addiction: Opioid agonists. In Schuster CR, Kuhar MJ (eds): Pharmacologic Aspects of Drug Dependence: Toward an Integrated Neurobehavioral Approach. Berlin, Springer, 1996, pp 95-114.

180. Naeye RL, Blanc W, Leblanc W, et al: Fetal complications of maternal heroin addiction: Abnormal growth, infections and episodes of stress. J Pediatr 1973;83:1055.

181. Lam SK, To WK, Duthie SJ, et al: Narcotic addiction in pregnancy with adverse maternal and perinatal outcome. Aust N Z J Obstet Gynaecol 1992;32:216.

182. Little BB, Snell LM, Klien VR, et al: Maternal and fetal effects of heroin addiction during pregnancy. J Reprod Med 1990;35:159.

183. Doberazak TM, Stephen KR, Wilets I: Neonatal opiate abstinence syndrome in term and preterm infants. J Pediatr 1991;118:933.

184. Alroom LG, Davidson J, Evans TJ, et al: Maternal narcotic abuse and the newborn. Arch Dis Child 1988;63:81.

185. Klonoff-Cohen H, Lam-Kruglick P: Maternal and paternal recreational drug use and sudden infant death syndrome. Arch Pediatr Adolesc Med 2001;155:765.

186. Illicit Drug Use. Trends in Initiation of Substance Use. Substance Abuse and Mental Health Services Administration 2001 National Household Survey on Drug Abuse, *http://www.samhsa.gov/oas/2k2/pregDU/pregDU.htm.*

187. Shiono P, Klebanoff M, Nugent R, et al: The impact of cocaine and marijuana use on low birth weight and preterm birth: a multicenter study. Am J Obstet Gyencol 1995;172:19027.

188. Wu T-C, Tashkin DP, Djahed B, et al: Pulmonary hazards of smoking marijuana as compared with tobacco. N Engl J Med 1988;318:347.

189. Abel E: Marijuana: The First Twelve Thousand Years. New York, Plenum Press, 1980.

190. Schneiderman J: Non-medical drug and chemical use in pregnancy. In Koren G (ed): Maternal-Fetal Toxicology: A Clinicians Guide, 2nd ed. New York, Marcel Dekker, 1994.

191. Sayle AE, Wilcox AJ, Weinberg CR: A prospective study of the onset of symptoms of pregnancy. J Clin Epidemiol 2002;55:676.

192. Kenney SP, Kekuda R, Prasad PD, et al: Cannabinoid receptors and their role in the regulation of the serotonin transporter in the human placenta. Am J Obstet Gynecol 1999;181:491.

193. Linn S, Schoenbaum SC, Manson RR, et al: The association of marijuana with outcome of pregnancy. Am J Pub Health 1983; 73:1161.

194. Hingson R, Alper JJ, Day N, et al: Effects of maternal drinking and marijuana use on fetal growth and development. Pediatrics 1982;70:539.

195. Fried PA, Makin JE: Neonatal behavioral correlates of prenatal exposure to marihuana, cigarettes and alcohol in a low risk population. Neurotoxicol Teratol 1987;9:1.

196. Scher MS, Richardson GA, Coble PA, et al: The effects of prenatal alcohol and marijuana exposure: Disturbances in neonatal sleep cycling and arousal. Pediatr Res 1988;24:101.

197. Dahl RE, Scher MS, Day NL, et al: The effects of prenatal marijuana exposure. Evidence of EEG-sleep disturbances. J Dev Behav Pediatr 1988;9:333.

198. Adolescents prenatally exposed to marijuana: Examination of facets of complex behaviors and comparisons with the influence of in utero cigarettes. J Clin Pharamcol 2002;42(11Suppl):97S.

199. Cornelius MD, Goldschmidt L, Day NL, Larkby C: Alcohol, tobacco and marijuana use among pregnant teenagers: 6-year follow-up of offspring growth effects. Neurol Teratol 2002;24:703.

200. Goldschmidt L, Day NL, Richardson GA: Effects of prenatal marijuana exposure on child behavior problems at age 10. Neurotoxicol Teratol 2000;22:325.

201. Milkovich L, Ban den Berg BJ: Effects of prenatal meprobamate and chlordiazepoxide hydrochloride on human embryonic and fetal development. N Engl J Med 1983;309:1282.

202. Kanto JH: Use of benzodiazepines during pregnancy, labor and lactation with particular reference to pharmacokinetic considerations. Drugs 1983;23:354.

203. Sutton LR, Hinderliter SA: Diazepam abuse in pregnant women on methadone maintenance: Implications for the neonate. Clin Pediatr 1990;29:108.

204. Gaily E, Granstrom M-L: A transient retardation of early postnatal growth in drug-exposed children of epileptic mothers. Epilepsy Res 1989;4:127.

205. Epidemiologic Trends in Drug Abuse: Proceedings of the Community Epidemiology Work Group—Highlights and Executive Summary, vol 1. Bethesda, Md, National Institute on Drug Abuse, Community Epidemiology Work Group, December 2001, p 57.

206. Kautman KR, Petrucha RA, Pitts FN: Phencyclidine in umbilical cord blood: Preliminary data. Am J Psychiatry 1983;140:450.

207. Mvula MM, Miller JM Jr, Ragan FA: Relationship of phencyclidine and pregnancy outcome. J Reprod Med 1999;44:1021.

208. Abruzzi W: Drug induced psychosis. Int J Addict 1977;12:183.

209. Johnston LD, O'Malley PM, Bachman JG: National survey results on drug use. In: The Monitoring the Future Study, 1975-1993, vol 1: Secondary School Students. Rockville, Md, U.S. Department of Health and Human Services, National Institutes of Health, 1994.

210. Wilkins-Haug L, Gabow PA: Toluene abuse during pregnancy: Obstetric outcomes and perinatal complications. Obstet Gynecol 1988;77:715.

211. Scheeres JJ, Chudley AE: Solvent abuse in pregnancy: A perinatal perspective. J Obstet Gynaecol Can 2002;24:22.

212. Costa LG, Guizzetti M, Burry M, et al: Developmental neurotoxicity: Do similar phenotypes indicate a common mode of action? A comparison of fetal alcohol syndrome, toluene embryopathy and maternal phenylketonuria. Toxicol Lett 2002;127:197.

213. Dawson N, Dadheech G, Speroff T, et al: The effect of gender on the prevalence and recognition of alcoholism in a general medicine inpatient service. J Gen Intern Med 1992;7:38.

214. Khals JH, Gfroerer J: Epidemiology and health consequences of drug abuse among pregnant women. Semin Perinatol 1991;15:265.

215. Russell M, Martier SS, Sokol RJ, et al: Screening for pregnancy risk drinking. Alcohol Clin Exp Res 1994;18:1156.

216. Mayfield D, McCleod G, Hall P: The CAGE questionnaire: Validation of a new alcoholism screening instrument. Am J Psychiatry 1974; 131:1121.

217. Midanik LT, Zahnd EG, Klein D: Alcohol and drug CAGE screeners for pregnant, low-income women: The California Perinatal Needs Assessment. Alcohol Clin Exp Res 1998;22:121.

218. Sokol RJ, Martier SS, Ager JW: The T-ACE questions: Practical prenatal detection of risk-drinking. Am J Obstet Gynecol 1989;160:863.

219. Kiekman ST, Floyd RL, Decoufle P, et al: A survey of obstetrician-gynecologists on their patients alcohol use during pregnancy. Obstet Gynecol 2000;95:756.

220. Cyr MG, Wartman SA: The effectiveness of routine screening questions in the detection of alcoholism. JAMA 1988;259:51.

221. Beckman RD, Amaro H: Patterns of women's use of alcohol treatment agencies. Alcohol Health Res World 1984-1985;9(2):14.

222. Connoly WB, Marshall AB: Drug addiction, pregnancy, and childbirth: Legal issues for the medical and social services communities. Clin Perinatal 1991;18:147.

223. Annas GJ: Testing poor pregnant women for cocaine—physicians as police investigators. N Engl J Med 2001;344:1729.

224. Knight EM, James H, Edwards CH, et al: Relationships of serum illicit drug concentrations during pregnancy to maternal nutritional status. J Nutr 1994;124:973S.

225. Tabor BL, Scoffi AR, Smith-Wallace T, et al: The effects of maternal cocaine use on the fetus: Changes in antepartum fetal heart tracings. Am J Obstet Gynecol 1991;165:1278.

226. Archie CC, Lee MI, Sokol RJ, et al: The effects of methadone treatment on the reactivity of the nonstress test. Obstet Gynecol 1989; 74:254.

227. Cejtin HE, Mills T, Swift EL: Effect of methadone on the biophysical profile. J Reprod Med 1996;41:819.

228. Richardson GA, Hamel SC, Goldschmidt L, Day NL: Growth of infants prenatally exposed to cocaine/crack: Comparison of a prenatal care and a no prenatal care sample. Pediatrics 1999; 104(2):E18.

229. Berenson AB, Wilkinson GS, Lopez LA: Effects of prenatal care on neonates born to drug-using women. Subst Use Misuse 1996; 31:1063.

230. Newschaffer CJ, Cocrof J, Hauck WW, et al: Improved birth outcomes associated with enhanced Medicaid prenatal care in drug-using women infected with the human immunodeficiency virus. Obstet Gynecol 1998;91:885.

231. Chazotte C, Youchah J, Freda MC: Cocaine use during pregnancy and low birth weight: The impact of prenatal care and drug treatment. Semin Perinatol 1995;19:293.

232. Committee on Drugs and the American Academy of Pediatrics: The transfer of drugs and other chemicals into human milk. Pediatrics 2001;108:776.

233. Ballard J: Treatment of neonatal abstinence syndrome with breast milk containing methadone. J Perinat Neonat Nurs 2002;15:76.

234. Scimeca MM, Savage SR, Portenoy R, Lowinson J: Treatment of pain in methadone maintained patients. Mt Sinai J Med 2000; 67:412.

235. Ramoska E, Sachetti AD: Propranolol-induced hypertension in treatment of cocaine intoxication. Ann Emerg Med 1985;13:1112.

236. Dusenbury SJ, Hicks MJ, Ferris CA, et al: Labetalol treatment of cocaine toxicity [Letter]. Ann Emerg Med 1985;16:142.

237. Zain AN, Mayes LC, Ferris CA, et al: Cocaine-abusing parturients undergoing cesarean section. A cohort study. Anesthesiology 1996; 85:1028.

238. Sullivan JT, Sykora K, Schneiderman J, et al: Assessment of alcohol withdrawal: The revised clinical institute withdrawal assessment for alcohol scale (CIWA-Ar). Br J Addict 1989;84:1353.

239. Saitz R, O'Malley SS: Pharmacotherapies for alcohol abuse. Med Clin North Am 1997;81:881.

240. Mitchell JL (consensus panel chair): Treatment Improvement Series (TIPS). Pregnant Substance Abusing Women. Rockville MD, U.S. Department of Health and Human Services, 1993.

241. Thorp JM Jr: Management of drug dependency, overdose, and withdrawal in the obstetric patient. Obstet Clin North Am 1995; 22:131.

242. Kandall SR, Doberczak TM, Jantunen M, et al: The methadone maintained pregnancy. Clin Perinatol 1999;26:173.

243. Hagopian GS, Wolfe IM, Sokol RJ, et al: Neonatal outcome following methadone exposure in utero. J Matern Fetal Med 1996; 5:348.

244. Doberczak TM, Kandall SR, Freidman P: Relationships between maternal methadone dosage, maternal-neonatal methadone levels and neonatal withdrawal. Obstet Gynecol 1993;81:936.

245. Brown HL, Britton KA, Mahaffery D, et al: Methadone maintenance in pregnancy: A reappraisal. Obstet Gynecol 1998;179:459.

246. Laken MP, McComish JF, Ager J: Predictors of prenatal substance use and birth weight during outpatient treatment. J Subst Abuse Treat 1997;14:359.

247. Pond SM, Kreek MJ, Tong TG, et al: Altered methadone pharmacokinetics in methadone-maintained pregnant women. J Pharmacol Exp Ther 1985;233:1.

248. Whittman BK, Segal S: A comparison of the effects of single and split dose methadone administration on the fetus: Ultrasound evaluation. Int J Addict 1991;26:231.

249. Drozdick J III, Berghella V, Hill MK, Kaltenbach K: Methadone trough levels in pregnancy. Obstet Gynecol 2002;187:1184.

250. Dashe JS, Sheffield JS, Olssher DA, et al: Relationship between maternal methadone dosage and neonatal withdrawal. Obstet Gyencol 2002;100:12444.

251. Hulse GK, O'Neill G: Methadone and the pregnant user: A matter for careful consideration. Aust N Z J Obstet Gynaecol 2001;41:329.

252. Dashe JS, Jackson GL, Olscher DA, et al: Opioid detoxification in pregnancy. Obstet Gyencol 1998;92:854.

253. Drug Dependence in Pregnancy: Clinical Management of Mother and Child. Services Research Monograph Series, DHEW Publication No. (ADM) 7-9-678. Rockville, Md, National Institute on Drug Abuse, Unites States Department of Health, Education, and Welfare, 1979, p 47.

254. Hulse GK, O'Neill G, Pereira C, et al: Obstetric and neonatal outcomes associated with maternal naltrexone exposure. Aust N Z J Obstet Gynaecol 2001;41:424.

255. Fischer F, Jagsch R, Eder H, et al: Comparison of methadone and slow-release morphine maintenance in pregnant addicts. Addiction 1999;94:231.

256. Johnson RE, Jones HE, Jasinski DR, et al: Buprenorphine treatment of pregnant opioid-dependent women: Maternal and neonatal outcomes. Drug and Alcohol Dep 2001;63:97.

257. Schindler SD, Eder H, Ortner R, et al: Neonatal outcome following buprenorphine maintenance during conception and throughout pregnancy. Addiction 2003;98:103.

258. Fischer G, Etzersdorfer P, Eder H, et al: Buprenorphine maintenance in pregnant opiate addicts. Eur Addict Res 1998; 4(Suppl 1):32.

259. Robinson SE: Buprenorphine: An analgesic with an expanding role in the treatment of opioid addiction. CNS Drug Rev 2002;8:377.

260. Eriksson M, Larsson G, Zetterstrom R: Amphetamine addiction and pregnancy. II. Pregnancy, delivery and the neonatal period: Socio-medical aspects. Acta Obstet Gynecol Scand 1981;60:253.

261. Schafer A, Eck M, Bell U: [Use of methadone in obstetric and gynecologic management of drug-dependent females with and without HIV infection.] Geburtshilfe Frauenheilkd 1991;51:595.

262. Institute of Medicine: Fetal alcohol syndrome: Diagnosis, epidemiology, prevention and treatment. Washington, D.C., National Academy Press, 1996.

263. Miller WR, Rollnick S: Motivational Interviewing. New York, Guilford Press, 1991.

264. Sweeney PJ, Schwartz RM, Mattis NG, et al: The effect of integrating substance abuse treatment with prenatal care on birth outcomes. J Perinatol 2000;20:219.

265. Daley M, Argeriou M, McCarty D, et al: The impact of substance abuse treatment modality on birth weight and health care expenditures. J Psychoactive Drugs 2001;33:57.

266. Whiteford L, Vitucci J: Pregnancy and addiction: Translating research into practice. Soc Sci Med 1997;44:1371.

267. Weisdorf T, Parran R, Graham A, et al: Comparison of pregnancy-specific interventions to a traditional treatment program for cocaine-addicted pregnant women. J Subst Abuse Treat 1998; 16:39.

268. McMurtie C, Rosenberg K, Kerker BD, et al: A unique drug treatment program for pregnant and postpartum substance-using women in New York City: Results of a pilot project, 1990-1995. Am J Drug Alcohol Abuse 1999;25:701.

269. Fiocchi FF, Kingree JB: Treatment retention and birth outcomes of crack users enrolled in a substance abuse treatment program for pregnant women. J Subst Abuse Treat 2001;20:137.

INDEX

Note: Page numbers followed by the letter f refer to figures, those followed by the letter t refer to tables.